Applied Clinical Pharmacokinetics

Third Edition

Larry A. Bauer, PharmD

Professor
Department of Pharmacy
School of Pharmacy

Adjunct Professor
Department of Laboratory Medicine
School of Medicine
University of Washington
Seattle, Washington

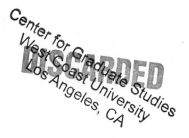

Center for Graduate Studies
West Coast University
Los Angeles, CA
DISCARDED

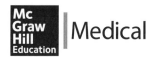 Medical

New York   Chicago   San Francisco   Athens   London   Madrid   Mexico City
Milan   New Delhi   Singapore   Sydney   Toronto

Applied Clinical Pharmacokinetics, 3rd edition

1 2 3 4 5 6 7 8 9 0   DOC/DOC   18 17 16 15 14

ISBN 978-0-07-179458-9
MHID 0-07-179458-1

This book was set in Times by Cenveo® Publisher Services.
The editors were Michael Weitz and Christina M. Thomas.
The production supervisor was Catherine Saggese
Project management was provided by Vastavikta Sharma, Cenveo Publisher Services.
RR Donnelley was printer and binder.

This book is printed on acid-free paper.

Library of Congress Cataloging-in-Publication Data
Bauer, Larry A., author.
Applied clinical pharmacokinetics / by Larry A. Bauer.—Third edition.
    p. ; cm.
Includes bibliographical references and index.
ISBN 978-0-07-179458-9 (hardcover : alk. paper)—ISBN 0-07-179458-1
(hardcover : alk. paper)
I. Title.
[DNLM: 1. Pharmacokinetics. 2. Pharmaceutical
Preparations—administration & dosage. QV 38]
RM301.5
615'.7—dc23
                                    2013029778

International Edition ISBN 978-1-25-925141-2; MHID 1-25-925141-1. Copyright © 2014. Exclusive rights by McGraw-Hill Education, for manufacture and export. This book cannot be re-exported from the country to which it is consigned by McGraw-Hill Education. The International Edition is not available in North America.

McGraw-Hill Education books are available at special quantity discounts to use premiums and sales promotions, or for use in corporate training programs. To contact a representative please visit the Contact Us pages at www.mhprofessional.com.

Dedication

Third time's a charm . . . right? Through the planned and unexpected, the little things and the big things, the pleasant side trips and trying travails, family are what make it all worthwhile. Thank you (S.P.B., L.A.B., and L.E.B.) for all of your love and support that helped make the third edition a reality.

Thanks for the huge amount of support and assistance from my colleagues. You guys help each and every day, whether it is insight on a new drug interaction, discussion of an interesting patient case, or the latest sports scores: John R. Horn, Douglas J. Black, Lingtak-Neander Chan, Danny D. Shen, and, of course, Philip D. Hansten.

"It's pretty far, but it doesn't seem like it."—Yogi Berra

—L.A.B.

Contents

viii   CONTENTS

About the Author

Larry A. Bauer, PharmD, is a Professor at the University of Washington School of Pharmacy and has been on the faculty since 1980. He also holds an adjunct appointment at the same rank in the Department of Laboratory Medicine where he is a toxicology consultant. He received a Bachelor of Science in Pharmacy degree (1977, Magna Cum Laude) from the University of Washington and a Doctor of Pharmacy degree (1980) from the University of Kentucky under the supervision of Dr. Robert Blouin. He also completed an ASHP-accredited hospital pharmacy residency (1980) specializing in clinical pharmacokinetics from A. B. Chandler Medical Center at the University of Kentucky under the preceptorship of Dr. Paul Parker. Dr. Bauer is a fellow of the American College of Clinical Pharmacology and the American College of Clinical Pharmacy.

Dr. Bauer's specialty area is in clinical pharmacokinetics, and he teaches courses and offers clinical clerkships in this area. His research interests include the pharmacokinetics and pharmacodynamics of drug interactions, the effects of liver disease and age on drug metabolism, and computer modeling of population pharmacokinetics. He has over 165 published research papers, abstracts, books and book chapters. Dr. Bauer is a member of several clinical pharmacology and clinical pharmacy professional organizations. He was Consulting Editor of Clinical Pharmacy (1981–1990), Field Editor of ASHP Signal (1981–1983), and a member of the Editorial Board of Clinical Pharmacology and Therapeutics. Recently, he completed an appointment to the Editorial Board of Antimicrobial Agents and Chemotherapy and, he reviews for many other scientific publications. Dr. Bauer has precepted three post-doctoral fellows in clinical pharmacokinetics who currently have faculty appointments in schools of pharmacy or positions in the pharmaceutical industry.

Foreword

As a pharmacist for 36 years, I am rarely surprised about most things that happen in my professional life. However, I continue to be amazed by the depth and breadth of both the practice and research efforts in the area of therapeutic drug monitoring. As I write this, it is baseball season, so perhaps that eternal philosopher says it best:

"In theory, there is no difference between theory and practice. In practice, there is."—Yogi Berra

Antibiotics usually take front-and-center attention in clinical pharmacokinetics. While the aminoglycosides continue to develop quietly, vancomycin is demanding more attention as pharmacokinetic/pharmacodynamic (PK/PD) relationships are uncovered and pathogen MICs push upward (short version: the bacteria are winning).

Immunosuppressants continue to be the number one category of monitored drugs in our health care system, and sirolimus makes its debut in this edition of the book. Of course, being a large transplant center contributes to this trend, but it is a rare clinician that doesn't encounter transplant patients and their medications on a routine basis.

While being a static area for quite some time, the next generation anticonvulsants are finally coming into their own. Updated treatment guidelines put these agents squarely in the spotlight, and the increase in serum concentration monitoring for these medications has been impressive. The challenge with these newer drugs is the role that therapeutic drug monitoring will play in their therapy because the concentration-response relationships are not as well defined for them compared to the older agents. Lamotrigine, levetiracetam, oxcarbazepine, and eslicarbazepine are included in this edition.

As for me, preparation for the fourth edition begins today.

Larry A. Bauer, PharmD
May 17, 2014

From *Applied Clinical Pharmacokinetics*, Second Edition

Upon beginning my thirtieth year as a pharmacist, the number of new approaches that continue to be developed for therapeutic drug monitoring impresses me. The second edition of *Applied Clinical Pharmacokinetics* includes new methods to dose immunosuppressants (2-hour postdose cyclosporine concentrations, area under the curve methods for cyclosporine and tacrolimus), and the elevation of what were new methods of dosing antibiotics to the mainstream (extended interval and area under the curve methods for aminoglycosides, trough-only monitoring for vancomycin). Other additions include more complete coverage of pediatric patients, dosing during hemoperfusion, an overview of methods preceding the initial and dosage adjustment sections, and a dosing strategies section that groups together initial and dosage adjustment techniques into a logical sequence. Of course, relevant sections, examples, problems, and references have been updated as needed for each chapter. However, one thing that remains unchanged is the general organization and philosophy of the book (please see the excerpt from the first edition following this section).

> Bernard of Chartres used to say that we are like dwarfs on the shoulders of giants, so that we can see more than they, and things at a greater distance, not by virtue of any sharpness of sight on our part, or any physical distinction, but because we are carried high and raised up by their giant size.—in Metalogicon (1159 A.D.), by John of Salisbury.

Depending on one's point of view, the discipline of therapeutic drug monitoring is entering its fifth decade. Some brilliant scientists and practitioners who have made significant contributions to the area (and whose names are in the reference list or attached to the methods recommended in this text) and changed the lives of countless patients are no longer with us. I extend my humble thanks to all of these exceptional individuals for making things a little bit clearer and a lot easier for the rest of us.

Larry A. Bauer, PharmD
June 2008

From *Applied Clinical Pharmacokinetics*, First Edition

The structure of this book is uniform for each chapter and is derived from my lectures in clinical pharmacokinetics. The introduction, which consists of a brief discussion of the clinical pharmacology and mechanism of action for the drug, is followed by sections that describe the therapeutic concentration range and anticipated adverse effects for the drug as well as a general monitoring scheme for the agent. Clinical monitoring parameters for therapeutic response and toxicity and basic clinical pharmacokinetic parameters for the compound are discussed next. The next sections describe the effects of disease states and conditions on the pharmacokinetics and dosing of the drug, and drug interactions that may occur with concurrent use of other agents. Each chapter concludes with a comprehensive presentation (with examples) of various methods to compute initial drug doses and to modify drug therapy regimens using serum concentrations to adjust doses. All dosing methods used in this text are ones that are published in peer-reviewed literature. Additionally, they are techniques that I have personal clinical experience with and have produced acceptable results in my practice and clinical clerkships. Finally, problems (with solutions) are included for each chapter so that the various dosing methods can be practiced. The problems are made up of brief clinical vignettes which, given a brief background, request that initial doses be computed or that dosage regimens be modified using drug concentrations.

This text is meant to teach clinical pharmacokinetic and therapeutic drug monitoring techniques to all clinical practitioners regardless of professional background. Pharmacists, physicians, nurse practitioners, and physician assistants are among the individuals who could benefit from the text. With the advent of the almost-universal Doctor of Pharmacy degree in colleges of pharmacy, this book could be used in a pharmaceutics, pharmacokinetics, therapeutics, or clinical pharmacy course sequence. It is also possible to use this textbook in a self-directed manner to teach oneself or review important concepts and techniques. Every effort was made to make the chapters "student-friendly." Abbreviations are held to an absolute minimum. When abbreviations are used, they are defined near the place where they are used. Rather than using appendices, important information is repeated in each drug section so that readers do not need to jump from section to section for critical data. Multiple dosage computation and adjustment techniques for each drug, ranging from the simplest to the sophisticated, are presented. The easiest pharmacokinetic equations that produce accurate results are used in each instance.

It is my strong belief that clinical pharmacokinetics cannot be practiced in a vacuum. Individuals interested in using these dosing techniques for their patients must also be excellent clinical practitioners. Although it is true that "kinetics = dose," clinicians must be able to select the best drug therapy among many choices and appropriately monitor patients for therapeutic response, adverse drug effects, potential drug interactions, disease states and conditions that alter drug dosage, and so on. Thus, it is not acceptable to simply suggest a dose and walk away from the patient, satisfied that the job has been done. It is my sincere hope that this book will help clinicians increase their knowledge in the area of therapeutic drug monitoring and improve care to their patients.

Larry A. Bauer, PharmD
May 17, 2014

BASIC CONCEPTS

1 Clinical Pharmacokinetic and Pharmacodynamic Concepts

INTRODUCTION

Clinical pharmacokinetics is the discipline that applies pharmacokinetic concepts and principles in humans in order to design individualized dosage regimens that optimize the therapeutic response of a medication while minimizing the chance of an adverse drug reaction. Pharmacokinetics is the study of the *absorption, distribution, metabolism,* and *excretion* of drugs.[1] When drugs are given extravascularly (eg, orally, intramuscularly, applied to the skin via a transdermal patch, etc), *absorption* must take place for the drug molecules to reach the systemic circulation. In order to be absorbed, the drug molecules must pass through several physiological barriers before reaching the vascular system. For example, when a medication is given orally, the drug dosage form must release drug molecules via dissolution, and the molecules must pass through the various layers of the gastrointestinal (GI) tract where they enter capillaries. *Distribution* occurs when drug molecules that have entered the vascular system pass from the bloodstream into various tissues and organs such as the muscle or heart. *Metabolism* is the chemical conversion of the drug molecule, usually by an enzymatically mediated reaction, into another chemical entity referred to as a *metabolite*. The metabolite may have the same, or different, pharmacological effect as the parent drug, or even cause toxic side effects. *Excretion* is the irreversible removal of drug from the body and commonly occurs via the kidney or biliary tract.

Pharmacodynamics is the relationship between drug concentration and pharmacological response. It is extremely important for clinicians to realize that the change in drug effect is usually not proportional to the change in drug dose or concentration (Figure 1-1). For example, when a drug dose or concentration is increased from a baseline value, the increase in pharmacological effect is greater when the initial dose or concentration is low compared to the change in drug effect observed when the initial dose or concentration is high. Thus, the increase in pharmacological effect that one observes in a patient as the dose is incremented is subject to the law of diminishing returns and will eventually reach a maximum. The reason that most drugs follow this pattern is because their pharmacological effect is produced by forming a complex with a drug receptor. Once the drug-receptor complex is formed, the pharmacological effect is expressed. Often, toxic side effects of drugs follow the same type of dose- or concentration-response relationship, albeit shifted to the right on the dose or concentration axis. In clinical situations, patients may need to tolerate some drug side effects in order to obtain the maximal pharmacological effect of the agent.

LINEAR VERSUS NONLINEAR PHARMACOKINETICS

When drugs are given on a constant basis, such as a continuous intravenous infusion or an oral medication given every 12 hours, serum drug concentrations increase until the rate of drug administration equals the rate of drug metabolism and excretion. At that point, serum drug concentrations become constant during a continuous intravenous infusion or exhibit a repeating pattern over each dosage interval for medications given at a scheduled time (Figure 1-2). For example, if theophylline is given as a continuous infusion at a rate of 50 mg/h, theophylline serum concentrations will increase until the removal of theophylline via hepatic

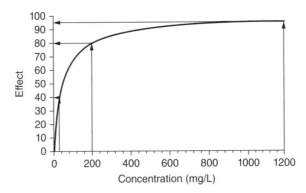

FIGURE 1-1   The relationship between drug concentration and response is usually a hyperbolic function: Effect $= (E_{max} \cdot C)/$ $(EC_{50} + C)$, where E_{max} is the maximum effect and EC_{50} is the drug concentration where the drug effect equals $E_{max}/2$. After a dosage change is made and drug concentrations increase, the drug effect does not change proportionally. Further, the increase in pharmacological effect is greater when the initial concentration is low compared to the change in drug effect observed when the initial concentration is high. In this graph, the drug effect changes ~50% (from ~40 to 80 units) with a fivefold increase in concentrations at low levels (from ~40 to 200 mg/L), but only ~20% (from ~80 to 95 units) when the same fivefold increase in concentrations is made at high concentrations (from ~200 to 1000 mg/L).

metabolism and renal excretion equals 50 mg/h. If cyclosporine is given orally at a dose of 300 mg every 12 hours, cyclosporine blood concentrations will follow a repeating pattern over the dosage interval that will increase after a dose is given (because of drug absorption from the GI tract) and decrease after absorption is complete. This repeating pattern continues and eventually drug concentrations for each dosage interval become superimposable when the amount of cyclosporine absorbed into the body from the GI tract equals the amount removed by hepatic metabolism over each dosage interval. Regardless of the mode of drug administration, when the rate of drug administration equals the rate of drug removal, the amount of drug contained in the body reaches a constant value. This equilibrium condition is known as *steady-state* and is extremely important in clinical pharmacokinetics because usually steady-state serum or blood concentrations are used to assess patient response and compute new dosage regimens.

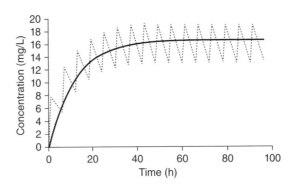

FIGURE 1-2   When medications are given on a continuous basis, serum concentrations increase until the rate of drug administration equals the elimination rate. In this case, the solid line shows serum concentrations in a patient receiving intravenous theophylline at a rate of 50 mg/h (*solid line*) and oral theophylline 300 mg every 6 hours (*dashed line*). Because the oral dosing rate (dose/dosage interval = 300 mg/6 h = 50 mg/h) equals the intravenous infusion rate, the drug accumulation patterns are similar. For the intravenous infusion, serum concentrations increase in a smooth pattern until steady-state is achieved. During oral dosing, the serum concentrations oscillate around the intravenous profile, increasing during drug absorption and decreasing after absorption is complete and elimination takes place.

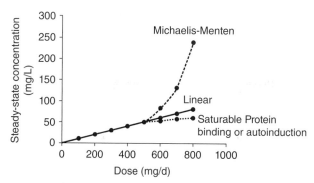

FIGURE 1-3   When doses are increased for most drugs, steady-state concentrations increase in a proportional fashion, leading to linear pharmacokinetics (*solid line*). However, in some cases proportional increases in steady-state concentrations do not occur after a dosage increase. When steady-state concentrations increase more than expected after a dosage increase (*upper dashed line*), Michaelis-Menten pharmacokinetics may be taking place. If steady-state concentrations increase less than expected after a dosage increase (*lower dashed line*), saturable plasma protein–binding or autoinduction are likely explanations.

If a patient is administered several different doses until steady-state is established and steady-state serum concentrations are obtained from the patient after each dosage level, it is possible to determine a pattern of drug accumulation (Figure 1-3). If a plot of steady-state concentration versus dose yields a straight line, the drug is said to follow *linear pharmacokinetics*. In this situation, steady-state serum concentrations increase or decrease proportionally with dose. Therefore, if a patient has a steady-state drug concentration of 10 µg/mL at a dosage rate of 100 mg/h, the steady-state serum concentration will increase to 15 µg/mL if the dosage rate is increased to 150 mg/h (eg, a 50% increase in dose yields a 50% increase in steady-state concentration).

While most drugs follow linear pharmacokinetics, in some cases drug concentrations do not change proportionally with dose. When steady-state concentrations change in a disproportionate fashion after the dose is altered, a plot of steady-state concentration versus dose is not a straight line and the drug is said to follow *nonlinear pharmacokinetics*. When steady-state concentrations increase more than expected after a dosage increase, the most likely explanation is that the processes removing the drug from the body have become saturated. This phenomenon is known as *saturable or Michaelis-Menten pharmacokinetics*. Both phenytoin[2] and salicylic acid[3] follow Michaelis-Menten pharmacokinetics. When steady-state concentrations increase less than expected after a dosage increase, there are two typical explanations. Some drugs, such as valproic acid[4] and disopyramide,[5] saturate plasma protein–binding sites so that as the dosage is increased, steady-state serum concentrations increase less than expected. Other drugs, such as carbamazepine,[6] increase their own rate of metabolism from the body as dose is increased so steady-state serum concentrations increase less than anticipated. This process is known as *autoinduction* of drug metabolism. In either case, the relationship between steady-state concentration and dose for drugs that follow nonlinear pharmacokinetics is fraught with significant intersubject variability. Drugs that exhibit nonlinear pharmacokinetics are often times very difficult to dose correctly.

Steady-state serum concentration/dose plots for medications are determined in humans early during the drug development process. Because of this, by the time a new drug is available for general use, it is usually known whether the drug follows linear or nonlinear pharmacokinetics, and it is not necessary to determine this relationship in individual patients. Thus, the clinician treating a patient knows whether to anticipate linear or nonlinear pharmacokinetics and can assume the appropriate situation when adjusting drug doses. Dealing with drugs that follow linear pharmacokinetics is more straightforward and relatively easy. If a patient has been taking a medication long enough for steady-state to have been established and it is determined that a dosage adjustment is necessary because of lack of drug effect or the presence of drug toxicity, steady-state drug concentrations will change in proportion to dose for drugs that follow linear pharmacokinetics. For example, if a patient is taking sustained-release procainamide 1000 mg every 12 hours for the treatment of a cardiac arrhythmia but is still having the arrhythmia, a clinician could obtain a steady-state procainamide serum concentration. If the procainamide concentration was too low (eg, 4 µg/mL before the next dose), a dosage increase could help suppress the arrhythmia. Using linear pharmacokinetic principles, one could determine that a dosage increase to 1500 mg every 12 hours would increase the steady-state procainamide serum concentration to 6 µg/mL (eg, new steady-state concentration = [new dose/old dose] × old steady-state concentration; new steady-state concentration = [1500 mg/1000 mg] × 4 µg/mL = 6 µg/mL).

CLEARANCE

Clearance (Cl) is the most important pharmacokinetic parameter because it determines the maintenance dose (MD) that is required to obtain a given steady-state serum concentration (Css): MD = Css • Cl. If one knows the clearance of a drug and wants to achieve a certain steady-state serum concentration, it is easy to compute the required maintenance dose. Target steady-state concentrations are usually chosen from previous studies in patients that have determined minimum effective concentrations and maximum concentrations that produce the desired pharmacological effect but avoid toxic side effects. This range of steady-state concentrations is known as the *therapeutic range* for the drug. The therapeutic range should be considered as an initial guideline for drug concentrations in a specific patient; drug dose and steady-state concentrations should then be titrated and individualized based on therapeutic response. For example, the therapeutic range for theophylline is generally accepted as 5-15 µg/mL for the treatment of asthma. If it were known that the theophylline clearance for a patient equaled 3 L/h and the desired steady-state theophylline serum concentration was 10 µg/mL, the theophylline maintenance dose to achieve this concentration would be 30 mg/h (10 µg/mL = 10 mg/L; MD = Css • Cl; MD = 10 mg/L • 3 L/h = 30 mg/h).

The definition of clearance is the volume of serum or blood completely cleared of the drug per unit time. Thus, the dimension of clearance is volume per unit time, such as L/h or mL/min. The liver is most often the organ responsible for drug metabolism while in most cases the kidney is responsible for drug elimination. The GI wall, lung, and kidney can also metabolize some drugs, and some medications are eliminated unchanged in the bile. Drug metabolism is characterized as Phase I reactions, which oxidize drug molecules, and Phase II reactions, which form glucuronide or sulfate esters with drug molecules. In either case, the resulting metabolite is more water soluble than the parent drug and is more likely to be eliminated in the urine.

The majority of drug metabolism is catalyzed by enzymes contained in the microsomes of hepatocytes known as the *cytochrome P-450 enzyme* system. This family of enzymes is very important to understand because specific enzymes are responsible for the metabolism of each drug entity. Once it is known that a patient is deficient in one of the enzymes, usually because the clearance of a known drug substrate is very low resulting in high steady-state serum concentrations for a low to moderate dose, it can be inferred that all drugs metabolized by that enzyme will have a low clearance and doses of other drugs that are substrates of the enzyme may be empirically reduced. If a metabolic drug interaction occurs between one medication and another known to be a substrate for a specific enzyme, it can be assumed that a drug interaction will occur between that drug and other substrates of the same enzyme. The enzymes are classified using a series of numbers and letters, and they indicate how closely related the enzymes are to each other using amino acid sequencing. As an example of the classification scheme, the enzyme known as *CYP3A4* is named because it is part of the cytochrome P-450 family (CYP), the major family group is "3," the subfamily group within the family is "A" and the specific, individual enzyme within the subfamily is "4." Thus, using this scheme, one can tell that CYP2C9 and CYP2E1 belong to the same family, and CYP2C9 and CYP2C19 belong to the same subfamily and are closely related, but they are different enzymes. Table 1-1 lists the cytochrome P-450 enzymes responsible for the majority of drug oxidative metabolism in humans along with examples of known substrates, inhibitors, and inducers.[7,8] Some ethnic groups are deficient in certain enzyme families to a varying extent, and this information is included.

TABLE 1-1   Cytochrome P-450 Enzymes, With Selected Substrates, Inhibitors, and Inducers[7,8]

Cytochrome P-450 Enzyme	Substrates	Inhibitors	Inducers
CYP1A2	Acetaminophen Caffeine Clomipramine Flutamide Frovatriptan Imipramine Leflunomide Mirtazapine Nortriptyline Olanzapine Ondansetron Phenacetin Pimozide Rasagiline Riluzone Roflumilast Ropinirole Ropivacaine Selegiline Tacrine Theophylline Tizanidine (R)-Warfarin Zileuton Zolmitriptan	Armodafinil Artemisinin Atazanavir Cimetidine Ciprofloxacin Enoxacin Erythromycin Fluvoxamine Interferon Mexiletine Tacrine Thiabendazole Ticlopidine Vemurafenib Zileuton	Barbiturates Carbamazepine Charcoal-broiled meat Omeprazole Phenobarbital Phenytoin Primidone Rifampin Tobacco/Marijuana Smoke
CYP2B6 PM: ~4% Caucasians	Bupropion Cyclophosphamide Ifosfamide	Thiotepa Ticlopidine	Phenobarbital Rifampin
CYP2C9 PM: ~7% Caucasians	Candesartan Celecoxib Chlorpropamide Diclofenac Dronabinol Glipizide Glyburide Ibuprofen Irbesartan Losartan Naproxen Phenytoin Piroxicam Sulfamethoxazole Tolbutamide Torsemide Valsartan (S)-Warfarin	Amiodarone Atazanavir Clopidogrel Cotrimoxazole Delavirdine Disulfiram Doxifluridine Efavirenz Fluconazole Fluvastatin Fluvoxamine Imatinib Isoniazid Leflunomide Metronidazole Miconazole Sulfamethoxazole Sulfinpyrazole Valproic acid Voriconazole Zafirlukast	Aminoglutethimide Barbiturates Carbamazepine Griseofulvin Phenobarbital Phenytoin Primidone Rifampin Rifapentine Ritonavir

(Continued)

TABLE 1-1   Cytochrome P-450 Enzymes, With Selected Substrates, Inhibitors, and Inducers[7,8] (Continued)

Cytochrome P-450 Enzyme	Substrates	Inhibitors	Inducers
CYP2C19 PM: ~4% Caucasians ~20% Japanese & Chinese	Amitriptyline Carisoprodol Citalopram Clomipramine Desmethyldiazepam Diazepam Hexobarbital Imipramine Lansoprazole (S)-Mephenytoin Nelfinavir Omeprazole Pantoprazole Phenytoin Primidone Propranolol Sertraline Voriconazole (R)-Warfarin	Chloramphenicol Cimetidine Clopidogrel Delavirdine Efavirenz Esomeprazole Fluconazole Felbamate Fluoxetine Fluvoxamine Isoniazid Moclobemide Modafinil Omeprazole Oxcarbazepine Ticlopidine Voriconazole	Barbiturates Phenobarbital Phenytoin Primidone Rifampin St. John's wort
CYP2D6 PM: ~8% Caucasians ~3% African Americans ~1% Japanese & Chinese	Amitriptyline Carvedilol Chlorpromazine Clomipramine Codeine Debrisoquin Desipramine Dextromethorphan Encainide Flecainide Fluoxetine Fluvoxamine Haloperidol Hydrocodone Imipramine Maprotiline Methamphetamine (S)-Metoprolol Mexiletine Nortriptyline Oxycodone Paroxetine Perhexiline Perphenazine Propafenone Propranolol Risperidone Sertraline Sparteine Thioridazine Timolol Tramadol Trazodone Venlafaxine	Abiraterone Amiodarone Bupropion Celecoxib Chloroquine Chlorpheniramine Chlorpromazine Cimetidine Cinacalcet Clemastine Darifenacin Diphenhydramine Dronedarone Duloxetine Flecainide Fluoxetine Haloperidol Hydroxyzine Imatinib Lumefantrine Moclobemide Paroxetine Perphenazine Promethazine Propafenone Propoxyphene Quinacrine Quinidine Quinine Ritonavir Sertraline Terbinafine Thioridazine Tripelennamine	

(Continued)

TABLE 1-1   Cytochrome P-450 Enzymes, With Selected Substrates, Inhibitors, and Inducers[7,8] (Continued)

Cytochrome P-450 Enzyme	Substrates	Inhibitors	Inducers
CYP2E1	Acetaminophen Chlorzoxazone Enflurane Ethanol Halothane Isoflurane Theophylline	Disulfiram	Ethanol Isoniazid
CYP3A group (includes 3A4, 3A5, 3A7)	Alfentanil Alprazolam Amiodarone Amlodipine Astemizole Atorvastatin Bepridil Bromocriptine Buspirone Carbamazepine Cerivastatin Chlorpheniramine Cilostazol Cisapride Clarithromycin Clonazepam Clopidogrel Cyclosporine Delavirdine Dexamethazone Diazepam Diltiazem Disopyramide Donepezil Doxorubicin Erythromycin Ethinyl Estradiol Etoposide Felodipine Fentanyl Finasteride Flurazepam Hydrocortisone Indinavir Isradipine Itraconazozle Ketoconazole Lansoprazole Lidocaine Loratadine Losartan Lovastatin Methylprednisolone Midazolam Nefazodone	Amiodarone Amprenavir Aprepitant Atazanavir Bocepravir Clarithromycin Conivaptan Crizotinib Cyclosporine Danazole Darunavir Delavirdine Desatinib Diltiazem Dronedarone Erythromycin Fluconazole Fluvoxamine Fosamprenavir Grapefruit Juice Imatinib Indinavir Isoniazid Itraconazole Ketoconazole Lapatinib Mifepristone Miconazole Nafcillin Nefazodone Nelfinavir Norfloxacin Quinupristin Ritonavir Saquinavir Tamoxifen Telaprevir Telithromycin Troleandomycin Verapamil Voriconazole Zafirlukast	Aminoglutethimide Armodafinil Artemether Barbiturates Bexarotene Bosentan Carbamazepine Dexamethasone Efavirenz Mitotane Modafinil Nefazodone Nevirapine Oxcarbazepine Phenobarbital Phenytoin Primidone Rifabutin Rifampin St. John's wort Troglitazone Vemurafenib

(Continued)

TABLE 1-1   Cytochrome P-450 Enzymes, With Selected Substrates, Inhibitors, and Inducers[7,8] (Continued)

Cytochrome P-450 Enzyme	Substrates	Inhibitors	Inducers
CYP3A group (includes 3A4, 3A5, 3A7) (Cont.)	Nelfinavir Nicardipine Nifedipine Nimodipine Nisoldipine Nitrendipine Oxycodone Pioglitazone Prednisolone Prednisone Progesterone Quinidine Quinine Rifabutin Ritonavir Salmeterol Saquinavir Sildenafil Simvastatin Sirolimus Sufentanil Tacrolimus Telithromycin Teniposide Terfenadine Testosterone Theophylline Topiramate Triazolam Troleandomycin Vardenafil Verapamil Vinblastine Vincristine Voriconazole Zalepion Ziprasidone Zolpidem Zonisamide		

Membrane transporters are proteins involved in the active transport of drug molecules across cell membranes, and this movement results in the transfer of drugs either into or out of cells.[9,10] Transporters have been identified in the intestinal epithelia, hepatocytes, kidney proximal tubules, and the cells comprising the blood-brain barrier. If a membrane transporter results in drug elimination from the body, the process can contribute toward drug clearance. In some cases, transporters may work in tandem with drug metabolizing enzymes by enhancing delivery of drug molecules to the enzyme. P-glycoprotein (PGP) is a transport protein responsible for the active secretion of drugs into the bile, urine, and GI tract. Many other drug transporters may be involved in the clearance of specific drug molecules. General classifications include the Organic Cation Transporters (OCT family), Organic Anion Transporters (OAT family), and the Organic Anion Transporting Polypeptides (OATP family). Table 1-2 lists selected membrane transporter substrates, inhibitors, and inducers.[7,9,10]

TABLE 1-2   Membrane Transporters, With Selected Substrates, Inhibitors, and Inducers[7,9,10]

Membrane Transporter	Substrates	Inhibitors	Inducers
P-Glycoprotein (PGP) Sites: intestinal enterocytes, kidney proximal tubule, hepatocytes (canalicular), brain endothelia	Alfentanil Aliskiren Ambrisentan Amprenavir Atorvastatin Azithromycin Boceprevir Budesonide Cetirizine Citalopram Clopidogrel Cyclosporine Daunorubicin Desloratadine Dexamethasone Digoxin Diltiazem Doxorubicin Eletriptan Erythromycin Etoposide Fexofenadine Glyburide Indinavir Imatinib Linagliptin Loperamide Loratadine Lovastatin Morphine Nelfinavir Olanzapine Ondansetron Paclitaxel Plicamycin Posaconazole Quinidine Raltegravir Ranolazine Rifampin Risperidone Ritonavir Saquinavir Tacrolimus Telaprevir Verapamil Vinblastine Vincristine	Alfentanil Amiodarone Bepridil Carvedilol Conivaptan Clarithromycin Cyclosporine Diltiazem Dronedarone Duloxetine Erythromycin Fenofibrate Grapefruit juice Indinavir Itraconazole Ketoconazole Lapatinib Lovastatin Mifepristone Nicardipine Nelfinavir Posaconazole Propafenone Quinidine Ritonavir Saquinavir Tacrolimus Tamoxifen Telaprevir Testosterone Ticagrelor Verapamil	Barbiturates Carbamazepine Dexamethasone Rifampin St. John's wort

(Continued)

TABLE 1-2   Membrane Transporters, With Selected Substrates, Inhibitors, and Inducers[7,9,10] (Continued)

Membrane Transporter	Substrates	Inhibitors	Inducers
OAT1B1 Site: hepatocytes (sinusoidal)	Bosentan Olmesartan Repaglinide Statins Valsartan	Cyclosporine Lopinavir Rifampicin Ritonavir Saquinavir	
OAT1 Sites: kidney proximal tubule, placenta	Acyclovir Cephradine Ciprofloxacin Methotrexate Zidovudine	Novobiocin Probenecid	
OAT3 Sites: kidney proximal tubule, choroid plexus, brain endothelia	Bumetanide Cefaclor Ceftizoxime Furosemide NSAIDs	Novobiocin Probenecid	
OCT1 Sites: hepatocytes (sinusoidal), intestinal enterocytes	Metformin Oxaliplatin	Disopyramide Quinidine Quinine	
OCT2 Sites: kidney proximal tubule, neurons	Amantadine Amiloride Metformin Pindolol Procainamide Ranitidine	Cetirizine Cimetidine Quinidine Testosterone	

NSAIDs, nonsteroidal anti-inflammatory drugs; OAT, Organic Anion Transporter, OCT, Organic Cation Transporter.

The kidney eliminates drugs by glomerular filtration and tubular secretion in the nephron. Once drug molecules have entered the urine by either of these processes, it is possible that the molecules may reenter the blood via a process known as *tubular reabsorption*. Glomerular filtration and, usually, tubular reabsorption are passive processes. Tubular secretion is an active process usually mediated by a membrane transporter, which facilitates the transfer of drug across the kidney tubule. The majority of drug tubular secretion takes place in the proximal tubule of the nephron while tubular reabsorption usually takes place in the distal tubule of the nephron.

The clearance for an organ, such as the liver or kidney, that metabolizes or eliminates drugs is determined by the blood flow to the organ and the ability of the organ to metabolize or eliminate the drug.[11] Liver blood flow (LBF) and renal blood flow (RBF) are each ~ 1-1.5 L/min in adults with normal cardiovascular function. The ability of an organ to remove or extract the drug from the blood or serum is usually measured by determining the extraction ratio (ER), which is the fraction of drug removed by the organ, and is computed by measuring the concentrations of the drug entering (C_{in}) and leaving (C_{out}) the organ: $ER = (C_{in} - C_{out})/C_{in}$. Liver or renal blood flow and the extraction ratio for a drug are rarely measured in patients. However, the extraction ratio is often times determined during the drug development process, and knowledge of this parameter can be extremely useful in determining how the pharmacokinetics of a drug will change during a drug interaction or whether a patient develops hepatic, renal, or cardiac failure. The drug clearance for an organ is equal to the product of the blood flow to the organ and the extraction ratio of the drug. Therefore, hepatic clearance (Cl_H) for a drug would be determined by taking the product of liver blood flow and the hepatic

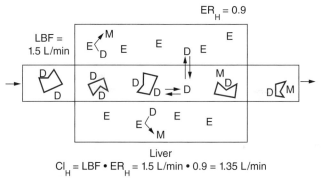

FIGURE 1-4   This schematic depicts the liver (*large box*) with the blood vessel supplying blood to it. When drug molecules (D) enter an organ (blood flows from left to right) that clears the drug, they may be bound to plasma proteins (*trapezoid shapes*) or exist in the unbound state. The unbound or "free" drug molecules are in equilibrium with the bound drug in the blood and unbound drug in the tissue. Drug-protein complexes are usually too big to diffuse across biologic membranes into tissues. Drug molecules that have entered hepatic tissue may encounter an enzyme (E) that metabolizes the drug. When this occurs, the drug is chemically converted to a metabolite (M) that can diffuse back into the blood and leave the liver along with drug molecules that were not metabolized. The clearance of drug is equal to the liver blood flow (LBF) times the extraction ratio (ER_H) for the organ.

extraction ratio (ER_H) for the drug ($Cl_H = LBF \cdot ER_H$), and renal clearance (Cl_R) for a medication would be determined by multiplying renal blood flow and the renal extraction ratio for the agent ($Cl_R = RBF \cdot ER_R$). For example, verapamil has a hepatic extraction ratio of 90% ($ER_H = 0.90$). For patients with normal liver blood flow (LBF = 1.5 L/min), hepatic clearance would be expected to equal 1.35 L/min ($Cl_H = LBF \cdot ER_H$, $Cl_H = 1.5$ L/min • 0.90 = 1.35 L/min; Figure 1-4). The total clearance for a drug is the sum of the individual clearances for each organ that extracts the medication. For example, the total clearance (Cl) for a drug that is metabolized by the liver and eliminated by the kidney is the sum of hepatic and renal clearance for the agent: $Cl = Cl_H + Cl_R$.

Hepatic clearance

The physiologic determinates of hepatic clearance have been extensively studied.[11-13] Another way to think of hepatic clearance is to recognize that its value is a function of the intrinsic ability of the enzyme to metabolize a drug (intrinsic clearance); the fraction of drug present in the bloodstream that is not bound to cells or proteins, such as albumin, α_1-acid glycoprotein, or lipoproteins, but is present in the unbound, or "free," state (unbound fraction of drug); and liver blood flow. The intrinsic clearance (Cl'_{int}) is the inherent ability of the enzyme to metabolize the drug and is the quotient of the Michaelis-Menten constants V_{max} (maximum rate of drug metabolism) and K_m (drug concentration at which the metabolic rate equals $V_{max}/2$; $Cl'_{int} = V_{max}/K_m$) for the unbound drug. The unbound fraction of drug in the blood or serum (f_B) is the unbound drug concentration divided by the total (bound + unbound) drug concentration. The relationship between the three physiological factors and hepatic drug clearance is

$$Cl_H = \frac{LBF \cdot (f_B \cdot Cl'_{int})}{LBF + (f_B \cdot Cl'_{int})}$$

Fortunately, most drugs have a large hepatic extraction ratio ($ER_H \geq 0.7$) or a small hepatic extraction ratio ($ER_H \leq 0.3$), and the relationship is simplified in these situations. For drugs with a low hepatic extraction ratio, hepatic clearance is mainly a product of the free fraction of the drug in the blood or serum and intrinsic clearance: $Cl_H = f_B \cdot Cl'_{int}$. In this case, drug interactions that displace drug molecules bound to proteins will increase the fraction of unbound drug in the blood ($\uparrow f_B$); more unbound drug molecules will be able to leave the vascular system (drug-protein complexes are far too big to exit the vascular system) and enter hepatocytes where the additional unbound drug will be metabolized and hepatic drug clearance will increase. Additionally, drug interactions that inhibit or induce the cytochrome P-450 enzyme system (decreasing or increasing Cl'_{int}, respectively) will change the hepatic clearance of the medication accordingly. The hepatic clearance of drugs with low extraction ratios does not change much when liver blood flow decreases secondary to liver or cardiac disease. Examples of drugs with low hepatic extraction ratios include valproic acid, phenytoin, and warfarin.

For drugs with a high hepatic extraction ratio, hepatic clearance is mainly a function of liver blood flow: $Cl_H = LBF$. The rate-limiting step for drug metabolism in this case is how much drug can be delivered to the liver because the capacity to metabolize drug is very large. In this case, hepatic clearance is very sensitive to changes in liver blood flow due to congestive heart failure or liver disease. However, the hepatic clearance of drugs with high extraction ratios does not change much when protein-binding displacement or enzyme induction or inhibition occurs due to drug interactions. Examples of drugs with high hepatic extraction ratios include lidocaine, morphine, and most tricyclic antidepressants.

Renal clearance

The physiologic determinants of renal clearance include glomerular filtration rate (GFR), the free fraction of drug in the blood or serum (f_B), the clearance of drug via renal tubular secretion (Cl_{sec}), and the fraction of drug reabsorbed in the kidney (FR): $Cl_R = [(f_B \cdot GFR) + Cl_{sec}](1 - FR)$.[14,15] Average glomerular filtration rates in adults with normal renal function are 100-120 mL/min. Because tubular secretion is an active process, it has been described by an equation similar to that used to explain liver metabolism: $Cl_{sec} = [RBF \cdot (f_B Cl'_{sec})]/[RBF + (f_B Cl'_{sec})]$, where Cl'_{sec} is the intrinsic clearance due to active tubular secretion. Thus, the entire equation is

$$Cl_R = \left[(f_B \cdot GFR) + \frac{RBF \cdot (f_B Cl'_{sec})}{RBF + (f_B Cl'_{sec})} \right](1 - FR)$$

If the renal clearance of a drug is greater than glomerular filtration rate, it is likely that the drug was eliminated, in part, by active tubular secretion. The aminoglycoside antibiotics and vancomycin are eliminated primarily by glomerular filtration. Digoxin, procainamide, ranitidine, and ciprofloxacin are eliminated by both glomerular filtration and active tubular secretion.

In some cases, glomerular filtration rate and renal tubular section function may be measured in patients with renal disease. However, for the purposes of drug dosing, glomerular filtration rate is approximated by measuring or estimating creatinine clearance for a patient. Creatinine is a by-product of muscle metabolism that is eliminated primarily by glomerular filtration.

VOLUME OF DISTRIBUTION

Volume of distribution (V) is an important pharmacokinetic parameter because it determines the loading dose (LD) that is required to achieve a particular steady-state drug concentration immediately after the dose is administered: $LD = Css \cdot V$ (Figure 1-5). However, it is rare to know the exact volume of distribution for a patient because it is necessary to administer a dose on a previous occasion in order to have computed the volume of distribution. Thus, usually an average volume of distribution measured in other patients with similar demographics (age, weight, gender, etc) and medical conditions (renal failure, liver failure, heart failure, etc) is used to estimate a loading dose (Figure 1-6). Because of this, most patients will not actually attain

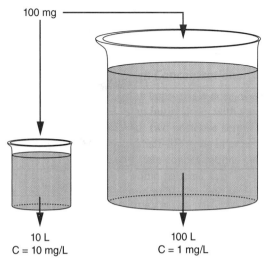

FIGURE 1-5 The volume of distribution (V) is a hypothetical volume that is the proportionality constant which relates the concentration of drug in the blood or serum (C) and the amount of drug in the body (A_B): $A_B = C \cdot V$. It can be thought of as a beaker of fluid representing the entire space that drug distributes into. In this case, one beaker, representing a patient with a small volume of distribution, contains 10 L while the other beaker, representing a patient with a large volume of distribution, contains 100 L. If 100 mg of drug is given to each patient, the resulting concentration will be 10 mg/L in the patient with the smaller volume of distribution but 1 mg/L in the patient with the larger volume of distribution. If the minimum concentration needed to exert the pharmacological effect of the drug is 5 mg/L, one patient will receive a benefit from the drug while the other will have a subtherapeutic concentration.

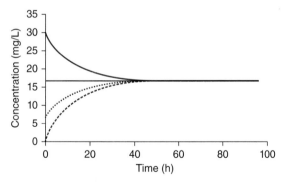

FIGURE 1-6 If the volume of distribution (V) is known for a patient, it is possible to administer a loading dose (LD) that will attain a specified steady-state drug concentration (Css): $LD = Css \cdot V$. This example depicts the ideal loading dose given as an intravenous bolus dose followed by a continuous intravenous infusion (*black solid line*) so steady-state is achieved immediately and maintained. If a loading dose was not given and a continuous infusion started (*dashed line*), it would take time to reach steady-state concentrations and the patient may not experience an effect from the drug until a minimum effect concentration is achieved. This situation would not be acceptable for many clinical situations where a quick onset of action is needed. Because the volume of distribution is not known for a patient before a dose is given, clinicians use an average volume of distribution previously measured in patients with similar demographics and disease states to compute loading doses. When this is done, the patient's volume of distribution may be smaller than average and result in higher than expected concentrations (*blue solid line*) or larger than average and result in lower than expected concentrations (*dotted line*). In these cases, it still takes 3-5 half-lives to reach steady-state, but therapeutic drug concentrations are achieved much sooner than giving the drug by intravenous infusion only.

steady-state after a loading dose, but, hopefully, serum drug concentrations will be high enough so that the patient will experience the pharmacological effect of the drug.

The volume of distribution is a hypothetical volume that relates drug serum concentrations to the amount of drug in the body. Thus, the dimension of volume of distribution is in volume units, such as L or mL. At any given time after drug has been absorbed from extravascular sites and the serum and tissue drug concentrations are in equilibrium, the serum concentration for a drug (C) is equal to the quotient of the amount of drug in the body (A_B) and the volume of distribution: $C = A_B/V$. The volume of distribution can be very small if the drug is primarily contained in the blood (warfarin V = 5-7 L), or very large if the drug distributes widely in the body and is mostly bound to bodily tissues (digoxin V = 500 L).

The physiologic determinates of volume of distribution are the actual volume of blood (V_B) and size (measured as a volume) of the various tissues and organs of the body (V_T). Therefore, a larger person, such as a 160-kg football player, would be expected to have a larger volume of distribution for a drug than a smaller person, such as a 40-kg grandmother. How the drug binds in the blood or serum compared to the binding in tissues is also an important determinate of the volume of distribution for a drug. For example, the reason warfarin has such a small volume of distribution is that it is highly bound to serum albumin so that the free fraction of drug in the blood (f_B) is very small. Digoxin has a very large volume of distribution because it is very highly bound to tissues (primarily muscle) so that the free fraction of drug in the tissues (f_T; f_T = unbound drug concentration in the tissue/total tissue drug concentration) is very small. The equation that relates all of these physiologic determinates to the volume of distribution is[16]

$$V = V_B + \frac{f_B}{f_T} V_T$$

This equation can help clinicians understand why a drug has a large or small volume of distribution or why the volume of distribution might change under various circumstances. An example is how the volume of distribution changes when a plasma protein binding drug interactions occurs. If a drug that is highly bound to plasma proteins is given to a patient and then a second drug that is also highly bound to the same plasma protein is given concurrently, the second drug will compete for plasma protein–binding sites and displace the first drug from the protein. In this case, the free fraction in the serum of the first drug will increase ($\uparrow f_B$), resulting in an increased volume of distribution: $\uparrow V = V_B + (\uparrow f_B/f_T)V_T$. While diffusion of drug molecules across a concentration gradient is a major driving force for drug distribution, membrane transporters are also involved in the distribution of agents in the body.[10]

HALF-LIFE AND ELIMINATION RATE CONSTANT

When drugs that follow linear pharmacokinetics are given to humans, serum concentrations decline in a curvilinear fashion (Figure 1-7). When the same data is plotted on a semilogarithmic axis, serum concentrations decrease in a linear fashion after drug absorption and distribution phases are complete (Figure 1-8). This part of the curve is known as the *elimination phase*. The time that it takes for serum concentrations to decrease by ½ in the elimination phase is a constant and is called the *half-life* ($t_{1/2}$). The half-life describes how quickly drug serum concentrations decrease in a patient after a medication is administered, and the dimension of half-life is time (h, min, d, etc). Another common measurement used to denote how quickly drug serum concentrations decline in a patient is the elimination rate constant (k_e). The dimension for the elimination rate constant is reciprocal time (h^{-1}, min^{-1}, d^{-1}, etc). If the amount of drug in the body is known, the elimination rate for the drug can be computed by taking the product of the elimination rate constant and the amount of drug in the body (A_B): elimination rate = $A_B \cdot k_e$. The half-life and elimination rate constant are related to each other by

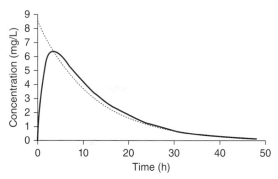

FIGURE 1-7   Serum concentration/time profile for a patient receiving 300 mg of theophylline orally (*solid line*) and by intravenous bolus (*dashed line*). If these data are plotted on rectilinear axes, serum concentrations decline in a curvilinear fashion in both cases. When the drug is given orally, serum concentrations initially increase while the drug is being absorbed and decline after drug absorption is complete.

the following equation, so it is easy to compute one once the other is known: $t_{1/2} = 0.693/k_e$. The elimination rate constant can also be measured graphically by computing the slope of the log concentration versus time graph during the elimination phase: using $\log_{10}$, $k_e/2.303 = -(\log C_1 - \log C_2)/(t_1 - t_2)$; or using natural logarithms, $k_e = -(\ln C_1 - \ln C_2)/(t_1 - t_2)$.

The half-life is important because it determines the time to steady-state during the continuous dosing of a drug and the dosage interval. The approach to steady-state serum concentrations is an exponential function. If a drug is administered on a continuous basis for 3 half-lives, serum concentrations are ~90% of steady-state values; on a continuous basis for 5 half-lives, serum concentrations equal ~95% of steady-state values; or on a continuous basis for 7 half-lives, serum concentrations achieve ~99% of steady-state values (Figure 1-9). Generally, drug serum concentrations used for pharmacokinetic monitoring can be safely measured after 3-5 estimated half-lives because most drug assays have 5%-10% measurement error. It should be noted that the half-life for a drug in a patient is not usually known but is estimated using values previously measured during pharmacokinetic studies conducted in similar patients.

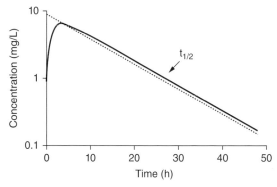

FIGURE 1-8   Serum concentration/time profile for a patient receiving 300 mg of theophylline orally (*solid line*) and by intravenous bolus (*dashed line*). If these data are plotted on semilogarithmic axes, serum concentrations decline in a straight line in both cases. When the drug is given orally, serum concentrations initially increase while the drug is being absorbed and decline after drug absorption is complete. This same data set is plotted in Figure 1-7 on rectilinear axes.

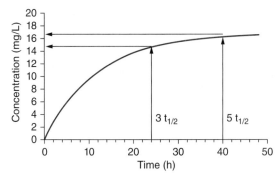

FIGURE 1-9   Serum concentration/time graph for a drug that has a half-life equal to 8 hours. The arrows indicate concentrations at 3 half-lives (24 h, ~90% of Css) and at 5 half-lives (40 hours, ~95% of Css). Because most drug assays have 5%-10% measurement error, serum concentrations obtained between 3 and 5 half-lives after dosing commenced can be considered to be at steady-state for clinical purposes and used to adjust drug doses.

The dosage interval for a drug is also determined by the half-life of the medication. For example, if the therapeutic range of a drug is 10-20 mg/L, the ideal dosage interval would not let maximum serum concentrations exceed 20 mg/L or allow the minimum serum concentration to go below 10 mg/L (Figure 1-10). In this case, the dosage interval that would produce this steady-state concentration/time profile would be every half-life. After a dose is given, the maximum serum concentration would be 20 mg/L. In 1 half-life the serum concentration would be 10 mg/L, and the next dose would be administered to the patient. At steady-state, this serum concentration/time profile would be repeated after each dose. During drug development, it is very common to use the drug half-life as the initial dosage interval for the new drug compound until the pharmacodynamics of the agent can be determined.

The half-life and elimination rate constant are known as *dependent parameters* because their values depend on the clearance (Cl) and volume of distribution (V) of the agent: $t_{1/2} = (0.693 \cdot V)/Cl$, $k_e = Cl/V$. The half-life and elimination rate constant for a drug can change either because of a change in clearance or a change in the volume of distribution. Because the values for clearance and volume of distribution depend solely on physiologic parameters and can vary independently of each other, they are known as *independent parameters*.

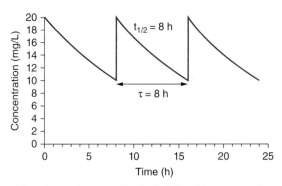

FIGURE 1-10   The dosage interval for a drug is determined by the half-life of the agent. In this case, the half-life of the drug is 8 hours, and the therapeutic range of the drug is 10-20 mg/L. In order to ensure that maximum serum concentrations never go above and minimum serum concentrations never go below the therapeutic range, it is necessary to give the drug every 8 hours (τ = dosage interval).

Mean residence time (MRT) is another parameter that describes persistence of drug in the body.[1] The mean residence time is the average amount of time during which drug molecules reside in the body. Half-life and elimination rate constant describe the elimination of drug only during the postabsorption and postdistribution phases, but the mean residence time covers the entire time during which the drug is in the body.

MICHAELIS-MENTEN OR SATURABLE PHARMACOKINETICS

Drugs that are metabolized by the cytochrome P-450 enzymes and other enzyme systems may undergo Michaelis-Menten or saturable pharmacokinetics. This is the type of nonlinear pharmacokinetics that occurs when the number of drug molecules overwhelms or saturates the ability of the enzymes to metabolize the drug.[2,3] When this occurs, steady-state drug serum concentrations increase in a disproportionate manner after an increase in dosage (see Figure 1-3). In this case the rate of drug removal is described by the classic Michaelis-Menten relationship that is used for all enzyme systems: rate of metabolism = $(V_{max} \cdot C)/(K_m + C)$, where V_{max} is the maximum rate of metabolism, C is the substrate concentration, and K_m is the substrate concentration where the rate of metabolism = $V_{max}/2$.

The clinical implication of Michaelis-Menten pharmacokinetics is that the clearance of a drug is not a constant as it is with linear pharmacokinetics, but it is concentration- or dose-dependent. As the dose or concentration increases, the clearance rate (Cl) decreases as the enzyme approaches saturable conditions: $Cl = V_{max}/(K_m + C)$. This is the reason concentrations increase disproportionately after a dosage increase. For example, phenytoin follows saturable pharmacokinetics with average Michaelis-Menten constants of V_{max} = 500 mg/d and K_m = 4 mg/L. The therapeutic range of phenytoin is 10-20 mg/L. As the steady-state concentration of phenytoin increases from 10 to 20 mg/L, clearance decreases from 36 to 21 L/d [Cl = V_{max}/ $(K_m + C)$; Cl = (500 mg/d)/(4 mg/L + 10 mg/L) = 36 L/d; Cl = (500 mg/d)/(4 mg/L + 20 mg/L) = 21 L/d]. Unfortunately, there is so much interpatient variability in Michaelis-Menten pharmacokinetic parameters for a drug (typically V_{max} = 100-1000 mg/d and K_m = 1-10 mg/L for phenytoin) that dosing drugs that follow saturable metabolism is extremely difficult.

The volume of distribution (V) is unaffected by saturable metabolism and is still determined by the physiologic volume of blood (V_B) and tissues (V_T) as well as the unbound concentration of drug in the blood (f_B) and tissues (f_T): V = V_B+ $(f_B/f_T)V_T$. Also, half-life ($t_{1/2}$) is still related to clearance and volume of distribution using the same equation as for linear pharmacokinetics: $t_{1/2}$ = (0.693 • V)/Cl. However, because clearance is dose- or concentration-dependent, half-life also changes with dosage or concentration changes. As doses or concentrations increase for a drug that follows Michaelis-Menten pharmacokinetics, clearance decreases and half-life becomes longer for the drug: $\uparrow t_{1/2}$ = (0.693 • V)/$\downarrow$Cl. The clinical implication of this finding is that the time to steady-state (3-5 $t_{1/2}$) is longer as the dose or concentration is increased for a drug that follows saturable pharmacokinetics.

Under steady-state conditions, the rate of drug administration equals the rate of drug removal. Therefore, for a drug that is solely removed by metabolism via one enzyme system, the Michaelis-Menten equation can be used to compute the maintenance dose (MD) required to achieve a target steady-state serum concentration (Css):

$$MD = \frac{V_{max} \cdot C_{SS}}{K_m + C_{SS}}$$

When the therapeutic range for a drug is far below the K_m value for the enzymes that metabolize the drug, this equation simplifies to: MD = (V_{max}/K_m)Css or, because V_{max}/K_m is a constant, MD = Cl • Css, where Cl = V_{max}/K_m. Therefore, when $K_m \gg$ Css, drugs that are metabolized follow linear pharmacokinetics. When the therapeutic range for a drug is far above the K_m value for the enzyme system that metabolizes the drug, the rate of metabolism becomes a constant equal to V_{max}. Under these conditions, only a fixed amount of drug is metabolized because the enzyme system is completely saturated and cannot increase its metabolic capacity. This situation is also known as *zero-order pharmacokinetics*. *First-order pharmacokinetics* is another name for linear pharmacokinetics.

Based on these facts, it can be seen that any drug that is metabolized by enzymes undergoes Michaelis-Menten pharmacokinetics. However, the therapeutic ranges of most drugs are far below the K_m for the enzymes that metabolize the agent. Because of this, most medications that are metabolized follow linear pharmacokinetics. However, even in these cases saturable drug metabolism can occur in drug overdose cases in which the drug concentration far exceeds the therapeutic range for the medication.

BIOAVAILABILITY

When a drug is administered extravascularly, the entire dose may not enter the systemic circulation. For example, an orally administered tablet may not completely dissolve so that part of the dose is eliminated in the stool, or a transdermal patch may not release the entire dose before it is removed from the skin. The fraction of the administered dose that is delivered to the systemic circulation is known as the *bioavailability* for the drug and dosage form. When medications are given orally, intramuscularly, subcutaneously, or by other extravascular routes, the drug must be absorbed across several biologic membranes before entering the vascular system. In these cases, drug serum concentrations rise while the drug is absorbed into the bloodstream, reach a maximum concentration (C_{max}) when the rate of drug absorption equals the rate of drug elimination, and eventually decrease according to the half-life of the drug. The phase of the curve over which absorption takes place is known as the *absorption phase*, and the time that the maximum concentration occurs is called T_{max} (Figure 1-11).

If a medication is given orally, drug molecules must pass through several organs before entering the systemic circulation. During absorption from the GI tract, the drug molecules will encounter enzymes that may metabolize the agent (primarily CYP3A4 substrates because ~90% of cytochrome P-450 contained in the gut wall is CYP3A4) or membrane transporters that may pump the drug back into the lumen and prevent absorption from taking place (primarily P-glycoprotein substrates). Once drug molecules are absorbed from the GI tract, they enter the portal vein. The portal vein and hepatic artery together supply blood to the liver, and the sum of portal vein (~2/3 total LBF) and hepatic artery (~1/3 total LBF) blood flows makes up liver blood flow (LBF) that equals ~1-1.5 L/min. If the drug is hepatically metabolized, part of the drug may be metabolized

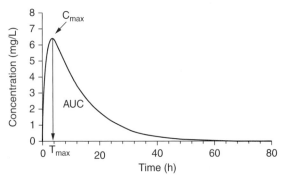

FIGURE 1-11   Area under the serum concentration/time curve (AUC), the maximum concentration (C_{max}), and the time that the maximum concentration occurs (T_{max}) are considered primary bioavailability parameters. When the AUC, C_{max}, and T_{max} are the same within statistical limits for two dosage forms of the same drug, the dosage forms are considered to be bioequivalent.

by the liver even though the majority of the drug was absorbed from the GI tract. Drugs that are substrates for CYP3A4 and CYP2D6 are particularly susceptible to presystemic metabolism by the liver. Blood leaving the liver via the hepatic vein enters the inferior vena cava and will eventually be pumped through the lung by the right side of the heart before entering the left side of the heart and being pumped into the arterial system. To a lesser extent, some drugs are metabolized by the lung or irreversibly eliminated into expired air.

The loss of drug from these combined processes is known as *presystemic metabolism* or the *first-pass effect*. Because the entire oral dose that was absorbed must take this route before entering the systemic vascular system, large amounts of drug can be lost via these processes. For example, the oral bioavailability of both propranolol (a substrate for CYP2D6 and CYP2C19) and verapamil (a substrate for CYP3A4 and P-glycoprotein) is about ~10% even though the oral dosage forms for each agent release 100% of the drug into the GI tract.

For drugs that follow linear pharmacokinetics, bioavailability is measured by comparing serum concentrations achieved after extravascular and intravenous doses in the same individual. Rather than compare drug concentrations at each time point, a composite of drug concentrations over time is derived by measuring the total area under the serum concentration time curve (AUC) for each route of administration (see Figure 1-11). If the extravascular and intravenous doses are the same, the bioavailability for a drug can be calculated by taking the ratio of the AUCs for each route of administration. For example, if 10 mg of a drug were administered to a subject on two separate occasions by intravenous (IV) and oral (PO) routes of administration, the bioavailability (F) would be computed by dividing the AUC after oral administration (AUC_{PO}) by the AUC after intravenous administration (AUC_{IV}): $F = AUC_{PO}/AUC_{IV}$. If it is not possible to administer the same dose intravenously and extravascularly because poor absorption or presystemic metabolism yields serum concentrations that are too low to measure, the bioavailability calculation can be corrected to allow for different size doses for the different routes of administration: $F = (AUC_{PO}/AUC_{IV})(D_{IV}/D_{PO})$, where D_{IV} is the intravenous dose and D_{PO} is the oral dose.

Bioequivalence

When the patent expires for drug entities, generic drugs are manufactured that are less expensive than brand name products. This is because the drug company manufacturing the generic drug does not have to prove that the drug is safe and effective as those studies were done by the pharmaceutical company producing the brand name drug. Although it is not a requirement for generic drug products to be marketed by a pharmaceutical company, a desirable attribute of a generic drug dosage form is that it produces the same serum concentration/time profile as its brand name counterpart. When it meets this requirement, the generic drug product is said to be *bioequivalent* to the brand name drug. In theory, it should be possible to substitute a bioequivalent generic drug dosage form for a brand name product without a change in steady-state drug serum concentrations or therapeutic efficacy.

Bioequivalence is achieved when the serum concentration/time curve for the generic and brand name drug dosage forms are deemed indistinguishable from each other using statistical tests. Concentration/time curves are superimposable when the area under the total serum concentration/time curve (AUC), maximum concentration (C_{max}), and time that the maximum concentration occurs (T_{max}) are identical within statistical limits. In order to achieve the Food and Drug Administration's (FDA) definition of oral bioequivalence and be awarded an "AB" rating in the FDA publication *Approved Drug Products With Therapeutic Equivalence Evaluations* (also known as *The Orange Book*), the pharmaceutical company producing a generic drug product must administer single doses or multiple doses of the drug until steady state is achieved of the both the generic and brand name drug dosage forms to a group of 18-24 humans, and prove that the AUC (from time = 0 to infinity after a single dose, or over the dosage interval at steady-state), C_{max}, and T_{max} values are statistically identical for the two dosage forms. The ratio of the area under the serum concentration/time curves for the generic ($AUC_{generic}$) and brand name (AUC_{brand}) drug dosage forms is known as the *relative bioavailability* ($F_{relative}$) as the reference AUC is derived from the brand name drug dosage form: $F_{relative} = AUC_{generic}/AUC_{brand}$. Many states allow the substitution of generic drugs for brand name drugs if the prescriber notes on the prescription order that generic substitution is acceptable, and the generic drug dosage form has an "AB" rating.

PROBLEMS

1. Define the following terms:
   a. absorption
   b. distribution
   c. metabolism
   d. elimination
   e. steady-state
   f. linear or first-order pharmacokinetics
   g. nonlinear pharmacokinetics
   h. saturable or Michaelis-Menten pharmacokinetics
   i. autoinduction
   j. therapeutic range
   k. zero-order pharmacokinetics
   l. bioavailability
   m. bioequivalent
   n. clearance
   o. volume of distribution
   p. half-life
   q. elimination rate constant
   r. mean residence time

2. Two new antibiotics are marketed by a pharmaceutical manufacture. Reading the package insert, you find the following information:

Dose	Curacillin Steady-State Concentrations (mg/L)	Bettermycin Steady-State Concentrations (mg/L)
0	0	0
100	15	25
250	37.5	62.5
500	75	190
1000	150	510

What type of pharmacokinetics does each of these drugs follow?

3. A patient with liver failure and a patient with heart failure need to be treated with a new antiarrhythmic drug. You find a research study that contains the following information for Stopabeat in patients similar to the ones you need to treat: Normal subjects: clearance = 45 L/h, volume of distribution = 175 L; Liver failure: clearance = 15 L/h, volume of distribution = 300 L; Heart failure: clearance = 30 L/h, volume of distribution = 100 L. Recommend an intravenous loading dose (LD) and continuous intravenous infusion maintenance dose (MD) to achieve a steady-state concentration of 10 mg/L for your two patients based on these data and estimate the time it will take to achieve steady-state conditions.

4. After the first dose of gentamicin is given to a patient with renal failure, the following serum concentrations are obtained:

Time After Dosage Administration (h)	Concentration (µg/mL)
1	7.7
24	5.6
48	4.0

Compute the half-life and the elimination rate constant for this patient.

5. Average values of Michaelis-Menten pharmacokinetic parameters for phenytoin in adults are $V_{max} = 500$ mg/d and $K_m = 4$ mg/L. What are the expected average doses of phenytoin that would produce steady-state concentrations at the lower and upper limits of the therapeutic range (10-20 mg/L)?

6. A new immunosuppressant, Noreject, is being studied in the renal transplant clinic where you work. Based on previous studies, the following area under the serum concentration/time curves (AUC) were measured after single doses of 10 mg in renal transplant patients: intravenous bolus AUC = 1530 mg • h/L, oral capsule AUC = 1220 mg · h/L, oral liquid AUC = 1420 mg • h/L. What is the bioavailability of the oral capsule and oral liquid? What is the relative bioavailability of the oral capsule compared to the oral liquid?

ANSWERS TO PROBLEMS

1. *Answer to Question 1.* The following are definitions for terms in problem 1:
   a. Passage of drug molecules through physiological/biological barriers before reaching the vascular system
   b. Passage of drug molecules from the bloodstream into tissues and organs
   c. Chemical conversion of a drug molecule into a metabolite
   d. Irreversible removal of drug from the body
   e. Rate of drug administration equals the rate of drug removal so that serum concentrations and amount of drug in the body are constant
   f. Situation where steady-state serum concentration or area under the serum concentration/time curve (AUC) changes proportionally with dosage changes
   g. Situation where steady-state serum concentration or area under the serum concentration/time curve (AUC) changes disproportionally with dosage changes
   h. Type of nonlinear pharmacokinetics where an increase in dose results in a disproportionally large increase in steady-state serum concentration or area under the serum concentration/time curve. Results from overwhelming or "saturating" the enzymes ability to metabolize the drug
   i. Situation where a drug increases its own rate of metabolism by inducing more drug metabolizing enzyme to be produced
   j. Minimum and maximum serum or blood concentrations that produce the desired pharmacological effect without producing unwanted adverse effects
   k. A constant amount of drug is eliminated per unit time usually due to complete saturation of the enzyme system responsible for the metabolism of the drug
   l. Fraction of administered dose that is delivered to the systemic circulation
   m. A dosage form for a drug that produces the same serum concentration/time profile as another dosage form of the same drug. Usually measured by showing that the two dosage forms have the same area

under the serum concentration/time curve (AUC), maximum serum concentration (C_{max}), and time that maximal serum concentration occurs (T_{max}) values within statistical limits

   n. Volume of serum or blood completely cleared of drug per unit time

   o. Proportionality constant that relates serum concentrations to amount of drug in the body

   p. Time required for serum concentrations to decrease by one-half after absorption and distribution phases are complete

   q. Terminal slope (using a ln C versus time plot) of the serum concentration/time curve after absorption and distribution phases are complete

   r. Average amount of time that drug molecules reside in the body

2. *Answer to Question 2.* A plot of steady-state concentration versus doses is a straight line for Curacillin, but a curved line for Bettermycin (see table for problem 2). Because this relationship is a straight line for Curacillin, it follows linear or first-order pharmacokinetics. Because the steady-state concentration versus dose plot is curved upward indicating disproportionally large increases in concentration after a dosage increase, Bettermycin follows nonlinear pharmacokinetics. The type of nonlinear pharmacokinetics is Michaelis-Menten or saturable pharmacokinetics.

3. *Answer to Question 3.* The liver failure patient would likely have pharmacokinetic parameters similar to the liver failure patients in the research study (Cl = 15 L/h, V = 300 L): LD = V • Css, LD = (300 L)(10 mg/L) = 3000 mg intravenous bolus; MD = Cl • Css, MD = (15 L/h)(10 mg/L) = 150 mg/h intravenous infusion. The half-life would be estimated using the clearance and volume of distribution: $t_{1/2}$ = (0.693V)/Cl, $t_{1/2}$ = [(0.693)(300 L)]/(15 L/h) = 13.9 hours. Steady-state would be achieved in 3-5 $t_{1/2}$ equal to 42-70 hours. The heart failure patient would likely have pharmacokinetic parameters similar to the heart failure patients in the research study (Cl = 30 L/h, V = 100 L): LD = V • Css, LD = (100 L)(10 mg/L) = 1000 mg intravenous bolus; MD = Cl · Css, MD = (30 L/h)(10 mg/L) = 300 mg/h intravenous infusion. The half-life would be estimated using the clearance and volume of distribution: $t_{1/2}$ = (0.693 V)/Cl, $t_{1/2}$ = [(0.693)(100 L)]/(30 L/h) = 2.3 hours. Steady-state would be achieved in 3-5 $t_{1/2}$ equal to 7-12 hours.

4. *Answer to Question 4.* The serum concentration/time profile is plotted on semilogarthimic paper (see table for problem 4), and the best straight line is drawn through the points. Because all of the concentrations fall on the straight line, any two concentration/time pairs can be used to compute the elimination rate constant (k_e): k_e = −(ln C_1 − ln C_2)/(t_1 − t_2), k_e = −(ln 7.7 − ln 4)/(1 h − 48 h) = 0.0139 h^{-1}. The elimination rate constant can be used to calculate the half-life for the patient: $t_{1/2}$ = 0.693/k_e, $t_{1/2}$ = 0.693/0.0139 h^{-1} = 50 hours.

5. *Answer to Question 5.* Because phenytoin follows saturable pharmacokinetics, the Michaelis-Menten equation can be used for concentrations of 10 mg/L and 20 mg/L: MD = (V_{max} • Css)/(K_m + Css); MD = [(500 mg/d)(10 mg/L)]/(4 mg/L + 10 mg/L) = 357 mg/d for Css = 10 mg/L; MD = [(500 mg/d)(20 mg/L)]/(4 mg/L + 20 mg/L) = 417 mg/d for Css = 20 mg/L.

6. *Answer to Question 6.* The bioavailability for the capsule and liquid are F = AUC_{PO}/AUC_{IV}; for capsule, F = (1220 mg • h/L)/(1530 mg • h/L) = 0.80 or 80%; for liquid, F = (1420 mg • h/L)/(1530 mg • h/L) = 0.93 or 93%. The relative bioavailability is $F_{relative}$ = $AUC_{CAPSULE}/AUC_{LIQUID}$; $F_{relative}$ = (1220 mg · h/L)/(1420 mg • h/L) = 0.86 or 86%.

REFERENCES

1. Shargel L, Yu A, Wu-Pong S. *Applied Biopharmaceutics and Pharmacokinetics.* 6th ed. New York, NY: McGraw-Hill; 2012.
2. Ludden TM, Allen JP, Valutsky WA, et al. Individualization of phenytoin dosage regimens. *Clin Pharmacol Ther.* 1977;21(3):287-293.
3. Levy G. Pharmacokinetics of salicylate elimination in man. *J Pharm Sci.* 1965;54(7):959-967.
4. Bowdle TA, Patel IH, Levy RH, Wilensky AJ. Valproic acid dosage and plasma protein binding and clearance. *Clin Pharmacol Ther.* 1980;28(4):486-492.

5. Lima JJ, Boudoulas H, Blanford M. Concentration-dependence of disopyramide binding to plasma protein and its influence on kinetics and dynamics. *J Pharmacol Exp Ther.* 1981;219(3):741-747.

6. Bertilsson L, Höjer B, Tybring G, Osterloh J, Rane A. Autoinduction of carbamazepine metabolism in children examined by a stable isotope technique. *Clin Pharmacol Ther.* 1980;27(1):83-88.

7. Hansten PD, Horn JR. *The Top 100 Drug Interactions—A Guide to Patient Management.* Freeland, WA: H & H Publications; 2014.

8. Flockhart D. Drug interactions—cytochrome P450 drug-interaction table. http://medicine.iupui.edu/clinpharm/ddis/table.aspx. Accessed October 6, 2013.

9. Zhang L, Huang SM, Lesko LJ. Transporter-mediated drug-drug interactions. *Clin Pharmacol Ther.* Apr 2011;89(4):481-484.

10. Giacomini KM, Huang SM, Tweedie DJ, et al. Membrane transporters in drug development. *Nat Rev Drug Discov.* Mar 2010;9(3): 215-236.

11. Rowland M, Benet LZ, Graham GG. Clearance concepts in pharmacokinetics. *J Pharmacokinet Biopharm.* 1973;1:123-136.

12. Wilkinson GR, Shand DG. A physiological approach to hepatic drug clearance. *Clin Pharmacol Ther.* 1975;18:377-390.

13. Nies AS, Shand DG, Wilkinson GR. Altered hepatic blood flow and drug disposition. *Clin Pharmacokinet.* 1976;1:131-155.

14. Levy G. Effect of plasma protein binding on renal clearance of drugs. *J Pharm Sci.* 1980;69:482-491.

15. Øie S, Bennet LZ. Altered drug disposition in disease states. *Annu Rep Med Chem.* 1980;15:277-296.

16. Gibaldi M, McNamara PJ. Apparent volumes of distribution and drug binding to plasma proteins and tissues. *Eur J Clin Pharmacol* 1978;13:373-378.

2

Clinical Pharmacokinetic Equations and Calculations

INTRODUCTION

Clinical pharmacokinetic dosage calculations are conducted using the easiest possible equations and methods that produce acceptable results. This is because there are usually only a few (sometimes as little as 1-2) drug serum concentrations on which to base the calculations. Drug serum concentrations are expensive (typically $35-100 each), and obtaining them can cause minor discomfort and trauma to the patient. This situation is much different than that found in pharmacokinetic research studies where there may be 10-15 drug serum concentrations used to calculate pharmacokinetic parameters and more complex equations can be used to describe the pharmacokinetics of the drug. Because the goal of therapeutic drug monitoring in patients is to individualize the drug dose and serum concentrations in order to produce the desired pharmacological effect and avoid adverse effects, it may not be possible, or even necessary, to compute pharmacokinetic parameters for every patient or clinical situation.

ONE-COMPARTMENT MODEL EQUATIONS FOR LINEAR PHARMACOKINETICS

When medications are administered to humans, the body acts as if it is a series of compartments[1] (Figure 2-1). In many cases, the drug distributes from the blood into the tissues quickly, and a psuedoequilibrium of drug movement between blood and tissues is established rapidly. When this occurs, a one-compartment model can be used to describe the serum concentrations of a drug.[2,3] In some clinical situations, it is possible to use a one-compartment model to compute doses for a drug even if drug distribution takes time to complete.[4,5] In this case, drug serum concentrations are not obtained in a patient until after the distribution phase is over.

Intravenous Bolus Equation

When a drug is given as an intravenous bolus and the drug distributes from the blood into the tissues quickly, the serum concentrations often decline in a straight line when plotted on semilogarithmic axes (Figure 2-2). In this case, a one-compartment model intravenous bolus equation can be used: $C = (D/V)e^{-k_e t}$, where t is the time after the intravenous bolus was given (t = 0 at the time the dose was administered), C is the concentration at time = t, V is the volume of distribution, and k_e is the elimination rate constant. Most drugs given intravenously cannot be given as an actual intravenous bolus because of side effects related to rapid injection. A short infusion of 5-30 minutes can avoid these types of adverse effects, and if the intravenous infusion time is very short compared to the half-life of the drug so that a large amount of drug is not eliminated during the infusion time, intravenous bolus equations can still be used.

For example, a patient is given a theophylline loading dose of 400 mg intravenously over 20 minutes. Because the patient received theophylline during previous hospitalizations, it is known that the volume of distribution is 30 L, the elimination rate constant equals 0.115 h^{-1}, and the half-life ($t_{1/2}$) is 6 hours

One-compartment model

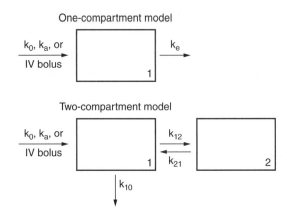

Two-compartment model

FIGURE 2-1   Using compartment models, the body can be represented as a series of discrete sections. The simplest model is the one-compartment model that depicts the body as one large container in which drug distribution between blood and tissues occurs instantaneously. Drug is introduced into the compartment, distributes immediately into a volume of distribution (V), and is removed from the body via metabolism and elimination via the elimination rate constant (k_e). The simplest multicompartment model is a two-compartment model that represents the body as a central compartment into which drug is administered and a peripheral compartment into which drug distributes. The central compartment 1 is composed of blood and tissues that equilibrate rapidly with blood. The peripheral compartment 2 represents tissues that equilibrate slowly with blood. Rate constants represent the transfer between compartments (k_{12}, k_{21}) and elimination from the body (k_{10}).

($t_{1/2} = 0.693/k_e = 0.693/0.115 \text{ h}^{-1} = 6 \text{ h}$). To compute the expected theophylline concentration 4 hours after the dose was given, a one-compartment model intravenous bolus equation can be used: $C = (D/V)e^{-k_e t} = (400 \text{ mg}/30\text{L})e^{-(0.115 \text{ h}^{-1})(4 \text{ h})} = 8.4 \text{ mg/L}$.

   If drug distribution is not rapid, it is still possible to use a one-compartment model intravenous bolus equation if the duration of the distribution phase and infusion time is small compared to the half-life of the drug and only a small amount of drug is eliminated during the infusion and distribution phases.[6] The strategy

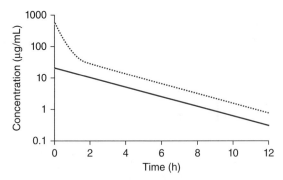

FIGURE 2-2   The solid line shows the serum concentration/time graph for a drug that follows one-compartment model pharmacokinetics after intravenous bolus administration. Drug distribution occurs instantaneously, and serum concentrations decline in a straight line on semilogarithmic axes. The dashed line represents the serum concentration/time plot for a drug that follows two-compartment model pharmacokinetics after an intravenous bolus is given. Immediately after the dose is given, serum concentrations decline rapidly. This portion of the curve is known as the *distribution phase*. During the distribution phase, drug is distributing between blood and tissues and is removed from the body via hepatic metabolism and renal elimination. Later, serum concentrations decline more slowly during the elimination phase. During the elimination phase, drug is primarily being removed from the body.

used in this situation is to infuse the medication and wait for the distribution phase to be over before obtaining serum concentrations in the patient. For instance, vancomycin must be infused slowly over 1 hour in order to avoid hypotension and red flushing around the head and neck areas. Additionally, vancomycin distributes slowly to tissues with a ½- to 1-hour distribution phase. Because the half-life of vancomycin in patients with normal renal function is approximately 8 hours, a one-compartment model intravenous bolus equation can be used to compute concentrations in the postinfusion, postdistribution phase without a large amount of error. As an example of this approach, a patient is given an intravenous dose of vancomycin 1000 mg. Because the patient has received this drug before, it is known that the volume of distribution equals 50 L, the elimination rate constant is 0.077 h^{-1}, and the half-life equals 9 hours ($t_{1/2} = 0.693/k_e = 0.693/0.077$ h^{-1} = 9 h). To calculate the expected vancomycin concentration 12 hours after the dose was given, a one-compartment model intravenous bolus equation can be used: $C = (D/V)e^{-k_e t} = (1000$ mg/50 L$)e^{-(0.077\ h^{-1})(12\ h)} = 7.9$ mg/L.

Pharmacokinetic parameters for patients can also be computed for use in the equations. If two or more serum concentrations are obtained after an intravenous bolus dose, the elimination rate constant, half-life and volume of distribution can be calculated (Figure 2-3). For example, a patient was given an intravenous loading dose of phenobarbital 600 mg over a period of about 1 hour. One day and 4 days after the dose was administered, phenobarbital serum concentrations were 12.6 mg/L and 7.5 mg/L, respectively. By plotting the serum concentration/time data on semilogarithmic axes, the time it takes for serum concentrations to decrease by ½ can be determined and is equal to 4 days. The elimination rate constant can be computed using the following relationship: $k_e = 0.693/t_{1/2} = 0.693/4$ d $= 0.173$ d^{-1}. The concentration/time line can be extrapolated to the y-axis where time = 0. Because this was the first dose of phenobarbital and the predose concentration was zero, the extrapolated concentration at time = 0 ($C_0 = 15$ mg/L in this case) can be used to calculate the volume of distribution (Figure 2-4): $V = D/C_0 = 600$ mg/(15 mg/L) $= 40$ L.

Alternatively, these parameters could be obtained by calculation without plotting the concentrations. The elimination rate constant can be computed using the following equation: $k_e = -(\ln C_1 - \ln C_2)/(t_1 - t_2)$, where t_1 and C_1 are the first time/concentration pair and t_2 and C_2 are the second time/concentration pair; $k_e = -[\ln (12.6$ mg/L$) - \ln (7.5$ mg/L$)]/(1$ d $- 4$ d$) = 0.173$ d^{-1}. The elimination rate constant can be converted into the half-life using the following equation: $t_{1/2} = 0.693/k_e = 0.693/0.173$ d^{-1} = 4 d. The volume of distribution can be calculated by dividing the dose by the serum concentration at time = 0. The serum concentration at time = zero (C_0) can be computed using a variation of the intravenous bolus equation: $C_0 = C/e^{-k_e t}$, where t and C are a time/concentration pair that occur after the intravenous bolus dose. Either phenobarbital concentration can

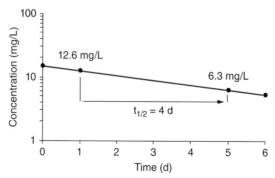

FIGURE 2-3   Phenobarbital concentrations are plotted on semilogarithmic axes, and a straight line is drawn connecting the concentrations. Half-life ($t_{1/2}$) is determined by measuring the time needed for serum concentrations to decline by ½ (ie, from 12.6 to 6.3 mg/L) and is converted to the elimination rate constant ($k_e = 0.693/t_{1/2} = 0.693/4$ d $= 0.173$ d^{-1}). The concentration/time line can be extrapolated to the concentration axis to derive the concentration at time zero ($C_0 = 15$ mg/L) and used to compute the volume of distribution ($V = D/C_0$).

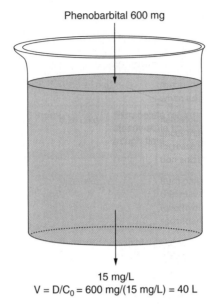

Phenobarbital 600 mg

15 mg/L
$V = D/C_0 = 600 \text{ mg}/(15 \text{ mg/L}) = 40 \text{ L}$

FIGURE 2-4   For a one-compartment model, the body can be thought of as a beaker containing fluid. If 600 mg of phenobarbital is added to a beaker of unknown volume and the resulting concentration is 15 mg/L, the volume can be computed by taking the quotient of the amount placed into the beaker and the concentration: $V = D/C_0 = 600 \text{ mg}/(15 \text{ mg/L}) = 40 \text{ L}$.

be used to compute C_0. In this case, the time/concentration pair on day 1 will be used (time = 1 d, concentration = 12.6 mg/L): $C_0 = C/e^{-k_e t} = (12.6 \text{ mg/L})/e^{-(0.173 \text{ d}^{-1})(1 \text{ d})} = 15.0 \text{ mg/L}$. The volume of distribution (V) is then computed: $V = D/C_0 = 600 \text{ mg}/(15 \text{ mg/L}) = 40 \text{ L}$.

Continuous and Intermittent Intravenous Infusion Equations

Some drugs are administered using a continuous intravenous infusion, and if the infusion is discontinued, the serum concentration/time profile decreases in a straight line when graphed on semilogarithmic axes (Figure 2-5).

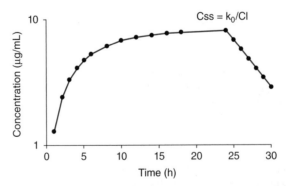

FIGURE 2-5   If a drug is given as a continuous intravenous infusion, serum concentrations increase until a steady-state concentration (Css) is achieved in 5-7 half-lives. The steady-state concentration is determined by the quotient of the infusion rate (k_0) and drug clearance (Cl): $Css = k_0/Cl$. When the infusion is discontinued, serum concentrations decline in a straight line if the graph is plotted on semilogarithmic axes. When $\log_{10}$ graph paper is used, the elimination rate constant (k_e) can be computed using the following formula: slope = $-k_e/2.303$.

In this case, a one-compartment model intravenous infusion equation can be used to compute concentrations (C) while the infusion is running: $C = (k_0/Cl)(1 - e^{-k_e t}) = [k_0/(k_e V)](1 - e^{-k_e t})$, where k_0 is the drug infusion rate (in amount per unit time, such as mg/h or μg/min), Cl is the drug clearance (since $Cl = k_e V$, this substitution was made in the second version of the equation), k_e is the elimination rate constant, and t is the time that the infusion has been running. If the infusion is allowed to continue until steady-state is achieved, the steady-state concentration (Css) can be calculated easily: $Css = k_0/Cl = k_0/(k_e V)$.

If the infusion is stopped, postinfusion serum concentrations ($C_{postinfusion}$) can be computed by calculating the concentration when the infusion ended (C_{end}) using the appropriate equation in the preceding paragraph, and the following equation: $C_{postinfusion} = C_{end}e^{-k_e t_{postinfusion}}$, where k_e is the elimination rate constant and $t_{postinfusion}$ is the postinfusion time ($t_{postinfusion} = 0$ at end of infusion and increases from that point).

For example, a patient is administered 60 mg/h of theophylline. It is known from previous hospital admissions that the patient has the following pharmacokinetic parameters for theophylline: V = 40 L and $k_e = 0.139$ h^{-1}. The serum concentration of theophylline in this patient after receiving the drug for 8 hours and at steady-state can be calculated: $C = [k_0/(k_e V)](1 - e^{-k_e t}) = [(60 \text{ mg/h})/(0.139 \text{ h}^{-1} \cdot 40 \text{ L})](1 - e^{-(0.139 \text{ h}^{-1})(8 \text{ h})}) = 7.2$ mg/L; $Css = k_0/(k_e V) = (60 \text{ mg/h})/(0.139 \text{ h}^{-1} \cdot 40 \text{ L}) = 10.8$ mg/L. It is possible to compute the theophylline serum concentration 6 hours after the infusion stopped in either circumstance. If the infusion only ran for 8 hours, the serum concentration 6 hours after the infusion stopped would be: $C_{postinfusion} = C_{end}e^{-k_e t_{postinfusion}} = (7.2 \text{ mg/L})e^{-(0.139 \text{ h}^{-1})(6 \text{ h})} = 3.1$ mg/L. If the infusion ran until steady-state was achieved, the serum concentration 6 hours after the infusion ended would be: $C_{postinfusion} = C_{end}e^{-k_e t_{postinfusion}} = (10.8 \text{ mg/L})e^{-(0.139 \text{ h}^{-1})(6 \text{ h})} = 4.7$ mg/L.·

Even if serum concentrations exhibit a distribution phase after the drug infusion has ended, it is still possible to use one-compartment model intravenous infusion equations for the drug without a large amount of error.[4,5] The strategy used in this instance is to infuse the medication and wait for the distribution phase to be over before measuring serum drug concentrations in the patient. For example, gentamicin, tobramycin, and amikacin are usually infused over ½ hour. When administered this way, these aminoglycoside antibiotics have distribution phases that last about ½ hour. Using this strategy, aminoglycoside serum concentrations are obtained no sooner than ½ hour after a 30-minute infusion in order to avoid the distribution phase. If aminoglycosides are infused over 1 hour, the distribution phase is very short and serum concentrations can be obtained immediately. For example, a patient is given an intravenous infusion of gentamicin 100 mg over 60 minutes. Because the patient received gentamicin before, it is known that the volume of distribution is 20 L, the elimination rate constant equals 0.231 h^{-1}, and the half-life equals 3 hours ($t_{1/2} = 0.693/k_e = 0.693/0.231$ h$^{-1} = 3$ h). To compute the gentamicin concentration at the end of infusion, a one-compartment model intravenous infusion equation can be used: $C = [k_0/(k_e V)](1 - e^{-k_e t}) = [(100 \text{ mg/1 h})/(0.231 \text{ h}^{-1} \cdot 20 \text{ L})](1 - e^{-(0.231 \text{ h}^{-1})(1 \text{ h})}) = 4.5$ mg/L.

Pharmacokinetic constants can also be calculated for use in the equations. If a steady-state concentration is obtained after a continuous intravenous infusion as been running uninterrupted for 3-5 half-lives, the drug clearance (Cl) can be calculated by rearranging the steady-state infusion formula: $Cl = k_0/Css$. For example, a patient receiving procainamide via intravenous infusion ($k_0 = 5$ mg/min) has a steady-state procainamide concentration measured as 8 mg/L. Procainamide clearance can be computed using the following expression: $Cl = k_0/Css = (5 \text{ mg/min})/(8 \text{ mg/L}) = 0.625$ L/min.

If the infusion did not run until steady-state was achieved, it is still possible to compute pharmacokinetic parameters from postinfusion concentrations. In the following example, a patient was given a single 120 mg dose of tobramycin as a 60 minute infusion, and concentrations at the end of infusion (6.2 mg/L) and 4 hours after the infusion ended (1.6 mg/L) were obtained. By plotting the serum concentration/time information on semilogarithmic axes, the half-life can be determined by measuring the time it takes for serum concentrations to decline by ½ (Figure 2-6), and equals 2 hours in this case. The elimination rate constant (k_e) can be calculated using the following formula: $k_e = 0.693/t_{1/2} = 0.693/2$ h $= 0.347$ h^{-1}. Alternatively, the elimination rate constant can be calculated without plotting the concentrations using the following equation: $k_e = -(\ln C_1 - \ln C_2)/(t_1 - t_2)$, where t_1 and C_1 are the first time/concentration pair and t_2 and C_2 are the second time/

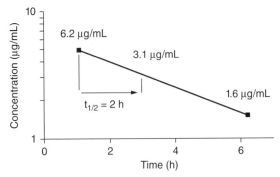

FIGURE 2-6   Tobramycin concentrations are plotted on semilogarithmic axes, and a straight line is drawn connecting the concentrations. Half-life ($t_{1/2}$) is determined by measuring the time needed for serum concentrations to decline by ½ (ie, from 6.2 to 3.1 mg/L) and is converted to the elimination rate constant ($k_e = 0.693/t_{1/2} = 0.693/2\ h = 0.347\ h^{-1}$). Volume of distribution is computed using the equation given in the text.

concentration pair; $k_e = -[\ln (6.2\ \text{mg/L}) - \ln (1.6\ \text{mg/L})]/(1\ h - 5\ h) = 0.339\ h^{-1}$ (note the slight difference in k_e is due to rounding errors). The elimination rate constant can be converted into the half-life using the following equation: $t_{1/2} = 0.693/k_e = 0.693/0.339\ h^{-1} = 2\ h$.

The volume of distribution (V) can be computed using the following equation[4]:

$$V = \frac{k_0 (1 - e^{-k_e t'})}{k_e [C_{max} - (C_{predose} e^{-k_e t'})]}$$

where k_0 is the infusion rate, k_e is the elimination rate constant, $t' = $ infusion time, C_{max} is the maximum concentration at the end of infusion, and $C_{predose}$ is the predose concentration. In this example, the volume of distribution is

$$V = \frac{(120\ \text{mg}\ /\ 1\ h)(1 - e^{-(0.339\ h^{-1})(1\ h)})}{0.339\ h^{-1}[(6.2\ \text{mg}\ /\ L) - (0\ \text{mg}\ /\ L \cdot e^{-(0.339\ h^{-1})(1\ h)})]} = 16.4\ L$$

Extravascular Equation

When a drug is administered extravascularly (eg, orally, intramuscularly, subcutaneously, transdermally, etc), absorption into the systemic vascular system must take place (Figure 2-7). If serum concentrations decrease in a straight line when plotted on semilogarithmic axes after drug absorption is complete, a one-compartment model extravascular equation can be used to describe the serum concentration/time curve: $C = \{(Fk_a D)/[V(k_a - k_e)]\}(e^{-k_e t} - e^{-k_a t})$, where t is the time after the extravascular dose was given ($t = 0$ at the time the dose was administered), C is the concentration at time $= t$, F is the bioavailability fraction, k_a is the absorption rate constant, D is the dose, V is the volume of distribution, and k_e is the elimination rate constant. The absorption rate constant describes how quickly drug is absorbed with a large number indicating fast absorption and a small number indicating slow absorption (see Figure 2-7).

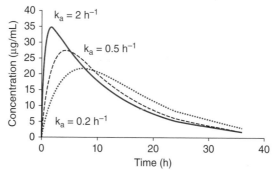

FIGURE 2-7   Serum concentration/time curves for extravascular drug administration for agents following a one-compartment pharmacokinetics. The absorption rate constant (k_a) controls how quickly the drug enters the body. A large absorption rate constant allows drug to enter the body quickly while a small elimination rate constant permits drug to enter the body more slowly. The solid line shows the concentration/time curve on semilogarithmic axes for an elimination rate constant equal to 2 h^{-1}. The dashed and dotted lines depict serum concentration/time plots for elimination rate constants of 0.5 h^{-1} and 0.1 h^{-1}, respectively.

An example of the use of this equation would be a patient who is administered 500 mg of oral procainamide as a capsule. It is known from prior clinic visits that the patient has a half-life equal to 4 hours, an elimination rate constant of 0.173 h^{-1} ($k_e = 0.693/t_{1/2} = 0.693/4$ h = 0.173 h^{-1}), and a volume of distribution of 175 L. The capsule that is administered to the patient has an absorption rate constant equal to 2 h^{-1} and an oral bioavailability fraction of 0.85. The procainamide serum concentration 4 hours after a single dose would be equal to

$$C = \frac{Fk_a D}{V(k_a - k_e)}(e^{-k_e t} - e^{-k_a t})$$

$$C = \frac{(0.85)(2\ h^{-1})(500\ mg)}{(175\ L)(2\ h^{-1} - 0.173\ h^{-1})}(e^{-(0.173\ h^{-1})(4\ h)} - e^{-(2\ h^{-1})(4\ h)})$$

$$C = 1.3\ mg/L$$

If the serum concentration/time curve displays a distribution phase, it is still possible to use one-compartment model equations after an extravascular dose is administered. In order to do this, serum concentrations are obtained only in the postdistribution phase. Because the absorption rate constant is also hard to measure in patients, it is also desirable to avoid drawing drug serum concentrations during the absorption phase in clinical situations. When only postabsorption, postdistribution serum concentrations are obtained for a drug that is administered extravascularly, the equation simplifies to: $C = [(FD)/V]e^{-k_e t}$, where C is the concentration at any postabsorption, postdistribution time; F is the bioavailability fraction; D is the dose, V is the volume of distribution, k_e is the elimination rate constant, and t is any postabsorption, postdistribution time. This approach works very well when the extravascular dose is rapidly absorbed and not a sustained- or extended-release dosage form. An example would be a patient receiving 24 mEq of lithium ion as lithium carbonate capsules. From previous clinic visits, it is known that the patient has a volume of distribution of 60 L and an elimination rate constant equal to 0.058 h^{-1}. The bioavailability of the capsule is known to be 0.90. The serum lithium concentration 12 hours after a single dose would be: $C = [(FD)/V]e^{-k_e t} = [(0.90 \bullet 24\ mEq)/60\ L]e^{-(0.058\ h^{-1})(12\ h)} = 0.18$ mEq/L.

Pharmacokinetic constants can also be calculated and used in these equations. If two or more postabsorption, postdistribution serum concentrations are obtained after an extravascular dose, the volume of distribution,

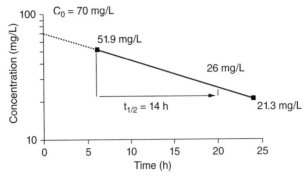

FIGURE 2-8   Valproic acid concentrations are plotted on semilogarithmic axes, and a straight line is drawn connecting the concentrations. Half-life ($t_{1/2}$) is determined by measuring the time needed for serum concentrations to decline by ½ (ie, from 51.9 to 26 mg/L) and is converted to the elimination rate constant ($k_e = 0.693/t_{1/2} = 0.693/14\ h = 0.0495\ h^{-1}$). The concentration/time line can be extrapolated to the concentration axis to derive the concentration at time zero ($C_0 = 70$ mg/L) and used to compute the hybrid constant volume of distribution/bioavailability fraction ($V/F = D/C_0$).

elimination rate constant, and half-life can be computed (Figure 2-8). For example, a patient is given an oral dose of valproic acid 750 mg as capsules. Six and 24 hours after the dose, the valproic acid serum concentrations are 51.9 and 21.3 mg/L, respectively. After the serum concentration/time data are graphed on semilogarithmic axes, the time it takes for serum concentrations to decrease by ½ can be measured and equals to 14 hours. The elimination rate constant is calculated using the following equation: $k_e = 0.693/t_{1/2} = 0.693/14$ h = 0.0495 h^{-1}. The concentration/time line can be extrapolated to the y-axis where time = 0. Because this was the first dose of valproic acid, the extrapolated concentration at time = 0 ($C_0 = 70$ mg/L) is used to estimate the hybrid volume of distribution/bioavailability (V/F) parameter: $V/F = D/C_0 = 750$ mg/70 L = 10.7 L. Even though the absolute volume of distribution and bioavailability cannot be computed without the administration of intravenous drug, the hybrid constant can be used in extravascular equations in place of V/F.

An alternative approach is to directly calculate the parameters without plotting the concentrations. The elimination rate constant (k_e) is computed using the following relationship: $k_e = -(\ln C_1 - \ln C_2)/(t_1 - t_2)$, where C_1 is the first concentration at time = t_1, and C_2 is the second concentration at time = t_2; $k_e = -[\ln (51.9\ \text{mg/L}) - \ln (21.3\ \text{mg/L})]/(6\ h - 24\ h) = 0.0495\ h^{-1}$. The elimination rate constant can be translated into the half-life using the following equation: $t_{1/2} = 0.693/k_e = 0.693/0.0495\ h^{-1} = 14$ h. The hybrid constant volume of distribution/bioavailability (V/F) is computed by taking the quotient of the dose and the extrapolated serum concentration at time = 0. The extrapolated serum concentration at time = zero (C_0) is calculated using a variation of the intravenous bolus equation: $C_0 = C/e^{-k_e t}$, where t and C are a time/concentration pair that occur after administration of the extravascular dose in the postabsorption and postdistribution phases. Either valproic acid concentration can be used to compute C_0. In this situation, the time/concentration pair at 24 hours will be used (time = 24 h, concentration = 21.3 mg/L): $C_0 = C/e^{-k_e t} = (21.3\ \text{mg/L})/e^{-(0.0495h^{-1})(24\ h)} = 70$ mg/L. The hybrid volume of distribution/bioavailability constant (V/F) is then computed: $V/F = D/C_0 = 750$ mg/(70 mg/L) = 10.7 L.

Multiple Dose and Steady-State Equations

In most cases, medications are administered to patients as multiple doses, and drug serum concentrations for therapeutic drug monitoring are not obtained until steady-state is achieved. For these reasons, multiple dose equations that reflect steady-state conditions are usually more useful in clinical settings than single-dose equations. Fortunately, it is simple to convert single-dose compartment model equations to their multiple-dose and steady-state counterparts.[7] In order to change a single-dose equation to the multiple dose version, it is necessary to multiply each exponential term in the equation by the multiple dosing factor: $(1 - e^{-nk_i\tau})/(1 - e^{-k_i\tau})$, where n is the number of doses administered, k_i is the rate constant found in the exponential of the single-dose equation, and τ is the dosage interval. At steady-state, the number of doses is large, the exponential term in the numerator of the multiple dosing factor ($-nk_i\tau$) becomes a large negative number, and the exponent approaches zero. Therefore, the steady-state version of the multiple dosing factor becomes the following: $1/(1 - e^{-k_i\tau})$, where k_i is the appropriate rate constant and τ is the dosage interval. Whenever the multiple dosing factor is used to change a single-dose equation to the multiple-dose or steady-state versions, the time variable in the equation resets to zero at the beginning of each dosage interval.

As an example of the conversion of a single-dose equation to the steady-state variant, the one-compartment model intravenous bolus equation is: $C = (D/V)e^{-k_e t}$, where C is the concentration at time = t, D is the dose, V is the volume of distribution, k_e is the elimination rate constant, and t is time after the dose is administered. Because there is only one exponential in the equation, the multiple dosing factor at steady-state is multiplied into the expression at only one place, substituting the elimination rate constant (k_e) for the rate constant in the multiple dosing factor: $C = (D/V)[e^{-k_e t}/(1 - e^{-k_e\tau})]$, where C is the steady-state concentration at any postdose time (t) after the dose (D) is given, V is the volume of distribution, k_e is the elimination rate constant, and τ is the dosage interval. Table 2-1 lists the one-compartment model equations for the different routes of administration under single-dose, multiple-dose, and steady-state conditions.

The following are examples of steady-state one-compartment model equations for intravenous, intermittent intravenous infusions, and extravascular routes of administration:

Intravenous Bolus

A patient with tonic-clonic seizures is given phenobarbital 100 mg intravenously daily until steady-state occurs. Pharmacokinetic constants for phenobarbital in the patient are: $k_e = 0.116\ d^{-1}$, V = 75 L. The steady-state concentration 23 hours [(23 h)/(24 h/d) = 0.96 d] after the last dose equals: $C = (D/V)[e^{-k_e t}/(1 - e^{-k_e\tau})] = (100\ mg/75\ L)[e^{-(0.116\ d^{-1})(0.96\ d)}/(1 - e^{-(0.116\ d^{-1})(1\ d)})] = 10.9\ mg/L$.

Intermittent Intravenous Infusion

A patient with gram-negative pneumonia is administered tobramycin 140 mg every 8 hours until steady-state is achieved. Pharmacokinetic parameters for tobramycin in the patient are: V = 16 L, $k_e = 0.30\ h^{-1}$.

TABLE 2-1   Single Dose, Multiple Dose, and Steady-State One-Compartment Model Equations

Route of Administration	Single Dose	Multiple Dose	Steady-State
Intravenous bolus	$C = (D/V)e^{-k_e t}$	$C = (D/V)e^{-k_e t}[(1 - e^{-nk_e\tau})/(1 - e^{-k_e\tau})]$	$C = (D/V)[e^{-k_e t}/(1 - e^{-k_e\tau})]$
Continuous intravenous infusion	$C = [k_0/(k_e V)](1 - e^{-k_e t})$	N/A	$Css = k_0/Cl = k_0/(k_e V)$
Intermittent intravenous infusion	$C = [k_0/(k_e V)](1 - e^{-k_e t'})$	$C = [k_0/(k_e V)](1 - e^{-k_e t'})[(1 - e^{-nk_e\tau})/(1 - e^{-k_e\tau})]$	$C = [k_0/(k_e V)][(1 - e^{-k_e t'})/(1 - e^{-k_e\tau})]$
Extravascular (postabsorption, postdistribution)	$C = [(FD)/V]e^{-k_e t}$	$C = [(FD)/V]e^{-k_e t}[(1 - e^{-nk_e\tau})/(1 - e^{-k_e\tau})]$	$C = (FD/V)[e^{-k_e t}/(1 - e^{-k_e\tau})]$
Average steady-state concentration (any route of administration)	N/A	N/A	$Css = [F(D/\tau)]/Cl$

C, drug serum concentration at time = t; Cl, clearance; D, dose; k_0, infusion rate; k_e, elimination rate constant; n, number of administered doses; τ, dosage interval; t', infusion time; V, volume of distribution.

The steady-state concentration immediately after a 1-hour infusion equals: $C = [k_0/(k_e V)][(1 - e^{-k_e t'})/(1 - e^{-k_e \tau})] = [(140 \text{ mg/h})/(0.30 \text{ h}^{-1} \cdot 16 \text{ L})][(1 - e^{(-0.30 \text{ h}^{-1} \cdot 1 \text{ h})})/(1 - e^{(-0.30 \text{ h}^{-1} \cdot 8 \text{ h})})] = 8.3 \text{ mg/L}$.

Extravascular

A patient with an arrhythmia is administered 250 mg of quinidine orally (as 300 mg quinidine sulfate tablets) every 6 hours until steady-state occurs. Pharmacokinetic constants for quinidine in the patient are: $V = 180$ L, $k_e = 0.0693 \text{ h}^{-1}$, F = 0.7. The postabsorption, postdistribution steady-state concentration just before the next dose (t = 6 h) equals:

$$C = (FD/V)[e^{-k_e t}/(1 - e^{-k_e \tau})]$$

$$C = [(0.7 \cdot 250 \text{ mg})/180 \text{ L}][e^{(-0.0693 \text{ h}^{-1} \cdot 6 \text{ h})}/(1 - e^{(-0.0693 \text{ h}^{-1} \cdot 6 \text{ h})})]$$

$$C = 1.9 \text{ mg/L}.$$

It is also possible to compute pharmacokinetic parameters under multiple-dose and steady-state conditions. Table 2-2 lists the methods to compute pharmacokinetic constants, using a one-compartment model for different routes of administration under single-dose, multiple-dose, and steady-state conditions. The main difference between single-dose and multiple-dose calculations is in the computation of the volume of distribution.

TABLE 2-2   Single Dose, Multiple Dose, and Steady-State Pharmacokinetic Constant Computations utilizing a One-Compartment Model

Route of Administration	Single Dose	Multiple Dose	Steady-State
Intravenous bolus	$k_e = -(\ln C_1 - \ln C_2)/(t_1 - t_2)$ $t_{1/2} = 0.693/k_e$ $V = D/C_0$ $Cl = k_e V$	$k_e = -(\ln C_1 - \ln C_2)/(t_1 - t_2)$ $t_{1/2} = 0.693/k_e$ $V = D/(C_0 - C_{predose})$ $Cl = k_e V$	$k_e = -(\ln C_1 - \ln C_2)/(t_1 - t_2)$ $t_{1/2} = 0.693/k_e$ $V = D/(C_0 - C_{predose})$ $Cl = k_e V$
Continuous intravenous infusion	N/A	N/A	$Cl = k_0/Css$
Intermittent intravenous infusion	$k_e = -(\ln C_1 - \ln C_2)/(t_1 - t_2)$ $t_{1/2} = 0.693/k_e$ $V = [k_0(1 - e^{-k_e t'})]/$ $\{k_e[C_{max} - (C_{predose}e^{-k_e t'})]\}$ $Cl = k_e V$	$k_e = -(\ln C_1 - \ln C_2)/(t_1 - t_2)$ $t_{1/2} = 0.693/k_e$ $V = [k_0(1 - e^{-k_e t'})]/$ $\{k_e[C_{max} - (C_{predose}e^{-k_e t'})]\}$ $Cl = k_e V$	$k_e = -(\ln C_1 - \ln C_2)/(t_1 - t_2)$ $t_{1/2} = 0.693/k_e$ $V = [k_0(1 - e^{-k_e t'})]/$ $\{k_e[C_{max} - (C_{predose}e^{-k_e t'})]\}$ $Cl = k_e V$
Extravascular (postabsorption, postdistribution)	$k_e = -(\ln C_1 - \ln C_2)/(t_1 - t_2)$ $t_{1/2} = 0.693/k_e$ $V/F = D/C_0$ $Cl/F = k_e(V/F)$	$k_e = -(\ln C_1 - \ln C_2)/(t_1 - t_2)$ $t_{1/2} = 0.693/k_e$ $V/F = D/(C_0 - C_{predose})$ $Cl/F = k_e(V/F)$	$k_e = -(\ln C_1 - \ln C_2)/(t_1 - t_2)$ $t_{1/2} = 0.693/k_e$ $V/F = D/(C_0 - C_{predose})$ $Cl/F = k_e(V/F)$
Average steady-state concentration (any route of administration)	N/A	N/A	$Cl/F = (D/\tau)/Css$

C_0, concentration at time = 0; C_1, drug serum concentration at time = t_1; C_2, drug serum concentration at time = t_2; Cl, drug clearance; Cl/F, hybrid constant clearance/bioavailability fraction; $C_{predose}$, predose concentration; Css, steady-state concentration; D, dose; k_0, continuous infusion rate; k_e, elimination rate constant; t', infusion time; $t_{1/2}$, half-life; V, volume of distribution; V/F, hybrid constant volume of distribution/bioavailability fraction.

When a single dose of medication is given, the predose concentration is assumed to be zero. However, when multiple doses are given, the predose concentration is not usually zero, and the volume of distribution equation (V) needs to have the baseline, predose concentration ($C_{predose}$) subtracted from the extrapolated drug concentration at time = 0 (C_0) for the intravenous bolus ($V = D/[C_0 - C_{predose}]$, where D is dose) and extravascular ($V/F = D/[C_0 - C_{predose}]$, where F is the bioavailability fraction and D is dose) cases. In the case of intermittent intravenous infusions, the volume of distribution equation already has a parameter for the predose concentration in it[4]:

$$V = \frac{k_0(1 - e^{-k_e t'})}{k_e[C_{max} - (C_{predose}e^{-k_e t'})]}$$

where k_0 is the infusion rate, k_e is the elimination rate constant, t' = infusion time, C_{max} is the maximum concentration at the end of infusion, and $C_{predose}$ is the predose concentration. For each route of administration, the elimination rate constant (k_e) is computed using the same equation as the single-dose situation: $k_e = -(\ln C_1 - \ln C_2)/(t_1 - t_2)$, where C_1 is the first concentration at time = t_1 and C_2 is the second concentration at time = t_2.

The following are examples of multiple-dose and steady-state computations of pharmacokinetic parameters using a one-compartment model for intravenous, intermittent intravenous infusions, and extravascular routes of administration:

Intravenous Bolus

A patient receiving theophylline 300 mg intravenously every 6 hours has a predose concentration equal to 2.5 mg/L and postdose concentrations of 9.2 mg/L 1 hour and 4.5 mg/L 5 hours after the second dose is given. The patient has an elimination rate constant (k_e) equal to: $k_e = -(\ln C_1 - \ln C_2)/(t_1 - t_2) = -[(\ln 9.2 \text{ mg/L}) - (\ln 4.5 \text{ mg/L})]/(1 \text{ h} - 5 \text{ h}) = 0.179 \text{ h}^{-1}$. The volume of distribution (V) of theophylline for the patient is: $C_0 = C/e^{-k_e t} = (9.2 \text{ mg/L})/e^{(-0.179 \text{ h}^{-1})(1 \text{ h})} = 11.0 \text{ mg/L}$ and $V = D/[C_0 - C_{predose}] = (300 \text{ mg})/(11.0 \text{ mg/L} - 2.5 \text{ mg/L}) = 35.3 \text{ L}$.

Intermittent Intravenous Infusion

A patient is prescribed gentamicin 100 mg infused over 60 minutes every 12 hours. A predose steady-state concentration ($C_{predose}$) is drawn and equals 2.5 mg/L. After the 1-hour infusion, a steady-state maximum concentration (C_{max}) is obtained and equals 7.9 mg/L. Because the patient is at steady-state, it can be assumed that all predose steady-state concentrations are equal. Thus, the predose steady-state concentration 12 hours after the dose can also be considered equal to 2.5 mg/L and used to compute the elimination rate constant (k_e) of gentamicin for the patient: $k_e = -(\ln C_1 - \ln C_2)/(t_1 - t_2) = -[(\ln 7.9 \text{ mg/L}) - (\ln 2.5 \text{ mg/L})]/(1 \text{ h} - 12 \text{ h}) = 0.105 \text{ h}^{-1}$. The volume of distribution (V) of gentamicin for the patient is

$$V = \frac{k_0(1 - e^{-k_e t'})}{k_e[C_{max} - (C_{predose}e^{-k_e t'})]}$$

where k_0 is the infusion rate, k_e is the elimination rate constant, t' = infusion time, C_{max} is the maximum concentration at the end of infusion, and $C_{predose}$ is the predose concentration. In this example, volume of distribution is

$$V = \frac{(100 \text{ mg} / 1 \text{ h})(1 - e^{-(0.105 \text{ h}^{-1})(1 \text{ h})})}{0.105 \text{ h}^{-1}[(7.9 \text{ mg} / \text{L}) - (2.5 \text{ mg} / \text{L} \cdot e^{-(0.105 \text{ h}^{-1})(1 \text{ h})})]} = 16.8 \text{ L}$$

Extravascular

A patient is given procainamide capsules 750 mg every 6 hours. The following concentrations are obtained before and after the second dose: $C_{predose}$ = 1.1 mg/L, concentrations 2 hours and 6 hours postdose equal 4.6 mg/L and 2.9 mg/L, respectively. The patient has an elimination rate constant (k_e) equal to: k_e = −(ln C_1 − ln C_2)/(t_1 − t_2) = −[(ln 4.6 mg/L) − (ln 2.9 mg/L)]/(2 h − 6 h) = 0.115 h^{-1}. The hybrid volume of distribution/bioavailability constant (V/F) of procainamide for the patient is: C_0 = C/e^{-ket} = (2.9 mg/L)/$e^{(-0.115 \, h^{-1})(6 \, h)}$ = 5.8 mg/L and V/F = D/[C_0 − $C_{predose}$] = (750 mg)/(5.8 mg/L − 1.1 mg/L) = 160 L.

Average Steady-State Concentration Equation

A very useful and easy equation can be used to compute the average steady-state concentration (Css) of a drug: Css = [F(D/τ)]/Cl, where F is the bioavailability fraction, D is the dose, τ is the dosage interval, and Cl is the drug clearance.[8] This equation works for any single- or multiple-compartment model, and because of this, it is deemed a model-independent equation. The steady-state concentration computed by this equation is the concentration that would have occurred if the dose, adjusted for bioavailability, was given as a continuous intravenous infusion. For example, 600 mg of theophylline tablets given orally every 12 hours (F = 1.0) would be equivalent to a 50 mg/h (600 mg/12 h = 50 mg/h) continuous intravenous infusion of theophylline. The average steady-state concentration equation is very useful when the half-life of the drug is long compared to the dosage interval or if a sustained-release dosage form is used. Examples of both situations follow:

Long Half-Life Compared to Dosage Interval

A patient is administered 250 μg of digoxin tablets daily for heart failure until steady-state. The pharmacokinetic constants for digoxin in the patient are: F = 0.7, Cl = 120 L/d. The average-steady-state concentration would equal: Css = [F(D/τ)]/Cl = [0.7(250 μg/d)]/(120 L/d) = 1.5 μg/L.

Sustained-Release Dosage Form

A patient is given 1500 mg of procainamide sustained-release tablets every 12 hours until steady-state for the treatment of an arrhythmia. The pharmacokinetic parameters for procainamide in the patient are: F = 0.85, Cl = 30 L/h. The average steady-state concentration would be: Css = [F(D/τ)]/Cl = [0.85(1500 mg/12 h)]/(30 L/h) = 3.5 mg/L.

If an average steady-state concentration (Css) is known for a drug, the hybrid pharmacokinetic constant clearance/bioavailability (Cl/F) can be computed: Cl/F = (D/τ)/Css, where D is dose and τ is the dosage interval. For example, a patient receiving 600 mg of sustained-release theophylline every 12 hours has a steady-state concentration equal to 11.2 mg/L. The clearance/bioavailability constant for theophylline in this patient would equal: Cl/F = (D/τ)/Css = (600 mg/12 h)/11.2 mg/L = 4.5 L/h.

DESIGNING INDIVIDUALIZED DOSAGE REGIMENS USING ONE-COMPARTMENT MODEL EQUATIONS

The goal of therapeutic drug monitoring is to customize medication doses that provide the optimal drug efficacy without adverse reactions. One-compartment model equations can be used to compute initial drug doses employing population pharmacokinetic parameters that estimate the constants for a patient.[4,5,9] The patient's own, unique pharmacokinetic parameters can be computed once doses have been administered and drug serum concentrations measured. At that time, individualized dosage regimens at steady-state can be designed for a patient. Table 2-3 lists the equations used to customize doses for the various routes of administration.

TABLE 2-3 Equations Used to Compute Individualized Dosage Regimens for Various Routes of Administration

Route of Administration	Dosage Interval (τ), Maintenance Dose (D or k_0), and Loading Dose (LD) Equations
Intravenous bolus	$\tau = (\ln Css_{max} - \ln Css_{min})/k_e$ $D = Css_{max}V(1 - e^{-k_e\tau})$ $LD = Css_{max}V$
Continuous intravenous infusion	$k_0 = CssCl = Cssk_eV$ $LD = CssV$
Intermittent intravenous infusion	$\tau = [(\ln Css_{max} - \ln Css_{min})/k_e] + t'$ $k_0 = Css_{max}k_eV[(1 - e^{-k_e\tau})/(1 - e^{-k_e t'})]$ $LD = k_0/(1 - e^{-k_e\tau})$
Extravascular (postabsorption, postdistribution)	$\tau = [(\ln Css_{max} - \ln Css_{min})/k_e] + T_{max}$ $D = [(Css_{max}V)/F][(1 - e^{-k_e\tau})/e^{-k_e T_{max}}]$ $LD = (Css_{max}V)/F$
Average steady-state concentration (any route of administration)	$D = (CssCl\tau)/F = (Cssk_eV\tau)/F$ $LD = (CssV)/F$

Css, steady-state concentration; Css_{min}, minimum steady-state concentration; Css_{max}, maximum steady-state concentration; F, bioavailability fraction; k_e, elimination rate constant; k_0, continuous infusion rate; t′, infusion time; T_{max}, time that Css_{max} occurs; V, volume of distribution.

Intravenous Bolus

If the volume of distribution and elimination rate constant can be estimated for a patient, a loading dose and initial maintenance dose can be computed. To design these doses, estimates of pharmacokinetic constants are obtained using patient characteristics such as weight, age, gender, renal and liver function, and other disease states and conditions that are known to affect the disposition and elimination of the drug. When the actual elimination rate constant and volume of distribution are measured for the medication, a maintenance dose to achieve any target steady-state concentrations can be designed.

Desired maximum and minimum steady-state concentrations are chosen for the patient. If the patient has never received the drug before, the therapeutic range can be used to choose starting concentrations. If the patient has taken the drug on previous occasions, safe and effective concentrations may be known. The dosage interval (τ) can be computed using the desired maximum (Css_{max}) and minimum (Css_{min}) steady-state concentrations: $\tau = (\ln Css_{max} - \ln Css_{min})/k_e$, where k_e is the elimination rate constant. The maintenance dose is then computed using the one-compartment model equation for intravenous bolus administration at the time Css_{max} occurs (t = 0 h after the bolus is given) solved for dose: $D = [Css_{max} V(1 - e^{-k_e\tau})]/e^{-ke(0\ h)} = Css_{max} V(1 - e^{-k_e\tau})$. If a loading dose (LD) is necessary, it is computed using the following equation: $LD = Css_{max} V$.

An example of this approach is a patient that needs to be treated for complex partial seizures with intravenous phenobarbital. An initial dosage regimen is designed using population pharmacokinetic parameters ($k_e = 0.139$ d^{-1}, V = 50 L) to achieve maximum (Css_{max}) and minimum (Css_{min}) steady-state concentrations equal to 30 mg/L and 25 mg/L, respectively: $\tau = (\ln Css_{max} - \ln Css_{min})/k_e = [\ln (30\ mg/L) - \ln (25\ mg/L)]/0.139$ $d^{-1} = 1.3$ d, round to a practical dosage interval of 1 d; $D = Css_{max} V(1 - e^{-k_e\tau}) = (30\ mg/L \cdot 50\ L)(1 - e^{(-0.139\ d^{-1})(1\ d)}) = 195$ mg, round to a practical dose of 200 mg. The patient would be prescribed intravenous phenobarbital 200 mg daily.

Continuous and Intermittent Intravenous Infusion

The dosage regimen for a continuous intravenous infusion is computed using the following equation: $k_0 = CssCl = Cssk_eV$, where k_0 is the infusion rate, Css is the steady-state drug concentration, Cl is the drug clearance, k_e is the elimination rate constant, and V is the volume of distribution. A loading dose (LD) is computed using the following expression: $LD = CssV$. An example using this method is a patient with a ventricular arrhythmia after a myocardial infarction needing treatment with lidocaine (population pharmacokinetic parameters used: $V = 50$ L, $Cl = 1.0$ L/min): $LD = CssV = (3$ mg/L)$(50$ L$) = 150$ mg; $k_0 = CssCl = (3$ mg/L$)$ $(1.0$ L/min$) = 3$ mg/min. The patient would be prescribed lidocaine 150 mg intravenously followed by a 3-mg/min continuous infusion.

For intermittent intravenous infusions the dosage interval (τ) is computed by choosing minimum (Css_{min}) and maximum (Css_{max}) steady-state concentrations: $\tau = [(\ln Css_{max} - \ln Css_{min})/k_e] + t'$, where k_e is the elimination rate constant and t' is the infusion time. The maintenance dose is calculated using the one-compartment model equation for intermittent intravenous infusions at the time Css_{max} occurs solved for infusion rate (k_0): $k_0 = Css_{max}k_eV[(1 - e^{-k_e\tau})/(1 - e^{-k_et'})]$, where k_e is the elimination rate constant and V is the volume of distribution. A loading dose (LD) can be calculated using the following formula that takes into account the amount of drug eliminated during the infusion time: $LD = k_0/(1 - e^{-k_e\tau})$.

An example using these techniques is a patient receiving tobramycin for the treatment of intra-abdominal sepsis. Using pharmacokinetic parameters ($V = 20$ L, $k_e = 0.087$ h^{-1}) previously measured in the patient using serum concentrations, compute a tobramycin dose (infused over 1 h) that would provide maximum (Css_{max}) and minimum (Css_{min}) steady-state concentrations of 6 mg/L and 1 mg/L, respectively: $\tau = [(\ln Css_{max} - \ln Css_{min})/k_e] + t' = [(\ln 6$ mg/L $- \ln 1$ mg/L$)/0.087$ h$^{-1}] + 1$ h $= 22$ h, round to practical dosage interval of 24 h; $k_0 = Css_{max}k_eV[(1 - e^{-k_e\tau})/(1 - e^{-k_et'})] = [(6$ mg/L$)(0.087$ h$^{-1})(20$ L$)][(1 - e^{(-0.087 h^{-1})(24 h)})/(1 - e^{(-0.087 h^{-1})(1 h)})] = 110$ mg. The patient would be prescribed tobramycin 110 mg infused over 1 hour every 24 hours.

Extravascular

The dosage regimen for extravascular doses is determined by choosing maximum (Css_{max}) and minimum (Css_{min}) steady-state concentrations: $\tau = [(\ln Css_{max} - \ln Css_{min})/k_e] + T_{max}$, where k_e is the elimination rate constant and T_{max} is the time that the maximum concentration occurs. The maintenance dose is computed using the one-compartment model equation for extravascular doses at the time Css_{max} occurs ($t = T_{max}$) solved for dose (D): $D = [(Css_{max}V)/F][(1 - e^{-k_e\tau})/e^{-k_eT_{max}}]$ where V is the volume of distribution and F is the bioavailability fraction. A loading dose (LD) can be computed using the following equation: $LD = (Css_{max}V)/F$.

An example of these computations is a patient with simple partial seizures that needs to receive valproic acid capsules (population pharmacokinetic parameters are $V = 12$ L, $k_e = 0.05$ h^{-1}, $T_{max} = 3$ h, $F = 1.0$) and maintain steady-state maximum (Css_{max}) and minimum (Css_{min}) concentrations of 80 mg/L and 50 mg/L, respectively: $\tau = [(\ln Css_{max} - \ln Css_{min})/k_e] + T_{max} = [(\ln 80$ mg/L $- \ln 50$ mg/L$)/0.05$ h$^{-1}] + 3$ h $= 12.4$ h, round to practical dosage interval of 12 h; $D = [(Css_{max}V)/F][(1 - e^{-k_e\tau})/e^{-k_eT_{max}}] = [(80$ mg/L $\cdot 12$ L$)/1.0]$ $[(1 - e^{(-0.05 h^{-1})(12 h)})/e^{(-0.05 h^{-1})(3 h)}] = 503$ mg, round to practical dose of 500 mg. The patient would be prescribed valproic acid capsules 500 mg orally every 12 hours.

Average Steady-State Concentration

If the drug is administered as a sustained-release dosage form or the half-life is long compared to the dosage interval, it is possible to use the average steady-state concentration equation to individualize doses. The dosage regimen is computed using the following equation: $D = (CssCl\tau)/F = (Cssk_eV\tau)/F$, where D is the dose, Css is the steady-state drug concentration, Cl is the drug clearance, τ is the dosage interval, k_e is the elimination rate constant, and V is the volume of distribution. A loading dose (LD) is computed using the following expression: $LD = (CssV)/F$.

An example of this technique is a patient with an atrial arrhythmia needing treatment with procainamide sustained-release tablets (clearance equals 24 L/h based on current procainamide continuous infusion; $F = 0.85$, $\tau = 12$ h for sustained-release tablet) and an average steady-state procainamide concentration equal to 5 mg/L: $D = (C_{ss}Cl\tau)/F = (5 \text{ mg/L} \cdot 24 \text{ L/h} \cdot 12 \text{ h})/0.85 = 1694$ mg, round to a practical dose of 1500 mg. The patient would be prescribed procainamide sustained-release tablets 1500 mg orally every 12 hours.

MULTICOMPARTMENT MODELS

When serum concentrations decrease in a rapid fashion initially and then decline at a slower rate later (see Figure 2-2), a multicompartment model can be used to describe the serum concentration/time curve[1] (see Figure 2-1). The reason serum concentrations drop so rapidly after the dose is given is that all of the drug is in the bloodstream initially, and drug is leaving the vascular system by distribution to tissues and by hepatic metabolism and/or renal elimination. This portion of the curve is called the *distribution phase*. After this phase of the curve is finished, drug distribution is nearly complete and a psuedoequilibrium is established between the blood and tissues. During the final part of the curve, serum concentrations drop more slowly as only metabolism and/or elimination are taking place. This portion of the curve is called the *elimination phase*, and the elimination half-life of the drug is measured in this part of the serum concentration/time graph. Digoxin, vancomycin, and lidocaine are examples of drugs that follow multicompartment pharmacokinetics.

A two-compartment model is the simplest of the multicompartment models. The equation that describes a two-compartment model after an intravenous bolus is: $C = \{[D(\alpha - k_{21})]/[V_1(\alpha - \beta)]\}e^{-\alpha t} + \{[D(k_{21} - \beta)]/[V_1(\alpha - \beta)]\}e^{-\beta t}$, where C is the drug serum concentration, D is the intravenous bolus dose, k_{21} is the rate constant that describes the transfer of drug from compartment 2 to compartment 1, α is the distribution rate constant, β is the elimination rate constant, V_1 is the volume of distribution for compartment 1, and t is the time after the dose was administered. Similar equations for a two-compartment model are available for intravenous infusions and extravascular doses. In order to get accurate values for the pharmacokinetic constants in the equation, three to five serum concentrations for each phase of the curve need to be obtained after a dose is given to a patient. Because of the cost and time involved to collect 6-10 serum concentrations after a dose, multicompartment models are rarely used in patient care situations. If a drug follows multicompartment pharmacokinetics, serum concentrations are usually not drawn for clinical use until the distribution phase is over and the elimination phase has been established. In these cases, it is possible to use simpler one-compartment model equations to compute doses with an acceptable degree of accuracy.

MICHAELIS-MENTEN EQUATIONS FOR SATURABLE PHARMACOKINETICS

When the dose of a drug is increased and steady-state serum concentrations do not increase in a proportional fashion, but instead increase more than expected, Michaelis-Menten or saturable pharmacokinetics may be taking place. This situation occurs when the serum concentration of the drug approaches or exceeds the K_m value for the enzyme system that is responsible for its metabolism. The Michaelis-Menten expression describes the dose required to attain a given steady-state drug concentration: $D = (V_{max} \cdot C_{ss})/(K_m + C_{ss})$, where D is the dose, Css is the steady-state drug concentration, V_{max} is the maximum rate of drug metabolism, and K_m is the concentration where the rate of metabolism equals $V_{max}/2$. Phenytoin is an example of a drug that follows saturable pharmacokinetics.[10]

Computing the Michaelis-Menten constants for a drug is not as straightforward as the calculation of pharmacokinetic parameters for a One-Compartment Linear Pharmacokinetic model. The calculation of V_{max} and K_m requires a graphical solution.[10] The Michaelis-Menten equation is rearranged to the following formula: $D = V_{max} - [K_m(D/C_{ss})]$. This version of the function takes the form of the equation of a straight line: $y = y\text{-intercept} + [(\text{slope})x]$.

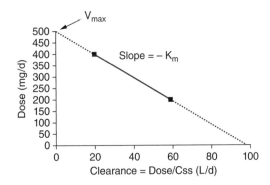

FIGURE 2-9   Michaelis-Menten plot for phenytoin. Dose (D) is plotted versus the ratio of dose and steady-state concentration (D/Css) for two or more different doses, and a straight line is drawn connecting the points. The slope of the line is $-K_m$, and the y-intercept is V_{max}. The Michaelis-Menten constants are then used to compute the dose needed to achieve a new desired steady-state concentration.

A plot of dose (D) versus dose divided by the steady-state concentration (D/Css) will yield a straight line with a slope equal to $-K_m$ and a y-intercept of V_{max}. In order to use this approach, a patient is placed on an initial dose (D_1) of the medication, a steady-state concentration is obtained (Css_1), and the dose/steady-state concentration ratio determined (D_1/Css_1). The dose of the medication is changed (D_2), a second steady-state concentration is measured (Css_2), and the new dose/steady-state concentration ratio is computed (D_2/Css_2). The dose and dose/steady-state concentration pairs are plotted on a graph so that V_{max} (the y-intercept) and K_m (the slope) can be determined (Figure 2-9). If additional doses are administered until steady-state has been achieved, they can also be added to the same plot and the best straight line computed using linear regression. Once V_{max} and K_m are known, the Michaelis-Menten expression can be used to compute a dose to reach any steady-state concentration.

An example is a patient receiving phenytoin for the treatment of tonic-clonic seizures. The patient received a dose of 300 mg/d with a steady-state concentration of 8 mg/L and a dose of 500 mg/d with a steady-state concentration equal to 22 mg/L. The dose/steady-state concentration ratios are 37.5 L/d and 22.7 L/d for the first and second doses, respectively ([300 mg/d]/8 mg/L = 37.5 L/d; [500 mg/d]/22 mg/L = 22.7 L/d). A plot of this data yields a V_{max} = 807 mg/d and a K_m = 13.5 mg/L (see Figure 2-9). The phenytoin dose to reach a steady-state concentration equal to 13 mg/L is: D = (V_{max} • Css)/(K_m + Css) = (807 mg/d • 13 mg/L)/(13.5 mg/L + 13 mg/L) = 396 mg/d, rounded to a practical dose of 400 mg/d.

CALCULATION OF CLEARANCE, VOLUME OF DISTRIBUTION, AND HALF-LIFE IN PHARMACOKINETIC RESEARCH STUDIES

It is important to understand the methods used to compute the three principal pharmacokinetic parameters in research studies as these will be used by clinicians to determine population pharmacokinetic parameters for initial dosage regimen design.[11] The typical pharmacokinetic research study administers a single dose of the medication and measures 10-15 serum concentrations for an estimated 3-5 half-lives or gives the drug until steady-state is achieved and obtains 10-15 serum concentrations over a dosage interval. In either case, the serum concentration/time plot is used to compute the area under the serum concentration/time curve (AUC). For drugs that follow linear pharmacokinetics, the AUC extrapolated to infinity after a single dose equals the AUC over the dosage interval at steady-state for a dose of the same size, so either can be used to compute pharmacokinetic constants.

Clearance (Cl) is computed by taking the ratio of the dose (D) and area under the serum concentration/time curve (AUC) for a drug that is administered intravenously: Cl = D/AUC. If the dose is administered extravascularly, the bioavailability fraction (F) must be included to compensate for drug that does not reach the systemic vascular system: Cl = (FD)/AUC.

Of the three volumes of distribution typically computed in a pharmacokinetic experiment, the one most useful in clinical situations is the volume of distribution (V) calculated using the area under the serum concentration/time curve (AUC): $V = D/(k_e AUC)$, where k_e is the elimination rate constant. For doses administered extravascularly, the bioavailability fraction (F) must be included to compensate for drug that does not reach the systemic vascular system: $V = (FD)/(k_e AUC)$.

Half-life is determined by plotting the serum concentration/time curve and computing the time it takes for serum concentrations to decrease by ½ in the postabsorption, postdistribution phase of the graph. In order to get the most accurate measurement of half-life, five to seven serum concentrations are usually measured during the terminal portion of the curve, and nonlinear regression is used to compute the best value for the parameter. Alternatively, the data can be plotted on semilogarithmic axes and linear regression utilized to compute the terminal half-life.

PROBLEMS

1. PZ is a 35-year-old, 60-kg female with a *Staphylococcus aureus* wound infection. While receiving vancomycin 1 g every 12 hours (infused over one hour), the steady-state peak concentration (obtained ½ hour after the end of infusion) was 35 mg/L, and the steady-state trough concentration (obtained immediately predose) was 15 mg/L. (A) Using one-compartment IV bolus equations, compute the pharmacokinetic parameters for this patient. (B) Using the patient-specific pharmacokinetic parameters calculated in part A, compute a new vancomycin dose that would achieve $Css_{max} = 30$ mg/L and $Css_{min} = 7.5$ mg/L.

2. Negamycin is a new antibiotic with an average volume of distribution of 0.35 L/kg and a half-life of 2 hours in patients with cystic fibrosis. Compute a dosage regimen for JM, a 22-year-old, 45-kg female cystic fibrosis patient with *Pseudomonas aeruginosa* in her sputum, that will achieve steady-state peak concentrations of 10 mg/L and trough concentrations of 0.6 mg/L using one-compartment model IV bolus equations (assume that the drug is given as an IV bolus).

3. KL is a 65-year-old, 60-kg female being treated for septic shock. Among other antibiotics, she is being treated with tobramycin 60 mg every 8 hours (infused over 1 hour). Steady-state serum concentrations are: $Css_{max} = 7.1$ mg/L, $Css_{min} = 3.1$ mg/L. Using one-compartment intermittent intravenous infusion equations, compute the pharmacokinetic parameters for this patient and use them to individualize the tobramycin dose to achieve $Css_{max} = 8$ mg/L and $Css_{min} = 1.0$ mg/L.

4. JB is a 52-year-old, 72-kg male being treated for gram negative pneumonia. Assuming a V = 18 L and a $t_{1/2} = 8$ h, design a gentamicin dosage (infused over 1 hour) to achieve $Css_{max} = 10$ mg/L and $Css_{min} = 1.2$ mg/L using one-compartment intermittent intravenous infusion equations.

5. EV is a 42-year-old, 84 kg male suffering from an acute asthmatic attack. Using one-compartment model equations, compute a theophylline IV bolus loading dose (to be administered over 20 minutes) and continuous infusion to achieve a Css = 12 mg/L. Assume a V = 40 L and $t_{1/2} = 5$ h.

6. BJ is a 62-year-old, 70-kg female with a ventricular arrhythmia. Assuming a V = 33 L and Cl = 0.5 L/min, use one-compartment model equations to compute a lidocaine IV bolus loading dose (to be administered over 1-2 minutes) and continuous infusion to achieve a Css = 3 mg/L.

7. MM is a 54-year-old, 68-kg male being treated with procainamide 750 mg regular release capsules every 6 hours for arrhythmia. The following steady-state concentration is available: Css_{min} = 1.5 mg/L (obtained immediately predose). Calculate a dose that will achieve a Css_{min} = 2.5 mg/L.

8. LM is a 59-year-old, 85-kg male needing treatment with oral quinidine for an arrhythmia. Assuming $F = 0.7$, T_{max} = 2 h, V = 200 L, and $t_{1/2}$ = 8 h, compute Css_{min} for a dose of oral quinidine 400 mg every 6 hours.

9. JB is a 78-year-old, 100-kg male being treated with digoxin for heart failure. While receiving digoxin tablets 125 µg daily, a steady-state digoxin concentration equal to 0.6 µg/L is obtained. (A) Assuming $F = 0.7$, compute digoxin clearance for the patient using the average steady-state concentration equation. (B) Compute a new digoxin tablet dose for the patient that will achieve Css = 1.2 µg/L.

10. QJ is a 67-year-old, 80-kg male being treated for chronic obstructive pulmonary disease. Sustained-release oral theophylline is being added to his drug regimen. Assuming $F = 1.0$, V = 40 L, and $t_{1/2}$ = 5 h, compute an oral theophylline dose to be administered every 12 hours that would achieve a Css = 8 mg/L using the average steady-state concentration equation.

11. TD is a 32-year-old, 70-kg male with generalized tonic-clonic seizures. Assuming Michaelis-Menten parameters of V_{max} = 500 mg/d and K_m = 4 mg/L, calculate a dose of phenytoin that will achieve Css = 15 mg/L.

12. OP is a 28-year-old, 55-kg female with complex partial seizures. She has the following information available: Css = 8 mg/L while receiving phenytoin 300 mg at bedtime and Css = 22 mg/L while receiving phenytoin 400 mg at bedtime. Compute the patient's Michaelis-Menten parameters for phenytoin and the phenytoin dose that would achieve Css = 15 mg/L.

ANSWERS TO PROBLEMS

1. *Answer to Question 1.*

   Part A:

   $k_e = -(\ln C_1 - \ln C_2)/(t_1 - t_2) = -[(\ln 35 \text{ mg/L}) - (\ln 15 \text{ mg/L})]/(1.5 \text{ h} - 12 \text{ h}) = 0.081 \text{ h}^{-1}$

   $t_{1/2} = 0.693/k_e = 0.693/0.081 \text{ h}^{-1} = 8.6 \text{ h}$

   $C_0 = C/e^{-ket} = (35 \text{ mg/L})/e^{(-0.081 \text{ h}^{-1})(1.5 \text{ h})} = 39.5 \text{ mg/L}$

   $V = D/[C_0 - C_{predose}] = (1000 \text{ mg})/(39.5 \text{ mg/L} - 15 \text{ mg/L}) = 41 \text{ L}$

   Part B:

   $\tau = [(\ln Css_{max} - \ln Css_{min})/k_e] = [\ln (30 \text{ mg/L}) - \ln (7.5 \text{ mg/L})]/0.081 \text{ h}^{-1} = 17.1 \text{ h}$, round to a dosage interval of 18 h.

   $D = Css_{max} V(1 - e^{-ke\tau}) = (30 \text{ mg/L} \cdot 41 \text{ L})(1 - e^{(-0.081 \text{ h}^{-1})(18 \text{ h})}) = 944 \text{ mg}$, round to a dose of 1000 mg.

   Recommended dose: 1000 mg every 18 hours

2. *Answer to Question 2.* Estimated V = 0.35 L/kg (45 kg) = 15.8 L

   Estimated $k_e = 0.693/t_{1/2} = 0.693/2 \text{ h} = 0.347 \text{ h}^{-1}$

   $\tau = [(\ln Css_{max} - \ln Css_{min})/k_e] = [\ln (10 \text{ mg/L}) - \ln (0.6 \text{ mg/L})]/0.347 \text{ h}^{-1} = 8.1 \text{ h}$, round to a dosage interval of 8 h.

$D = Css_{max} V(1 - e^{-k_e\tau}) = (10\ mg/L \cdot 15.8\ L)(1 - e^{(-0.347\ h^{-1})(8\ h)}) = 148$ mg, round to a dose of 150 mg.

Recommended dose: 150 mg every 8 hours

If desired a loading dose can be calculated: $LD = Css_{max} V = (10\ mg/L)(15.8\ L) = 158$ mg, round to a dose of 160 mg.

3. *Answer to Question 3.* $k_e = -(\ln C_1 - \ln C_2)/(t_1 - t_2) = -[(\ln 7.1\ mg/L) - (\ln 3.1\ mg/L)]/(1\ h - 8\ h) = 0.118\ h^{-1}$

$$V = \frac{k_0(1 - e^{-k_e t'})}{k_e[C_{max} - (C_{predose} e^{-k_e t'})]}$$

$$V = \frac{(60\ mg\ /\ 1\ h)(1 - e^{-(0.118 h^{-1})(1\ h)})}{0.118\ h^{-1}[(7.1\ mg\ /\ L) - (3.1\ mg\ /\ L \cdot e^{-(0.118 h^{-1})(1\ h)})]} = 13\ L$$

$\tau = [(\ln Css_{max} - \ln Css_{min})/k_e] + t' = [(\ln 8\ mg/L - \ln 1\ mg/L)/0.118\ h^{-1}] + 1\ h = 18.6$ h, round to dosage interval of 18 h.

$k_0 = Css_{max} k_e V[(1 - e^{-k_e\tau})/(1 - e^{-k_e t'})] = [(8\ mg/L)(0.118\ h^{-1})(13\ L)][(1 - e^{(-0.118\ h^{-1})(18\ h)})/(1 - e^{(-0.118\ h^{-1})(1\ h)})] = 97$ mg, round to dose of 100 mg

Recommended dose: 100 mg every 18 hours

4. *Answer to Question 4.* $k_e = 0.693/t_{1/2} = 0.693/8\ h = 0.087\ h^{-1}$, $V = 18\ L$

$\tau = [(\ln Css_{max} - \ln Css_{min})/k_e] + t' = [(\ln 10\ mg/L - \ln 1.2\ mg/L)/0.087\ h^{-1}] + 1\ h = 25.4$ h, round to dosage interval of 24 h.

$k_0 = Css_{max} k_e V[(1 - e^{-k_e\tau})/(1 - e^{-k_e t'})] = [(10\ mg/L)(0.087\ h^{-1})(18\ L)][(1 - e^{(-0.087\ h^{-1})(24\ h)})/(1 - e^{(-0.087\ h^{-1})(1\ h)})] = 165$ mg

Recommended dose: 165 mg every 24 hours

5. *Answer to Question 5.* $k_e = 0.693/t_{1/2} = 0.693/5\ h = 0.139\ h^{-1}$

$$V = 40\ L,\ Cl = k_e V = (0.139\ h^{-1})(40\ L) = 5.56\ L/h$$

$$LD = Css\ V = (12\ mg/L)(40\ L) = 480\ mg,\ \text{round to 500 mg IV over 20 min}$$

$$k_0 = Css\ Cl = (12\ mg/L)(5.56\ L/h) = 67\ mg/h,\ \text{round to 70 mg/h}$$

6. *Answer to Question 6.* $LD = Css\ V = (3\ mg/L)(33\ L) = 99$ mg, round to 100 mg IV over 2 min

$$k_0 = Css\ Cl = (3\ mg/L)(0.5\ L/min) = 1.5\ mg/min$$

7. *Answer to Question 7.* $D_{new}/D_{old} = Css_{new}/Css_{old}$

$$D_{new} = D_{old}(Css_{new}/Css_{old}) = 750\ mg\ [(2.5\ mg/L)/(1.5\ mg/L)] = 1250\ mg$$

Recommended dose: 1250 mg every 6 hours

8. *Answer to Question 8.* $k_e = 0.693/t_{1/2} = 0.693/8\ h = 0.087\ h^{-1}$

$$Css_{max} = [(FD)/V][e^{-k_e Tmax}/(1 - e^{-k_e\tau})]$$

$$Css_{max} = [(0.7 \cdot 400\ mg)/200\ L][e^{-(0.087\ h^{-1})(2\ h)}/(1 - e^{-(0.087\ h^{-1})(6\ h)})] = 2.9\ mg/L$$

$$Css_{min} = Css_{max} e^{-k_e(\tau - Tmax)} = (2.9\ mg/L)e^{-(0.087\ h^{-1})(6\ h - 2\ h)} = 2.0\ mg/L$$

9. *Answer to Question 9.*

Part A:

$$Css = F(D/\tau)/Cl$$

$$Cl = F(D/\tau)/Css = [0.7(125\ \mu g/1\ d)]/(0.6\ \mu g/L) = 146\ L/d$$

Part B:

$$D_{new} = D_{old}(Css_{new}/Css_{old}) = 125\ \mu g\ [(1.2\ \mu g/L)/(0.6\ \mu g/L)] = 250\ \mu g$$

Recommended dose: 250 μg daily

10. *Answer to Question 10.* $k_e = 0.693/t_{1/2} = 0.693/5\ h = 0.139\ h^{-1}$

$$Cl = k_e V = (0.139\ h^{-1})(40\ L) = 5.56\ L/h$$

$$Css = F(D/\tau)/Cl$$

$$D = (Css \cdot Cl \cdot \tau)/F = (8\ mg/L \cdot 5.56\ L/h \cdot 12\ h)/1.0 = 534\ mg,\ round\ to\ 500\ mg$$

Recommended dose: 500 mg every 12 hours

11. *Answer to Question 11.* $D = (V_{max} \cdot Css)/(K_m + Css) = (500\ mg/d \cdot 15\ mg/L)/(4\ mg/L + 15\ mg/L) = 395\ mg$, round to 400 mg

Recommended dose: 400 mg daily at bedtime

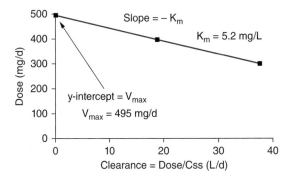

12. *Answer to Question 12.* Graph data (see attached graph): $K_m = 5.2\ mg/L$, $V_{max} = 495\ mg/d$

$$D = (V_{max} \cdot Css)/(K_m + Css) = (495\ mg/d \cdot 15\ mg/L)/(5.2\ mg/L + 15\ mg/L) = 367\ mg,\ round\ to\ 375\ mg$$

Recommended dose: 375 mg daily at bedtime

REFERENCES

1. Riegelman S, Loo JCK, Rowland M. Shortcomings in pharmacokinetic analysis by conceiving the body to exhibit properties of a single compartment. *J Pharm Sci.* 1968;57(1):117-123.

2. Teorell T. Kinetics of distribution of substances administered to the body. I. The extravascular modes of administration. *Archs Int Pharmacodyn Ther.* 1937;57:205-225.

3. Teorell T. Kinetics of distribution of substances administered to the body. II. The intravascular modes of administration. *Archs Int Pharmacodyn Ther.* 1937;57:226-240.

4. Sawchuk RJ, Zaske DE, Cipolle RJ, Wargin WA, Strate RG. Kinetic model for gentamicin dosing with the use of individual patient parameters. *Clin Pharmacol Ther.* 1977;21:362-365.

5. Matzke GR, McGory RW, Halstenson CE, Keane WF. Pharmacokinetics of vancomycin in patients with various degrees of renal function. *Antimicrob Agents Chemother.* 1984;25:433-437.

6. Murphy JE, Winter ME. Clinical pharmacokinetics pearls: bolus versus infusion equations. *Pharmacotherapy.* 1996;16(4):698-700.

7. Benet LZ. General treatment of linear mammillary models with elimination from any compartment as used in pharmacokinetics. *J Pharm Sci.* 1972;61(4):536-541.

8. Wagner JG, Northam JI, Alway CD, Carpenter OS. Blood levels of drug at the equilibrium state after multiple dosing. *Nature.* 1965;207:1301-1302.

9. Jusko WJ, Koup JR, Vance JW, Schentag JJ, Kuritzky P. Intravenous theophylline therapy: nomogram guidelines. *Ann Intern Med.* 1977;86(4):400-404.

10. Ludden TM, Allen JP, Valutsky WA, et al. Individualization of phenytoin dosage regimens. *Clin Pharmacol Ther.* 1977;21(3):287-293.

11. Shargel L, Yu A, Wu-Pong S. *Applied Biopharmaceutics and Pharmacokinetics.* 6th ed. New York, NY: McGraw-Hill; 2012.

3 Drug Dosing in Special Populations: Renal and Hepatic Disease, Dialysis, Heart Failure, Obesity, and Drug Interactions

INTRODUCTION

All medications have specific disease states and conditions that change the pharmacokinetics of the drug and warrant dosage modification. However, the dosing of most drugs will be altered by one or more of the important factors discussed in this chapter. Renal or hepatic disease will decrease the elimination or metabolism of the majority drugs and change the clearance of the agent. Dialysis procedures, conducted using artificial kidneys in patients with renal failure, removes some medications from the body while the pharmacokinetics of other drugs are not changed. Heart failure results in low cardiac output which decreases blood flow to eliminating organs, and the clearance rate of drugs with moderate-to-high extraction ratios are particularly sensitive to alterations in organ blood flow. Obesity adds excessive adipose tissue to the body, which may change the way that drugs distribute in the body and alter the volume of distribution for the medication. Finally, drug interactions can inhibit or induce drug metabolism, alter drug protein binding, or change blood flow to organs that eliminate or metabolize the drug.

RENAL DISEASE

Most water-soluble drugs are eliminated unchanged to some extent by the kidney. In addition to this, drug metabolites that were made more water soluble via oxidation or conjugation are typically removed by renal elimination. The nephron is the functional unit of the kidney that is responsible for waste product removal from the body and also eliminates drug molecules (Figure 3-1). Unbound drug molecules that are relatively small are filtered at the glomerulus. Glomerular filtration is the primary elimination route for many medications. Drugs can be actively secreted into the urine, and this process usually takes place in the proximal tubules. Tubular secretion is an active process conducted by relatively specific carriers or pumps that move the drug from blood vessels in close proximity to the nephron into the proximal tubule. Additionally, some medications may be reabsorbed from the urine back into the blood by the kidney. Reabsorption is usually a passive process and requires a degree of lipid solubility for the drug molecule. Thus, tubular reabsorption is influenced by the pH of the urine, the pKa of the drug molecule, and the resulting extent of molecular ionization. Compounds that are not ionized in the urine are more lipid soluble, better able to pass through lipid membranes, and more prone to renal tubular reabsorption. The equation that describes these various routes of renal elimination is

$$Cl_R = [(f_B \cdot GFR) + \frac{RBF \cdot (f_B Cl'_{sec})}{RBF + (f_B Cl'_{sec})}](1 - FR)$$

where f_B is the free fraction of drug in the blood, GFR is glomerular filtration rate, RBF is renal blood flow, Cl'_{sec} is the intrinsic clearance for tubular secretion of unbound drug, and FR is the fraction reabsorbed.[1]

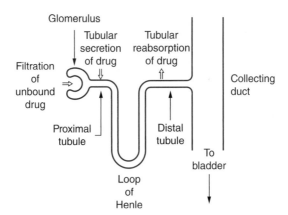

FIGURE 3-1   The nephron is the functional unit of the kidney responsible for drug elimination. Unbound drug is filtered freely at the glomerulus (shown by arrow). Active tubular secretion of drug (denoted by arrow into nephron) usually occurs in the proximal tubule of the nephron. Passive tubular reabsorption (denoted by *arrow* out of nephron) usually occurs in the distal tubule of the nephron. Tubular reabsorption requires un-ionized drug molecules so that the molecules can pass through the lipid membranes of the nephron and surrounding capillaries.

When infants are born, renal function is not yet completely developed in full-term neonates (~ 40 weeks' gestational age). Kidney development is complete and renal function stabilizes 3-6 months after birth. In premature infants (<35 weeks), kidney development may take even longer during the postpartum period. Kidney function, as measured by glomerular filtration rate, typically averages ~ 120-140 mL/min in young, healthy adults aged 18-22 years. As humans age, there is a gradual decline in glomerular function so that by 65 years of age, the average glomerular filtration rate is ~ 50-60 mL/min. The expected glomerular filtration rate for otherwise healthy, normal 80-year-old adults is ~ 30-40 mL/min. A glomerular filtration rate of 80-120 mL/min is usually considered the normal range by most clinical laboratories.

In patients with renal disease, there is a functional loss of nephrons. Depending on the etiology of the renal disease, patients with acute kidney failure may recoup their baseline renal function after a period of supportive care and dialysis long enough for their kidneys to recover. Patients with acute renal failure due to a sudden decrease in renal blood flow, such as that seen during hypotension, shock, or hypovolemia, or due to nephrotoxic drug therapy such as aminoglycoside antibiotics or vancomycin, often have their kidney function return to its preinsult level if they survive the underlying causes of their renal dysfunction. Patients with chronic renal failure sustain permanent loss of functional nephrons due to irreversible damage and do not recover lost kidney function.

Measurement and Estimation of Glomerular Filtration Rate and Creatinine Clearance

Glomerular filtration rate (GFR) can be determined by administration of special test compounds such as inulin or ^{125}I-iothalamate; this is sometimes done for patients by nephrologists when precise determination of renal function is needed. Glomerular filtration rate can be estimated using the modified Modification of Diet in Renal Disease (MDRD) equation: GFR (in mL/min/1.73 m^2) = 186 • $S_{Cr}^{-1.154}$ • Age$^{-0.203}$ • (0.742, if female) • (1.212, if African-American).[2,3] For example, the estimated GFR for a 53-year-old African-American male with a S_{Cr} = 2.7 mg/dL would be computed as follows: GFR = 186 • (2.7 mg/dL)$^{-1.154}$ • (53 y)$^{-0.203}$ • 1.212 = 32 mL/min/1.73 m^2. If standardized serum creatinine laboratory values are used in the calculation, a formula similar to the original equation is used: GFR (in mL/min/1.73 m^2) = 175 • $S_{Cr}^{-1.154}$ • Age$^{-0.203}$ • (0.742, if female) • (1.212, if African-American).[4]

In response to some limitations noted in the MDRD equations, the Chronic Kidney Disease–Epidemiology Collaboration (CKD-EPI) group developed another widely used equation to estimate glomerular filtration rate: GFR (in mL/min/1.73 m^2) = 141 • min(S_{Cr}/κ, 1)$^\alpha$ • max(S_{Cr}/κ, 1)$^{-1.209}$ • 0.993^{Age} • (1.018, if female) • (1.159, if black), where κ is 0.7 for females or 0.9 for males, α is −0.329 for females or −0.411 for males, min indicates the minimum of Scr/κ or 1, and max indicates the maximum of Scr/κ or 1.[5] There are other versions of both the MDRD and CKD-EPI equations, which include additional variables such as blood urea nitrogen and cystatin C.[6]

The methods recommended by the Food and Drug Administration (FDA) and others to determine renal function for the purposes of drug dosing are estimated creatinine clearance (CrCl)[7-13] or estimated glomerular filtration rate.[11,14,15] Creatinine is a by-product of muscle metabolism that is primarily eliminated by glomerular filtration. Because of this property, creatinine clearance is used as a surrogate measurement of glomerular filtration rate. Because creatinine is also eliminated by other routes, CrCl does not equal GFR, so the two parameters are not interchangeable.[3,8] In the case of drugs that were approved by the FDA prior to 2010, only creatinine clearance measurements may have been used to determine drug dosing requirements for patients with decreased renal function.

Creatinine clearance rates can be measured by collecting urine for a specified period and collecting a blood sample for determination of serum creatinine at the midpoint of the concurrent urine collection time: CrCl (in mL/min) = (U_{Cr} • V_{urine})/(S_{Cr} • T), where U_{Cr} is the urine creatinine concentration in mg/dL, V_{urine} is the volume of urine collected in mL, S_{Cr} is the serum creatinine collected at the midpoint of the urine collection in mg/dL, and T is the time in minutes of the urine collection. Because creatinine renal secretion exhibits diurnal variation, most nephrologists use a 24-hour urine collection period for the determination of creatinine clearance. For example, a 24-hour urine was collected for a patient with the following results: U_{Cr} = 55 mg/dL, V_{urine} = 1000 mL, S_{Cr} = 1.0 mg/dL, T = 24 h × 60 min/h = 1440 min, and CrCl (in mL/min) = (U_{Cr} • V_{urine})/(S_{Cr} • T) = (55 mg/dL • 1000 mL)/(1.0 mg/dL • 1440 min) = 38 mL/min. However, for the purpose of drug dosing, collection periods of 8-12 hours have been sufficient, and they provide a quicker turnaround time in emergent situations. Also, if renal function is stable, the blood sample for determination of serum creatinine may not need to be collected at the precise midpoint of the urine collection.

Routine measurement of creatinine clearances in patients has been fraught with problems. Incomplete urine collections, serum creatinine concentrations obtained at incorrect times, and collection time errors can produce erroneous measured creatinine clearance values. This realization has prompted investigators to derive methods that estimate creatinine clearance from serum creatinine values and other patient characteristics in various populations. The most widely used of these formulas for adults aged 18 years and older is the method suggested by Cockcroft and Gault[16]: for males, CrCl$_{est}$ = [(140 − age)BW]/(72 • S_{Cr}); for females, CrCl$_{est}$ = [0.85(140 − age)BW]/(72 • S_{Cr}); where CrCl$_{est}$ is estimated creatinine clearance in mL/min, age is in years, BW is body weight in kg, S_{Cr} is serum creatinine in mg/dL. The Cockcroft-Gault method should only be used in patients aged 18 years or older, actual weight within 30% of their ideal body weight [IBW$_{males}$ (in kg) = 50 + 2.3(Ht −60) or IBW$_{females}$ (in kg) = 45 + 2.3(Ht −60), where Ht is height in inches], and stable serum creatinine concentrations. The 0.85 correction factor for females is present because they have smaller muscle mass than men and, therefore, produce less creatinine per day. For example, a 55-year-old, 80-kg, 5-ft 11-in male has a serum creatinine equal to 1.9 mg/dL. The estimated creatinine clearance would be: IBW$_{males}$ = 50 + 2.3(Ht −60) = 50 + 2.3(71 in − 60 in) = 75 kg, so the patient is within 30% of his ideal body weight (IBW) and the Cockcroft-Gault method can be used; CrCl$_{est}$ = [(140 − age)BW]/(72 • S_{Cr}) = [(140 − 55 y)80 kg]/(72 • 1.9 mg/dL) = 50 mL/min.

Some patients have decreased muscle mass due to disease states and conditions that affect muscle or prevent exercise. Patients with spinal cord injury, cancer patients with muscle wasting, human immunodeficiency virus (HIV)–infected patients, cachectic patients, and patients with poor nutrition are examples of situations where muscle mass may be very small resulting in low creatinine production. In these cases, serum creatinine concentrations are low due to the low creatinine production rate and not due to high renal clearance of creatinine. In these cases, investigators have suggested that if serum creatinine values are less than 1.0 mg/dL for a patient, an arbitrary value of 1 mg/dL be used in the Cockcroft-Gault formula to estimate creatinine clearance.[17-19] While it appears that the resulting estimate of creatinine clearance is closer to the actual creatinine clearance in these patients, it can still result in misestimates. It may be necessary to measure creatinine clearance in these types of patients if an accurate reflection of glomerular filtration rate is needed.

If serum creatinine values are not stable, but increasing or decreasing in a patient, the Cockcroft-Gault equation cannot be used to estimate creatinine clearance. In this case, an alternative method must be used that was suggested by Jelliffe and Jelliffe.[20] The first step in this method is to estimate creatinine production. The formula for this is different for males and females due to gender-dependent differences in muscle mass: Ess_{male} = IBW[29.3 − (0.203 • Age)]; Ess_{female} = IBW[25.1 − (0.175 • Age)], where Ess is the excretion of creatinine, IBW is ideal body weight in kg, and age is in years. The remainder of the equations correct creatinine production for renal function and adjust the estimated creatinine clearance value according to whether the renal function is getting better or worse:

$$Ess_{corrected} = Ess[1.035 − (0.0337 • Scr_{ave})]$$

$$E = Ess_{corrected} − \frac{[4IBW(Scr_2 − Scr_1)]}{\Delta t}$$

$$CrCl \text{ (in mL/min/1.73 m}^2) = E/(14.4 • Scr_{ave})$$

where Scr_{ave} is the average of the two serum creatinine determinations in mg/dL, Scr_1 is the first serum creatinine and Scr_2 is the second serum creatinine both in mg/dL, and Δt is the time that expired between the measurement of Scr_1 and Scr_2 in minutes.

If patients are not within 30% of their ideal body weight, other methods to estimate creatinine clearance should be used.[21,22] It has been suggested that use of ideal body weight or adjusted body weight (ideal body weight plus 40% of obese weight) instead of actual body weight in the Cockcroft-Gault equation gives an adequate estimate of creatinine clearance for obese individuals.[23-25] However, Salazar and Corcoran[26] derived a method for estimating creatinine clearance specifically for obese patients, and it is recommended for use in this population[21,27]:

$$CrCl_{est(males)} = \frac{(137 − age)[(0.285 • Wt) + (12.1 \cdot Ht^2)]}{(51 • S_{Cr})}$$

$$CrCl_{est(females)} = \frac{(146 − age)[(0.287 • Wt) + (9.74 • Ht^2)]}{(60 • S_{Cr})}$$

where age is in years, Wt is weight in kg, Ht is height in m, and S_{Cr} is serum creatinine in mg/dL.

Methods to estimate creatinine clearance for children and young adults are also available according to their age[28]: age 0-1 year, $CrCl_{est}$ (in mL/min/1.73 m^2) = (0.45 • Ht)/S_{Cr}; age 1-20 years, $CrCl_{est}$ (in mL/min/1.73 m^2) = (0.55 • Ht)/S_{Cr}, where Ht is in cm and S_{Cr} is in mg/dL. Note that for these formulas, estimated creatinine clearance is normalized to 1.73 m^2, which is the body surface area of an adult male with a height and weight of approximately 5 ft 10 in and 70 kg, respectively.

Estimation of Drug Dosing and Pharmacokinetic Parameters Using Creatinine Clearance

It is common to base initial doses of drugs that are renally eliminated on creatinine clearance even though glomerular filtration rate is the physiologic parameter that directly measures renal function. There are several methods that reliably estimate creatinine clearance for a variety of disparate patient populations; methods to estimate glomerular filtration rate are relatively new and limited to a few patient groups. The basis for using creatinine clearance for renal drug dosing is that renal clearance of the drug is smaller in patients with a reduced glomerular filtration rate, and measured or estimated creatinine clearance is a surrogate marker for glomerular filtration rate. An implicit assumption made in this approach is that all drug excreting processes of the kidney, including tubular section and reabsorption, decline in parallel with glomerular filtration. The basis of this assumption is the intact nephron theory. While tubular secretion and reabsorption may not always decline in proportion to glomerular filtration, this approach approximates the decline in tubular function and is a useful approach to initial drug dosing in patients with renal dysfunction. However, clinicians should bear in mind that the suggested doses for patients with renal impairment are an initial guideline only, and doses may need to be increased in patients who exhibit suboptimal drug response and decreased in patients with adverse effects.

Breakpoints to consider altering drug doses are useful for clinicians to keep in mind.[7,9-11] Generally, one should consider a possible, modest decrease in drug doses when creatinine clearance is less than 50-60 mL/min, a moderate decrease in drug doses when creatinine clearance is less than 25-30 mL/min, and a substantial decrease in drug doses when creatinine clearance is 15 mL/min or less. In order to modify doses for patients with renal impairment, it is possible to decrease the drug dose and retain the usual dosage interval, retain the usual dose and increase the dosage interval, or simultaneously decrease the dosage and prolong the dosage interval. The approach used depends on the route of administration, the dosage forms available, and the pharmacodynamic response to the drug. For example, if the drug is prescribed orally and only a limited number of solid dosage forms are available, one will usually administer the usual dose and increase the dosage interval. If the drug is given parenterally, a smaller dose can be administered, and it is more likely that the usual dosage interval will be retained. Finally, for drugs with narrow therapeutic ranges such as aminoglycoside antibiotics and vancomycin in which target serum concentrations for maximum and minimum steady-state concentrations are established, both the dose and dosage interval can be manipulated to achieve the targeted drug levels. If the drug dose is reduced and the dosage interval remains unaltered in patients with decreased renal function, maximum drug concentrations are usually lower and minimum drug concentrations higher than that encountered in patients with normal renal function receiving the typical drug dose (Figure 3-2). If the dosage interval

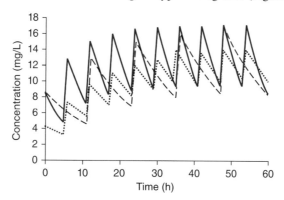

FIGURE 3-2   Serum concentration versus time profile for a patient with normal kidney function receiving a renally eliminated drug at the dose of 300 mg every 6 hours (*solid line*). In a patient with renal dysfunction, it is possible to give the same dose and prolong the dosage interval (300 mg every 12 hours, *dashed line*), or a reduced dose at the same dosage interval (150 mg every 6 hours, dotted line). Giving the same dose at a longer dosage interval in the patient with renal disease usually results in a concentration/time profile similar to that seen in a normal patient receiving the normal dose. However, giving a smaller dose and keeping the dosage interval the same usually produces a concentration/time profile with a lower peak steady-state concentration and a higher trough steady-state concentration. Note that because the total daily dose is the same for both renal disease dosage regimens (600 mg/d), the average steady-state concentration is identical for both dosage schemes. The same dosage options are available for liver metabolized drugs for patients with hepatic dysfunction.

TABLE 3-1   Manufacturer's Recommended Dosing Schedule for Renal Dysfunction and Hemodialysis Patients Receiving Gabapentin[64]

CrCl (mL/min)	Daily Dose (mg/d)	Dosage (mg)				
≥60	900-3600	300 TID	400 TID	600 TID	800 TID	1200 TID
30-59	400-1400	200 BID	300 BID	400 BID	500 BID	700 BID
15-29	200-700	200 QD	300 QD	400 QD	500 QD	700 QD
15[a]	100-300	100 QD	125 QD	150 QD	200 QD	300 QD

Supplemental posthemodialysis dose (mg)[b]					
Hemodialysis	125[b]	150[b]	200[b]	250[b]	350[b]

BID, twice daily; QD, once daily; TID, three times daily.

[a] For patients with creatinine clearance <15 mL/min, reduce daily dose in proportion to creatinine clearance (eg, patients with a creatinine clearance of 7.5 mL/min should receive ½ the daily dose that patients with a creatinine clearance of 15 mL/min receive).

[b] Patients on hemodialysis should receive maintenance doses based on estimates of creatinine clearance as indicated in the upper portion of the table and a supplemental posthemodialysis dose administered after each 4 hours of hemodialysis as indicated in the lower portion of the table.

is prolonged and the drug dosage remains the same, maximum and minimum drug concentrations are usually about the same as in patients with good renal function receiving the usual drug dose.

Since the mid-1980s, the FDA has required pharmacokinetic studies to be done for agents that are renally eliminated in patients with decreased creatinine clearances or glomerular filtration rates before receiving agency approval.[11] In these cases, the package insert for the drug probably contains reasonable initial dosage guidelines. For example, the manufacture's suggested guidelines for the dosing of gabapentin in patients with renal dysfunction are listed in Table 3-1. Guidelines to change drug doses for patients with decreased renal function are available for older drugs as well as updated guidelines for newer drugs that may not be included in the package insert.[7,9,10,29-31] Also, the primary literature should be consulted to ensure that the newest guidelines are used for all drugs. If no specific information is available for a medication, it is possible to calculate modified initial drug doses using the method described by Dettli.[32]

For drugs with narrow therapeutic indexes, measured or estimated creatinine clearance may be used to estimate pharmacokinetic parameters for a patient based on prior studies conducted in other patients with renal dysfunction. Estimated pharmacokinetic parameters are then used in pharmacokinetic dosing equations to compute initial doses for patients. Clearance is the best pharmacokinetic parameter to estimate using creatinine clearance because it is an independent parameter that deals solely with drug elimination. The relationship between drug clearance and creatinine clearance is usually approximated by a straight line with a slope that is a function of the renal clearance for the drug and an intercept that is related to the nonrenal clearance of the drug (Figure 3-3). For digoxin, the equation that describes the relationship between digoxin clearance (Cl) and creatinine clearance (CrCl in mL/min) is: Cl (in mL/min) $= 1.303 \bullet CrCl + Cl_{NR}$, where Cl_{NR} is nonrenal clearance and equals 20 mL/min in patients with moderate-severe heart failure and 40 mL/min in patients with no or mild heart failure.[33] The equation using glomerular filtration rate (GFR in mL/min) instead of creatinine clearance as an index for renal function is: Cl (in mL/min) $= 1.101 \bullet GFR + Cl_{NR}$, where Cl_{NR} is nonrenal clearance and equals 20 mL/min in patients with moderate-severe heart failure and 40 mL/min in patients with no or mild heart failure.[33] Digoxin is one of the few drugs marketed before 2010 in which the relationship between drug clearance and both creatinine clearance and glomerular filtration rate is known.

Elimination rate constant (k_e) can also be estimated using creatinine clearance, but it is a dependent pharmacokinetic parameter whose result is reliant on the relative values of clearance and volume of distribution

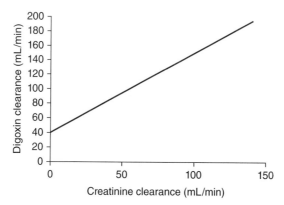

FIGURE 3-3 Relationship between creatinine clearance and digoxin clearance used to estimate initial digoxin clearance when no drug concentrations are available. The y-axis intercept (40 mL/min) is nonrenal clearance for digoxin in patients with no or mild heart failure. If the patient has moderate-severe heart failure, nonrenal clearance is set to a value of 20 mL/min.

$(k_e = Cl/V)$. Because of this, changes in elimination rate constant may not always be due to changes in the renal elimination of the drug. The relationship between elimination rate constant and creatinine clearance is usually approximated by a straight line with a slope that is a function of renal elimination for the agent and an intercept that is related to the elimination of drug in functionally anephric patients (GFR ≈ 0; Figure 3-4). For the aminoglycoside antibiotics, an equation that represents the relationship between aminoglycoside antibiotic elimination rate constant (k_e) and creatinine clearance (CrCl in mL/min) is: k_e (in h^{-1}) = 0.00293 • CrCl + 0.014.[34]

Volume of distribution can also change in patients with decreased renal function. Plasma protein–binding displacement of drug by endogenous or exogenous substances that would normally be eliminated by the kidney but accumulate in the blood of patients with poor kidney function can increase the volume of distribution of drugs. Conversely, the volume of distribution of a drug can decrease if compounds normally excreted by the kidney accumulate to the extent that displacement of drug from tissue binding sites occurs. Digoxin volume

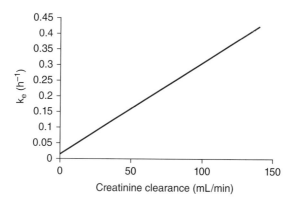

FIGURE 3-4 Relationship between creatinine clearance and aminoglycoside elimination rate constant (k_e) used to estimate initial aminoglycoside elimination when no drug concentrations are available. The y-axis intercept (0.014 h^{-1}) is nonrenal elimination for aminoglycosides.

of distribution decreases in patients with decreased renal function according to the following equation[35]: V (in L) = 226 + [(298 • CrCl)/(29.1 + CrCl)] where CrCl is in mL/min. The decline in volume of distribution presumably occurs because of displacement of tissue-bound digoxin.

HEPATIC DISEASE

Most lipid-soluble drugs are metabolized to some degree by the liver. Phase I–type reactions, such as oxidation, hydrolysis, and reduction, are often mediated by the cytochrome P-450 enzyme system (CYP) that is bound to the membrane of the endoplasmic reticulum inside hepatocytes. Phase II–type reactions, including conjugation to form glucuronides, acetates, or sulfates, may also be mediated in the liver by cytosolic enzymes contained in hepatocytes. Phases I and II drug metabolism generally results in metabolites that are more water soluble and prone to elimination by the kidney. Transport proteins, such as P-glycoprotein, actively secrete drug molecules into the bile.

The liver receives its blood supply via the hepatic artery, which contains oxygenated blood from the aorta via the superior mesenteric artery, and the portal vein, which drains the gastrointestinal tract (Figure 3-5). Liver blood flow averages 1-1.5 L/min in adults with about 1/3 coming from the hepatic artery and about 2/3 coming from the portal vein. Orally administered medications must pass through the liver before entering the systemic circulation, so if the drug is metabolized by the liver, a portion of the dose may be inactivated by the hepatic first-pass effect before having a chance to exert a pharmacologic effect. In addition to hepatic metabolism, drugs can be eliminated unchanged by liver in the bile. The equation that describes hepatic drug metabolism is[36]:

$$Cl_H = \frac{LBF \cdot (f_B \cdot Cl'_{int})}{LBF + (f_B \cdot Cl'_{int})}$$

where LBF is liver blood flow, f_B is the fraction of unbound drug in the blood, and Cl'_{int} is intrinsic clearance.

Hepatic metabolism of drugs is not completely developed in neonates (~ 40 weeks' gestational age) and continues to increase so that by age 3-6 months it is stable. In premature infants (<35 weeks), hepatic metabolism may take even longer to develop in the postpartum period. On a per kilogram basis, drug metabolism is more rapid in children until puberty. At that point, metabolic rate gradually decreases to adult values.

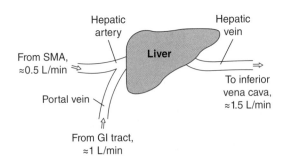

FIGURE 3-5   Schematic representation of the liver. Liver blood flow to the organ is supplied by the hepatic artery and the portal vein. The hepatic artery branches off of the superior mesenteric artery and provides oxygenated blood to the liver at the rate of ~ 0.5 L/min. The portal vein drains blood from the gastrointestinal tract at the rate of ~ 1 L/min and passes its contents to the liver. Any chemicals, including orally administered drugs, must pass through the liver before it enters the systemic circulation. The hepatic vein drains the liver of blood and empties into the inferior vena cava.

The effect of advanced age on hepatic drug metabolism is quite variable. Patients older than 65 years may have decreased hepatic clearance of some drugs, but often times concurrent disease states and conditions that affect drug pharmacokinetics obscure the influence of age in these older individuals. Elderly individuals have decreased liver mass, and it appears that hepatocytes which are still present have decreased ability to metabolize drugs.

There are two major types of liver disease: hepatitis and cirrhosis. Patients with hepatitis experience an inflammation of the liver, and as a result, hepatocytes may experience decreased ability to function or die. Patients with acute hepatitis usually experience mild, transient decreases in drug metabolism that require no or minor changes in drug dosing. If the patient develops chronic hepatitis, it is likely that irreversible hepatocyte damage will be more widespread and drug dosage changes will be required at some point. In patients with hepatic cirrhosis, there is a permanent loss of functional hepatocytes. Drug dosage schedules usually need to be modified in patients with severe cirrhosis. With sufficient long-term hepatocyte damage, patients with chronic hepatitis can progress to hepatic cirrhosis.

When hepatocytes are damaged, they are no longer able to metabolize drugs efficiently, and intrinsic clearance decreases, which reduces the hepatic clearance of the drug. If the drug experiences a hepatic first-pass effect, less drug will be lost by presystemic metabolism and bioavailability will increase. A simultaneous decrease in hepatic clearance and liver first-pass effect results in extremely large increases in steady-state concentrations for orally administered drugs. Liver blood flow also decreases in patients with cirrhosis because hepatocytes are replaced by nonfunctional connective tissue which increases intraorgan pressure causing portal vein hypertension and shunting of blood flow around the liver. The decrease in liver blood flow results in less drug delivery to still-functioning hepatocytes and depresses hepatic drug clearance even further. The liver produces albumin and, probably, α_1-acid glycoprotein, the two major proteins that bind acidic and basic drugs, respectively, in the blood. In patients with cirrhosis, the production of these proteins declines. When this is the case, the free fraction of drugs in the blood increases because of a lack of binding proteins. Additionally, high concentrations of endogenous substances in the blood that are normally eliminated by the liver, such as bilirubin, can displace drugs from plasma protein–binding sites. The increased free fraction in the blood will alter hepatic and renal drug clearance as well as the volume of distribution for drugs that are highly protein bound ($V = V_B + (f_B/f_T)V_T$, where V is the volume of distribution, V_B and V_T are the physiologic volume of blood and tissues, respectively, and f_B and f_T are the free fraction of drug in the blood and tissues, respectively). Because clearance typically decreases and volume of distribution usually increases or does not appreciably change for a drug in patients with liver disease, the elimination rate constant (k_e) almost always increases in patients with decreased liver function (k_e = Cl/V, where Cl is clearance and V is volume of distribution).

Determination of Child-Pugh Scores

Unfortunately, there is no single laboratory test that can be used to assess liver function in the same way that measured or estimated creatinine clearance is used to measure renal function. The most common way to estimate the ability of the liver to metabolize drug is to determine the Child-Pugh score for a patient.[37] The Child-Pugh score consists of five laboratory tests or clinical symptoms. The five areas include serum albumin, total bilirubin, prothrombin time, ascites, and hepatic encephalopathy. Each of these areas is given a score of 1 (normal) to 3 (severely abnormal; Table 3-2), and the scores for the five areas are summed. The Child-Pugh score for a patient with normal liver function is 5 while the score for a patient with grossly abnormal serum albumin, total bilirubin, and prothrombin time values in addition to severe ascites and hepatic encephalopathy is 15. A Child-Pugh score equal to 8-9 is grounds for a moderate decrease (~ 25%) in initial daily drug dose for agents that are primarily (≥60%) hepatically metabolized, and a score of 10 or greater indicates that a significant decrease in initial daily dose (~ 50%) is required for drugs that are mostly liver metabolized. As in

TABLE 3-2   Child-Pugh Scores for Patients With Liver Disease[37]

Test/Symptom	Score 1 Point	Score 2 Points	Score 3 Points
Total bilirubin (mg/dL)	<2.0	2.0-3.0	>3.0
Serum albumin (g/dL)	>3.5	2.8-3.5	<2.8
Prothrombin time (seconds prolonged over control)	<4	4-6	>6
Ascites	Absent	Slight	Moderate
Hepatic encephalopathy	None	Moderate	Severe

any patient with or without liver dysfunction, initial doses are meant as starting points for dosage titration based on patient response and avoidance of adverse effects.

For example, the usual dose of a medication that is 95% liver metabolized is 500 mg every 6 hours, and the total daily dose is 2000 mg/d. For a hepatic cirrhosis patient with a Child-Pugh score of 12, an appropriate initial dose would be 50% of the usual dose or 1000 mg/d. The drug could be prescribed to the patient as 250 mg every 6 hours or 500 mg every 12 hours. The patient would be closely monitored for pharmacologic and toxic effects due to the medication, and the dose would be modified as needed.

Estimation of Drug Dosing and Pharmacokinetic Parameters for Liver Metabolized Drugs

For drugs that are primarily liver metabolized, pharmacokinetic parameters are assigned to patients with liver disease by assessing values previously measured in patients with the same type of liver disease (eg, hepatitis or cirrhosis) and a similar degree of liver dysfunction. Table 3-3 gives values for theophylline clearance in a variety of patients, including patients with cirrhosis.[38] The dose and dosing interval needed to achieve steady-state concentrations in the lower end of the therapeutic range using pharmacokinetic parameters measured in patients with liver disease are computed using pharmacokinetic equations. For example, the theophylline dosage rates listed in Table 3-3 are designed to produce steady-state theophylline concentrations between 8 and 12 mg/L. They were computed by multiplying theophylline clearance and the desired steady-state concentration ($MD = Css \cdot Cl$, where MD is the maintenance dose, Css is the steady-state concentration, and Cl is drug

TABLE 3-3   Theophylline Clearance and Dosage Rates for Patients With Various Disease States and Conditions[38]

Disease State/Condition	Mean Clearance (mL/min/kg)	Mean Dose (mg/kg/h)
Children 1-9 y	1.4	0.8
Children 9-12 y or adults smokers	1.25	0.7
Adolescents 12-16 y or elderly smokers (> 65 y)	0.9	0.5
Adults nonsmokers	0.7	0.4
Elderly nonsmokers (> 65 y)	0.5	0.3
Decompensated CHF, cor pulmonale, cirrhosis	0.35	0.2

Mean volume of distribution = 0.5 L/kg.

clearance). Average theophylline clearance is about 50% less in adults with liver cirrhosis compared to adults with normal hepatic function. Because of this, initial theophylline doses for patients with hepatic cirrhosis are ½ the usual dose for adult patients with normal liver function.

When prescribing medications that are principally eliminated by the liver in patients with liver dysfunction, it is possible to decrease the dose while retaining the normal dosage interval, retain the normal dose and prolong the dosage interval, or modify both the dose and dosage interval. Compared to individuals with normal liver function receiving a drug at the usual dose and dosage interval, patients with hepatic disease who receive a normal dose but a prolonged dosage interval will have similar maximum and minimum steady-state serum concentrations (see Figure 3-2). However, if the dose is decreased but the dosage interval kept at the usual frequency, maximum steady-state concentrations will be lower and minimum steady-state concentrations will be higher for patients with liver disease than for patients with normal hepatic function. The actual method used to reduce the dose for patients with liver dysfunction will depend on the route of administration and the available dosage forms. For example, if the medication is only available as an oral capsule, it is likely that the usual dose will be given to a patient with liver disease, but the dosage interval will be prolonged. However, if the drug is given parenterally, it may be possible to simultaneously modify the dose and dosage interval to attain the same maximum and minimum steady-state concentrations in patients with hepatic dysfunction as those encountered in patients with normal liver function.

Implications of Hepatic Disease on Serum Drug Concentration Monitoring and Drug Effects

The pharmacokinetic alterations that occur with hepatic disease result in complex changes for total and unbound steady-state concentrations and drug response. The changes that occur depend on whether the drug has a low or high hepatic extraction ratio. As previously discussed, hepatic drug metabolism is described by the following equation:[36]

$$Cl_H = \frac{LBF \cdot (f_B \cdot Cl'_{int})}{LBF + (f_B \cdot Cl'_{int})}$$

where LBF is liver blood flow, f_B is the fraction of unbound drug in the blood, and Cl'_{int} is intrinsic clearance. For drugs with a low hepatic extraction ratio ($\leq 30\%$), the numeric value of liver blood flow is much greater than the product of unbound fraction of drug in the blood and the intrinsic clearance of the compound ($LBF \gg f_B \cdot Cl'_{int}$), and the sum in the denominator of the hepatic clearance equation is almost equal to liver blood flow [$LBF \approx LBF + (f_B \cdot Cl'_{int})$]. When this substitution is made into the hepatic clearance equation, hepatic clearance is equal to the product of free fraction in the blood and the intrinsic clearance of the drug for a drug with a low hepatic extraction ratio:

$$Cl_H = \frac{LBF \cdot (f_B \cdot Cl'_{int})}{LBF} = f_B \cdot Cl'_{int}$$

Similarly, for drugs with a high hepatic extraction ratio ($\geq 70\%$), the numeric value of liver blood flow is much less than the product of unbound fraction of drug in the blood and the intrinsic clearance of the agent ($LBF \ll f_B \cdot Cl'_{int}$), and the sum in the denominator of the hepatic clearance equation is almost equal to the product of free fraction of drug in the blood and intrinsic clearance [$f_B \cdot Cl'_{int} \approx LBF + (f_B \cdot Cl'_{int})$]. When this substitution is made into the hepatic clearance equation, hepatic clearance is equal to liver blood flow for a drug with a high hepatic extraction ratio:

$$Cl_H = \frac{LBF \cdot (f_B \cdot Cl'_{int})}{f_B \cdot Cl'_{int}} = LBF$$

For drugs with intermediate hepatic extraction ratios, the entire liver clearance equation must be used, and all three factors, liver blood flow, free fraction of drug in the blood, and intrinsic clearance, are important parameters that must be taken into account. An extremely important point for clinicians to understand is that the factors that are important determinants of hepatic clearance are different depending on the liver extraction ratio for the drug.

In order to illustrate the differences that may occur in steady-state drug concentrations and pharmacologic effects for patients with liver disease, a graphical technique is used (Figure 3-6). The example assumes that a low hepatic extraction ratio drug (100% liver metabolized) is being given to a patient as a continuous intravenous infusion and that all physiologic, pharmacokinetic, and drug effect parameters (shown on the y-axis) are initially stable. On the x-axis, an arrow indicates that intrinsic clearance decreases due to the development of hepatic cirrhosis in the patient; an assumption made for this illustration is that any changes in the parameters are instantaneous. An increase in the parameter is denoted as an uptick in the line while a decrease in the parameter is shown as a downtick in the line. The first three parameters are physiologic values (LBF, f_B, and Cl'_{int}) that will change in response to the development of hepatic dysfunction. In this case, only intrinsic clearance decreased due to the destruction of hepatocytes, and liver blood flow and free fraction of drug in the blood was not altered (see Figure 3-6). This change will decrease the hepatic clearance of the drug, volume of distribution will not be modified because blood and tissue volume or plasma protein and tissue binding did not change, and half-life will increase because of the decrease in clearance [$t_{1/2} = (0.693 \cdot V)/Cl$, where $t_{1/2}$ is half-life, Cl is clearance, and V is volume of distribution]. Total and unbound steady-state drug concentrations

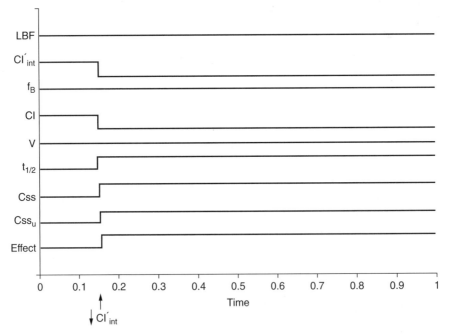

FIGURE 3-6 Changes in physiologic parameters (LBF, liver blood flow; Cl'_{int}, intrinsic clearance; f_B, free fraction of drug in the blood), pharmacokinetic parameters (Cl, clearance; V, volume of distribution; $t_{1/2}$, half-life), and drug concentration and effect (Css, total steady-state concentration; Css_u, unbound steady-state concentration; effect = pharmacologic effect) for a low hepatic extraction ratio drug if intrinsic clearance decreases (indicated by *arrow*). An uptick in the line indicates an increase in the value of the parameter, while a downtick in the line indicates a decrease in the value of the parameter. Intrinsic clearance could decrease due to loss of functional hepatocytes secondary to liver cirrhosis or a drug interaction that inhibits drug metabolizing enzymes.

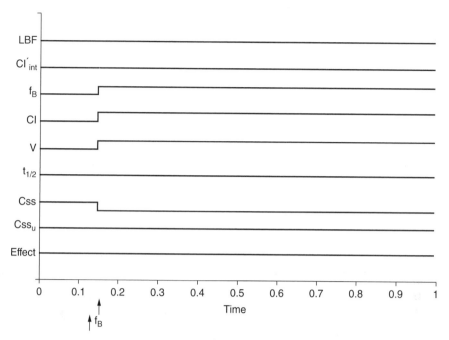

FIGURE 3-7 Changes in physiologic parameters (LBF, liver blood flow; Cl'_{int}, intrinsic clearance; f_B, free fraction of drug in the blood), pharmacokinetic parameters (Cl, clearance; V, volume of distribution; $t_{1/2}$, half-life), and drug concentration and effect (Css, total steady-state concentration; Css_u, unbound steady-state concentration; effect, pharmacologic effect) for a low hepatic extraction ratio drug if decreased protein binding occurred ($\uparrow f_B$, indicated by *arrow*). An uptick in the line indicates an increase in the value of the parameter, while a downtick in the line indicates a decrease in the value of the parameter. Increased free fraction of drug in the blood secondary to decreased plasma protein binding could happen during liver dysfunction because of hypoalbuminemia or hyperbilirubinemia. Increased free fraction of drug can occur in patients with normal liver function secondary to a plasma protein–binding displacement drug interaction.

will increase in tandem, and the pharmacologic response will increase because of the increase in unbound serum concentration.

Using the same baseline conditions as in the previous example, it is possible to examine what would happen if the major change in a similar patient receiving the same drug was decreased plasma protein binding due to hypoalbuminemia and hyperbilirubinemia (Figure 3-7). Under these circumstances, liver blood flow and intrinsic clearance would not change, but free fraction of drug in the blood would increase. Because of the increased free fraction of drug in the blood, both clearance and volume of distribution would simultaneously increase. Clearance increases for a low hepatic extraction ratio drug because more is free to leave the bloodstream and enter hepatocytes where it can be metabolized. Volume of distribution increases because more drug is free to leave the vascular system and enter various tissues. Depending on the relative changes in clearance and volume of distribution, half-life could increase, decrease, or not change; for the purpose of this example the assumption is made that alterations in these independent parameters are similar so half-life does not change. The total steady-state concentration would decrease because total clearance increased, but the unbound steady-state concentration would remain unchanged because the decrease in total concentration is offset by the increase in free fraction of unbound drug. Finally, the pharmacologic effect of the drug is the same because free steady-state concentrations of the drug did not change. This can be an unexpected outcome for the decrease in protein binding, especially because the total steady-state concentration of the drug decreased. Clinicians need to be on the outlook for situations like this because the total drug concentration (bound + unbound) can be misleading and cause an unwarranted increase in drug dosage. Unbound drug concentrations are available for several agents that are highly plasma protein bound, such as phenytoin, valproic acid, and carbamazepine, and are valuable tools to guide drug dosage in liver disease patients.

Finally, decreases in liver blood flow need to be considered for drugs with low hepatic extraction ratios. A decrease in liver blood flow will not change intrinsic clearance, plasma protein binding, clearance or volume of distribution under usual circumstances and, thus, will not change total steady-state concentrations, unbound steady-state concentrations, or the pharmacologic effects of the drug. However, a drastic decrease in liver blood flow can effectively stop delivery of drug to the liver and change liver clearance even for compounds with a low hepatic extraction ratios.

For drugs with high hepatic extraction ratios, the pattern of changes using the aforementioned model is entirely different. If intrinsic clearance changes due to hepatocyte destruction for a high hepatic extraction ratio drug, liver blood flow and unbound fraction of drug in the blood remain unaltered (Figure 3-8). Pharmacokinetic constants also do not change, because none are influenced by intrinsic clearance. Because of this, unbound and total steady-state drug concentrations and pharmacologic effect are unchanged. If the drug were administered orally, the hepatic first-pass effect would be decreased, which would increase the bioavailability of the drug. Because this is effectively an increase in drug dosage, average total and unbound drug concentrations and pharmacologic effect would increase for this route of administration (Css = [F(D/τ)/Cl],

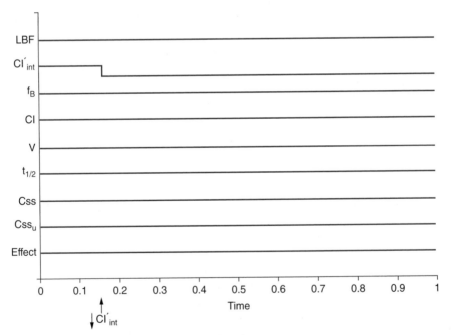

FIGURE 3-8   Changes in physiologic parameters (LBF, liver blood flow; Cl'$_{int}$, intrinsic clearance; f$_B$, free fraction of drug in the blood), pharmacokinetic parameters (Cl, clearance; V, volume of distribution; t$_{1/2}$, half-life), and drug concentration and effect (Css, total steady-state concentration; Css$_u$, unbound steady-state concentration; effect, pharmacologic effect) for a high hepatic extraction ratio drug if intrinsic clearance decreases (indicated by *arrow*). An uptick in the line indicates an increase in the value of the parameter, while a downtick in the line indicates a decrease in the value of the parameter. Intrinsic clearance could decrease due to loss of functional hepatocytes secondary to liver cirrhosis or a drug interaction that inhibits drug metabolizing enzymes.

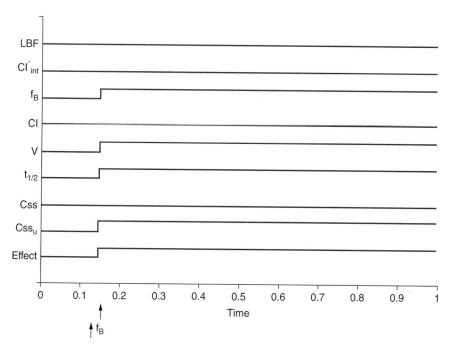

FIGURE 3-9   Changes in physiologic parameters (LBF, liver blood flow; Cl'_{int}, intrinsic clearance; f_B, free fraction of drug in the blood), pharmacokinetic parameters (Cl, clearance; V, volume of distribution; $t_{1/2}$, half-life), and drug concentration and effect (Css, total steady-state concentration; Css_u, unbound steady-state concentration; effect, pharmacologic effect) for a high hepatic extraction ratio drug if decreased protein binding occurred ($\uparrow f_B$, indicated by *arrow*). An uptick in the line indicates an increase in the value of the parameter, while a downtick in the line indicates a decrease in the value of the parameter. Increased free fraction of drug in the blood secondary to decreased plasma protein binding could happen during liver dysfunction because of hypoalbuminemia or hyperbilirubinemia. Increased free fraction of drug can occur in patients with normal liver function secondary to a plasma protein–binding displacement drug interaction.

where F is the bioavailability fraction, Css it the total steady-state drug concentration, D is dose, τ is the dosage interval, and Cl is clearance).

A decrease in plasma protein binding due to lack of binding protein or displacement from binding sites causes severe problems for high hepatic extraction ratio drugs (Figure 3-9). Decreased plasma protein binding results in an increased free fraction of drug in the blood, but no change in liver blood flow or intrinsic clearance. Because clearance is a function of liver blood flow, it does not change. However, a higher free fraction of drug in the blood increases the volume of distribution and this change causes a longer half-life for the drug. Total steady-state concentration does not change because clearance did not change. However, unbound steady-state concentration increases because of the increased free fraction of drug in the blood. Pharmacologic effect increases due to the increased unbound steady-state concentration. This is a very subtle change in drug metabolism, because total steady-state concentrations do not change, but the pharmacologic effect is augmented. Clinicians need to keep this possible change in mind and order unbound drug concentrations, if available, when they suspect that this phenomenon may be taking place. If unbound drug concentrations (or no drug concentrations) are available, a trial decrease in dose may be warranted. Orally administered drug would result in a similar pattern of change, but the increased free fraction of drug in the blood would result in a larger hepatic first-pass effect and an effective reduction in dose, which would partially offset the increase in unbound steady-state concentration.

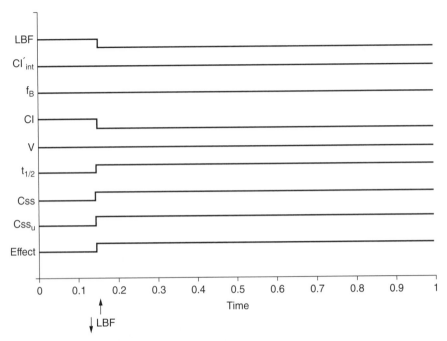

FIGURE 3-10 Changes in physiologic parameters (LBF, liver blood flow; Cl'_{int}, intrinsic clearance; f_B, free fraction of drug in the blood), pharmacokinetic parameters (Cl, clearance; V, volume of distribution; $t_{1/2}$, half-life), and drug concentration and effect (Css, total steady-state concentration; Css_u, unbound steady-state concentration; effect, pharmacologic effect) for a high hepatic extraction ratio drug if liver blood flow decreases ($\downarrow$LBF, indicated by *arrow*). An uptick in the line indicates an increase in the value of the parameter, while a downtick in the line indicates a decrease in the value of the parameter. Decreased liver blood flow could happen due to portal hypertension secondary to hepatic cirrhosis. Decreased liver blood flow can occur in patients with normal liver function secondary to a drug interaction with an agent that decreases cardiac output such as β-blockers.

If liver blood flow decreases, the pharmacokinetic and pharmacologic changes are more straightforward for medications with large hepatic extraction ratios (Figure 3-10). Decreased liver blood flow does not change intrinsic clearance or the unbound fraction of drug in the blood. Clearance decreases because it is dependent on liver blood flow for drugs with a high hepatic extraction ratio. Volume of distribution remains constant, but half-life increases because of the decrease in clearance. Total steady-state concentration increases because of the decrease in clearance, free steady-state concentration rises due to the increase in total steady-state concentration, and the increase in pharmacologic effect tracks the change in free concentration. If the drug is given orally, the first-pass effect would increase, and bioavailability would decrease, partially offsetting the increase in total and unbound steady-state concentrations.

HEART FAILURE

Heart failure is accompanied by a decrease in cardiac output which results in lower liver and renal blood flow. Changes in drug pharmacokinetics due to decreased renal blood flow are not widely reported. However, declines in hepatic clearance, especially for compounds with moderate-to-high hepatic extraction ratios, are reported for many drugs. Additionally, decreased drug bioavailability has been reported in patients with heart failure. The proposed mechanisms for decreased bioavailability are collection of edema fluid in the gastrointestinal tract which makes absorption of drug molecules more difficult and decreased blood flow to the gastrointestinal tract. The volume of distribution for some drugs decreases in patients with heart failure. Because clearance and volume of distribution may or may not simultaneously change, the alteration in half-life, if any, is difficult to predict in patients with heart failure.

DIALYSIS

Dialysis is a process whereby substances move via a concentration gradient across a semipermeable membrane (Figure 3-11). Artificial kidneys (also known as *dialysis coils* or *filters*) that use a synthetic semipermeable membrane to remove waste products from the blood are available for use in hemodialysis. Also, physiologic membranes, such as those present in the peritoneal cavity in the lower abdomen, can be used with peritoneal dialysis as an endogenous semipermeable membrane. Substances that are small enough to pass through the pores in the semipermeable membrane will pass out of the blood into the dialysis fluid. Once in the dialysis fluid, waste products and other compounds can be removed from the body. In some cases, dialysis is used to remove drugs from the bodies of patients who have taken drug overdoses or experience severe adverse effects from the drug. However, in most cases drug molecules are removed from the blood coincidental to the removal of toxic waste products that would usually be eliminated by the kidney.

Because drugs can be removed by dialysis, it is important to understand when drug dosing needs to be modified in renal failure patients undergoing the procedure. Often, dialysis removes enough drug from a patient's body that supplemental doses need to be given after dialysis has been completed (Figure 3-12). In a renal failure patient, the only clearance mechanism available to remove drugs from the body is nonrenal ($Cl = Cl_{NR}$, where Cl is total clearance and Cl_{NR} is nonrenal clearance). When the patient receives dialysis, clearance from both nonrenal routes and dialysis are present, which will accelerate drug removal from the body during the dialysis procedure if the compound is significantly removed by dialysis ($Cl = Cl_{NR} + Cl_D$, where Cl_D is dialysis clearance). In order to determine if dialysis clearance is significant, one should consider the absolute value of dialysis clearance and the relative contribution of dialysis clearance to total clearance. Additionally, if dialysis clearance is 30% or greater of total clearance or if the total amount of drug removed

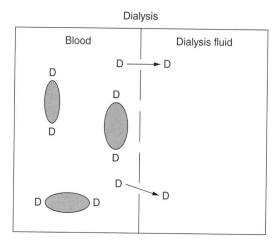

FIGURE 3-11 Dialysis removal of drug can occur when a patient's blood comes in contact with a semipermeable membrane that has drug-free dialysis fluid on the other side. In this schematic, the semipermeable membrane has pores in it large enough for unbound drug to pass through (represented by D), but not for protein-bound drug to pass through (denoted by Ds attached to ovals representing plasma proteins).

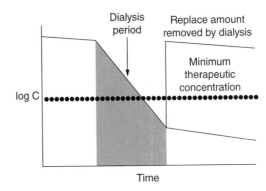

FIGURE 3-12   Concentration/time graph for a drug removed by dialysis. The shaded area indicates the time period that a dialysis procedure was conducted. Because extra drug was removed from the blood during dialysis, concentrations dropped much faster during that period. After dialysis is finished, the concentrations again drop at the predialysis rate. If drug concentrations drop below the minimum therapeutic concentration (shown by the *dark, dotted horizontal line*), it may be necessary to give a supplemental dose to retain the pharmacologic effect of the drug (indicated by increase in drug concentration after dialysis).

by the dialysis procedure is enough to warrant a postdialysis replacement dose, dialysis clearance is considered to be significant.

Drug Characteristics That Effect Dialysis Removal
Molecular Size

Molecular size relative to pore size in the semipermeable membrane is a factor that influences dialysis clearance of a compound. Many hemodialysis procedures are conducted using "low-flux" artificial kidneys that have relatively small pores in the semipermeable membranes. However, "high-flux" filters are now available and widely used in some patients. The semipermeable membranes of these artificial kidneys have much larger pore sizes and larger surface areas so large drug molecules, such as vancomycin, that were previously considered unable to be removed by hemodialysis can be cleared by high-flux filters. It is important that clinicians know which type of artificial kidney is used for a patient before assessing its potential to remove drug molecules.

For low-flux filters, small drug molecules (molecular weight <500 Da, such as theophylline, lidocaine, procainamide) relative to the pore size of the semipermeable membrane tend to be readily eliminated by dialysis and have high extraction ratios for the artificial kidney. In this case, dialyzability of the drug is influenced by blood flow to the artificial kidney, dialysis fluid flow rate to the artificial kidney, and the surface area of the semipermeable membrane inside the artificial kidney. Increased blood flow delivers more drug to the dialysis coil, increased dialysis fluid flow rate removes drug that entered the dialysis fluid more quickly from the artificial kidney and increases the concentration gradient across the semipermeable membrane, and increased semipermeable membrane surface area increases the number of pores that a drug molecule will encounter making it easier for drug molecules to pass from the blood into the dialysis fluid.

Drug molecules with moderate molecular weights [molecular weight 500-1000 Da, such as aminoglycoside antibiotics (~ 400-500 Da) and digoxin] have a decreased ability to pass through the semipermeable membrane contained in low-flux filters. However, many drugs that fall in this intermediate category have sufficient dialysis clearances to require postdialysis replacement doses. Large drug molecules (molecular weight >1000 Da, such as vancomycin) are not removed to a significant extent when low-flux filters are used for dialysis because pore sizes in these artificial kidneys are too small for the molecules to fit through. However, many large molecular weight drugs can be removed by dialysis when high-flux filters arc used, and, in some of these cases, supplemental postdialysis drug doses will be needed to maintain therapeutic amounts of drug in the body.

Water/Lipid Solubility

Drugs that have a high degree of water solubility will tend to partition into the water-based dialysis fluid, while lipid-soluble drugs tend to remain in the blood.

Plasma Protein Binding

Only unbound drug molecules are able to pass through the pores in the semipermeable membrane; drug-plasma protein complexes are too large to pass through the pores and gain access to the dialysis fluid side of the semipermeable membrane. Drugs that are not highly plasma protein bound have high free fractions of drug in the blood and are prone to better dialysis clearance. Drugs that are highly bound to plasma proteins have low free fractions of drug in the blood and poor dialysis clearance rates.

Volume of Distribution

The volume of distribution for a drug is a function of blood volume (V_B), organ size (V_T), drug plasma protein binding (f_B, free fraction of drug in the blood), and drug tissue binding [f_T, free fraction of drug in the tissues; $V = V_B + (f_B/f_T)V_T$]. Medications with large volumes of distribution are principally located at tissue binding sites and not in the blood where dialysis can remove the drug. Because of this, agents with large volumes of distribution are not easily removed from the body. In fact, some compounds such as digoxin, have good hemodialysis clearance rates, and drug contained in the bloodstream is very effectively eliminated. However, in this case the majority of the drug is present in the tissues and only a small amount of the total drug present in the body is removed. If serum concentrations of these types of drugs are followed closely during hemodialysis, the concentrations decrease by a substantial amount. However, when dialysis is completed, the blood and tissues have a chance to reequilibrate and serum concentrations increase, sometimes to their predialysis concentration. This "rebound" in serum concentration has been reported for several drugs.

Compounds with small volumes of distribution (<1 L/kg, such as the aminoglycoside antibiotics and theophylline) usually demonstrate high dialysis clearance rates. Drugs with moderate volumes of distribution (1-2 L/kg) have intermediate dialysis clearance values, while agents with large volumes of distribution (>2 L/kg, such as digoxin and tricyclic antidepressants) have poor dialysis characteristics.

HEMODIALYSIS

Hemodialysis is a very efficient procedure for removing toxic waste from the blood of renal failure patients (Figure 3-13). Blood is pumped out of the patient at the rate of 300-400 mL/min and through one side of the semipermeable membrane of the artificial kidney by the hemodialysis machine. Cleansed blood is then pumped back into the vascular system of the patient. In acute situations, vascular access can be obtained through centrally placed catheters. For patients with chronic renal failure, vascular shunts made of synthetic materials will be surgically placed between a high blood flow artery and vein in the arm or other site for the purpose of conducting hemodialysis. Dialysis fluid is pumped through the artificial kidney at a rate of 400-600 mL/min on the other side of the semipermeable membrane, in the opposite direction of blood flow. This "counter-current" flow is more efficient in removing waste products than running the blood and dialysis fluid in parallel to each other. Dialysis fluid is electrolyte and osmotically balanced for the individual patient. It is possible to increase or decrease serum electrolytes by increasing or decreasing the concentration of the ion in the dialysis fluid compared to the concurrent serum value. Also, by adding solutes in order to increase the

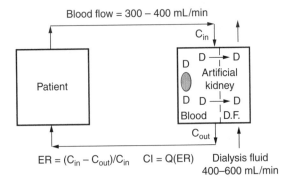

FIGURE 3-13   Hemodialysis removes blood from the patient's body (indicated by *arrows* from patient to artificial kidney) and passes it through an artificial kidney that contains a semipermeable membrane. Inside the artificial kidney, waste products pass into the dialysis fluid and are eliminated from the body. If drug molecules can pass through the pores in the semipermeable membrane, they will also be eliminated from the body. The extraction ratio of the artificial kidney can be computed using the concentration into (C_{in}) and out of (C_{out}) the device. Dialysis clearance can be calculated by taking the product of the dialysis extraction ratio and blood flow to the dialysis machine. D, drug molecule; D.F., dialysis fluid.

osmolality of the dialysis fluid relative to the blood, it is possible to remove fluid from the patient's body by osmotic pressure across the semipermeable membrane of the artificial kidney. This process is known as *ultrafiltration*. Using low-flux filters, hemodialysis is usually performed for 3-4 hours three times weekly. Using high-flux filters (hemofilters with larger pore sizes that allow larger molecules to move or "flux" across the semipermeable membrane), blood and dialysis fluid flow rates may be higher, and the procedure may be conducted 1-2 hours three times weekly.

Traditional hemodialysis can be used to treat acute renal failure but is most often used for patients with chronic renal failure. For patients with acute renal failure, sustained low-efficiency dialysis (SLED) is often preferred. This hemodialysis variant uses lower blood flow (~ 200 mL/min) and dialysis fluid flow (~ 300 mL/min) rates for 6- to 12-hour periods during 5-6 days a week. Because of the slower flow rates, drug clearances (in mL/min) are often times lower, but the longer and more frequent dialysis periods may result in more drug lost from the body.

The FDA has required pharmacokinetic studies to be done for renally eliminated drugs in patients receiving chronic hemodialysis since the mid-1980s. Because of this, the package insert for the drug may include manufacturer recommended doses to be administered to patients in the posthemodialysis period (see Table 3-1). Guidelines for the administration of posthemodialysis replacement doses are available for older drugs as well as updated guidelines for newer drugs that may not be included in the package insert.[7,9,10] Also, the primary literature should be consulted to ensure that the newest guidelines are used for all drugs. When the hemodialysis removal characteristics of a drug and the need for postdialysis replacement doses are assessed, it should be recognized that the majority of information available is for traditional hemodialysis using low-flux artificial kidneys. If a high-flux dialysis coil is used or sustained low-efficiency dialysis is the treatment technique, the primary literature is probably the best source of information. However, in many cases drug dialysis clearance studies have not been conducted using these newer technologies.

Computation of Initial Doses and Modification of Doses Using Drug Serum Concentrations

Initial drug doses of patients with renal failure undergoing hemodialysis can be based on expected pharmacokinetic parameters for this population when published information for a drug is inadequate or the agent has a very narrow therapeutic index. For example, an initial dosage regimen for tobramycin needs to be computed for a patient to achieve peak concentrations of 6-7 mg/L and postdialysis concentrations 1-2 mg/L. The patient is a 62-year-old, 5-ft 8-in male who weighs 65 kg, has chronic renal failure, and receives hemodialysis three times weekly with a low-flux dialysis filter. Patients with renal failure are prone to having poor fluid balance because their kidneys are not able to provide this important function. Because of this, the patient should be assessed for overhydration (due to renal failure) or underhydration (due to renal failure and increased loss due to fever). Weight is a good indication of fluid status, and this patient's weight is less than his ideal weight [IBW_{male} = 50 kg + 2.3(Ht − 60) = 50 kg + 2.3(68 in − 60) = 68 kg]. Other indications of state of hydration (skin turgor, etc) indicate that the patient has normal fluid balance at this time. Because of this, the average volume of distribution for aminoglycoside antibiotics equal to 0.26 L/kg can be used.

A loading dose of tobramycin would be appropriate for this patient because the expected half-life is long (~ 50 hours); administration of maintenance doses only might not result in therapeutic maximum concentrations for a considerable time period while drug accumulation is occurring. The loading dose is to be given after hemodialysis ends at 1300 H on Monday (hemodialysis conducted on Monday, Wednesday, and Friday from 0900 to 1300 H). Because the patient is expected to have a long half-life compared to the infusion time of the drug (½-1 hours), little drug will be eliminated during the infusion period, and IV bolus one-compartment model equations can be used. The loading dose for this patient would be based on the expected volume of distribution: V = 0.26 L/kg • 65 kg = 16.9 L; LD = C_{max} • V = 6 mg/L • 16.9 L = 101 mg, rounded to 100 mg (LD is loading dose, C_{max} is the maximum concentration after drug administration). This loading dose was given at 1400 H (Figure 3-14). Until the next dialysis period at 0900 H on Wednesday, tobramycin is cleared only by the patient's own body mechanisms. The expected elimination rate constant (k_e) for a patient with a creatinine clearance of approximately zero is: k_e (in h^{-1}) = 0.00293 • CrCl + 0.014 = 0.00293 (0 mL/min) + 0.014 = 0.014 h^{-1}. The expected concentration at 0900 H on Wednesday is: C = $C_0 e^{-k_e t}$, where C is the concentration at t hours after the initial concentration of C_0; C = (6 mg/L)e$^{-(0.014\ h^{-1})(43\ h)}$ = 3.3 mg/L.

While the patient receives hemodialysis, tobramycin is eliminated by the patient's own mechanisms plus dialysis clearance. During hemodialysis with a low-flux filter, the average half-life for aminoglycosides

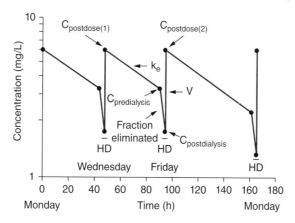

FIGURE 3-14   Concentration/time graph for tobramycin in a hemodialysis patient using estimated, population pharmacokinetic parameters. The initial dose was given postdialysis at 1400 H on Monday (time = 0 hour). Hemodialysis periods are shown by small horizontal bars labeled with HD, and days are indicated on the time line. In order to compute patient-specific pharmacokinetic parameters, four serum concentrations are measured. The elimination rate constant (k_e) is computed using two concentrations after dosage administration ($C_{postdose(1)}$ and $C_{predialysis}$), the fraction eliminated by dialysis by two concentrations ($C_{predialysis}$ and $C_{postdialysis}$) before and after dialysis, and the volume of distribution using two concentrations ($C_{postdialysis}$ and $C_{postdose(2)}$) after another dosage administration.

is 4 hours. Because the patient is dialyzed for 4 hours, the tobramycin serum concentration should decrease by ½, to a value of 1.7 mg/L, or using formal computations: $k_e = 0.693/(t_{1/2}) = 0.693/4\ h = 0.173\ h^{-1}$; $C = C_0 e^{-k_e t} = (3.3\ mg/L)e^{-(0.173\ h^{-1})(4\ h)} = 1.7\ mg/L$. At this time, a postdialysis replacement dose could be given to increase the maximum concentration to its original value of 6 mg/L: Replacement dose $= (C_{max} - C_{baseline})V = (6\ mg/L - 1.7\ mg/L)16.9\ L = 73\ mg$, round to 75 mg (where C_{max} is the maximum postdose concentration and $C_{baseline}$ is the predose concentration). The postdialysis replacement dose of 75 mg was administered at 1400 H on Wednesday. Because all time frames and pharmacokinetic parameters are the same for Monday to Wednesday and Wednesday to Friday, the postdialysis replacement dose on Friday at 1400 H would also be 75 mg. However, more time elapses from Friday after drug administration to Monday before dialysis (67 h), the next day for hemodialysis to be conducted in the patient and this needs to be accounted for: $C = C_0 e^{-k_e t} = (6\ mg/L)e^{-(0.014\ h^{-1})(67\ h)} = 2.3\ mg/L$. Again, a 4-hour hemodialysis period would decrease serum concentrations by ½, to a value of 1.2 mg/L: $C = C_0 e^{-k_e t} = (2.3\ mg/L)e^{-(0.173\ h^{-1})(4\ h)} = 1.2\ mg/L$. At this time, a postdialysis replacement dose could be given to increase the maximum concentration to the original value of 6 mg/L: Replacement dose $= (C_{max} - C_{baseline})V = (6\ mg/L - 1.2\ mg/L)16.9\ L = 81\ mg$, round to 80 mg (where C_{max} is the maximum postdose concentration and $C_{baseline}$ is the predose concentration). The postdialysis replacement dose of 80 mg was administered at 1400 H on Monday. Because all time frames and pharmacokinetic parameters repeat during subsequent weeks, the following postdialysis replacement doses would be prescribed postdialysis at 1400 H: Wednesday and Friday 75 mg, Monday 80 mg. In this particular example, recommended daily doses are within 5 mg of each other, and if the clinician wished, the same postdialysis dose could be given on each day. However, this will not be true in every case.

Because the initial dosage scheme outlined for this patient used average, estimated pharmacokinetic parameters, it is likely that the patient has different pharmacokinetic characteristics. It is possible to measure the patient's own unique pharmacokinetic parameters using four serum concentrations (see Figure 3-14). The intradialysis elimination rate constant can be determined by obtaining postdose ($C_{postdose(1)}$) and predialysis ($C_{predialysis}$) concentrations [$k_e = (\ln C_{postdose(1)} - \ln C_{predialysis})/\Delta t$, where Δt is the time between the two concentrations], the fraction of drug eliminated by dialysis can be computed using pre- and postdialysis ($C_{postdialysis}$) concentrations (fraction eliminated $= [(C_{predialysis} - C_{postdialysis})/C_{predialysis}]$, and the volume of distribution can be calculated using postdialysis and postdose concentrations ($V = D/(C_{postdose(2)} - C_{postdialysis})$). Note that if the drug has a postdialysis "rebound" in drug concentrations, postdialysis serum samples should be obtained after blood and tissue have had the opportunity to reequilibrate. In the case of aminoglycosides, postdialysis samples should be collected no sooner than 3-4 hours after the end of dialysis. Once individualized pharmacokinetic parameters have been measured, they can be used in the same equations used to compute initial doses in the previous section in place of average, population pharmacokinetic parameters and to calculate individualized doses for dialysis patients. It is also possible to use a mixture of measured and population-estimated pharmacokinetic parameters. For instance, a clinician may wish to measure the elimination rate constant or volume of distribution for a patient, but elect to use an average population estimate for fraction of drug removed by the artificial kidney.

The same initial dosage strategies and individualization techniques can be used to construct dosage schedules for patients receiving sustained low-efficiency dialysis (SLED). The only differences compared to traditional hemodialysis are that dialysis periods are longer and that drug elimination is decreased while the patient is receiving dialysis. This results in a lower drug clearance rate and a longer drug half-life during SLED.

Methods to Measure Hemodialysis Clearance

If needed, hemodialysis clearance can be measured in patients. The extraction ratio method measures the extraction of drug across the artificial kidney by obtaining simultaneous blood samples on input (C_{in}) and

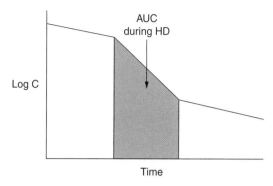

FIGURE 3-15   One method to measure hemodialysis clearance is to take the quotient of the amount of drug eliminated by the dialysis procedure ($A_{Dialysis}$) and the area under the concentration/time curve (AUC) during the dialysis time period (HD, indicated by the *shaded area*).

outlet (C_{out}) side of the dialysis coil (see Figure 3-13). The tubing carrying blood to and from the patient usually has injection ports that can be used as access points to get the necessary blood samples. The artificial kidney extraction ratio (ER) can be computed using serum concentrations measured from the blood samples: $ER = (C_{in} - C_{out})/C_{in}$. Blood flow from the hemodialysis machine (HDBF) is available as a continuous read out on the pump, and hemodialysis clearance (Cl_{HD}) can be computed by taking the product of the extraction ratio and blood flow parameters: $Cl_{HD} = HDBF \cdot ER$. The advantage to this technique is that it is methodologically simple. The disadvantage is that if the dialysis extraction ratio is low, serum concentration differences between C_{in} and C_{out} will be small and difficult for the drug assay to determine.

Another method is to collect the waste dialysis fluid used during the dialysis procedure and measure several serum drug concentrations during the same time interval (Figure 3-15). The amount of drug eliminated in the dialysis fluid ($A_{Dialysis}$) is determined by multiplying the volume of dialysis fluid ($V_{Dialysis}$), and the concentration of drug in the dialysis fluid ($C_{Dialysis}$): $A_{Dialysis} = V_{Dialysis} \cdot C_{Dialysis}$. Hemodialysis clearance (Cl_{HD}) is computed by dividing the amount of drug eliminated in the dialysis fluid by the area under the serum concentration/time curve during the dialysis period ($AUC_{Dialysis}$, calculated using the serum concentrations obtained during hemodialysis): $Cl_{HD} = A_{Dialysis}/AUC_{Dialysis}$. An advantage of this method is that it is determined using multiple serum concentrations and may be more accurate. Disadvantages include collection of a large volume of dialysis fluid (~ 120 L) and the large number of serum concentrations needed to determine $AUC_{Dialysis}$.

The final method is to collect all the waste dialysis fluid used during the dialysis period and measure a single serum drug concentration at the midpoint of the procedure. Using this information, hemodialysis clearance (Cl_{HD}) can be computed using the following equation: $Cl_{HD} = (C_{Dialysis} \cdot V_{Dialysis})/(C_{Serum} \cdot T_{Dialysis})$, where $C_{Dialysis}$ is the drug concentration in the dialysis fluid, $V_{Dialysis}$ is the volume of dialysis fluid, C_{Serum} is the drug serum concentration, and $T_{Dialysis}$ is the duration of the hemodialysis procedure. An advantage of this technique is that it requires only one serum concentration. The chief disadvantage is the all dialysis fluid used during hemodialysis must be collected.

HEMOFILTRATION

Hemofiltration comprises a family of techniques that have some similarities and some differences compared to hemodialysis.[39] The hemofilter used in hemofiltration is similar to the artificial kidney used in hemodialysis. The pore size in hemofilters is large, which allows drug molecules up to 20,000 Da to cross its semipermeable membrane.

Continuous arteriovenous hemofiltration (CAVH) and continuous venovenous hemofiltration (CVVH) use an extracorporeal circuit that runs from an artery to a vein or from a vein to a vein, respectively. These processes do not use a dialysis fluid, so plasma water that passes through the hemofilter is collected and discarded. Continuous arteriovenous hemodialysis with filtration (CAVHD) and continuous venovenous hemodialysis with filtration (CVVHD) is a hybrid of conventional hemodialysis and CAVH or CVVH, respectively. The hemofilter has hemodialysis fluid on the other side of the semipermeable membrane containing the patient's blood. For CVVH and CVVHD, a mechanical pump is used to propel blood through the hemofilter. For CAVH and CAVHD, the patient's own blood pressure usually provides the propulsion of blood through the hemofilter.

The sieving coefficient is the ratio of the drug concentration in the hemofiltrate to the drug concentration in the serum. Table 3-4 lists sieving coefficients for a variety of drugs.[40,41] The ultrafiltration rate (UFR) is the filtration provided by the specific hemofiltration technique. Typical ranges for UFR are 10-16 mL/min for procedures that do not use extracorporeal blood pumps and 20-30 mL/min for procedures that use extracorporeal blood pumps. When hemofiltration procedures that incorporate dialysis fluid are used, an additional 15-20 mL/min is added to these values.[40,41]

TABLE 3-4   Hemofiltration Sieving Coefficients for Selected Drugs[40,41]

Drug	Sieving Coefficient	Drug	Sieving Coefficient
Antibiotics		Streptomycin	0.30
Amikacin	0.95	Sulfamethoxazole	0.30
Amphotericin B	0.35	Teicoplanin	0.05
Amphotericin B (liposomal)	0.10	Ticarcillin	0.83
Ampicillin	0.69	Tobramycin	0.90
Cefepime	0.72	Vancomycin	0.80
Cefoperazone	0.27	**Other drugs**	
Cefotaxime	1.06	Amrinone	0.80
Cefoxitin	0.83	Chlordiazepoxide	0.05
Ceftazidime	0.90	Cisplatin	0.10
Ceftriaxone	0.20	Clofibrate	0.06
Cephapirin	1.48	Cyclosporine	0.58
Cilastatin	0.75	Diazepam	0.02
Ciprofloxacin	0.58	Digoxin	0.70
Clavulanic acid	1.69	Digitoxin	0.15
Clindamycin	0.49	Famotidine	0.73
Doxycycline	0.40	Glyburide	0.60
Erythromycin	0.37	Glutethimide	0.02
Fluconazole	1.00	Lidocaine	0.14
Flucytosine	0.80	Lithium	0.90
Ganciclovir	0.84	Metamizole	0.40
Gentamicin	0.81	N-acetylprocainamide	0.92
Imipenem	0.90	Nizatidine	0.59
Meropenem	1.00	Nitrazepam	0.08
Metronidazole	0.84	Nomifensine	0.70
Mezlocillin	0.71	Oxazepam	0.10
Nafcillin	0.55	Phenobarbital	0.80
Netilmicin	0.93	Phenytoin	0.45
Oxacillin	0.02	Procainamide	0.86
Pefloxacin	0.80	Ranitidine	0.78
Penicillin	0.68	Tacrolimus	0.26
Piperacillin	0.82	Theophylline	0.80

Several different methods of calculating additional doses during hemofiltration have been suggested[40,41]:

1. Based on the expected UFRs noted just previously, hemofiltration is usually equivalent to a glomerular filtration rate (GFR) of 10-50 mL/min. In lieu of specific recommendations for a drug, clinicians can use this GFR rate with FDA or renal drug dosing guidelines to suggest an adjusted dose.[7,9,10]
2. A supplemental dose (SD) can be estimated using a measured or estimated steady-state drug concentration (Css), unbound fraction in the serum (f_B), ultrafiltration rate (UFR), and drug dosing interval (τ): SD = Css • f_B • UFR • τ. Supplemental doses are given in addition to maintenance doses of the drug.
3. A booster dose (BD) can be computed using an actual measured concentration (C_{actual}), a desired concentration ($C_{desired}$), and an estimated or actual volume of distribution (V): BD = ($C_{desired}$ − C_{actual})V. Booster doses are given in addition to maintenance doses of the drug.

Additionally, drug dosing tables have been published for antibiotics that include hemofiltration characteristics and basic pharmacokinetic information.[42]

PERITONEAL DIALYSIS

Peritoneal dialysis involves the surgical insertion of a catheter in the lower abdomen into the peritoneal cavity (Figure 3-16). The peritoneal membrane covering the internal organs is highly vascularized, so when dialysis fluid (1-3 L) is introduced into the peritoneal cavity using the catheter, waste products move from the blood vessels of the peritoneal membrane (a semipermeable membrane) into the dialysis fluid along a concentration gradient. The dialysis fluid is periodically removed from the peritoneal cavity and discarded. Outpatients undergoing chronic ambulatory peritoneal dialysis have dialysis fluid present in their peritoneal cavities all day or most hours of a day.

Compared to hemodialysis, peritoneal dialysis removes drug much less efficiently. Therefore, it is less likely that replacement drug doses will need to be given during intermittent peritoneal dialysis and that drug dosages will need to be increased while patients receive chronic peritoneal dialysis. For instance, in patients with end-stage renal disease, the half-life of aminoglycoside antibiotics is ~ 50 hours. During hemodialysis, the half-life reduces to ~ 4 hours, but, during peritoneal dialysis in patients without peritonitis, the half-life

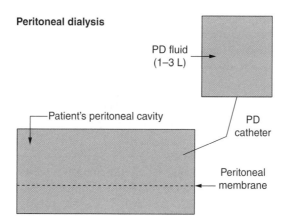

FIGURE 3-16   Schematic of peritoneal dialysis procedure. A catheter (labeled *PD catheter*) is surgically inserted into the patient's peritoneal cavity and used to introduce 1-3 L of dialysis fluid (labeled *PD fluid*). The dialysis fluid comes into contact with capillaries in the peritoneal membrane where waste products and drugs pass from the blood into the fluid. After the dwell time has concluded, the dialysis fluid is removed from the peritoneal cavity via the catheter and discarded.

only decreases to ~ 36 hours. In patients receiving chronic peritoneal dialysis, dialysis removal of drug is simply another clearance mechanism taking place in the patient body, so the usual methods of measuring serum concentrations and dosage adjustment require little or no modification. For patients undergoing peritoneal dialysis, clinicians should consult the manufacture's package insert for drugs recently marketed (mid-1980s or later), reviews listing the peritoneal dialysis removal of older drugs and updated information on newer agents,[7,9,10] and the primary literature for the newest guidelines for all compounds.

Drugs can also be added to peritoneal dialysis fluid. If the agent is absorbed from the dialysis fluid into the body, systemic effects due to the drug may occur. Epoetin and insulin have been administered in this fashion to patients receiving peritoneal dialysis. Because the development of peritonitis is a common problem in patients receiving peritoneal dialysis, antibiotics have been administered intraperitoneally for local treatment of the infection using dialysis fluid as the delivery vehicle.[43] In most cases, antibiotics are absorbed into the body when given this way, but therapeutic serum concentrations may not be achieved for all agents making systemically administered doses necessary. Clinicians should pay particular attention to whether studies measuring peritoneal dialysis removal or absorption of drugs were conducted in patients with peritonitis. Peritonitis involves inflammation of the peritoneal membrane and increases its permeability. Increased permeability allows for greater flux of drug across the membrane which allows more drug removal during dialysis or more drug absorption if the drug is added to the peritoneal dialysis fluid.

Methods to Measure Peritoneal Dialysis Clearance

If necessary, peritoneal dialysis clearance can be measured in patients. One method is to collect the waste dialysis fluid used during a peritoneal dialysis period and measure several serum drug concentrations during the same time interval (see Figure 3-15). The amount of drug eliminated in the dialysis fluid ($A_{Dialysis}$) is calculated by multiplying the volume of dialysis fluid ($V_{Dialysis}$) and the concentration of drug in the dialysis fluid ($C_{Dialysis}$): $A_{Dialysis} = V_{Dialysis} \cdot C_{Dialysis}$. Peritoneal clearance ($Cl_{PD}$) is computed by dividing the amount of drug eliminated in the dialysis fluid by the area under the serum concentration/time curve during the dialysis period ($AUC_{Dialysis}$, calculated using the serum concentrations obtained during peritoneal dialysis): $Cl_{PD} = A_{Dialysis}/AUC_{Dialysis}$. An advantage of this method is that the dialysate volume is relatively small. Disadvantages are the large number of serum concentrations needed to determine $AUC_{Dialysis}$, and if only a small amount of drug is removed via dialysis, the drug assay may not be sensitive enough to measure a small concentration.

Another method is to collect all the waste dialysis fluid used during a dialysis period and measure a single serum drug concentration at the midpoint of the procedure. Using this information, peritoneal clearance (Cl_{PD}) can be computed using the following equation: $Cl_{PD} = (C_{Dialysis} \cdot V_{Dialysis})/(C_{Serum} \cdot T_{Dialysis})$, where $C_{Dialysis}$ is the drug concentration in the dialysis fluid, $V_{Dialysis}$ is the volume of dialysis fluid, C_{Serum} is the drug serum concentration, and $T_{Dialysis}$ is the duration that dialysis fluid remained in the peritoneal cavity. Advantages of this technique are that it requires only one serum concentration and the volume of dialysis fluid is relatively small. A disadvantage is that if only a small amount of drug is removed via dialysis, the drug assay may not be sensitive enough to measure a low concentration.

OBESITY

The presence of excessive adipose tissue can alter the pharmacokinetics of drugs by changing the volume of distribution. The general physiologic equation for volume of distribution can be broken down into separate parameters for individual tissue types:

$$V = V_B + \frac{f_B}{f_T} V_T = V_B + \frac{f_B}{f_{heart}} V_{heart} + \frac{f_B}{f_{muscle}} V_{muscle} + \frac{f_B}{f_{fat}} V_{fat} + \ldots + \frac{f_B}{f_n} V_n$$

Because of this, the sheer amount of adipose tissue will be a primary determinant of how much obesity will affect the volume of distribution of the drug. Also, the magnitude of effect that adipose tissue has on the volume of distribution for a drug is dependent on the binding of drug in the tissue itself. If the drug has a large affinity for adipose tissue and is highly bound there, the free fraction in adipose tissue will be small ($\downarrow f_{fat}$) and a large amount of drug will accumulate in that tissue. Medications that have high lipid solubility tend to partition into adipose tissue, and the volume of distribution in obese patients for these drugs can be dramatically larger than that in normal-weight patients. Examples of lipophilic drugs with larger volume of distribution values in obese individuals include diazepam,[44] carbamazepine,[45] and trazodone.[46] However, hydrophilic drugs tend to not distribute into adipose tissue so that the volume of distribution for many water-soluble drugs is not significantly different in obese and normal-weight patients. The volumes of distribution for digoxin,[47] cimetidine,[48] and ranitidine[49] are similar in overweight and normal-weight subjects.

Although the presence of excessive adipose tissue is the most obvious change that occurs in obese individuals, other physiologic changes are present. While adipose cells contain more than 90% fat, there are additional supportive tissues, extracellular fluid, and blood present in adipose tissue. Also, some lean tissues hypertrophy in obese individuals. The net result of these changes is that hydrophilic drugs with small volumes of distribution may experience distribution alterations in obese patients. For example, the aminoglycoside antibiotics are water-soluble molecules that have relatively small volumes of distribution similar to the value of extracellular fluid (V = 0.26 L/kg). Because the volume of distribution is so small (~ 18 L in a 70-kg person), the addition of just a few liters of extracellular fluid can alter the pharmacokinetics of these antibiotics. The additional extracellular fluid contained in excessive adipose tissue and other organs that hypertrophy in obese individuals causes larger volumes of distribution for the aminoglycoside antibiotics in overweight patients. Formulas that correct aminoglycoside volume of distribution for obese individuals are available.[50-53] However, if the volume of distribution for a hydrophilic drug is intermediate or large, the additional extracellular fluid contained in adipose tissue and other sources in obese individuals may not significantly alter the distribution of the agent. Examples are of medications with larger and intermediate volumes of distribution are digoxin (V = 500 L) and vancomycin (V = 50 L); the addition of a few extra liters of extracellular fluid due to obesity will not substantially change the volume of distribution for these agents.[47,54,55]

Another change that is found in obese individuals is increased glomerular filtration rates. This alteration primarily affects hydrophilic drug compounds that are renally eliminated and will increase the renal clearance of the agent. Vancomycin,[54,55] the aminoglycosides,[50-52] and cimetidine[48] all have higher clearance rates in obese patients compared to normal-weight individuals. Special methods are used to estimate creatinine clearance for obese patients, as previously noted in the Measurement and Estimation of Glomerular Filtration Rate and Creatinine Clearance section of this chapter.[21,22,26]

Obesity has variable effects on the metabolism of drugs. For many agents, such as carbamazepine[45] and cyclosporine,[56] obesity does not significantly affect hepatic clearance. While for other drugs, obesity increases hepatic clearance, as with diazepam,[44] or decreases metabolic clearance, as with methylprednisolone.[57] Clinicians should be aware of this variability and dose hepatically metabolized drugs cautiously in obese individuals in the absence of specific recommendations.

Half-life changes vary according to the relative alterations in clearance (Cl) and volume of distribution (V): $t_{1/2} = (0.693 \cdot V)/Cl$, where $t_{1/2}$ is half-life. In the case of the aminoglycoside antibiotics, clearance and volume of distribution increases are about the same magnitude in obese patients, so half-life does not change.[50-52] If the volume of distribution increases with obesity but clearance is unaffected, half-life can increase dramatically as with carbamazepine.[45] Finally, if clearance changes and volume of distribution remain constant, obesity may also cause a change in the half-life of a drug as is the case for methylprednisolone.[57]

DRUG INTERACTIONS

Pharmacokinetic drug interactions occur between drugs when one agent changes the clearance or volume of distribution of another medication. There are several drug interaction mechanisms that result in altered drug clearance. A drug can inhibit or induce the enzymes responsible for the metabolism of other drugs, or it can inhibit or induce membrane transporters of other drugs. Enzyme inhibition decreases intrinsic clearance, and enzyme induction increases intrinsic clearance. If two drugs are eliminated by the same enzyme, they may compete for the metabolic pathway and decrease the clearance of one or both compounds. Two drugs eliminated by the same active renal tubular secretion mechanism can compete for the pathway and decrease the renal clearance of one or both agents. Induction or inhibition of membrane transporters by one drug can also increase or decrease the volume of distribution of another drug. Another type of drug interaction displaces a drug from plasma protein–binding sites because the two compounds share the same binding site, and the two compete for the same area on plasma proteins. By virtue of its pharmacologic effect, a drug may increase or decrease blood flow to an organ that eliminates or metabolizes another medication and thereby decrease the clearance of the medication.

Changes in plasma protein binding also cause alterations in volume of distribution. If two drugs share the same tissue binding sites, it is possible for tissue-binding displacement drug interactions to occur and change the volume of distribution for one of the medications. Half-life may change as a result of drug interactions, or, if clearance and volume of distribution alterations are about equal, half-life may remain constant even though a major drug interaction has occurred.

The same graphical scheme introduced in the hepatic disease section of this chapter can be used to understand the clinical impact of drug interactions (see Figures 3-6 to 3-10). To use these charts, it is necessary to know whether the drug under discussion has a low extraction ratio or high extraction ratio. The hepatic clearance of drugs with low hepatic extraction ratios equals the product of free fraction in the blood and intrinsic clearance ($Cl_H = f_B Cl'_{int}$), while the hepatic clearance of drugs with high hepatic extraction ratios equals liver blood flow ($Cl_H = LBF$). Whether a drug has a high or low extraction ratio, the volume of distribution ($V = V_B + [f_B/f_T]V_T$) and half-life ($t_{1/2} = [0.693 \cdot V]/Cl$) relationships are the same. The unbound steady-state concentration of drug in the blood equals the product of the total steady-state concentration and the unbound fraction of drug in the blood: $Css_u = f_B Css$. The effect of the drug increases when the unbound steady-state concentration increases and decreases when Css_u declines.

Plasma Protein–Binding Displacement Drug Interactions

For a drug with a low hepatic extraction ratio, plasma protein–binding displacement drug interactions cause major pharmacokinetic alterations, but these interactions are not clinically significant because the pharmacologic effect of the drug does not change (see Figure 3-7). Because the clearance of the drug is dependent on the fraction of unbound drug in the blood and intrinsic clearance for a low hepatic extraction ratio agent, addition of a plasma protein–binding displacing compound will increase clearance ($\uparrow Cl = \uparrow f_B Cl'_{int}$) and volume of distribution ($\uparrow V = V_B + [\uparrow f_B/f_T]V_T$). Because half-life depends on clearance and volume of distribution, it is likely that because both increase, half-life will not substantially change ($t_{1/2} = [0.693 \cdot \uparrow V]/\uparrow Cl$). However, it is possible that if either clearance or volume of distribution changes disproportionately, half-life will change. The total steady-state concentration will decline because of the increase in clearance ($\downarrow Css = k_0/\uparrow Cl$, where k_0 is the infusion rate of drug). However, the unbound steady-state concentration will remain unaltered because the free fraction of drug in the blood is higher than it was before the drug interaction occurred ($Css_u = \uparrow f_B \downarrow Css$). The pharmacologic effect of the drug does not change because the free concentration of drug in the blood is unchanged. An example of this drug interaction is the addition of diflunisal to patients stabilized on warfarin therapy.[58] Diflunisal displaces warfarin from plasma protein–binding sites but does not augment the anticoagulant effect of warfarin. If drug concentrations are available for the medication, it can be difficult to convince clinicians that a drug dosage increase is not needed even though total concentrations decline as a result of this interaction. When available, unbound drug concentrations can be used to document that no change in drug dosing is needed.

For drugs with high hepatic extraction ratios given intravenously, plasma protein–binding displacement drug interactions cause both major pharmacokinetic and pharmacodynamic changes (see Figure 3-9). Because the clearance of the drug is dependent solely on liver blood flow for an agent of this type, total clearance does not change. However, both volume of distribution $[\uparrow V = V_B + (\uparrow f_B/f_T)V_T]$ and half-life $[\uparrow t_{1/2} = (0.693 \cdot \uparrow V)/Cl]$ will increase because of plasma protein–binding displacement of the drug. Because total clearance did not change, the total steady-state concentration remains unaltered. However, the free concentration $(\uparrow Css_u = \uparrow f_B Css)$ and pharmacologic effect $(\uparrow effect \propto \uparrow Css_u)$ of the drug will both increase. Currently, there are no clinically significant drug interactions of this type. However, clinicians should be on the outlook for this profile for highly protein-bound drugs with high hepatic extraction ratios given intravenously because the interaction is very subtle. Most noteworthy is the fact that although total concentrations remain unchanged, the pharmacologic effect of the drug is augmented. If available, unbound drug concentration could be used to document the drug interaction.

If a drug with a high hepatic extraction ratio is given orally, a plasma protein–binding displacement drug interaction will cause a simultaneous increase in the unbound fraction of drug in the blood $(\uparrow f_B)$ and the hepatic presystemic metabolism of the drug. Hepatic presystemic metabolism increases because the higher unbound fraction of drug in the blood allows more drug molecules to enter the liver where they are ultimately metabolized. The increase in hepatic presystemic metabolism leads to an increased first-pass effect and decreased drug bioavailability $(\downarrow F)$. Total steady-state drug concentrations will be lower because of decreased drug bioavailability $[\downarrow Css = (\downarrow F[D/t])/Cl]$. However, the unbound steady-state drug concentration and pharmacologic effect remain unchanged due to this type of drug interaction because the increase in unbound fraction is offset by the decrease in the total steady-state concentration $(\sim Css_u = \uparrow f_B \downarrow Css)$. Route of administration plays an important role in how important plasma protein–binding displacement drug interactions are for agents with high hepatic extraction ratios.

Inhibition Drug Interactions

Inhibition of hepatic drug metabolism is probably the most common drug interaction encountered in patients. For drugs with low hepatic extraction ratios, this type of drug interaction produces clinically significant changes in drug pharmacokinetics and effect (see Figure 3-6). The addition of a hepatic enzyme inhibitor will decrease intrinsic clearance and total clearance for the drug $(\downarrow Cl = f_B \downarrow Cl'_{int})$. Because volume of distribution remains unaltered, the half-life of the drug will increase $(\uparrow t_{1/2} = [0.693 \cdot V]/ \downarrow Cl)$. As a result of the total clearance decrease, total steady-state drug concentrations will increase $(\uparrow Css = k_0/\downarrow Cl)$. The rise in unbound steady-state drug concentration will mirror that seen with total drug concentration, and the effect of the drug will increase in proportion to unbound concentration. An example of this drug interaction is the addition of ciprofloxacin to a patient stabilized on theophylline therapy.[59]

For drugs with high hepatic extraction ratios, this category of drug interaction produces variable effects depending on the route of administration for the drug. If the drug is given intravenously and an enzyme inhibitor is added, the decrease in intrinsic clearance is usually not substantial enough to cause major pharmacokinetic and pharmacodynamic effects because clearance is a function of liver blood flow (see Figure 3-8). However, if the drug is given orally and an enzyme inhibitor is added to therapy, presystemic metabolism of the medication may be greatly depressed and the first-pass effect can decrease dramatically leading to improved drug bioavailability. This effective increase in administered oral dose will increase the total and unbound steady-state drug concentrations, and lead to an increase in the pharmacologic effect of the drug.

Induction Drug Interactions

Drugs with low hepatic extraction ratios exhibit clinically significant drug interactions that alter drug pharmacokinetics and pharmacologic response when hepatic enzyme inducers are coadministered (Figure 3-17). Enzyme inducers increase intrinsic clearance of the drug and thereby increase the total clearance of

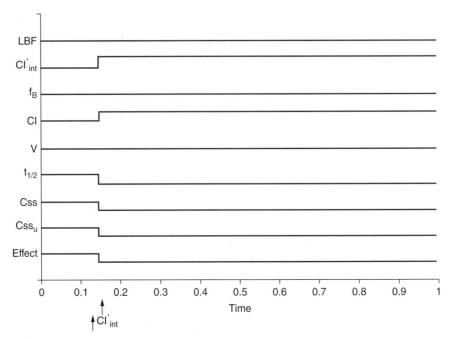

FIGURE 3-17   Changes in physiologic parameters (LBF, liver blood flow; Cl'$_{int}$, intrinsic clearance; f$_B$, free fraction of drug in the blood), pharmacokinetic parameters (Cl, clearance; V, volume of distribution; t$_{1/2}$, half-life), and drug concentration and effect (Css, total steady-state concentration; Css$_u$, unbound steady-state concentration; effect, pharmacologic effect) for a low hepatic extraction ratio drug if intrinsic clearance increases (indicated by *arrow*). An uptick in the line indicates an increase in the value of the parameter, while a downtick in the line indicates a decrease in the value of the parameter. Intrinsic clearance could increase due to a drug interaction that induces drug metabolizing enzymes.

the medication ($\uparrow$Cl = f$_B$$\uparrow$Cl'$_{int}$). The increase in total clearance will cause a shorter half-life as volume of distribution remains unchanged ($\downarrow$t$_{1/2}$ = [0.693 • V]/$\uparrow$Cl). Increased total clearance will also cause decreased total steady-state concentration ($\downarrow$Css = k$_0$/$\uparrow$Cl), unbound steady-state concentration ($\downarrow$Css$_u$ = f$_B$$\downarrow$Css), and pharmacologic effect ($\downarrow$effect $\propto$ $\downarrow$Css$_u$). Carbamazepine is a potent enzyme inducer that, when added to a patient's therapy, can cause this type of drug interaction with many other medications such as warfarin.[60]

For drugs with high hepatic extraction ratios, this type of drug interaction results in variable effects depending on the route of administration for the drug. If the drug is given intravenously and an enzyme inducer is added, the increase in intrinsic clearance is usually not large enough to cause major pharmacokinetic and pharmacologic effect alterations because total clearance is a function of liver blood flow (Figure 3-18). However, if the drug is given orally and an enzyme inducer is added to the treatment regimen, presystemic metabolism of the medication may be increased and the first-pass effect augmented leading to decreased drug bioavailability. This effective decrease in administered oral dose will decrease the total and unbound steady-state drug concentrations and lead to a decrease in the pharmacologic effect of the agent.

Alteration in Organ Blood Flow

By virtue of the pharmacologic effect for a drug, it may be possible for an agent to change liver blood flow. For instance, β-blockers can decrease heart rate and cardiac output which decreases liver blood flow. Because liver blood flow is the predominate factor that determines clearance for high hepatic extraction ratio drugs, this type of interaction is only important for this category of medication. β-Blockers decrease lidocaine clearance by decreasing liver blood flow.[61]

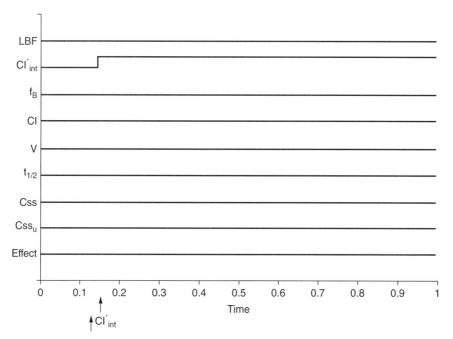

FIGURE 3-18   Changes in physiologic parameters (LBF, liver blood flow; Cl′$_{int}$, intrinsic clearance; f$_B$, free fraction of drug in the blood), pharmacokinetic parameters (Cl, clearance; V, volume of distribution; t$_{1/2}$, half-life), and drug concentration and effect (Css, total steady-state concentration; Css$_u$, unbound steady-state concentration; effect, pharmacologic effect) for a high hepatic extraction ratio drug if intrinsic clearance increases (indicated by *arrow*). An uptick in the line indicates an increase in the value of the parameter, while a downtick in the line indicates a decrease in the value of the parameter. Intrinsic clearance could increase due to a drug interaction that induces drug metabolizing enzymes.

If a drug with a high hepatic extraction ratio is administered to a patient and another agent that decreases liver blood flow is then added to the patient's therapy, total clearance will decrease (see Figure 3-10). Because volume of distribution remains unaltered, the half-life of the drug will increase [$\uparrow$t$_{1/2}$ = (0.693 • V)/ $\downarrow$Cl]. As a result of the total clearance decrease, total steady-state drug concentrations will increase ($\uparrow$Css = k$_0$/$\downarrow$Cl). The rise in unbound steady-state drug concentration will mirror that seen with total drug concentration, and the effect of the drug will increase in proportion to unbound concentration. If the coadministered drug increases liver blood flow, as can be the case with vasodilators such as the calcium channel blockers,[62,63] all of the aforementioned changes will occur in the opposite direction [$\uparrow$Cl = $\uparrow$LBF; $\downarrow$t$_{1/2}$ = (0.693 • V)/ $\uparrow$Cl; $\downarrow$Css = k$_0$/$\uparrow$Cl; $\downarrow$Css$_u$ = f$_B$$\downarrow$Css] and the decline in unbound steady-state concentration will cause a decrease in pharmacologic effect of the drug.

PROBLEMS

1. A creatinine clearance is measured in a 75-year-old Caucasian male patient with multiple myeloma to monitor changes in renal function. The serum creatinine, measured at the midpoint of the 24-hour urine collection, was 2.1 mg/dL. Urine creatinine concentration was 50 mg/dL, and urine volume was 1400 mL. (A) Calculate this patient's creatinine clearance. (B) Estimate the patient's glomerular filtration rate using the modified MDRD equation.

2. A 52-year-old, 65-kg, 5-ft 3-in-tall female patient with a methicillin-resistant *Staphylococcus aureus* (MRSA) infection needs to have an initial vancomycin dose computed. In order to do this, an estimated creatinine clearance needs to be calculated. This patient has a serum creatinine value equal to 1.8 mg/dL. Calculate her estimated creatinine clearance and estimated vancomycin clearance [assume vancomycin clearance is Cl (in mL/min/kg) = 0.695 (CrCl in mL/min/kg) + 0.05].

3. A 70-year-old, 80-kg, 5-ft 11-in-tall male with a *Pseudomonas aeruginosa* infection needs to have an initial tobramycin dose computed. In order to do this, an estimated creatinine clearance must be calculated. This patient's current serum creatinine equals 2.5 mg/dL and is stable. Compute his estimated creatinine clearance and estimated tobramycin elimination rate constant and half-life [assume tobramycin elimination rate constant is k_e(in h^{-1}) = 0.00293(CrCl in mL/min) + 0.014].

4. A 51-year-old, 54-kg, 5-ft 4-in female with worsening renal function needs to have her renal function assessed for drug dosage adjustment. Yesterday at 0800 H, her serum creatinine was 1.3 mg/dL. Today at 0800 H, her serum creatinine was 2.1 mg/dL. Compute her estimated creatinine clearance.

5. A 66-year-old, 120-kg, 5-ft 2-in-tall female has a serum creatinine equal to 3.1 mg/dL. Compute an estimated creatinine clearance for this patient.

6. A 59-year-old, 140-kg, 5-ft 8-in-tall male with severe heart failure has a serum creatinine equal to 2.4 mg/dL. Compute an estimated creatinine clearance, digoxin clearance, and digoxin volume of distribution for this patient. Assume estimated digoxin clearance in severe heart failure: Cl (in mL/min) = 1.303(CrCl in mL/min) + 20; estimated digoxin volume of distribution: V (in L) = 226 + [(298 • CrCl)/ (29.1 + CrCl)].

7. A 62-year-old, 65-kg male with hepatic cirrhosis (total bilirubin = 2.6 mg/dL, serum albumin = 2.5 mg/ dL, prothrombin time prolonged over normal by 8 seconds, slight amount of ascitic fluid, no hepatic encephalopathy) and severe chronic obstructive pulmonary disease needs to have an initial theophylline dose computed. The patient is not a tobacco smoker and does not have heart failure. Compute the patient's Child-Pugh score, estimated theophylline clearance, and theophylline dose to achieve a steady-state concentration equal to 10 mg/L.

8. A 32-year-old, 70-kg, 5-ft 8in-tall female with chronic renal failure receiving hemodialysis developed atrial fibrillation. She is to receive a new antiarrhythmic, Defibfast, for the treatment of atrial fibrillation. In patients with chronic renal failure, the following average pharmacokinetic parameters were measured in six subjects: V = 0.5 L/kg, $t_{1/2}$ = 36 h. When these subjects received hemodialysis, the hemodialysis extraction ratio was 33%. The patient just completed a hemodialysis run (Monday, 0800-1200 H). Compute a posthemodialysis loading dose to achieve a peak concentration of 50 mg/L. The next dialysis period is Wednesday at the same time. Calculate a posthemodialysis dose that will raise this patient's concentration to 50 mg/L.

9. A 47-year-old, 75-kg, 5-ft 9-in-tall male hemodialysis patient with chronic renal failure has a serious gram negative infection being treated with a new antibiotic, Bactocidal. The following concentrations were obtained: Monday, @ 1200 H (posthemodialysis) = 15 mg/L; Monday, @ 1205 H (post-IV bolus 1000-mg dose) = 65 mg/L; Wednesday, @0800 H (prehemodialysis) = 32 mg/L; Wednesday, @1200 H (posthemodialysis for 4 hours) = 8 mg/L. Compute volume of distribution, elimination rate constant and half-life for the interdialysis period, and the hemodialysis extraction ratio. What posthemodialysis dose on Wednesday would achieve a postdose concentration of 100 mg/L? What would be the pre- and post-hemodialysis concentrations on Friday (hemodialysis from 0800 to 1200 H) if that dose was given?

10. A patient receiving hemodialysis has the following concentrations obtained during a hemodialysis run: concentration into artificial kidney = 75 mg/L, concentration leaving artificial kidney = 25 mg/L. Blood flow through the artificial kidney is 400 mL/min. Compute the hemodialysis extraction ratio and clearance.

11. A patient receiving peritoneal dialysis has the following drug concentrations obtained: concentration in the dialysis fluid = 35 mg/L, concentration in serum at midpoint of peritoneal dialysis = 50 mg/L. The volume of dialysis fluid is 2 L, and the dwell time in the peritoneal cavity is 6 hours. Compute peritoneal dialysis for the drug.

12. A patient is receiving phenytoin (a low hepatic extraction ratio drug) for the treatment of tonic-clonic seizures. Because of continued seizure activity, valproic acid is added to the patient's drug regimen. Valproic acid inhibits the clearance of phenytoin and displaces phenytoin from plasma protein–binding sites. Assuming that these changes occur instantaneously with the institution of valproic acid therapy, diagram how the following parameters will change for phenytoin: liver blood flow, intrinsic clearance, free fraction of drug in the blood, clearance, volume of distribution, half-life, total steady-state concentration, unbound steady-state concentration, and drug effect.

ANSWERS TO PROBLEMS

1. *Answer to Question 1.*
   (A) $CrCl = (U_{Cr} \cdot V_{urine})/(S_{Cr} \cdot T) = (50 \text{ mg/dL} \cdot 1400 \text{ mL})/(2.1 \text{ mg/dL} \cdot 1440 \text{ min}) = 23 \text{ mL/min}$

   (B) This patient is a Caucasian male, so none of the modifying factors are needed.

   $$GFR = 186 \cdot S_{Cr}^{-1.154} \cdot Age^{-0.203} = 186 \cdot (2.1 \text{ mg/dL})^{-1.154} \cdot (75 \text{ y})^{-0.203} = 33 \text{ mL/min/1.73 m}^2$$

2. *Answer to Question 2.* Check IBW for patient to see if she is obese:

   $IBW = 45 \text{ kg} + (Ht - 60) = 45 \text{ kg} + 2.3(63 - 60) = 52 \text{ kg}$; patient is within 30% of IBW (52 ± 16 kg)

   Calculate estimated creatinine clearance:

   $$CrCl_{est} = [0.85(140 - age)BW]/(72 \cdot S_{Cr}) = [0.85(140 - 52 \text{ y})65 \text{ kg}]/(72 \cdot 1.8 \text{ mg/dL}) = 37 \text{ mL/min}$$
   $$CrCl_{est} = (37 \text{ mL/min})/65 \text{ kg} = 0.569 \text{ mL/min/kg}$$

   Calculate estimated vancomycin clearance:

   $$Cl \text{ (in mL/min/kg)} = 0.695 \text{ (Cr Cl in mL/min/kg)} + 0.05 = 0.695(0.569 \text{ mL/min/kg}) + 0.05$$
   $$= 0.446 \text{ mL/min/kg}$$
   $$Cl = 0.446 \text{ mL/min/kg}(65 \text{ kg}) = 29 \text{ mL/min}$$

3. *Answer to Question 3.* Check IBW for patient to see if he is obese:

   $IBW = 50 \text{ kg} + (Ht - 60) = 50 \text{ kg} + 2.3(71 - 60) = 75 \text{ kg}$; patient is within 30% of IBW (75 ± 23 kg)

   Calculate estimated creatinine clearance:

   $$CrCl_{est} = [(140 - age)BW]/(72 \cdot S_{Cr}) = [(140 - 70 \text{ y})80 \text{ kg}]/(72 \cdot 2.5 \text{ mg/dL}) = 31 \text{ mL/min}$$

   Calculate estimated tobramycin elimination rate constant and half-life:

   $$k_e (\text{in h}^{-1}) = 0.00293(CrCl \text{ in mL/min}) + 0.014 = 0.00293(31 \text{ mL/min}) + 0.014 = 0.105 \text{ h}^{-1}$$
   $$t_{1/2} = 0.693/k_e = 0.693/0.105 \text{ h}^{-1} = 6.6 \text{ h}$$

4. *Answer to Question 4.* The Jelliffe method is used to estimate creatinine clearance in patients with changing renal function:

   Ideal body weight is calculated: $IBW = 45 \text{ kg} + (Ht - 60) = 45 \text{ kg} + 2.3(64 - 60) = 54 \text{ kg}$

   $$Ess_{female} = IBW[25.1 - (0.175 \cdot Age)] = 54 \text{ kg}[25.1 - (0.175 \cdot 51 \text{ y})] = 873.5$$

   Average serum creatinine is computed: $Scr_{ave} = (1.3 \text{ mg/dL} + 2.1 \text{ mg/dL})/2 = 1.7 \text{ mg/dL}$

$$\text{Ess}_{\text{corrected}} = \text{Ess}[1.035 - (0.0337 \bullet \text{Scr}_{\text{ave}})] = 873.5[1.035 - (0.0337 \bullet 1.7 \text{ mg/dL})] = 854.0$$

$$E = \text{Ess}_{\text{corrected}} - \frac{[4\text{IBW}(\text{Scr}_2 - \text{Scr}_1)]}{\Delta t} = 854 - \frac{[4 \bullet 54 \text{ kg}(2.1 \text{ mg/dL} - 1.3 \text{ mg/dL})]}{24 \text{ h} \bullet 60 \text{ min/h}} = 853.9$$

$$\text{CrCl} = E/(14.4 \bullet \text{Scr}_{\text{ave}}) = 853.9/(14.4 \bullet 1.7 \text{ mg/dL}) = 35 \text{ mL/min/1.73 m}^2$$

5. *Answer to Question 5.* This patient is obese, so the Salazar-Corcoran method is used:

Height is converted from inches to meters: Ht = (62 in • 2.54 cm/in)/(100 cm/m) = 1.57 m

$$\text{CrCl}_{\text{est(females)}} = \frac{(146 - \text{age})[(0.287 \bullet \text{Wt}) + (9.74 \bullet \text{Ht}^2)]}{(60 \bullet \text{S}_{\text{Cr}})}$$

$$\text{CrCl}_{\text{est(females)}} = \frac{(146 - 66 \text{ y})[(0.287 \bullet 120 \text{ kg}) + (9.74 \bullet \{1.57 \text{ m}\}^2)]}{(60 \bullet 3.1 \text{ mg/dL})} = 25 \text{ mL/min}$$

6. *Answer to Question 6.* This patient is obese, so the Salazar-Corcoran method is used to estimate creatinine clearance:

Height is converted from inches to meters: Ht = (68 in • 2.54 cm/in)/(100 cm/m) = 1.73 m

$$\text{CrCl}_{\text{est(males)}} = \frac{(137 - \text{age})[(0.285 \bullet \text{Wt}) + (12.1 \bullet \text{Ht}^2)]}{(51 \bullet \text{S}_{\text{Cr}})}$$

$$\text{CrCl}_{\text{est(males)}} = \frac{(137 - 59 \text{ y})[(0.285 \bullet 140 \text{ kg}) + (12.1 \bullet \{1.73 \text{ m}\}^2)]}{(51 \bullet 2.4 \text{ mg/dL})} = 49 \text{ mL/min}$$

Calculate estimated digoxin pharmacokinetic parameters:

Cl (in mL/min) = 1.303(CrCl in mL/min) + 20 = 1.303(49 mL/min) + 20 = 84 mL/min

V (in L) = 226 + [(298 • CrCl)/(29.1 + CrCl)] = 226 + [(298 • 49 mL/min)/(29.1 + 49 mL/min)] = 413 L

7. *Answer to Question 7.* Child-Pugh score (from Table 3-2): total bilirubin = 2 points, albumin = 3 points, prothrombin time = 3 points, ascites = 2 points, encephalopathy = 1 point. Total = 11 points, severe hepatic dysfunction.

Theophylline clearance (from Table 3-3): Cl = 0.35 mL/min/kg (65 kg) = 22.8 mL/min

Cl = (22.8 mL/min • 60 min/h)/1000 mL/L = 1.37 L/h

Theophylline dose: MD = Css • Cl = (10 mg/L)(1.37 L/h) = 14 mg/h of theophylline

8. *Answer to Question 8.* Calculate pharmacokinetic parameters:

$$V = 0.5 \text{ L/kg (70 kg)} = 35 \text{ L}$$
$$k_e = 0.693/t_{1/2} = 0.693/36 \text{ h} = 0.0193 \text{ h}^{-1}$$

Calculate loading dose: LD = C • V = (50 mg/L)(35 L) = 1750 mg

Calculate predialysis concentration: $C = C_0 e^{-k_e t} = (50 \text{ mg/L})e^{-(0.0193h^{-1})(44 \text{ h})} = 21 \text{ mg/L}$

Calculate posthemodialysis concentration: $C_{\text{postdialysis}} = C_{\text{predialysis}}(1 - \text{ER}_{\text{HD}}) = (21 \text{ mg/L})(1 - 0.33) = 14 \text{ mg/L}$

Calculate postdialysis dose: $D = V(C_{\text{postdose}} - C_{\text{predose}}) = (35 \text{ L})(50 \text{ mg/L} - 14 \text{ mg/L}) = 1260 \text{ mg}$

9. *Answer to Question 9.* Compute pharmacokinetic parameters:

$$V = D/(C_{postdose} - C_{predose}) = 1000 \text{ mg}/(65 \text{ mg/L} - 15 \text{ mg/L}) = 20 \text{ L}$$

$$k_e = (\ln C_1 - \ln C_2)/\Delta t = (\ln 65 \text{ mg/L} - \ln 32 \text{ mg/L})/44 \text{ h} = 0.0161 \text{ h}^{-1}$$

$$t_{1/2} = 0.693/k_e = 0.693/0.0161 \text{ h}^{-1} = 43 \text{ h}$$

Calculate hemodialysis extraction ratio: $ER_{HD} = (C_{predialysis} - C_{postdialysis})/C_{predialysis} = (32 \text{ mg/L} - 8 \text{ mg/L})/$ 32 mg/L = 0.75 or 75%

Compute postdialysis dose for Wednesday: $D = V (C_{postdose} - C_{predose}) = (20 \text{ L})(100 \text{ mg/L} - 8 \text{ mg/L}) =$ 1840 mg

Calculate predialysis concentration for Friday: $C = C_0 e^{-k_e t} = (100 \text{ mg/L})e^{-(0.0161 h^{-1})(44 \text{ h})} = 49 \text{ mg/L}$

Calculate postdialysis concentration for Friday: $C_{postdialysis} = C_{predialysis}(1 - ER_{HD}) = (49 \text{ mg/L})(1 - 0.75) =$ 12 mg/L

10. *Answer to Question 10.* $ER_{HD} = (C_{predialysis} - C_{postdialysis})/C_{predialysis} = (75 \text{ mg/L} - 25 \text{ mg/L})/75 \text{ mg/L} =$ 0.67 or 67%

$$Cl_{HD} = HDBF \bullet ER_{HD} = (400 \text{ mL/min})(0.67) = 268 \text{ mL/min}$$

11. *Answer to Question 11.* $Cl_{PD} = (C_{Dialysis} \bullet V_{Dialysis})/(C_{Serum} \bullet T_{Dialysis}) = (35 \text{ mg/L} \bullet 2000 \text{ mL})/(50 \text{ mg/L} \bullet$ 360 min) = 3.9 mL/min

12. *Answer to Question 12.* Please see Figure 3-19 for diagram. Addition of valproic acid will increase the free fraction of phenytoin in the blood and decrease phenytoin intrinsic clearance. Because phenytoin

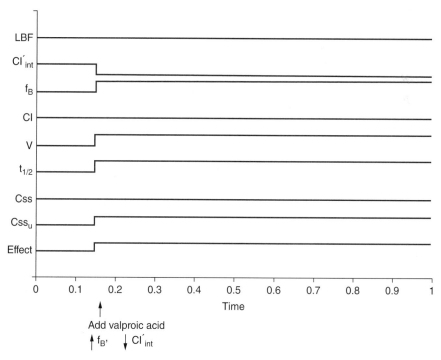

FIGURE 3-19   Solution for problem 12.

is a low hepatic extraction ratio drug, clearance will not change ($Cl = \uparrow f_B \downarrow Cl'_{int}$). However, phenytoin volume of distribution will increase ($\uparrow V = V_B + [\uparrow f_B/f_T]V_T$), resulting in an increased half-life ($\uparrow t_{1/2} = [0.693 \cdot \uparrow V]/Cl$). Total phenytoin concentration is unchanged because clearance is stable. However, because of the increase in free fraction, the unbound steady-state concentration rises ($\uparrow Css_u = \uparrow f_B Css$) and drug effect increases.

REFERENCES

1. Gibaldi M, Perrier D. *Pharmacokinetics*. Vol 15. 2nd ed. New York, NY: Marcel Dekker; 1982.
2. Bailie GR, Uhlig K, Levey AS. Clinical practice guidelines in nephrology: evaluation, classification, and stratification of chronic kidney disease. *Pharmacotherapy*. Apr 2005;25(4):491-502.
3. Levey AS, Bosch JP, Lewis JB, Greene T, Rogers N, Roth D. A more accurate method to estimate glomerular filtration rate from serum creatinine: a new prediction equation. Modification of Diet in Renal Disease Study Group. *Ann Intern Med*. Mar 16, 1999;130(6):461-470.
4. Levey AS, Coresh J, Greene T, et al. Using standardized serum creatinine values in the modification of diet in renal disease study equation for estimating glomerular filtration rate. *Ann Intern Med*. Aug 15, 2006;145(4):247-254.
5. Levey AS, Stevens LA, Schmid CH, et al. A new equation to estimate glomerular filtration rate. *Ann Intern Med*. May 5, 2009;150(9):604-612.
6. Stevens LA, Padala S, Levey AS. Advances in glomerular filtration rate-estimating equations. *Curr Opin Nephrol Hypertens*. May 2010;19(3):298-307.
7. Aronoff GR, Bennett WM, Berns JS, et al. *Drug Prescribing in Renal Failure*. 5th ed. Philadelphia, PA: American College of Physicians; 2007.
8. Bauer L. Creatinine clearance versus glomerular filtration rate for the use of renal drug dosing in patients with kidney dysfunction. *Pharmacotherapy*. Sep 2005;25(9):1286-1287; discussion 1287.
9. Bennett WM. Guide to drug dosage in renal failure. *Clin Pharmacokinet*. 1988;15(5):326-354.
10. Bennett WM, Aronoff GR, Golper TA. *Drug Prescribing in Renal Failure: Dosing Guidelines for Adults*. 3rd ed. Philadelphia, PA: American College of Physicians; 1994.
11. FDA. Guidance for industry: pharmacokinetics in patients with impaired renal function—study design, data analysis, and impact on dosing and labeling (draft guidance). *Food and Drug Administration*. http://www.fda.gov/downloads/Drugs/GuidanceComplianceRegulatoryInformation/Guidances/UCM204959.pdf. Accessed February 24, 2014.
12. Wolowich WR, Raymo L, Rodriguez JC. Problems with the use of the modified diet in renal disease formula to estimate renal function. *Pharmacotherapy*. Sep 2005;25(9):1283-1284; discussion 1284-1285.
13. Dowling TC, Matzke GR, Murphy JE, Burckart GJ. Evaluation of renal drug dosing: prescribing information and clinical pharmacist approaches. *Pharmacotherapy*. Aug 2010;30(8):776-786.
14. Matzke GR, Aronoff GR, Atkinson AJ Jr, et al. Drug dosing consideration in patients with acute and chronic kidney disease-a clinical update from Kidney Disease: Improving Global Outcomes (KDIGO). *Kidney Int*. Dec 2011;80(11):1122-1137.
15. Nyman HA, Dowling TC, Hudson JQ, Peter WL, Joy MS, Nolin TD. Comparative evaluation of the Cockcroft-Gault Equation and the Modification of Diet in Renal Disease (MDRD) study equation for drug dosing: an opinion of the Nephrology Practice and Research Network of the American College of Clinical Pharmacy. *Pharmacotherapy*. Nov 2011;31(11):1130-1144.
16. Cockcroft DW, Gault MH. Prediction of creatinine clearance from serum creatinine. *Nephron*. 1976;16:31-41.
17. Mohler JL, Barton SD, Blouin RA, Cowen DL, Flanigan RC. The evaluation of creatinine clearance in spinal cord injury patients. *J Urol*. 1986;136(2):366-369.
18. Reichley RM, Ritchie DJ, Bailey TC. Analysis of various creatinine clearance formulas in predicting gentamicin elimination in patients with low serum creatinine. *Pharmacotherapy*. 1995;15(5):625-630.
19. Smythe M, Hoffman J, Kizy K, Dmuchowski C. Estimating creatinine clearance in elderly patients with low serum creatinine concentrations. *Am J Hosp Pharm*. 1994;51(2):198-204.
20. Jelliffe RW, Jelliffe SM. A computer program for estimation of creatinine clearance from unstable serum creatinine levels, age, sex, and weight. *Mathematical Biosciences*. 1972;14:17-24.
21. Verhave JC, Fesler P, Ribstein J, du Cailar G, Mimran A. Estimation of renal function in subjects with normal serum creatinine levels: influence of age and body mass index. *Am J Kidney Dis*. Aug 2005;46(2):233-241.
22. Dionne RE, Bauer LA, Gibson GA, Griffen WO, Blouin RA. Estimating creatinine clearance in morbidly obese patients. *Am J Hosp Pharm*. 1981;38:841-844.
23. Park EJ, Pai MP, Dong T, et al. The influence of body size descriptors on the estimation of kidney function in normal weight, overweight, obese, and morbidly obese adults. *Ann Pharmacother*. Mar 2012;46(3):317-328.

24. Winter MA, Guhr KN, Berg GM. Impact of various body weights and serum creatinine concentrations on the bias and accuracy of the Cockcroft-Gault equation. *Pharmacotherapy*. Jul 2012;32(7):604-612.

25. Demirovic JA, Pai AB, Pai MP. Estimation of creatinine clearance in morbidly obese patients. *Am J Health Syst Pharm*. Apr 1, 2009;66(7):642-648.

26. Salazar DE, Corcoran GB. Predicting creatinine clearance and renal drug clearance in obese patients from estimated fat-free body mass. *Am J Med*. 1988;84:1053-1060.

27. Spinler SA, Nawarskas JJ, Boyce EG, Connors JE, Charland SL, Goldfarb S. Predictive performance of ten equations for estimating creatinine clearance in cardiac patients. Iohexol Cooperative Study Group. *Ann Pharmacother*. Dec 1998;32(12):1275-1283.

28. Traub SL, Johnson CE. Comparison of methods of estimating creatinine clearance in children. *Am J Hosp Pharm*. 1980;37:195-201.

29. Fillastre JP, Singlas E. Pharmacokinetics of newer drugs in patients with renal impairment (Part I). *Clin Pharmacokinet*. 1991;20(4):293-310.

30. Singlas E, Fillastre JP. Pharmacokinetics of newer drugs in patients with renal impairment (Part II). *Clin Pharmacokinet*. 1991;20(5):389-410.

31. Lam YW, Banerji S, Hatfield C, Talbert RL. Principles of drug administration in renal insufficiency. *Clin Pharmacokinet*. 1997;32(1):30-57.

32. Dettli L. Drug dosage in renal disease. *Clin Pharmacokinet*. 1976;1(2):126-134.

33. Koup JR, Jusko WJ, Elwood CM, Kohli RK. Digoxin pharmacokinetics: role of renal failure in dosage regimen design. *Clin Pharmacol Ther*. 1975;18:9-21.

34. DiPiro JT, Spruill WJ, Wade WE, Blouin RA, Pruemer JM. *Concepts in Clinical Pharmacokinetics*. 5th ed. Bethesda, MD: American Society of Hospital Pharmacists, Inc.; 2010.

35. Jusko WJ, Szefler SJ, Goldfarb AL. Pharmacokinetic design of digoxin dosage regimens in relation to renal function. *J Clin Pharmacol*. 1974;14(10):525-535.

36. Wilkinson GR, Shand DG. A physiological approach to hepatic drug clearance. *Clin Pharmacol Ther*. 1975;18(4):377-390.

37. Pugh RN, Murray-Lyon IM, Dawson JL, Pietroni MC, Williams R. Transection of the oesophagus for bleeding oesophageal varices. *Br J Surg*. 1973;60(8):646-649.

38. Edwards DJ, Zarowitz BJ, Slaughter RL. Theophylline. In: Evans WE, Schentag JJ, Jusko WJ, eds. *Applied Pharmacokinetics: Principles of Therapeutic Drug Monitoring*. 3rd ed. Vancouver, WA: Applied Therapeutics, Inc.; 1992:557.

39. Forni LG, Hilton PJ. Continuous hemofiltration in the treatment of acute renal failure. *N Engl J Med*. May 1, 1997;336(18):1303-1309.

40. Golper TA, Marx MA. Drug dosing adjustments during continuous renal replacement therapies. *Kidney Int Suppl*. May 1998;66:S165-S168.

41. Golper TA. Update on drug sieving coefficients and dosing adjustments during continuous renal replacement therapies. *Contrib Nephrol*. 2001;(132):349-353.

42. Choi G, Gomersall CD, Tian Q, Joynt GM, Li AM, Lipman J. Principles of antibacterial dosing in continuous renal replacement therapy. *Blood Purif*. 2010;30(3):195-212.

43. Gilbert DN, Moellering RC, Eliopoulos GM, Chambers HF, Saag MS. *The Sanford Guide to Antimicrobial Therapy*. 44th ed. Sperryville, VA: Antimicrobial Therapy; 2014.

44. Abernethy DR, Greenblatt DJ, Divoll M, Harmatz JS, Shader RI. Alterations in drug distribution and clearance due to obesity. *J Pharmacol Exp Ther*. 1981;217:681-685.

45. Caraco Y, Zylber-Katz E, Berry EM, Levy M. Significant weight reduction in obese subjects enhances carbamazepine elimination. *Clin Pharmacol Therap*. 1992;51:501-506.

46. Greenblatt DJ, Friedman H, Burstein ES, Scavone JM, Blyden GT. Trazodone kinetics: effect of age, gender, and obesity. *Clin Pharmacol Ther*. 1987;42:193-200.

47. Abernethy DR, Greenblatt DJ, Smith TW. Digoxin disposition in obesity: clinical pharmacokinetic investigation. *Am Heart J*. 1981;102:740-744.

48. Bauer LA, Wareing-Tran C, Edwards WAD, Raisys V, Ferrer L. Cimetidine clearance in the obese. *Clin Pharmacol Therap*. 1985;37:425-430.

49. Davis RL, Quenzer RW. Ranitidine pharmacokinetics in morbid obesity. *Clin Pharmacol Ther*. 1990;47:154.

50. Blouin RA, Mann HJ, Griffen WO, Bauer LA, Record KE. Tobramycin pharmacokinetics in morbidly obese patients. *Clin Pharmacol Therap*. 1979;26:508-512.

51. Bauer LA, Blouin RA, Griffen WO, Record KE, Bell RM. Amikacin pharmacokinetics in morbidly obese patients. *Am J Hosp Pharm*. 1980;37:519-522.

52. Bauer LA, Edwards WAD, Dellinger EP, Simonowitz DA. Influence of weight on aminoglycoside pharmacokinetics in normal weight and morbidly obese patients. *Eur J Clin Pharmacol*. 1983;24:643-647.

53. Schwartz SN, Pazin GJ, Lyon JA, Ho M, Pasculle AW. A controlled investigation of the pharmacokinetics of gentamicin and tobramycin in obese subjects. *J Infect Dis*. Oct 1978;138(4):499-505.

54. Bauer LA, Black DJ, Lill JS. Vancomycin dosing in morbidly obese patients. *Eur J Clin Pharmacol.* Oct 1998;54(8):621-625.

55. Blouin RA, Bauer LA, Miller DD, Record KE, Griffen WO. Vancomycin pharmacokinetics in normal and morbidly obese subjects. *Antimicrob Agents Chemother.* 1982;21:575-580.

56. Flechner SM, Kolbeinsson ME, Tam J, Lum B. The impact of body weight on cyclosporine pharmacokinetics in renal transplant recipients. *Transplantation.* 1989;47:806-810.

57. Dunn TE, Ludwig EA, Slaughter RI, Carara DJ, Jusko WJ. Pharmacokinetics and pharmacodynamics of methylprednisolone in obesity. *Clin Pharmacol Ther.* 1991;49:536-549.

58. Serlin MJ, Mossman S, Sibeon RG, Tempero KF, Breckenridge AM. Interaction between diflunisal and warfarin. *Clin Pharmacol Ther.* 1980;28(4):493-498.

59. Loi CM, Parker BM, Cusack BJ, Vestal R. Individual and combined effects of cimetidine and ciprofloxacin on theophylline metabolism in male nonsmokers. *Br J Clin Pharmacol.* 1993;36(3):195-200.

60. Massey EW. Effect of carbamazepine on Coumadin metabolism. *Ann Neurol.* 1983;13(6):691-692.

61. Schneck DW, Luderer JR, Davis D, Vary J. Effects of nadolol and propranolol on plasma lidocaine clearance. *Clin Pharmacol Ther.* 1984;36(5):584-587.

62. Bauer LA, Stenwall M, Horn JR, Davis R, Opheim K, Greene HL. Changes in antipyrine and indocyanine green kinetics during nifedipine, verapamil, and diltiazem therapy. *Clin Pharmacol Ther.* 1986;40(2):239-242.

63. Reiss WG, Bauer LA, Horn JR, Zierler BK, Easterling TR, Strandness DE. The effects of oral nifedipine on hepatic blood flow in humans. *Clin Pharmacol Ther.* 1991;50(4):379-384.

64. Pfizer. Product information for Neurontin. http://labeling.pfizer.com/ShowLabeling.aspx?id=630. Accessed February 24, 2014.

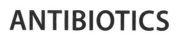

II

ANTIBIOTICS

4 The Aminoglycoside Antibiotics

INTRODUCTION

The aminoglycoside antibiotics are widely used for the treatment of severe gram-negative infections such as pneumonia or bacteremia, often in combination with a β-lactam antibiotic. Aminoglycosides are also used for gram-positive infections such as infective endocarditis in combination with penicillins when antibiotic synergy is required for optimal killing. Aminoglycoside antibiotics available in the United States that are in common use include gentamicin, tobramycin, netilmicin, and amikacin.

Aminoglycoside antibiotics are bactericidal, and the drugs exhibit concentration-dependent bacterial killing. Antibiotics with concentration-dependent killing characteristically kill bacteria at a faster rate when drug concentrations are higher. Also, aminoglycosides have a concentration-dependent postantibiotic effect. The postantibiotic effect is the phenomenon of continued bacterial killing even though serum concentrations have fallen below the minimum inhibitory concentration (MIC). Because the postantibiotic effect is concentration-dependent for the aminoglycosides, higher drug concentrations lead to a longer postantibiotic effect. The mechanisms of action for aminoglycosides are binding to the 30S ribosomal subunit inhibiting protein synthesis and misreading of messenger RNA (mRNA) causing dysfunctional protein production.[1]

THERAPEUTIC AND TOXIC CONCENTRATIONS

The MIC for susceptible bacteria is higher for amikacin than it is for the other aminoglycosides. Because the pharmacokinetics are similar for all these drugs, higher doses of amikacin are needed to treat infections. The *conventional method* of dosing aminoglycoside antibiotics is to administer multiple daily doses (usually every 8 hours, with normal renal function).[2] This method of dosing is most often used for the treatment of infective endocarditis, but it can also be considered for other patients, especially those with poor renal function.

In order to take advantage of concentration-dependent bacterial killing and the postantibiotic effect, *extended-interval* (usually the total daily dose given once per day) aminoglycoside administration is another dosing option.[3] This dosing method is now the predominate mode of administration, except for the treatment of endocarditis where aminoglycosides are used for their synergistic effect with penicillins or vancomycin. Because these two different methods of dosage administration have very different target concentrations, it is important to identify which is being used when discussing serum concentration monitoring.

Conventional Dosing

Aminoglycoside antibiotics are given as short-term (½-1 hour) infusions. If a 1-hour infusion is used, maximum end of infusion "peak" concentrations are measured when the infusion is completed (Figure 4-1). If a one-half hour infusion is used, serum concentrations exhibit a distribution phase so that drug in the blood and in the tissues are not yet in equilibrium. Because of this, a one-half hour waiting period is allowed for distribution to finish if a one-half hour infusion is used before peak concentrations are measured. Therapeutic

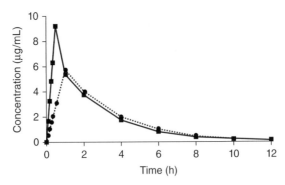

FIGURE 4-1   Concentration/time plot for gentamicin 120 mg given as a ½-hour infusion (*squares with solid line*) and as a 1-hour infusion (*circles with dashed line*). When given as a ½-hour infusion, end of infusion concentrations are higher because the serum and tissues are not in equilibrium. A ½-hour waiting time for aminoglycoside distribution to tissues is allowed before peak concentrations are measured. If aminoglycosides are given as 1-hour infusions, distribution has an opportunity to occur during the infusion time and peak concentrations can be obtained immediately. In either case, concentrations 1 hour after the infusion was initiated are similar.

steady-state peak concentrations for gentamicin, tobramycin, and netilmicin are generally 5-10 μg/mL for gram-negative infections. Infection sites with more susceptible bacteria, such as intra-abdominal infections usually can be treated with steady-state peak concentrations at the lower end of this range (typically 5-7 μg/mL). Infection sites that are difficult to penetrate and with bacteria that have higher MIC values, such as pseudomonal pneumonia, usually require steady-state peak concentrations in the higher end of the range (typically 8-10 μg/mL). When gentamicin, tobramycin, or netilmicin are used synergistically with penicillins or other antibiotics for the treatment of gram-positive infections such as infective endocarditis, steady-state peak concentrations of 3-4 μg/mL are often times adequate. Therapeutic peak concentrations for amikacin are 15-30 μg/mL.

Exceeding peak steady-state concentrations of 12-14 μg/mL for gentamicin, tobramycin, or netilmicin or 35-40 μg/mL for amikacin when using conventional dosing leads to an increased risk of ototoxicity.[4] The types of ototoxicity that aminoglycosides cause are auditory and vestibular, and the damage is permanent. Aminoglycosides accumulate in the lymph of the inner ear causing ongoing damage to cochlear or vestibular sensory cells.[1] Auditory ototoxicity usually is first noted at high frequencies (>4000 Hz) and is difficult to detect using clinical means. Audiometry is required to detect high tone hearing loss and is seldom done in patient care areas. Older patients may have lost the ability to hear in this range for other reasons. If aminoglycoside treatment is not discontinued in individuals with high-frequency auditory ototoxicity, hearing loss will progress to lower frequencies. As a result, aminoglycoside-induced hearing losses are not usually detected until the patient is unable to detect sounds in the conversational frequency zone (<4000 Hz). Often, the first sign of auditory ototoxicity is tinnitus. Vestibular ototoxicity results in the loss of balance. Again, this type of ototoxicity is difficult to detect because many patients treated with aminoglycosides are bed-bound. Besides loss of equilibrium, headache, ataxia, nausea, vomiting, nystagmus, and vertigo can all be signs of vestibular ototoxicity. Although this version of ototoxicity is also permanent, patients can often times compensate using visual cues, such as use of the horizon, to maintain balance and avoid ataxia. In some studies, predose ("trough") steady-state concentrations have been found to be related to ototoxicity.[5,6] However, peak steady-state concentrations have also been elevated in these patients, which clouds the relationship between serum concentrations and this type of drug-induced adverse effect.

Trough steady-state concentrations (predose or minimum concentrations usually obtained within 30 minutes of the next dose) above 2-3 μg/mL for tobramycin, gentamicin, or netilmicin or 10 μg/mL for amikacin predispose patients to an increased risk of nephrotoxicity.[7,8] Aminoglycoside antibiotics accumulate in the proximal tubular cells of the kidney, decrease the ability of the kidney to concentrate urine, and, ultimately, decrease glomerular filtration.[9-11] Nephrotoxicity due to aminoglycoside therapy is unlikely to occur before 3-5 days of therapy with proper dosing of the antibiotic. However, aminoglycoside nephrotoxicity can occur even with the low-intensity, synergistic treatment that is used during the therapy of endocarditits.[12] Because many patients receiving aminoglycosides are critically ill, other sources of nephrotoxicity, such as hypotension or other nephrotoxic drug therapy, should be ruled out before a diagnosis of aminoglycoside renal damage is made in a patient. Unlike ototoxicity, aminoglycoside-induced nephrotoxicity is usually reversible with little, if any, residual damage if the antibiotic is withdrawn soon after renal function tests change. With proper patient monitoring, mild renal dysfunction resulting in serum creatinine increases of 0.5-2 mg/dL may be the only result of aminoglycoside nephrotoxicity. However, if the patient develops renal failure, the cost of maintaining the patient on dialysis until kidney function returns can exceed $50,000-100,000 and, if the patient is critically ill, may contribute to his or her death. In some investigations, peak concentrations have been related to nephrotoxicity.[13] However, trough concentrations have also been high in these patients, which obscures the relationship between serum concentrations and nephrotoxicity.

Keeping peak and trough concentrations within the suggested ranges does not completely avoid nephrotoxicity and ototoxicity in patients but, hopefully, decreases the likelihood that patients will experience these serious adverse effects.[14] Also, even though serum concentrations are controlled within the suggested ranges, duration of therapy exceeding 14 days, large total cumulative doses, and concurrent therapy with other nephrotoxic drugs such as vancomycin can predispose patients to these side effects of the aminoglycoside antibiotics.[15-18]

Extended-Interval Dosing

Beginning in the mid-1990s, infectious disease specialists began to recognize the importance of pharmacodynamic principles when treating infections. Measures such as C_{max}/MIC for concentration-dependent antibiotics (where C_{max} is the maximum antibiotic concentration), t > MIC for time-dependent antibiotics (time when antibiotic concentrations are above MIC), and AUC/MIC (where AUC is the area under the concentration-time curve for the antibiotic) were recognized as parameters that could be used to help define the response to antibiotic treatment as a combination of exposure to the antibiotic (C_{max} or AUC) and bacterial sensitivity (MIC).[19-22]

Because aminoglycoside antibiotics exhibit concentration-dependent bacterial killing and the postantibiotic effect is longer with higher concentrations, investigators studied the possibility of giving a higher dose of aminoglycoside once daily.[3,23,24] Generally, these studies have shown comparable microbiologic and clinical cure rates for most infections and about the same rate of nephrotoxicity (~5%-10%) as with conventional dosing. Auditory ototoxicity has not been monitored using audiometry in most of these investigations, but loss of hearing in the conversational range as well as signs and symptoms of vestibular toxicity have usually been assessed and found to be similar to aminoglycoside therapy dosed conventionally. Based on this data, clinicians are using extended-interval dosing for most patients. An exception to this is the treatment of infective endocarditis where the aminoglycoside is used at a lower dose for its synergistic effect in combination with a penicillin or vancomycin. This indication is treated solely with conventional dosing when an aminoglycoside is required.

In order to optimize the treatment of serious gram-negative infections with aminoglycosides, a C_{max}/MIC ratio of greater than 8-10 is considered necessary to affect a clinical cure.[25-28] For *Pseudomonas aeruginosa* infections where the organism has an expected MIC ≈ 2 μg/mL, peak concentrations between 20 and 30 μg/mL and trough concentrations of less than 1 μg/mL have been suggested.[3] At the present time, there is not a consensus on how to approach concentration monitoring using this mode of administration.[29-35]

Some clinicians measure steady-state peak and trough concentrations while others measure two steady-state postdose concentrations or a single steady-state postdose concentration.[36] Other clinicians suggest that individualizing the aminoglycoside C_{max}/MIC, AUC, or AUC_{24}/MIC (where AUC_{24} is the area under the concentration-time curve for the antibiotic for a duration of 24 hours) is the best approach.[25-28,30,32,37–41]

Because of the extremely high peak concentrations obtained during extended-interval dosing of aminoglycosides, it can be difficult to understand why increased toxicity is not seen in patients. The hypothesized reason is that both nephrotoxicity and ototoxicity are due to accumulation of aminoglycoside in the relevant tissue. Because the dosage interval is prolonged in extended-interval administration, aminoglycoside concentrations are low for a long period of time and may allow for diffusion of drug out of tissue and into the blood, which avoids drug accumulation in the ear and kidney. Also, some of the uptake mechanisms into the ear and kidney may be saturable, so that high peak serum concentrations of aminoglycosides may not result in high renal or ear tissue concentrations.

Because large doses of aminoglycoside are given as a single dose with this mode of administration, two additional adverse effects become of concern. Because of the manufacturing process used to produce aminoglycoside antibiotics, very low residual amounts of gram-negative endotoxin are sometimes present in the commercial product. Reports of infusion-related hypotension in patients receiving extended-interval aminoglycosides during the late 1990s have been attributed to the amount of toxin administered at one time.[42,43] Acute neuromuscular blockade, usually associated with concurrent administration of anesthetics or neuromuscular blockers, is also a possible adverse effect of aminoglycosides associated with high drug concentrations. Because of the high peak concentrations achieved using extended-interval dosing, surgical and intensive care patients should be monitored for this possible adverse effect.

Differential Toxicity Among Aminoglycosides

Studies are available that attempt to determine nephrotoxicity differences among antibiotics. Gentamicin accumulates to a greater extent in kidney tissue when compared to tobramycin.[11,1417] Because doses of amikacin are larger than those for gentamicin and tobramycin, amikacin renal accumulation must be adjusted for dosage differences.[9,14] When this is done, amikacin accumulation patterns are similar to gentamicin. Based on these accumulation profiles and associated clinical data and other trials, some clinicians believe that tobramycin is less nephrotoxic than gentamicin or amikacin.[44] There is less conclusive data for netilmicin. Other clinical trials that compare the nephrotoxicity potential of gentamicin and tobramycin indicate that the two drugs are similar in this area.[45,46] Generally, gentamicin is the most widely used aminoglycoside, followed by tobramycin and netilmicin. This usage pattern is due, in part, to the fact that gentamicin was the first aminoglycoside available generically and was much less expensive than the other drugs for a number of years. Amikacin is usually reserved for use in infections where the organism is resistant to other aminoglycosides.

CLINICAL MONITORING PARAMETERS

Clinicians should always consult the patient's chart to confirm that antibiotic therapy is appropriate for current microbiologic cultures and sensitivities. Also, it should be confirmed that the patient is receiving other appropriate concurrent antibiotic therapy, such as β-lactam or anaerobic agents, when necessary to treat the infection. Patients with severe infections usually have elevated white blood cell counts and body temperatures. Measurement of serial white blood cell counts and body temperatures are useful to determine the efficacy of antibiotic therapy. A white blood cell count with a differential will identify the types of white blood cells that are elevated. A large number of neutrophils and immature neutrophils, clinically known as a "shift to the left," can also be observed in patients with severe bacterial infections. Favorable response to antibiotic treatment is usually indicated by high white blood cell counts decreasing toward the normal range, the trend of body temperatures (plotted as body temperature vs time, also known as the "fever curve") approaching normal, and any specific infection site tests or procedures resolving. For instance, in pneumonia patients the chest x-ray should be resolving, in patients with an intra-abdominal infection abdominal pain and tenderness should be decreasing, or in patients with a wound infection the wound should be less inflamed with less purulent discharge. Clinicians should also be aware that immunocompromised patients with a bacterial infection may not be able to mount a fever or elevated white blood cell count.

Aminoglycoside steady-state peak and trough serum concentrations should be measured in 3–5 estimated half-lives when the drug is given using conventional dosage approaches. Methods to estimate this parameter are given in the initial dose calculation portion of this chapter. Because prolongation of the dosage interval is often used in patients with decreased elimination, a useful clinical rule is to measure serum concentrations after the third dose. If this approach is used, the dosage interval is increased in tandem with the increase in half-life so that 3-5 half-lives have elapsed by the time the third dose is administered. Additionally, the third dose typically occurs 1-3 days after dosing has commenced and this is a good time to also assess clinical efficacy of the treatment. Steady-state serum concentrations, in conjunction with clinical response, are used to adjust the antibiotic dose, if necessary. Methods for adjusting aminoglycoside doses using serum concentrations are discussed later in this chapter. If the dosage is adjusted, aminoglycoside elimination changes or laboratory and clinical monitoring indicate that the infection is not resolving or worsening, clinicians should consider rechecking steady-state drug concentrations.

When extended-interval aminoglycoside therapy is used, several different monitoring techniques can be used.[36] Some clinicians measure steady-state peak and trough concentrations while others measure two steady-state postdose concentrations. Other approaches include obtaining only a steady-state trough concentration, measuring a single aminoglycoside serum concentration 6-14 hours after a dose and using a dosage nomogram to adjust the dosage interval, or individualizing the aminoglycoside C_{max}/MIC, AUC, or AUC_{24}/MIC for each patient (where AUC_{24} is the area under the concentration-time curve for the antibiotic for a duration of 24 hours; please see dosing section later in this chapter for details on each methodology).[25-28,30,32,37-41]

Serial monitoring of serum creatinine concentrations should be used to detect nephrotoxicity. Ideally, a baseline serum creatinine concentration is obtained before aminoglycoside therapy is initiated and three times weekly during treatment. An increasing serum creatinine test on two or more consecutive measurement occasions indicates that more intensive monitoring of serum creatinine values, such as daily, is needed. If serum creatinine measurements increase more than 0.5 mg/dL over the baseline value (or >25%-30% over baseline for serum creatinine values >2 mg/dL) and other causes of declining renal function have been ruled out (other nephrotoxic drugs or agents, hypotension, etc), alternatives to aminoglycoside therapy or, if that option is not possible, intensive aminoglycoside serum concentration monitoring should be initiated to ensure that excessive amounts of aminoglycoside do not accumulate in the patient. In the clinical setting, audiometry is rarely used to detect ototoxicity because it is difficult to accomplish in severely ill patients. Instead, clinical signs and symptoms of auditory (decreased hearing acuity in the conversational range, feeling of fullness or pressure in the ears, tinnitus) or vestibular (loss of equilibrium, headache, nausea, vomiting, vertigo, nystagmus, ataxia) ototoxicity are monitored at the same time intervals as serum creatinine determination. Because coadministration of an aminoglycoside with vancomycin can increase adverse drug reactions by twofold or more, patients taking both of these antibiotics concurrently should be monitored daily for the development of nephrotoxicity or ototoxicity.

BASIC CLINICAL PHARMACOKINETIC PARAMETERS

The aminoglycosides are eliminated almost completely (≥90%) unchanged in the urine primarily by glomerular filtration (Table 4-1).[10,1417] These antibiotics are usually given by short-term (½-1 hour)

TABLE 4-1   Disease States and Conditions That Alter Aminoglycoside Pharmacokinetics

Disease State/Condition	Half-Life	Volume of Distribution	Comment
Adult, normal renal function	2 h (range: 1.5-3 h)	0.26 L/kg (range: 0.2-0.3 L/kg)	Usual doses 3-5 mg/kg/d for gentamicin, tobramycin, netilmicin or 15 mg/kg/d for amikacin when using conventional dosing
Adult, renal failure	50 h (range: 36-72 h)	0.26 L/kg	Renal failure patients commonly have fluid imbalances that may decrease (underhydration) or increase (overhydration) the volume of distribution and secondarily change half-life
Burns	1.5 h	0.26 L/kg	Burn patients commonly have fluid imbalances that may decrease (underhydration) or increase (overhydration) the volume of distribution and secondarily change half-life
Critically ill patients with sepsis	Increased (variable)	Increased (variable)	Decreased blood pressure lowers renal blood flow and damages nephrons due to hypoxia which decreases the renal clearance. Vigorous intravenous fluid therapy used to treat hypotension increases the volume of distribution. Half-life increases due to clearance and volume of distribution changes ($\uparrow\uparrow t_{1/2} = (0.693 \cdot \uparrow V)/\downarrow Cl$)
Penicillin therapy (patients with creatinine clearance <30 mL/min)	Variable	0.26 L/kg	Some penicillins (penicillin G, ampicillin, nafcillin, carbenicillin, ticarcillin) can bind and inactivate aminoglycosides in vivo
Obesity (>30% over IBW) with normal renal function	2-3 h	V (in L) = 0.26 [IBW + 0.4 (TBW − IBW)]	Aminoglycosides enter the extracellular fluid contained in adipose tissue requiring a correction factor to estimate volume of distribution
Cystic fibrosis	1.5 h	0.35 L/kg	Larger volume of distribution and shorter half-life usually result in larger daily doses
Ascites/overhydration	Variable	V (in L) = (0.26 · DBW) + (TBW − DBW)	Aminoglycosides distribute to excess extracellular fluid; correction equation assumes that weight gain is due to fluid accumulation. Alterations in volume of distribution can cause secondary changes in half-life
Hemodialysis	3-4 h	0.26 L/kg	While receiving hemodialysis, aminoglycoside half-life will decrease from ~50 h to ~4 h. Renal failure patients commonly have fluid imbalances that may decrease (underhydration) or increase (overhydration) the volume of distribution and secondarily change half-life
Peritoneal dialysis	36 h	0.26 L/kg	While receiving peritoneal dialysis, aminoglycoside half-life will decrease from ~50 h to ~36 h. Renal failure patients commonly have fluid imbalances that may decrease (underhydration) or increase (overhydration) the volume of distribution and secondarily change half-life

DBW, dry body weight; IBW, ideal body weight; TBW, total body weight.

intermittent intravenous infusions, although they can be given intramuscularly. When aminoglycosides are given intramuscularly, they exhibit very good bioavailability of ~100% and are rapidly absorbed with maximal concentrations occurring about 1 hour after injection. Exceptions to this situation are patients who are hypotensive or obese. Hypotensive patients shunt blood flow away from peripheral tissues, such as muscle, to provide maximal blood flow to internal organs. As a result, intramuscularly administered drugs may be malabsorbed in hypotensive patients, such as those with gram-negative sepsis. Care must be taken with obese individuals to use a long enough needle to penetrate subcutaneous fat and enter muscle tissue when administering aminoglycoside antibiotics. Drug injected into poorly perfused fatty tissue will likely be malabsorbed. Oral bioavailability is poor (<10%) so systemic infections cannot be treated by this route of administration. Plasma protein binding is low (<10%).

Manufacturer recommended doses for conventional dosing in patients with normal renal function are 3-5 mg/kg/d for gentamicin and tobramycin, 4-6 mg/kg/d for netilmicin, and 15 mg/kg/d for amikacin. These amounts are divided into three equal daily doses for gentamicin, tobramycin, or netilmicin, or two or three equal daily doses for amikacin. Extended-interval doses obtained from the literature for patients with normal renal function are 4-7 mg/kg/d for gentamicin, tobramycin, or netilmicin, and 11-20 mg/kg/d for amikacin.[3,24,29-35,47-53]

EFFECTS OF DISEASE STATES AND CONDITIONS ON AMINOGLYCOSIDE PHARMACOKINETICS AND DOSING

Nonobese adults with normal renal function (creatinine clearance >80 mL/min, Table 4-1) have an average aminoglycoside half-life of 2 hours (range: 1.5-3 hours), and the average aminoglycoside volume of distribution is 0.26 L/kg (range: 0.2-0.3 L/kg) in this population.[54-57] The volume of distribution is similar to extracellular fluid content of the body, and fluid balance will be an important factor when estimating the aminoglycoside volume of distribution for a patient. Patients who have been febrile due to their infections for 24 hours or more may be significantly dehydrated and have lower volumes of distribution until rehydrated.

Because aminoglycosides are eliminated primarily by glomerular filtration, renal dysfunction is the most important disease state that affects aminoglycoside pharmacokinetics.[58,59] The elimination rate constant decreases in proportion to creatinine clearance because of the decline in drug clearance (Figure 4-2).[60,61] This relationship between renal function and aminoglycoside elimination will form the basis for initial dosage

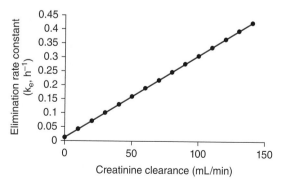

FIGURE 4-2   The elimination rate constant (k_e) for aminoglycoside antibiotics increases in proportion with creatinine clearance (CrCl). The equation for this relationship is k_e (in h^{-1}) = 0.00293(CrCl in mL/min) + 0.014. This equation is used to estimate the aminoglycoside elimination rate constant in patients for initial dosing purposes.

computation later in this chapter. Because the kidney is the organ responsible for maintaining fluid and electrolyte balance in the body, patients with renal failure are sometimes overhydrated. Body weight can be an effective way for detecting overhydration in a patient. If the usual weight of the patient is 70 kg when they are in normal fluid balance, known as the patient's "dry weight," and the patient is currently 75 kg with signs and symptoms of overhydration (pedal edema, extended neck veins, etc), the additional 5 kg of weight could be considered extra fluid and added to the estimated volume of distribution for the patient. Because 1 L of water weights 1 kg, the estimated volume of distribution for this patient would be 18.2 L using the patient's dry weight (V = 0.26 L/kg • 70 kg = 18.2 L) plus 5 L to account for the additional 5 kg of extra fluid yielding a total volume of distribution equal to 23.2 L (V = 18.2 L + 5 L = 23.2 L). Care would be needed to alter the estimated volume of distribution toward normal as the excess fluid was lost and the patient's weight returned to its usual value.

A major body burn (>40% body surface area) can cause large changes in aminoglycoside pharmacokinetics.[62-65] Forty-eight to 72 hours after a major burn, the basal metabolic rate of the patient increases to facilitate tissue repair. Because of the increase in basal metabolic rate, glomerular filtration rate (GFR) increases, which increases aminoglycoside clearance. Because of the increase in drug clearance, the average half-life for aminoglycosides in burn patients is ~1.5 hours. If the patient is in normal fluid balance, the average volume of distribution will be the same as in normal adults (0.26 L/kg). However, because the skin is the organ that prevents fluid evaporation from the body and the integrity of the skin has been violated by thermal injury, these patients can be dehydrated, especially if they have had a fever for more than 24 hours. The result is a lower volume of distribution for aminoglycosides. Alternatively, some burn patients may be overhydrated due to vigorous fluid therapy used to treat hypotension. This will result in a larger than expected aminoglycoside volume of distribution. Unfortunately, there is no precise way to correct for fluid balance in these patients. Frequent use of aminoglycoside serum concentrations are used to guide therapy in this population.

Critically ill patients with sepsis can have higher volumes of distribution, lower clearances, and longer half-lives for aminoglycosides due to the physiologic changes induced by sepsis and the treatment of any resulting hypotension. Decreased blood pressure causes lower end-organ perfusion, which includes the kidneys. Both lower renal blood flow and primary damage to nephrons in the functional kidney tissue due to hypoxia decrease the renal clearance of aminoglycosides. Hypotension is often treated with vigorous intravenous fluid therapy, which increases the volume of distribution of the antibiotics. When clearance decreases and volume of distribution simultaneously increases, the half-life of a drug responds by increasing its value ($\uparrow\uparrow t_{1/2} = (0.693 • \uparrow V)/\downarrow Cl$).[66-68]

Concurrent therapy with some penicillins can increase aminoglycoside clearance by chemically inactivating both the penicillin and aminoglycoside via formation of a covalent bond between the two antibiotic molecules.[69-73] Penicillin G, ampicillin, nafcillin, carbenicillin, and ticarcillin are the penicillins most likely to cause this interaction. Piperacillin and mezlocillin, as well as cephalosporins, do not inactivate aminoglycosides to an appreciable extent. This in vivo interaction is most likely to occur in patients with poor renal function (creatinine clearance <30 mL/min) so that the elimination of both the aminoglycoside and penicillin is slower. Under these conditions, serum concentrations of both antibiotics will be higher for a longer period of time and facilitate the inactivation process. In patients with renal failure receiving an aminoglycoside alone, the addition of one of the interacting penicillins can decrease the aminoglycoside half-life from ~50 hours when given alone to ~12 hours when given in combination and result in a dosage increase for the aminoglycoside. Another place where this interaction is important to note is when patients are receiving concurrent therapy with one of the interacting penicillins and an aminoglycoside antibiotic, and serum concentration monitoring of the aminoglycoside is planned. When a blood sample is obtained for measurement of the aminoglycoside serum concentration, penicillin contained in the blood collection tube can continue to inactivate aminoglycoside. This will lead to a spuriously low aminoglycoside concentration results which can lead to dosing adjustment errors. For example, a peak gentamicin serum concentration is obtained in a patient receiving concurrent gentamicin and penicillin G therapy. When the blood sample is drawn from the patient, the gentamicin concentration was 8 μg/mL. By the time the sample is processed by the laboratory, 6 hours expire because of transportation, etc. Because of this, penicillin G inactivates aminoglycoside molecules, and the concentration of gentamicin decreases to 4 μg/mL. The laboratory measures this concentration and reports it to the clinicians caring for the patient. Because the desired peak concentration is 8 μg/mL, the dose of gentamicin is doubled so that the reported peak concentration of 4 μg/mL will increase to the target concentration. Of course, because the actual peak concentration is 8 μg/mL in the patient all along, the new peak concentration resulting from the dosage increase will be 16 μg/mL. In order to prevent this in vitro inactivation interaction in patients receiving concurrent penicillin and aminoglycoside treatment when the drug assay will not be run for longer than 1-2 hours after specimen collection, blood samples should have the serum separated using centrifugation. The serum is removed and placed in a separate tube then frozen to prevent the chemical reaction from occurring. Alternatively, a small amount of β-lactamase (<5% of total blood volume to prevent sample dilution) can be added to break the β-lactam bond of the penicillin and avoid inactivation of the aminoglycoside antibiotic.

Aminoglycosides are relatively polar molecules with good water solubility. Because of this, they do not enter adipose cells to any significant extent. However, in patients who weigh more than 30% over their ideal body weight, the volume of distribution for aminoglycosides increases because of the additional extracellular fluid contained in adipose tissue (Figure 4-3).[74-76] The reason why aminoglycoside volume of distribution is affected by this relatively small amount of additional extracellular fluid in adipose tissue is that the baseline volume of distribution for these drugs is relatively small to begin with (0.26 L/kg or ~18 L for a 70-kg person). For other water-soluble drugs with larger volumes of distribution, the additional extracellular fluid

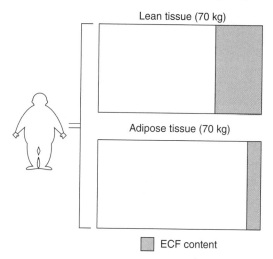

140-kg obese patient with ideal body weight of 70 kg

FIGURE 4-3   Schematic of extracellular fluid content of lean and adipose tissue in a morbidly obese patient with an actual body weight of 140 kg and an ideal body weight of 70 kg. Lean tissue contains about 0.26 L/kg extracellular fluid, but adipose tissue has about 40% of the extracellular fluid content that lean tissue does. The equation that estimates volume of distribution for aminoglycosides in obese patients normalizes adipose tissue extracellular content into lean tissue equivalents.

contained in adipose tissue may not be a significant factor. Adipose tissue contains ~40% of the extracellular fluid that is present in lean tissue. To compensate for the increased extracellular fluid of adipose tissue and the greater volume of distribution found in obese patients (>30% over ideal body weight), the following formula can be used to estimate aminoglycoside volume of distribution (V in L) for initial dosing purposes: $V = 0.26 \cdot [IBW + 0.4(TBW - IBW)]$, where IBW is ideal body weight and TBW is the patient's actual total body weight. In morbidly obese (>90% above ideal body weight) patients with normal serum creatinine concentrations, the clearance of aminoglycoside antibiotics is also increased.[74-76] The reason for the increased drug clearance is larger kidneys which result in larger creatinine clearance rates. Because both volume of distribution and clearance simultaneously change in obese patients to about the same extent, the aminoglycoside half-life value is appropriate for the patient's renal function ($t_{1/2} = [0.693 \cdot V]/Cl$).

Cystic fibrosis is a disease state that affects exocrine glands. In the lung, the result is the production of thick, tenacious sputum that predisposes patients to pulmonary infections. Patients with cystic fibrosis have larger aminoglycoside volumes of distribution (0.35 L/kg) because body composition is altered.[47-50,77-82] Generally cystic fibrosis patients have decreased adipose tissue and increased extracellular fluid due to disease-state–induced gastrointestinal malabsorption. These patients also have higher aminoglycoside clearance values due to increased glomerular filtration rates. Because clearance rates tend to increase more than volume of distribution values, the average aminoglycoside half-life is typically shorter in patients with cystic fibrosis ($t_{1/2} = 1.5$ hours). Extended-interval dosing can be used to treat pulmonary exacerbations in cystic fibrosis patients.[47,49,83,84] Aminoglycosides can also be administered via inhalation at a dose of 300 mg twice daily in a cyclic fashion (4 weeks on, 4 weeks off) for patients with cystic fibrosis.[85] If cystic fibrosis patients receive a lung transplant for the treatment of their disease, aminoglycoside clearance may decrease, volume of distribution may increase, and half-life may increase in the postsurgical time period.[86,87]

Liver disease patients with ascites have additional extracellular fluid due to accumulation of ascitic fluid.[88-90] Because aminoglycosides pass into ascitic fluid, the volume of distribution is increased in these patients. The approach to estimating an initial volume of distribution is similar to that used in renal failure patients who are fluid overloaded. The weight of the patient when ascitic fluid is not present is known as the patient's *dry weight*. If this value is not known and the patient is not obese, ideal body weight can be used as an estimate of the dry weight. A reasonable estimate of the volume of distribution (V in L) for a patient with ascites, or who is overhydrated for other reasons, can be estimated using the following equation: $V = (0.26 \cdot DBW) + (TBW - DBW)$, where DBW is the patient's dry body weight and TBW is the patient's actual total body weight. Because of the large amount of variation in aminoglycoside, volume of distribution for patients with ascites or overhydration, dosing should be guided by aminoglycoside serum concentrations. Also, as excess fluid is lost, clinicians should anticipate a decrease in the volume of distribution for these drugs.

Premature infants (gestational age ≤34 weeks) have a larger amount of body water compared to adults.[51,91-94] Aminoglycoside volume of distribution is larger (0.5-0.6 L/kg) because of this physiologic difference. Additionally, kidneys are not completely developed either so glomerular filtration and aminoglycoside clearance are decreased. A larger volume of distribution and lower clearance rate result in a prolonged average half-life equal to 6-10 hours. Full-term neonates (gestational age ~40 weeks) also have a larger volume of distribution (mean V = 0.4-0.5 L/kg) and lower aminoglycoside clearance, resulting in longer half-life values ($t_{1/2} = 4-5$ h). By about 6 months, the mean volume of distribution is still large (V = 0.3-0.4 L/kg), but kidney development is complete, aminoglycoside clearance increases, and half-life is shorter ($t_{1/2} = 2-3$ h). These values remain relatively constant until about 2 years of age. At that time, aminoglycoside volume of distribution, clearance, and half-life gradually approach adult values at puberty (~12-14 years old). Initial doses for neonates aged 28 days or younger are based on weight and age.[95]

Aminoglycoside	Route	Body Weight ≤2 kg		Body Weight >2 kg	
		≤ 7 d old	8–28 d old[a]	≤ 7 d old	8–28 d old
Amikacin	IV, IM	15 mg/kg every 48 h	15 mg/kg every 24-48 h	15 mg/kg every 24 h	15 mg/kg every 12-24 h
Gentamicin or Tobramycin	IV, IM	5 mg/kg every 48 h	4-5 mg/kg every 24-48 h	4 mg/kg every 24 h	4 mg/kg every 12-24 h

[a]For extremely low-birth-weight neonates (<1 kg), 48-hour dosage interval may be used for up to 2 weeks old.

Doses for infants and children with severe infections include amikacin 15-22.5 mg/kg/d IV or IM given every 8 hours, gentamicin or tobramycin 3-7.5 mg/kg/d IV or IM given every 8 hours, and tobramycin 8-10 mg/kg/d IV or IM given every 8 hours for cystic fibrosis pulmonary exacerbations.[95] Extended-interval aminoglycoside dosing can be conducted in pediatric patients.[96,97] Suggested extended-interval doses for infants and children with severe infections and normal renal function include amikacin 15-20 mg/kg every 24 hours and gentamicin or tobramycin 4.5-7.5 mg/kg every 24 hours.[95] After initial doses are started, steady-state aminoglycoside serum concentrations are used to individualize doses for either conventional or extended-interval dosing.

Therapeutic hypothermia is used in both neonates and older patients as a neuroprotective measure. For neonates, it can be used to treat hypoxic ischemic encephalopathy. For adults, it can be used as a therapy for intracranial hypertension unresponsive to other treatments. In both cases, body temperature is decreased to ~33°C, and hypothermia causes several changes in the pharmacokinetics of aminoglycosides. Principal factors among the physiologic alterations that cause these pharmacokinetic changes are decreased cardiac output and vasoconstriction, which cause decreased renal blood flow and glomerular filtration rate, and an overall decreased metabolic rate. These changes decrease clearance and increase half-life for the aminoglycoside antibiotics in a variable fashion, depending of the baseline renal function of the patient.[98-100]

Hemodialysis efficiently removes aminoglycoside antibiotics from the body.[101-107] Gentamicin, tobramycin, netilmicin, and amikacin are relatively small molecules that are water soluble and have a small volume of distribution and low plasma protein binding. All of these characteristics lead to very good hemodialysis removal. The average aminoglycoside half-life in a renal failure patient is 50 hours. During hemodialysis with a "low-flux" artificial kidney, half-life decreases to 4 hours and results in about 50% of the drug being removed during a typical dialysis period (3-4 hours). Similarly, hemodialysis performed with a "high-flux" filter decreases aminoglycoside half-life to 2 hours, and short-daily hemodialysis (2 h/d, 6 d/wk with a high-flux filter) has a dialysis clearance of 134 mL/min.[108,109] If the patient is properly hydrated, the volume of distribution for aminoglycosides is 0.26 L/kg. Hemodialysis procedures, such as ultrafiltration, can be used to assist in the maintenance of proper fluid balance in patients. Because kidneys provide fluid and electrolyte balance, it is not unusual for patients with renal failure receiving hemodialysis to be over- or underhydrated. As previously discussed in the renal failure section in the above paragraphs, body weight is an effective way to assess hydration status and can be used to adjust initial volume of distribution estimates.

Peritoneal dialysis is much less efficient in removing aminoglycosides from the body.[110-112] Peritoneal dialysis will decrease the half-life of aminoglycosides in a renal failure patient from about 50 hours to about 36 hours during the dialysis procedure. If the patient is receiving peritoneal dialysis on a chronic, ongoing basis, such as continuous ambulatory peritoneal dialysis (CAPD), aminoglycoside half-life will be shorter all of the time because of the additional dialysis clearance. Patients receiving continuous ambulatory peritoneal dialysis sometimes develop peritonitis that can be treated by adding aminoglycoside (or other) antibiotics to the peritoneal dialysis fluid. While about one-half of the intraperitoneal aminoglycoside dose is systemically absorbed during a 5- to 6-hour dwell time, if a patient with peritonitis develops secondary bacteremia, it may be necessary to use parenteral antibiotics to cure the infection.[110-112] Peritonitis causes inflammation of the peritoneal membrane, which facilitates absorption of aminoglycoside administered via dialysis fluid and elimination of aminoglycoside present in the body.

Continuous renal replacement therapy (CRRT) consists of a family of techniques that provides removal of toxic metabolic substances in patients with acute renal failure.[113-115] A large amount of variability exists in aminoglycoside removal depending on the type of CRRT used in a patient. Average hemofilter sieving coefficients for the aminoglycoside antibiotics are[116,117] gentamicin 0.81, tobramycin 0.90, netilmicin 0.93, and amikacin 0.95. Because continuous arteriovenous hemofiltration (CAVH) and continuous venovenous hemofiltration (CVVH) provide an average creatinine clearance of ~30 mL/min, this value is typically used to initiate therapy in patients. Then, aminoglycoside serum concentration monitoring is used to individualize dosing early in therapy.[53,118] Clearance rates for continuous venovenous hemodiafiltration (CVVHDF) are typically two to three times higher than hemofiltration (~60-90 mL/min).[119,120]

DRUG INTERACTIONS

Most important drug interactions are pharmacodynamic, and not pharmacokinetic, in nature. Vancomycin,[15,18,121] amphotericin B,[18] cyclosporin,[122] and furosemide[13,17,18] enhance the nephrotoxicity potential of the aminoglycosides. Each of these agents can cause nephrotoxicity when administered alone. When these drugs are administered concurrently with an aminoglycoside, serum creatinine concentrations should be monitored on a daily basis. Additionally, serum concentrations of vancomycin or cyclosporin, as well as the aminoglycoside, should be measured. Loop diuretics,[123,124] including furosemide, bumetanide, and ethacrynic acid, can cause ototoxicity, and an increased incidence of this adverse effect has been reported when aminoglycosides have been coadministered. If aminoglycoside antibiotics are administered with loop diuretics, clinical signs and symptoms of ototoxicity (auditory: decreased hearing acuity in the conversational range, feeling of fullness or pressure in the ears, tinnitus; vestibular: loss of equilibrium, headache, nausea, vomiting, nystagmus, vertigo, ataxia) should be monitored daily.

Aminoglycosides have intrinsic nondepolarizing neuromuscular blocking activity and may prolong the effects of neuromuscular blocking agents such as succinylcholine.[125] Surgical and intensive care patients receiving neuromuscular blockers and aminoglycosides should be monitored for this potential adverse effect. As previously discussed, penicillins (primarily penicillin G, ampicillin, nafcillin, carbenicillin, ticarcillin) can inactivate aminoglycosides in vivo and in blood specimen tubes intended for the measurement of aminoglycoside serum concentrations.[69-73] These two classes of drugs can also inactivate each other in intravenous administration bags and syringes, and they should not be mixed together.

INITIAL DOSAGE DETERMINATION METHODS

Several methods to initiate aminoglycoside therapy are available. The *Pharmacokinetic Dosing method* is the most flexible of the techniques. It allows for individualized target serum concentrations to be chosen for a patient, so it can be used for both conventional and extended-interval dosing. Also, each pharmacokinetic parameter can be customized to reflect specific disease states and conditions present in the patient. However, it is computationally intensive. The *Hull and Sarubbi nomogram* uses the dosing concepts in the Pharmacokinetic Dosing method. However, in order to simplify calculations, it makes simplifying assumptions: target concentration ranges consistent with conventional dosing only, fixed volume of distribution parameter in the normal range, limited dosage interval selection (no longer than 24 hours). Thus, it should be used only in patients who only have renal dysfunction and/or obesity as complicating factors and only when conventional dosing is to be used. The *Hartford nomogram* has similar strengths and weaknesses when compared to the Hull and Sarubbi nomogram, but it is designed for use when extended-interval dosing is desired. This nomogram also incorporates a method to adjust aminoglycoside doses based on serum concentration feedback. *Literature-based recommended dosing* is a commonly used method to prescribe initial doses of aminoglycosides to pediatric patients. Doses are based on those that commonly produce steady-state concentrations within the therapeutic range, although there is a wide variation in the actual concentrations for a specific patient.

Pharmacokinetic Dosing Method

The goal of initial dosing of aminoglycosides is to compute the best dose possible for the patient given their set of disease states and conditions that influence aminoglycoside pharmacokinetics and the site and severity of the infection. In order to do this, pharmacokinetic parameters for the patient will be estimated using average parameters measured in other patients with similar disease state and condition profiles (Table 4-1).

Elimination Rate Constant Estimate

Aminoglycosides are almost totally eliminated unchanged in the urine, and there is a good relationship between creatinine clearance and aminoglycoside elimination rate constant (see Figure 4-2). This relationship allows the estimation of the aminoglycoside elimination rate constant for a patient, which can be used to compute an initial dose of the antibiotic. Mathematically, the equation for the straight line shown in Figure 4-2 is: $k_e = 0.00293(CrCl) + 0.014$, where k_e is the aminoglycoside elimination rate constant in h^{-1} and CrCl is creatinine clearance in mL/min. A limitation in using elimination rate constant as the elimination parameter in this relationship is that it is a hybrid pharmacokinetic constant whose value can be influenced by either clearance or volume of distribution ($k_e = Cl/V$). Because gentamicin, tobramycin, netilmicin, and amikacin have similar pharmacokinetic properties, the same elimination rate constant versus creatinine clearance relationship can be used for all of the antibiotics. For example, the estimated elimination rate constant for an individual with a creatinine clearance of 10 mL/min is 0.043 h^{-1} which yields an estimated half-life of 16 hours [$k_e = 0.00293(CrCl) + 0.014 = 0.00293(10 \text{ mL/min}) + 0.014 = 0.043 \text{ h}^{-1}$; $t_{1/2} = 0.693/(0.043 \text{ h}^{-1}) = 16 \text{ h}$]. Taking the patient's renal function into account, when deriving initial doses of aminoglycoside antibiotics, is the single most important characteristic to assess. However, note that the relationship between k_e and renal function is based on CrCl and not estimated glomerular filtration rate (eGFR). Because eGFR is typically greater than CrCl, systematic errors can be made in the calculation of the aminoglycoside elimination rate for a patient if the correct renal function parameter is not selected.[126]

Volume of Distribution Estimate

The average volume of distribution for patients without disease states and conditions that change this parameter is 0.26 L/kg. Thus, for a nonobese 70-kg patient, the estimated volume of distribution would be 18.2 L ($V = 0.26 \text{ L/kg} \cdot 70 \text{ kg} = 18.2 \text{ L}$). If a patient weights less than their ideal body weight, actual body weight is used to estimate volume of distribution. For patients whose weight is between their ideal body weight and 30% over ideal weight, actual body weight can be used to compute estimated volume of distribution, although some clinicians prefer to use ideal body weight for these individuals. In patients who are more than 30% above their ideal body weight, volume of distribution (V) estimates should include both ideal and actual total body weights using the following equation: $V = 0.26[IBW + 0.4(TBW - IBW)]$, where V is in L, IBW is ideal body weight in kg, and TBW is total body weight in kg (see Figure 4-3). For an obese patient whose ideal body weight is 55 kg and total body weight is 95 kg, the estimated volume of distribution would be 18.5 L: $V = 0.26[IBW + 0.4(TBW - IBW)] = 0.26[55 \text{ kg} + 0.4(95 \text{ kg} - 55 \text{ kg})] = 18.5 \text{ L}$. In patients who are overhydrated or with ascites, their dry body weight (weight without the extra fluid) can be used to provide an improved volume of distribution estimate (V in L) using the following formula: $V = (0.26 \cdot DBW) + (TBW - DBW)$, where DBW is the patient's dry body weight and TBW is the patient's actual total body weight. For example, a patient with a significant of ascitic fluid currently weighs 80 kg. It is known from previous clinic visits and history that the patient usually weighs 70 kg without the additional fluid. The estimated volume of distribution for this patient would be 28.2 L: $V = (0.26 \cdot DBW) + (TBW - DBW) = (0.26 \cdot 70 \text{ kg}) + (80 \text{ kg} - 70 \text{ kg}) = 28.2$ L. Other disease states and conditions also influence aminoglycoside volume of distribution, and the values of this parameter given in Table 4-1 will be used when necessary. For instance, the average volume of distribution for cystic fibrosis patients is 0.35 L/kg. Therefore, the estimated volume of distribution for a 55-kg patient with cystic fibrosis is 19.3 L: $V = 0.35$ L/kg (55 kg) = 19.3 L.

Selection of Appropriate Pharmacokinetic Model and Equations

When given by intravenous injection over less than 1 hour, aminoglycosides follow a three-compartment pharmacokinetic model (Figure 4-4). After the end of infusion, serum concentrations drop rapidly because of distribution of drug from blood to tissues (α or distribution phase). If aminoglycosides are infused over 1 hour, the distribution phase is not usually observed. By about 1 hour after the beginning of the antibiotic infusion, drug concentrations decline more slowly, and the elimination rate constant for this segment of the concentration/time curve is the one that varies with renal function (β or elimination phase). Finally, at very low serum concentrations not detected by aminoglycoside concentration assays in clinical use (≤ 0.5 µg/mL), drug that was tissue-bound to various organs (especially the kidney) is released from tissue-binding sites and eliminated (γ or tissue-release phase). While this model was instrumental in advancing current ideas regarding aminoglycoside tissue accumulation and nephrotoxicity, it cannot easily be used clinically because of its mathematical complexity.[9-11,14,17] Because of this, the simpler one-compartment model is widely used and allows accurate dosage calculation.[2,3,36,60,61,63,64,127]

Intravenously administered aminoglycosides are given over ½-1 hour as intermittent continuous infusions. Because drug is eliminated during the infusion time (and any waiting time that is necessary to allow for distribution to finish), pharmacokinetic equations that take into account this loss are preferred in patients with

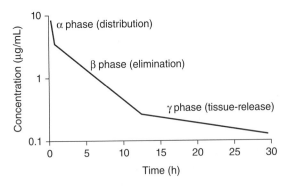

FIGURE 4-4   Multicompartment model characteristics of aminoglycosides. If aminoglycoside antibiotics are given as an intravenous bolus injection, the serum concentration/time curve declines in three distinct phases. The first phase (α or distribution phase) occurs as antibiotic in the blood distributes into tissues, although drug is also cleared from the blood during this time, too. The second phase (β or elimination phase) begins when blood and tissues are in near equilibrium, and the predominate process is elimination from the body. The half-life for this phase of the curve is dramatically influenced by the patient's renal function ($t_{1/2} = 2$ hours for normal renal function, $t_{1/2} = 50$ hours for renal failure). The final phase (γ or tissue-release phase) occurs at very low serum concentrations (<0.5 µg/mL) and represents the release of tissue-bound aminoglycoside into the blood where it will be cleared from the body.

good renal function. If this is not done, a large amount of drug may be eliminated during infusion and waiting periods, and the peak concentration will be miscalculated. Generally, infusion equations should be used if the patient has a creatinine clearance greater than 30 mL/min. For creatinine clearances of 30 mL/min or less, very little aminoglycoside is eliminated during infusion and waiting period times, and intravenous bolus equations accurately compute peak concentrations.[128] Aminoglycoside steady-state peak ($Cmax_{ss}$) and trough ($Cmin_{ss}$) serum concentrations are chosen to treat the patient based on the type, site, and severity of infection as well as the infecting organism. Steady-state versions of one-compartment model intermittent intravenous infusion $\{Cmax_{ss} = [k_0/(k_e V)][(1 - e^{-k_e t'})/(1 - e^{-k_e \tau})]$, $Cmin_{ss} = Cmax_{ss} e^{-[k_e(\tau - t')]}$, where k_0 is the infusion rate, k_e is the elimination rate constant, V is the volume of distribution, t' is the drug infusion time, and τ is the dosage interval} or intravenous bolus $\{Cmax_{ss} = (D/V)[e^{-k_e t}/(1 - e^{-k_e \tau})]$, $Cmin_{ss} = Cmax_{ss} e^{-k_e \tau}$, where D is the antibiotic dose, V is the volume of distribution, k_e is the elimination rate constant, t is the time $Cmax_{ss}$ was measured, and τ is the dosage interval} equations are chosen based on the patient's renal function to compute the required doses needed to achieve desired aminoglycoside concentrations. Note that intermittent intravenous infusion equations will work well regardless of the patient's creatinine clearance. However, the intravenous bolus equations are easier to solve, save time, and are less likely to invoke a computational error. Because of these reasons, some clinicians prefer this simpler approach.

Steady-State Concentration Selection

Aminoglycoside peak steady-state concentrations are selected based on site and severity of infection as well as the infecting organism. Severe infections, such as gram-negative pneumonia or septicemia, or infections with organisms that have a high minimum inhibitory concentration (MIC) such as *Pseudomonas aeruginosa* (typical MIC ≈ 2 µg/mL for gentamicin, tobramycin, or netilmicin), generally require peak steady-state serum concentrations of 8-10 µg/mL for gentamicin, tobramycin, or netilmicin or 25-30 µg/mL for amikacin when using conventional dosing. Moderate infections at sites that are easier to penetrate or with organisms that display lower MIC values, such as intra-abdominal infections, are usually treated with peak gentamicin, tobramycin, or netilmicin steady-state serum concentrations equal to 5-7 µg/mL or with amikacin peak steady-state serum concentrations equal to 15-25 µg/mL. When treating urinary tract infections due to susceptible organisms or using aminoglycosides for synergy in combination with penicillins or other antibiotics for the treatment of gram-positive infections such as infective endocarditis, steady-state peak concentrations of 3-4 µg/mL are usually adequate for gentamicin, tobramycin, or netilmicin or 12-15 µg/mL for amikacin. Pyelonephritis is considered a soft-tissue infection, not a urinary tract infection, and it requires higher peak steady-state concentrations to achieve a cure. Similar target peak steady-state concentrations for extended-interval aminoglycoside dosing are less established, although concentrations of 20-30 µg/mL for gentamicin, tobramycin, and netilmicin or 55-65 µg/mL for amikacin have been suggested for *Pseudomonas aeruginosa* and other serious infections, including pulmonary exacerbations in cystic fibrosis patients. These peak concentrations are designed to attain optimal C_{max}/MIC ratios that are 8-10 or greater. Desirable concentrations for steady-state trough concentrations are chosen based on avoidance of potential toxicity. For conventional dosing, steady-state trough concentrations should be maintained less than 2 µg/mL for tobramycin, gentamicin, and netilmicin or less than 5-7 µg/mL for amikacin. Using extended-interval dosing, steady-state trough concentrations should be less than 1 µg/mL for gentamicin, tobramycin, netilmicin, or amikacin.

Dosage Computation

The equations given in Table 4-2 are used to compute aminoglycoside doses depending on the renal function of the patient (intermittent intravenous infusion for any creatinine clearance value; if desired, intravenous bolus for creatinine clearances ≤30 mL/min may optionally be used).

TABLE 4-2A   One-Compartment Model Equations Used With Aminoglycoside Antibiotics

Route of Administration	Single Dose	Multiple Dose	Steady-State
Intravenous bolus	$C = (D/V)e^{-k_e t}$	$C = (D/V)e^{-k_e t}[(1 - e^{-nk_e \tau})/(1 - e^{-k_e \tau})]$	$C = (D/V)[e^{-k_e t}/(1 - e^{-k_e \tau})]$
Intermittent intravenous infusion	$C = [k_0/(k_e V)](1 - e^{-k_e t'})$	$C = [k_0/(k_e V)](1 - e^{-k_e t'})[(1 - e^{-nk_e \tau})/(1 - e^{-k_e \tau})]$	$C = [k_0/(k_e V)][(1 - e^{-k_e t'})/(1 - e^{-k_e \tau})]$

C, drug serum concentration at time = t; D, dose; k_0, infusion rate; k_e, elimination rate constant; n, number of administered doses; t', infusion time; τ, dosage interval; V, volume of distribution.

TABLE 4-2B   Pharmacokinetic Constant Computations Utilizing a One-Compartment Model Used With Aminoglycoside Antibiotics

Route of Administration	Single Dose	Multiple Dose	Steady-State
Intravenous bolus	$k_e = -(\ln C_1 - \ln C_2)/(t_1 - t_2)$	$k_e = -(\ln C_1 - \ln C_2)/(t_1 - t_2)$	$k_e = -(\ln C_1 - \ln C_2)/(t_1 - t_2)$
	$t_{1/2} = 0.693/k_e$	$t_{1/2} = 0.693/k_e$	$t_{1/2} = 0.693/k_e$
	$V = D/C_0$	$V = D/(C_0 - C_{predose})$	$V = D/(C_0 - C_{predose})$
	$Cl = k_e V$	$Cl = k_e V$	$Cl = k_e V$
Intermittent intravenous infusion	$k_e = -(\ln C_1 - \ln C_2)/(t_1 - t_2)$	$k_e = -(\ln C_1 - \ln C_2)/(t_1 - t_2)$	$k_e = -(\ln C_1 - \ln C_2)/(t_1 - t_2)$
	$t_{1/2} = 0.693/k_e$	$t_{1/2} = 0.693/k_e$	$t_{1/2} = 0.693/k_e$
	$V = [k_0(1 - e^{-k_e t'})]/\{k_e[C_{max} - (C_{predose} e^{-k_e t'})]\}$	$V = [k_0(1 - e^{-k_e t'})]/\{k_e[C_{max} - (C_{predose} e^{-k_e t'})]\}$	$V = [k_0(1 - e^{-k_e t'})]/\{k_e[C_{max} - (C_{predose} e^{-k_e t'})]\}$
	$Cl = k_e V$	$Cl = k_e V$	$Cl = k_e V$

C_0, concentration at time = 0; C_1, drug serum concentration at time = t_1; C_2, drug serum concentration at time = t_2; Cl, drug clearance; $C_{predose}$, predose concentration; D, dose; k_0, continuous infusion rate; k_e, elimination rate constant; $t_{1/2}$, half-life; t', infusion time; V, volume of distribution.

TABLE 4-2C   Equations Used to Compute Individualized Dosage Regimens for Various Routes of Administration Used With Aminoglycoside Antibiotics

Route of Administration	Dosage Interval (τ), Maintenance Dose (D or k_0), and Loading Dose (LD) Equations
Intravenous bolus	$\tau = (\ln Css_{max} - \ln Css_{min})/k_e$
	$D = Css_{max} V(1 - e^{-k_e \tau})$
	$LD = Css_{max} V$
Intermittent intravenous infusion	$\tau = [(\ln Css_{max} - \ln Css_{min})/k_e] + t'$
	$k_0 = Css_{max} k_e V[(1 - e^{-k_e \tau})/(1 - e^{-k_e t'})]$
	$LD = k_0/(1 - e^{-k_e \tau})$

Css_{min}, minimum steady-state concentration; Css_{max}, maximum steady-state concentration; k_0, continuous infusion rate; k_e, elimination rate constant; t', infusion time; V, volume of distribution.

EXAMPLE 1 ▶▶▶

JM is a 50-year-old, 70-kg (height = 5 ft 10 in) male with gram-negative pneumonia. His current serum creatinine is 0.9 mg/dL, and it has been stable over the last 5 days since admission. Compute a gentamicin dose for this patient using conventional dosing.

1. *Estimate creatinine clearance.*

    This patient has a stable serum creatinine and is not obese. The Cockcroft-Gault equation can be used to estimate creatinine clearance:

    $$CrCl_{est} = [(140 - age)BW]/(72 \cdot S_{Cr}) = [(140 - 50 \text{ y})70 \text{ kg}]/(72 \cdot 0.9 \text{ mg/dL})$$
    $$CrCl_{est} = 97 \text{ mL/min}$$

2. *Estimate elimination rate constant (k_e) and half-life ($t_{1/2}$).*

    The elimination rate constant versus creatinine clearance relationship is used to estimate the gentamicin elimination rate for this patient:

    $$k_e = 0.00293(CrCl) + 0.014 = 0.00293(97 \text{ mL/min}) + 0.014 = 0.298 \text{ h}^{-1}$$
    $$t_{1/2} = 0.693/k_e = 0.693/0.298 \text{ h}^{-1} = 2.3 \text{ h}$$

3. *Estimate volume of distribution (V).*

    The patient has no disease states or conditions that would alter the volume of distribution from the normal value of 0.26 L/kg:

    $$V = 0.26 \text{ L/kg } (70 \text{ kg}) = 18.2 \text{ L}$$

4. *Choose desired steady-state serum concentrations.*

    Gram-negative pneumonia patients treated with aminoglycoside antibiotics require steady-state peak concentrations ($Cmax_{ss}$) equal to 8–10 µg/mL; steady-state trough ($Cmin_{ss}$) concentrations should be less than 2 µg/mL to avoid toxicity. Set $Cmax_{ss} = 9$ µg/mL and $Cmin_{ss} = 1$ µg/mL.

5. *Use intermittent intravenous infusion equations to compute dose (see Table 4-2).*

    Calculate required dosage interval (τ), using a 1-hour infusion:

    $$\tau = [(\ln Css_{max} - \ln Css_{min})/k_e] + t' = [(\ln 9 \text{ µg/mL} - \ln 1 \text{ µg/mL})/0.298 \text{ h}^{-1}] + 1 \text{ h} = 8.4 \text{ h}$$

    Dosage intervals should be rounded to clinically acceptable intervals of 8, 12, 18, 24, 36, 48, and 72 hours, and multiples of 24 hours thereafter, whenever possible. In this case, the dosage interval would be rounded to 8 hours. Also, steady-state peak concentrations are similar if drawn immediately after a 1-hour infusion or ½ hour after a ½-hour infusion, so the dose could be administered either way.

    $$k_0 = Css_{max}k_eV[(1 - e^{-k_e\tau})/(1 - e^{-k_et'})]$$
    $$k_0 = (9 \text{ mg/L} \cdot 0.298 \text{ h}^{-1} \cdot 18.2 \text{ L}) \{[1 - e^{-(0.298 \text{ h}^{-1})(8 \text{ h})}]/[1 - e^{-(0.298 \text{ h}^{-1})(1 \text{ h})}]\} = 172 \text{ mg}$$

    Aminoglycoside doses should be rounded to the nearest 5-10 mg. This dose would be rounded to 170 mg. (Note: µg/mL = mg/L and this concentration unit was substituted for Css_{max} so that unnecessary unit conversion was not required.)

    The prescribed maintenance dose would be: 170 mg every 8 hours.

6. *Compute loading dose (LD), if needed.*

    Loading doses should be considered for patients with creatinine clearance values less than 60 mL/min. The administration of a loading dose in these patients will allow achievement of therapeutic peak concentrations quicker than if maintenance doses alone are given. However, because the pharmacokinetic parameters used to compute these initial doses are only *estimated* values and not *actual* values, the patient's own parameters may be much different than the estimated constants and steady state will not be achieved until 3-5 half-lives have passed.

    $$LD = k_0/(1 - e^{-k_e\tau}) = 170 \text{ mg}/[1 - e^{-(0.298 \text{ h}^{-1})(8 \text{ h})}] = 187 \text{ mg}$$

    As noted, this loading dose is only about 10% greater than the maintenance dose and would not be given to the patient. As the expected half-life is 2.3 hour, the patient should be at steady state after the second dose is given.

EXAMPLE 2 ▶ ▶ ▶

Same patient profile as in example 1, but serum creatinine is 3.5 mg/dL indicating renal impairment. *(Note: Intravenous bolus equations are used to illustrate differences with intermittent intravenous infusion equations.)*

1. *Estimate creatinine clearance.*
   This patient has a stable serum creatinine and is not obese. The Cockcroft-Gault equation can be used to estimate creatinine clearance:

   $$CrCl_{est} = [(140 - age)BW]/(72 \cdot S_{Cr}) = [(140 - 50 \text{ y})70 \text{ kg}]/(72 \cdot 3.5 \text{ mg/dL})$$
   $$CrCl_{est} = 25 \text{ mL/min}$$

2. *Estimate elimination rate constant (k_e) and half-life ($t_{1/2}$).*
   The elimination rate constant versus creatinine clearance relationship is used to estimate the gentamicin elimination rate for this patient:

   $$k_e = 0.00293(CrCl) + 0.014 = 0.00293(25 \text{ mL/min}) + 0.014 = 0.087 \text{ h}^{-1}$$
   $$t_{1/2} = 0.693/k_e = 0.693/0.087 \text{ h}^{-1} = 8 \text{ h}$$

3. *Estimate volume of distribution (V).*
   The patient has no disease states or conditions that would alter the volume of distribution from the normal value of 0.26 L/kg:

   $$V = 0.26 \text{ L/kg} (70 \text{ kg}) = 18.2 \text{ L}$$

4. *Choose desired steady-state serum concentrations.*
   Gram-negative pneumonia patients treated with aminoglycoside antibiotics require steady-state peak concentrations ($Cmax_{ss}$) equal to 8–10 µg/mL; steady-state trough ($Cmin_{ss}$) concentrations should be less than 2 µg/mL to avoid toxicity. Set $Cmax_{ss} = 9$ µg/mL and $Cmin_{ss} = 1$ µg/mL.

5. *Use intravenous bolus equations to compute dose (see Table 4-2).*
   Calculate required dosage interval (τ):

   $$\tau = [(\ln Css_{max} - \ln Css_{min})/k_e] = (\ln 9 \text{ µg/mL} - \ln 1 \text{ µg/mL})/0.087 \text{ h}^{-1} = 25 \text{ h}$$

   Dosage intervals should be rounded to clinically acceptable intervals of 8, 12, 18, 24, 36, 48, and 72 hours, and multiples of 24 hours thereafter, whenever possible. In this case, the dosage interval would be rounded to 24 hours. Also, steady-state peak concentrations are similar if drawn immediately after a 1-hour infusion or ½ hour after a ½-hour infusion, so the dose could be administered either way.

   $$D = Css_{max} V(1 - e^{-k_e \tau})$$
   $$D = 9 \text{ mg/L} \cdot 18.2 \text{ L}[1 - e^{-(0.087 \text{ h}^{-1})(24 \text{ h})}] = 143 \text{ mg}$$

   Aminoglycoside doses should be rounded to the nearest 5-10 mg. This dose would be rounded to 145 mg. (Note: µg/mL = mg/L and this concentration unit was substituted for Css_{max} so that unnecessary unit conversion was not required.)
   The prescribed maintenance dose would be: 145 mg every 24 hours.

   Note: Although this dose is given once daily, it is not extended-interval dosing because desired serum concentrations are within the conventional range.

6. *Compute loading dose (LD), if needed.*
   Loading doses should be considered for patients with creatinine clearance values less than 60 mL/min. The administration of a loading dose in these patients will allow achievement of therapeutic peak concentrations quicker than if maintenance doses alone are given. However, because the pharmacokinetic parameters used

to compute these initial doses are only *estimated* values and not *actual* values, the patient's own parameters may be much different than the estimated constants and steady state will not be achieved until 3-5 half-lives have passed.

$$LD = Css_{max} V = 9 \text{ mg/L} \cdot 18.2 \text{ L} = 164 \text{ mg}$$

Round loading dose to 165 mg. It would be given as the first dose. The next dose would be a maintenance dose given a dosage interval away from the loading dose, in this case 24 hours later.

EXAMPLE 3 ▶▶▶

ZW is a 35-year-old, 150-kg (height = 5 ft 5 in) female with an intra-abdominal infection. Her current serum creatinine is 1.1 mg/dL and is stable. Compute a tobramycin dose for this patient using conventional dosing.

1. *Estimate creatinine clearance.*

This patient has a stable serum creatinine and is obese [$IBW_{females}$ (in kg) = 45 + 2.3(Ht − 60) = 45 + 2.3(65 in − 60) = 57 kg]. The Salazar and Corcoran equation can be used to estimate creatinine clearance:

$$CrCl_{est(females)} = \frac{(146 - age)[(0.287 \cdot Wt) + (9.74 \cdot Ht^2)]}{(60 \cdot S_{Cr})}$$

$$CrCl_{est(females)} = \frac{(146 - 35 \text{ y})\{(0.287 \cdot 150 \text{ kg}) + [9.74 \cdot (1.65 \text{ m})^2]\}}{(60 \cdot 1.1 \text{ mg/dL})} = 117 \text{ mL/min}$$

Note: Height is converted from inches to meters: Ht = (65 in · 2.54 cm/in)/(100 cm/m) = 1.65 m.

2. *Estimate elimination rate constant (k_e) and half-life ($t_{1/2}$).*

The elimination rate constant versus creatinine clearance relationship is used to estimate the gentamicin elimination rate for this patient:

$$k_e = 0.00293(CrCl) + 0.014 = 0.00293(117 \text{ mL/min}) + 0.014 = 0.357 \text{ h}^{-1}$$

$$t_{1/2} = 0.693/k_e = 0.693/0.357 \text{ h}^{-1} = 1.9 \text{ h}$$

3. *Estimate volume of distribution (V).*

The patient is obese, so the volume of distribution would be estimated using the following formula:

$$V = 0.26[IBW + 0.4(TBW - IBW)] = 0.26[57 \text{ kg} + 0.4(150 \text{ kg} - 57 \text{ kg})] = 24.5 \text{ L}$$

4. *Choose desired steady-state serum concentrations.*

Intra-abdominal infection patients treated with aminoglycoside antibiotics require steady-state peak concentrations ($Cmax_{ss}$) equal to 5-7 µg/mL; steady-state trough ($Cmin_{ss}$) concentrations should be less than 2 µg/mL to avoid toxicity. Set $Cmax_{ss} = 6$ µg/mL and $Cmin_{ss} = 0.5$ µg/mL.

5. *Use intermittent intravenous infusion equations to compute dose (see Table 4-2).*

Calculate required dosage interval (τ) using a 1-hour infusion:

$$\tau = [(\ln Css_{max} - \ln Css_{min})/k_e] + t' = [(\ln 6 \text{ µg/mL} - \ln 0.5 \text{ µg/mL})/0.357 \text{ h}^{-1}] + 1 \text{ h} = 8 \text{ h}$$

Dosage intervals should be rounded to clinically acceptable intervals of 8, 12, 18, 24, 36, 48, and 72 hours, and multiples of 24 hours thereafter, whenever possible. In this case, the dosage interval is 8 hours. Also, steady-state peak concentrations are similar if drawn immediately after a 1-hour infusion or ½ hour after a ½-hour infusion, so the dose could be administered either way.

$$k_0 = Css_{max} k_e V[(1 - e^{-k_e \tau})/(1 - e^{-k_e t'})]$$

$$k_0 = (6 \text{ mg/L} \cdot 0.357 \text{ h}^{-1} \cdot 24.5 \text{ L})\{[1 - e^{-(0.357 \text{ h}^{-1})(8 \text{ h})}]/[1 - e^{-(0.357 \text{ h}^{-1})(1 \text{ h})}]\} = 165 \text{ mg}$$

Aminoglycoside doses should be rounded to the nearest 5-10 mg. This dose does not need to be rounded. (Note: μg/mL = mg/L and this concentration unit was substituted for Css_{max} so that unnecessary unit conversion was not required.)

The prescribed maintenance dose would be: 165 mg every 8 hours.

6. *Compute loading dose (LD), if needed.*
Loading doses should be considered for patients with creatinine clearance values less than 60 mL/min. The administration of a loading dose in these patients will allow achievement of therapeutic peak concentrations quicker than if maintenance doses alone are given. However, because the pharmacokinetic parameters used to compute these initial doses are only *estimated* values and not *actual* values, the patient's own parameters may be much different than the estimated constants and steady state will not be achieved until 3–5 half-lives have passed.

$$LD = k_0/(1 - e^{-k_e \tau}) = 165 \text{ mg}/[1 - e^{-(0.357 \text{ h}^{-1})(8 \text{ h})}] = 175 \text{ mg}$$

As noted, this loading dose is less than 10% greater than the maintenance dose and would not be given to the patient. Because the expected half-life is 1.9 hours, the patient should be at steady state after the second dose is given.

EXAMPLE 4 ▶ ▶ ▶

JM is a 20-year-old, 76-kg (height = 5 ft 8 in) male with a gram-negative pneumonia. His current serum creatinine is 1.1 mg/dL and is stable. Compute a tobramycin dose for this patient using extended-interval dosing.

1. *Estimate creatinine clearance.*
This patient has a stable serum creatinine and is not obese {IBW_{males} = 50 + 2.3(Ht − 60) = 50 + 2.3(68 in − 60) = 68 kg; % overweight = [100(76 kg − 68 kg)]/68 kg = 12%}. The Cockcroft-Gault equation can be used to estimate creatinine clearance:

$$CrCl_{est} = [(140 - age)BW]/(72 \cdot S_{Cr}) = [(140 - 20 \text{ y})76 \text{ kg}]/(72 \cdot 1.1 \text{ mg/dL})$$

$$CrCl_{est} = 115 \text{ mL/min}$$

2. *Estimate elimination rate constant (k_e) and half-life ($t_{1/2}$).*
The elimination rate constant versus creatinine clearance relationship is used to estimate the gentamicin elimination rate for this patient:

$$k_e = 0.00293(CrCl) + 0.014 = 0.00293(115 \text{ mL/min}) + 0.014 = 0.351 \text{ h}^{-1}$$

$$t_{1/2} = 0.693/k_e = 0.693/0.351 \text{ h}^{-1} = 2.0 \text{ h}$$

3. *Estimate volume of distribution (V).*
The patient has no disease states or conditions that would alter the volume of distribution from the normal value of 0.26 L/kg:

$$V = 0.26 \text{ L/kg} (76 \text{ kg}) = 19.8 \text{ L}$$

4. *Choose desired steady-state serum concentrations.*
Gram-negative pneumonia patients treated with extended-interval aminoglycoside antibiotics require steady-state peak concentrations ($Cmax_{ss}$) equal to 20-30 μg/mL; steady-state trough ($Cmin_{ss}$) concentrations should be less than 1 μg/mL to avoid toxicity. Set $Cmax_{ss}$ = 30 μg/mL and $Cmin_{ss}$ = 0.1 μg/mL.

5. *Use intermittent intravenous infusion equations to compute dose (see Table 4–2).*

Calculate required dosage interval (τ) using a 1-hour infusion:

$$\tau = [(\ln Css_{max} - \ln Css_{min})/k_e] + t' = [(\ln 30\ \mu g/mL - \ln 0.1\ \mu g/mL)/0.351\ h^{-1}] + 1\ h = 17.3\ h$$

Dosage intervals for extended-interval dosing should be rounded to clinically acceptable intervals of 24, 36, 48, 60, and 72 hours, and multiples of 24 hours thereafter, whenever possible. Some clinicians prefer to avoid the use of extended-interval dosing beyond a dosage interval of 48 hours because serum concentrations can be below the MIC far beyond the time frame afforded by the postantibiotic effect. For these situations, they revert to conventional dosing for the patient. In this case, the patient's dosage interval will be rounded to 24 hours. Because of this, the steady-state trough concentration would be expected to fall below 0.1 $\mu g/mL$. Also, steady-state peak concentrations are similar if drawn immediately after a 1-hour infusion or ½ hour after a ½-hour infusion, so the dose could be administered either way.

$$k_0 = Css_{max} k_e V[(1 - e^{-k_e \tau})/(1 - e^{-k_e t'})]$$
$$k_0 = (30\ mg/L \cdot 0.351\ h^{-1} \cdot 19.8\ L)\{[1 - e^{-(0.351\ h^{-1})(24\ h)}]/[1 - e^{-(0.351\ h^{-1})(1\ h)}]\} = 704\ mg$$

Aminoglycoside doses should be rounded to the nearest 10-50 mg for extended-interval dosing. This dose would be rounded to 700 mg. (Note: $\mu g/mL = mg/L$, and this concentration unit was substituted for Css_{max} so that unnecessary unit conversion was not required.)

The prescribed maintenance dose would be: 700 mg every 24 hours.

6. *Compute loading dose (LD), if needed.*

Loading doses should be considered for patients with creatinine clearance values less than 60 mL/min. The administration of a loading dose in these patients will allow achievement of therapeutic peak concentrations quicker than if maintenance doses alone are given. However, because the pharmacokinetic parameters used to compute these initial doses are only *estimated* values and not *actual* values, the patient's own parameters may be much different than the estimated constants and steady state will not be achieved until 3–5 half-lives have passed.

$$LD = k_0/(1 - e^{-k_e \tau}) = 700\ mg/[1 - e^{-(0.351\ h^{-1})(24\ h)}] = 700\ mg$$

As noted, this loading dose is less than 10% greater than the maintenance dose and would not be given to the patient. Because the expected half-life is 2.0 hours, the patient should be at steady state after the first dose is given.

EXAMPLE 5 ▶▶▶

JM is an 80-year-old, 80-kg (height = 5 ft 8 in) male with Streptococcus viridans endocarditis. His current serum creatinine is 1.5 mg/dL, and it has been stable. Ampicillin and gentamicin will be used to treat the infection. Compute a gentamicin dose for this patient using conventional dosing.

1. *Estimate creatinine clearance.*

This patient has a stable serum creatinine and is not obese {$IBW_{males} = 50 + 2.3(Ht - 60) = 50 + 2.3(68\ in - 60) = 68$ kg; % overweight = [100(80 − 68 kg)]/68 kg = 18%}. The Cockcroft-Gault equation can be used to estimate creatinine clearance:

$$CrCl_{est} = [(140 - age)BW]/(72 \cdot S_{Cr}) = [(140 - 80\ y)80\ kg]/(72 \cdot 1.5\ mg/dL)$$

$$CrCl_{est} = 44\ mL/min$$

2. *Estimate elimination rate constant (k_e) and half-life ($t_{1/2}$).*
The elimination rate constant versus creatinine clearance relationship is used to estimate the gentamicin elimination rate for this patient:

$$k_e = 0.00293(CrCl) + 0.014 = 0.00293(44 \text{ mL/min}) + 0.014 = 0.143 \text{ h}^{-1}$$
$$t_{1/2} = 0.693/k_e = 0.693/0.143 \text{ h}^{-1} = 4.8 \text{ h}$$

3. *Estimate volume of distribution (V).*
The patient has no disease states or conditions that would alter the volume of distribution from the normal value of 0.26 L/kg:

$$V = 0.26 \text{ L/kg } (80 \text{ kg}) = 20.8 \text{ L}$$

4. *Choose desired steady-state serum concentrations.*
S. viridans endocarditis patients treated with aminoglycoside antibiotics require steady-state peak concentrations ($Cmax_{ss}$) equal to 3-4 µg/mL; steady-state trough ($Cmin_{ss}$) concentrations should be less than 2 µg/mL to avoid toxicity. Set $Cmax_{ss} = 4$ µg/mL and $Cmin_{ss} = 1$ µg/mL.

5. *Use intermittent intravenous infusion equations to compute dose (see Table 4-2).*
Calculate required dosage interval (τ) using a 1-hour infusion:

$$\tau = [(\ln Css_{max} - \ln Css_{min})/k_e] + t' = [(\ln 4 \text{ µg/mL} - \ln 1 \text{ µg/mL})/0.143 \text{ h}^{-1}] + 1 \text{ h} = 11 \text{ h}$$

Dosage intervals should be rounded to clinically acceptable intervals of 8, 12, 18, 24, 36, 48, and 72 hours, and multiples of 24 hours thereafter, whenever possible. In this case, the dosage interval would be rounded to 12 hours. Also, steady-state peak concentrations are similar if drawn immediately after a 1-hour infusion or ½ hour after a ½-hour infusion, so the dose could be administered either way.

$$k_0 = Css_{max} k_e V[(1 - e^{-k_e\tau})/(1 - e^{-k_e t'})]$$
$$k_0 = (4 \text{ mg/L} \cdot 0.143 \text{ h}^{-1} \cdot 20.8 \text{ L})\{[1 - e^{-(0.143 \text{ h}^{-1})(12 \text{ h})}]/[1 - e^{-(0.143 \text{ h}^{-1})(1 \text{ h})}]\} = 73 \text{ mg}$$

Aminoglycoside doses should be rounded to the nearest 5-10 mg. This dose would be rounded to 70 mg. (Note: µg/mL = mg/L, and this concentration unit was substituted for Css_{max} so that unnecessary unit conversion was not required.)
The prescribed maintenance dose would be: 70 mg every 12 hours.
Because the patient is receiving concurrent treatment with ampicillin, care would be taken to avoid in vitro inactivation in blood sample tubes intended for the determination of aminoglycoside serum concentrations.

6. *Compute loading dose (LD), if needed.*
Loading doses should be considered for patients with creatinine clearance values less than 60 mL/min. The administration of a loading dose in these patients will allow achievement of therapeutic peak concentrations quicker than if maintenance doses alone are given. However, because the pharmacokinetic parameters used to compute these initial doses are only *estimated* values and not *actual* values, the patient's own parameters may be much different than the estimated constants and steady state will not be achieved until 3–5 half-lives have passed.

$$LD = k_0/(1 - e^{-k_e\tau}) = 70 \text{ mg}/[1 - e^{-(0.143 \text{ h}^{-1})(12 \text{ h})}] = 85 \text{ mg}$$

The loading dose would be given as the first dose. The next dose would be a maintenance dose given a dosage interval away from the loading dose, in this case 12 hours later.

EXAMPLE 6 ▶ ▶ ▶

Same patient profile as in example 2, but extended-interval dosing is used.

1. *Estimate creatinine clearance.*

This patient has a stable serum creatinine and is not obese. The Cockcroft-Gault equation can be used to estimate creatinine clearance:

$$CrCl_{est} = [(140 - age)BW]/(72 \cdot S_{Cr}) = [(140 - 50 \text{ y})70 \text{ kg}]/(72 \cdot 3.5 \text{ mg/dL})$$

$$CrCl_{est} = 25 \text{ mL/min}$$

2. *Estimate elimination rate constant (k_e) and half-life ($t_{1/2}$).*

The elimination rate constant versus creatinine clearance relationship is used to estimate the gentamicin elimination rate for this patient:

$$k_e = 0.00293(CrCl) + 0.014 = 0.00293(25 \text{ mL/min}) + 0.014 = 0.087 \text{ h}^{-1}$$

$$t_{1/2} = 0.693/k_e = 0.693/0.087 \text{ h}^{-1} = 8 \text{ h}$$

3. *Estimate volume of distribution (V).*

The patient has no disease states or conditions that would alter the volume of distribution from the normal value of 0.26 L/kg:

$$V = 0.26 \text{ L/kg} (70 \text{ kg}) = 18.2 \text{ L}$$

4. *Choose desired steady-state serum concentrations.*

Gram-negative pneumonia patients treated with aminoglycoside antibiotics require steady-state peak concentrations ($Cmax_{ss}$) of more than 20 µg/mL; steady-state trough ($Cmin_{ss}$) concentrations should be less than 1 µg/mL to avoid toxicity. Set $Cmax_{ss} = 20$ µg/mL and $Cmin_{ss} = 0.5$ µg/mL.

5. *Use intermittent intravenous infusion equations to compute dose (see Table 4–2).*

Calculate required dosage interval (τ):

$$\tau = [(\ln Css_{max} - \ln Css_{min})/k_e] = (\ln 20 \text{ µg/mL} - \ln 0.5 \text{ µg/mL})/0.087 \text{ h}^{-1} = 42 \text{ h}$$

Dosage intervals for extended-interval dosing should be rounded to clinically acceptable intervals of 24, 36, 48, 60, and 72 hours, and multiples of 24 hours thereafter, whenever possible. Some clinicians prefer to avoid the use of extended-interval dosing beyond a dosage interval of 48 hours because serum concentrations can be below the MIC far beyond the time frame afforded by the postantibiotic effect. For these situations, they revert to conventional dosing for the patient. In this case, the dosage interval would be rounded to 48 hours. Also, steady-state peak concentrations are similar if drawn immediately after a 1-hour infusion or ½ hour after a ½-hour infusion, so the dose could be administered either way.

$$D = Css_{max} V(1 - e^{-k_e\tau})$$

$$D = 20 \text{ mg/L} \cdot 18.2 \text{ L}[1 - e^{-(0.087 \text{ h}^{-1})(48 \text{ h})}] = 358 \text{ mg}$$

For extended-interval dosing, aminoglycoside doses should be rounded to the nearest 10–50 mg. This dose would be rounded to 350 mg. (Note: µg/mL = mg/L and this concentration unit was substituted for Css_{max} so that unnecessary unit conversion was not required.)

The prescribed maintenance dose would be: 350 mg every 48 hours.

6. *Compute loading dose (LD), if needed.*

Loading doses should be considered for patients with creatinine clearance values less than 60 mL/min. The administration of a loading dose in these patients will allow achievement of therapeutic peak concentrations quicker than if maintenance doses alone are given. However, because the pharmacokinetic parameters used to compute these initial doses are only *estimated* values and not *actual* values, the patient's own parameters may be much different than the estimated constants and steady state will not be achieved until 3-5 half-lives have passed.

$$LD = Css_{max} V = 20 \text{ mg/L} \cdot 18.2 \text{ L} = 364 \text{ mg}$$

As noted, this loading dose is about 10% greater than the maintenance dose and would not be given to the patient. Because the expected half-life is 8 hours, the patient should be at steady state after the first dose is given.

EXAMPLE 7 ▶ ▶ ▶

DQ is a 20-year-old, 61-kg (height = 5 ft 8 in) male with a pulmonary exacerbation due to cystic fibrosis. His current serum creatinine is 0.7 mg/dL and is stable. Compute a tobramycin dose for this patient using extended-interval dosing.

1. *Estimate creatinine clearance.*
   This patient has a stable serum creatinine and is not obese. The Cockcroft-Gault equation can be used to estimate creatinine clearance:

$$CrCl_{est} = [(140 - age)BW]/(72 \cdot S_{Cr}) = [(140 - 20 \text{ y}) 61 \text{ kg}]/(72 \cdot 0.7 \text{ mg/dL})$$
$$CrCl_{est} = 145 \text{ mL/min}$$

2. *Estimate elimination rate constant (k_e) and half-life ($t_{1/2}$).*
   The elimination rate constant versus creatinine clearance relationship is used to estimate the gentamicin elimination rate for this patient:

$$k_e = 0.00293(CrCl) + 0.014 = 0.00293(145 \text{ mL/min}) + 0.014 = 0.439 \text{ h}^{-1}$$
$$t_{1/2} = 0.693/k_e = 0.693/0.439 \text{ h}^{-1} = 1.6 \text{ h}$$

3. *Estimate volume of distribution (V).*
   The patient has cystic fibrosis, so the volume of distribution equals 0.35 L/kg:

$$V = 0.35 \text{ L/kg} (61 \text{ kg}) = 21.4 \text{ L}$$

4. *Choose desired steady-state serum concentrations.*
   Cystic fibrosis patients treated with extended-interval aminoglycoside antibiotics require steady-state peak concentrations ($Cmax_{ss}$) equal to 20-30 µg/mL; steady-state trough ($Cmin_{ss}$) concentrations should be less than 1 µg/mL to avoid toxicity. Set $Cmax_{ss} = 30$ µg/mL and $Cmin_{ss} = 0.01$ µg/mL.

5. *Use intermittent intravenous infusion equations to compute dose (see Table 4-2).*
   Calculate required dosage interval (τ) using a 1-hour infusion:

$$\tau = [(\ln Css_{max} - \ln Css_{min})/k_e] + t' = [(\ln 30 \text{ µg/mL} - \ln 0.01 \text{ µg/mL})/0.439 \text{ h}^{-1}] + 1 \text{ h} = 19.2 \text{ h}$$

Dosage intervals for extended-interval dosing should be rounded to clinically acceptable intervals of 24, 36, 48, 60, and 72 hours, and multiples of 24 hours thereafter, whenever possible. Some clinicians prefer to avoid the use of extended-interval dosing beyond a dosage interval of 48 hours because serum concentrations can be below the MIC far beyond the time frame afforded by the postantibiotic effect. For these situations, they revert to conventional dosing for the patient. In this case, the patient's dosage interval will be rounded to 24 hours. Because of this, the steady-state trough concentration would be expected to fall below 0.01 µg/mL. Also, steady-state peak concentrations are similar if drawn immediately after a 1-hour infusion or ½ hour after a ½-hour infusion, so the dose could be administered either way.

$$k_0 = Css_{max}k_eV[(1 - e^{-k_e\tau})/(1 - e^{-k_e t'})]$$

$$k_0 = (30 \text{ mg/L} \cdot 0.439 \text{ h}^{-1} \cdot 21.4 \text{ L})\{[1 - e^{-(0.439 \text{ h}^{-1})(24 \text{ h})}]/[1 - e^{-(0.439 \text{ h}^{-1})(1 \text{ h})}]\} = 793 \text{ mg}$$

Aminoglycoside doses should be rounded to the nearest 10–50 mg for extended-interval dosing. This dose would be rounded to 800 mg. (Note: μg/mL = mg/L, and this concentration unit was substituted for Css_{max} so that unnecessary unit conversion was not required.)

The prescribed maintenance dose would be: 800 mg every 24 hours.

6. *Compute loading dose (LD), if needed.*

Loading doses should be considered for patients with creatinine clearance values less than 60 mL/min. The administration of a loading dose in these patients will allow achievement of therapeutic peak concentrations quicker than if maintenance doses alone are given. However, because the pharmacokinetic parameters used to compute these initial doses are only *estimated* values and not *actual* values, the patient's own parameters may be much different than the estimated constants and steady state will not be achieved until 3–5 half-lives have passed.

$$LD = k_0/(1 - e^{-k_e\tau}) = 800 \text{ mg}/[1 - e^{-(0.439 \text{ h}^{-1})(24 \text{ h})}] = 800 \text{ mg}$$

As noted, this loading dose is within 10% of the maintenance dose and would not be given to the patient. Because the expected half-life is 1.6 hours, the patient should be at steady state after the first dose is given.

Hull and Sarubbi Nomogram Method

For patients who do not have disease states or conditions that alter volume of distribution, the only two patient-specific factors that change when using the Pharmacokinetic Dosing method is patient weight and creatinine clearance. Because of this, it is possible to make a simple nomogram to handle uncomplicated patients with a standard volume of distribution (Table 4-3). The Hull and Sarubbi aminoglycoside dosing nomogram is a quick and efficient way to apply pharmacokinetic dosing concepts without using complicated pharmacokinetic equations.[60,61] With a simple modification, it can also be used for obese patients. If the patient is greater than or equal to 30% above ideal body weight, an adjusted body weight (ABW) can be calculated and used as the weight factor [ABW (in kg) = IBW + 0.4(TBW – IBW), where IBW is ideal body weight in kg and TBW is actual total body weight in kg].[74-76] As can be seen, this equation is derived from the computation for volume of distribution in obese patients. Also, the Salazar and Corcoran method of estimating creatinine clearance in obese patients should be used to compute renal function in these individuals.[129-132]

Steady-state peak concentrations are selected as discussed in the Pharmacokinetic Dosing method section and used to determine a loading dose from the nomogram (see Table 4-3). Logically, lower loading doses produce lower expected peak concentrations, and higher loading doses result in higher expected peak concentrations. Once the loading dose is found, the patient's creatinine clearance is used to estimate the half-life, dosage interval, and maintenance dose (as a percent of the administered loading dose). The maintenance dose supplied by the nomogram is the percent of the loading dose that was eliminated during the different dosage interval time frames, and will, therefore, provide the same estimated peak concentration at steady state as that supplied by the loading dose. To illustrate how the nomogram is used, the same conventional-dosing patient examples used in the previous section will be repeated for this dosage approach using the same example number. Because the nomogram uses slightly different estimates for volume of distribution and elimination rate constant, some minor differences in suggested doses are expected. Because the cystic fibrosis example requires a different volume of distribution (0.35 L/kg), the Hull and Sarubbi nomogram cannot be used.

TABLE 4-3   Aminoglycoside Dosage Chart (Adapted From Sarubbi and Hull[60])

1. Compute patient's creatinine clearance (CrCl) using Cockcroft-Gault method: $CrCl = [(140 - age)BW]/(Scr \times 72)$. Multiply by 0.85 for females. Use Salazar-Cocoran method if weight > 30% over IBW.
2. Use patient's weight if within 30% of IBW; otherwise use adjusted dosing weight = IBW + [0.40(TBW − IBW)].
3. Select loading dose in mg/kg to provide peak serum concentrations in range listed below for the desired aminoglycoside antibiotic:

Aminoglycoside	Usual Loading Doses (mg/kg)	Expected Peak Serum Concentrations (µg/mL)
Tobramycin Gentamicin Netilmicin	1.5-2.0	4-10
Amikacin Kanamycin	5.0-7.5	15-30

4. Select Maintenance Dose (as percentage of loading dose) to continue peak serum concentrations indicated above according to desired dosage interval and the patient's creatinine clearance. To maintain usual peak/trough ratio, use dosage intervals in clear areas. *Note: Dosing for patients with CrCl ≤ 10 mL/min should be assisted by measuring serum concentrations

Percentage of Loading Dose Required for Dosage Interval Selected

CrCl (mL/min)	Est. Half-Life (h)	8 h	12 h	24 h
>90	2–3	90%	—	—
90	3.1	84	—	—
80	3.4	80	91%	—
70	3.9	76	88	—
60	4.5	71	84	—
50	5.3	65	79	—
40	6.5	57	72	92%
30	8.4	48	63	86
25	9.9	43	57	81
20	11.9	37	50	75
17	13.6	33	46	70
15	15.1	31	42	67
12	17.9	27	37	61
10*	20.4	24	34	56
7*	25.9	19	28	47
5*	31.5	16	23	41
2*	46.8	11	16	30
0*	69.3	8	11	21

EXAMPLE 1 ▶ ▶ ▶

JM is a 50-year-old, 70-kg (height = 5 ft 10 in) male with gram-negative pneumonia. His current serum creatinine is 0.9 mg/dL, and it has been stable over the last 5 days since admission. Compute a gentamicin dose for this patient using conventional dosing.

1. *Estimate creatinine clearance.*

   This patient has a stable serum creatinine and is not obese. The Cockcroft-Gault equation can be used to estimate creatinine clearance:

   $$CrCl_{est} = [(140 - age)BW]/(72 \cdot S_{Cr}) = [(140 - 50 \text{ y})70 \text{ kg}]/(72 \cdot 0.9 \text{ mg/dL})$$
   $$CrCl_{est} = 97 \text{ mL/min}$$

2. *Choose desired steady-state serum concentrations.*

   Gram-negative pneumonia patients treated with aminoglycoside antibiotics require steady-state peak concentrations ($Cmax_{ss}$) equal to 8-10 µg/mL.

3. *Select loading dose (see Table 4-3).*

   A loading dose (LD) of 2 mg/kg will provide a peak concentration of 8–10 µg/mL.

   $$LD = 2 \text{ mg/kg}(70 \text{ kg}) = 140 \text{ mg}$$

4. *Determine estimated half-life, maintenance dose, and dosage interval.*

   From the nomogram the estimated half-life is 2-3 hours, the maintenance dose (MD) is 90% of the loading dose [MD = 0.90(140 mg) = 126 mg], and the dosage interval is 8 hours.

   Aminoglycoside doses should be rounded to the nearest 5-10 mg. Steady-state peak concentrations are similar if drawn immediately after a 1-hour infusion or ½ hour after a ½-hour infusion, so the dose could be administered either way.

   The prescribed maintenance dose would be: 125 mg every 8 hours.

EXAMPLE 2 ▶ ▶ ▶

Same patient profile as in example 1, but serum creatinine is 3.5 mg/dL indicating renal impairment.

1. *Estimate creatinine clearance.*

   This patient has a stable serum creatinine and is not obese. The Cockcroft-Gault equation can be used to estimate creatinine clearance:

   $$CrCl_{est} = [(140 - age)BW]/(72 \cdot S_{Cr}) = [(140 - 50 \text{ y})70 \text{ kg}]/(72 \cdot 3.5 \text{ mg/dL})$$
   $$CrCl_{est} = 25 \text{ mL/min}$$

2. *Choose desired steady-state serum concentrations.*

   Gram-negative pneumonia patients treated with aminoglycoside antibiotics require steady-state peak concentrations ($Cmax_{ss}$) equal to 8-10 µg/mL.

3. *Select loading dose (see Table 4-3).*

   A loading dose (LD) of 2 mg/kg will provide a peak concentration of 8-10 µg/mL.

   $$LD = 2 \text{ mg/kg}(70 \text{ kg}) = 140 \text{ mg}$$

4. *Determine estimated half-life, maintenance dose, and dosage interval.*

   From the nomogram the estimated half-life is 9.9 hours, the maintenance dose (MD) is 81% of the loading dose [MD = 0.81(140 mg) = 113 mg], and the dosage interval is 24 hours. Note: Because of the $Cmax_{ss}$ and $Cmin_{ss}$ chosen for this patient, the 24-hour dosage interval is used to allow enough time to attain target concentrations.

   Aminoglycoside doses should be rounded to the nearest 5-10 mg. Steady-state peak concentrations are similar if drawn immediately after a 1-hour infusion or ½ hour after a ½-hour infusion, so the dose could be administered either way.

   The prescribed maintenance dose would be: 115 mg every 24 hours.

EXAMPLE 3 ▶ ▶ ▶

ZW is a 35-year-old, 150-kg (height = 5 ft 5 in) female with an intra-abdominal infection. Her current serum creatinine is 1.1 mg/dL and is stable. Compute a tobramycin dose for this patient using conventional dosing.

1. *Estimate creatinine clearance.*
   This patient has a stable serum creatinine and is obese [IBW$_{females}$ (in kg) = 45 + 2.3(Ht − 60) = 45 + 2.3 (65 in − 60) = 57 kg]. The Salazar and Corcoran equation can be used to estimate creatinine clearance:

$$CrCl_{est(females)} = \frac{(146 - age)[(0.287 \cdot Wt) + (9.74 \cdot Ht^2)]}{(60 \cdot S_{Cr})}$$

$$CrCl_{est(females)} = \frac{(146 - 35 \text{ y})\{(0.287 \cdot 150 \text{ kg}) + [9.74 \cdot (1.65 \text{ m})^2]\}}{(60 \cdot 1.1 \text{ mg/dL})} = 117 \text{ mL/min}$$

   Note: Height is converted from inches to meters: Ht = (65 in · 2.54 cm/in)/(100 cm/m) = 1.65 m.

2. *Choose desired steady-state serum concentrations.*
   Intra-abdominal infection patients treated with aminoglycoside antibiotics require steady-state peak concentrations (Cmax$_{ss}$) equal to 5-7 µg/mL.

3. *Select loading dose (see Table 4-3).*
   A loading dose (LD) of 1.7 mg/kg will provide a peak concentration of 5-7 µg/mL.
   Because the patient is obese, adjusted body weight (ABW) will be used to compute the dose:

$$ABW = IBW + 0.4(TBW - IBW) = 57 \text{ kg} + 0.4(150 \text{ kg} - 57 \text{ kg}) = 94 \text{ kg}$$

$$LD = 1.7 \text{ mg/kg}(94 \text{ kg}) = 160 \text{ mg}$$

4. *Determine estimated half-life, maintenance dose, and dosage interval.*
   From the nomogram the estimated half-life is 2-3 hours, the maintenance dose (MD) is 90% of the loading dose [MD = 0.90(160 mg) = 144 mg], and the dosage interval is 8 hours.
   Aminoglycoside doses should be rounded to the nearest 5-10 mg. Steady-state peak concentrations are similar if drawn immediately after a 1-hour infusion or ½ hour after a ½-hour infusion, so the dose could be administered either way.
   The prescribed maintenance dose would be: 145 mg every 8 hours.

EXAMPLE 4 ▶ ▶ ▶

JM is an 80-year-old, 80-kg (height = 5 ft 8 in) male with S. viridans endocarditis. His current serum creatinine is 1.5 mg/dL, and it has been stable. Ampicillin and gentamicin will be used to treat the infection. Compute a gentamicin dose for this patient using conventional dosing.

1. *Estimate creatinine clearance.*
   This patient has a stable serum creatinine and is not obese [IBW$_{males}$ = 50 + 2.3(Ht − 60) = 50 + 2.3(68 in − 60) = 68 kg; % overweight = [100(80 kg − 68 kg)]/68 kg = 18%}. The Cockcroft-Gault equation can be used to estimate creatinine clearance:

$$CrCl_{est} = [(140 - age)BW]/(72 \cdot S_{Cr}) = [(140 - 80 \text{ y})80 \text{ kg}]/(72 \cdot 1.5 \text{ mg/dL})$$

$$CrCl_{est} = 44 \text{ mL/min}$$

2. *Choose desired steady-state serum concentrations.*

S. viridans endocarditis patients treated with aminoglycoside antibiotics require steady-state peak concentrations ($Cmax_{ss}$) equal to 3-4 µg/mL.

3. *Select loading dose (see Table 4-3).*

A loading dose (LD) of 1.5 mg/kg will provide a peak concentration of 5-7 µg/mL. This is the lowest dose suggested by the nomogram and will be used in this example. However, some clinicians may substitute a loading dose of 1-1.2 mg/kg designed to produce a steady-state peak concentration equal to 3-4 µg/mL.

$$LD = 1.5 \text{ mg/kg } (80 \text{ kg}) = 120 \text{ mg or } LD = 1.2 \text{ mg/kg } (80 \text{ kg}) = 96 \text{ mg, rounded to 95 mg}$$

4. *Determine estimated half-life, maintenance dose, and dosage interval.*

From the nomogram the estimated half-life is 6.5 hours, suggesting that a 12 hour dosage interval is appropriate. The maintenance dose (MD) is 72% of the loading dose [MD = 0.72(120 mg) = 86 mg or MD = 0.72 (95 mg) = 68 mg], and the dosage interval is 12 hours.

Aminoglycoside doses should be rounded to the nearest 5-10 mg. Steady-state peak concentrations are similar if drawn immediately after a 1-hour infusion or ½ hour after a ½-hour infusion, so the dose could be administered either way.

The prescribed maintenance dose would be: 85 mg every 12 hours or 70 mg every 12 hours, depending on the loading dose chosen.

Because the patient is receiving concurrent treatment with ampicillin, care would be taken to avoid in vitro inactivation in blood sample tubes intended for the determination of aminoglycoside serum concentrations.

Hartford Nomogram Method for Extended-Interval Dosing

Extended-interval dosing is now the mainstream method used to administer aminoglycoside antibiotics. Conventional dosing is still preferred for endocarditis patients because the aminoglycoside is usually used for antibiotic synergy. Extended-interval doses obtained from the literature for patients with normal renal function are 4-7 mg/kg/d for gentamicin, tobramycin, or netilmicin and 11-20 mg/kg/d for amikacin.[3,24,29-35,47-53] The most-widely used extended-interval aminoglycoside dosage nomogram for patients with renal dysfunction is the Hartford nomogram which uses a 7-mg/kg dose (Table 4-4).[3] This nomogram is designed to achieve an optimal C_{max}/MIC of more than 10 for serious gram-negative infections (bacterial MIC ≈ 2 µg/mL, C_{max} ≈ 20-30 µg/mL). Because the nomogram is essentially the concentration-time graph for gentamicin after a single dose of 7 mg/kg, it cannot be used for other dosage rates. The initial dose is 7 mg/kg of gentamicin (although it was not derived using tobramycin or netilmicin, because of the pharmacokinetic similarity among the antibiotics it should be possible to use these aminoglycosides as well). The dosage interval is set according to the patient's creatinine clearance (see Table 4-4).

The Hartford nomogram includes a method to adjust doses based on gentamicin serum concentrations. This portion of the nomogram contains average serum concentration/time lines for gentamicin in patients with creatinine clearances of 60 mL/min, 40 mL/min, and 20 mL/min. A gentamicin serum concentration is measured 6-14 hours after the first dose is given, and this concentration/time point is plotted on the graph (see Table 4-4). The suggested dosage interval is indicated by which zone the serum concentration/time point falls in. To illustrate how the nomogram is used, the same patient examples utilized in the pharmacokinetic dosing section will be repeated for this dosage approach using the same example number. Because the cystic fibrosis example requires a different volume of distribution (0.35 L/kg) and extended-interval dosing has not been adequately tested in patients with endocarditis, the Hartford nomogram should not be used in these situations.

TABLE 4–4   Hartford Nomogram for Extended Interval Aminoglycosides (Adapted from Nicolau et al[3])

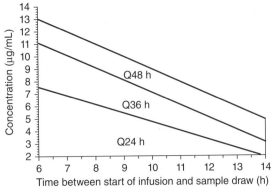

1. Administer 7 mg/kg gentamicin or tobramycin with initial dosage interval:

Estimated CrCl (mL/min)	Initial Dosage Interval
≥60	q24h
40–59	q36h
20–39	q48h
<20	Monitor serial concentrations & administer next dose when <1 µg/mL

2. Obtain timed serum concentration, 6-14 hours after dose (ideally first dose).
3. Alter dosage interval to that indicated by the nomogram zone (above q48h zone, monitor serial concentrations and administer next dose when <1 µg/mL).

Note: Refer to original nomogram for actual patient dosing.

EXAMPLE 1 ▶ ▶ ▶

JM is a 50-year-old, 70-kg (height = 5 ft 10 in) male with gram-negative pneumonia. His current serum creatinine is 0.9 mg/dL, and it has been stable over the last 5 days since admission. Compute a gentamicin dose for this patient using conventional dosing.

1. *Estimate creatinine clearance.*

   This patient has a stable serum creatinine and is not obese. The Cockcroft-Gault equation can be used to estimate creatinine clearance:

   $$CrCl_{est} = [(140 - age)BW]/(72 \cdot S_{Cr}) = [(140 - 50 \text{ y})70 \text{ kg}]/(72 \cdot 0.9 \text{ mg/dL})$$

   $$CrCl_{est} = 97 \text{ mL/min}$$

2. *Compute initial dose and dosage interval (see Table 4-4).*

   A dose (D) of 7 mg/kg will provide a peak concentration of more than 20 µg/mL.

   $$D = 7 \text{ mg/kg} (70 \text{ kg}) = 490 \text{ mg}$$

   Dosage interval would be 24 hours using the nomogram. Extended-interval aminoglycoside doses should be rounded to the nearest 10-50 mg.

   The prescribed maintenance dose would be: 500 mg every 24 hours.

3. *Determine dosage interval using serum concentration monitoring.*

A gentamicin serum concentration measured 10 hours after the dose equals 3 μg/mL. Based on the nomogram, a dosage interval of 24 hours is the correct value and does not need to be altered.

EXAMPLE 2 ▶ ▶ ▶

Same patient profile as in example 1, but serum creatinine is 3.5 mg/dL indicating renal impairment.

1. *Estimate creatinine clearance.*

This patient has a stable serum creatinine and is not obese. The Cockcroft-Gault equation can be used to estimate creatinine clearance:

$$CrCl_{est} = [(140 - age)BW]/(72 \cdot S_{Cr}) = [(140 - 50 \text{ y})70 \text{ kg}]/(72 \cdot 3.5 \text{ mg/dL})$$

$$CrCl_{est} = 25 \text{ mL/min}$$

2. *Compute initial dose and dosage interval (see Table 4-4).*

A dose (D) of 7 mg/kg will provide a peak concentration of more than 20 μg/mL.

$$D = 7 \text{ mg/kg } (70 \text{ kg}) = 490 \text{ mg}$$

Dosage interval would be 48 hours using the nomogram. Extended-interval aminoglycoside doses should be rounded to the nearest 10-50 mg.

The prescribed maintenance dose would be: 500 mg every 48 hours.

3. *Determine dosage interval using serum concentration monitoring.*

A gentamicin serum concentration measured 13 hours after the dose equals 9 μg/mL. Based on the nomogram, a dosage interval of 48 hours is too short and serial concentrations should be monitored. When the gentamicin serum concentration is less than 1 μg/mL, the next dose can be given. Based on the patient's estimated elimination rate constant [$k_e = 0.00293(CrCl) + 0.014 = 0.00293(25 \text{ mL/min}) + 0.014 = 0.087 \text{ h}^{-1}$; $t_{1/2} = 0.693/k_e = 0.693/0.087 \text{ h}^{-1} = 8 \text{ h}$], it will take approximately 3-4 half-lives or about an additional 24-32 hours after the gentamicin serum concentration for the value to drop below 1 μg/mL.

Some clinicians prefer to avoid the use of extended-interval dosing beyond a dosage interval of 48 hours because serum aminoglycoside concentrations can be below the MIC far beyond the time frame afforded by the postantibiotic effect. For these situations, they revert to conventional dosing for the patient.

EXAMPLE 3 ▶ ▶ ▶

ZW is a 35-year-old, 150-kg (height = 5 ft 5 in) female with an intra-abdominal infection. Her current serum creatinine is 1.1 mg/dL and is stable. Compute a tobramycin dose for this patient using conventional dosing.

1. *Estimate creatinine clearance.*

This patient has a stable serum creatinine and is obese [$IBW_{females}$ (in kg) = 45 + 2.3(Ht − 60) = 45 + 2.3(65 in − 60) = 57 kg]. The Salazar and Corcoran equation can be used to estimate creatinine clearance:

$$CrCl_{est(females)} = \frac{(146 - age)[(0.287 \cdot Wt) + (9.74 \cdot Ht^2)]}{(60 \cdot S_{Cr})}$$

$$CrCl_{est(females)} = \frac{(146 - 35\ y)\{(0.287 \cdot 150\ kg) + [9.74 \cdot (1.65\ m)^2]\}}{(60 \cdot 1.1\ mg/dL)} = 117\ mL/min$$

Note: Height is converted from inches to meters: Ht = (65 in • 2.54 cm/in)/(100 cm/m) = 1.65 m.

2. *Compute initial dose and dosage interval (see Table 4-4).*

A dose (D) of 7 mg/kg will provide a peak concentration of more than 20 µg/mL. Because the patient is obese, adjusted body weight (ABW) will be used to compute the dose:

$$ABW = IBW + 0.4(TBW - IBW) = 57\ kg + 0.4(150\ kg - 57\ kg) = 94\ kg$$
$$D = 7\ mg/kg\ (94\ kg) = 658\ mg$$

Dosage interval would be 24 hours using the nomogram. Extended-interval aminoglycoside doses should be rounded to the nearest 10-50 mg.

The prescribed maintenance dose would be: 650 mg every 24 hours.

3. *Determine dosage interval using serum concentration monitoring.*

A gentamicin serum concentration measured 8 hours after the dose equals 4 µg/mL. Based on the nomogram, a dosage interval of 24 hours is the correct value and does not need to be altered.

Assuming linear pharmacokinetics, clinicians have begun to use the Hartford nomogram for doses other than 7 mg/kg. Because this approach has not been formally evaluated, care should be exercised when using this approach. For example, if the clinical situation warrants it (such as a bacteria with an MIC ≤1 µg/mL, so that an optimal Cmax/MIC of more than 8–10 still can be attained), a dose of 5 mg/kg could be administered to a patient, the initial dosage intervals suggested in the Hartford nomogram used, and a serum concentration measured to confirm the dosage interval. Assuming linear pharmacokinetics, the critical concentrations for changing dosage intervals on the y-axis of the Hartford nomogram graph would be decreased by 5/7 (the ratio of the 5-mg/kg dose administered to the 7-mg/kg dose suggested by the nomogram). Additionally, a similar nomogram for gentamicin or tobramycin doses of 5 mg/kg is also available.[133,134]

Literature-Based Recommended Dosing

Because of the large amount of variability in aminoglycoside pharmacokinetics, even when concurrent disease states and conditions are identified, many clinicians believe that the use of standard aminoglycoside doses for pediatric patients is warranted. The original computation of these doses was based on the Pharmacokinetic Dosing methods described in the previous section, and subsequently modified based on clinical experience. In general, the expected aminoglycoside steady-state serum concentrations used to compute these doses were similar to those for adults given conventional dosing. Suggested initial aminoglycoside doses for various pediatric patients are listed in the Effects of Disease States and Conditions on Aminoglycoside Pharmacokinetics and Dosing section. Doses for neonates that are less than 10 mg are usually rounded to the nearest 10th of a milligram. If serum creatinine values are available, estimated creatinine clearance can be computed using equations that are specific for pediatric patients [age 0-1 year, $CrCl_{est}$ (in mL/min/1.73 m^2) = (0.45 • Ht)/S_{Cr}; age 1-20 years, $CrCl_{est}$ (in mL/min/1.73 m^2) = (0.55 • Ht)/S_{Cr}, where Ht is in cm and S_{Cr} is in mg/dL].[135]

EXAMPLE 1 ▶ ▶ ▶

MM is a 3-day-old, 1015-g male with suspected neonatal sepsis. His serum creatinine has not been measured, but it is assumed that it is typical for his age and weight. Compute an initial gentamicin dose for this patient.

1. *Compute initial dose and dosage interval.*

   Often, serum creatinine measurements are not available for initial dosage computation in neonates. The dosage recommendations for this population assume typical renal function, so it is important to verify that the assumption is valid.

   From the pediatrics dosage recommendations given earlier in this chapter, a patient in this age and weight category should receive gentamicin 5 mg/kg every 48 hours. (Note: Gram will be converted to kilograms before the computation is made.)

$$\text{Dose} = 5 \text{ mg/kg} \, (1.015 \text{ kg}) = 5.1 \text{ mg}$$

The prescribed dose will be 5.1 mg every 48 hours.

USE OF AMINOGLYCOSIDE SERUM CONCENTRATIONS TO ALTER DOSAGES

Because of pharmacokinetic variability among patients, it is likely that doses computed using patient population characteristics will not always produce aminoglycoside serum concentrations that are expected. Because of this, aminoglycoside serum concentrations are measured in most patients to ensure that therapeutic, nontoxic levels are present. However, not all patients may require serum concentration monitoring. For example, if it is expected that only a limited number of doses will be administered as is the case for surgical prophylaxis or an appropriate dose for the renal function and concurrent disease states of the patient is prescribed [eg, 1 mg/kg every 8 hours for 3-5 days in a patient with a creatinine clearance of 80-120 mL/min for antibiotic synergy in the treatment of methicillin-sensitive *Staphylococcus aureus* (MSSA) aortic or mitral valve endocarditis], aminoglycoside serum concentration monitoring may not be necessary. Whether or not aminoglycoside concentrations are measured, important patient parameters (fever curves, white blood cell counts, serum creatinine concentrations, etc) should be followed to confirm that the patient is responding to treatment and not developing adverse drug reactions.

When aminoglycoside serum concentrations are measured in patients and a dosage change is necessary, clinicians should seek to use the simplest, most straightforward method available to determine a dose that will provide safe and effective treatment. Generally, this involves choosing aminoglycoside serum concentrations that will not only avoid toxicities but will also achieve target C_{max}/MIC values for the infection. In most cases, a simple dosage ratio can be used to change aminoglycoside doses as these antibiotics follow *linear pharmacokinetics*. Sometimes, it is not possible to simply change the dose, and the dosage interval must also be changed to achieve desired serum concentrations. In this case, it may be possible to use *pharmacokinetic concepts* to alter the aminoglycoside dose that the patient needs. In some situations, it may be necessary to compute the aminoglycoside pharmacokinetic parameters for the patient using the *Sawchuk-Zaske method* and utilize these to calculate the best drug dose. Some clinicians advocate using individualized *area under the concentration-time curve* determinations to individualize aminoglycoside doses. Finally, computerized methods that incorporate expected population pharmacokinetic characteristics (*Bayesian pharmacokinetic computer programs*) can be used in difficult cases where renal function is changing, serum concentrations are obtained at suboptimal times, or the patient was not at steady state when serum concentrations were measured.

Linear Pharmacokinetics Method

Because aminoglycoside antibiotics follow linear, dose-proportional pharmacokinetics, steady-state serum concentrations change in proportion to dose according to the following equation: $D_{new}/C_{ss,new} = D_{old}/C_{ss,old}$ or $D_{new} = (C_{ss,new}/C_{ss,old})D_{old}$, where D is the dose, Css is the steady-state peak or trough concentration, old indicates the dose that produced the steady-state concentration that the patient is currently receiving, and new denotes the dose necessary to produce the desired steady-state concentration. The advantages of this method are that it is quick and simple. The disadvantages are that steady-state concentrations are required and that it may not be possible to attain desired serum concentrations by only changing the dose.

EXAMPLE 1 ▶ ▶ ▶

JM is a 50-year-old, 70-kg (height = 5 ft 10 in) male with gram-negative pneumonia. His current serum creatinine is 0.9 mg/dL, and it has been stable over the last 5 days since admission. A gentamicin dose of 170 mg every 8 hours was prescribed and expected to achieve steady-state peak and trough concentrations equal to 9 µg/mL and 1 µg/mL, respectively. After the third dose, steady-state peak and trough concentrations were measured and were 12 µg/mL and 1.4 µg/mL, respectively. Calculate a new gentamicin dose that would provide a steady-state peak of 9 µg/mL.

1. *Estimate creatinine clearance.*
   This patient has a stable serum creatinine and is not obese. The Cockcroft-Gault equation can be used to estimate creatinine clearance:

   $$CrCl_{est} = [(140 - age)BW]/(72 \cdot S_{Cr}) = [(140 - 50 \text{ y})70 \text{ kg}]/(72 \cdot 0.9 \text{ mg/dL})$$

   $$CrCl_{est} = 97 \text{ mL/min}$$

2. *Estimate elimination rate constant (k_e) and half-life ($t_{1/2}$).*
   The elimination rate constant versus creatinine clearance relationship is used to estimate the gentamicin elimination rate for this patient:

   $$k_e = 0.00293(CrCl) + 0.014 = 0.00293(97 \text{ mL/min}) + 0.014 = 0.298 \text{ h}^{-1}$$

   $$t_{1/2} = 0.693/k_e = 0.693/0.298 \text{ h}^{-1} = 2.3 \text{ h}$$

   Because the patient has been receiving gentamicin for more than 3-5 estimated half-lives, it is likely that the measured serum concentrations are steady-state values.

3. *Compute new dose to achieve desired serum concentration.*
   Using linear pharmacokinetics, the new dose to attain the desired concentration should be proportional to the old dose that produced the measured concentration:

   $$D_{new} = (C_{ss,new}/C_{ss,old})D_{old} = (9 \text{ µg/mL} / 12 \text{ µg/mL}) \, 170 \text{ mg} = 128 \text{ mg, round to } 130 \text{ mg}$$

   The new suggested dose would be 130 mg every 8 hours to be started at next scheduled dosing time.

4. *Check steady-state trough concentration for new dosage regimen.*
   Using linear pharmacokinetics, the new steady-state concentration can be estimated and should be proportional to the old dose that produced the measured concentration:

   $$C_{ss,new} = (D_{new}/D_{old})C_{ss,old} = (130 \text{ mg}/170 \text{ mg}) \, 1.4 \text{ µg/mL} = 1.1 \text{ µg/mL}$$

   This steady-state trough concentration should be safe and effective for the infection that is being treated.

EXAMPLE 2 ▶ ▶ ▶

ZW is a 35-year-old, 150-kg (height = 5 ft 5 in) female with an intra-abdominal infection. Her current serum creatinine is 1.1 mg/dL and is stable. A tobramycin dose of 165 mg every 8 hours was prescribed and expected to achieve steady-state peak and trough concentrations equal to 6 µg/mL and 0.5 µg/mL, respectively. After the fifth dose, steady-state peak and trough concentrations were measured and were 4 µg/mL and less than 0.5 µg/mL (eg, below assay limits), respectively. Calculate a new tobramycin dose that would provide a steady-state peak of 6 µg/mL.

1. *Estimate creatinine clearance.*

   This patient has a stable serum creatinine and is obese [$IBW_{females}$ (in kg) = 45 + 2.3(Ht – 60) = 45 + 2.3(65 in – 60) = 57 kg]. The Salazar and Corcoran equation can be used to estimate creatinine clearance:

   $$CrCl_{est(females)} = \frac{(146 - age)[(0.287 \cdot Wt) + (9.74 \cdot Ht^2)]}{(60 \cdot S_{Cr})}$$

   $$CrCl_{est(females)} = \frac{(146 - 35\ y)\{(0.287 \cdot 150\ kg) + [9.74 \cdot (1.65\ m)^2]\}}{(60 \cdot 1.1\ mg/dL)} = 117\ mL/min$$

   Note: Height is converted from inches to meters: Ht = (65 in · 2.54 cm/in)/(100 cm/m) = 1.65 m.

2. *Estimate elimination rate constant (k_e) and half-life ($t_{1/2}$).*

   The elimination rate constant versus creatinine clearance relationship is used to estimate the gentamicin elimination rate for this patient:

   $$k_e = 0.00293(CrCl) + 0.014 = 0.00293(117\ mL/min) + 0.014 = 0.357\ h^{-1}$$
   $$t_{1/2} = 0.693/k_e = 0.693/0.357\ h^{-1} = 1.9\ h$$

   Because the patient has been receiving tobramycin for more than 3-5 estimated half-lives, it is likely that the measured serum concentrations are steady-state values.

3. *Compute new dose to achieve desired serum concentration.*

   Using linear pharmacokinetics, the new dose to attain the desired concentration should be proportional to the old dose that produced the measured concentration:

   $$D_{new} = (C_{ss,new}/C_{ss,old})D_{old} = (6\ µg/mL\ /\ 4\ µg/mL)\ 165\ mg = 247\ mg,\ round\ to\ 250\ mg$$

   The new suggested dose would be 250 mg every 8 hours to be started at next scheduled dosing time.

4. *Check steady-state trough concentration for new dosage regimen.*

   Using linear pharmacokinetics, the new steady-state concentration can be estimated and should be proportional to the old dose that produced the measured concentration. However, in this situation the trough concentration is below assay limits and was reported as less than 0.5 µg/mL. Because of this, the maximum value that the steady-state trough could possibly be is 0.5 µg/mL, and this value can be used to compute a rough approximation of the expected concentration:

   $$C_{ss,new} = (D_{new}/D_{old})C_{ss,old} = (250\ mg/165\ mg)\ 0.5\ µg/mL = 0.8\ µg/mL$$

   Thus, the steady-state trough concentration should be no greater than 0.8 µg/mL. This steady-state trough concentration should be safe and effective for the infection that is being treated.

EXAMPLE 3 ▶ ▶ ▶

QZ is a 50-year-old, 70-kg (height = 5 ft 10 in) male with gram-negative pneumonia. His current serum creatinine is 0.9 mg/dL, and it has been stable over the last 3 days since admission. A gentamicin dose of 550 mg every 24 hours was prescribed and expected to achieve steady-state peak and trough concentrations equal to 30 μg/mL and less than 1 μg/mL, respectively. After the third dose, steady-state peak and trough concentrations were measured and were 37 μg/mL and 1 μg/mL, respectively. Calculate a new gentamicin dose that would provide a steady-state peak of 30 μg/mL and a steady-state trough of less than 1.

1. *Estimate creatinine clearance.*

This patient has a stable serum creatinine and is not obese. The Cockcroft-Gault equation can be used to estimate creatinine clearance:

$$CrCl_{est} = [(140 - age)BW]/(72 \cdot S_{Cr}) = [(140 - 50 \text{ y})70 \text{ kg}]/(72 \cdot 0.9 \text{ mg/dL})$$

$$CrCl_{est} = 97 \text{ mL/min}$$

2. *Estimate elimination rate constant (k_e) and half-life ($t_{1/2}$).*

The elimination rate constant versus creatinine clearance relationship is used to estimate the gentamicin elimination rate for this patient:

$$k_e = 0.00293(CrCl) + 0.014 = 0.00293(97 \text{ mL/min}) + 0.014 = 0.298 \text{ h}^{-1}$$

$$t_{1/2} = 0.693/k_e = 0.693/0.298 \text{ h}^{-1} = 2.3 \text{ h}$$

Because the patient has been receiving gentamicin for more than 3–5 estimated half-lives, it is likely that the measured serum concentrations are steady-state values.

3. *Compute new dose to achieve desired serum concentration.*

Using linear pharmacokinetics, the new dose to attain the desired concentration should be proportional to the old dose that produced the measured concentration:

$$D_{new} = (C_{ss,new}/C_{ss,old})D_{old} = (30 \text{ μg/mL} / 37 \text{ μg/mL}) \text{ 550 mg} = 446 \text{ mg, round to 450 mg}$$

The new suggested dose would be 450 mg every 24 hours to be started at next scheduled dosing time.

4. *Check steady-state trough concentration for new dosage regimen.*

Using linear pharmacokinetics, the new steady-state concentration can be estimated and should be proportional to the old dose that produced the measured concentration:

$$C_{ss,new} = (D_{new}/D_{old})C_{ss,old} = (450 \text{ mg}/550 \text{ mg}) \text{ 1 μg/mL} = 0.8 \text{ μg/mL}$$

This steady-state trough concentration should be safe and effective for the infection that is being treated.

Pharmacokinetic Concepts Method

As implied by the name, this technique derives alternate doses by estimating actual pharmacokinetic parameters or surrogates for pharmacokinetic parameters.[136] It is a very useful way to calculate drug doses when the Linear Pharmacokinetic method is not sufficient because a dosage change that will produce a proportional change in steady-state peak and trough concentrations is not appropriate. The only requirement is a steady-state peak and trough aminoglycoside serum concentration pair obtained before and after a dose (Figure 4-5). This method can be used to adjust doses for either conventional dosing or extended-interval dosing. The following steps are used to compute new aminoglycoside doses:

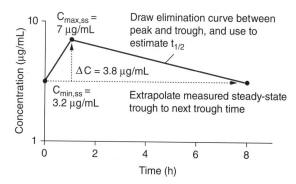

FIGURE 4-5   Graphical representation of the Pharmacokinetic Concepts method where a steady-state peak (Css_{max}) and trough (Css_{min}) concentration pair is used to individualize aminoglycoside therapy. Because the patient is at steady state, consecutive trough concentrations will be identical, so the trough concentration can be extrapolated to the next predose time. The change in concentration after a dose is given (ΔC) is a surrogate measure of the volume of distribution and will be used to compute the new dose for the patient.

1. *Draw a rough sketch of the serum log concentration/time curve by hand, keeping track of the relative time between the serum concentrations (see Figure 4-5).*

2. *Because the patient is at steady state, the trough concentration can be extrapolated to the next trough value time (see Figure 4-5).*

3. *Draw the elimination curve between the steady-state peak concentration and the extrapolated trough concentration. Use this line to estimate half-life.* For example, a patient receives a gentamicin dose of 80 mg given every 8 hours that produces a steady-state peak equal to 7 µg/mL and a steady-state trough equal to 3.2 µg/mL, and the dose is infused over ½ hour and the peak concentration is drawn ½ hour later (see Figure 4-5). The time between the measured steady-state peak and the extrapolated trough concentration is 7 hours (the 8 hour dosage interval minus the 1-hour combined infusion and waiting time). The definition of half-life is the time needed for serum concentrations to decrease by ½. Because the serum concentration declined by approximately ½ from the peak concentration to the trough concentration, the aminoglycoside half-life for this patient is approximately 7 hours. This information will be used to set the new dosage interval for the patient.

4. *Determine the difference in concentration between the steady-state peak and trough concentrations. The difference in concentration will change proportionally with the dose size.* In the current example the patient is receiving a gentamicin dose equal to 80 mg every 8 hours, which produced steady-state peak and trough concentrations of 7 µg/mL and 3.2 µg/mL, respectively. The difference between the peak and trough values is 3.8 µg/mL. The change in serum concentration is proportional to the dose, and this information will be used to set a new dose for the patient.

5. *Choose new steady-state peak and trough concentrations.* For the purposes of this example, the desired steady-state peak and trough concentrations will be approximately 7 µg/mL and 1 µg/mL, respectively.

6. *Determine the new dosage interval for the desired concentrations.* In this example, the patient currently has the desired peak concentration of 7 µg/mL. In 1 half-life, the serum concentration will decline to 3.5 µg/mL, in an additional half-life the gentamicin concentration will decrease to 1.8 µg/mL, and in 1 more half-life the concentration will decline to 0.9 µg/mL (Figure 4-6). Because the approximate half-life is 7 hours and 3 half-lives are required for serum concentrations to decrease from the desired peak

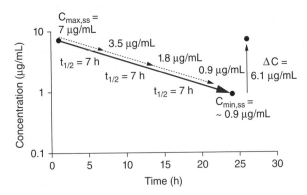

FIGURE 4-6   The Pharmacokinetic Concept method uses the estimated half-life to graphically compute the new dosage interval and the change in concentration to calculate the dose for a patient.

concentration to the desired trough concentration, the dosage interval should be 21 hours (7 hours × 3 half-lives). This value would be rounded off to the clinically acceptable value of 24 hours, and the actual trough concentration would be expected to be slightly lower than 0.9 µg/mL.

7. *Determine the new dose for the desired concentrations.* The desired peak concentration is 7 µg/mL, and the expected trough concentration is 0.9 µg/mL. The change in concentration between these values is 6.1 µg/mL. It is known from measured serum concentrations that administration of 80 mg changes serum concentrations by 3.8 µg/mL and that the change in serum concentration between the peak and trough values is proportional to the size of the dose. Therefore, a simple ratio will be used to compute the required dose: $D_{new} = (\Delta C_{new}/\Delta C_{old})D_{old}$, where D_{new} and D_{old} are the new and old doses, respectively; ΔC_{new} is the change in concentration between the peak and trough for the new dose; and ΔC_{old} is the change in concentration between the peak and trough for the old dose. (Note: This relationship is appropriate because doses are given into a fixed, constant volume of distribution; it is not because the drug follows linear pharmacokinetics so this method will work whether the agent follows nonlinear or linear pharmacokinetics.) For this example: $D_{new} = (6.1 \text{ µg/mL}/3.8 \text{ µg/mL})$ 80 mg = 128 mg, which would be rounded to 130 mg. Gentamicin 130 mg every 24 hours would be started 24 hours after the last dose of the previous dosage regimen.

Once this method is mastered, it can be used without the need for a calculator. The following are examples that use the Pharmacokinetic Concepts method to change aminoglycoside doses.

EXAMPLE 1 ▶ ▶ ▶

JM is a 50-year-old, 70-kg (height = 5 ft 10 in) male with gram-negative pneumonia. His current serum creatinine is 3.5 mg/dL, and it has been stable over the last 5 days since admission. A gentamicin dose of 115 mg every 24 hours was prescribed and expected to achieve steady-state peak and trough concentrations equal to 8-10 µg/mL and less than 2 µg/mL, respectively. After the third dose, steady-state peak and trough concentrations were measured and were 12 µg/mL and 3.5 µg/mL, respectively. Calculate a new gentamicin dose that would provide a steady-state peak of 9 µg/mL and a trough of less than 2 µg/mL.

1. *Estimate creatinine clearance.*

   This patient has a stable serum creatinine and is not obese. The Cockcroft-Gault equation can be used to estimate creatinine clearance:

   $$CrCl_{est} = [(140 - age)BW]/(72 \cdot S_{Cr}) = [(140 - 50 \text{ y})70 \text{ kg}]/(72 \cdot 3.5 \text{ mg/dL})$$

   $$CrCl_{est} = 25 \text{ mL/min}$$

2. *Estimate elimination rate constant (k_e) and half-life $(t_{1/2})$.*

   The elimination rate constant versus creatinine clearance relationship is used to estimate the gentamicin elimination rate for this patient:

   $$k_e = 0.00293(CrCl) + 0.014 = 0.00293(25 \text{ mL/min}) + 0.014 = 0.087 \text{ h}^{-1}$$

   $$t_{1/2} = 0.693/k_e = 0.693/0.087 \text{ h}^{-1} = 8 \text{ h}$$

   Because the patient has been receiving gentamicin for more than 3–5 estimated half-lives, it is likely that the measured serum concentrations are steady-state values.

3. *Use Pharmacokinetics Concept method to compute a new dose.*

   1. *Draw a rough sketch of the serum log concentration/time curve by hand, keeping track of the relative time between the serum concentrations (Figure 4-7).*

   2. *Because the patient is at steady state, the trough concentration can be extrapolated to the next trough value time (see Figure 4-7).*

   3. *Draw the elimination curve between the steady-state peak concentration and the extrapolated trough concentration. Use this line to estimate half-life.* The patient is receiving a gentamicin dose of 115 mg given every 24 hours that produces a steady-state peak equal to 12 µg/mL and a steady-state trough equal to 3.5 µg/mL, and the dose is infused over ½ hour and the peak concentration is drawn ½ hour later (see Figure 4-7). The time between the measured steady-state peak and the extrapolated trough concentration is 23 hours (the 24-hour dosage interval minus the 1-hour combined infusion and waiting time). The definition of half-life is the time needed for serum concentrations to decrease by ½. It would take 1 half-life for the peak serum concentration to decline from 12 to 6 µg/mL, and an additional half-life for the serum concentration to decrease from 6 to 3 µg/mL. The concentration of 3 µg/mL is very close to the

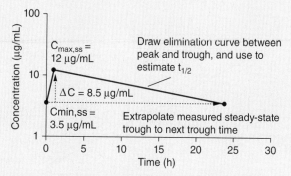

FIGURE 4-7 Graphical representation of the Pharmacokinetic Concept method where a steady-state peak (Css_{max}) and trough (Css_{min}) concentration pair is used to individualize aminoglycoside therapy. Because the patient is at steady state, consecutive trough concentrations will be identical, so the trough concentration can be extrapolated to the next predose time. The change in concentration after a dose is given (ΔC) is a surrogate measure of the volume of distribution and will be used to compute the new dose for the patient.

extrapolated trough value of 3.5 µg/mL. Therefore, 2 half-lives expired during the 23-hour time period between the peak concentration and extrapolated trough concentration, and the estimated half-life is 12 hours (23 hours/2 half-lives = ~12 hours). This information will be used to set the new dosage interval for the patient

4. *Determine the difference in concentration between the steady-state peak and trough concentrations. The difference in concentration will change proportionally with the dose size.* In the current example the patient is receiving a gentamicin dose equal to 115 mg every 24 hours, which produced steady-state peak and trough concentrations of 12 µg/mL and 3.5 µg/mL, respectively. The difference between the peak and trough values is 8.5 µg/mL. The change in serum concentration is proportional to the dose, and this information will be used to set a new dose for the patient.

5. *Choose new steady-state peak and trough concentrations.* For the purposes of this example, the desired steady-state peak and trough concentrations will be approximately 9 µg/mL and less than 2 µg/mL, respectively.

6. *Determine the new dosage interval for the desired concentrations (Figure 4-8).* Using the desired concentrations, it will take 1 half-life for the peak concentration of 9 µg/mL to decrease to 4.5 µg/mL, 1 more half-life for the serum concentration to decrease to 2.3 µg/mL, and an additional half-life for serum concentrations to decline to 1.2 µg/mL. Therefore, the dosage interval will need to be approximately 3 half-lives or 36 hours (12 hours × 3 half-live = 36 hours). When a dosage interval such as 36 hours is used, care must be taken to ensure that the scheduled doses are actually administered as the drug will only be given every other day, and sometimes this type of administration schedule is overlooked and doses are missed.

7. *Determine the new dose for the desired concentrations (see Figure 4-8).* The desired peak concentration is 9 µg/mL, and the expected trough concentration is 1.2 µg/mL. The change in concentration between these values is 7.8 µg/mL. It is known from measured serum concentrations that administration of 115 mg changes serum concentrations by 8.5 µg/mL and that the change in serum concentration between the peak and trough values is proportional to the size of the dose. In this case: $D_{new} = (\Delta C_{new}/\Delta C_{old})D_{old} = (7.8 \, \mu g/mL \, / \, 8.5 \, \mu g/mL) \, 115 \, mg = 105 \, mg$. Gentamicin 105 mg every 36 hours would be started 36 hours after the last dose of the previous dosage regimen.

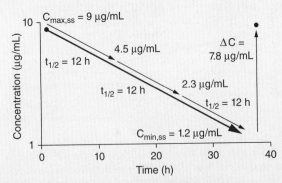

FIGURE 4-8   The Pharmacokinetic Concept method uses the estimated half-life to graphically compute the new dosage interval and the change in concentration to calculate the dose for a patient.

EXAMPLE 2 ▶▶▶

ZW is a 35-year-old, 150-kg (height = 5 ft 5 in) female with an intra-abdominal infection. Her current serum creatinine is 1.1 mg/dL and is stable. A tobramycin dose of 165 mg every 8 hours was prescribed and expected to achieve steady-state peak and trough concentrations equal to 6 μg/mL and 0.5 μg/mL, respectively. After the fifth dose, steady-state peak and trough concentrations were measured and were 5 μg/mL and 2.6 μg/mL, respectively. Calculate a new tobramycin dose that would provide a steady-state peak of 6 μg/mL and a steady-state trough of 1 or less.

1. *Estimate creatinine clearance.*

This patient has a stable serum creatinine and is obese [IBW$_{females}$ (in kg) = 45 + 2.3(Ht − 60) = 45 + 2.3(65 in − 60) = 57 kg]. The Salazar and Corcoran equation can be used to estimate creatinine clearance:

$$CrCl_{est(females)} = \frac{(146 - age)[(0.287 \cdot Wt) + (9.74 \cdot Ht^2)]}{(60 \cdot S_{Cr})}$$

$$CrCl_{est(females)} = \frac{(146 - 35\ y)\{(0.287 \cdot 150\ kg) + [9.74 \cdot (1.65\ m)^2]\}}{(60 \cdot 1.1\ mg/dL)} = 117\ mL/min$$

Note: Height is converted from inches to meters: Ht = (65 in · 2.54 cm/in)/(100 cm/m) = 1.65 m.

2. *Estimate elimination rate constant (k_e) and half-life ($t_{1/2}$).*

The elimination rate constant versus creatinine clearance relationship is used to estimate the tobramycin elimination rate for this patient:

$$k_e = 0.00293(CrCl) + 0.014 = 0.00293(117\ mL/min) + 0.014 = 0.357\ h^{-1}$$

$$t_{1/2} = 0.693/k_e = 0.693/0.357\ h^{-1} = 1.9\ h$$

Because the patient has been receiving tobramycin for more than 3–5 estimated half-lives, it is likely that the measured serum concentrations are steady-state values.

3. *Use Pharmacokinetics Concept Method to compute a new dose.*

1. *Draw a rough sketch of the serum log concentration/time curve by hand, keeping track of the relative time between the serum concentrations (Figure 4-9).*

2. *Because the patient is at steady state, the trough concentration can be extrapolated to the next trough value time (see Figure 4-9).*

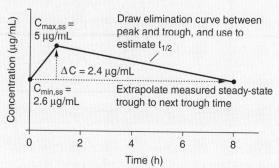

FIGURE 4-9   Graphical representation of the Pharmacokinetic Concept method where a steady-state peak (Css$_{max}$) and trough (Css$_{min}$) concentration pair is used to individualize aminoglycoside therapy. Because the patient is at steady state, consecutive trough concentrations will be identical, so the trough concentration can be extrapolated to the next predose time. The change in concentration after a dose is given (ΔC) is a surrogate measure of the volume of distribution and will be used to compute the new dose for the patient.

3. *Draw the elimination curve between the steady-state peak concentration and the extrapolated trough concentration. Use this line to estimate half-life.* The patient is receiving a tobramycin dose of 165 mg given every 8 hours that produces a steady-state peak equal to 5 µg/mL and a steady-state trough equal to 2.6 µg/mL, and the dose is infused over ½ hour and the peak concentration is drawn ½ hour later (see Figure 4-9). The time between the measured steady-state peak and the extrapolated trough concentration is 7 hours (the 8-hour dosage interval minus the 1-hour combined infusion and waiting time). The definition of half-life is the time needed for serum concentrations to decrease by ½. It would take 1 half-life for the peak serum concentration to decline from 5 to 2.5 µg/mL. The concentration of 2.6 µg/mL is very close to the extrapolated trough value of 2.5 µg/mL. Therefore, 1 half-life expired during the 7-hour time period between the peak concentration and extrapolated trough concentration, and the estimated half-life is 7 hours. This information will be used to set the new dosage interval for the patient

4. *Determine the difference in concentration between the steady-state peak and trough concentrations. The difference in concentration will change proportionally with the dose size.* In the current example the patient is receiving a tobramycin dose equal to 165 mg every 8 hours, which produced steady-state peak and trough concentrations of 5 µg/mL and 2.6 µg/mL, respectively. The difference between the peak and trough values is 2.4 µg/mL. The change in serum concentration is proportional to the dose, and this information will be used to set a new dose for the patient.

5. *Choose new steady-state peak and trough concentrations.* For the purposes of this example, the desired steady-state peak and trough concentrations will be approximately 6 µg/mL and 1 µg/mL or less, respectively.

6. *Determine the new dosage interval for the desired concentrations.* Using the desired concentrations, it will take 1 half-life for the peak concentration of 6 µg/mL to decrease to 3 µg/mL, 1 more half-life for the serum concentration to decrease to 1.5 µg/mL, and an additional half-life for serum concentrations to decline to 0.8 µg/mL. Therefore, the dosage interval will need to be approximately 3 half-lives or 21 hours (7 hours × 3 half-lives = 21 hours), which would be rounded to 24 hours.

7. *Determine the new dose for the desired concentrations.* The desired peak concentration is 6 µg/mL, and the expected trough concentration is 0.8 µg/mL. The change in concentration between these values is 5.2 µg/mL. It is known from measured serum concentrations that administration of 165 mg changes serum concentrations by 2.4 µg/mL and that the change in serum concentration between the peak and trough values is proportional to the size of the dose. In this case: $D_{new} = (\Delta C_{new}/\Delta C_{old})D_{old} = (5.2 \text{ µg/mL}/2.4 \text{ µg/mL})$ 165 mg = 358 mg, rounded to 360 mg. Tobramycin 360 mg every 24 hours would be started 24 hours after the last dose of the previous dosage regimen.

EXAMPLE 3 ▶ ▶ ▶

SD is a 57-year-old, 75-kg (height = 5 ft 9 in) male with gram-negative pneumonia. His current serum creatinine is 1.4 mg/dL, and it has been stable over the last 5 days since admission. A tobramycin dose of 500 mg every 24 hours was prescribed and expected to achieve steady-state peak and trough concentrations equal to 20 µg/mL and less than 1 µg/mL, respectively. After the third dose, steady-state peak and trough concentrations were measured and were 20 µg/mL and 2.5 µg/mL, respectively. Calculate a new tobramycin dose that would provide a steady-state peak of 25 µg/mL and a trough of less than 1 µg/mL.

1. *Estimate creatinine clearance.*

This patient has a stable serum creatinine and is not obese. The Cockcroft-Gault equation can be used to estimate creatinine clearance:

$$CrCl_{est} = [(140 - age)BW]/(72 \cdot S_{Cr}) = [(140 - 57\ y)75\ kg]/(72 \cdot 1.4\ mg/dL)$$

$$CrCl_{est} = 62\ mL/min$$

2. *Estimate elimination rate constant (k_e) and half-life ($t_{1/2}$).*

The elimination rate constant versus creatinine clearance relationship is used to estimate the tobramycin elimination rate for this patient:

$$k_e = 0.00293(CrCl) + 0.014 = 0.00293(62\ mL/min) + 0.014 = 0.195\ h^{-1}$$

$$t_{1/2} = 0.693/k_e = 0.693/0.195\ h^{-1} = 3.6\ h$$

Because the patient has been receiving tobramycin for more than 3–5 estimated half-lives, it is likely that the measured serum concentrations are steady-state values.

3. *Use Pharmacokinetics Concept method to compute a new dose.*

   1. *Draw a rough sketch of the serum log concentration/time curve by hand, keeping track of the relative time between the serum concentrations.*

   2. *Because the patient is at steady state, the trough concentration can be extrapolated to the next trough value time.*

   3. *Draw the elimination curve between the steady-state peak concentration and the extrapolated trough concentration. Use this line to estimate half-life.* The patient is receiving an tobramycin dose of 500 mg given every 24 hours that produces a steady-state peak equal to 20 µg/mL and a steady-state trough equal to 2.5 µg/mL, and the dose is infused over ½ hour and the peak concentration is drawn ½ hour later. The time between the measured steady-state peak and the extrapolated trough concentration is 23 hours (the 24-hour dosage interval minus the 1-hour combined infusion and waiting time). The definition of half-life is the time needed for serum concentrations to decrease by ½. It would take 1 half-life for the peak serum concentration to decline from 20 to 10 µg/mL, an additional half-life for the serum concentration to decrease from 10 to 5 µg/mL, and another half-life for the serum concentration to decline from 5 to 2.5 µg/mL. The concentration of 2.5 µg/mL is identical to the extrapolated trough value of 2.5 µg/mL. Therefore, 3 half-lives expired during the 23-hour time period between the peak concentration and extrapolated trough concentration, and the estimated half-life is 8 hours (23 hours/3 half-lives = ~8 hours). This information will be used to set the new dosage interval for the patient

   4. *Determine the difference in concentration between the steady-state peak and trough concentrations. The difference in concentration will change proportionally with the dose size.* In the current example the patient is receiving a tobramycin dose equal to 500 mg every 24 hours, which produced steady-state peak and trough concentrations of 20 µg/mL and 2.5 µg/mL, respectively. The difference between the peak and trough values is 17.5 µg/mL. The change in serum concentration is proportional to the dose, and this information will be used to set a new dose for the patient.

   5. *Choose new steady-state peak and trough concentrations.* For the purposes of this example, the desired steady-state peak and trough concentrations will be approximately 25 µg/mL and less than 1 µg/mL, respectively.

   6. *Determine the new dosage interval for the desired concentrations.* Using the desired concentrations, it will take 1 half-life for the peak concentration of 25 µg/mL to decrease to 12.5 µg/mL, 1 more half-life for the serum concentration to decrease to 6 µg/mL, an additional half-life for serum concentrations to decline to 3 µg/mL, and 2 additional half-lives for them to fall to 1.5 µg/mL and 0.75 µg/mL, respectively. Therefore,

the dosage interval will need to be approximately 5 half-lives or 36 hours (8 hours × 5 half-live = 40 hours, round to 36 hours). When a dosage interval such as 36 hours is used, care must be taken to ensure that the scheduled doses are actually administered as the drug will only be given every other day, and sometimes this type of administration schedule is overlooked and doses are missed.

7. *Determine the new dose for the desired concentrations.* The desired peak concentration is 25 μg/mL, and the expected trough concentration is less than 1 μg/mL. The change in concentration between these values is 24 μg/mL. It is known from measured serum concentrations that administration of 500 mg changes serum concentrations by 17.5 μg/mL and that the change in serum concentration between the peak and trough values is proportional to the size of the dose. In this case: $D_{new} = (\Delta C_{new}/\Delta C_{old})D_{old} = (24\ \mu g/mL\ /\ 17.5\ \mu g/mL)$ 500 mg = 685 mg, round to 675. Tobramycin 675 mg every 36 hours would be started 36 hours after the last dose of the previous dosage regimen.

Sawchuk-Zaske Method

The Sawchuk-Zaske method of adjusting aminoglycoside doses was among the first techniques available to change doses using serum concentrations.[2,62-64,127] It allows the computation of an individual's own, unique pharmacokinetic constants and uses those to calculate a dose to achieve desired aminoglycoside concentrations. The standard Sawchuk-Zaske method conducts a small pharmacokinetic experiment using three to four aminoglycoside serum concentrations obtained during a dosage interval and does not require steady-state conditions. The modified Sawchuk-Zaske methods assume that steady state has been achieved and require only a pair of steady-state concentrations obtained during a dosage interval. This method can be utilized to adjust doses for either conventional or extended-interval dosing. The Sawchuk-Zaske method has also been successfully used to dose vancomycin and theophylline.

Standard Sawchuk-Zaske Method

The standard version of the Sawchuk-Zaske method does not require steady-state concentrations. A trough aminoglycoside concentration is obtained before a dose, a peak aminoglycoside concentration is obtained after the dose is infused (immediately after a 1-hour infusion or ½ hour after a ½-hour infusion), and one to two additional postdose serum aminoglycoside concentrations are obtained (Figure 4-10). Ideally, the one to two postdose concentrations should be obtained at least 1 estimated half-life from each other to minimize the influence of assay error. The postdose serum concentrations are used to calculate the aminoglycoside elimination rate constant and half-life (see Figure 4-10). The half-life can be computed by graphing the postdose concentrations on semilogrithmic paper, drawing the best straight line through the data points, and determining the time needed for serum concentrations to decline by one-half. Once the half-life is known, the elimination rate constant (k_e) can be computed: $k_e = 0.693/t_{1/2}$. Alternatively, the elimination rate constant can be directly calculated using the postdose serum concentrations [$k_e = (\ln C_1 - \ln C_2)/\Delta t$, where C_1 and C_2 are postdose serum concentrations and Δt is the time that expired between the times that C_1 and C_2 were obtained, and the half-life can be computed using the elimination rate constant ($t_{1/2} = 0.693/k_e$). The volume of distribution (V) is calculated using the following equation:

$$V = \frac{D/t'(1 - e^{-k_e t'})}{k_e[C_{max} - (C_{min}e^{-k_e t'})]}$$

where D is the aminoglycoside dose, t′ is the infusion time, k_e is the elimination rate constant, C_{max} is the peak concentration, and C_{min} is the trough concentration. The elimination rate constant and volume of distribution measured in this fashion are the patient's own, unique aminoglycoside pharmacokinetic constants and can be

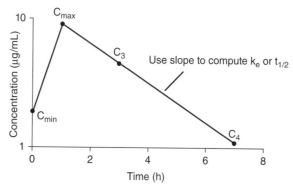

FIGURE 4-10   The Sawchuk-Zaske method for individualization of aminoglycoside doses uses a trough (C_{min}), peak (C_{max}), and one or two additional postdose concentrations (C_3, C_4) to compute a patient's own, unique pharmacokinetic parameters. This version of the Sawchuk-Zaske method does not require steady-state conditions. The peak and trough concentrations are used to calculate the volume of distribution, and the postdose concentrations (C_{max}, C_3, C_4) are used to compute half-life. Once volume of distribution and half-life have been measured, they can be used to compute the exact dose needed to achieve desired aminoglycoside concentrations.

used in one-compartment model intravenous infusion equations to compute the required dose to achieve any desired serum concentration.

Steady-State Sawchuk-Zaske Method: Peak/Trough Version

If a steady-state peak and trough aminoglycoside concentration pair is available for a patient, the Sawchuk-Zaske method can be used to compute patient pharmacokinetic parameters and aminoglycoside doses (Figure 4-11). Because the patient is at steady state, the measured trough concentration obtained before the dose was given can be extrapolated to the next dosage time and used to compute the aminoglycoside elimination rate constant [$k_e = (\ln C_{max,ss} - \ln C_{min,ss})]/\tau - t'$, where Css_{max} and Css_{min} are the steady-state peak and trough serum concentrations and t' and τ are the infusion time and dosage interval, and the half-life can be

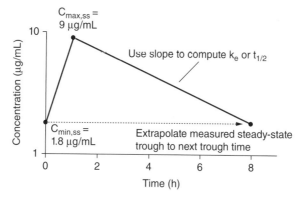

FIGURE 4-11   The steady-state peak/trough version of the Sawchuk-Zaske method uses a steady-state peak (Css_{max}) and trough (Css_{min}) concentration pair to individualize aminoglycoside therapy. Because the patient is at steady state, consecutive trough concentrations will be identical, so the trough concentration can be extrapolated to the next predose time. The steady-state peak and trough concentrations are used to calculate the volume of distribution and half-life. Once volume of distribution and half-life have been measured, they can be used to compute the exact dose needed to achieve desired aminoglycoside concentrations.

computed using the elimination rate constant ($t_{1/2}$ = 0.693/k_e). The volume of distribution (V) is calculated using the following equation:

$$V = \frac{D/t'(1 - e^{-k_e t'})}{k_e[Css_{max} - (Css_{min}e^{-k_e t'})]}$$

where D is the aminoglycoside dose, t' is the infusion time, k_e is the elimination rate constant, Css_{max} is the steady-state peak concentration, and Css_{min} is the steady-state trough concentration. The elimination rate constant and volume of distribution measured in this way are the patient's own, unique aminoglycoside pharmacokinetic constants and can be used in one-compartment model intravenous infusion equations to compute the required dose to achieve any desired serum concentration. The dosage calculations are similar to those done in the initial dosage section of this chapter, except that the patient's real pharmacokinetic parameters are used in the equations instead of population pharmacokinetic estimates.

Steady-State Sawchuk-Zaske Method: Two Post-Dose Concentrations Version

Sometimes, steady-state trough concentrations will be below the assay limit or it is not possible to measure a predose concentration. Trough concentrations that are too low to accurately measure occur especially during therapy with extended-interval aminoglycoside dosing. In these cases, it may be preferable to measure two postdose steady-state concentrations and use these to compute values that can be used in the Sawchuk-Zaske method (Figure 4-12).

The two postdose steady-state concentrations should be drawn at least 1 estimated half-life apart in order to minimize the effect of assay error on the calculations. While one of the two steady-state concentrations can be a peak concentration, it is not a requirement. During extended-interval dosing, some patients may have longer distribution phases so many clinicians suggest that the first postdose concentration be obtained at least

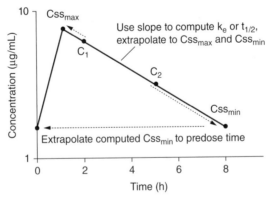

FIGURE 4-12   The steady-state two postdose concentration version of the Sawchuk-Zaske method uses two postdose concentrations (C_1 and C_2) to individualize aminoglycoside therapy. Once the concentrations are obtained, they are extrapolated either mathematically or graphically to determine steady-state peak (Css_{max}) and trough (Css_{min}) values. The elimination rate constant is calculated using the measured concentrations: $k_e = (\ln C_1 - \ln C_2)/\Delta t$, where C_1 and C_2 are the first and second steady-state postdose concentrations, respectively, and Δt is the time that expired between the two concentrations. Steady-state peak and trough concentrations are calculated using the following equations: $Css_{max} = C_1/(e^{-k_e t})$, where C_1 is the first measured steady-state concentration, k_e is the elimination rate constant, and t is the time between C_1 and Css_{max}; $Css_{min} = C_2 e^{-k_e t}$, where C_2 is the second measured steady-state concentration, k_e is the elimination rate constant, and t is the time between C_2 and Css_{min}.

1 hour after the completion of the infusion for this method of administration. The second postdose concentration should be drawn early enough in the dosage interval so that it is not below assay limits (typically no later than 14-16 hours postdose during extended-interval or 4-6 hours postdose during conventional dosing for patients with CrCl >60 mL/min).

Once the concentrations are obtained, they are extrapolated either mathematically or graphically (see Figure 4-12) to determine peak and trough values. The elimination rate constant is calculated using the measured concentrations: $k_e = (\ln C_1 - \ln C_2)/\Delta t$, where C_1 and C_2 are the first and second steady-state postdose concentrations and Δt is the time that expired between the two concentrations. If one of the concentrations is a peak concentration, it is unnecessary to extrapolate it and only the trough concentration needs to be computed. However, if neither concentration is a peak, both steady-state peak and trough concentrations need to be calculated: $Css_{max} = C_1/(e^{-k_e t})$, where C_1 is the first measured steady-state concentration, k_e is the elimination rate constant, and t is the time between C_1 and Css_{max}; $Css_{min} = C_2 e^{-k_e t}$, where C_2 is the second measured steady-state concentration, k_e is the elimination rate constant, and t is the time between C_2 and Css_{min}.

The volume of distribution (V) is calculated using the following equation:

$$V = \frac{D/t'(1 - e^{-k_e t'})}{k_e [Css_{max} - (Css_{min} e^{-k_e t'})]}$$

where D is the aminoglycoside dose, t' is the infusion time, k_e is the elimination rate constant, Css_{max} is the steady-state peak concentration, and Css_{min} is the steady-state trough concentration. The elimination rate constant and volume of distribution measured in this fashion are the patient's own, unique aminoglycoside pharmacokinetic constants and can be used in one-compartment model intravenous infusion equations to compute the required dose to achieve any desired serum concentration. The dosage calculations are similar to those done in the initial dosage section of this chapter, except that the patient's real pharmacokinetic parameters are used in the equations instead of population pharmacokinetic estimates.

To illustrate the similarities and differences between the Pharmacokinetic Concepts and the Sawchuk-Zaske methods, some of the same cases used in the previous section will be used as examples here.

EXAMPLE 1 ▶▶▶

JH is a 24-year-old, 70-kg (height = 6 ft 0 in) male with gram-negative pneumonia. His current serum creatinine is 1.0 mg/dL, and it has been stable over the last 7 days since admission. An amikacin dose of 400 mg every 8 hours was prescribed. After the third dose, the following amikacin serum concentrations were obtained:

Time	Amikacin concentration (μg/mL)
0800 H	2.0
0800–0900 H	Amikacin 400 mg
0900 H	22.1
1100 H	11.9
1600 H	2.5

Medication administration sheets were checked, and the previous dose was given 2 hours early (2200 H the previous day). Because of this, it is known that the patient is not at steady state. Calculate a new amikacin dose that would provide a steady-state peak of 28 μg/mL and a trough between 3 μg/mL.

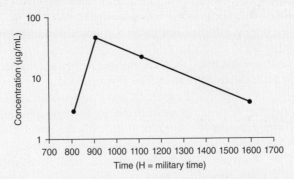

FIGURE 4-13   Graph of amikacin serum concentrations used in Sawchuk-Zaske method example.

Use Sawchuk-Zaske method to compute a new dose.

1. *Plot serum concentration/time data (Figure 4-13). Because serum concentrations decrease in a straight line, use any two postdose concentrations to compute the patient's elimination rate constant and half-life.*

$$k_e = (\ln Css_{max} - \ln Css_{min})/\tau - t' = (\ln 22.1\ \mu g/mL - \ln 2.5\ \mu g/mL)/(16\ H - 09\ H) = 0.311\ h^{-1}$$

$$t_{1/2} = 0.693/k_e = 0.693/0.311\ h^{-1} = 2.2\ h$$

Compute the patient's volume of distribution.

$$V = \frac{D/t'(1-e^{-k_e t'})}{k_e[Css_{max} - (Css_{min}e^{-k_e t'})]} = \frac{(400\ mg/1h)(1-e^{-(0.311\ h^{-1})(1\ h)})}{0.311\ h^{-1}[22.1\ mg/L - (2.5\ mg/L\ e^{-(0.311\ h^{-1})(1\ h)})]}$$

$$V = 17.0\ L$$

2. *Choose new steady-state peak and trough concentrations.* For the purposes of this example, the desired steady-state peak and trough concentrations will be 28 μg/mL and 3 μg/mL, respectively.

3. *Determine the new dosage interval for the desired concentrations.* As in the initial dosage section of this chapter, the dosage interval (τ) is computed using the following equation using a 1-hour infusion time (t′):

$$\tau = [(\ln Css_{max} - \ln Css_{min})/k_e] + t' = [(\ln 28\ \mu g/mL - \ln 3\ \mu g/mL)/0.311\ h^{-1}] + 1\ h = 8\ h$$

4. *Determine the new dose for the desired concentrations.* The dose is computed using the one-compartment model intravenous infusion equation used in the initial dosing section of this chapter:

$$k_0 = Css_{max}k_e V[(1 - e^{-k_e \tau})/(1 - e^{-k_e t'})]$$

$$k_0 = (28\ mg/L \cdot 0.311\ h^{-1} \cdot 17\ L)[(1 - e^{-(0.311\ h^{-1})(8\ h)})/(1 - e^{-(0.311\ h^{-1})(1\ h)})] = 508\ mg,\ rounded\ to\ 500\ mg$$

A dose of amikacin 500 mg every 8 hours would be prescribed to begin 8 hours after the last dose of the previous regimen.

EXAMPLE 2 ▶▶▶

JM is a 50-year-old, 70-kg (height = 5 ft 10 in) male with gram-negative pneumonia. His current serum creatinine is 3.5 mg/dL, and it has been stable over the last 5 days since admission. A gentamicin dose of 115 mg every 24 hours was prescribed and expected to achieve steady-state peak and trough concentrations equal to 8-10 μg/mL and less than 2 μg/mL, respectively. After the third dose, steady-state peak and trough concentrations were measured and were 12 μg/mL and 3.5 μg/mL, respectively. Calculate a new gentamicin dose that would provide a steady-state peak of 9 μg/mL and a trough of less than 2 μg/mL.

1. *Estimate creatinine clearance.*

   This patient has a stable serum creatinine and is not obese. The Cockcroft-Gault equation can be used to estimate creatinine clearance:

   $$CrCl_{est} = [(140 - age)BW]/(72 \cdot S_{Cr}) = [(140 - 50 \text{ y})70 \text{ kg}]/(72 \cdot 3.5 \text{ mg/dL})$$

   $$CrCl_{est} = 25 \text{ mL/min}$$

2. *Estimate elimination rate constant (k_e) and half-life ($t_{1/2}$).*

   The elimination rate constant versus creatinine clearance relationship is used to estimate the gentamicin elimination rate for this patient:

   $$k_e = 0.00293(CrCl) + 0.014 = 0.00293(25 \text{ mL/min}) + 0.014 = 0.087 \text{ h}^{-1}$$

   $$t_{1/2} = 0.693/k_e = 0.693/0.087 \text{ h}^{-1} = 8 \text{ h}$$

   Because the patient has been receiving gentamicin for more than 3-5 estimated half-lives, it is likely that the measured serum concentrations are steady-state values.

3. *Use Steady-State Sawchuk-Zaske method to compute a new dose.*

   Compute the patient's elimination rate constant and half-life. (Note: For infusion times less than 1 hour, t′ is considered to be the sum of the infusion and waiting times.)

   $$k_e = (\ln Css_{max} - \ln Css_{min})/\tau - t' = (\ln 12 \text{ μg/mL} - \ln 3.5 \text{ μg/mL})/(24 \text{ h} - 1 \text{ h}) = 0.054 \text{ h}^{-1}$$

   $$t_{1/2} = 0.693/k_e = 0.693/0.054 \text{ h}^{-1} = 12.8 \text{ h}$$

   Compute the patient's volume of distribution.

   $$V = \frac{D/t'(1 - e^{-k_e t'})}{k_e[Css_{max} - (Css_{min}e^{-k_e t'})]} = \frac{(115 \text{ mg/1h})(1 - e^{-(0.054 h^{-1})(1 h)})}{0.054 \text{ h}^{-1}[12 \text{ mg/L} - (3.5 \text{ mg/L } e^{-(0.054 h^{-1})(1 h)})]}$$

   $$V = 12.9 \text{ L}$$

4. *Choose new steady-state peak and trough concentrations.* For the purposes of this example, the desired steady-state peak and trough concentrations will be approximately 9 μg/mL and 1.5 μg/mL, respectively.

5. *Determine the new dosage interval for the desired concentrations.* As in the initial dosage section of this chapter, the dosage interval (τ) is computed using the following equation using a 1-hour infusion time (t′):

   $$\tau = [(\ln Css_{max} - \ln Css_{min})/k_e] + t' = [(\ln 9 \text{ μg/mL} - \ln 1.5 \text{ μg/mL})/0.054 \text{ h}^{-1}] + 1 \text{ h} = 34 \text{ h, rounded to 36 h}$$

6. *Determine the new dose for the desired concentrations.* The dose is computed using the one-compartment model intravenous infusion equation used in the initial dosing section of this chapter:

   $$k_0 = Css_{max}k_eV[(1 - e^{-k_e \tau})/(1 - e^{-k_e t'})]$$

   $$k_0 = (9 \text{ mg/L} \cdot 0.054 \text{ h}^{-1} \cdot 12.9 \text{ L})\{[1 - e^{-(0.054 h^{-1})(36 h)}]/[(1 - e^{-(0.054 h^{-1})(1 h)})]\} = 102 \text{ mg, rounded to 100 mg}$$

   A dose of gentamicin 100 mg every 36 hours would be prescribed to begin 36 hours after the last dose of the previous regimen. This dose is very similar to that derived for the patient using the Pharmacokinetic Concepts method (105 mg every 36 hours).

EXAMPLE 3 ▶▶▶

ZW is a 35-year-old, 150-kg (height = 5 ft 5 in) female with an intra-abdominal infection. Her current serum creatinine is 1.1 mg/dL and is stable. A tobramycin dose of 165 mg every 8 hours was prescribed and expected to achieve steady-state peak and trough concentrations equal to 6 µg/mL and 0.5 µg/mL, respectively. After the fifth dose, steady-state peak and trough concentrations were measured and were 5 µg/mL and 2.6 µg/mL, respectively. Calculate a new tobramycin dose that would provide a steady-state peak of 6 µg/mL and a steady-state trough of 1 µg/mL or less.

1. *Estimate creatinine clearance.*
   This patient has a stable serum creatinine and is obese [IBW$_{females}$ (in kg) = 45 + 2.3(Ht − 60) = 45 + 2.3(65 in − 60) = 57 kg]. The Salazar and Corcoran equation can be used to estimate creatinine clearance:

$$CrCl_{est(females)} = \frac{(146 - age)[(0.287 \cdot Wt) + (9.74 \cdot Ht^2)]}{(60 \cdot S_{Cr})}$$

$$CrCl_{est(females)} = \frac{(146 - 35\ y)\{(0.287 \cdot 150\ kg) + [9.74 \cdot (1.65\ m)^2]\}}{(60 \cdot 1.1\ mg/dL)} = 117\ mL/min$$

   Note: Height is converted from inches to meters: Ht = (65 in • 2.54 cm/in)/(100 cm/m) = 1.65 m.

2. *Estimate elimination rate constant (k_e) and half-life ($t_{1/2}$).*
   The elimination rate constant versus creatinine clearance relationship is used to estimate the tobramycin elimination rate for this patient:

$$k_e = 0.00293(CrCl) + 0.014 = 0.00293(117\ mL/min) + 0.014 = 0.357\ h^{-1}$$

$$t_{1/2} = 0.693/k_e = 0.693/0.357\ h^{-1} = 1.9\ h$$

   Because the patient has been receiving tobramycin for more than 3-5 estimated half-lives, it is likely that the measured serum concentrations are steady-state values.

3. *Use Steady-State Sawchuk-Zaske method to compute a new dose.*
   Compute the patient's elimination rate constant and half-life. (Note: For infusion times less than 1 hour, t′ is considered to be the sum of the infusion and waiting times.)

$$k_e = (\ln Css_{max} - \ln Css_{min})/\tau - t' = (\ln 5\ µg/mL - \ln 2.6\ µg/mL)/(8\ h - 1\ h) = 0.093\ h^{-1}$$

$$t_{1/2} = 0.693/k_e = 0.693/0.093\ h^{-1} = 7.5\ h$$

   Compute the patient's volume of distribution.

$$V = \frac{D/t'(1 - e^{-k_e t'})}{k_e[Css_{max} - (Css_{min}e^{-k_e t'})]} = \frac{(165\ mg/1\ h)[1 - e^{-(0.093\ h^{-1})(1\ h)}]}{0.093\ h^{-1}[5\ mg/L - (2.6\ mg/L\ e^{-(0.093\ h^{-1})(1\ h)})]}$$

$$V = 59.9\ L$$

4. *Choose new steady-state peak and trough concentrations.* For the purposes of this example, the desired steady-state peak and trough concentrations will be 6 µg/mL and 0.8 µg/mL, respectively.

5. *Determine the new dosage interval for the desired concentrations.* As in the initial dosage section of this chapter, the dosage interval (τ) is computed using the following equation using a 1-hour infusion time (t′):

$$\tau = [(\ln Css_{max} - \ln Css_{min})/k_e] + t' = [(\ln 6\ µg/mL - \ln 0.8\ µg/mL)/0.093\ h^{-1}] + 1\ h = 23\ h, \text{rounded to 24 h}$$

6. *Determine the new dose for the desired concentrations.* The dose is computed using the one-compartment model intravenous infusion equation used in the initial dosing section of this chapter:

$$k_0 = Css_{max}k_eV[(1 - e^{-k_e\tau})/(1 - e^{-k_et'})]$$

$$k_0 = (6 \text{ mg/L} \cdot 0.093 \text{ h}^{-1} \cdot 59.9 \text{ L})\{[1 - e^{-(0.093 \text{ h}^{-1})(24 \text{ h})}]/[1 - e^{-(0.093 \text{ h}^{-1})(1 \text{ h})}]\} = 336 \text{ mg, rounded to } 335 \text{ mg}$$

A dose of gentamicin 335 mg every 24 hours would be prescribed to begin 24 hours after the last dose of the previous regimen. This dose is very similar to that derived for the patient using the Pharmacokinetic Concepts method (360 mg every 24 hours).

EXAMPLE 4 ▶ ▶ ▶

PL is a 52-year-old, 67-kg (height = 5 ft 6 in) female with neutropenia and gram-negative sepsis. His current serum creatinine is 1.5 mg/dL, and it has been stable over the last 5 days. A gentamicin dose of 110 mg every 12 hours was prescribed and expected to achieve steady-state peak and trough concentrations equal to 8–10 μg/mL and less than 2 μg/mL, respectively. After the third dose, steady-state concentrations were measured and were 3.8 μg/mL 1 hour after the end of a 1-hour infusion and 1.6 μg/mL 4 hours after the first concentration. Calculate a new gentamicin dose that would provide a steady-state peak of 9 μg/mL and a trough less than 2 μg/mL.

1. *Estimate creatinine clearance.*

This patient has a stable serum creatinine and is not obese. The Cockcroft-Gault equation can be used to estimate creatinine clearance:

$$CrCl_{est} = \{[(140 - age)BW]0.85\}/(72 \cdot S_{Cr}) = \{[(140 - 52 \text{ y})67 \text{ kg}]0.85\}/(72 \cdot 1.5 \text{ mg/dL})$$

$$CrCl_{est} = 46 \text{ mL/min}$$

2. *Estimate elimination rate constant (k_e) and half-life ($t_{1/2}$).*

The elimination rate constant versus creatinine clearance relationship is used to estimate the gentamicin elimination rate for this patient:

$$k_e = 0.00293(CrCl) + 0.014 = 0.00293(46 \text{ mL/min}) + 0.014 = 0.149 \text{ h}^{-1}$$

$$t_{1/2} = 0.693/k_e = 0.693/0.149 \text{ h}^{-1} = 4.7 \text{ h}$$

Because the patient has been receiving gentamicin for more than 3-5 estimated half-lives, it is likely that the measured serum concentrations are steady-state values.

3. *Use Steady-State Sawchuk-Zaske method to compute a new dose.*

Compute the patient's actual elimination rate constant and half-life. (Note: For infusion times less than 1 hour, t' is considered to be the sum of the infusion and waiting times.)

$$k_e = (\ln C_1 - \ln C_2)/\Delta t = (\ln 3.8 \text{ μg/mL} - \ln 1.6 \text{ μg/mL})/(4 \text{ h}) = 0.216 \text{ h}^{-1}$$

$$t_{1/2} = 0.693/k_e = 0.693/0.216 \text{ h}^{-1} = 3.2 \text{ h}$$

Extrapolate measured concentrations to steady-state peak and trough values.

$$Css_{max} = C_1/(e^{-k_et}) = (3.8 \text{ μg/mL})/[e^{-(0.216 \text{ h}^{-1})(1 \text{ h})}] = 4.7 \text{ μg/mL}$$

$$Css_{min} = C_2e^{-k_et} = (1.6 \text{ μg/mL})[e^{-(0.216 \text{ h}^{-1})(6 \text{ h})}] = 0.4 \text{ μg/mL}$$

Compute the patient's volume of distribution.

$$V = \frac{D/t'(1 - e^{-k_e t'})}{k_e[Css_{max} - (Css_{min} e^{-k_e t'})]} = \frac{(110 \text{ mg}/1 \text{ h})[1 - e^{-(0.216 \text{ h}^{-1})(1 \text{ h})}]}{0.216 \text{ h}^{-1}[4.7 \text{ mg/L} - (0.4 \text{ mg/L } e^{-(0.216 \text{ h}^{-1})(1 \text{ h})})]}$$

$$V = 22.6 \text{ L}$$

4. *Choose new steady-state peak and trough concentrations.* For the purposes of this example, the desired steady-state peak and trough concentrations will be 9 µg/mL and 1.5 µg/mL, respectively.

5. *Determine the new dosage interval for the desired concentrations.* As in the initial dosage section of this chapter, the dosage interval (τ) is computed using the following equation using a 1-hour infusion time (t'):

$$\tau = [(\ln Css_{max} - \ln Css_{min})/k_e] + t' = [(\ln 9 \text{ µg/mL} - \ln 1.5 \text{ µg/mL})/0.216 \text{ h}^{-1}] + 1 \text{ h} = 9.3 \text{ h, rounded to 8 h}$$

6. *Determine the new dose for the desired concentrations.* The dose is computed using the one-compartment model intravenous infusion equation used in the initial dosing section of this chapter:

$$k_0 = Css_{max} k_e V[(1 - e^{-k_e \tau})/(1 - e^{-k_e t'})]$$

$$k_0 = (9 \text{ mg/L} \cdot 0.216 \text{ h}^{-1} \cdot 22.6 \text{ L})\{[1 - e^{-(0.216 \text{ h}^{-1})(8 \text{ h})}]/[1 - e^{-(0.216 \text{ h}^{-1})(1 \text{ h})}]\} = 186 \text{ mg, rounded to 185 mg}$$

A dose of gentamicin 185 mg every 8 hours would be prescribed to begin approximately 8 hours after the last dose of the current regimen.

EXAMPLE 5 ▶ ▶ ▶

KE is a 67-year-old, 81-kg (height = 5 ft 11 in) male with a hepatic abscess. His current serum creatinine is 1.9 mg/dL, and it has been stable over the last 5 days. A gentamicin dose of 400 mg every 24 hours was prescribed and expected to achieve steady-state peak and trough concentrations equal to 20 µg/mL and less than 1 µg/mL, respectively. After the third dose, steady-state concentrations were measured and were 17.5 µg/mL 2 hours after the end of a 1-hour infusion and 4.8 µg/mL 16 hours after the end of infusion. Calculate a new gentamicin dose that would provide a steady-state peak of 20 µg/mL and a trough of less than 1 µg/mL.

1. *Estimate creatinine clearance.*
   This patient has a stable serum creatinine and is not obese. The Cockcroft-Gault equation can be used to estimate creatinine clearance:

$$CrCl_{est} = [(140 - age)BW]/(72 \cdot S_{Cr}) = [(140 - 67 \text{ y})81 \text{ kg}]/(72 \cdot 1.9 \text{ mg/dL})$$

$$CrCl_{est} = 43 \text{ mL/min}$$

2. *Estimate elimination rate constant (k_e) and half-life ($t_{1/2}$).*
   The elimination rate constant versus creatinine clearance relationship is used to estimate the gentamicin elimination rate for this patient:

$$k_e = 0.00293(CrCl) + 0.014 = 0.00293(43 \text{ mL/min}) + 0.014 = 0.140 \text{ h}^{-1}$$

$$t_{1/2} = 0.693/k_e = 0.693/0.140 \text{ h}^{-1} = 5.0 \text{ h}$$

Because the patient has been receiving gentamicin for more than 3-5 estimated half-lives, it is likely that the measured serum concentrations are steady-state values.

3. Use Steady-State Sawchuk-Zaske method to compute a new dose.

   Compute the patient's actual elimination rate constant and half-life. (Note: For infusion times less than 1 hour, t′ is considered to be the sum of the infusion and waiting times.)

   $$k_e = (\ln C_1 - \ln C_2)/\Delta t = (\ln 17.5\ \mu g/mL - \ln 4.8\ \mu g/mL)/(14\ h) = 0.092\ h^{-1}$$

   $$t_{1/2} = 0.693/k_e = 0.693/0.092\ h^{-1} = 7.5\ h$$

   Extrapolate measured concentrations to steady-state peak and trough values.

   $$Css_{max} = C_1/(e^{-k_e t}) = (17.5\ \mu g/mL)/[e^{-(0.092\ h^{-1})(2\ h)}] = 21.0\ \mu g/mL$$

   $$Css_{min} = C_2 e^{-k_e t} = (4.8\ \mu g/mL)[e^{-(0.092\ h^{-1})(7\ h)}] = 2.5\ \mu g/mL$$

   Compute the patient's volume of distribution.

   $$V = \frac{D/t'(1 - e^{-k_e t'})}{k_e[Css_{max} - (Css_{min} e^{-k_e t'})]} = \frac{(400\ mg/1\ h)[1 - e^{-(0.092\ h^{-1})(1\ h)}]}{0.092\ h^{-1}\{21\ mg/L - [2.5\ mg/L\ e^{-(0.092\ h^{-1})(1\ h)}]\}}$$

   $$V = 20.4\ L$$

4. *Choose new steady-state peak and trough concentrations.* For the purposes of this example, the desired steady-state peak and trough concentrations will be 20 μg/mL and 0.5 μg/mL, respectively.

5. *Determine the new dosage interval for the desired concentrations.* As in the initial dosage section of this chapter, the dosage interval (τ) is computed using the following equation using a 1-hour infusion time (t′):

   $$\tau = [(\ln Css_{max} - \ln Css_{min})/k_e] + t' = [(\ln 20\ \mu g/mL - \ln 0.5\ \mu g/mL)/0.092\ h^{-1}] + 1\ h = 41\ h,\ \text{rounded to 36 h}$$

6. *Determine the new dose for the desired concentrations.* The dose is computed using the one-compartment model intravenous infusion equation used in the initial dosing section of this chapter:

   $$k_0 = Css_{max} k_e V[(1 - e^{-k_e \tau})/(1 - e^{-k_e t'})]$$

   $$k_0 = (20\ mg/L \cdot 0.092\ h^{-1} \cdot 20.4\ L)\{[1 - e^{-(0.092\ h^{-1})(36\ h)}]/[1 - e^{-(0.092\ h^{-1})(1\ h)}]\} = 411\ mg,\ \text{rounded to 400 mg}$$

   A dose of gentamicin 400 mg every 36 hours would be prescribed to begin approximately 12 hours after the last dose of the current regimen.

EXAMPLE 6 ▶ ▶ ▶

SD is a 57-year-old, 75-kg (height = 5 ft 9 in) male with neutropenia and gram-negative sepsis. His current serum creatinine is 1.4 mg/dL, and it has been stable over the last 5 days since admission. A tobramycin dose of 500 mg every 24 hours was prescribed and expected to achieve steady-state peak and trough concentrations equal to 25 μg/mL and 1 μg/mL, respectively. After the third dose, steady-state peak and trough concentrations were measured and were 20 μg/mL and 2.5 μg/mL, respectively. Calculate a new tobramycin dose that would provide a steady-state peak of 25 μg/mL and a trough 1 μg/mL.

1. *Estimate creatinine clearance.*

   This patient has a stable serum creatinine and is not obese. The Cockcroft-Gault equation can be used to estimate creatinine clearance:

   $$CrCl_{est} = [(140 - age)BW]/(72 \cdot S_{Cr}) = [(140 - 57\ y)75\ kg]/(72 \cdot 1.4\ mg/dL)$$

   $$CrCl_{est} = 62\ mL/min$$

2. *Estimate elimination rate constant (k_e) and half-life ($t_{1/2}$).*

The elimination rate constant versus creatinine clearance relationship is used to estimate the tobramycin elimination rate for this patient:

$$k_e = 0.00293(CrCl) + 0.014 = 0.00293(62 \text{ mL/min}) + 0.014 = 0.195 \text{ h}^{-1}$$

$$t_{1/2} = 0.693/k_e = 0.693/0.195 \text{ h}^{-1} = 3.6 \text{ h}$$

Because the patient has been receiving tobramycin for more than 3-5 estimated half-lives, it is likely that the measured serum concentrations are steady-state values.

3. *Use steady-state Sawchuk-Zaske method to compute a new dose.*

Compute the patient's elimination rate constant and half-life. (Note: For infusion times less than 1 hour, t′ is considered to be the sum of the infusion and waiting times.)

$$k_e = (\ln Css_{max} - \ln Css_{min})/\tau - t' = (\ln 20 \text{ μg/mL} - \ln 2.5 \text{ μg/mL})/(24 \text{ h} - 1 \text{ h}) = 0.0904 \text{ h}^{-1}$$

$$t_{1/2} = 0.693/k_e = 0.693/0.0904 \text{ h}^{-1} = 7.7 \text{ h}$$

Compute the patient's volume of distribution.

$$V = \frac{D/t'(1 - e^{-k_e t'})}{k_e[Css_{max} - (Css_{min} e^{-k_e t'})]} = \frac{(500 \text{ mg}/1 \text{ h})[1 - e^{-(0.0904 \text{ h}^{-1})(1 \text{ h})}]}{0.0904 \text{ h}^{-1}\{20 \text{ mg/L} - [2.5 \text{ mg/L } e^{-(0.0904 \text{ h}^{-1})(1 \text{ h})}]\}}$$

$$V = 27.0 \text{ L}$$

4. *Choose new steady-state peak and trough concentrations.* For the purposes of this example, the desired steady-state peak and trough concentrations will be approximately 25 μg/mL and 1 μg/mL, respectively.

5. *Determine the new dosage interval for the desired concentrations.* As in the initial dosage section of this chapter, the dosage interval (τ) is computed using the following equation using a 1-hour infusion time (t′):

$$\tau = [(\ln Css_{max} - \ln Css_{min})/k_e] + t' = [(\ln 25 \text{ μg/mL} - \ln 1 \text{ μg/mL})/0.0904 \text{ h}^{-1}] + 1 \text{ h} = 37 \text{ h, rounded to } 36 \text{ h}$$

6. *Determine the new dose for the desired concentrations.* The dose is computed using the one-compartment model intravenous infusion equation used in the initial dosing section of this chapter:

$$k_0 = Css_{max} k_e V[(1 - e^{-k_e \tau})/(1 - e^{-k_e t'})]$$

$$k_0 = (25 \text{ mg/L} \cdot 0.0904 \text{ h}^{-1} \cdot 27.0 \text{ L})\{[1 - e^{-(0.0904 \text{ h}^{-1})(36 \text{ h})}]/[1 - e^{-(0.0904 \text{ h}^{-1})(1 \text{ h})}]\} = 678 \text{ mg, rounded to } 675 \text{ mg}$$

A dose of gentamicin 675 mg every 36 hours would be prescribed to begin 36 hours after the last dose of the previous regimen.

Area Under the Curve Method

Area under the concentration-time curve (AUC) is the best measurement of total exposure to a drug, and some clinicians recommend adjustment of aminoglycoside doses so that target steady-state AUC values are achieved instead of altering doses to attain target steady-state peak and trough concentrations. Most often, the AUC method is used with extended-interval aminoglycoside dosing. Different therapeutic AUC values have been suggested by various investigations studying this dosing method. A target AUC equal to 70-120 (mg • h)/L for gentamicin or tobramycin will be used in examples and problems for this section (~5 mg/kg ≈ 72 (mg • h)/L,

6 mg/kg ≈ 86 (mg • h)/L, and 7 mg/kg ≈ 101 (mg • h)/L for patients with normal renal function).[30,32,37-41] Steady-state peak and trough concentrations should also be evaluated when a dosage change is made to ensure that they are in the appropriate range.

Measured AUC Using Steady-State Peak and Trough Concentrations

To make use of this approach, the patient is started on an appropriate dose of extended-interval gentamicin or tobramycin. Typical doses of 5-7 mg/kg/d are used as an initial dose, with the dosage interval determined by renal function.[3,134] After steady state has been achieved, two postdose serum concentrations are drawn. The two concentrations should be drawn at least 1 estimated half-life apart in order to minimize the effect of assay error on the calculations. While one of the two steady-state concentrations can be a peak concentration, it is not a requirement. During extended-interval dosing, some patients may have longer distribution phases so many clinicians suggest that the first postdose concentration be obtained several hours after the completion of the infusion. The second postdose concentration should be drawn early enough in the dosage interval so that it is not below assay limits (typically no later than 14-16 hours post dose for patients with CrCl >60 mL/min).

Once the concentrations are obtained, they are extrapolated either mathematically or graphically (Figure 4-14) to determine steady-state peak and trough values. The elimination rate constant is calculated using the measured concentrations: $k_e = (\ln C_1 - \ln C_2)/\Delta t$, where C_1 and C_2 are the first and second steady-state postdose concentrations, respectively, and Δt is the time that expired between the two concentrations. If one of the concentrations is a peak concentration, it is unnecessary to extrapolate it, and only the trough concentration needs to be computed. However, if neither concentration is a peak, both steady-state peak and trough concentrations need to be calculated: $Css_{max} = C_1/(e^{-k_e t})$, where C_1 is the first measured steady-state

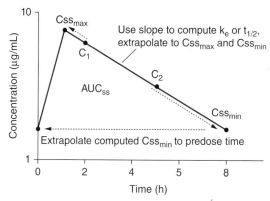

FIGURE 4-14   The Area Under the Curve (AUC) method uses two postdose concentrations (C_1 and C_2) to individualize aminoglycoside therapy. Once the concentrations are obtained, they are extrapolated either mathematically or graphically to determine steady-state peak and trough values. The elimination rate constant is calculated using the measured concentrations: $k_e = (\ln C_1 - \ln C_2)/\Delta t$, where C_1 and C_2 are the first and second steady-state postdose concentrations and Δt is the time that expired between the two concentrations. Steady-state peak and trough concentrations are calculated using the following equations: $Css_{max} = C_1/(e^{-k_e t})$, where C_1 is the first measured steady-state concentration, k_e is the elimination rate constant, and t is the time between C_1 and Css_{max}; $Css_{min} = C_2 e^{-k_e t}$, where C_2 is the second measured steady-state concentration, k_e is the elimination rate constant, and t is the time between C_2 and Css_{min}. The steady-state area under the concentration-time curve during the dosage interval (AUC_{ss}) is computed using the following equation:

$$AUC_{ss} = \frac{Css_{max} - Css_{min}}{k_e} + \left(0.065 \cdot \frac{Css_{max} - Css_{min}}{k_e} \right)$$

concentration, k_e is the elimination rate constant, and t is the time between C_1 and Css_{max}; $Css_{min} = C_2e^{-k_et}$, where C_2 is the second measured steady-state concentration, k_e is the elimination rate constant, and t is the time between C_2 and Css_{min}.

The steady-state area under the concentration-time curve during the dosage interval (AUC_{ss}) is computed using the following equation:[30,32,37-39]

$$AUC_{ss} = \frac{Css_{max} - Css_{max}}{k_e} + \left(0.065 \cdot \frac{Css_{max} - Css_{min}}{k_e}\right)$$

The dose is adjusted to attain the target AUC_{ss} using linear pharmacokinetics: $D_{new} = (AUC_{ss,new}/AUC_{ss,old})$ D_{old}, where D_{new} denotes the new computed dose and D_{old} the original dose, and $AUC_{ss,new}$ and $AUC_{ss,old}$ are the new target AUC_{ss} and the old original AUC_{ss}, respectively. Once the new dose has been determined, Css_{max} and Css_{min} should be calculated to ensure that their values are also appropriate for the infection that is being treated: $C_{ss,new} = (D_{new}/D_{old})C_{ss,old}$, where D_{new} denotes the new computed dose and D_{old} the original dose, and $C_{ss,new}$ and $C_{ss,old}$ are the new target C_{ss} and the old original C_{ss}, respectively. This calculation is repeated separately for both Css_{max} and Css_{min}.

EXAMPLE 1 ▶▶▶

KE is a 23-year-old, 59-kg (height = 5 ft 4 in) female with salpingitis. Her current serum creatinine is 0.6 mg/dL, and it has been stable over the last 3 days. A gentamicin dose of 250 mg every 24 hours was prescribed and expected to achieve steady-state peak and trough concentrations equal to 25 µg/mL and less than 1 µg/mL, respectively. After the third dose, steady-state concentrations were measured and equaled 9.6 µg/mL 2 hours after the end of a 1-hour infusion and 2.6 µg/mL 6 hours after the end of infusion. Calculate a new gentamicin dose that would provide a steady-state AUC of 81 (mg • h)/L.

1. *Estimate creatinine clearance.*
   This patient has a stable serum creatinine and is not obese. The Cockcroft-Gault equation can be used to estimate creatinine clearance:

   $$CrCl_{est} = \{[(140 - age)BW]0.85\}/(72 \cdot S_{Cr}) = \{[(140 - 23 \text{ y})59 \text{ kg}]0.85\}/(72 \cdot 0.6 \text{ mg/dL})$$

   $$CrCl_{est} = 136 \text{ mL/min}$$

2. *Estimate elimination rate constant (k_e) and half-life ($t_{1/2}$).*
   The elimination rate constant versus creatinine clearance relationship is used to estimate the gentamicin elimination rate for this patient:

   $$k_e = 0.00293(CrCl) + 0.014 = 0.00293(136 \text{ mL/min}) + 0.014 = 0.413 \text{ h}^{-1}$$

   $$t_{1/2} = 0.693/k_e = 0.693/0.413 \text{ h}^{-1} = 1.7 \text{ h}$$

   Because the patient has been receiving gentamicin for more than 3-5 estimated half-lives, it is likely that the measured serum concentrations are steady-state values.

3. *Use Steady-State AUC method to compute a new dose.*
   Compute the patient's actual elimination rate constant and half-life. (Note: For infusion times less than 1 hour, t' is considered to be the sum of the infusion and waiting times.)

   $$k_e = (\ln C_1 - \ln C_2)/\Delta t = (\ln 9.6 \text{ µg/mL} - \ln 2.6 \text{ µg/mL})/(4 \text{ h}) = 0.327 \text{ h}^{-1}$$

   $$t_{1/2} = 0.693/k_e = 0.693/0.327 \text{ h}^{-1} = 2.1 \text{ h}$$

Extrapolate measured concentrations to steady-state peak and trough values.

$$Css_{max} = C_1/(e^{-k_e t}) = (9.6 \, \mu g/mL)/(e^{-(0.327 \, h^{-1})(2 \, h)}) = 18.5 \, \mu g/mL$$

$$Css_{min} = C_2 e^{-k_e t} = (2.6 \, \mu g/mL)(e^{-(0.327 \, h^{-1})(17 \, h)}) = 0.01 \, \mu g/mL$$

Compute the patient's AUC_{ss}. (Note: mg/L = µg/mL and this substitution was made to aid the calculation.)

$$AUC_{ss} = \frac{Css_{max} - Css_{min}}{k_e} + \left(0.065 \cdot \frac{Css_{max} - Css_{min}}{k_e} \right)$$

$$AUC_{ss} = \frac{18.5 \, mg/L - 0.01 \, mg/L}{0.327 \, h^{-1}} + \left(0.065 \cdot \frac{18.5 \, mg/L - 0.01 \, mg/L}{0.327 \, h^{-1}} \right)$$

$$AUC_{ss} = 60.2 \, (mg \cdot h)/L$$

4. *Choose new target AUC_{ss}.* For the purposes of this example, a desired steady-state of AUC of 81 (mg • h)/L was chosen.

5. *Determine the new dose for the desired AUC_{ss}.*

$$D_{new} = (AUC_{ss,new}/AUC_{ss,old})D_{old} = \{[81 \, (mg \cdot h)/L]/[60.2 \, (mg \cdot h)/L]\}250 \, mg = 336 \, mg, \text{ rounded to } 350 \, mg$$

6. *Determine the new steady-state peak and trough concentrations.*

$$C_{ss,new} = (D_{new}/D_{old})C_{ss,old} = (350 \, mg/250 \, mg) \, 18.5 \, \mu g/mL = 25.9 \, \mu g/mL \text{ for the peak}$$

$$C_{ss,new} = (D_{new}/D_{old})C_{ss,old} = (350 \, mg/250 \, mg) \, 0.01 \, \mu g/mL = 0.01 \, \mu g/mL \text{ for the trough}$$

These steady-state peak and trough concentrations are acceptable for the infection being treated and the new prescribed dose would be 350 mg every 24 hours.

Measured AUC Using Concentration(s) and Bayesian Pharmacokinetic Computer Program

Bayesian pharmacokinetic computer programs can compute pharmacokinetic values using one or more drug concentrations, and the concentrations do not need to be at steady state (please see next major section of this chapter for more information). Once the program has computed gentamicin clearance, it can be used to compute AUC for the dose (AUC = D/Cl, where D is the gentamicin dose), or the program may report AUC directly.

EXAMPLE 2 ▶ ▶ ▶

KE is a 23-year-old, 59-kg (height = 5 ft 4 in) female with salpingitis. Her current serum creatinine is 0.6 mg/dL, and it has been stable over the last 3 days. A gentamicin dose of 250 mg every 24 hours was prescribed and expected to achieve steady-state peak and trough concentrations equal to 25 µg/mL and less than 1 µg/mL, respectively. After the third dose, steady-state concentrations were measured and equaled 9.6 µg/mL 2 hours after the end of a 1-hour infusion and 2.6 µg/mL 6 hours after the end of infusion. Calculate a new gentamicin dose that would provide a steady-state AUC of 81 (mg • h)/L.

1. *Calculate AUC using the Bayesian pharmacokinetic computer program.*
   The pharmacokinetic parameters computed by the program are a volume of distribution of 12.7 L, a half-life equal to 2.2 hours, and clearance of 3.95 L/h.
   The AUC for a dose is: $AUC = D/Cl = (250 \text{ mg})/(3.95 \text{ L/h}) = 63.3 \text{ (mg} \cdot \text{h)/L}$.

2. *Compute new dose based on AUC target.*
   Gentamicin follows linear pharmacokinetics, so the AUC and steady-state trough concentrations change proportionally with dose.

   $$\text{Dose}_{new} = (AUC_{new}/AUC_{old})\text{Dose}_{old} = (81/63.3)(250 \text{ mg/d}) = 320 \text{ mg/d, round to } 325 \text{ mg/d}$$

   Check new steady-state gentamicin trough and peak concentrations for this AUC: the Bayesian pharmacokinetic computer program computes steady-state gentamicin trough and peak concentrations of 0.02 µg/mL and 22.1 µg/mL, respectively, for the new dose. These would provide a C_{max}/MIC of more than 10 for bacteria up to a MIC = 2 µg/mL.

EXAMPLE 3 ▶ ▶ ▶

KE is a 23-year-old, 59-kg (height = 5 ft 4 in) female with salpingitis. Her current serum creatinine is 0.6 mg/dL, and it has been stable over the last 3 days. A gentamicin dose of 250 mg every 24 hours was prescribed and expected to achieve steady-state peak and trough concentrations equal to 25 µg/mL and less than 1 µg/mL, respectively. After the third dose, a steady-state concentration was measured and equaled 9.6 µg/mL 2 hours after the end of a 1-hour infusion. Calculate a new gentamicin dose that would provide a steady-state AUC of 81 (mg · h)/L. *(Note: This is the same case as Example 2, but only one serum concentration is available.)*

1. *Calculate AUC using the Bayesian pharmacokinetic computer program.*
   The pharmacokinetic parameters computed by the program are a volume of distribution of 13.6 L, a half-life equal to 2.5 hours, and clearance of 3.76 L/h.
   The AUC for a dose is: $AUC = D/Cl = (250 \text{ mg})/(3.76 \text{ L/h}) = 66.5 \text{ (mg} \cdot \text{h)/L}$.

2. *Compute new dose based on AUC target.*
   Gentamicin follows linear pharmacokinetics, so the AUC and steady-state trough concentrations change proportionally with dose.

   $$\text{Dose}_{new} = (AUC_{new}/AUC_{old})\text{Dose}_{old} = (81/66.5)(250 \text{ mg/d}) = 305 \text{ mg/d, round to } 300 \text{ mg/d}$$

   Check new steady-state gentamicin trough and peak concentrations for this AUC: the Bayesian pharmacokinetic computer program computes steady-state gentamicin trough and peak concentrations of 0.03 µg/mL and 19.3 µg/mL, respectively, for the new dose. These would provide a Cmax/MIC of more than 10 for bacteria up to a MIC = ~2 µg/mL.

BAYESIAN PHARMACOKINETIC COMPUTER PROGRAMS

Computer programs are available that can assist in the computation of pharmacokinetic parameters for patients.[137-141] The most reliable computer programs use a nonlinear regression algorithm that incorporates components of Bayes theorem. Nonlinear regression is a statistical technique that uses an iterative process to compute the best pharmacokinetic parameters for a concentration/time data set. Briefly, the patient's drug dosage schedule and serum concentrations are input into the computer. The computer program has a pharmacokinetic equation preprogrammed for the drug and administration method (oral, intravenous bolus, intravenous infusion, etc). Typically, a one-compartment model is used, although some programs allow the user to choose among several different equations. Using population estimates based on demographic information for the patient (age, weight, gender, renal function, etc) supplied by the user, the computer program then computes estimated serum concentrations at each time there are actual serum concentrations. Kinetic parameters are then changed by the computer program, and a new set of estimated serum concentrations are computed. The pharmacokinetic parameters that generated the estimated serum concentrations closest to the actual values are remembered by the computer program, and the process is repeated until the set of pharmacokinetic parameters that result in estimated serum concentrations that are statistically closest to the actual serum concentrations are generated. These pharmacokinetic parameters can then be used to compute improved dosing schedules for patients. Bayes theorem is used in the computer algorithm to balance the results of the computations between values based solely on the patient's serum drug concentrations and those based only on patient population parameters. Results from studies that compare various methods of dosage adjustment have consistently found that these types of computer dosing programs perform at least as well as experienced clinical pharmacokineticists and clinicians and better than inexperienced clinicians.

Some clinicians use Bayesian pharmacokinetic computer programs exclusively to alter drug doses based on serum concentrations. An advantage of this approach is that consistent dosage recommendations are made when several different practitioners are involved in therapeutic drug monitoring programs. However, because simpler dosing methods work just as well for patients with stable pharmacokinetic parameters and steady-state drug concentrations, many clinicians reserve the use of computer programs for more difficult situations. Those situations include serum concentrations that are not at steady state, serum concentrations not obtained at the specific times needed to employ simpler methods, and unstable pharmacokinetic parameters. When only a limited number of aminoglycoside concentrations are available, Bayesian pharmacokinetic computer programs can be used to compute a complete patient pharmacokinetic profile that includes clearance, volume of distribution, and half-life. Many Bayesian pharmacokinetic computer programs are available to users, and most should provide answers similar to the one used in the following examples. The program used to solve problems in this book is DrugCalc written by Dr Dennis Mungall.[142]

EXAMPLE 1 ▶ ▶ ▶

JM is a 50-year-old, 70-kg (height = 5 ft 10 in) male with gram-negative pneumonia. His current serum creatinine is 0.9 mg/dL, and it has been stable over the last 5 days since admission. A gentamicin dose of 170 mg every 8 hours was prescribed and expected to achieve steady-state peak and trough concentrations equal to 9 μg/mL and 1 μg/mL, respectively. After the third dose, steady-state peak and trough concentrations were measured and were 12 μg/mL and 1.4 μg/mL, respectively. Calculate a new gentamicin dose that would provide a steady-state peak of 9 μg/mL and steady-state trough of 1 μg/mL.

1. *Enter patient demographic, drug dosing, and serum concentration/time data into the computer program.*

2. *Compute pharmacokinetic parameters for the patient using Bayesian pharmacokinetic computer program.*
   The pharmacokinetic parameters computed by the program are a volume of distribution of 13.5 L, a half-life equal to 2.1 hours, and an elimination rate constant of 0.326 h^{-1}.

3. *Compute dose required to achieve desired aminoglycoside serum concentrations.*
   The one-compartment model intravenous infusion equations used by the program to compute doses indicate that a dose of 135 mg every 8 hours will produce a steady-state peak concentration of 9.2 μg/mL and a steady-state trough concentration of 0.9 μg/mL. Using the Simpler Linear Pharmacokinetics method previously described in this chapter, a similar dose of 140 mg every 8 hours was computed.

EXAMPLE 2 ▶ ▶ ▶

JM is a 50-year-old, 70-kg (height = 5 ft 10 in) male with gram-negative pneumonia. His current serum creatinine is 3.5 mg/dL, and it has been stable over the last 5 days since admission. A gentamicin dose of 115 mg every 24 hours was prescribed and expected to achieve steady-state peak and trough concentrations equal to 8-10 µg/mL and less than 2 µg/mL, respectively. After the third dose, steady-state peak and trough concentrations were measured and were 12 µg/mL and 3.5 µg/mL, respectively. Calculate a new gentamicin dose that would provide a steady-state peak of 9 µg/mL and a steady-state trough equal to 1.5 µg/mL.

1. *Enter patient demographic, drug dosing, and serum concentration/time data into the computer program.*

2. *Compute pharmacokinetic parameters for the patient using Bayesian pharmacokinetic computer program.*
   The pharmacokinetic parameters computed by the program are a volume of distribution of 14.6 L, a half-life equal to 14.7 hours, and an elimination rate constant of 0.047 h^{-1}. These values are slightly different than those computed using the steady-state Sawchuk-Zaske method (V = 12.9 L, $t_{1/2}$ = 12.8 h, k_e = 0.054 h^{-1}) because the patient probably was not at steady state when the serum concentrations were drawn.

3. *Compute dose required to achieve desired aminoglycoside serum concentrations.*
   The one-compartment model intravenous infusion equations used by the program to compute doses indicate that a dose of 110 mg every 36 hours will produce a steady-state peak concentration of 9 µg/mL and a steady-state trough concentration of 1.7 µg/mL. Using the steady-state Sawchuk-Zaske and Pharmacokinetic Concepts methods previously described in this chapter, a similar doses of 100 mg every 36 hours and 105 mg every 36 hours, respectively, were computed.

EXAMPLE 3 ▶ ▶ ▶

KE is a 23-year-old, 59-kg (height = 5 ft 4 in) female with salpingitis. Her current serum creatinine is 0.6 mg/dL, and it has been stable over the last 3 days. A gentamicin dose of 250 mg every 24 hours was prescribed and expected to achieve steady-state peak and trough concentrations equal to 25 µg/mL and less than 1 µg/mL, respectively. After the third dose, steady-state concentrations were measured and equaled 9.6 µg/mL 2 hours after the end of a 1-hour infusion and 2.6 µg/mL 6 hours after the end of infusion. Calculate a new gentamicin dose that would provide a steady-state peak of 25 µg/mL and a steady-state trough of less than 1 µg/mL.

1. *Enter patient demographic, drug dosing, and serum concentration/time data into the computer program.*

2. *Compute pharmacokinetic parameters for the patient using Bayesian pharmacokinetic computer program.*
   The pharmacokinetic parameters computed by the program are a volume of distribution of 12.7 L, a half-life equal to 2.2 hours, an elimination rate constant of 0.315 h^{-1}, and a clearance of 3.95 L/h.

3. *Compute dose required to achieve desired aminoglycoside serum concentrations.*
   The one-compartment model intravenous infusion equations used by the program to compute doses indicate that a dose of 350 mg every 24 hours will produce a steady-state peak concentration of 24 µg/mL and a steady-state trough concentration of 0.02 µg/mL.

EXAMPLE 4 ▶▶▶

JH is a 24-year-old, 70-kg (height = 6 ft 0 in) male with gram-negative pneumonia. His current serum creatinine is 1.0 mg/dL, and it has been stable over the last 7 days since admission. An amikacin dose of 400 mg every 8 hours was prescribed. After the third dose, the following amikacin serum concentrations were obtained:

Time	Amikacin concentration (μg/mL)
0800 H	2.0
0800–0900 H	Amikacin 400 mg
0900 H	22.1
1100 H	11.9
1600 H	2.5

Medication administration sheets were checked, and the previous dose was given 2 hours early (2200 H the previous day). Because of this, it is known that the patient is not at steady state. Calculate a new amikacin dose that would provide a steady-state peak of 28 μg/mL and a trough between 3 μg/mL.

1. *Enter patient demographic, drug dosing, and serum concentration/time data into the computer program.*

2. *Compute pharmacokinetic parameters for the patient using Bayesian pharmacokinetic computer program.*
   The pharmacokinetic parameters computed by the program are a volume of distribution of 17.1 L, a half-life equal to 2.4 hours, and an elimination rate constant of 0.292 h^{-1}. These values are similar to those computed using the Sawchuk-Zaske method (V = 17.0 L, t$_{1/2}$ = 2.2 h, k$_e$ = 0.311 h^{-1}).

3. *Compute dose required to achieve desired aminoglycoside serum concentrations.*
   The one-compartment model intravenous infusion equations used by the program to compute doses indicate that a dose of 500 mg every 8 hours will produce a steady-state peak concentration of 28 μg/mL and a steady-state trough concentration of 3.6 μg/mL. Using the Sawchuk-Zaske method previously described in this chapter, the identical dose of 500 mg every 8 hours was computed.

DOSING STRATEGIES

Initial dose and dosage adjustment techniques using serum concentrations can be used in any combination as long as the limitations of each method are observed. Some dosing approaches link together logically when considered according to their basic approaches or philosophies. Dosage strategies that follow similar pathways are given in Tables 4-5A and 4-5B.

TABLE 4-5A   Conventional Dosing Schemes

Dosing Approach/Philosophy	Initial Dosing	Use of Serum Concentrations to Alter Doses
Pharmacokinetic parameters/equations	Pharmacokinetic Dosing method	Sawchuk-Zaske method
Nomogram/pharmacokinetic concepts	Hull and Sarubbi Nomogram (adults) or Literature-based Recommended Dosing (pediatrics)	Pharmacokinetic Concepts method
Computerized	Bayesian computer program	Bayesian computer program

TABLE 4-5B   Extended-Interval Dosing Schemes

Dosing Approach/Philosophy	Initial Dosing	Use of Serum Concentrations to Alter Doses
Pharmacokinetic parameters/equations	Pharmacokinetic Dosing method	Sawchuk-Zaske method or Area Under the Curve (AUC) method
Nomogram/Concepts	Hartford nomogram	Hartford nomogram (1 concentration) or Pharmacokinetic Concepts method (≥2 concentrations)
Computerized	Bayesian computer program	Bayesian computer program

SPECIAL DOSING CONSIDERATIONS

Hemodialysis Dosing

Aminoglycoside antibiotics are eliminated by dialysis, so renal failure patients receiving hemodialysis must have aminoglycoside dosage regimens that take dialysis clearance into account. Note that these techniques can be used with either conventional dosing or extended-interval dosing target steady-state serum concentrations. Hemodialysis and other extracorporeal methods of drug removal are completely discussed in Chapter 3 (Computation of Initial Doses and Modification of Doses Using Drug Serum Concentrations section).

EXAMPLE 1 ▶ ▶ ▶

A 62-year-old, 5-ft 8-in male who weighs 65 kg has chronic renal failure and receives hemodialysis three times weekly with a low-flux dialysis filter. An initial dosage regimen for tobramycin needs to be computed for a patient to achieve peak concentrations of 6-7 mg/L and postdialysis concentrations 1-2 mg/L.

Initial Dosage Determination

1. Patients with renal failure are prone to having poor fluid balance because their kidneys are not able to provide this important function. Because of this, the patient should be assessed for overhydration (due to renal failure) or underhydration (due to renal failure and increased loss due to fever).

Weight is a good indication of fluid status, and this patient's weight is less than his ideal weight [IBW_{male} = 50 kg + 2.3(Ht − 60) = 50 kg + 2.3(68 in − 60) = 68 kg]. Other indications of state of hydration (skin turgor, etc) indicate that the patient has normal fluid balance at this time. Because of this, the average volume of distribution for aminoglycoside antibiotics equal to 0.26 L/kg can be used.

2. A loading dose of tobramycin would be appropriate for this patient because the expected half-life is long (~50 hours); administration of maintenance doses only might not result in therapeutic maximum concentrations for a considerable time period while drug accumulation is occurring. The loading dose is to be given after hemodialysis ends at 1300 H on Monday (hemodialysis conducted on Monday, Wednesday, and Friday from 0900 to 1300 H).

Because the patient is expected to have a long half-life compared to the infusion time of the drug (1/2-1 h), little drug will be eliminated during the infusion period, and IV bolus one-compartment model equations can be used. The loading dose for this patient would be based on the expected volume of distribution: $V = 0.26$ L/kg • 65 kg = 16.9 L; LD = C_{max} • V = 6 mg/L • 16.9 L = 101 mg, rounded to 100 mg (LD is loading dose, C_{max} is the maximum concentration after drug administration). This loading dose was given at 1400 H (see Figure 4-15).

Until the next dialysis period at 0900 H on Wednesday, tobramycin is cleared only by the patient's own body mechanisms. The expected elimination rate constant (k_e) for a patient with a creatinine clearance of approximately zero is: k_e (in h^{-1}) = 0.00293 • CrCl + 0.014 = 0.00293 (0 mL/min) + 0.014 = 0.014 h^{-1}. The expected concentration at 0900 H on Wednesday is: $C = C_0 e^{-k_e t}$, where C is the concentration at t hours after the initial concentration of C_0; $C = (6 \text{ mg/L})e^{-(0.014 \text{ h}^{-1})(43 \text{ h})} = 3.3$ mg/L.

3. While the patient is receiving hemodialysis, tobramycin is eliminated by the patient's own mechanisms plus dialysis clearance. During hemodialysis with a low-flux filter, the average half-life for aminoglycosides is 4 hours. Because the patient is dialyzed for 4 hours, the tobramycin serum concentration should decrease by ½ to 1.7 mg/L, or using formal computations: $k_e = 0.693/(t_{1/2}) = 0.693/4$ h = 0.173 h^{-1}; $C = C_0 e^{-k_e t} = (3.3 \text{ mg/L})e^{-(0.173 \text{ h}^{-1})(4 \text{ h})} = 1.7$ mg/L.

At this time, a postdialysis replacement dose could be given to increase the maximum concentration to its original value of 6 mg/L: Replacement dose = $(C_{max} - C_{baseline})V = (6 \text{ mg/L} - 1.7 \text{ mg/L})16.9$ L = 73 mg, round to 75 mg (where C_{max} is the maximum postdose concentration and $C_{baseline}$ is the predose concentration). The postdialysis replacement dose of 75 mg was administered at 1400 H on Wednesday. Because all time frames and pharmacokinetic parameters are the same for Monday to Wednesday and Wednesday to Friday, the postdialysis replacement dose on Friday at 1400 H would also be 75 mg.

However, more time elapses from Friday after drug administration to Monday before dialysis (67 hours), the next day for hemodialysis to be conducted in the patient and this needs to be accounted for: $C = C_0 e^{-k_e t} = (6 \text{ mg/L})e^{-(0.014 \text{ h}^{-1})(67 \text{ h})} = 2.3$ mg/L. Again, a 4-hour hemodialysis period would decrease serum concentrations by ½ to 1.2 mg/L: $C = C_0 e^{-k_e t} = (2.3 \text{ mg/L})e^{-(0.173 \text{ h}^{-1})(4 \text{ h})} = 1.2$ mg/L. At this time, a postdialysis replacement dose could be given to increase the maximum concentration to the original value of 6 mg/L: Replacement dose = $(C_{max} - C_{baseline})V = (6 \text{ mg/L} - 1.2 \text{ mg/L})16.9$ L = 81 mg, round to 80 mg (where C_{max} is the maximum postdose concentration and $C_{baseline}$ is the predose concentration). The postdialysis replacement dose of 80 mg was administered at 1400 H on Monday.

Because all time frames and pharmacokinetic parameters subsequent weeks, the following postdialysis replacement doses would be prescribed postdialysis at 1400: Wednesday and Friday 75 mg, Monday 80 mg. In this particular example, recommended daily doses are within 5 mg of each other, and if the clinician wished, the same postdialysis dose could be given on each day. However, this will not be true in every case.

Use of Aminoglycoside Serum Concentrations to Alter Dosages

1. Because the initial dosage scheme outlined for this patient used average, estimated pharmacokinetic parameters, it is likely that the patient has different pharmacokinetic characteristics. It is possible to measure the patient's own unique pharmacokinetic parameters using four serum concentrations (Figure 4-15).

The intradialysis elimination rate constant can be determined by obtaining postdose ($C_{postdose(1)}$) and predialysis ($C_{predialysis}$) concentrations [$k_e = (C_{postdose(1)} - C_{predialysis})/\Delta t$, where Δt is the time between the two concentrations], the fraction of drug eliminated by dialysis can be computed using predialysis and postdialysis ($C_{postdialysis}$) concentrations {fraction eliminated = $[(C_{predialysis} - C_{postdialysis})/C_{predialysis}]$}, and the volume of distribution can be calculated using postdialysis and postdose concentrations [$V = D/(C_{postdose(2)} - C_{predialysis})$].

Note that if the drug has a postdialysis "rebound" in drug concentrations, postdialysis serum samples should be obtained after blood and tissue have had the opportunity to reequilibrate. In the case of aminoglycosides, postdialysis samples should be collected no sooner than 3-4 hours after the end of dialysis.

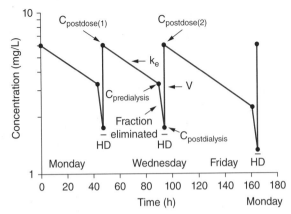

FIGURE 4-15   Concentration/time graph for tobramycin in a hemodialysis patient using estimated, population pharmacokinetic parameters. The initial dose was given postdialysis at 1400 H on Monday (time = 0 hour). Hemodialysis periods are shown by small horizontal bars labeled with HD, and days are indicated on the time line. In order to compute patient-specific pharmacokinetic parameters, four serum concentrations are measured. The elimination rate constant (k_e) is computed using two concentrations after dosage administration ($C_{postdose(1)}$ and $C_{predialysis}$), the fraction eliminated by dialysis by two concentrations ($C_{predialysis}$ and $C_{postdialysis}$) before and after dialysis, and the volume of distribution using two concentrations ($C_{postdialysis}$ and $C_{postdose(2)}$) after another dosage administration.

2. Once individualized pharmacokinetic parameters have been measured, they can be used in the same equations used to compute initial doses in the previous section in place of average, population pharmacokinetic parameters and used to calculate individualized doses for dialysis patients. It is also possible to use a mixture of measured and population-estimated pharmacokinetic parameters. For instance, a clinician may wish to measure the elimination rate constant or volume of distribution for a patient but elect to use an average population estimate for fraction of drug removed by the artificial kidney.

PROBLEMS

The following problems are intended to emphasize the computation of initial and individualized doses using clinical pharmacokinetic techniques. Clinicians should always consult the patient's chart to confirm that antibiotic therapy is appropriate for current microbiologic cultures and sensitivities. Also, it should be confirmed that the patient is receiving other appropriate concurrent antibiotic therapy, such as β-lactam or anaerobic agents, when necessary to treat the infection.

1. PQ is a 75-year-old, 62-kg (height = 5 ft 9 in) male with gram-negative sepsis. His current serum creatinine is 1.3 mg/dL, and it has been stable since admission. Compute a gentamicin dose for this patient to provide a steady-state peak concentration of 8 μg/mL and a steady-state trough concentration of 1.5 μg/mL using conventional dosing.

2. Patient PQ (see problem 1) was prescribed gentamicin 110 mg every 12 hours. Steady-state gentamicin concentrations were obtained before and after the fourth dose, and the peak concentration (obtained ½ hour after a ½-hour infusion of gentamicin) was 9.5 μg/mL while the trough concentration (obtained within ½ hour before dosage administration) was 3.0 μg/mL. Compute a revised gentamicin dose for this patient to provide a steady-state peak concentration of 8 μg/mL and a steady-state trough concentration of 1 μg/mL using conventional dosing.

3. ZW is a 35-year-old, 75-kg (height = 5 ft 7 in) female with gram-negative pneumonia and chronic renal failure. Her current serum creatinine is 3.7 mg/dL, and it has been stable since admission. Compute a gentamicin dose for this patient to provide a steady-state peak concentration of 10 μg/mL and a steady-state trough concentration of 1.0 μg/mL using conventional dosing.

4. Patient ZW (see problem 3) was prescribed gentamicin 120 mg every 24 hours. Steady-state gentamicin concentrations were obtained before and after the fourth dose, and the peak concentration (obtained ½ hour after a ½-hour infusion of gentamicin) was 7 μg/mL while the trough concentration (obtained within ½ hour before dosage administration) was less than 0.5 μg/mL. Compute a revised gentamicin dose for this patient to provide a steady-state peak concentration of 10 μg/mL and a steady-state trough concentration of less than 2 μg/mL using conventional dosing.

5. JK is a 55-year-old, 140-kg (height = 5 ft 8 in) male with an intra-abdominal infection secondary to a knife wound. His current serum creatinine is 0.9 mg/dL, and it has been stable since admission. Compute a gentamicin dose for this patient to provide a steady-state peak concentration of 6 μg/mL and a steady-state trough concentration of 0.5 μg/mL using conventional dosing.

6. Patient JK (see problem 5) was prescribed gentamicin 120 mg every 8 hours. Steady-state gentamicin concentrations were obtained before and after the fourth dose, and the peak concentration (obtained ½ hour after a ½-hour infusion of gentamicin) was 5.9 μg/mL while the trough concentration (obtained within ½ hour before dosage administration) was 2.5 μg/mL. Compute a revised gentamicin dose for this patient to provide a steady-state peak concentration of 6 μg/mL and a steady-state trough concentration of less than 1 μg/mL using conventional dosing.

7. AF is a 45-year-old, 140-kg (5 ft 2 in) female with an S. viridans endocarditis. Her current serum creatinine is 2.4 mg/dL and is stable. Compute a tobramycin dose for this patient to provide a steady-state peak concentration of 4 μg/mL, and a steady-state trough concentration of 0.5 μg/mL using conventional dosing.

8. Patient AF (see problem 7) was prescribed tobramycin 100 mg every 12 hours. Steady-state tobramycin concentrations were obtained before and after the fourth dose, and the peak concentration (obtained ½ hour after a ½-hour infusion of tobramycin) was 6.2 μg/mL while the trough concentration (obtained within ½ hour before dosage administration) was 1.5 μg/mL. Compute a revised tobramycin dose for this patient to provide a steady-state peak concentration of 4 μg/mL and a steady-state trough concentration of 1 μg/mL or less using conventional dosing.

9. FH is a 24-year-old, 60-kg (5 ft 7 in) male with cystic fibrosis and *Pseudomonas aeruginosa* cultured from a sputum culture. He was hospitalized due to worsening pulmonary function tests. His current serum creatinine is 0.7 mg/dL. Compute a tobramycin dose for this patient to provide a steady-state peak concentration of 10 μg/mL, and a steady-state trough concentration of less than 2 μg/mL using conventional dosing.

10. Patient FH (see problem 9) was prescribed tobramycin 250 mg every 8 hours. Steady-state tobramycin concentrations were obtained before and after the fourth dose, and the peak concentration (obtained ½ hour after a ½-hour infusion of tobramycin) was 7.9 μg/mL while the trough concentration (obtained within ½ hour before dosage administration) was 1 μg/mL. Compute a revised tobramycin dose for this patient to provide a steady-state peak concentration of 10 μg/mL and a steady-state trough concentration of 1-2 μg/mL using conventional dosing.

11. TY is a 66-year-old, 65-kg (5 ft 5 in) female with a suspected tubo-ovarian abscess secondary to hysterectomy surgery. While in the hospital, she developed ascites due to preexisting liver cirrhosis and her current weight is 72 kg. Her current serum creatinine is 1.4 mg/dL. Compute a gentamicin dose for this patient to provide a steady-state peak concentration of 6 μg/mL, and a steady-state trough concentration of less than 2 μg/mL using conventional dosing.

12. Patient TY (see problem 11) was prescribed gentamicin 120 mg every 12 hours. Steady-state gentamicin concentrations were obtained before and after the fourth dose, and the peak concentration (obtained ½ hour after a ½-hour infusion of gentamicin) was 4 μg/mL while the trough concentration (obtained within ½ hour before dosage administration) was 0.8 μg/mL. Compute a revised gentamicin dose for this patient to provide a steady-state peak concentration of 6 μg/mL and a steady-state trough concentration of 1 μg/mL using conventional dosing.

13. UQ is a 27-year-old, 85-kg (6 ft 2 in) male trauma patient with a gram-negative pneumonia and is currently on a respirator. He sustained multiple injuries secondary to a motor vehicle accident 2 weeks ago and lost a large amount of blood at the accident site. He developed acute renal failure because of prolonged hypotension and poor perfusion of his kidneys (current postdialysis serum creatinine is 5.3 mg/dL). He is receiving hemodialysis on Mondays, Wednesdays, and Fridays from 0800 to 1200 H, using a low-flux dialysis filter. Recommend a gentamicin dosage regimen that will achieve peak concentrations of 8 μg/mL and postdialysis concentrations of ~2 μg/mL. The first dose of the regimen will be given immediately after hemodialysis is finished on Wednesday at 1200 H.

14. Patient UQ (see problem 13) was prescribed gentamicin 180 mg loading dose and 130 mg after each dialysis. The following serum concentrations were obtained:

Date/Time	Description	Concentration (μg/mL)
Friday at 1200 H	Postdose (130 mg)	6.4
Monday at 0800 H	Predialysis	2.2
Monday at 1300 H	Postdialysis (1 h after end of dialysis to allow for rebound in serum concentrations)	0.7
Monday at 1400 H	Postdose (130 mg)	6.9

Use these serum concentrations to compute the patient's own pharmacokinetic parameters for gentamicin and a new dosage schedule that will achieve peak concentrations of 8 μg/mL and postdialysis concentrations of less than 2 μg/mL.

15. LS is a 67-year-old, 60-kg (5 ft 2 in) female with a serum creatinine equal to 1.8 mg/dL placed on tobramycin for a hospital-acquired gram-negative pneumonia. The prescribed dose was tobramycin 80 mg every 8 hours (infused over 1 hour) and two doses have been given at 0800 and 1600 hours. A trough concentration of 2.9 μg/mL was obtained at 1530 hours (½ hour before the second dose) and a peak concentration of 5.2 μg/mL was obtained at 1705 hours (5 minutes after infusion of the second dose). Compute the dose to give $Css_{max} = 8$ μg/mL and $Css_{min} = 1.5$ μg/mL.

16. KK is a 52-year-old, 87-kg (6 ft 2 in) male status postappendectomy who developed a fever, elevated white blood cell count, and abdominal pain 24 hours after surgery. His current serum creatinine is 1.4 mg/dL and stable. (A) Compute an initial extended-interval gentamicin dose for this patient. (B) Nine hours after the second dose of gentamicin 610 mg every 24 hours, a gentamicin serum concentration equal to 8.2 μg/mL is measured. Compute a revised gentamicin dose for this patient to provide steady-state peak concentrations of greater than 20 μg/mL and steady-state trough concentrations of less than 1 μg/mL.

17. XS is a 45-year-old, 65-kg (5 ft 4 in) female bone marrow transplant recipient who develops a neutropenic fever. Her current serum creatinine is 1.1 mg/dL. She is administered tobramycin 5 mg/kg daily (325 mg) as part of her antibiotic therapy. A tobramycin serum concentration was obtained 5 hours after the first dose and equaled 19 μg/mL. Compute a revised tobramycin dose for this patient to provide

steady-state peak concentrations of greater than 25 μg/mL and steady-state trough concentrations of less than 1 μg/mL.

18. DT is a 3-day-old, 2050-g female with suspected neonatal sepsis. Her serum creatinine has not been measured, but it is assumed that it is typical for her age and weight. Compute an initial tobramycin dose for this patient.

19. Patient DT (see problem 18) was prescribed tobramycin 5 mg every 12 hours. Steady-state tobramycin concentrations were obtained, and the peak concentration (obtained ½ hour after a ½-hour infusion of tobramycin) was 4.5 μg/mL while the trough concentration (obtained within ½ hour before dosage administration) was 0.9 μg/mL. Compute a revised tobramycin dose for this patient to provide a steady-state peak concentration of 6 μg/mL and a steady-state trough concentration of 1.5 μg/mL, using conventional dosing.

20. UL is a 7-year-old, 24-kg, 3-ft 11-in male with gram-negative sepsis. His serum creatinine is 0.5 mg/dL, and it has been stable for the last 2 days. Compute an initial gentamicin dose for this patient.

21. Patient UL (see problem 20) was prescribed gentamicin 60 mg every 8 hours and was expected to achieve steady-state peak and trough concentrations equal to 8 μg/mL and less than 2 μg/mL, respectively. Steady-state concentrations were measured and were 4.5 μg/mL 1 hour after the end of a 1-hour infusion and 1.5 μg/mL 4 hours after the end of infusion. Calculate a new gentamicin dose that would provide a steady-state peak of 9 μg/mL and a trough 1 μg/mL.

22. RD is a 59-year-old, 79-kg (height = 5 ft 11 in) male with a gram-negative pneumonia. His current serum creatinine is 1.5 mg/dL, and it has been stable over the last 3 days. A gentamicin dose of 450 mg every 24 hours was prescribed and expected to achieve steady-state peak and trough concentrations equal to 30 μg/mL and less than 1 μg/mL, respectively. After the second dose, steady-state concentrations were measured and were 16.1 μg/mL 2 hours after the end of a 1-hour infusion and 2.5 μg/mL 16 hours after the end of infusion. Calculate a new gentamicin dose that would provide a steady-state peak of 30 μg/mL and a trough less than 1 μg/mL.

23. DH is a 56-year-old, 69-kg (height = 5 ft 7 in) female with gram-negative sepsis. Her current serum creatinine is 1.2 mg/dL, and it has been stable over the last 5 days since admission. A tobramycin dose of 500 mg every 24 hours was prescribed. After the third dose, steady-state peak and trough concentrations were measured and were 19 μg/mL and 1.9 μg/mL, respectively. Calculate a new tobramycin dose that would provide a steady-state peak of 25 μg/mL and a trough 1 μg/mL.

24. NM is a 55-year-old, 135-kg (height = 5 ft 8 in) male with an intra-abdominal infection secondary to a knife wound. His current serum creatinine is 1.3 mg/dL, and it has been stable since admission. He was prescribed gentamicin 500 mg every 24 hours infused over 1 hour. Steady-state gentamicin concentrations were obtained after the third dose, and the concentration 2 hours after the infusion ended was 10.2 μg/mL while the concentration 10 hours after the infusion ended was 1.1 μg/mL. Compute a revised gentamicin dose for this patient to provide a steady-state peak concentration of 25 μg/mL and a steady-state trough concentration of less than 1 μg/mL using extended-interval dosing.

25. MI is a 27-year-old, 68-kg (height = 5 ft 4 in) female with salpingitis. Her current serum creatinine is 1.4 mg/dL, and it has been stable over the last 3 days. Compute a tobramycin dose for this patient to provide a steady-state peak concentration of 25 μg/mL and a steady-state trough of less than 1 μg/mL using extended-interval dosing.

26. Patient MI (see problem 25) was prescribed tobramycin 475 mg every 24 hours. After the third dose, steady-state concentrations were measured and equaled 17.0 μg/mL 1 hour after the end of a 1-hour infusion and 9.8 μg/mL 6 hours after end of infusion. Calculate a new tobramycin dose that would provide a steady-state peak concentration of 25 μg/mL and a steady-state trough of 1 μg/mL.

27. EK is a 23-year-old, 67-kg (height = 5 ft 8 in) male with peritonitis. His current serum creatinine is 0.8 mg/dL, and it has been stable over the last 3 days. A tobramycin dose of 350 mg every 24 hours

was prescribed and expected to achieve steady-state peak and trough concentrations equal to 25 µg/mL and less than 1 µg/mL, respectively. After the second-dose, steady-state concentrations were measured and equaled 9.6 µg/mL 2 hours after the end of a 1-hour infusion and 2.6 µg/mL 6 hours after the end of infusion. Calculate a new tobramycin dose that would provide a steady-state AUC of 81 (mg • h)/L.

ANSWERS TO PROBLEMS

1. *Solution to problem 1.* The initial gentamicin dose for patient PQ using the Pharmacokinetic Dosing method would be calculated as follows:

1. *Estimate creatinine clearance.*

This patient has a stable serum creatinine and is not obese. The Cockcroft-Gault equation can be used to estimate creatinine clearance:

$$CrCl_{est} = [(140 - age)BW]/(72 • S_{Cr}) = [(140 - 75\ y)62\ kg]/(72 • 1.3\ mg/dL)$$

$$CrCl_{est} = 43\ mL/min$$

2. *Estimate elimination rate constant (k_e) and half-life ($t_{1/2}$).*

The elimination rate constant versus creatinine clearance relationship is used to estimate the gentamicin elimination rate for this patient:

$$k_e = 0.00293(CrCl) + 0.014 = 0.00293(43\ mL/min) + 0.014 = 0.140\ h^{-1}$$

$$t_{1/2} = 0.693/k_e = 0.693/0.140\ h^{-1} = 4.9\ h$$

3. *Estimate volume of distribution (V).*

The patient has no disease states or conditions that would alter the volume of distribution from the normal value of 0.26 L/kg:

$$V = 0.26\ L/kg\ (62\ kg) = 16.1\ L$$

4. *Choose desired steady-state serum concentrations.*

Gram-negative sepsis patients treated with aminoglycoside antibiotics require steady-state peak concentrations ($Cmax_{ss}$) equal to 8-10 µg/mL; steady-state trough ($Cmin_{ss}$) concentrations should be less than 2 µg/mL to avoid toxicity. Set $Cmax_{ss} = 8$ µg/mL and $Cmin_{ss} = 1.5$ µg/mL.

5. *Use intermittent intravenous infusion equations to compute dose.*

Calculate required dosage interval (τ) using a 1-hour infusion:

$$\tau = [(ln\ Css_{max} - ln\ Css_{min})/k_e] + t' = [(ln\ 8\ µg/mL - ln\ 1.5\ µg/mL)/0.140\ h^{-1}] + 1\ h = 12.9\ h$$

Dosage intervals should be rounded to clinically acceptable intervals of 8, 12, 18, 24, 36, 48, 72 hours, and multiples of 24 hours thereafter, whenever possible. In this case, the dosage interval would be rounded to 12 hours. Also, steady-state peak concentrations are similar if drawn immediately after a 1-hour infusion or ½ hour after a ½-hour infusion, so the dose could be administered either way.

$$k_0 = Css_{max}k_eV[(1 - e^{-k_e\tau})/(1 - e^{-k_et'})]$$

$$k_0 = (8\ mg/L • 0.140\ h^{-1} • 16.1\ L)\{[1 - e^{-(0.140\ h^{-1})(12\ h)}]/[1 - e^{-(0.140\ h^{-1})(1\ h)}]\} = 112\ mg$$

Aminoglycoside doses should be rounded to the nearest 5-10 mg. This dose would be rounded to 110 mg. (Note: µg/mL = mg/L and this concentration unit was substituted for Css_{max} so that unnecessary unit conversion was not required.)

The prescribed maintenance dose would be: 110 mg every 12 hours.

6. *Compute loading dose (LD), if needed.*

Loading doses should be considered for patients with creatinine clearance values less than 60 mL/min. The administration of a loading dose in these patients will allow achievement of therapeutic peak concentrations quicker than if maintenance doses alone are given. However, because the pharmacokinetic parameters used to compute these initial doses are only *estimated* values and not *actual* values, the patient's own parameters may be much different than the estimated constants and steady state will not be achieved until 3-5 half-lives have passed.

$$LD = k_0/(1 - e^{-k_e \tau}) = 110 \text{ mg}/[1 - e^{-(0.140 \text{ h}^{-1})(12 \text{ h})}] = 135 \text{ mg}$$

The gentamicin dose computed using the Hull and Sarubbi nomogram would be:

1. *Estimate creatinine clearance.*

This patient has a stable serum creatinine and is not obese. The Cockcroft-Gault equation can be used to estimate creatinine clearance:

$$CrCl_{est} = [(140 - age)BW]/(72 \cdot S_{Cr}) = [(140 - 75 \text{ y})62 \text{ kg}]/(72 \cdot 1.3 \text{ mg/dL})$$
$$CrCl_{est} = 43 \text{ mL/min}$$

2. *Choose desired steady-state serum concentrations.*

Gram-negative sepsis patients treated with gentamicin require steady-state peak concentrations ($Cmax_{ss}$) equal to 8-10 µg/mL.

3. *Select loading dose (see Table 4-3).*

A loading dose (LD) of 2 mg/kg will provide a peak concentration of 8-10 µg/mL.

$$LD = 2 \text{ mg/kg}(62 \text{ kg}) = 124 \text{ mg, rounded to } 125 \text{ mg}$$

4. *Determine estimated half-life, maintenance dose, and dosage interval.*

From the nomogram the estimated half-life is 6.5 hours (suggesting that a 12-hour dosage interval is appropriate), the maintenance dose (MD) is 72% of the loading dose [MD = 0.72(125 mg) = 90 mg], and the dosage interval is 12 hours.

Aminoglycoside doses should be rounded to the nearest 5-10 mg. Steady-state peak concentrations are similar if drawn immediately after a 1-hour infusion or ½ hour after a ½-hour infusion, so the dose could be administered either way.

The prescribed maintenance dose would be: 90 mg every 12 hours.

2. *Solution to problem 2.* The revised gentamicin dose for patient PQ using the Pharmacokinetics Concept method would be calculated as follows:

1. *Draw a rough sketch of the serum log concentration/time curve by hand, keeping track of the relative time between the serum concentrations (Figure 4-16).*
2. *Because the patient is at steady state, the trough concentration can be extrapolated to the next trough value time (see Figure 4-16).*
3. *Draw the elimination curve between the steady-state peak concentration and the extrapolated trough concentration. Use this line to estimate half-life.* The patient is receiving a gentamicin dose of 110 mg given every 12 hours that produces a steady-state peak equal to 9.5 µg/mL and a steady-state trough equal to 3.0 µg/mL, and the dose is infused over ½ hour and the peak concentration is drawn ½ hour later (see Figure 4-16). The time between the measured steady-state peak and the extrapolated trough concentration is 11 hours (the 12-hour dosage interval minus the

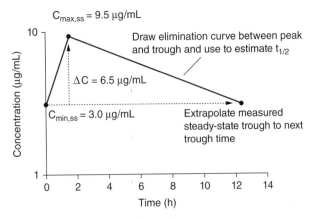

FIGURE 4-16   Solution to Problem 2 using Pharmacokinetic Concept method.

1-hour combined infusion and waiting time). The definition of half-life is the time needed for serum concentrations to decrease by ½. It would take 1 half-life for the peak serum concentration to decline from 9.5 to 4.8 μg/mL, and an additional half-life for the serum concentration to decrease from 4.8 to 2.4 μg/mL. The concentration of 3.0 μg/mL is close to, but slightly more than, the extrapolated trough value of 2.4 μg/mL. Therefore, 1.75 half-lives expired during the 11-hour time period between the peak concentration and extrapolated trough concentration, and the estimated half-life is 7 hours (11 hours/1.75 half-lives = ~7 hours). This information will be used to set the new dosage interval for the patient.

4. *Determine the difference in concentration between the steady-state peak and trough concentrations. The difference in concentration will change proportionally with the dose size.* In the current example the patient is receiving a gentamicin dose equal to 110 mg every 12 hours, which produced steady-state peak and trough concentrations of 9.5 μg/mL and 3 μg/mL, respectively. The difference between the peak and trough values is 6.5 μg/mL. The change in serum concentration is proportional to the dose, and this information will be used to set a new dose for the patient.

5. *Choose new steady-state peak and trough concentrations.* For the purposes of this example, the desired steady-state peak and trough concentrations will be approximately 8 μg/mL and 1 μg/mL, respectively.

6. *Determine the new dosage interval for the desired concentrations.* Using the desired concentrations, it will take 1 half-life for the peak concentration of 8 μg/mL to decrease to 4 μg/mL, 1 more half-life for the serum concentration to decrease to 2 μg/mL, and an additional half-life for serum concentrations to decline to 1 μg/mL. Therefore, the dosage interval will need to be approximately 3 half-lives or 21 hours (7 hours × 3 half-lives = 21 hours). The dosage interval would be rounded to the clinically acceptable value of 24 hours.

7. *Determine the new dose for the desired concentrations.* The desired peak concentration is 8 μg/mL, and the expected trough concentration is 1 μg/mL. The change in concentration between these values is 7 μg/mL. It is known from measured serum concentrations that administration of 110 mg changes serum concentrations by 6.5 μg/mL and that the change in serum concentration between the peak and trough values is proportional to the size of the dose. In this case: $D_{new} = (\Delta C_{new}/\Delta C_{old})$ $D_{old} = (7\ \mu g/mL / 6.5\ \mu g/mL)\ 110\ mg = 118\ mg$, rounded to 120 mg. Gentamicin 120 mg every 24 hours would be started 24 hours after the last dose of the previous dosage regimen.

The revised gentamicin dose for patient PQ using the steady-state Sawchuk-Zaske method would be calculated as follows:

1. *Compute the patient's elimination rate constant and half-life. (Note: For infusion times less than 1 hour, t′ is considered to be the sum of the infusion and waiting times.)*

$$k_e = (\ln Css_{max} - \ln Css_{min})/\tau - t' = (\ln 9.5 \ \mu g/mL - \ln 3 \ \mu g/mL)/(12 \ h - 1 \ h) = 0.105 \ h^{-1}$$
$$t_{1/2} = 0.693/k_e = 0.693/0.105 \ h^{-1} = 6.6 \ h$$

2. *Compute the patient's volume of distribution.*

$$V = \frac{D/t'(1 - e^{-k_e t'})}{k_e[Css_{max} - (Css_{min}e^{-k_e t'})]} = \frac{(110 \ mg/1 \ h)[1 - e^{-(0.105 \ h^{-1})(1 \ h)}]}{0.105 \ h^{-1}[9.5 \ mg/L - (3 \ mg/L \ e^{-(0.105 \ h^{-1})(1 \ h)}]}$$
$$V = 15.4 \ L$$

3. *Choose new steady-state peak and trough concentrations.* For the purposes of this example, the desired steady-state peak and trough concentrations will be approximately 8 µg/mL and 1 µg/mL, respectively.

4. *Determine the new dosage interval for the desired concentrations.* As in the initial dosage section of this chapter, the dosage interval (τ) is computed using the following equation using a 1-hour infusion time (t′):

$$\tau = [(\ln Css_{max} - \ln Css_{min})/k_e] + t' = [(\ln 8 \ \mu g/mL - \ln 1 \ \mu g/mL)/0.105 \ h^{-1}] + 1 \ h = 21 \ h, \text{ round to } 24 \ h$$

5. *Determine the new dose for the desired concentrations.* The dose is computed using the one-compartment model intravenous infusion equation used in the initial dosing section of this chapter:

$$k_0 = Css_{max}k_e V[(1 - e^{-k_e \tau})/(1 - e^{-k_e t'})]$$
$$k_0 = (8 \ mg/L \bullet 0.105 \ h^{-1} \bullet 15.4 \ L)\{[1 - e^{-(0.105 \ h^{-1})(24 \ h)}]/[1 - e^{-(0.105 \ h^{-1})(1 \ h)}]\}$$
$$= 119 \ mg, \text{ rounded to } 120 \ mg$$

A dose of gentamicin 120 mg every 24 hours would be prescribed to begin 24 hours after the last dose of the previous regimen. This dose is identical to that derived for the patient using the Pharmacokinetic Concepts method (120 mg every 24 hours).

3. **Solution to problem 3.** The initial gentamicin dose for patient ZW using the Pharmacokinetic Dosing method would be calculated as follows:

1. *Estimate creatinine clearance.*

This patient has a stable serum creatinine and is not obese. The Cockcroft-Gault equation can be used to estimate creatinine clearance:

$$CrCl_{est} = \{[(140 - age)BW]/(72 \bullet S_{Cr})\}0.85 = \{[(140 - 35 \ y)75 \ kg]/(72 \bullet 3.7 \ mg/dL)\}0.85$$
$$CrCl_{est} = 25 \ mL/min$$

2. *Estimate elimination rate constant (k_e) and half-life ($t_{1/2}$).*

The elimination rate constant versus creatinine clearance relationship is used to estimate the gentamicin elimination rate for this patient:

$$k_e = 0.00293(CrCl) + 0.014 = 0.00293(25 \ mL/min) + 0.014 = 0.088 \ h^{-1}$$
$$t_{1/2} = 0.693/k_e = 0.693/0.088 \ h^{-1} = 7.9 \ h$$

3. *Estimate volume of distribution (V).*

The patient has no disease states or conditions that would alter the volume of distribution from the normal value of 0.26 L/kg:

$$V = 0.26 \text{ L/kg } (75 \text{ kg}) = 19.5 \text{ L}$$

4. *Choose desired steady-state serum concentrations.*

Gram-negative pneumonia patients treated with aminoglycoside antibiotics require steady-state peak concentrations ($Cmax_{ss}$) equal to 8-10 µg/mL; steady-state trough ($Cmin_{ss}$) concentrations should be less than 2 µg/mL to avoid toxicity. Set $Cmax_{ss} = 10$ µg/mL and $Cmin_{ss} = 1$ µg/mL.

5. *Use intermittent intravenous infusion equations to compute dose.*

Calculate required dosage interval (τ), using a 1-hour infusion:

$$\tau = [(\ln Css_{max} - \ln Css_{min})/k_e] + t' = [(\ln 10 \text{ µg/mL} - \ln 1 \text{ µg/mL})/0.088 \text{ h}^{-1}] + 1 \text{ h} = 27 \text{ h}$$

Dosage intervals should be rounded to clinically acceptable intervals of 8, 12, 18, 24, 36, 48, 72 hours, and multiples of 24 hours thereafter, whenever possible. In this case, the dosage interval would be rounded to 24 hours. Also, steady-state peak concentrations are similar if drawn immediately after a 1-hour infusion or ½ hour after a ½-hour infusion, so the dose could be administered either way.

$$k_0 = Css_{max}k_eV[(1 - e^{-k_e\tau})/(1 - e^{-k_et'})]$$

$$k_0 = (10 \text{ mg/L} \bullet 0.088 \text{ h}^{-1} \bullet 19.5 \text{ L})\{[1 - e^{-(0.088 \text{ h}^{-1})(24 \text{ h})}]/[1 - e^{-(0.088 \text{ h}^{-1})(1 \text{ h})}]\} = 179 \text{ mg}$$

Aminoglycoside doses should be rounded to the nearest 5-10 mg. This dose would be rounded to 180 mg. (Note: µg/mL = mg/L, and this concentration unit was substituted for Css_{max} so that unnecessary unit conversion was not required.)

The prescribed maintenance dose would be: 180 mg every 24 hours.

6. *Compute loading dose (LD), if needed.*

Loading doses should be considered for patients with creatinine clearance values less than 60 mL/min. The administration of a loading dose in these patients will allow achievement of therapeutic peak concentrations quicker than if maintenance doses alone are given. However, because the pharmacokinetic parameters used to compute these initial doses are only *estimated* values and not *actual* values, the patient's own parameters may be much different than the estimated constants and steady state will not be achieved until 3-5 half-lives have passed.

$$LD = k_0/(1 - e^{-k_e\tau}) = 180 \text{ mg}/[1 - e^{-(0.088 \text{ h}^{-1})(24 \text{ h})}] = 205 \text{ mg}$$

The gentamicin dose computed using the Hull and Sarubbi nomogram would be:

1. *Estimate creatinine clearance.*

This patient has a stable serum creatinine and is not obese. The Cockcroft-Gault equation can be used to estimate creatinine clearance:

$$CrCl_{est} = \{[(140 - \text{age})BW]/(72 \bullet S_{Cr})\}0.85 = \{[(140 - 35 \text{ y})75 \text{ kg}]/(72 \bullet 3.7 \text{ mg/dL})\}0.85$$

$$CrCl_{est} = 25 \text{ mL/min}$$

2. *Choose desired steady-state serum concentrations.*

Gram-negative sepsis patients treated with gentamicin require steady-state peak concentrations ($Cmax_{ss}$) equal to 8-10 µg/mL.

3. *Select loading dose (see Table 4-3).*

A loading dose (LD) of 2 mg/kg will provide a peak concentration of 8-10 μg/mL.

$$LD = 2 \text{ mg/kg}(75 \text{ kg}) = 150 \text{ mg}$$

4. *Determine estimated half-life, maintenance dose, and dosage interval.*

From the nomogram the estimated half-life is 9.9 hours (suggesting that a 24-hour dosage interval is appropriate), the maintenance dose (MD) is 81% of the loading dose (MD = 0.81[150 mg] = 122 mg), and the dosage interval is 24 hours. Note: 24-hour dosage interval chosen because longer time period is needed for concentrations to drop from desired peak to desired trough concentration.

Aminoglycoside doses should be rounded to the nearest 5-10 mg. Steady-state peak concentrations are similar if drawn immediately after a 1-hour infusion or ½ hour after a ½-hour infusion, so the dose could be administered either way.

The prescribed maintenance dose would be: 120 mg every 24 hours.

4. *Solution to problem 4.* Compute modified dose for ZW using linear pharmacokinetics:

1. *Compute new dose to achieve desired serum concentration.*

Using linear pharmacokinetics, the new dose to attain the desired concentration should be proportional to the old dose that produced the measured concentration:

$$D_{new} = (C_{ss,new}/C_{ss,old})D_{old} = (10 \text{ μg/mL}/7 \text{ μg/mL}) \, 120 \text{ mg} = 171 \text{ mg, round to } 170 \text{ mg}$$

The new suggested dose would be 170 mg every 24 hours to be started at next scheduled dosing time.

2. *Check steady-state trough concentration for new dosage regimen.*

Using linear pharmacokinetics, the new steady-state concentration can be estimated and should be proportional to the old dose that produced the measured concentration. The measured trough concentration was below assay limits (<0.5 μg/mL), so the maximum value it could be is 0.5 μg/mL:

$$C_{ss,new} = (D_{new}/D_{old})C_{ss,old} = (170 \text{ mg}/120 \text{ mg}) \, 0.5 \text{ μg/mL} = 0.7 \text{ μg/mL}$$

The steady-state trough concentration would be expected to be no greater than 0.7 μg/mL, and should be safe and effective for the infection that is being treated.

5. *Solution to problem 5.* The initial gentamicin dose for patient JK using the Pharmacokinetic Dosing method would be calculated as follows:

1. *Estimate creatinine clearance.*

This patient has a stable serum creatinine and is obese [IBW_{males} (in kg) = 50 + 2.3(Ht – 60) = 50 + 2.3(68 in – 60) = 68.4 kg]. The Salazar and Corcoran equation can be used to estimate creatinine clearance:

$$CrCl_{est(males)} = \frac{(137 - age)[(0.285 \bullet Wt) + (12.1 \bullet Ht^2)]}{(51 \bullet S_{Cr})}$$

$$CrCl_{est(males)} = \frac{(137 - 55 \text{ y})\{(0.285 \bullet 140 \text{ kg}) + [12.1 \bullet (1.73 \text{ m})^2]\}}{(51 \bullet 0.9 \text{ mg/dL})} = 136 \text{ mL/min}$$

Note: Height is converted from inches to meters: Ht = (68 in • 2.54 cm/in)/(100 cm/m) = 1.73 m.

2. *Estimate elimination rate constant (k_e) and half-life ($t_{1/2}$).*

The elimination rate constant versus creatinine clearance relationship is used to estimate the gentamicin elimination rate for this patient:

$$k_e = 0.00293(CrCl) + 0.014 = 0.00293(136 \text{ mL/min}) + 0.014 = 0.412 \text{ h}^{-1}$$

$$t_{1/2} = 0.693/k_e = 0.693/0.412 \text{ h}^{-1} = 1.7 \text{ h}$$

3. *Estimate volume of distribution (V).*

The patient is overweight so the volume of distribution is estimated using the equation that corrects for obesity:

$$V = 0.26 \text{ L/kg [IBW} + 0.4(\text{TBW} - \text{IBW})] = 0.26 \text{ L/kg}[68.4 \text{ kg} + 0.4(140 \text{ kg} - 68.4 \text{ kg})] = 25.2 \text{ L}$$

4. *Choose desired steady-state serum concentrations.*

Intra-abdominal sepsis patients treated with aminoglycoside antibiotics require steady-state peak concentrations ($Cmax_{ss}$) equal to 5-6 µg/mL; steady-state trough ($Cmin_{ss}$) concentrations should be less than 2 µg/mL to avoid toxicity. Set $Cmax_{ss} = 6$ µg/mL and $Cmin_{ss} = 0.5$ µg/mL.

5. *Use intermittent intravenous infusion equations to compute dose.*

Calculate required dosage interval (τ) using a 1-hour infusion:

$$\tau = [(\ln Css_{max} - \ln Css_{min})/k_e] + t' = [(\ln 6 \text{ µg/mL} - \ln 0.5 \text{ µg/mL})/0.412 \text{ h}^{-1}] + 1 \text{ h} = 7 \text{ h}$$

Dosage intervals should be rounded to clinically acceptable intervals of 8, 12, 18, 24, 36, 48, 72 hours, and multiples of 24 hours thereafter, whenever possible. In this case, the dosage interval would be rounded to 8 hours. Also, steady-state peak concentrations are similar if drawn immediately after a 1-hour infusion or ½ hour after a ½-hour infusion, so the dose could be administered either way.

$$k_0 = Css_{max}k_eV[(1 - e^{-k_e\tau})/(1 - e^{-k_et'})]$$
$$k_0 = (6 \text{ mg/L} \bullet 0.412 \text{ h}^{-1} \bullet 25.2 \text{ L})\{[1 - e^{-(0.412 \text{ h}^{-1})(8 \text{ h})}]/[1 - e^{-(0.412 \text{ h}^{-1})(1 \text{ h})}]\} = 178 \text{ mg}$$

Aminoglycoside doses should be rounded to the nearest 5-10 mg. This dose would be rounded to 180 mg. (Note: µg/mL = mg/L, and this concentration unit was substituted for Css_{max} so that unnecessary unit conversion was not required.)

The prescribed maintenance dose would be: 180 mg every 8 hours.

6. *Compute loading dose (LD), if needed.*

Loading doses should be considered for patients with creatinine clearance values less than 60 mL/min. The administration of a loading dose in these patients will allow achievement of therapeutic peak concentrations quicker than if maintenance doses alone are given. However, because the pharmacokinetic parameters used to compute these initial doses are only *estimated* values and not *actual* values, the patient's own parameters may be much different than the estimated constants and steady state will not be achieved until 3-5 half-lives have passed.

$$LD = k_0/(1 - e^{-k_e\tau}) = 180 \text{ mg}/(1 - e^{-(0.412 \text{ h}^{-1})(8 \text{ h})}) = 187 \text{ mg}$$

Because the patient has a short aminoglycoside half-life, the loading dose is similar to the maintenance dose and the loading dose would be omitted.

The gentamicin dose computed using the Hull and Sarubbi nomogram would be:

1. *Estimate creatinine clearance.*

This patient has a stable serum creatinine and is obese [IBW_{males} (in kg) = 50 + 2.3(Ht − 60) = 50 + 2.3(68 in − 60) = 68.4 kg]. The Salazar and Corcoran equation can be used to estimate creatinine clearance:

$$CrCl_{est(males)} = \frac{(137 - age)[(0.285 \bullet Wt) + (12.1 \bullet Ht^2)]}{(51 \bullet S_{Cr})}$$

$$CrCl_{est(males)} = \frac{(137 - 55 \text{ y})\{(0.285 \cdot 140 \text{ kg}) + [12.1 \cdot (1.73 \text{ m})^2]\}}{(51 \cdot 0.9 \text{ mg/dL})} = 136 \text{ mL/min}$$

Note: Height is converted from inches to meters: Ht = (68 in • 2.54 cm/in)/(100 cm/m) = 1.73 m.

2. *Choose desired steady-state serum concentrations.*

Gram-negative sepsis patients treated with gentamicin require steady-state peak concentrations ($Cmax_{ss}$) equal to 5-6 µg/mL.

3. *Select loading dose (see Table 4-3).*

A loading dose (LD) of 1.5 mg/kg will provide a peak concentration of 5-6 µg/mL. The patient is obese, so the patient's adjusted body weight (ABW) will be used as the weight factor in the nomogram.

$$ABW \text{ (in kg)} = IBW + 0.4(TBW - IBW) = 68.4 \text{ kg} + 0.4(140 \text{ kg} - 68.4 \text{ kg}) = 97 \text{ kg}$$
$$LD = 1.5 \text{ mg/kg}(97 \text{ kg}) = 146 \text{ mg, rounded to } 145 \text{ mg}$$

4. *Determine estimated half-life, maintenance dose, and dosage interval.*

From the nomogram the estimated half-life is 2-3 hours (suggesting that an 8-hour dosage interval is appropriate), the maintenance dose (MD) is 90% of the loading dose [MD = 0.90(145 mg) = 131 mg], and the dosage interval is 8 hours.

Aminoglycoside doses should be rounded to the nearest 5-10 mg. Steady-state peak concentrations are similar if drawn immediately after a 1-hour infusion or ½ hour after a ½-hour infusion, so the dose could be administered either way.

The prescribed maintenance dose would be: 130 mg every 8 hours.

6. *Solution to problem 6.* The revised gentamicin dose for patient JK using the Pharmacokinetics Concept Method would be calculated as follows:

1. *Draw a rough sketch of the serum log concentration/time curve by hand, keeping track of the relative time between the serum concentrations (Figure 4-17).*
2. *Because the patient is at steady state, the trough concentration can be extrapolated to the next trough value time (see Figure 4-17).*

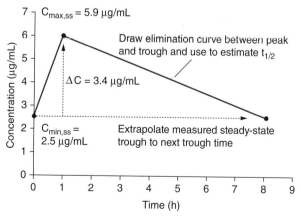

FIGURE 4-17   Solution to Problem 6 using Pharmacokinetic Concept method.

3. *Draw the elimination curve between the steady-state peak concentration and the extrapolated trough concentration. Use this line to estimate half-life.* The patient is receiving a gentamicin dose of 120 mg given every 8 hours that produces a steady-state peak equal to 5.9 µg/mL and a steady-state trough equal to 2.5 µg/mL, and the dose is infused over ½ hour and the peak concentration is drawn ½ hour later (see Figure 4-17). The time between the measured steady-state peak and the extrapolated trough concentration is 7 hours (the 8-hour dosage interval minus the 1-hour combined infusion and waiting time). The definition of half-life is the time needed for serum concentrations to decrease by ½. It would take 1 half-life for the peak serum concentration to decline from 5.9 to 3.0 µg/mL, and about ¼ of an additional half-life for the serum concentration to decrease from 3.0 to 2.5 µg/mL. Therefore, 1.25 half-lives expired during the 7-hour time period between the peak concentration and extrapolated trough concentration, and the estimated half-life is 6 hours (7 hours/1.25 half-lives = ~6 hours). This information will be used to set the new dosage interval for the patient

4. *Determine the difference in concentration between the steady-state peak and trough concentrations. The difference in concentration will change proportionally with the dose size.* In the current example the patient is receiving a gentamicin dose equal to 120 mg every 8 hours, which produced steady-state peak and trough concentrations of 5.9 µg/mL and 2.5 µg/mL, respectively. The difference between the peak and trough values is 3.4 µg/mL. The change in serum concentration is proportional to the dose, and this information will be used to set a new dose for the patient.

5. *Choose new steady-state peak and trough concentrations.* For the purposes of this example, the desired steady-state peak and trough concentrations will be approximately 6 µg/mL and less than 1 µg/mL, respectively.

6. *Determine the new dosage interval for the desired concentrations.* Using the desired concentrations, it will take 1 half-life for the peak concentration of 6 µg/mL to decrease to 3 µg/mL, 1 more half-life for the serum concentration to decrease to 1.5 µg/mL, and an additional half-life for serum concentrations to decline to 0.8 µg/mL. Therefore, the dosage interval will need to be approximately 3 half-lives or 18 hours (6 hours × 3 half-lives = 18 hours).

7. *Determine the new dose for the desired concentrations.* The desired peak concentration is 6 µg/mL, and the expected trough concentration is 0.8 µg/mL. The change in concentration between these values is 5.2 µg/mL. It is known from measured serum concentrations that administration of 120 mg changes serum concentrations by 3.4 µg/mL and that the change in serum concentration between the peak and trough values is proportional to the size of the dose. In this case: $D_{new} = (\Delta C_{new}/\Delta C_{old})D_{old} =$ (5.2 µg/mL/3.4 µg/mL) 120 mg = 184 mg. Gentamicin 185 mg every 18 hours would be started 18 hours after the last dose of the previous dosage regimen.

The revised gentamicin dose for patient JK using the steady-state Sawchuk-Zaske method would be calculated as follows:

1. *Compute the patient's elimination rate constant and half-life. (Note: For infusion times less than 1 hour, t′ is considered to be the sum of the infusion and waiting times.)*

$$k_e = (\ln Css_{max} - \ln Css_{min})/\tau - t' = (\ln 5.9 \text{ µg/mL} - \ln 2.5 \text{ µg/mL})/(8 \text{ h} - 1 \text{ h}) = 0.123 \text{ h}^{-1}$$

$$t_{1/2} = 0.693/k_e = 0.693/0.123 \text{ h}^{-1} = 5.6 \text{ h}$$

2. *Compute the patient's volume of distribution.*

$$V = \frac{D/t'(1 - e^{-k_e t'})}{k_e[Css_{max} - (Css_{min}e^{-k_e t'})]} = \frac{(120 \text{ mg/1 h})[1 - e^{-(0.123 \text{ h}^{-1})(1 \text{ h})}]}{0.123 \text{ h}^{-1}\{5.9 \text{ mg/L} - [2.5 \text{ mg/L } e^{-(0.123 \text{ h}^{-1})(1 \text{ h})}]\}}$$

$$V = 30.6 \text{ L}$$

3. *Choose new steady-state peak and trough concentrations.* For the purposes of this example, the desired steady-state peak and trough concentrations will be approximately 6 µg/mL and 0.8 µg/mL, respectively.

4. *Determine the new dosage interval for the desired concentrations.* As in the initial dosage section of this chapter, the dosage interval (τ) is computed using the following equation using a 1-hour infusion time (t′):

$$\tau = [(\ln Css_{max} - \ln Css_{min})/k_e] + t' = [(\ln 6\ \mu g/mL - \ln 0.8\ \mu g/mL)/0.123\ h^{-1}] + 1\ h$$
$$= 17\ h,\ \text{round to } 18\ h$$

5. *Determine the new dose for the desired concentrations.* The dose is computed using the one-compartment model intravenous infusion equation used in the initial dosing section of this chapter:

$$k_0 = Css_{max}k_e V[(1 - e^{-k_e\tau})/(1 - e^{-k_e t'})]$$
$$k_0 = (6\ mg/L \bullet 0.123\ h^{-1} \bullet 30.6\ L)\{[1 - e^{-(0.123\ h^{-1})(18\ h)}]/[1 - e^{-(0.123\ h^{-1})(1\ h)}]\}$$
$$= 174\ mg,\ \text{rounded to } 175\ mg$$

A dose of gentamicin 175 mg every 18 hours would be prescribed to begin 18 hours after the last dose of the previous regimen. This dose is very similar to that derived for the patient using the Pharmacokinetic Concepts method (185 mg every 18 hours).

7. *Solution to problem 7.* The initial tobramycin dose for patient AF using the Pharmacokinetic Dosing method would be calculated as follows:

1. *Estimate creatinine clearance.*

This patient has a stable serum creatinine and is obese [$IBW_{females}$ (in kg) = 45 + 2.3(Ht − 60) = 45 + 2.3(62 in − 60) = 50 kg]. The Salazar and Corcoran equation can be used to estimate creatinine clearance:

$$CrCl_{est(females)} = \frac{(146 - age)[(0.287 \bullet Wt) + (9.74 \bullet Ht^2)]}{(60 \bullet S_{Cr})}$$

$$CrCl_{est(females)} = \frac{(146 - 45\ y)\{(0.287 \bullet 140\ kg) + [9.74 \bullet (1.57\ m)^2]\}}{(60 \bullet 2.4\ mg/dL)} = 45\ mL/min$$

Note: Height is converted from inches to meters: Ht = (62 in • 2.54 cm/in)/(100 cm/m) = 1.57 m.

2. *Estimate elimination rate constant (k_e) and half-life ($t_{1/2}$).*
The elimination rate constant versus creatinine clearance relationship is used to estimate the tobramycin elimination rate for this patient:

$$k_e = 0.00293(CrCl) + 0.014 = 0.00293(45\ mL/min) + 0.014 = 0.146\ h^{-1}$$
$$t_{1/2} = 0.693/k_e = 0.693/0.146\ h^{-1} = 4.7\ h$$

3. *Estimate volume of distribution (V).*

The patient is obese, so the volume of distribution would be estimated using the following formula:

$$V = 0.26[IBW + 0.4(TBW - IBW)] = 0.26[50\ kg + 0.4(140\ kg - 50\ kg)] = 22.3\ L$$

4. *Choose desired steady-state serum concentrations.*

Endocarditis patients treated with aminoglycoside antibiotics for gram-positive synergy require steady-state peak concentrations ($Cmax_{ss}$) equal to 3-4 µg/mL; steady-state trough ($Cmin_{ss}$) concentrations should be less than 1 µg/mL to avoid toxicity. Set $Cmax_{ss}$ = 4 µg/mL and $Cmin_{ss}$ = 0.5 µg/mL.

5. *Use intermittent intravenous infusion equations to compute dose (see Table 4-2).*

Calculate required dosage interval (τ) using a 1-hour infusion:

$$\tau = [(\ln Css_{max} - \ln Css_{min})/k_e] + t' = [(\ln 4\ \mu g/mL - \ln 0.5\ \mu g/mL)/0.146\ h^{-1}] + 1\ h = 15\ h$$

Dosage intervals should be rounded to clinically acceptable intervals of 8, 12, 18, 24, 36, 48, and 72 hours, and multiples of 24 hours thereafter, whenever possible. In this case, the dosage interval is rounded to 12 hours. Also, steady-state peak concentrations are similar if drawn immediately after a 1-hour infusion or ½ hour after a ½-hour infusion, so the dose could be administered either way.

$$k_0 = Css_{max}k_e V[(1 - e^{-k_e\tau})/(1 - e^{-k_e t'})]$$

$$k_0 = (4\ mg/L \bullet 0.146\ h^{-1} \bullet 22.3\ L)\{[1 - e^{-(0.146\ h^{-1})(12\ h)}]/[1 - e^{-(0.146\ h^{-1})(1\ h)}]\} = 79\ mg$$

Aminoglycoside doses should be rounded to the nearest 5-10 mg. This dose would be rounded to 80 mg. (Note: $\mu g/mL = mg/L$, and this concentration unit was substituted for Css_{max} so that unnecessary unit conversion was not required.)

The prescribed maintenance dose would be: 80 mg every 12 hours.

6. *Compute loading dose (LD), if needed.*

Loading doses should be considered for patients with creatinine clearance values less than 60 mL/min. The administration of a loading dose in these patients will allow achievement of therapeutic peak concentrations quicker than if maintenance doses alone are given. However, because the pharmacokinetic parameters used to compute these initial doses are only *estimated* values and not *actual* values, the patient's own parameters may be much different than the estimated constants and steady state will not be achieved until 3-5 half-lives have passed.

$$LD = k_0/(1 - e^{-k_e\tau}) = 80\ mg/[1 - e^{-(0.146\ h^{-1})(12\ h)}] = 97\ mg$$

This loading dose would be rounded to 100 mg and would be given as the first dose. The first maintenance dose would be given 12 hours later.

The tobramycin dose computed using the Hull and Sarubbi nomogram would be:

1. *Estimate creatinine clearance.*

This patient has a stable serum creatinine and is obese [$IBW_{females}$ (in kg) = 45 + 2.3(Ht −60) = 45 + 2.3(62 in −60) = 50 kg]. The Salazar and Corcoran equation can be used to estimate creatinine clearance:

$$CrCl_{est(females)} = \frac{(146 - age)[(0.287 \bullet Wt) + (9.74 \bullet Ht^2)]}{(60 \bullet S_{Cr})}$$

$$CrCl_{est(females)} = \frac{(146 - 45\ y)\{(0.287 \bullet 140\ kg) + [9.74 \bullet (1.57\ m)^2]\}}{(60 \bullet 2.4\ mg/dL)} = 45\ mL/min$$

Note: Height is converted from inches to meters: Ht = (62 in $\bullet$ 2.54 cm/in)/(100 cm/m) = 1.57 m.

2. *Choose desired steady-state serum concentrations.*

Gram-positive endocarditis patients treated with aminoglycoside antibiotics for synergy require steady-state peak concentrations ($Cmax_{ss}$) equal to 3-4 µg/mL.

3. *Select loading dose (see Table 4-3).*

A loading dose (LD) of 1.5 mg/kg will provide a peak concentration of 5-7 µg/mL. This is the lowest dose suggested by the nomogram and will be used in this example. However, some clinicians may substitute a loading dose of 1-1.2 mg/kg designed to produce a steady-state peak concentration equal to 3-4 µg/mL.

Because the patient is obese, adjusted body weight (ABW) will be used to compute the dose:

$$ABW = IBW + 0.4(TBW - IBW) = 50 \text{ kg} + 0.4(140 \text{ kg} - 50 \text{ kg}) = 86 \text{ kg}$$
$$LD = 1.5 \text{ mg/kg} (86 \text{ kg}) = 129 \text{ mg, rounded to } 130 \text{ mg or}$$
$$LD = 1.2 \text{ mg/kg} (86 \text{ kg}) = 103 \text{ mg, rounded to } 100 \text{ mg}$$

4. *Determine estimated half-life, maintenance dose, and dosage interval.*

From the nomogram the estimated half-life is ~6 hours, suggesting that a 12-dosage interval is appropriate. The maintenance dose (MD) is 72% of the loading dose [MD = 0.72(130 mg) = 94 mg or MD = 0.72(100 mg) = 72 mg], and the dosage interval is 12 hours.

Aminoglycoside doses should be rounded to the nearest 5-10 mg. Steady-state peak concentrations are similar if drawn immediately after a 1-hour infusion or ½ hour after a ½-hour infusion, so the dose could be administered either way.

The prescribed maintenance dose would be: 95 mg every 12 hours or 70 mg every 12 hours, depending on the loading dose chosen.

8. *Solution to problem 8.* Compute modified dose for AF using linear pharmacokinetics:

1. *Compute new dose to achieve desired serum concentration.*

Using linear pharmacokinetics, the new dose to attain the desired concentration should be proportional to the old dose that produced the measured concentration:

$$D_{new} = (C_{ss,new}/C_{ss,old})D_{old} = (4 \text{ µg/mL} / 6.2 \text{ µg/mL}) \, 100 \text{ mg} = 65 \text{ mg}$$

The new suggested dose would be 65 mg every 12 hours to be started at next scheduled dosing time.

2. *Check steady-state trough concentration for new dosage regimen.*

Using linear pharmacokinetics, the new steady-state concentration can be estimated and should be proportional to the old dose that produced the measured concentration.

$$C_{ss,new} = (D_{new}/D_{old})C_{ss,old} = (65 \text{ mg}/100 \text{ mg}) \, 1.5 \text{ µg/mL} = 1 \text{ µg/mL}$$

This steady-state trough concentration should be safe and effective for the infection that is being treated.

The revised tobramycin dose for patient AF using the Pharmacokinetics Concept method would be calculated as follows:

1. *Draw a rough sketch of the serum log concentration/time curve by hand, keeping track of the relative time between the serum concentrations (Figure 4-18).*

2. *Because the patient is at steady state, the trough concentration can be extrapolated to the next trough value time (see Figure 4-18).*

3. *Draw the elimination curve between the steady-state peak concentration and the extrapolated trough concentration. Use this line to estimate half-life.* The patient is receiving a tobramycin dose of 100 mg given every 12 hours that produces a steady-state peak equal to 6.2 µg/mL and a steady-state trough

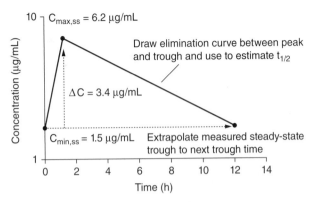

FIGURE 4-18   Solution to Problem 8 using Pharmacokinetic Concept method.

equal to 1.5 µg/mL, and the dose is infused over ½ hour and the peak concentration is drawn ½ hour later (see Figure 4-18). The time between the measured steady-state peak and the extrapolated trough concentration is 11 hours (the 12-hour dosage interval minus the 1-hour combined infusion and waiting time). The definition of half-life is the time needed for serum concentrations to decrease by ½. It would take 1 half-life for the peak serum concentration to decline from 6.2 to 3.1 µg/mL, and an additional half-life for the concentration to decrease from 3.1 to 1.6 µg/mL. The concentration of 1.5 µg/mL is very close to the extrapolated trough value of 1.6 µg/mL. Therefore, 2 half-lives expired during the 11-hour time period between the peak concentration and extrapolated trough concentration, and the estimated half-life is ~6 hours. This information will be used to set the new dosage interval for the patient.

4. *Determine the difference in concentration between the steady-state peak and trough concentrations. The difference in concentration will change proportionally with the dose size.* In the current example the patient is receiving a tobramycin dose equal to 100 mg every 12 hours, which produced steady-state peak and trough concentrations of 6.2 µg/mL and 1.5 µg/mL, respectively. The difference between the peak and trough values is 4.7 µg/mL. The change in serum concentration is proportional to the dose, and this information will be used to set a new dose for the patient.

5. *Choose new steady-state peak and trough concentrations.* For the purposes of this example, the desired steady-state peak and trough concentrations will be approximately 4 µg/mL and less than or equal to 1 µg/mL, respectively.

6. *Determine the new dosage interval for the desired concentrations.* Using the desired concentrations, it will take 1 half-life for the peak concentration of 4 µg/mL to decrease to 2 µg/mL, and 1 more half-life for the serum concentration to decrease to 1 µg/mL. Therefore, the dosage interval will need to be approximately 2 half-lives or 12 hours (6 hours × 2 half-lives = 12 hours).

7. *Determine the new dose for the desired concentrations.* The desired peak concentration is 4 µg/mL, and the expected trough concentration is 1 µg/mL. The change in concentration between these values is 3.0 µg/mL. It is known from measured serum concentrations that administration of 100 mg changes serum concentrations by 4.7 µg/mL and that the change in serum concentration between the peak and trough values is proportional to the size of the dose. In this case: $D_{new} = (\Delta C_{new}/\Delta C_{old}) D_{old} = (3.0 \text{ µg/mL}/4.7 \text{ µg/mL}) 100 \text{ mg} = 64 \text{ mg}$, rounded to 65 mg. Tobramycin 65 mg every 12 hours would be started 12 hours after the last dose of the previous dosage regimen.

The revised tobramycin dose for patient AF using the steady-state Sawchuk-Zaske method would be calculated as follows:

1. *Compute the patient's elimination rate constant and half-life. (Note: For infusion times less than 1 hour, t' is considered to be the sum of the infusion and waiting times.)*

$$k_e = (\ln Css_{max} - \ln Css_{min})/\tau - t' = (\ln 6.2\ \mu g/mL - \ln 1.5\ \mu g/mL)/(12\ h - 1\ h) = 0.129\ h^{-1}$$

$$t_{1/2} = 0.693/k_e = 0.693/0.129\ h^{-1} = 5.4\ h$$

2. *Compute the patient's volume of distribution.*

$$V = \frac{D/t'(1 - e^{-k_e t'})}{k_e[Css_{max} - (Css_{min}e^{-k_e t'})]} = \frac{(100\ mg/1\ h)[1 - e^{-(0.129 h^{-1})(1\ h)}]}{0.129\ h^{-1}\{6.2\ mg/L - [1.5\ mg/L\ e^{-(0.129\ h^{-1})(1\ h)}]\}}$$

$$V = 19.2\ L$$

3. *Choose new steady-state peak and trough concentrations.* For the purposes of this example, the desired steady-state peak and trough concentrations will be 4 µg/mL and less than or equal to 1 µg/mL, respectively.

4. *Determine the new dosage interval for the desired concentrations.* As in the initial dosage section of this chapter, the dosage interval (τ) is computed using the following equation using a 1-hour infusion time (t'):

$$\tau = [(\ln Css_{max} - \ln Css_{min})/k_e] + t' = [(\ln 4\ \mu g/mL - \ln 1\ \mu g/mL)/0.129\ h^{-1}] + 1\ h = 12\ h$$

5. *Determine the new dose for the desired concentrations.* The dose is computed using the one-compartment model intravenous infusion equation used in the initial dosing section of this chapter:

$$k_0 = Css_{max}k_e V[(1 - e^{-k_e \tau})/(1 - e^{-k_e t'})]$$

$$k_0 = (4\ mg/L \bullet 0.129\ h^{-1} \bullet 19.2\ L)\{[1 - e^{-(0.129\ h^{-1})(12\ h)}]/[1 - e^{-(0.129\ h^{-1})(1\ h)}]\} = 65\ mg$$

A dose of tobramycin 65 mg every 12 hours would be prescribed to begin 12 hours after the last dose of the previous regimen. This dose is identical to that derived for the patient using the Linear Pharmacokinetics method and the Pharmacokinetic Concepts method (65 mg every 12 hours).

9. *Solution to problem 9.* The initial tobramycin dose for patient FH using the Pharmacokinetic Dosing method would be calculated as follows:

1. *Estimate creatinine clearance.*

This patient has a stable serum creatinine and is not obese. The Cockcroft-Gault equation can be used to estimate creatinine clearance:

$$CrCl_{est} = [(140 - age)BW]/(72 \bullet S_{Cr}) = [(140 - 24\ y)60\ kg]/(72 \bullet 0.7\ mg/dL)$$

$$CrCl_{est} = 138\ mL/min$$

2. *Estimate elimination rate constant (k_e) and half-life ($t_{1/2}$).*

The elimination rate constant versus creatinine clearance relationship is used to estimate the tobramycin elimination rate for this patient:

$$k_e = 0.00293(CrCl) + 0.014 = 0.00293(138\ mL/min) + 0.014 = 0.419\ h^{-1}$$

$$t_{1/2} = 0.693/k_e = 0.693/0.419\ h^{-1} = 1.7\ h$$

3. *Estimate volume of distribution (V).*

The patient has no disease states or conditions that would alter the volume of distribution from the normal value of 0.35 L/kg for cystic fibrosis patients:

$$V = 0.35 \text{ L/kg } (60 \text{ kg}) = 21 \text{ L}$$

4. *Choose desired steady-state serum concentrations.*

Cystic fibrosis patients with a sputum culture positive for *P. aeruginosa* and a pulmonary exacerbation treated with aminoglycoside antibiotics require steady-state peak concentrations ($Cmax_{ss}$) equal to 8-10 µg/mL; steady-state trough ($Cmin_{ss}$) concentrations should be less than 2 µg/mL to avoid toxicity. Set $Cmax_{ss} = 10$ µg/mL and $Cmin_{ss} = 1$ µg/mL.

5. *Use intermittent intravenous infusion equations to compute dose.*

Calculate required dosage interval (τ) using a 1-hour infusion:

$$\tau = [(\ln Css_{max} - \ln Css_{min})/k_e] + t' = [(\ln 10 \text{ µg/mL} - \ln 1 \text{ µg/mL})/0.419 \text{ h}^{-1}] + 1 \text{ h} = 6.5 \text{ h}$$

Dosage intervals should be rounded to clinically acceptable intervals of 8, 12, 18, 24, 36, 48, and 72 hours, and multiples of 24 hours thereafter, whenever possible. In this case, the dosage interval would be rounded to 8 hours. Also, steady-state peak concentrations are similar if drawn immediately after a 1-hour infusion or ½ hour after a ½-hour infusion, so the dose could be administered either way.

$$k_0 = Css_{max} k_e V[(1 - e^{-k_e\tau})/(1 - e^{-k_e t'})]$$

$$k_0 = (10 \text{ mg/L} \bullet 0.419 \text{ h}^{-1} \bullet 21 \text{ L})\{[1 - e^{-(0.419 \text{ h}^{-1})(8 \text{ h})}]/[1 - e^{-(0.419 \text{ h}^{-1})(1 \text{ h})}]\} = 248 \text{ mg}$$

Aminoglycoside doses should be rounded to the nearest 5-10 mg. This dose would be rounded to 250 mg. (Note: µg/mL = mg/L, and this concentration unit was substituted for Css_{max} so that unnecessary unit conversion was not required.)

The prescribed maintenance dose would be: 250 mg every 8 hours.

6. *Compute loading dose (LD), if needed.*

Loading doses for patients with creatinine clearance values more than 60 mL/min are usually close to maintenance doses, so are often not given to this patient population.

$$LD = k_0/(1 - e^{-k_e\tau}) = 250 \text{ mg}/[1 - e^{-(0.419 \text{ h}^{-1})(8 \text{ h})}] = 259 \text{ mg, rounded to } 260 \text{ mg}$$

10. *Solution to problem 10.* Compute modified dose for FH using linear pharmacokinetics:

1. *Compute new dose to achieve desired serum concentration.*

Using linear pharmacokinetics, the new dose to attain the desired concentration should be proportional to the old dose that produced the measured concentration:

$$D_{new} = (C_{ss,new}/C_{ss,old})D_{old} = (10 \text{ µg/mL }/7.9 \text{ µg/mL}) 250 \text{ mg} = 316 \text{ mg}$$

The new suggested dose would be 315 mg every 8 hours to be started at next scheduled dosing time.

2. *Check steady-state trough concentration for new dosage regimen.*

Using linear pharmacokinetics, the new steady-state concentration can be estimated and should be proportional to the old dose that produced the measured concentration:

$$C_{ss,new} = (D_{new}/D_{old})C_{ss,old} = (315 \text{ mg}/250 \text{ mg}) 1 \text{ µg/mL} = 1.3 \text{ µg/mL}$$

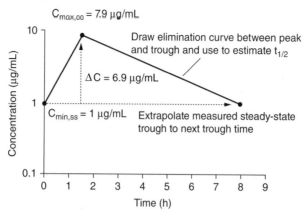

FIGURE 4-19 Solution to Problem 10 using Pharmacokinetic Concept method.

This steady-state trough concentration should be safe and effective for the infection that is being treated.

The revised tobramycin dose for patient FH using the Pharmacokinetics Concept method would be calculated as follows:

1. *Draw a rough sketch of the serum log concentration/time curve by hand, keeping track of the relative time between the serum concentrations (Figure 4-19).*
2. *Because the patient is at steady state, the trough concentration can be extrapolated to the next trough value time (see Figure 4-19).*
3. *Draw the elimination curve between the steady-state peak concentration and the extrapolated trough concentration. Use this line to estimate half-life.* The patient is receiving a tobramycin dose of 250 mg given every 8 hours that produces a steady-state peak equal to 7.9 µg/mL and a steady-state trough equal to 1 µg/mL, and the dose is infused over ½ hour and the peak concentration is drawn ½ hour later (see Figure 4-19). The time between the measured steady-state peak and the extrapolated trough concentration is 7 hours (the 8-hour dosage interval minus the 1-hour combined infusion and waiting time). The definition of half-life is the time needed for serum concentrations to decrease by ½. It would take 1 half-life for the peak serum concentration to decline from 7.9 to 4 µg/mL, an additional half-life for the serum concentration to decrease from 4 to 2 µg/mL, and another half-life for the concentration to decline from 2 to 1 µg/mL. Therefore, 3 half-lives expired during the 7-hour time period between the peak concentration and extrapolated trough concentration, and the estimated half-life is 2 hours (7 hours/3 half-lives = ~2 hours). This information will be used to set the new dosage interval for the patient
4. *Determine the difference in concentration between the steady-state peak and trough concentrations. The difference in concentration will change proportionally with the dose size.* In the current example the patient is receiving a tobramycin dose equal to 250 mg every 8 hours, which produced steady-state peak and trough concentrations of 7.9 µg/mL and 1 µg/mL, respectively. The difference between the peak and trough values is 6.9 µg/mL. The change in serum concentration is proportional to the dose, and this information will be used to set a new dose for the patient.
5. *Choose new steady-state peak and trough concentrations.* For the purposes of this example, the desired steady-state peak and trough concentrations will be approximately 10 µg/mL and 1 µg/mL, respectively.

6. *Determine the new dosage interval for the desired concentrations.* Using the desired concentrations, it will take 1 half-life for the peak concentration of 10 μg/mL to decrease to 5 μg/mL, 1 more half-life for the serum concentration to decrease to 2.5 μg/mL, an additional half-life for serum concentrations to decline from 2.5 to 1.3 μg/mL, and a final half-life for serum concentrations to reach 0.7 μg/mL. Therefore, the dosage interval will need to be approximately 4 half-lives or 8 hours (2 hours × 4 half-lives = 8 hours).

7. *Determine the new dose for the desired concentrations.* The desired peak concentration is 10 μg/mL, and the expected trough concentration is 0.7 μg/mL. The change in concentration between these values is 9.3 μg/mL. It is known from measured serum concentrations that administration of 250 mg changes serum concentrations by 6.9 μg/mL and that the change in serum concentration between the peak and trough values is proportional to the size of the dose. In this case: $D_{new} = (\Delta C_{new}/\Delta C_{old})D_{old}$ = (9.3 μg/mL / 6.9 μg/mL) 250 mg = 336 mg, rounded to 335 mg. Tobramycin 335 mg every 8 hours would be started 8 hours after the last dose of the previous dosage regimen.

The revised tobramycin dose for patient FH using the steady-state Sawchuk-Zaske method would be calculated as follows:

1. *Compute the patient's elimination rate constant and half-life. (Note: For infusion times less than 1 hour, t′ is considered to be the sum of the infusion and waiting times.)*

$$k_e = (\ln Css_{max} - \ln Css_{min})/\tau - t' = (\ln 7.9 \text{ μg/mL} - \ln 1 \text{ μg/mL})/(8 \text{ h} - 1 \text{ h}) = 0.295 \text{ h}^{-1}$$

$$t_{1/2} = 0.693/k_e = 0.693/0.295 \text{ h}^{-1} = 2.3 \text{ h}$$

2. *Compute the patient's volume of distribution.*

$$V = \frac{D/t'(1 - e^{-k_e t'})}{k_e[Css_{max} - (Css_{min}e^{-k_e t'})]} = \frac{(250 \text{ mg}/1 \text{ h})[1 - e^{-(0.295 \text{ h}^{-1})(1 \text{ h})}]}{0.295 \text{ h}^{-1}\{7.9 \text{ mg/L} - [1 \text{ mg/L } e^{-(0.295 \text{ h}^{-1})(1 \text{ h})}]\}}$$

$$V = 30.3 \text{ L}$$

3. *Choose new steady-state peak and trough concentrations.* For the purposes of this example, the desired steady-state peak and trough concentrations will be 10 μg/mL and 1 μg/mL, respectively.

4. *Determine the new dosage interval for the desired concentrations.* As in the initial dosage section of this chapter, the dosage interval (τ) is computed using the following equation using a 1-hour infusion time (t′):

$$\tau = [(\ln Css_{max} - \ln Css_{min})/k_e] + t' = [(\ln 10 \text{ μg/mL} - \ln 1 \text{ μg/mL})/0.295 \text{ h}^{-1}] + 1 \text{ h}$$

$$= 8.8 \text{ h, round to 8 h}$$

5. *Determine the new dose for the desired concentrations.* The dose is computed using the one-compartment model intravenous infusion equation used in the initial dosing section of this chapter:

$$k_0 = Css_{max}k_e V[(1 - e^{-k_e \tau})/(1 - e^{-k_e t'})]$$

$$k_0 = (10 \text{ mg/L} \cdot 0.295 \text{ h}^{-1} \cdot 30.3 \text{ L})\{[1 - e^{-(0.295 \text{ h}^{-1})(8 \text{ h})}]/[1 - e^{-(0.295 \text{ h}^{-1})(1 \text{ h})}]\}$$

$$= 316 \text{ mg, rounded to 315 mg}$$

A dose of tobramycin 315 mg every 8 hours would be prescribed to begin 8 hours after the last dose of the previous regimen. This dose is identical to that derived for the patient using the Linear Pharmacokinetics method (315 mg every 8 hours) and is very similar to that calculated by the Pharmacokinetic Concepts method (335 mg every 8 hours).

11. *Solution to problem 11.* The initial gentamicin dose for patient TY would be calculated as follows:

1. *Estimate creatinine clearance.*

This patient has a stable serum creatinine and is not obese. The Cockcroft-Gault equation can be used to estimate creatinine clearance:

$$CrCl_{est} = \{[(140 - age)BW] \cdot 0.85\}/(72 \cdot S_{Cr}) = \{[(140 - 66 \text{ y})65 \text{ kg}] \cdot 0.85\}/(72 \cdot 1.4 \text{ mg/dL})$$

$$CrCl_{est} = 41 \text{ mL/min}$$

2. *Estimate elimination rate constant (k_e) and half-life ($t_{1/2}$).*
The elimination rate constant versus creatinine clearance relationship is used to estimate the gentamicin elimination rate for this patient:

$$k_e = 0.00293(CrCl) + 0.014 = 0.00293(41 \text{ mL/min}) + 0.014 = 0.133 \text{ h}^{-1}$$
$$t_{1/2} = 0.693/k_e = 0.693/0.133 \text{ h}^{-1} = 5.2 \text{ h}$$

3. *Estimate volume of distribution (V).*

The patient has excess extracellular fluid due to ascites, and the formula used to take this into account will be used. The patient's dry body weight (DBW) before ascitic fluid accumulated was 65 kg, and her current weight (TBW) has increased to 72 kg:

$$V = (0.26 \cdot DBW) + (TBW - DBW) = (0.26 \cdot 65 \text{ kg}) + (72 \text{ kg} - 65 \text{ kg}) = 23.9 \text{ L}$$

4. *Choose desired steady-state serum concentrations.*

For the purposes of this example, a steady-state peak concentration ($Cmax_{ss}$) equal to 6 µg/mL and steady-state trough ($Cmin_{ss}$) concentration equal to 1 µg/mL will be used to design the dosage regimen.

5. *Use intermittent intravenous infusion equations to compute dose.*

Calculate required dosage interval (τ) using a 1-hour infusion:

$$\tau = [(\ln Css_{max} - \ln Css_{min})/k_e] + t' = [(\ln 6 \text{ µg/mL} - \ln 1 \text{ µg/mL})/0.133 \text{ h}^{-1}] + 1 \text{ h} = 14.5 \text{ h}$$

Dosage intervals should be rounded to clinically acceptable intervals of 8, 12, 18, 24, 36, 48, and 72 hours, and multiples of 24 hours thereafter, whenever possible. In this case, the dosage interval would be rounded to 12 hours. Also, steady-state peak concentrations are similar if drawn immediately after a 1-hour infusion or ½ hour after a ½-hour infusion, so the dose could be administered either way.

$$k_0 = Css_{max}k_eV[(1 - e^{-k_e\tau})/(1 - e^{-k_et'})]$$
$$k_0 = (6 \text{ mg/L} \cdot 0.133 \text{ h}^{-1} \cdot 23.9 \text{ L})\{[1 - e^{-(0.133 \text{ h}^{-1})(12 \text{ h})}]/[1 - e^{-(0.133 \text{ h}^{-1})(1 \text{ h})}]\} = 122 \text{ mg}$$

Aminoglycoside doses should be rounded to the nearest 5-10 mg. This dose would be rounded to 120 mg. (Note: µg/mL = mg/L and this concentration unit was substituted for Css_{max} so that unnecessary unit conversion was not required.)

The prescribed maintenance dose would be: 120 mg every 12 hours.

6. *Compute loading dose (LD), if needed.*

Loading doses for patients with creatinine clearance values below 60 mL/min can be given:

$$LD = k_0/(1 - e^{-k_e\tau}) = 120 \text{ mg}/[1 - e^{-(0.133 \text{ h}^{-1})(12 \text{ h})}] = 151 \text{ mg, rounded to 150 mg}$$

The loading dose would be given as the first dose and subsequent doses would be maintenance doses.

12. *Solution to problem 12.* Compute modified dose for TY using linear pharmacokinetics:

1. *Compute new dose to achieve desired serum concentration.*

Using linear pharmacokinetics, the new dose to attain the desired concentration should be proportional to the old dose that produced the measured concentration:

$$D_{new} = (C_{ss,new}/C_{ss,old})D_{old} = (6 \text{ µg/mL} /4 \text{ µg/mL}) \ 120 \text{ mg} = 180 \text{ mg}$$

The new suggested dose would be 180 mg every 12 hours to be started at next scheduled dosing time.

2. *Check steady-state trough concentration for new dosage regimen.*

Using linear pharmacokinetics, the new steady-state concentration can be estimated and should be proportional to the old dose that produced the measured concentration:

$$C_{ss,new} = (D_{new}/D_{old})C_{ss,old} = (180 \text{ mg}/120 \text{ mg}) \ 0.8 \text{ µg/mL} = 1.2 \text{ µg/mL}$$

This steady-state trough concentration should be safe and effective for the infection that is being treated.

The revised gentamicin dose for patient TY using the Pharmacokinetics Concept method would be calculated as follows:

1. *Draw a rough sketch of the serum log concentration/time curve by hand, keeping track of the relative time between the serum concentrations (Figure 4-20).*
2. *Because the patient is at steady state, the trough concentration can be extrapolated to the next trough value time (see Figure 4-20).*
3. *Draw the elimination curve between the steady-state peak concentration and the extrapolated trough concentration. Use this line to estimate half-life.* The patient is receiving a gentamicin dose of 120 mg given every 12 hours that produces a steady-state peak equal to 4 µg/mL and a steady-state trough equal to 0.8 µg/mL, and the dose is infused over ½ hour and the peak concentration is drawn ½ hour later (see Figure 4-20). The time between the measured steady-state peak and the extrapolated trough concentration is 11 hours (the 12-hour dosage interval minus the 1-hour combined infusion and waiting time). The definition of half-life is the time needed for serum concentrations to decrease by ½. It would take 1 half-life for the peak serum concentration to decline from 4 to 2 µg/mL, and an additional half-life for the serum concentration to decrease from 2 to 1 µg/mL. The concentration of 1 µg/mL is close to the observed value of 0.8 µg/mL. Therefore, 2 half-lives

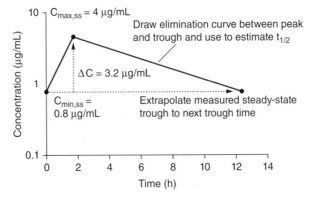

FIGURE 4-20   Solution to Problem 12 using Pharmacokinetic Concept method.

expired during the 11-hour time period between the peak concentration and extrapolated trough concentration, and the estimated half-life is 6 hours (11 hours/2 half-lives = ~6 hours). This information will be used to set the new dosage interval for the patient.

4. *Determine the difference in concentration between the steady-state peak and trough concentrations. The difference in concentration will change proportionally with the dose size.* In the current example, the patient is receiving a gentamicin dose equal to 120 mg every 12 hours, which produced steady-state peak and trough concentrations of 4 μg/mL and 0.8 μg/mL, respectively. The difference between the peak and trough values is 3.2 μg/mL. The change in serum concentration is proportional to the dose, and this information will be used to set a new dose for the patient.

5. *Choose new steady-state peak and trough concentrations.* For the purposes of this example, the desired steady-state peak and trough concentrations will be approximately 6 μg/mL and 1 μg/mL, respectively.

6. *Determine the new dosage interval for the desired concentrations.* Using the desired concentrations, it will take 1 half-life for the peak concentration of 6 μg/mL to decrease to 3 μg/mL, and an additional half-life for serum concentrations to decline from 3 to 1.5 μg/mL. This concentration is close to the desired trough concentration of 1 μg/mL. Therefore, the dosage interval will need to be approximately 2 half-lives or 12 hours (6 hours × 2 half-lives = 12 hours).

7. *Determine the new dose for the desired concentrations.* The desired peak concentration is 6 μg/mL, and the expected trough concentration is 1.5 μg/mL. The change in concentration between these values is 4.5 μg/mL. It is known from measured serum concentrations that administration of 120 mg changes serum concentrations by 3.2 μg/mL and that the change in serum concentration between the peak and trough values is proportional to the size of the dose. In this case: $D_{new} = (\Delta C_{new}/\Delta C_{old})D_{old} = (4.5 \ \mu g/mL / 3.2 \ \mu g/mL) \ 120 \ mg = 168 \ mg$, rounded to 170 mg. Gentamicin 170 mg every 12 hours would be started 12 hours after the last dose of the previous dosage regimen.

The revised gentamicin dose for patient TY using the steady-state Sawchuk-Zaske method would be calculated as follows:

1. *Compute the patient's elimination rate constant and half-life. (Note: For infusion times less than 1 hour, t′ is considered to be the sum of the infusion and waiting times.)*

$$k_e = (\ln Css_{max} - \ln Css_{min})/\tau - t' = (\ln 4 \ \mu g/mL - \ln 0.8 \ \mu g/mL)/(12 \ h - 1 \ h) = 0.146 \ h^{-1}$$

$$t_{1/2} = 0.693/k_e = 0.693/0.146 \ h^{-1} = 4.7 \ h$$

2. *Compute the patient's volume of distribution.*

$$V = \frac{D/t'(1-e^{-k_e t'})}{k_e[Css_{max} - (Css_{min}e^{-k_e t'})]} = \frac{(120 \ mg/1 \ h)[1 - e^{-(0.146 \ h^{-1})(1 \ h)}]}{0.146 \ h^{-1}\{4 \ mg/L - [0.8 \ mg/L \ e^{-(0.146 \ h^{-1})(1 \ h)}]\}}$$

$$V = 33.7 \ L$$

3. *Choose new steady-state peak and trough concentrations.* For the purposes of this example, the desired steady-state peak and trough concentrations will be 6 μg/mL and 1 μg/mL, respectively.

4. *Determine the new dosage interval for the desired concentrations.* As in the initial dosage section of this chapter, the dosage interval (τ) is computed using the following equation using a 1-hour infusion time (t′):

$$\tau = [(\ln Css_{max} - \ln Css_{min})/k_e] + t' = [(\ln 6 \ \mu g/mL - \ln 1.0 \ \mu g/mL)/0.146 \ h^{-1}] + 1 \ h$$
$$= 13.3 \ h, \text{ round to } 12 \ h$$

5. *Determine the new dose for the desired concentrations.* The dose is computed using the one-compartment model intravenous infusion equation used in the initial dosing section of this chapter:

$$k_0 = Css_{max} k_e V[(1 - e^{-k_e \tau})/(1 - e^{-k_e t'})]$$

$$k_0 = (6 \text{ mg/L} \bullet 0.146 \text{ h}^{-1} \bullet 33.7 \text{ L})\{[1 - e^{-(0.146 \text{ h}^{-1})(12 \text{ h})}]/[1 - e^{-(0.146 \text{ h}^{-1})(1 \text{ h})}]\} = 180 \text{ mg}$$

A dose of gentamicin 180 mg every 12 hours would be prescribed to begin 12 hours after the last dose of the previous regimen. This dose is identical to that derived for the patient using the Linear Pharmacokinetics method (180 mg every 12 hours) and is very similar to that derived by the Pharmacokinetic Concepts method (170 mg every 12 hours).

13. *Solution to problem 13.* The initial gentamicin dose for patient UQ would be calculated as follows:

1. *Estimate creatinine clearance.*

This patient is not obese. The patient is in acute renal failure and receiving hemodialysis. Because dialysis removes creatinine, the serum creatinine cannot be used to estimate creatinine clearance for the patient. Because the patient's renal function is poor enough to require dialysis, the creatinine clearance will be assumed to equal zero.

2. *Estimate elimination rate constant (k_e) and half-life ($t_{1/2}$).*

The elimination rate constant versus creatinine clearance relationship is used to estimate the gentamicin elimination rate for this patient:

$$k_e = 0.00293(CrCl) + 0.014 = 0.00293(0 \text{ mL/min}) + 0.014 = 0.014 \text{ h}^{-1}$$

$$t_{1/2} = 0.693/k_e = 0.693/0.014 \text{ h}^{-1} = 50 \text{ h}$$

3. *Estimate volume of distribution (V).*

The patient has renal failure and would need to be assessed for volume status to rule out over- and underhydration. In this case, the patient is in good fluid balance, and the volume of distribution from the normal value of 0.26 L/kg would be used:

$$V = 0.26 \text{ L/kg (85 kg)} = 22.1 \text{ L}$$

4. *Choose desired steady-state serum concentrations.*

Gram-negative pneumonia patients treated with aminoglycoside antibiotics require steady-state peak concentrations ($Cmax_{ss}$) equal to 8-10 µg/mL; steady-state trough ($Cmin_{ss}$) concentrations should be less than 2 µg/mL to avoid toxicity. Set $Cmax_{ss}$ = 8 µg/mL and $Cmin_{ss}$ ~2 µg/mL.

5. *Compute first dose.*

Because the patient has renal failure with a gentamicin half-life ~50 hours, very little antibiotic is eliminated during the ½- to 1-hour infusion time. Simple intravenous bolus equations can be used to compute doses in this case.

$$LD = C_{max} V = 8 \text{ mg/L} \bullet 22.1 \text{ L} = 177 \text{ mg}$$

Aminoglycoside doses should be rounded to the nearest 5-10 mg. This dose would be rounded to 180 mg. (Note: µg/mL = mg/L, and this concentration unit was substituted for Cmax so that unnecessary unit conversion was not required.)

The prescribed maintenance dose would be: 180 mg postdialysis at 1200 H on Wednesday.

6. *Estimate pre- and postdialysis aminoglycoside concentration.*

The next dialysis session will occur on Friday at 0800 H. The time expired between the dose given on Wednesday at 1200 H and this hemodialysis period is 44 hours (Figure 4-21). During the interdialysis

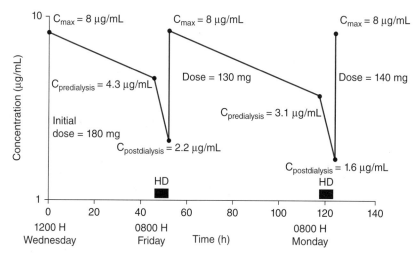

FIGURE 4-21   Solution to Problem 13.

time period only the patient's own, endogenous clearance will eliminate gentamicin. The predialysis serum concentration will be:

$$C = C_0 e^{-k_e t} = (8 \ \mu g/mL)e^{-(0.014 \ h^{-1})(44 \ h)} = 4.3 \ \mu g/mL$$

The average half-life of aminoglycosides during hemodialysis with a low-flux membrane is 4 hours. Because the usual dialysis time is 3-4 hours with a low-flux filter, intradialysis elimination can be computed:

$$k_e = 0.693/t_{1/2} = 0.693/4 \ h = 0.173 \ h^{-1}$$
$$C = C_0 e^{-k_e t} = (4.3 \ \mu g/mL)e^{-(0.173 \ h^{-1})(4 \ h)} = 2.2 \ \mu g/mL$$

Alternatively, because aminoglycoside half-life on dialysis is 4 hours and the dialysis period is 4 hours, one can deduce that the postdialysis serum concentration will be ½ the predialysis value.

7. *Calculate postdialysis replacement dose.*

The postdialysis serum concentration of 2.2 µg/mL is an estimate of the actual serum concentration and is close enough to the target concentration that a postdialysis dose will be administered immediately at the end of the procedure.

Replacement dose = $(C_{max} - C_{baseline})V$ = (8 mg/L − 2.2 mg/L) 22.1 L = 128 mg, rounded to 130 mg

8. *Compute pre- and postdialysis concentrations plus postdialysis dose for next dialysis cycle.*

The Friday-to-Monday dialysis cycle includes an extra day, so the concentration profile for that time period will be estimated (see Figure 4-21). The time between the gentamicin dose given at 1200 H on Friday and the next dialysis period at 0800 H on Monday is 68 hours.

$$C = C_0 e^{-k_e t} = (8 \ \mu g/mL)e^{-(0.014 \ h^{-1})(68 \ h)} = 3.1 \ \mu g/mL \text{ predialysis on Monday}$$

$$C = C_0 e^{-k_e t} = (3.1 \ \mu g/mL)e^{-(0.173 \ h^{-1})(4 \ h)} = 1.6 \ \mu g/mL \text{ postdialysis on Monday}$$

Replacement dose = $(C_{max} - C_{baseline})V$ = (8 mg/L − 1.6 mg/L) 22.1 L = 141 mg, rounded to 140 mg. The dialysis periods for this patient are scheduled, and because the dosage recommendation is based on estimated pharmacokinetic parameters, a postdialysis dose of 130 mg could be suggested so that all doses were uniform.

14. *Solution to problem 14.* The revised gentamicin dose for patient UQ using intravenous bolus equations would be calculated as follows:

1. *Compute the patient's elimination rate constant and half-life.*

$$k_e = (\ln C_{postdose(1)} - \ln C_{predialysis})/\Delta t = (\ln 6.4 \ \mu g/mL - \ln 2.2 \ \mu g/mL)/(68 \ h) = 0.0157 \ h^{-1}$$
$$t_{1/2} = 0.693/k_e = 0.693/0.0157 \ h^{-1} = 44 \ h$$

2. *Compute the patient's volume of distribution.*

$$V = \frac{D}{C_{postdose(2)} - C_{postdialysis}} = \frac{130 \ mg}{6.9 \ mg/L - 0.7 \ mg/L}$$
$$V = 21 \ L$$

3. *Compute the fraction of drug eliminated by the dialysis procedure.*

$$\text{Fraction eliminated} = (C_{predialysis} - C_{postdialysis})/C_{predialysis} = (2.2 \ \mu g/mL - 0.7 \ \mu g/mL)/2.2 \ \mu g/mL = 0.68 \text{ or } 68\%$$

The fraction remaining after hemodialysis is $1 - $ fraction eliminated or $1 - 0.68 = 0.32$ or 32%.

4. *Compute pre- and postdialysis concentrations plus postdialysis dose for next dialysis cycle using patient's own pharmacokinetic parameters.*

The time between the gentamicin concentration obtained at 1400 H on Monday and the next dialysis period at 0800 H on Wednesday is 42 hours.

$$C = C_0 e^{-k_e t} = (6.9 \ \mu g/mL)e^{-(0.0157 \ h^{-1})(42 \ h)} = 3.6 \ \mu g/mL \text{ predialysis on Wednesday}$$

The fraction remaining after hemodialysis is $1 - $ fraction eliminated or $1 - 0.68 = 0.32$ or 32%.

$$\text{Fraction remaining} = 0.32 \bullet 3.6 \ \mu g/mL = 1.2 \ \mu g/mL$$

$$\text{Replacement dose} = (C_{max} - C_{baseline})V = (8 \ mg/L - 1.2 \ mg/L) \ 21 \ L = 143 \ mg, \text{ rounded to } 145 \ mg.$$

15. *Solution to problem 15.* This patient is an older individual with poor renal function ($CrCl_{est} = \{[(140 - age)BW] \bullet 0.85\}/(72 \bullet S_{Cr}) = \{[(140 - 67 \ y)60 \ kg] \bullet 0.85\}/(72 \bullet 1.8 \ mg/dL) = 29 \ mL/min$) and is not at steady-state when the serum concentrations were obtained. Because of this, a Bayesian pharmacokinetic computer program is the best method to compute revised doses for this individual.

1. *Enter patient demographic, drug dosing, and serum concentration/time data into the computer program.*
2. *Compute pharmacokinetic parameters for the patient using Bayesian pharmacokinetic computer program.*

The pharmacokinetic parameters computed by the program are a volume of distribution of 21.4 L, a half-life equal to 13.5 hours, and an elimination rate constant of $0.051 \ h^{-1}$.

3. *Compute dose required to achieve desired aminoglycoside serum concentrations.*

The one-compartment model intravenous infusion equations used by the program to compute doses indicate that a dose of 150 mg every 36 hours will produce a steady-state peak concentration of 8.1 μg/mL and a steady-state trough concentration of 1.3 μg/mL.

16. *Solution to problem 16.* This patient could receive an extended-interval gentamicin dose between 5 and 7 mg/kg.
   a. Using the Hartford nomogram initial dosing guidelines:
      1. *Estimate creatinine clearance.*

This patient has a stable serum creatinine and is not obese. The Cockcroft-Gault equation can be used to estimate creatinine clearance:

$$CrCl_{est} = [(140 - age)BW]/(72 \cdot S_{Cr}) = [(140 - 52 \text{ y})87 \text{ kg}]/(72 \cdot 1.4 \text{ mg/dL})$$
$$CrCl_{est} = 76 \text{ mL/min}$$

2. *Compute initial dose and dosage interval (see Table 4-4).*
   A dose (D) of 7 mg/kg will provide a peak concentration more than 20 μg/mL.

$$D = 7 \text{ mg/kg}(87 \text{ kg}) = 609 \text{ mg, round to 600 mg}$$

Because the patient's estimated creatinine clearance is more than 60 mL/min, a dosage interval of 24 hours is chosen.

The prescribed maintenance dose would be: 600 mg every 24 hours.

b. Using the Hartford nomogram to individualize dosage interval:
   1. *Determine dosage interval using serum concentration monitoring (see Table 4-4).*
      A gentamicin serum concentration measured 9 hours after the dose equals 8.2 μg/mL. Based on the nomogram, a dosage interval of 36 hours is the correct value and would be instituted with the next dose: 600 mg every 36 hours.

c. Using a Bayesian pharmacokinetic computer dosing program to individualize dose and dosage interval:
   1. *Enter patient demographic, drug dosing, and serum concentration/time data into the computer program.*
   2. *Compute pharmacokinetic parameters for the patient using Bayesian pharmacokinetic computer program.*

The pharmacokinetic parameters computed by the program are a volume of distribution of 21.5 L, a half-life equal to 4.7 hours, and an elimination rate constant of 0.149 h^{-1}.

   3. *Compute dose required to achieve desired aminoglycoside serum concentrations.*

The one-compartment model intravenous infusion equations used by the program to compute doses indicate that a dose of 550 mg every 24 hours will produce a steady-state peak concentration of 24.4 μg/mL and a steady-state trough concentration of 0.8 μg/mL.

17. *Solution to problem 17.* This patient had extended-interval tobramycin therapy instituted by other clinicians at a rate of 5 mg/kg/d. The tobramycin dose is less than 7 mg/kg, and the serum concentration was not obtained 6-14 hours after the dose. Because of these reasons, the Hartford nomogram cannot be used, and a Bayesian pharmacokinetic computer program is the best method to compute revised doses for this individual.

   1. *Enter patient demographic, drug dosing, and serum concentration/time data into the computer program.*
   2. *Compute pharmacokinetic parameters for the patient using Bayesian pharmacokinetic computer program.*

The pharmacokinetic parameters computed by the program are a volume of distribution of 11.6 L, a half-life equal to 6.6 hours, and an elimination rate constant of 0.105 h^{-1}.

   3. *Compute dose required to achieve desired aminoglycoside serum concentrations.*

If the patient continued to receive the prescribed dose, the estimated steady-state peak and trough concentrations are 28.9 μg/mL and 2.6 μg/mL. The one-compartment model intravenous infusion equations used by the program to compute doses indicate that a dose of 300 mg every 36 hours will produce a steady-state peak concentration of 25.1 μg/mL and a steady-state trough concentration of 0.6 μg/mL.

18. *Solution to problem 18.* The initial tobramycin dose for patient DT would be calculated as follows:

1. *Compute initial dose and dosage interval.*

Often, serum creatinine measurements are not available for initial dosage computation in neonates. The dosage recommendations for this population assume typical renal function, so it is important to verify that the assumption is valid.

From the pediatric dosage recommendations given earlier in this chapter, a patient in this age and weight category should receive tobramycin 4 mg/kg every 24 hours. (*Note: Grams will be converted to kilograms before the computation is made.*)

$$\text{Dose} = 4 \text{ mg/kg}(2.050 \text{ kg}) = 8.2 \text{ mg}$$

The prescribed dose will be 8.2 mg every 24 hours.

19. *Solution to problem 19.* Compute modified dose for DT using linear pharmacokinetics:

1. *Compute new dose to achieve desired serum concentration.*

Using linear pharmacokinetics, the new dose to attain the desired concentration should be proportional to the old dose that produced the measured concentration:

$$D_{new} = (C_{ss,new}/C_{ss,old})D_{old} = (6 \text{ μg/mL}/4.5 \text{ μg/mL}) \, 5 \text{ mg} = 6.7 \text{ mg}$$

The new suggested dose would be 6.7 mg every 12 hours to be started at next scheduled dosing time.

2. *Check steady-state trough concentration for new dosage regimen.*

Using linear pharmacokinetics, the new steady-state concentration can be estimated and should be proportional to the old dose that produced the measured concentration.

$$C_{ss,new} = (D_{new}/D_{old})C_{ss,old} = (6.7 \text{ mg/5 mg}) \, 0.9 \text{ μg/mL} = 1.2 \text{ μg/mL}$$

20. *Solution to problem 20.*

1. *Estimate creatinine clearance.*

This patient has a stable serum creatinine and is not obese. The pediatric CrCl equation from Chapter 3 can be used to estimate creatinine clearance. (*Note: Height converted from inches to centimeters, 47 in • 2.54 cm/in = 119 cm.*)

$$CrCl_{est} = (0.55 \bullet Ht)/S_{Cr} = (0.55 \bullet 119 \text{ cm})/(0.5 \text{ mg/dL})$$
$$CrCl_{est} = 131 \text{ mL/min/1.73 m}^2$$

The patient has normal renal function, so typical initial doses can be used.

2. *Compute initial dose and dosage interval, using literature-based recommended dosing for pediatric patients.*

The dosage recommendations for this population assume typical renal function, so it is important to verify that the assumption is valid.

From the pediatrics dosage recommendations given earlier in this chapter, a patient in this age and weight category should receive gentamicin 7.5 mg/kg/d given as divided doses every 8 hours.

$$\text{Dose} = 7.5 \text{ mg/kg/d}(24 \text{ kg}) = 180 \text{ mg/d}$$
$$(180 \text{ mg/d})/(3 \text{ doses/d}) = 60 \text{ mg/dose}$$

The prescribed dose will be 60 mg every 8 hours.

21. *Solution to problem 21.*

1. *Use Steady-State Sawchuk-Zaske method to compute a new dose.*

Compute the patient's actual elimination rate constant and half-life. (Note: For infusion times less than 1 hour, t′ is considered to be the sum of the infusion and waiting times.)

$$k_e = (\ln C_1 - \ln C_2)/\Delta t = (\ln 4.5 \text{ µg/mL} - \ln 1.5 \text{ µg/mL})/(3 \text{ h}) = 0.366 \text{ h}^{-1}$$

$$t_{1/2} = 0.693/k_e = 0.693/0.366 \text{ h}^{-1} = 1.9 \text{ h}$$

Extrapolate measured concentrations to steady-state peak and trough values.

$$Css_{max} = C_1/(e^{-k_e t'}) = (4.5 \text{ µg/mL})/(e^{-(0.366 \text{ h}^{-1})(1 \text{ h})}) = 6.5 \text{ µg/mL}$$

$$Css_{min} = C_2 e^{-k_e t} = (1.5 \text{ µg/mL})(e^{-(0.366 \text{ h}^{-1})(3 \text{ h})}) = 0.5 \text{ µg/mL}$$

Compute the patient's volume of distribution.

$$V = \frac{D/t'(1 - e^{-k_e t'})}{k_e[Css_{max} - (Css_{min}e^{-k_e t'})]} = \frac{(60 \text{ mg}/1 \text{ h})[1 - e^{-(0.366 \text{ h}^{-1})(1 \text{ h})}]}{0.366 \text{ h}^{-1}[6.5 \text{ mg/L} - (0.5 \text{ mg/L } e^{-(0.366 \text{ h}^{-1})(1 \text{ h})})]}$$

$$V = 8.2 \text{ L}$$

2. *Choose new steady-state peak and trough concentrations.* The desired steady-state peak and trough concentrations will be 9 µg/mL and 1 µg/mL, respectively.

3. *Determine the new dosage interval for the desired concentrations.* As in the initial dosage section of this chapter, the dosage interval (τ) is computed using the following equation using a 1-hour infusion time (t′):

$$\tau = [(\ln Css_{max} - \ln Css_{min})/k_e] + t' = [(\ln 9 \text{ µg/mL} - \ln 1 \text{ µg/mL})/0.366 \text{ h}^{-1}] + 1 \text{ h} = 7 \text{ h, rounded to 8 hours}$$

4. *Determine the new dose for the desired concentrations.* The dose is computed using the one-compartment model intravenous infusion equation used in the initial dosing section of this chapter:

$$k_0 = Css_{max}k_e V[(1 - e^{-k_e \tau})/(1 - e^{-k_e t'})]$$

$$k_0 = (9 \text{ mg/L} \bullet 0.366 \text{ h}^{-1} \bullet 8.2 \text{ L})[(1 - e^{-(0.366 \text{ h}^{-1})(8 \text{ h})})/(1 - e^{-(0.366 \text{ h}^{-1})(1 \text{ h})})] = 83 \text{ mg, rounded to 85 mg}$$

A dose of gentamicin 85 mg every 8 hours would be prescribed to begin approximately 8 hours after the last dose of the current regimen.

22. *Solution to problem 22.*

Steady-State Sawchuk-Zaske Method

1. *Estimate creatinine clearance.*

This patient has a stable serum creatinine and is not obese. The Cockcroft-Gault equation can be used to estimate creatinine clearance:

$$CrCl_{est} = [(140 - \text{age})BW]/(72 \bullet S_{Cr}) = [(140 - 59 \text{ y})79 \text{ kg}]/(72 \bullet 1.5 \text{ mg/dL})$$

$$CrCl_{est} = 59 \text{ mL/min}$$

2. *Estimate elimination rate constant (k_e) and half-life ($t_{1/2}$).*

The elimination rate constant versus creatinine clearance relationship is used to estimate the gentamicin elimination rate for this patient:

$$k_e = 0.00293(CrCl) + 0.014 = 0.00293(59 \text{ mL/min}) + 0.014 = 0.187 \text{ h}^{-1}$$

$$t_{1/2} = 0.693/k_e = 0.693/0.187 \text{ h}^{-1} = 3.7 \text{ h}$$

Because the patient has been receiving gentamicin for more than 3-5 estimated half-lives, it is likely that the measured serum concentrations are steady-state values.

3. *Use Steady-State Sawchuk-Zaske method to compute a new dose.*

Compute the patient's actual elimination rate constant and half-life. (Note: For infusion times less than 1 hour, t′ is considered to be the sum of the infusion and waiting times.)

$$k_e = (\ln C_1 - \ln C_2)/\Delta t = (\ln 16.1 \ \mu g/mL - \ln 2.5 \ \mu g/mL)/(14 \ h) = 0.133 \ h^{-1}$$

$$t_{1/2} = 0.693/k_e = 0.693/0.133 \ h^{-1} = 5.2 \ h$$

Extrapolate measured concentrations to steady-state peak and trough values.

$$Css_{max} = C_1/(e^{-k_e t}) = (16.1 \ \mu g/mL)/[e^{-(0.133 \ h^{-1})(2 \ h)}] = 21.0 \ \mu g/mL$$

$$Css_{min} = C_2 e^{-k_e t} = (2.5 \ \mu g/mL)[e^{-(0.133 \ h^{-1})(7 \ h)}] = 1.0 \ \mu g/mL$$

Compute the patient's volume of distribution.

$$V = \frac{D/t'(1-e^{-k_e t'})}{k_e[Css_{max} - (Css_{min}e^{-k_e t'})]} = \frac{(450 \ mg/1 \ h)[1 - e^{-(0.133 \ h^{-1})(1 \ h)}]}{0.133 \ h^{-1}[21 \ mg/L - [1 \ mg/L \ e^{-(0.133 \ h^{-1})(1 \ h)}]\}}$$

$$V = 20.9 \ L$$

4. *Choose new steady-state peak and trough concentrations.* For the purposes of this example, the desired steady-state peak and trough concentrations will be 30 μg/mL and 0.3 μg/mL, respectively.

5. *Determine the new dosage interval for the desired concentrations.* The dosage interval (τ) is computed using the following equation using a 1-hour infusion time (t'):

$$\tau = [(\ln Css_{max} - \ln Css_{min})/k_e] + t' = [(\ln 30 \ \mu g/mL - \ln 0.3 \ \mu g/mL)/0.133 \ h^{-1}] + 1 \ h = 36 \ h$$

6. *Determine the new dose for the desired concentrations.* The dose is computed using the one-compartment model intravenous infusion equation used in the initial dosing section of this chapter:

$$k_0 = Css_{max} k_e V[(1 - e^{-k_e \tau})/(1 - e^{-k_e t'})]$$

$$k_0 = (30 \ mg/L \cdot 0.133 \ h^{-1} \cdot 20.9 \ L)\{[1 - e^{-(0.133 \ h^{-1})(36 \ h)}]/[1 - e^{-(0.133 \ h^{-1})(1 \ h)}]\} = 664 \ mg, \text{ rounded to } 650 \ mg$$

A dose of gentamicin 650 mg every 36 hours would be prescribed to begin after the last dose of the current regimen.

Bayesian Pharmacokinetic Computer Dosing Program Method

1. *Enter patient demographic, drug dosing, and serum concentration/time data into the computer program.*
2. *Compute pharmacokinetic parameters for the patient using Bayesian pharmacokinetic computer program.*

The pharmacokinetic parameters computed by the program are a volume of distribution of 20.7 L, a half-life equal to 5.2 hours, and an elimination rate constant of 0.133 h^{-1}.

3. *Compute dose required to achieve desired aminoglycoside serum concentrations.*

The one-compartment model intravenous infusion equations used by the program to compute doses indicate that a dose of 650 mg every 36 hours will produce a steady-state peak concentration of 29.7 μg/mL and a steady-state trough concentration of 0.3 μg/mL.

23. *Solution to problem 23.*

Pharmacokinetic Concepts Method

1. *Estimate creatinine clearance.*

This patient has a stable serum creatinine and is not obese. The Cockcroft-Gault equation can be used to estimate creatinine clearance:

$$CrCl_{est} = \{[(140 - age)BW]\,0.85\}/(72 \bullet S_{Cr}) = \{[(140 - 56\text{ y})69\text{ kg}]0.85\}/(72 \bullet 1.2\text{ mg/dL})$$

$$CrCl_{est} = 57\text{ mL/min}$$

2. *Estimate elimination rate constant (k_e) and half-life ($t_{1/2}$).*

The elimination rate constant versus creatinine clearance relationship is used to estimate the tobramycin elimination rate for this patient:

$$k_e = 0.00293(CrCl) + 0.014 = 0.00293(57\text{ mL/min}) + 0.014 = 0.181\text{ h}^{-1}$$

$$t_{1/2} = 0.693/k_e = 0.693/0.181\text{ h}^{-1} = 3.8\text{ h}$$

Because the patient has been receiving tobramycin for more than 3–5 estimated half-lives, it is likely that the measured serum concentrations are steady-state values.

3. *Use Pharmacokinetics Concept method to compute a new dose.*

   1. *Draw a rough sketch of the serum log concentration/time curve by hand, keeping track of the relative time between the serum concentrations.*

   2. *Because the patient is at steady state, the trough concentration can be extrapolated to the next trough value time.*

   3. *Draw the elimination curve between the steady-state peak concentration and the extrapolated trough concentration. Use this line to estimate half-life.* The patient is receiving a tobramycin dose of 500 mg given every 24 hours that produces a steady-state peak equal to 19 µg/mL and a steady-state trough equal to 1.9 µg/mL, and the dose is infused over ½ hour and the peak concentration is drawn ½ hour later. The time between the measured steady-state peak and the extrapolated trough concentration is 23 hours (the 24-hour dosage interval minus the 1-hour combined infusion and waiting time). The definition of half-life is the time needed for serum concentrations to decrease by ½. It would take 1 half-life for the peak serum concentration to decline from 19 to 9 µg/mL, an additional half-life for the serum concentration to decrease from 9 to 4.5 µg/mL, and another half-life for the serum concentration to decline from 4.5 to 2.25 µg/mL. The concentration of 1.9 µg/mL is close to the extrapolated trough value of 2.25 µg/mL. Therefore, 3 half-lives expired during the 23-hour time period between the peak concentration and extrapolated trough concentration, and the estimated half-life is 8 hours (23 hours/3 half-lives = ~8 hours). This information will be used to set the new dosage interval for the patient.

   4. *Determine the difference in concentration between the steady-state peak and trough concentrations. The difference in concentration will change proportionally with the dose size.* In the current example the patient is receiving a tobramycin dose equal to 500 mg every 24 hours, which produced steady-state peak and trough concentrations of 19 µg/mL and 1.9 µg/mL, respectively. The difference between the peak and trough values is 17.1 µg/mL. The change in serum concentration is proportional to the dose, and this information will be used to set a new dose for the patient.

   5. *Choose new steady-state peak and trough concentrations.* For the purposes of this example, the desired steady-state peak and trough concentrations will be approximately 25 µg/mL and 1 µg/mL, respectively.

6. *Determine the new dosage interval for the desired concentrations.* Using the desired concentrations, it will take 1 half-life for the peak concentration of 25 µg/mL to decrease to 12.5 µg/mL, 1 more half-life for the serum concentration to decrease to 6 µg/mL, an additional half-life for serum concentrations to decline to 3 µg/mL, and 2 additional half-lives for them to fall to 1.5 µg/mL and 0.75 µg/mL, respectively. Therefore, the dosage interval will need to be approximately 5 half-lives or 36 hours (8 hours × 5 half-live = 40 hours, round to 36 hours). When a dosage interval such as 36 hours is used, care must be taken to ensure that the scheduled doses are actually administered as the drug will only be given every other day and sometimes this type of administration schedule is overlooked and doses are missed.

7. *Determine the new dose for the desired concentrations.* The desired peak concentration is 25 µg/mL, and the expected trough concentration is 1 µg/mL. The change in concentration between these values is 24 µg/mL. It is known from measured serum concentrations that administration of 500 mg changes serum concentrations by 17.1 µg/mL and that the change in serum concentration between the peak and trough values is proportional to the size of the dose. In this case: $D_{new} = (\Delta C_{new}/\Delta C_{old})$ $D_{old} = (24$ µg/mL$/17.1$ µg/mL$) 500$ mg $= 702$ mg, round to 700. Tobramycin 700 mg every 36 hours would be started 36 hours after the last dose of the previous dosage regimen.

Steady-State Sawchuk-Zaske Method

1. *Estimate creatinine clearance.*

This patient has a stable serum creatinine and is not obese. The Cockcroft-Gault equation can be used to estimate creatinine clearance:

$$CrCl_{est} = \{[(140 - age)BW]0.85\}/(72 \cdot S_{Cr}) = \{[(140 - 56 \text{ y})69 \text{ kg}]0.85\}/(72 \cdot 1.2 \text{ mg/dL})$$
$$CrCl_{est} = 57 \text{ mL/min}$$

2. *Estimate elimination rate constant (k_e) and half-life ($t_{1/2}$).*

The elimination rate constant versus creatinine clearance relationship is used to estimate the tobramycin elimination rate for this patient:

$$k_e = 0.00293(CrCl) + 0.014 = 0.00293(57 \text{ mL/min}) + 0.014 = 0.181 \text{ h}^{-1}$$
$$t_{1/2} = 0.693/k_e = 0.693/0.181 \text{ h}^{-1} = 3.8 \text{ h}$$

Because the patient has been receiving tobramycin for more than 3-5 estimated half-lives, it is likely that the measured serum concentrations are steady-state values.

3. *Use Steady-State Sawchuk-Zaske method to compute a new dose.*

Compute the patient's elimination rate constant and half-life. (Note: For infusion times less than 1 hour, t′ is considered to be the sum of the infusion and waiting times.)

$$k_e = (\ln Css_{max} - \ln Css_{min})/\tau - t' = (\ln 19 \text{ µg/mL} - \ln 1.9 \text{ µg/mL})/(24 \text{ h} - 1 \text{ h}) = 0.100 \text{ h}^{-1}$$
$$t_{1/2} = 0.693/k_e = 0.693/0.100 \text{ h}^{-1} = 6.9 \text{ h}$$

Compute the patient's volume of distribution.

$$V = \frac{D/t'(1-e^{-k_e t'})}{k_e[Css_{max} - (Css_{min}e^{-k_e t'})]} = \frac{(500 \text{ mg}/1\text{h})(1 - e^{-(0.100 \text{ h}^{-1})(1 \text{ h})})}{0.100 \text{ h}^{-1}[19 \text{ mg/L} - (1.9 \text{ mg/L } e^{-(0.100 \text{ h}^{-1})(1 \text{ h})})]}$$
$$V = 27.5 \text{ L}$$

4. *Choose new steady-state peak and trough concentrations.* For the purposes of this example, the desired steady-state peak and trough concentrations will be approximately 25 µg/mL and 1 µg/mL, respectively.

5. *Determine the new dosage interval for the desired concentrations.* As in the initial dosage section of this chapter, the dosage interval (τ) is computed using the following equation using a 1-hour infusion time (t'):

$$\tau = [(\ln Css_{max} - \ln Css_{min})/k_e] + t' = [(\ln 25 \; \mu g/mL - \ln 1 \; \mu g/mL)/0.100 \; h^{-1}] + 1 \; h$$
$$= 33 \; h, \; \text{rounded to 36 hours}$$

6. *Determine the new dose for the desired concentrations.* The dose is computed using the one-compartment model intravenous infusion equation used in the initial dosing section of this chapter:

$$k_0 = Css_{max}k_eV[(1 - e^{-k_e\tau})/(1 - e^{-k_et'})]$$

$$k_0 = (25 \; mg/L \bullet 0.100 \; h^{-1} \bullet 27.5 \; L)[(1 - e^{-(0.100 \; h^{-1})(36 \; h)})/(1 - e^{-(0.100 \; h^{-1})(1 \; h)})] = 704 \; mg, \; \text{rounded to 700 mg}$$

A dose of tobramycin 700 mg every 36 hours would be prescribed to begin 36 hours after the last dose of the previous regimen.

Bayesian Pharmacokinetic Computer Dosing Program Method

1. *Enter patient demographic, drug dosing, and serum concentration/time data into the computer program.*
2. *Compute pharmacokinetic parameters for the patient using Bayesian pharmacokinetic computer program.*

The pharmacokinetic parameters computed by the program are a volume of distribution of 25.7 L, a half-life equal to 6.7 hours, and an elimination rate constant of 0.103 h^{-1}.

3. *Compute dose required to achieve desired aminoglycoside serum concentrations.*

The one-compartment model intravenous infusion equations used by the program to compute doses indicate that a dose of 700 mg every 36 hours will produce a steady-state peak concentration of 26.6 $\mu g/mL$ and a steady-state trough concentration of 0.7 $\mu g/mL$.

24. *Solution to problem 24.*

Steady-State Sawchuk-Zaske Method

1. *Estimate creatinine clearance.*

This patient has a stable serum creatinine and is obese [IBW_{males} (in kg) = 50 + 2.3(Ht −60) = 50 + 2.3(68 in − 60) = 68.4 kg]. The Salazar and Corcoran equation can be used to estimate creatinine clearance:

$$CrCl_{est(males)} = \frac{(137 - age)[(0.285 \bullet Wt) + (12.1 \bullet Ht^2)]}{(51 \bullet S_{Cr})}$$

$$CrCl_{est(males)} = \frac{(137 - 55 \; y)\{(0.285 \bullet 135 \; kg) + [12.1 \bullet (1.73 \; m)^2]\}}{(51 \bullet 1.3 \; mg/dL)} = 92 \; mL/min$$

Note: Height is converted from inches to meters: Ht = (68 in $\bullet$ 2.54 cm/in)/(100 cm/m) = 1.73 m.

2. *Estimate elimination rate constant (k_e) and half-life ($t_{1/2}$).*

The elimination rate constant versus creatinine clearance relationship is used to estimate the gentamicin elimination rate for this patient:

$$k_e = 0.00293(CrCl) + 0.014 = 0.00293(92 \; mL/min) + 0.014 = 0.284 \; h^{-1}$$
$$t_{1/2} = 0.693/k_e = 0.693/0.284 \; h^{-1} = 2.4 \; h$$

Because the patient has been receiving gentamicin for more than 3-5 estimated half-lives, it is likely that the measured serum concentrations are steady-state values.

3. *Use Steady-State Sawchuk-Zaske method to compute a new dose.*

Compute the patient's actual elimination rate constant and half-life. (Note: For infusion times less than 1 hour, t′ is considered to be the sum of the infusion and waiting times.)

$$k_e = (\ln C_1 - \ln C_2)/\Delta t = (\ln 10.2\ \mu g/mL - \ln 1.1\ \mu g/mL)/(8\ h) = 0.278\ h^{-1}$$

$$t_{1/2} = 0.693/k_e = 0.693/0.278\ h^{-1} = 2.5\ h$$

Extrapolate measured concentrations to steady-state peak and trough values.

$$Css_{max} = C_1/(e^{-k_e t}) = (10.2\ \mu g/mL)/[e^{-(0.278\ h^{-1})(2\ h)}] = 17.8\ \mu g/mL$$

$$Css_{min} = C_2 e^{-k_e t} = (1.1\ \mu g/mL)[e^{-(0.278\ h^{-1})(13\ h)}] = 0.03\ \mu g/mL$$

Compute the patient's volume of distribution.

$$V = \frac{D/t'(1-e^{-k_e t'})}{k_e[Css_{max} - (Css_{min}e^{-k_e t'})]} = \frac{(500\ mg/1\ h)[1 - e^{-(0.278\ h^{-1})(1\ h)}]}{0.278\ h^{-1}\{17.8\ mg/L - [0.03\ mg/L\ e^{-(0.278\ h^{-1})(1\ h)}]\}}$$

$$V = 24.6\ L$$

4. *Choose new steady-state peak and trough concentrations.* For the purposes of this example, the desired steady-state peak and trough concentrations will be 25 µg/mL and 0.1 µg/mL, respectively.

5. *Determine the new dosage interval for the desired concentrations.* The dosage interval (τ) is computed using the following equation using a 1-hour infusion time (t′):

$$\tau = [(\ln Css_{max} - \ln Css_{min})/k_e] + t' = [(\ln 25\ \mu g/mL - \ln 0.1\ \mu g/mL)/0.278\ h^{-1}] + 1\ h$$

$$= 21\ h,\ \text{round to 24 hours}$$

6. *Determine the new dose for the desired concentrations.* The dose is computed using the one-compartment model intravenous infusion equation used in the initial dosing section of this chapter:

$$k_0 = Css_{max} k_e V[(1 - e^{-k_e \tau})/(1 - e^{-k_e t'})]$$

$$k_0 = (25\ mg/L \bullet 0.278\ h^{-1} \bullet 24.6\ L)\{[1 - e^{-(0.278\ h^{-1})(24\ h)}]/[1 - e^{-(0.278\ h^{-1})(1\ h)}]\} = 704\ mg,\ \text{rounded to 700 mg}$$

A dose of gentamicin 700 mg every 24 hours would be prescribed to begin after the last dose of the current regimen.

Bayesian Pharmacokinetic Computer Dosing Program Method

1. *Enter patient demographic, drug dosing, and serum concentration/time data into the computer program.*
2. *Compute pharmacokinetic parameters for the patient using Bayesian pharmacokinetic computer program.*

The pharmacokinetic parameters computed by the program are a volume of distribution of 23.7 L, a half-life equal to 2.5 hours, and an elimination rate constant of 0.277 h^{-1}.

3. *Compute dose required to achieve desired aminoglycoside serum concentrations.*

The one-compartment model intravenous infusion equations used by the program to compute doses indicate that a dose of 700 mg every 24 hours will produce a steady-state peak concentration of 25.8 µg/mL and a steady-state trough concentration of 0.04 µg/mL.

25. *Solution for problem 25.*

Hartford Nomogram

1. *Estimate creatinine clearance.*

This patient has a stable serum creatinine and is not obese (<30% over IBW). The Cockcroft-Gault equation can be used to estimate creatinine clearance:

$$CrCl_{est} = \{[(140 - age)BW]0.85\}/(72 \cdot S_{Cr}) = \{[(140 - 27\ y)68\ kg]0.85\}/(72 \cdot 1.4\ mg/dL)$$

$$CrCl_{est} = 65\ mL/min$$

2. *Compute initial dose and dosage interval (see Table 4-4).*

A dose (D) of 7 mg/kg will provide a peak concentration more than 20 µg/mL.

$$D = 7\ mg/kg(68\ kg) = 476\ mg, \text{ round to } 475\ mg$$

Dosage interval would be 24 hours using the nomogram. Extended-interval aminoglycoside doses should be rounded to the nearest 10-50 mg.

The prescribed maintenance dose would be: 475 mg every 24 hours.

Pharmacokinetic Dosing Method

1. *Estimate creatinine clearance.*

This patient has a stable serum creatinine and is not obese (<30% over IBW). The Cockcroft-Gault equation can be used to estimate creatinine clearance:

$$CrCl_{est} = \{[(140 - age)BW]0.85\}/(72 \cdot S_{Cr}) = \{[(140 - 27\ y)68\ kg]0.85\}/(72 \cdot 1.4\ mg/dL)$$

$$CrCl_{est} = 65\ mL/min$$

2. *Estimate elimination rate constant (k_e) and half-life ($t_{1/2}$).*

The elimination rate constant versus creatinine clearance relationship is used to estimate the tobramycin elimination rate for this patient:

$$k_e = 0.00293(CrCl) + 0.014 = 0.00293(65\ mL/min) + 0.014 = 0.204\ h^{-1}$$
$$t_{1/2} = 0.693/k_e = 0.693/0.204\ h^{-1} = 3.4\ h$$

3. *Estimate volume of distribution (V).*

The patient has no disease states or conditions that would alter the volume of distribution from the normal value of 0.26 L/kg:

$$V = 0.26\ L/kg\ (68\ kg) = 17.7\ L$$

4. *Choose desired steady-state serum concentrations.*

Steady-state peak concentrations ($Cmax_{ss}$) equal to 25 µg/mL and steady-state trough ($Cmin_{ss}$) concentrations of less than 1 µg/mL were chosen for this patient. Set $Cmax_{ss}$ = 25 µg/mL and $Cmin_{ss}$ = 1 µg/mL.

5. *Use intermittent intravenous infusion equations to compute dose (see Table 4-2).*

Calculate required dosage interval (τ) using a 1-hour infusion:

$$\tau = [(\ln Css_{max} - \ln Css_{min})/k_e] + t' = [(\ln 25\ \mu g/mL - \ln 1\ \mu g/mL)/0.204\ h^{-1}] + 1\ h = 17\ h, \text{ round to } 24\ hours$$

Dosage intervals should be rounded to clinically acceptable intervals of 8, 12, 18, 24, 36, 48, and 72 hours, and multiples of 24 hours thereafter, whenever possible. In this case, the dosage interval would be rounded to 24 hours. Also, steady-state peak concentrations are similar if drawn immediately after a 1-hour infusion or ½ hour after a ½-hour infusion, so the dose could be administered either way.

$$k_0 = Css_{max} k_e V[(1 - e^{-k_e \tau})/(1 - e^{-k_e t'})]$$

$$k_0 = (25 \text{ mg/L} \bullet 0.204 \text{ h}^{-1} \bullet 17.7 \text{ L})\{[1 - e^{-(0.204 \text{ h}^{-1})(24 \text{ h})}]/[1 - e^{-(0.204 \text{ h}^{-1})(1 \text{ h})}]\} = 485 \text{ mg, round to } 475 \text{ mg}$$

This dose would be rounded to 475 mg. (Note: µg/mL = mg/L and this concentration unit was substituted for Css_{max} so that unnecessary unit conversion was not required.)

The prescribed maintenance dose would be: 475 mg every 24 hours.

26. *Solution for problem 26.* The revised tobramycin dose for the patient would be calculated as follows:

Hartford Nomogram

1. *Estimate creatinine clearance.*

This patient has a stable serum creatinine and is not obese (<30% over IBW). The Cockcroft-Gault equation can be used to estimate creatinine clearance:

$$CrCl_{est} = \{[(140 - \text{age})BW]0.85\}/(72 \bullet S_{Cr}) = \{[(140 - 27 \text{ y})68 \text{ kg}]0.85\}/(72 \bullet 1.4 \text{ mg/dL})$$

$$CrCl_{est} = 65 \text{ mL/min}$$

2. *Estimate elimination rate constant (k_e) and half-life ($t_{1/2}$).*

The elimination rate constant versus creatinine clearance relationship is used to estimate the tobramycin elimination rate for this patient:

$$k_e = 0.00293(CrCl) + 0.014 = 0.00293(65 \text{ mL/min}) + 0.014 = 0.204 \text{ h}^{-1}$$

$$t_{1/2} = 0.693/k_e = 0.693/0.204 \text{ h}^{-1} = 3.4 \text{ h}$$

Because the patient has been receiving tobramycin for more than 3-5 estimated half-lives, it is likely that the measured serum concentrations are steady-state values.

3. *Determine dosage interval using serum concentration monitoring.*

A tobramycin serum concentration measured 7 hours (6 hours postinfusion + 1 hour infusion time) after the dose equals 9.8 µg/mL. Based on the nomogram, a dosage interval of 36 hours is the correct value and the new dose would be 475 mg every 36 hours.

Steady-State Sawchuk-Zaske Method: Two Postdose Concentrations Version

1. *Estimate creatinine clearance.*

This patient has a stable serum creatinine and is not obese (<30% over IBW). The Cockcroft-Gault equation can be used to estimate creatinine clearance:

$$CrCl_{est} = \{[(140 - \text{age})BW]0.85\}/(72 \bullet S_{Cr}) = \{[(140 - 27 \text{ y})68 \text{ kg}]0.85\}/(72 \bullet 1.4 \text{ mg/dL})$$

$$CrCl_{est} = 65 \text{ mL/min}$$

2. *Estimate elimination rate constant (k_e) and half-life ($t_{1/2}$).*

The elimination rate constant versus creatinine clearance relationship is used to estimate the tobramycin elimination rate for this patient:

$$k_e = 0.00293(CrCl) + 0.014 = 0.00293(65 \text{ mL/min}) + 0.014 = 0.204 \text{ h}^{-1}$$

$$t_{1/2} = 0.693/k_e = 0.693/0.204 \text{ h}^{-1} = 3.4 \text{ h}$$

Because the patient has been receiving tobramycin for more than 3-5 estimated half-lives, it is likely that the measured serum concentrations are steady-state values.

3. *Use Steady-State Sawchuk-Zaske method to compute a new dose.*

Compute the patient's actual elimination rate constant and half-life. (Note: For infusion times less than 1 hour, t′ is considered to be the sum of the infusion and waiting times.)

$$k_e = (\ln C_1 - \ln C_2)/\Delta t = (\ln 17 \text{ μg/mL} - \ln 9.8 \text{ μg/mL})/(5 \text{ h}) = 0.110 \text{ h}^{-1}$$

$$t_{1/2} = 0.693/k_e = 0.693/0.110 \text{ h}^{-1} = 6.3 \text{ h}$$

Extrapolate measured concentrations to steady-state peak and trough values.

$$Css_{max} = C_1/(e^{-k_e t'}) = (17.0 \text{ μg/mL})/[e^{-(0.110 \text{ h}^{-1})(1 \text{ h})}] = 19.0 \text{ μg/mL}$$

$$Css_{min} = C_2 e^{-k_e t} = (9.8 \text{ μg/mL})[e^{-(0.110 \text{ h}^{-1})(17 \text{ h})}] = 1.5 \text{ μg/mL}$$

Compute the patient's volume of distribution.

$$V = \frac{D/t'(1 - e^{-k_e t'})}{k_e[Css_{max} - \{Css_{min} e^{-k_e t'}\}]} = \frac{(475 \text{ mg/1 h})[1 - e^{-(0.110 \text{ h}^{-1})(1 \text{ h})}]}{0.110 \text{ h}^{-1}\{19.0 \text{ mg/L} - [1.5 \text{ mg/L } e^{-(0.110 \text{ h}^{-1})(1 \text{ h})}]\}}$$

$$V = 25.5 \text{ L}$$

4. *Choose new steady-state peak and trough concentrations.* For the purposes of this example, the desired steady-state peak and trough concentrations will be 25 μg/mL and 1 μg/mL, respectively.

5. *Determine the new dosage interval for the desired concentrations.* As in the initial dosage section of this chapter, the dosage interval (τ) is computed using the following equation using a 1-hour infusion time (t′):

$$\tau = [(\ln Css_{max} - \ln Css_{min})/k_e] + t' = [(\ln 25 \text{ μg/mL} - \ln 1 \text{ μg/mL})/0.110 \text{ h}^{-1}] + 1 \text{ h}$$
$$= 30 \text{ h, rounded to 36 hours (rounded to longer dosage interval to ensure trough} < 1 \text{ μg/mL})$$

6. *Determine the new dose for the desired concentrations.* The dose is computed using the one-compartment model intravenous infusion equation used in the initial dosing section of this chapter:

$$k_0 = Css_{max} k_e V[(1 - e^{-k_e \tau})/(1 - e^{-k_e t'})]$$

$$k_0 = (25 \text{ mg/L} \cdot 0.110 \text{ h}^{-1} \cdot 25.5 \text{ L})\{[1 - e^{-(0.110 \text{ h}^{-1})(36 \text{ h})}]/[1 - e^{-(0.110 \text{ h}^{-1})(1 \text{ h})}]\} = 660 \text{ mg, rounded to 650 mg}$$

A dose of tobramycin 650 mg every 36 hours would be prescribed to begin approximately 36 hours after the last dose of the current regimen.

Bayesian Pharmacokinetic Computer Program Method

1. *Enter patient demographic, drug dosing, and serum concentration/time data into the computer program.*
2. *Compute pharmacokinetic parameters for the patient using Bayesian pharmacokinetic computer program.*

The pharmacokinetic parameters computed by the program are a volume of distribution of 22.2 L, a half-life equal to 5.3 hours, and an elimination rate constant of 0.130 h^{-1}.

3. *Compute dose required to achieve desired aminoglycoside serum concentrations.*

The one-compartment model intravenous infusion equations used by the program to compute doses indicate that a dose of 650 mg every 36 hours will produce a steady-state peak concentration of 27.8 μg/mL and a steady-state trough concentration of 0.3 μg/mL.

27. *Solution to problem 27.* The revised tobramycin dose for the patient would be calculated as follows:

AUC Method Using Steady-State Peak and Trough Concentrations

1. *Estimate creatinine clearance.*

This patient has a stable serum creatinine and is not obese. The Cockcroft-Gault equation can be used to estimate creatinine clearance:

$$CrCl_{est} = [(140 - age)BW]/(72 \cdot S_{Cr}) = [(140 - 23 \text{ y})67 \text{ kg}]/(72 \cdot 0.8 \text{ mg/dL})$$
$$CrCl_{est} = 136 \text{ mL/min}$$

2. *Estimate elimination rate constant (k_e) and half-life ($t_{1/2}$).*

The elimination rate constant versus creatinine clearance relationship is used to estimate the tobramycin elimination rate for this patient:

$$k_e = 0.00293(CrCl) + 0.014 = 0.00293(136 \text{ mL/min}) + 0.014 = 0.413 \text{ h}^{-1}$$
$$t_{1/2} = 0.693/k_e = 0.693/0.413 \text{ h}^{-1} = 1.7 \text{ h}$$

Because the patient has been receiving tobramycin for more than 3-5 estimated half-lives, it is likely that the measured serum concentrations are steady-state values.

3. *Use Steady-State AUC method to compute a new dose.*

Compute the patient's actual elimination rate constant and half-life. (Note: For infusion times less than 1 hour, t′ is considered to be the sum of the infusion and waiting times.)

$$k_e = (\ln C_1 - \ln C_2)/\Delta t = (\ln 9.6 \text{ μg/mL} - \ln 2.6 \text{ μg/mL})/(4 \text{ h}) = 0.327 \text{ h}^{-1}$$
$$t_{1/2} = 0.693/k_e = 0.693/0.327 \text{ h}^{-1} = 2.1 \text{ h}$$

Extrapolate measured concentrations to steady-state peak and trough values.

$$Css_{max} = C_1/(e^{-k_e t}) = (9.6 \text{ μg/mL})/[e^{-(0.327 \text{ h}^{-1})(2 \text{ h})}] = 18.5 \text{ μg/mL}$$
$$Css_{min} = C_2 e^{-k_e t} = (2.6 \text{ μg/mL})[e^{-(0.327 \text{ h}^{-1})(17 \text{ h})}] = 0.01 \text{ μg/mL}$$

Compute the patient's AUC_{ss} (Note: mg/L = μg/mL and this substitution was made to aid the calculation.)

$$AUC_{ss} = \frac{Css_{max} - Css_{max}}{k_e} + \left(0.065 \cdot \frac{Css_{max} - Css_{min}}{k_e} \right)$$

$$AUC_{ss} = \frac{18.5 \text{ mg/L} - 0.01 \text{ m/L}}{0.327 \text{ h}^{-1}} + \left(0.065 \cdot \frac{18.5 \text{ mg/L} - 0.01 \text{ mg/L}}{0.327 \text{ h}^{-1}} \right)$$
$$AUC_{ss} = 60.2 \text{ (mg} \cdot \text{h)/L}$$

4. *Choose new target AUC_{ss}.* For the purposes of this example, a desired steady state of AUC of 81 (mg • h)/L was chosen.

5. *Determine the new dose for the desired AUC_{ss}.*

$$D_{new} = (AUC_{ss,new}/AUC_{ss,old})D_{old} = \{[81 \ (mg \bullet h)/L]/[60.2 \ (mg \bullet h)/L]\}350 \ mg = 471 \ mg, \text{ rounded to } 475 \ mg$$

6. *Determine the new steady-state peak and trough concentrations.*

$$C_{ss,new} = (D_{new}/D_{old})C_{ss,old} = (475 \ mg/350 \ mg) \ 18.5 \ \mu g/mL = 25.1 \ \mu g/mL \text{ for the peak}$$
$$C_{ss,new} = (D_{new}/D_{old})C_{ss,old} = (475 \ mg/350 \ mg) \ 0.01 \ \mu g/mL = 0.01 \ \mu g/mL \text{ for the trough}$$

These steady-state peak and trough concentrations are acceptable for the infection being treated and the new prescribed dose would be 475 mg every 24 hours.

AUC Method Using Concentration(s) and Bayesian Pharmacokinetic Computer Program

1. *Calculate AUC using the Bayesian pharmacokinetic computer program.*

The pharmacokinetic parameters computed by the program are a volume of distribution of 16.6 L, a half-life equal to 2.2 hours, and clearance of 5.36 L/h.

The AUC for a dose is: $AUC = D/Cl = (350 \ mg)/(5.36 \ L/h) = 65.3 \ (mg \bullet h)/L$.

2. *Compute new dose based on AUC target.*

Tobramycin follows linear pharmacokinetics, so the AUC and steady-state trough concentrations change proportionally with dose.

$$\text{Dose}_{new} = (AUC_{new}/AUC_{old})\text{Dose}_{old} = (81/65.3)(350 \ mg/d) = 434 \ mg/d, \text{ round to } 450 \ mg/d$$

Check new steady-state tobramycin trough and peak concentrations for this AUC: The Bayesian pharmacokinetic computer program computes steady-state tobramycin trough and peak concentrations of 0.01 $\mu g/mL$ and 23.2 $\mu g/mL$, respectively, for the new dose. These would provide a C_{max}/MIC of more than 10 for bacteria up to a MIC = 2 $\mu g/mL$.

REFERENCES

1. MacDougall C, Chambers HF. Aminoglycosides. In: Brunton L, Chabner B, Knollman B, eds. *The Pharmacological Basis of Therapeutics.* 12th ed. New York, NY: McGraw-Hill; 2011:1505-1520.
2. Zaske DE, Cipolle RJ, Rotschafer JC, Solem LD, Mosier NR, Strate RG. Gentamicin pharmacokinetics in 1,640 patients: method for control of serum concentrations. *Antimicrob Agents Chemother.* 1982;21:407-411.
3. Nicolau DP, Freeman CD, Belliveau PP, Nightingale CH, Ross JW, Quintilliani R. Experience with a once-daily aminoglycoside program administered to 2,184 adult patients. *Antimicrob Agents Chemother.* 1995;39:650-655.
4. Jackson GG, Arcieri G. Ototoxicity of gentamicin in man: a survey and controlled analysis of clinical experience in the United States. *J Infect Dis.* 1971;124 (suppl):130-137.
5. Black RE, Lau WK, Weinstein RJ, Young LS, Hewitt WL. Ototoxicity of amikacin. *Antimicrob Agents Chemother.* 1976;9(6):956-961.
6. Mawer GE, Ahmad R, Dobbs SM, Tooth JA. Prescribing aids for gentamicin. *Br J Clin Pharmacol.* 1974;1:45-50.
7. Smith CR, Maxwell RR, Edwards CQ, Rogers JF, Lietman PS. Nephrotoxicity induced by gentamicin and amikacin. *Johns Hopkins Med J.* 1978;142(3):85-90.
8. Dahlgren JG, Anderson ET, Hewitt WL. Gentamicin blood levels: a guide to nephrotoxicity. *Antimicrob Agents Chemother.* 1975;8:58-62.
9. French MA, Cerra FB, Plaut ME, Schentag JJ. Amikacin and gentamicin accumulation pharmacokinetics and nephrotoxicity in critically ill patients. *Antimicrob Agents Chemother.* 1981;19(1):147-152.
10. Schentag JJ, Jusko WJ. Renal clearance and tissue accumulation of gentamicin. *Clin Pharmacol Ther.* 1977;22:364-370.
11. Schentag JJ, Plaut ME, Cerra FB. Comparative nephrotoxicity of gentamicin and tobramycin: pharmacokinetic and clinical studies in 201 patients. *Antimicrob Agents Chemother.* 1981;19:859-866.

12. Cosgrove SE, Vigliani GA, Fowler VG Jr, et al. Initial low-dose gentamicin for *Staphylococcus aureus* bacteremia and endocarditis is nephrotoxic. *Clin Infect Dis.* Mar 15, 2009;48(6):713-721.

13. Moore RD, Smith CR, Lipsky JJ, Mellits ED, Lietman PS. Risk factors for nephrotoxicity in patients treated with aminoglycosides. *Ann Intern Med.* 1984;100(3):352-357.

14. Schentag JJ, Plaut ME, Cerra FB, Wels PB, Walczak P, Buckley RJ. Aminoglycoside nephrotoxicity in critically ill surgical patients. *J Surg Research.* 1979;26:270-279.

15. Rybak MJ, Albrecht LM, Boike SC, Chandrasekar PH. Nephrotoxicity of vancomycin, alone and with an aminoglycoside. *J Antimicrob Chemother.* 1990;25(4):679-687.

16. Lane AZ, Wright GE, Blair DC. Ototoxicity and nephrotoxicity of amikacin: an overview of phase II and phase III experience in the United States. *Am J Med.* 1977;62(6):911-918.

17. Schentag JJ, Cerra FB, Plaut ME. Clinical and pharmacokinetic characteristics of aminoglycoside nephrotoxicity in 201 critically ill patients. *Antimicrob Agents Chemother.* 1982;21(5):721-726.

18. Bertino JS Jr, Booker LA, Franck PA, Jenkins PL, Franck KR, Nafziger AN. Incidence of and significant risk factors for aminoglycoside-associated nephrotoxicity in patients dosed by using individualized pharmacokinetic monitoring [see comments]. *J Infect Dis.* 1993;167(1):173-179.

19. Drusano GL. Antimicrobial pharmacodynamics: critical interactions of "bug and drug." *Nat Rev Microbiol.* Apr 2004;2(4):289-300.

20. Craig WA. Basic pharmacodynamics of antibacterials with clinical applications to the use of beta-lactams, glycopeptides, and linezolid. *Infect Dis Clin North Am.* Sep 2003;17(3):479-501.

21. Craig WA. Pharmacokinetic/pharmacodynamic parameters: rationale for antibacterial dosing of mice and men. *Clin Infect Dis.* Jan 1998;26(1):1-10; quiz 11-12.

22. Hyatt JM, McKinnon PS, Zimmer GS, Schentag JJ. The importance of pharmacokinetic/pharmacodynamic surrogate markers to outcome. Focus on antibacterial agents. *Clin Pharmacokinet.* Feb 1995;28(2):143-160.

23. Prins JM, Buller HR, Kuijper EJ, Tange RA, Speelman P. Once versus thrice daily gentamicin in patients with serious infections [see comments]. *Lancet.* 1993;341(8841):335-339.

24. Maller R, Ahrne H, Holmen C, Lausen I, Nilsson LE, Smedjegard J. Once- versus twice-daily amikacin regimen: efficacy and safety in systemic gram-negative infections. Scandinavian Amikacin Once Daily Study Group. *J Antimicrob Chemother.* 1993;31(6):939-948.

25. Mohamed AF, Nielsen EI, Cars O, Friberg LE. Pharmacokinetic-pharmacodynamic model for gentamicin and its adaptive resistance with predictions of dosing schedules in newborn infants. *Antimicrob Agents Chemother.* Jan 2012;56(1):179-188.

26. Moore RD, Lietman PS, Smith CR. Clinical response to aminoglycoside therapy: importance of the ratio of peak concentration to minimal inhibitory concentration. *J Infect Dis.* Jan 1987;155(1):93-99.

27. Kashuba AD, Nafziger AN, Drusano GL, Bertino JS Jr. Optimizing aminoglycoside therapy for nosocomial pneumonia caused by gram-negative bacteria. *Antimicrob Agents Chemother.* Mar 1999;43(3):623-629.

28. Kashuba AD, Bertino JS Jr, Nafziger AN. Dosing of aminoglycosides to rapidly attain pharmacodynamic goals and hasten therapeutic response by using individualized pharmacokinetic monitoring of patients with pneumonia caused by gram-negative organisms. *Antimicrob Agents Chemother.* Jul 1998;42(7):1842-1844.

29. Barclay ML, Begg EJ, Hickling KG. What is the evidence for once-daily aminoglycoside therapy? *Clin Pharmacokinet.* 1994;27(1):32-48.

30. Barclay ML, Duffull SB, Begg EJ, Buttimore RC. Experience of once-daily aminoglycoside dosing using a target area under the concentration-time curve. *Aust N Z J Med.* 1995;25(3):230-235.

31. Barclay ML, Kirkpatrick CM, Begg EJ. Once daily aminoglycoside therapy. Is it less toxic than multiple daily doses and how should it be monitored? *Clin Pharmacokinet.* 1999;36(2):89-98.

32. Begg EJ, Barclay ML, Duffull SB. A suggested approach to once-daily aminoglycoside dosing. *Br J Clin Pharmacol.* 1995;39(6):605-609.

33. Blaser J, Konig C, Simmen HP, Thurnheer U. Monitoring serum concentrations for once-daily netilmicin dosing regimens. *J Antimicrob Chemother.* 1994;33(2):341-348.

34. Janknegt R. Aminoglycoside monitoring in the once- or twice-daily era. The Dutch situation considered. *Pharm World Sci.* 1993;15(4):151-155.

35. Prins JM, Koopmans RP, Buller HR, Kuijper EJ, Speelman P. Easier monitoring of aminoglycoside therapy with once-daily dosing schedules. *Eur J Clin Microbiol Infect Dis.* 1995;14(6):531-535.

36. Bauer LA. Comparison of four methods to adjust extended-interval aminoglycoside doses. *Clin Pharmacol Ther.* 2007;81(suppl 1):S53.

37. Dang L, Duffull S. Development of a semimechanistic model to describe the pharmacokinetics of gentamicin in patients receiving hemodialysis. *J Clin Pharmacol.* Jun 2006;46(6):662-673.

38. Teigen MM, Duffull S, Dang L, Johnson DW. Dosing of gentamicin in patients with end-stage renal disease receiving hemodialysis. *J Clin Pharmacol.* Nov 2006;46(11):1259-1267.

39. Stickland MD, Kirkpatrick CM, Begg EJ, Duffull SB, Oddie SJ, Darlow BA. An extended interval dosing method for gentamicin in neonates. *J Antimicrob Chemother.* Dec 2001;48(6):887-893.

40. Zelenitsky SA, Rubinstein E, Ariano RE, Zhanel GG. Integrating pharmacokinetics, pharmacodynamics and MIC distributions to assess changing antimicrobial activity against clinical isolates of *Pseudomonas aeruginosa* causing infections in Canadian hospitals (CANWARD). *J Antimicrob Chemother.* May 2013;68 (suppl 1):i67-72.

41. Zelenitsky SA, Harding GK, Sun S, Ubhi K, Ariano RE. Treatment and outcome of *Pseudomonas aeruginosa* bacteraemia: an antibiotic pharmacodynamic analysis. *J Antimicrob Chemother.* Oct 2003;52(4):668-674.

42. Anon. Endotoxin-like reactions associated with intravenous gentamicin—California, 1998. *MMWR Morb Mortal Wkly Rep.* 1998;47(41):877-880.

43. Krieger JA, Duncan L. Gentamicin contaminated with endotoxin [letter]. *N Engl J Med.* 1999;340(14):1122.

44. Smith CR, Lipsky JJ, Laskin OL, et al. Double-blind comparison of the nephrotoxicity and auditory toxicity of gentamicin and tobramycin. *N Engl J Med.* 1980;302(20):1106-1109.

45. Feig PU, Mitchell PP, Abrutyn E, et al. Aminoglycoside nephrotoxicity: a double blind prospective randomized study of gentamicin and tobramycin. *J Antimicrob Chemother.* 1982;10(3):217-226.

46. Kahlmeter G, Hallberg T, Kamme C. Gentamicin and tobramycin in patients with various infections—nephrotoxicity. *J Antimicrob Chemother.* 1978;4 (suppl A):47-52.

47. Vic P, Ategbo S, Turck D, et al. Efficacy, tolerance, and pharmacokinetics of once daily tobramycin for pseudomonas exacerbations in cystic fibrosis. *Arch Dis Child.* 1998;78(6):536-539.

48. Bragonier R, Brown NM. The pharmacokinetics and toxicity of once-daily tobramycin therapy in children with cystic fibrosis. *J Antimicrob Chemother.* 1998;42(1):103-106.

49. Bates RD, Nahata MC, Jones JW, et al. Pharmacokinetics and safety of tobramycin after once-daily administration in patients with cystic fibrosis. *Chest.* 1997;112(5):1208-1213.

50. Bass KD, Larkin SE, Paap C, Haase GM. Pharmacokinetics of once-daily gentamicin dosing in pediatric patients. *J Pediatr Surg.* 1998;33(7):1104-1107.

51. Weber W, Kewitz G, Rost KL, Looby M, Nitz M, Harnisch L. Population kinetics of gentamicin in neonates. *Eur J Clin Pharmacol.* 1993;44(suppl 1):S23-S25.

52. Demczar DJ, Nafziger AN, Bertino JS Jr. Pharmacokinetics of gentamicin at traditional versus high doses: implications for once-daily aminoglycoside dosing. *Antimicrob Agents Chemother.* 1997;41(5):1115-1119.

53. Gilbert DN, Chambers HF, Eliopoulos GM, Saag MS, Black D, Freedman DO, Pavia AT, Schwartz BS. *The Sanford Guide to Antimicrobial Therapy.* 44th ed. Sperryville, VA: Antimicrobial Therapy, Inc.; 2014.

54. Bauer LA, Blouin RA. Amikacin pharmacokinetics in young men with pneumonia. *Clin Pharm.* 1982;1(4):353-355.

55. Bauer LA, Blouin RA. Influence of age on tobramycin pharmacokinetics in patients with normal renal function. *Antimicrob Agents Chemother.* 1981;20(5):587-589.

56. Bauer LA, Blouin RA. Gentamicin pharmacokinetics: effect of aging in patients with normal renal function. *J Am Geriatr Soc.* 1982;30(5):309-311.

57. Bauer LA, Blouin RA. Influence of age on amikacin pharmacokinetics in patients without renal disease. Comparison with gentamicin and tobramycin. *Eur J Clin Pharmacol.* 1983;24(5):639-642.

58. Barza M, Brown RB, Shen D, Gibaldi M, Weinstein L. Predictability of blood levels of gentamicin in man. *J Infect Dis.* 1975;132(2):165-174.

59. Kaye D, Levison ME, Labovitz ED. The unpredictability of serum concentrations of gentamicin: pharmacokinetics of gentamicin in patients with normal and abnormal renal function. *J Infect Dis.* 1974;130(2):150-154.

60. Sarubbi FA Jr, Hull JH. Amikacin serum concentrations: prediction of levels and dosage guidelines. *Ann Intern Med.* 1978;89(5 Pt 1): 612-618.

61. Hull JH, Sarubbi FA Jr. Gentamicin serum concentrations: pharmacokinetic predictions. *Ann Intern Med.* 1976;85(2):183-189.

62. Bootman JL, Wertheimer AI, Zaske D, Rowland C. Individualizing gentamicin dosage regimens in burn patients with gram-negative septicemia: a cost-benefit analysis. *J Pharm Sci.* 1979;68(3):267-272.

63. Zaske DE, Sawchuk RJ, Gerding DN, Strate RG. Increased dosage requirements of gentamicin in burn patients. *J Trauma.* 1976;16(10):824-828.

64. Zaske DE, Sawchuk RJ, Strate RG. The necessity of increased doses of amikacin in burn patients. *Surgery.* 1978;84(5): 603-608.

65. Bracco D, Landry C, Dubois MJ, Eggimann P. Pharmacokinetic variability of extended interval tobramycin in burn patients. *Burns.* Sep 2008;34(6):791-796.

66. Mann HJ, Fuhs DW, Awang R, Ndemo FA, Cerra FB. Altered aminoglycoside pharmacokinetics in critically ill patients with sepsis. *Clin Pharm.* Feb 1987;6(2):148-153.

67. Tang GJ, Tang JJ, Lin BS, Kong CW, Lee TY. Factors affecting gentamicin pharmacokinetics in septic patients. *Acta Anaesthesiol Scand.* Aug 1999;43(7):726-730.

68. Delattre IK, Musuamba FT, Jacqmin P, et al. Population pharmacokinetics of four beta-lactams in critically ill septic patients come-dicated with amikacin. *Clin Biochem.* Jul 2010;45(10-11):780-786.

69. Tindula RJ, Ambrose PJ, Harralson AF. Aminoglycoside inactivation by penicillins and cephalosporins and its impact on drug-level monitoring. *Drug Intell Clin Pharm.* 1983;17(12):906-908.

70. Wallace SM, Chan LY. In vitro interaction of aminoglycosides with beta-lactam penicillins. *Antimicrob Agents Chemother.* 1985; 28(2):274-281.

71. Henderson JL, Polk RE, Kline BJ. In vitro inactivation of gentamicin, tobramycin, and netilmicin by carbenicillin, azlocillin, or mezlocillin. *Am J Hosp Pharm.* 1981;38(8):1167-1170.

72. Pickering LK, Rutherford I. Effect of concentration and time upon inactivation of tobramycin, gentamicin, netilmicin and amikacin by azlocillin, carbenicillin, mecillinam, mezlocillin and piperacillin. *J Pharmacol Exp Ther.* 1981;217(2):345-349.

73. Hale DC, Jenkins R, Matsen JM. In-vitro inactivation of aminoglycoside antibiotics by piperacillin and carbenicillin. *Am J Clin Pathol.* 1980;74(3):316-319.

74. Bauer LA, Blouin RA, Griffen WO Jr, Record KE, Bell RM. Amikacin pharmacokinetics in morbidly obese patients. *Am J Hosp Pharm.* 1980;37(4):519-522.

75. Bauer LA, Edwards WA, Dellinger EP, Simonowitz DA. Influence of weight on aminoglycoside pharmacokinetics in normal weight and morbidly obese patients. *Eur J Clin Pharmacol.* 1983;24(5):643-647.

76. Blouin RA, Mann HJ, Griffen WO Jr, Bauer LA, Record KE. Tobramycin pharmacokinetics in morbidly obese patients. *Clin Pharmacol Ther.* 1979;26(4):508-512.

77. Bauer LA, Piecoro JJ Jr, Wilson HD, Blouin RA. Gentamicin and tobramycin pharmacokinetics in patients with cystic fibrosis. *Clin Pharm.* 1983;2(3):262-264.

78. Bosso JA, Townsend PL, Herbst JJ, Matsen JM. Pharmacokinetics and dosage requirements of netilmicin in cystic fibrosis patients. *Antimicrob Agents Chemother.* 1985;28(6):829-831.

79. Kearns GL, Hilman BC, Wilson JT. Dosing implications of altered gentamicin disposition in patients with cystic fibrosis. *J Pediatr.* 1982;100(2):312-318.

80. Kelly HB, Menendez R, Fan L, Murphy S. Pharmacokinetics of tobramycin in cystic fibrosis. *J Pediatr.* 1982;100(2):318-321.

81. Hennig S, Standing JF, Staatz CE, Thomson AH. Population pharmacokinetics of tobramycin in patients with and without cystic fibrosis. *Clin Pharmacokinet.* Apr 2013;52(4):289-301.

82. Hennig S, Norris R, Kirkpatrick CM. Target concentration intervention is needed for tobramycin dosing in paediatric patients with cystic fibrosis—a population pharmacokinetic study. *Br J Clin Pharmacol.* Apr 2008;65(4):502-510.

83. Smyth A, Tan KH, Hyman-Taylor P, et al. Once versus three-times daily regimens of tobramycin treatment for pulmonary exacerba-tions of cystic fibrosis—the TOPIC study: a randomised controlled trial. *Lancet.* Feb 12-18, 2005;365(9459):573-578.

84. Master V, Roberts GW, Coulthard KP, et al. Efficacy of once-daily tobramycin monotherapy for acute pulmonary exacerbations of cystic fibrosis: a preliminary study. *Pediatr Pulmonol.* May 2001;31(5):367-376.

85. Ramsey BW, Pepe MS, Quan JM, et al. Intermittent administration of inhaled tobramycin in patients with cystic fibrosis. Cystic Fibrosis Inhaled Tobramycin Study Group. *N Engl J Med.* 1999;340(1):23-30.

86. Walsh KA, Davis GA, Hayes D Jr, Kuhn RJ, Weant KA, Flynn JD. Tobramycin pharmacokinetics in patients with cystic fibrosis before and after bilateral lung transplantation. *Transpl Infect Dis.* Dec 2011;13(6):616-621.

87. Dupuis RE, Sredzienski ES. Tobramycin pharmacokinetics in patients with cystic fibrosis preceding and following lung transplanta-tion. *Ther Drug Monit.* Apr 1999;21(2):161-165.

88. Lanao JM, Dominguez-Gil A, Macias JG, Diez JL, Nieto MJ. The influence of ascites on the pharmacokinetics of amikacin. *Int J Clin Pharmacol Ther Toxicol.* 1980;18(2):57-61.

89. Gill MA, Kern JW. Altered gentamicin distribution in ascitic patients. *Am J Hosp Pharm.* 1979;36(12):1704-1706.

90. Sampliner R, Perrier D, Powell R, Finley P. Influence of ascites on tobramycin pharmacokinetics. *J Clin Pharmacol.* 1984;24(1): 43-46.

91. Izquierdo M, Lanao JM, Cervero L, Jimenez NV, Dominguez-Gil A. Population pharmacokinetics of gentamicin in premature infants. *Ther Drug Monit.* 1992;14(3):177-183.

92. Hindmarsh KW, Nation RL, Williams GL, John E, French JN. Pharmacokinetics of gentamicin in very low birth weight preterm infants. *Eur J Clin Pharmacol.* 1983;24(5):649-653.

93. Rameis H, Popow C, Graninger W. Gentamicin monitoring in low-birth-weight newborns. *Biol Res Pregnancy Perinatol.* 1983;4(3):123-126.

94. Lingvall M, Reith D, Broadbent R. The effect of sepsis upon gentamicin pharmacokinetics in neonates. *Br J Clin Pharmacol.* Jan 2005;59(1):54-61.

95. Pickering LK, Baker CJ, Kimberlin DW, Long SS. *Red Book: 2012 Report of the Committee on Infectious Diseases.* 29th ed. Elk Grove Village, IL: American Academy of Pediatrics; 2012.

96. Contopoulos-Ioannidis DG, Giotis ND, Baliatsa DV, Ioannidis JP. Extended-interval aminoglycoside administration for children: a meta-analysis. *Pediatrics.* Jul 2004;114(1): e111-e118.

97. Dupuis LL, Sung L, Taylor T, et al. Tobramycin pharmacokinetics in children with febrile neutropenia undergoing stem cell transplantation: once-daily versus thrice-daily administration. *Pharmacotherapy.* May 2004;24(5):564-573.

98. Frymoyer A, Meng L, Bonifacio SL, Verotta D, Guglielmo BJ. Gentamicin Pharmacokinetics and dosing in neonates with hypoxic ischemic encephalopathy receiving hypothermia. *Pharmacotherapy.* Apr 1, 2013;33(7):718-726.

99. Mark LF, Solomon A, Northington FJ, Lee CK. Gentamicin pharmacokinetics in neonates undergoing therapeutic hypothermia. *Ther Drug Monit.* Apr 2013;35(2):217-222.

100. Mercer JM, Neyens RR. Aminoglycoside pharmacokinetic parameters in neurocritical care patients undergoing induced hypothermia. *Pharmacotherapy.* Jul 2010;30(7):654-660.

101. Madhavan T, Yaremchuk K, Levin N, et al. Effect of renal failure and dialysis on the serum concentration of the aminoglycoside amikacin. *Antimicrob Agents Chemother.* 1976;10(3):464-466.

102. Armstrong DK, Hodgman T, Visconti JA, Reilley TE, Garner WL, Dasta JF. Hemodialysis of amikacin in critically ill patients. *Crit Care Med.* 1988;16(5):517-520.

103. Herrero A, Rius Alarco F, Garcia Diez JM, Mahiques E, Domingo JV. Pharmacokinetics of netilmicin in renal insufficiency and hemodialysis. *Int J Clin Pharmacol Ther Toxicol.* 1988;26(2):84-87.

104. Halstenson CE, Berkseth RO, Mann HJ, Matzke GR. Aminoglycoside redistribution phenomenon after hemodialysis: netilmicin and tobramycin. *Int J Clin Pharmacol Ther Toxicol.* 1987;25(1):50-55.

105. Matzke GR, Halstenson CE, Keane WF. Hemodialysis elimination rates and clearance of gentamicin and tobramycin. *Antimicrob Agents Chemother.* 1984;25(1):128-130.

106. Dager WE, King JH. Aminoglycosides in intermittent hemodialysis: pharmacokinetics with individual dosing. *Ann Pharmacother.* Jan 2006;40(1):9-14.

107. Sowinski KM, Magner SJ, Lucksiri A, Scott MK, Hamburger RJ, Mueller BA. Influence of hemodialysis on gentamicin pharmacokinetics, removal during hemodialysis, and recommended dosing. *Clin J Am Soc Nephrol.* Mar 2008;3(2):355-361.

108. Basile C, Di Maggio A, Curino E, Scatizzi A. Pharmacokinetics of netilmicin in hypertonic hemodiafiltration and standard hemodialysis. *Clin Nephrol.* 1985;24(6):305-309.

109. Decker BS, Mohamed AN, Chambers M, Kraus MA, Moe SM, Sowinski KM. Gentamicin pharmacokinetics and pharmacodynamics during short-daily hemodialysis. *Am J Nephrol.* 2012;36(2):144-150.

110. Smeltzer BD, Schwartzman MS, Bertino JS Jr. Amikacin pharmacokinetics during continuous ambulatory peritoneal dialysis. *Antimicrob Agents Chemother.* 1988;32(2):236-240.

111. Pancorbo S, Comty C. Pharmacokinetics of gentamicin in patients undergoing continuous ambulatory peritoneal dialysis. *Antimicrob Agents Chemother.* 1981;19(4):605-607.

112. Bunke CM, Aronoff GR, Brier ME, Sloan RS, Luft FC. Tobramycin kinetics during continuous ambulatory peritoneal dialysis. *Clin Pharmacol Ther.* 1983;34(1):110-116.

113. Forni LG, Hilton PJ. Continuous hemofiltration in the treatment of acute renal failure. *N Engl J Med.* May 1, 1997;336(18):1303-1309.

114. Tolwani A. Continuous renal-replacement therapy for acute kidney injury. *N Engl J Med.* Dec 27, 2012;367(26):2505-2514.

115. Schneider AG, Bellomo R, Bagshaw SM, et al. Choice of renal replacement therapy modality and dialysis dependence after acute kidney injury: a systematic review and meta-analysis. *Intensive Care Med.* Jun 2013;39(6):987-997.

116. Golper TA, Marx MA. Drug dosing adjustments during continuous renal replacement therapies. *Kidney Int Suppl.* May 1998;66:S165-S168.

117. Golper TA. Update on drug sieving coefficients and dosing adjustments during continuous renal replacement therapies. *Contrib Nephrol.* 2001;(132):349-353.

118. Petejova N, Zahalkova J, Duricova J, et al. Gentamicin pharmacokinetics during continuous venovenous hemofiltration in critically ill septic patients. *J Chemother.* Apr 2012;24(2):107-112.

119. Taccone FS, de Backer D, Laterre PF, et al. Pharmacokinetics of a loading dose of amikacin in septic patients undergoing continuous renal replacement therapy. *Int J Antimicrob Agents.* Jun 2011;37(6):531-535.

120. D'Arcy DM, Casey E, Gowing CM, Donnelly MB, Corrigan OI. An open prospective study of amikacin pharmacokinetics in critically ill patients during treatment with continuous venovenous haemodiafiltration. *BMC Pharmacol Toxicol.* 2012;13(1):14.

121. Goetz MB, Sayers J. Nephrotoxicity of vancomycin and aminoglycoside therapy separately and in combination. *J Antimicrob Chemother.* Aug 1993;32(2):325-334.

122. Chandrasekar PH, Cronin SM. Nephrotoxicity in bone marrow transplant recipients receiving aminoglycoside plus cyclosporine or aminoglycoside alone. *J Antimicrob Chemother.* 1991;27(6):845-849.

123. Harpur ES. The pharmacology of ototoxic drugs. *Br J Audiol.* 1982;16(2):81-93.

124. Mathog RH, Klein WJ Jr. Ototoxicity of ethacrynic acid and aminoglycoside antibiotics in uremia. *N Engl J Med.* 1969;280(22):1223-1224.

125. Paradelis AG, Triantaphyllidis C, Giala MM. Neuromuscular blocking activity of aminoglycoside antibiotics. *Methods Find Exp Clin Pharmacol.* 1980;2(1):45-51.

126. Charhon N, Neely MN, Bourguignon L, Maire P, Jelliffe RW, Goutelle S. Comparison of four renal function estimation equations for pharmacokinetic modeling of gentamicin in geriatric patients. *Antimicrob Agents Chemother.* Apr 2012;56(4):1862-1869.

127. Sawchuk RJ, Zaske DE, Cipolle RJ, Wargin WA, Strate RG. Kinetic model for gentamicin dosing with the use of individual patient parameters. *Clin Pharmacol Ther.* 1977;21(3):362-369.

128. Murphy JE, Winter ME. Clinical pharmacokinetic pearls: bolus versus infusion equations. *Pharmacotherapy.* 1996;16(4):698-700.

129. Dionne RE, Bauer LA, Gibson GA, Griffen WO, Blouin RA. Estimating creatinine clearance in morbidly obese patients. *Am J Hosp Pharm.* 1981;38:841-844.

130. Verhave JC, Fesler P, Ribstein J, du Cailar G, Mimran A. Estimation of renal function in subjects with normal serum creatinine levels: influence of age and body mass index. *Am J Kidney Dis.* Aug 2005;46(2):233-241.

131. Spinler SA, Nawarskas JJ, Boyce EG, Connors JE, Charland SL, Goldfarb S. Predictive performance of ten equations for estimating creatinine clearance in cardiac patients. Iohexol Cooperative Study Group. *Ann Pharmacother.* 1998;32(12):1275-1283.

132. Salazar DE, Corcoran GB. Predicting creatinine clearance and renal drug clearance in obese patients from estimated fat-free body mass. *Am J Med.* 1988;84(6):1053-1060.

133. Wallace AW, Jones M, Bertino JS Jr. Evaluation of four once-daily aminoglycoside dosing nomograms. *Pharmacotherapy.* Sep 2002;22(9):1077-1083.

134. Anaizi N. Once-daily dosing of aminoglycosides. A consensus document. *Int J Clin Pharmacol Ther.* Jun 1997;35(6):223-226.

135. Traub SL, Johnson CE. Comparison of methods of estimating creatinine clearance in children. *Am J Hosp Pharm.* 1980;37:195-201.

136. McCormack JP, Carleton B. A simpler approach to pharmacokinetic dosage adjustments. *Pharmacotherapy.* 1997;17(6):1349-1351.

137. Burton ME, Brater DC, Chen PS, Day RB, Huber PJ, Vasko MR. A Bayesian feedback method of aminoglycoside dosing. *Clin Pharmacol Ther.* 1985;37(3):349-357.

138. Burton ME, Chow MS, Platt DR, Day RB, Brater DC, Vasko MR. Accuracy of Bayesian and Sawchuk-Zaske dosing methods for gentamicin. *Clin Pharm.* 1986;5(2):143-149.

139. Rodvold KA, Blum RA. Predictive performance of Sawchuk-Zaske and Bayesian dosing methods for tobramycin. *J Clin Pharmacol.* 1987;27(5):419-424.

140. Murray KM, Bauer LA, Koup JR. Predictive performance of computer dosing methods for tobramycin using two pharmacokinetic models and two weighting algorithms. *Clin Pharm.* 1986;5(5):411-414.

141. Koup JR, Killen T, Bauer LA. Multiple-dose non-linear regression analysis program. Aminoglycoside dose prediction. *Clin Pharmacokinet.* 1983;8(5):456-462.

142. Wandell M, Mungall D. Computer assisted drug interpretation and drug regimen optimization. *Am Assoc Clin Chem.* 1984;6:1-11.

5 Vancomycin

INTRODUCTION

Vancomycin is a glycopeptide antibiotic used to treat severe gram-positive infections due to organisms that are resistant to other antibiotics such as methicillin-resistant staphylococci and ampicillin-resistant enterococci. It is also used to treat infections caused by other sensitive gram-positive organisms in patients who are allergic to penicillins.

Vancomycin is bactericidal and exhibits time-dependent or concentration-independent bacterial killing.[1] Antibiotics with time-dependent killing characteristically kill bacteria most effectively when drug concentrations are a multiple (usually three to five times) of the minimum inhibitory concentration (MIC) for the bacteria.[1,2] The mechanism of action for vancomycin is inhibition of cell wall synthesis in susceptible bacteria by binding to the D-alanyl-D-alanine terminal end of cell wall precursor units.[3] Many strains of *Enterococcus* have high MIC values for vancomycin, and for these bacteria vancomycin may only demonstrate bacteriostatic properties.

THERAPEUTIC AND TOXIC CONCENTRATIONS

Vancomycin is administered as a short-term (1 hour) intermittent intravenous infusion for doses up to 1500 mg or as a 1.5- to 2-hour intermittent intravenous infusion for larger doses (>1500 mg). Infusion rate–related side effects have been noted when shorter infusion times (~30 minutes or less) have been used. Urticarial or erythematous reactions, intense flushing (known as the "red-man" or "red-neck" syndrome), tachycardia, and hypotension have all been reported and can be largely avoided with the longer infusion time. Even with a 1- to 2-hour infusion time, vancomycin serum concentrations exhibit a distribution phase so that drug in the blood and in the tissues are not yet in equilibrium (Figure 5-1). Because of this, a ½- to 1-hour waiting period is allowed for distribution to finish before maximum or "peak" concentrations are measured. Because vancomycin exhibits time-dependent killing, microbiologic or clinical cure rates are not closely associated with peak serum concentrations. However, ototoxicity has been reported when vancomycin serum concentrations exceed 80 μg/mL.[4,5] Because vancomycin does not enter the central nervous system in appreciable amounts when given intravenously,[3] steady-state peak concentrations of 50-60 μg/mL, steady-state trough concentrations of 15-20 μg/mL, or direct administration into the cerebral spinal fluid may be necessary.[6-8]

Trough concentrations (predose or minimum concentrations usually obtained within 30 minutes of the next dose) are usually related to therapeutic outcome for vancomycin because the antibiotic follows time-dependent bacterial killing.[1] Optimal bactericidal effects are found at concentrations three to five times the organism's MIC.[1,2] Because the average vancomycin MICs for *Staphylococcus aureus* and *Staphylococcus epidermidis* are 1-2 μg/mL, from a historic perspective minimum predose or trough steady-state concentrations equal to 5-10 μg/mL were usually adequate to resolve infections with susceptible organisms through the year 2000. Development of methicillin-resistant *Staphylococcus aureus* (MRSA) during the early 2000s with MICs of 1.5-2 μg/mL required higher steady-state trough concentrations to achieve a clinical cure.[9-12]

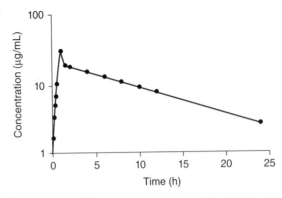

FIGURE 5-1   Concentration/time plot for vancomycin 1000 mg given as a 1-hour infusion (*circles* with *dashed line*). When given as a 1-hour infusion, end-of-infusion concentrations are higher because the serum and tissues are not in equilibrium. A ½- to 1-hour waiting time for vancomycin distribution to tissues is allowed before peak concentrations are measured.

The need for higher trough concentrations in institutions with antibiograms that included MRSA with higher MIC values lead to the expansion of the therapeutic trough concentration range to 5-15 µg/mL.

Vancomycin penetrates into lung tissue poorly (average serum:tissue ratio of 6:1, average epithelial lining fluid:plasma concentrations ratio of 0.68) and pulmonary concentrations are highly variable among patients.[13-15] Based on these findings and reports of therapeutic failures, current treatment guidelines recommend vancomycin steady-state trough concentrations equal to 10-15 µg/mL for lower-intensity dosing and 15-20 µg/mL for complicated infections due to MRSA, such as bacteremia, endocarditis, meningitis, osteomyelitis, severe skin infections, and hospital-acquired pneumonia.[16-18] Steady-state vancomycin trough levels less than 10 µg/mL are discouraged due to the possibility of lower levels contributing to treatment failure or to the development of resistance. The development of vancomycin intermediate-level–resistant *S. aureus* (VISA) and heterogeneously resistant isolates of MRSA (heterogeneous vancomycin-intermediate *S. aureus* [hVISA]), a mixed colony of sensitive and resistant MRSA subpopulations] during therapy with vancomycin appears to be an important factor in treatment failures.[9,19-21]

Beginning in the mid-1990s, infectious disease specialists began to recognize the importance of pharmacodynamic principles when treating infections.[22-25] Measures such as C_{max}/MIC for concentration-dependent antibiotics (where C_{max} is the maximum antibiotic concentration), t > MIC for time-dependent antibiotics (time when antibiotic concentrations are above MIC), and AUC/MIC (where AUC is the area under the concentration-time curve for the antibiotic) were recognized as parameters that could be used to help define the response to antibiotic treatment as a combination of exposure to the antibiotic (AUC) and bacterial sensitivity (MIC).

For the treatment of *S. aureus* pneumonia, this concept was put to the test with vancomycin. In two retrospective studies, it was found that the AUC_{24}/MIC > 400 corresponded to a statistically higher clinical cure rate for patients with MRSA or MSSA (methicillin-sensitive *S. aureus*).[26,27] AUC_{24} is the area under the concentration-time curve for 24 hours of antibiotic treatment. Thus, if the antibiotic is administered every 8 hours, AUC_{24} includes three dosage intervals, but if the antibiotic is administered every 24 hours, AUC_{24} includes only one dosage interval. For these investigations, AUC_{24} was not computed using patient vancomycin serum concentrations. Instead, it was calculated by taking the quotient of the daily vancomycin dose and an approximation of vancomycin clearance determined from an estimation of creatinine clearance ($CrCl_{est}$) using the Cockcroft-Gault equation ($AUC_{24} = D/\{[(CrCl_{est} \bullet 0.79) + 15.4] \bullet 0.06\}$, where D is the daily vancomycin dose).[28,29] However, computed AUC_{24} was validated in one of the later investigations by determining AUC_{24} using a Bayesian pharmacokinetic computer program in 30 patients and comparing the measured and estimated values. MIC was measured using a broth microdilution method. In the earlier trial, 70 pneumonia patients were studied (50% MSSA isolates, 50% MRSA isolates) with clinical success in 78% for AUC_{24}/MIC >345). In the later trial, 90 pneumonia patients were studied (57 MSSA infections, 33 MRSA infections) with clinical success in 78% for AUC_{24}/MIC >400). Among the patient risk factors for treatment failure were intensive care patients, ventilator support, low serum albumin, MRSA isolate as infecting organism, multilobe lung involvement, high baseline APACHE II (Acute Physiology and Chronic Health Evaluation, second edition) score.

Since the advent of these investigations, AUC_{24}/MIC > 400 has become an accepted standard for the treatment of all *S. aureus* infections.[16,17] Some studies have assessed this threshold for MRSA bacteremia and MRSA endocarditis, while others have derived their own AUC_{24}/MIC ratios using a variety of techniques to estimate or measure AUC_{24}. Either broth microdilution or Etest® has been used to determine MIC.[30-36] Obviously, different methodologies to determine AUC_{24} or MIC can influence the AUC_{24}/MIC value. Other studies are available that use simulations to study the impact of AUC_{24}/MIC > 400 for vancomycin on the treatment of staphylococcal infections.[37-44] Also obvious is the fact that the results of studies involving only simulations must be judged differently than retrospective or prospective clinical trials.

Of course, there are other important patient and bacterial factors (such as site of infection, intact host immunologic response, other concurrent patient disease states, bacteria-specific genetic and virulence differences, magnitude of bacterial load invoking an inoculum effect, etc) that need to be considered when assessing antibiotic response. Hopefully, future pharmacokinetic/pharmacodynamic (PK/PD) investigations with vancomycin will include prospective clinical trials for individual infection sites and specific pathogens where AUC_{24} is measured using drug serum concentrations and MIC values are measured using uniform laboratory methods. This critical information is needed in order to seriously contemplate using this approach in the clinical setting. In lieu of this data, there is some information that indicates achieving steady-state vancomycin trough concentrations of 15-20 µg/mL for serious invasive MRSA infections is effective for bacteria with a MIC 2 µg/mL or less.[11,12,45]

Vancomycin-associated ototoxicity is usually first noted by the appearance of tinnitus, dizziness, or high-frequency hearing loss (>4000 Hz).[4,7,46] Because the hearing loss is initially at high frequencies, the auditory deficit can be challenging to detect unless audiometry is conducted at baseline before drug is administered and during vancomycin treatment. Because audiometry is difficult to conduct in seriously ill patients, it is rarely done in patients receiving ototoxic drugs so clinicians should monitor for signs and symptoms that may indicate that ototoxicity is occurring in a patient (auditory: tinnitus, feeling of fullness or pressure in the ears, loss of hearing acuity in the conversational range; vestibular: loss of equilibrium, headache, nausea, vomiting, vertigo, dizziness, nystagmus, ataxia). Ototoxicity can be permanent if appropriate changes in vancomycin dosing are not made.[4,7,46,47] Steady-state trough vancomycin concentrations in excess of 20 µg/mL are associated with ototoxicity, and other patient risk factors include age more than 53 years and preexisting hearing loss. For this patient subgroup, the ototoxicity rate is 19%. While vancomycin ototoxicity usually occurs bilaterally, unilateral changes have been noted.[48] In some reports of vancomycin-induced ototoxicity, it is unclear when vancomycin serum concentrations were obtained during the dosage interval so the exact association between concentrations and ototoxicity is uncertain.

Trough vancomycin steady-state concentrations of more than 15 µg/mL are related to an increased incidence of nephrotoxicity, with reported rates as high as 30%-35%.[12,49-55] Coadministration of an aminoglycoside with vancomycin may double the risk of developing renal toxicity. Many patients receiving vancomycin are critically ill, so other sources of renal dysfunction, such as dehydration, hypotension, or other nephrotoxic drug therapy (such as aminoglycosides, amphotericin B, loop diuretics, or immunosuppressants) should be ruled out before the diagnosis of vancomycin-induced renal damage is made in a patient. Compared to aminoglycoside antibiotics, vancomycin is usually considered to have less nephrotoxicity potential, but this impression was formed when target steady-state trough levels for vancomycin were in the 5 to 10 μg/mL range.[56] In contrast to ototoxicity, vancomycin-related nephrotoxicity is usually reversible with a low incidence of residual damage if the antibiotic is withdrawn or doses appropriately adjusted soon after renal function tests change. With adequate patient monitoring and dosage adjustments, the only result of vancomycin nephrotoxicity may be transient serum creatinine increases of 0.5-2.0 mg/dL.[52,57] However, if kidney damage progresses to renal failure, the cost of maintaining the patient on dialysis until kidney function returns can exceed $50,000-100,000 and, if the patient is critically ill, may contribute to his or her death.

Nephrotoxicity and ototoxicity cannot be completely avoided when using vancomycin by keeping serum concentrations within the suggested ranges. However, by adjusting vancomycin dosage regimens so that potentially toxic serum concentrations are avoided, drug concentration–related adverse effects should be held to the absolute minimum.

CLINICAL MONITORING PARAMETERS

Clinicians should always consult the patient's chart to confirm that antibiotic therapy is appropriate for current microbiologic cultures and sensitivities. Antibiograms should be consulted regularly to note changes in resistance patterns and minimum inhibitory concentrations for pathogens. Also, it should be confirmed that the patient is receiving other appropriate concurrent antibiotic therapy, such as aminoglycosides, when necessary to treat the infection. Patients with severe infections usually have elevated white blood cell counts and body temperatures. Measurement of serial white blood cell counts and body temperatures is useful to determine the efficacy of antibiotic therapy. A white blood cell count with a differential will identify the types of white blood cells that are elevated. A large number of neutrophils and immature neutrophils, clinically known as a "shift to the left," can also be observed in patients with severe bacterial infections. Favorable response to antibiotic treatment is usually indicated by high white blood cell counts decreasing toward the normal range, the trend of body temperatures (plotted as body temperature vs time, also known as the "fever curve") approaching normal, and any specific infection site tests or procedures resolving. For instance, in pneumonia patients the chest x-ray should be resolving, in patients with infective endocarditis the size of the bacterial vegetation on the heart valve should be decreasing, or in patients with a wound infection the wound should be less inflamed with less purulent discharge. Clinicians should also be aware that immunocompromised patients with a bacterial infection may not be able to mount a fever or elevated white blood cell count.

Vancomycin steady-state serum concentrations should be measured in 3-5 estimated half-lives. Methods to estimate this parameter are given in the initial dose calculation portion of this chapter. Because prolongation of the dosage interval is often used in patients with decreased elimination, a useful clinical rule is to measure serum concentrations after the third dose. If this approach is used, the dosage interval is increased in tandem with the increase in half-life so that 3-5 half-lives have elapsed by the time the third dose is administered. Additionally, the third dose typically occurs 1-3 days after dosing has commenced and this is a good time to also assess clinical efficacy of the treatment. Steady-state serum concentrations, in conjunction with clinical response, are used to adjust the antibiotic dose, if necessary. Methods for adjusting vancomycin doses using serum concentrations are discussed later in this chapter. If the dosage is adjusted, vancomycin elimination changes or laboratory and clinical monitoring indicate that the infection is not resolving or worsening, or the patient exhibits a potential adverse drug reaction, clinicians should consider rechecking steady-state drug concentrations.

While some clinicians continue to monitor both steady-state peak and trough vancomycin serum concentrations, most individuals advocate the measurement of just a steady-state trough concentration.[11,12,18,58,59] The reasoning behind this approach is that vancomycin follows time-dependent bacterial killing, and the efficacy of the drug should be most closely related to the minimum serum concentration encountered over the dosage interval. Current treatment guidelines recommend vancomycin steady-state trough concentrations equal to

10-15 µg/mL for lower-intensity dosing and 15-20 µg/mL for complicated infections due to MRSA, such as bacteremia, endocarditis, meningitis, osteomyelitis, severe skin infections, and hospital-acquired pneumonia.[16-18] Steady-state vancomycin trough levels of less than 10 µg/mL are discouraged due to the possibility of lower levels contributing to treatment failure or to the development of resistance. There is some information that indicates achieving steady-state vancomycin trough concentrations of 15-20 µg/mL for serious invasive MRSA infections is effective for bacteria with a MIC of 2 µg/mL or less.[11,12,45] Because nephrotoxicity and ototoxicity are related to high trough concentrations, measurement of this value should ensure therapeutic, nontoxic drug concentrations as much as possible.

Vancomycin has a moderate-sized volume of distribution (~0.7 L/kg) and does not significantly change for most disease states or conditions. Based on this, the argument has been made that if a patient has a therapeutic steady-state trough concentration (15-20 µg/mL) and the dose is in the usual range (1000-2000 mg), it is difficult to produce a steady-state peak concentration that would be above the accepted toxic range (>80 µg/mL).[60] While these arguments are intellectually sound and appealing, one of the reasons to measure drug serum concentrations is pharmacokinetic variability. If a patient developed toxicity while receiving vancomycin, it could be difficult to prove that steady-state peak concentrations were in the acceptable range if no serum concentrations were obtained at that time. Clinicians should consider measuring peak concentrations for vancomycin when large doses are given (>1500 mg/dose), for infections that require high peak concentrations (such as central nervous system infections), or if the determination of a peak concentration could aid in the pharmacokinetic computation of the best dose.

Serial monitoring of serum creatinine concentrations should be used to detect nephrotoxicity. Ideally, a baseline serum creatinine concentration is obtained before vancomycin therapy is initiated and three times weekly during treatment. An increasing serum creatinine test on two or more consecutive measurement occasions indicates that more intensive monitoring of serum creatinine values, such as daily, is needed. If serum creatinine measurements increase more than 0.5 mg/dL over the baseline value (or >25%-30% over baseline for serum creatinine values >2 mg/dL) and other causes of declining renal function have been ruled out (other nephrotoxic drugs or agents, hypotension, etc), alternatives to vancomycin therapy or, if that option is not possible, intensive vancomycin serum concentration monitoring should be initiated to ensure that excessive amounts of vancomycin do not accumulate in the patient.

In the clinical setting, audiometry is rarely used to detect ototoxicity because it is difficult to accomplish in severely ill patients. Instead, clinical signs and symptoms of auditory (decreased hearing acuity in the conversational range, feeling of fullness or pressure in the ears, tinnitus) or vestibular (loss of equilibrium, headache, nausea, vomiting, vertigo, nystagmus, ataxia) ototoxicity are monitored at the same time intervals as serum creatinine determination. When high vancomycin concentrations are needed for therapeutic reasons (trough >20 µg/mL, peak >50-60 µg/mL), assessment of renal function and auditory/vestibular function should be conducted on a daily basis. Vancomycin can also cause allergic symptoms such as chills, fever, skin rashes, and anaphylactoid reactions.

BASIC CLINICAL PHARMACOKINETIC PARAMETERS

Vancomycin is almost completely eliminated unchanged in the urine primarily by glomerular filtration (≥90%; Table 5-1).[61] This antibiotic is given by short-term (1 hour) intermittent intravenous infusion. Intramuscular administration is usually avoided because this route has been reported to cause tissue necrosis at the site of injection. Oral bioavailability is poor (<10%) so systemic infections cannot be treated by this route of administration.[5] However, patients with renal failure who have been given oral vancomycin for the treatment of antibiotic-associated colitis have accumulated therapeutic concentrations because gut wall inflammation increased vancomycin bioavailability and renal dysfunction decreased drug clearance.[62-65] Plasma protein binding is ~55%.[66]

TABLE 5-1   Disease States and Conditions That Alter Vancomycin Pharmacokinetic

Disease State/ Condition	Half-Life	Volume of Distribution	Comment
Adult, normal renal function	8 h (range: 7-9 h)	0.7 L/kg (range: 0.5-1.0 L/kg)	Manufacturer recommended dose: 30 mg/kg/d in two divided doses
Adult, renal failure	130 h (range: 120-140 h)	0.7 L/kg (range: 0.5-1.0 L/kg)	Underhydration or overhydration does not affect the volume of distribution as much as with aminoglycosides
Burns	4 h	0.7 L/kg	Because of shorter half-life, some patients may need every 6 to 8 h dosage interval to maintain therapeutic trough concentrations
Hematological malignancies	variable	1.05 L/kg	Clearance increases to 1.43 mL/min/kg. Because the pharmacokinetic changes increase both physiologic pharmacokinetic parameters, the effect on half-life is variable, depending on whether the increase in volume of distribution or the increase in clearance predominates in an individual patient [$t_{1/2} = (0.693 \cdot V)/Cl$]
Obesity (>30% over IBW) with normal renal function	3-4 h	V = 0.7 IBW	Total daily doses are based on TBW, V estimates based on IBW. Because of shorter half-life, some patients may require every 8 h dosage interval to maintain therapeutic trough concentrations

IBW, ideal body weight; TBW, total body weight.

The manufacturer recommended dose for vancomycin in patients with normal renal function is 30 mg/kg/d given as two or four divided daily doses. In normal-weight adults, the dose is usually 2 g/d given as 1000 mg every 12 hours. However, these doses will not usually achieve recommended trough concentrations to treat serious infections for patients with normal renal function. Current guidelines recommend an initial maintenance dose of 15-20 mg/kg every 8-12 hours for patients with normal renal function, followed by dosage adjustment guided by steady-state vancomycin trough concentrations obtained just before the fourth dose. For seriously ill patients, a loading dose of 25-30 mg/kg can be administered.[17] Loading doses can be particularly useful to rapidly attain effective vancomycin concentrations for patients with poor renal function.

Because vancomycin follows time-dependent pharmacodynamics, some clinicians advocate administering vancomycin as a continuous intravenous infusion, usually preceded by an intravenous loading dose. In these cases, the steady-state vancomycin concentration is titrated by changing the infusion rate of the drug.[67-72]

EFFECTS OF DISEASE STATES AND CONDITIONS ON VANCOMYCIN PHARMACOKINETICS AND DOSING

Nonobese adults with normal renal function (creatinine clearance >80 mL/min, Table 5-1) have an average vancomycin half-life of 8 hours (range = 7-9 hours), and the average volume of distribution for vancomycin is 0.7 L/kg (range = 0.5-1.0 L/kg) in this population.[73,74] Because of the moderate size for volume of distribution, fluid balance (under- or overhydration) is less of an issue with vancomycin compared to the aminoglycoside antibiotics.

Because vancomycin is eliminated principally by glomerular filtration, renal dysfunction is the most important disease state that influences vancomycin pharmacokinetics.[75-77] Vancomycin total clearance decreases

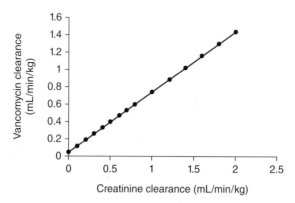

FIGURE 5-2   The clearance rate for vancomycin increases in proportion with creatinine clearance (CrCl). The equation for this relationship is Cl (in mL/min/kg) = 0.695(CrCl in mL/min/kg) + 0.05. This equation is used to estimate vancomycin clearance in patients for initial dosing purposes.

proportionally to decreases in creatinine clearance (Figure 5-2).[75] The relationship between renal function and vancomycin clearance forms the basis for initial dosage computation methods presented later in this chapter.

Major body burns (>30%-40% body surface area) can cause large changes in vancomycin pharmacokinetics.[78,79] Forty-eight to 72 hours after a major burn, the basal metabolic rate of the patient increases to facilitate tissue repair. The increase in basal metabolic rate causes an increase in glomerular filtration rate that increases vancomycin clearance. Because of the increase in drug clearance, the average half-life for vancomycin in burn patients is 4 hours.

Patients with hematological malignancies have higher clearance rates and larger volumes of distribution for vancomycin.[37,80-82] Because the changes increase both physiologic pharmacokinetic parameters simultaneously, the effect on half-life is variable, depending on whether the increase in volume of distribution or the increase in clearance predominates in an individual patient [$t_{1/2} = (0.693 \cdot V)/Cl$].

Unlike with aminoglycosides, vancomycin pharmacokinetics in adult cystic fibrosis patients are not significantly different than typical values found in normal individuals.[83]

Obese individuals with normal serum creatinine concentrations have increased vancomycin clearance secondary to increased glomerular filtration rate and are best dosed with vancomycin using total body weight (TBW).[73,74,84,85] The reason for the increased drug clearance is kidney hypertrophy that results in larger creatinine clearance rates. Volume of distribution does not significantly change with obesity and is best estimated using ideal body weight (IBW) in patients more than 30% overweight (>30% over IBW, V = 0.7 L/kg IBW).[73,74,85] Because the primary pharmacokinetic change for vancomycin in obesity is increased drug clearance with a negligible change in volume of distribution, average half-life decreases to 3.3 hours [$t_{1/2} = (0.693 \cdot V)/Cl$]. Some morbidly obese patients will require every 6- to 8-hour dosing to maintain vancomycin steady-state trough concentrations within the therapeutic range.[73]

Premature infants (gestational age 32 weeks) have a larger amount of body water compared to adults. However, vancomycin volume of distribution (V = 0.7 L/kg) is not greatly affected by these greater amounts of body water as is the case with aminoglycoside antibiotics. Kidneys are not completely developed at this early age so glomerular filtration and vancomycin clearance (15 mL/min) are decreased.[86-89] A lower clearance rate with about the same volume of distribution as adults results in a longer average half-life for vancomycin in premature babies (10 hours). Full-term neonates (gestational age ~40 weeks) have similar volumes of distribution for vancomycin compared to premature infants, but their vancomycin clearance rate is twice that found in infants born prematurely (30 mL/min). The increase in drug clearance is due to additional renal development that occurred in utero. The vancomycin half-life in full-term babies is about 7 hours. At about

3 months of age, vancomycin clearance has nearly doubled again (50 mL/min), resulting in a half-life of approximately 4 hours. The increase in vancomycin clearance continues through 4-8 years of age when clearance equals 130-160 mL/min while volume of distribution remains ~0.7 L/kg so that half-life is 2-3 hours. At that time, vancomycin clearance and half-life gradually approach adult values as puberty approaches in children (~12-14 years old).

Intravenous vancomycin doses for neonates are based on renal function, weight, and age.[90] Steady-state trough vancomycin serum concentrations are used to individualize doses:

Neonate ≤28 weeks Gestational age: Serum Creatinine (mg/dL)	Neonate >28 weeks Gestational age: Serum Creatinine (mg/dL)	Vancomycin Dose
<0.9	<0.7	15 mg/kg every 12 h
0.9-1.1	0.7-0.9	20 mg/kg every 24 h
1.2-1.4	1.0-1.2	15 mg/kg every 24 h
1.5-1.8	1.3-1.6	10 mg/kg every 24 h
>1.8	>1.6	15 mg/kg every 48 h

Intravenous doses for older infants and children are 40-45 mg/kg/d given as three to four divided doses for mild to moderate infections (maximum dose, 1000-2000 mg/d) and 45-60 mg/kg/d given as three to four divided doses for severe infections (maximum dose, 2000-4000 mg/d).[91] Steady-state trough vancomycin serum concentrations are used to individualize doses.

The effect that hemodialysis has on vancomycin pharmacokinetics depends on the type of artificial kidney used during the procedure. Vancomycin is a relatively large molecule with a moderate-sized volume of distribution and intermediate protein binding. These characteristics lead to poor hemodialysis removal from the body. The mean vancomycin half-life for patients with renal failure is 120-140 hours.[28,77,92-98] Using traditional "low-flux" hemodialysis filters, an insignificant amount (<10%) of the total vancomycin body stores is removed during a 3- to 4-hour dialysis period.[76,77] When hemodialysis is performed with a "high-flux" filter, vancomycin serum concentrations decrease with a half-life equal to 4-5 hours during the dialysis period, and 25%-45% of a vancomycin dose can be removed by the dialysis procedure. Compared to postdialysis values obtained immediately at the end of the procedure, serum concentrations of vancomycin can slowly increase or "rebound" over the next 2-6 hours by about 15%-35%. Postdialysis vancomycin serum concentrations to determine whether supplemental doses are needed should be measured after the rebound period in patients receiving hemodialysis with a high-flux filter.[93-99]

Because of the infusion rate–related side effects that occur with vancomycin, doses are sometimes given to hemodialysis patients directly into the dialysis tubing injection port 1-1.5 hours prior to the end of a session. In this case, it may be necessary to increase the vancomycin dose by 25%-35% if a high-flux hemofilter is used in order to compensate for the amount of drug removed during infusion.[96,97] However, if a low-flux hemodialysis filter is being used during the infusion of vancomycin using this technique, such a low amount of the drug is lost that a dosage adjustment is not necessary.[100]

For patients with hemodynamic instability, a variant of hemodialysis known as *sustained-low efficiency dialysis* (SLED) or *extended daily dialysis* (EDD) can be performed where reduced blood flow and dialysate flow rates are used. To compensate for the reduced blood flow and dialysate flow rates (~200 mL/min and ~300 mL/min, respectively), the duration of dialysis is extended to 6-12 hours per day, and a high-flux filter is utilized most of the time. As one might expect, vancomycin is eliminated by this type of procedure, but the half-life during a dialysis period is 9-11 hours, and the amount of vancomycin removed is 20%-30%.[94,101]

Peritoneal dialysis removes only a negligible amount of vancomycin.[102-104] Patients who develop peritonitis while receiving peritoneal dialysis can be treated by placing vancomycin into the dialysis fluid. Over a 6-hour dwell time, approximately 50% of a vancomycin dose (1000 mg in 2 L dialysis fluid) is absorbed from the peritoneal cavity in renal failure patients without peritonitis.[102] Peritonitis causes inflammation of the peritoneal membrane, which facilitates absorption of vancomycin placed in the peritoneal dialysis fluid (up to 90% absorbed) and dialysis elimination of vancomycin from the body.[104,105] Automated peritoneal dialysis is used at nighttime by some renal failure patients. This dialysis technique allows several exchanges of dialysis fluid during the night while the patient sleeps. In patients who use regular continuous ambulatory peritoneal dialysis (CAPD; dwell time 7-8 hours per exchange) augmented with automated peritoneal dialysis (dwell time 2-3 hours per exchange), vancomycin half-life is 12 hours during the automated procedure but 63 hours during CAPD.[106]

Continuous renal replacement therapy (CRRT) removes vancomycin from the body. The hemofiltration sieving coefficient for vancomycin is 0.80.[107,108] In general, continuous venovenous hemofiltration (CVVH) and continuous arteriovenous hemofiltration (CAVH) provide a vancomycin clearance rate of about 20-30 mL/min, while continuous venovenous hemodialysis (CVVHD) and continuous venovenous hemodiafiltration (CVVHDF) can provide higher clearance rates.[109-116] Recommended initial doses for critically ill patients with acute renal failure undergoing continuous venovenous hemofiltration (CVVH) are a loading dose of 15-20 mg/kg followed by 250-500 mg every 12 hours.[117] For patients undergoing continuous arteriovenous hemofiltration (CAVH), the recommended initial dose is 500 mg every 24-48 hours.[6] Because of pharmacokinetic variability, vancomycin concentrations should be measured in CRRT patients to ensure effective steady-state concentrations are maintained.

Extracorporeal membrane oxygenation (ECMO) is used in patients of all ages to aid in gas exchange for severe respiratory or cardiorespiratory failure. Vancomycin pharmacokinetics can be affected to a variable degree by ECMO, so steady-state vancomycin serum concentrations should be used to guide therapy in these patients.[118-120] Cardiopulmonary bypass does not significantly influence the pharmacokinetics of vancomycin.[121]

DRUG INTERACTIONS

The most important drug interactions with vancomycin are pharmacodynamic, not pharmacokinetic, in nature. Coadministration of aminoglycoside antibiotics enhances the nephrotoxicity potential of vancomycin by two-fold or more.[50,122,123] Aminoglycosides can cause nephrotoxicity when administered alone. When an aminoglycoside and vancomycin are administered concurrently, serum creatinine concentrations should be monitored on a daily basis. Additionally, serum concentrations of the aminoglycoside, as well as vancomycin, should be measured. Patients receiving other nephrotoxic or ototoxic agents while taking vancomycin should be carefully monitored for adverse effects.

When vancomycin is administered to patients stabilized on warfarin therapy, the hypoprothrombinemic effect of the anticoagulant may be augmented.[124] The mechanism of this interaction is unknown, but it resulted in a mean 45% increase in prothrombin time over baseline values when warfarin was given alone. Patients receiving warfarin therapy who require vancomycin treatment should have a baseline prothrombin time ratio (INR) measured before the antibiotic is administered and daily INR tests until it is certain that anticoagulation status is stable.

INITIAL DOSAGE DETERMINATION METHODS

Several methods to initiate vancomycin therapy are available. The *Pharmacokinetic Dosing method* is the most flexible of the techniques. It allows individualized target serum concentrations to be chosen for a patient, and each pharmacokinetic parameter can be customized to reflect specific disease states and conditions present in the patient. However, it is computationally intensive.[58,125]

Nomograms use the dosing concepts in the Pharmacokinetic Dosing method. However, in order to simplify calculations, they make simplifying assumptions. The *Moellering nomogram* is designed to achieve average steady-state concentrations equal to 15 µg/mL. Some clinicians find this approach confusing as target steady-state peak and trough concentrations are not stated by the nomogram. Because the computed dose provided by the nomogram is expressed in mg/kg/24 h, it can be difficult to determine the best dosage interval. However, once experience is gained with this approach, the Moellering nomogram computes doses similar, but not identical, to the Pharmacokinetic Dosing method. The *Matzke nomogram* is constructed to produce steady-state vancomycin peak and trough concentrations of 30 µg/mL and 7.5 µg/mL, respectively. When these target concentrations are acceptable, the Matzke nomogram computes doses that are very similar to those calculated by the Pharmacokinetic Dosing method. However, because the expected concentrations are below the contemporary therapeutic range for trough levels, the Matzke nomogram computes doses that may require some adjustment before administration to patients. To address the problem of a higher target steady-state target range, the *Rybak nomogram* was derived specifically to attain steady-state vancomycin trough concentrations of 15-20 µg/mL. However, its use is limited to $CrCl_{est}$ between 40 and 109 mL/min and body weights of 50-110 kg.

Literature-based recommended dosing is a commonly used method to prescribe initial doses of vancomycin to pediatric patients. Doses are based on those that commonly produce steady-state concentrations within the therapeutic range, although there is a wide variation in the actual concentrations for a specific patient.

Pharmacokinetic Dosing Method

The goal of initial dosing of vancomycin is to compute the best dose possible for the patient given their set of disease states and conditions that influence vancomycin pharmacokinetics and the site and severity of the infection. In order to do this, pharmacokinetic parameters for the patient will be estimated using mean parameters measured in other individuals with similar disease state and condition profiles.

Clearance Estimate

Vancomycin is almost completely eliminated unchanged by the kidney, and there is a good relationship between creatinine clearance and vancomycin clearance (see Figure 5-2).[75] This relationship permits the estimation of the vancomycin clearance for a patient, which can be used to calculate an initial dose of the drug. Mathematically, the equation for the straight line shown in Figure 5-2 is: Cl = 0.695(CrCl) + 0.05, where Cl is vancomycin clearance in mL/min/kg and CrCl is creatinine clearance in mL/min/kg. Because each clearance value is normalized for the patient's weight, the estimated or measured creatinine clearance must be divided by the patient's weight in kg before using it in the equation, and the resulting vancomycin clearance must be multiplied by the patient's weight if the answer is needed in the units of mL/min. The weight factor that is used for all individuals, including obese patients, is total body weight (TBW).[73,74,77,84,85] It is not possible to simply enter a patient's creatinine clearance in mL/min and expect the resulting vancomycin clearance to have the units of mL/min with the idea that dividing the creatinine clearance by weight, then multiplying the vancomycin clearance by weight, mathematically cancels the weight factor out of the equation. The reason this does not work is that the y-intercept of the creatinine clearance/vancomycin clearance equation, which represents nonrenal vancomycin clearance, is in terms of mL/min/kg so mathematical cancellation of the weight factor is not possible. For example, the estimated vancomycin clearance for an individual with a creatinine clearance of 100 mL/min who weighs 70 kg is 1.04 mL/min/kg or 73 mL/min: Cl = 0.695[(100 mL/min)/70kg] + 0.05 = 1.04 mL/min/kg or 1.04 mL/min/kg • 70 kg = 73 mL/min. Taking the patient's renal function into account when deriving an initial dose of vancomycin is the single most important characteristic to assess.

Volume of Distribution Estimate

The average volume of distribution of vancomycin is 0.7 L/kg for all patient groups except for those with hematologic malignancies, where the value is 1.05 L/kg.[37,73,74,80-82] The weight factor that is used to calculate vancomycin volume of distribution for obese patients is ideal body weight (IBW).[73,74,85] Thus, for an 80-kg patient, the estimated vancomycin volume of distribution would be 56 L: V = 0.7 L/kg • 80 kg = 56 L. For a 150-kg obese patient with an ideal body weight of 60 kg, the estimated vancomycin volume of distribution is 42 L: V = 0.7 L/kg • 60 kg = 42 L.

Elimination Rate Constant and Half-Life Estimates

The vancomycin elimination rate constant (k_e) is computed using the estimated clearance and volume of distribution values for the drug in the following equation: $k_e = Cl/V$. It is usually expressed using the unit of h^{-1}. For example, for a patient with a vancomycin clearance equal to 1.04 mL/min/kg and a vancomycin volume of distribution equal to 0.7 L/kg, the elimination rate constant (in h^{-1}) would be computed as follows: $k_e =$ (1.04 mL/min/kg • 60 min/h)/(0.7 L/kg • 1000 mL/L) = 0.089 h^{-1}, where 60 min/h and 1000 mL/L are used as unit conversion factors for time and volume, respectively. Vancomycin half-life would be calculated using the equation that relates elimination rate constant and half-life: $t_{1/2} = 0.693/k_e = 0.693/0.089\ h^{-1} = 7.8\ h$.

Selection of Appropriate Pharmacokinetic Model and Equations

When given by intravenous infusion over an hour, vancomycin serum concentrations follow a two- or three-compartment pharmacokinetic model (see Figure 5-1). After the end of infusion if a two-compartment model is followed, serum concentrations drop rapidly because of distribution of drug from blood to tissues (α or distribution phase). By about 30-60 minutes after the end of infusion, vancomycin serum concentrations decline more slowly, and the elimination rate constant for this portion of the concentration/time curve is one that varies with renal function (β or elimination phase). In patients whose vancomycin serum concentration/time curve follows a three-compartment model, an intermediate distribution phase is found between the α and β portions of the graph. While these models are important to understand conceptually, they cannot easily be used clinically because of their mathematical complexity. Because of this, the simpler one-compartment model is widely used and allows accurate dosage calculation when peak vancomycin serum concentrations are obtained after drug distribution is finished.[73,77]

Intravenously administered vancomycin is given over 1 hour as intermittent continuous infusions for doses between 1000-1500 mg. Because the drug has a long half-life relative to the infusion time (1 hour) and waiting time (0.5-1 hour) necessary to allow for distribution to complete before peak concentrations are obtained, little of the drug is eliminated during this 1.5- to 2-hour time period. Intravenous infusion pharmacokinetic equations that take into account the loss of drug during the infusion time are not generally needed because so little vancomycin is eliminated during the infusion and waiting time periods. Therefore, although the antibiotic is given as an intravenous infusion, intravenous bolus equations accurately predict peak vancomycin concentrations and are mathematically simpler.[126] Because of these reasons, intravenous bolus equations are preferred by many clinicians to compute vancomycin doses (Table 5-2). Vancomycin steady-state peak (Css_{max}) and trough (Css_{min}) serum concentrations are chosen to treat the patient based on the type, site, and severity of infection as well as the infecting organism. Steady-state versions of one-compartment model intravenous bolus equations are as follows (see Table 5-2): $Css_{max} = (D/V)/(1 - e^{-k_e\tau})$, $Css_{min} = Css_{max}e^{-k_e\tau}$, where D is the antibiotic dose, V is the volume of distribution, k_e is the elimination rate constant, t is time, and τ is the dosage interval.

Steady-State Concentration Selection

Vancomycin steady-state trough concentrations are selected based on site and severity of infection in addition to the infecting organism. Because of reports of therapeutic failures, current treatment guidelines recommend

TABLE 5-2A   One-Compartment Model Equations Used With Vancomycin

Route of Administration	Single Dose	Multiple Dose	Steady-State
Intravenous bolus	$C = (D/V)e^{-k_e t}$	$C = (D/V)e^{-k_e t}[(1 - e^{-nk_e \tau})/(1 - e^{-k_e \tau})]$	$C = (D/V)[e^{-k_e t}/(1 - e^{-k_e \tau})]$

C, drug serum concentration at time = t; D, dose; k_e, elimination rate constant; n, number of administered doses; τ, dosage interval; V, volume of distribution.

TABLE 5-2B   Pharmacokinetic Constant Computations Utilizing a One-Compartment Model Used With Vancomycin

Route of Administration	Single Dose	Multiple Dose	Steady-State
Intravenous bolus	$k_e = -(\ln C_1 - \ln C_2)/(t_1 - t_2)$	$k_e = -(\ln C_1 - \ln C_2)/(t_1 - t_2)$	$k_e = -(\ln C_1 - \ln C_2)/(t_1 - t_2)$
	$t_{1/2} = 0.693/k_e$	$t_{1/2} = 0.693/k_e$	$t_{1/2} = 0.693/k_e$
	$V = D/C_{max}$	$V = D/(C_{max} - C_{min})$	$V = D/(Css_{max} - Css_{min})$
	$Cl = k_e V$	$Cl = k_e V$	$Cl = k_e V$

C_0, concentration at time = 0; C_1, drug serum concentration at time = t_1; C_2, drug serum concentration at time = t_2; Cl, drug clearance; C_{min}, predose trough concentration; C_{max}, postdose peak concentration; D, dose; k_e, elimination rate constant; $t_{1/2}$, half-life; V, volume of distribution.

TABLE 5-2C   Equations Used to Compute Individualized Dosage Regimens for Vancomycin

Route of Administration	Dosage Interval (τ), Maintenance Dose (D), and Loading Dose (LD) Equations
Intravenous bolus	$\tau = (\ln Css_{max} - \ln Css_{min})/k_e$
	$D = Css_{max} V(1 - e^{-k_e \tau})$
	$LD = Css_{max} V$

Css_{max}, maximum steady-state concentration; Css_{min}, minimum steady-state concentration; k_0, continuous infusion rate; k_e, elimination rate constant; V, volume of distribution.

vancomycin steady-state trough concentrations equal to 10-15 µg/mL for lower-intensity dosing and 15-20 µg/mL for complicated infections due to MRSA, such as bacteremia, endocarditis, meningitis, osteomyelitis, severe skin infections, and hospital-acquired pneumonia.[16-18] Steady-state vancomycin trough levels less than 10 µg/mL are discouraged due to the possibility of lower levels contributing to treatment failure or to the development of resistance. Whenever vancomycin doses are used that exceed steady-state trough concentrations of 20 µg/mL, serum creatinine concentrations and signs or symptoms of hearing or vestibular disturbance should be monitored daily to detect early signs of toxicity.

Steady-state peak vancomycin concentrations are chosen to provide adequate antibiotic penetration to the site of infection and to avoid adverse drug reactions. A commonly used range for this value is 30-50 µg/mL. In severe, life-threatening infections of the central nervous system, peak vancomycin serum concentrations as high as 60 µg/mL may be necessary to facilitate drug penetration. Whenever doses of vancomycin are used that exceed steady-state peak concentrations of 50 µg/mL, the patient should be monitored daily for early signs of ototoxicity (decreased hearing acuity in the conversational range, feeling of fullness or pressure in the ears, tinnitus, loss of equilibrium, headache, nausea, vomiting, vertigo, nystagmus, ataxia) or nephrotoxicity (serum creatinine concentrations).

Dosage Computation

The equations given in Table 5-2 are used to compute vancomycin doses.

EXAMPLE 1 ▶▶▶

JM is a 50-year-old, 70-kg (height = 5 ft 11 in) male with an MRSA wound infection. His current serum creatinine is 0.9 mg/dL, and it has been stable over the last 5 days since admission. Compute a vancomycin dose for this patient.

1. *Estimate creatinine clearance.*

This patient has a stable serum creatinine and is not obese. The Cockcroft-Gault equation can be used to estimate creatinine clearance:

$$CrCl_{est} = [(140 - age)BW]/(72 \cdot S_{Cr}) = [(140 - 50 \text{ y})70 \text{ kg}]/(72 \cdot 0.9 \text{ mg/dL})$$

$$CrCl_{est} = 97 \text{ mL/min}$$

2. *Estimate vancomycin clearance.*

The vancomycin clearance versus creatinine clearance relationship is used to estimate the vancomycin clearance for this patient:

$$Cl = 0.695(CrCl) + 0.05 = 0.695[(97 \text{ mL/min})/70 \text{kg}] + 0.05 = 1.015 \text{ mL/min/kg}$$

3. *Estimate vancomycin volume of distribution.*

The average volume of distribution for vancomycin is 0.7 L/kg:

$$V = 0.7 \text{ L/kg} \cdot 70 \text{ kg} = 49 \text{ L}$$

4. *Estimate vancomycin elimination rate constant (k_e) and half-life ($t_{1/2}$).*

$$k_e = Cl/V = (1.015 \text{ mL/min/kg} \cdot 60 \text{ min/h})/(0.7 \text{ L/kg} \cdot 1000 \text{ mL/L}) = 0.087 \text{ h}^{-1}$$
$$t_{1/2} = 0.693/k_e = 0.693/0.087 \text{ h}^{-1} = 8 \text{ h}$$

5. *Choose desired steady-state serum concentrations.*

Patients with *S. aureus* wound infections need to be carefully assessed. This patient did not appear to be in acute distress, with a normal temperature and slightly elevated WBC. The wound was warm and red with a slight amount of purulent discharge. Because the infection was localized to the wound area, a $Css_{min} = 12 \mu g/mL$ and $Css_{max} = 30 \mu g/mL$ were chosen.

6. *Use intravenous bolus equations to compute dose (see Table 5-2).*

Calculate required dosage interval (τ):

$$\tau = (\ln Css_{max} - \ln Css_{min})/k_e = (\ln 30 \mu g/mL - \ln 12 \mu g/mL)/0.087 \text{ h}^{-1} = 10.5 \text{ h}$$

Dosage intervals should be rounded to clinically acceptable intervals of 8, 12, 18, 24, 36, 48, 72 hours, and multiples of 24 hours thereafter, whenever possible. In this case, the dosage interval would be rounded to 12 hours.

Calculate required dose (D):

$$D = Css_{max} V(1 - e^{-k_e\tau}) = 30 \text{ mg/L} \cdot 49 \text{ L} [1 - e^{-(0.087 \text{ h}^{-1})(12 \text{ h})}] = 953 \text{ mg}$$

Vancomycin doses should be rounded to the nearest 100–250 mg. This dose would be rounded to 1000 mg. (Note: μg/mL = mg/L, and this concentration unit was substituted for Css_{max} so that unnecessary unit conversion was not required.)

The prescribed maintenance dose would be 1000 mg every 12 hours.

7. *Compute loading dose (LD), if needed.*

Loading doses should be considered for patients with creatinine clearance values less than 60 mL/min. The administration of a loading dose in these patients will allow achievement of therapeutic concentrations quicker than if maintenance doses alone are given. However, because the pharmacokinetic parameters used to compute these initial doses are only *estimated* values and not *actual* values, the patient's own parameters may be much different than the estimated constants and steady state will not be achieved until 3-5 half-lives have passed.

$$LD = Css_{max} V = 30 \text{ mg/L} \cdot 49 \text{ L} = 1470 \text{ mg, rounded to } 1500 \text{ mg}$$

As noted, this patient has good renal function (CrCl ≥60 mL/min) so a loading dose would not be prescribed for this patient.

EXAMPLE 2 ▶ ▶ ▶

The same patient profile as in example 1, but serum creatinine is 3.5 mg/dL indicating renal impairment.

1. *Estimate creatinine clearance.*

This patient has a stable serum creatinine and is not obese. The Cockcroft-Gault equation can be used to estimate creatinine clearance:

$$CrCl_{est} = [(140 - age)BW]/(72 \cdot S_{Cr}) = [(140 - 50 \text{ y})70 \text{ kg}]/(72 \cdot 3.5 \text{ mg/dL})$$
$$CrCl_{est} = 25 \text{ mL/min}$$

2. *Estimate vancomycin clearance.*

The vancomycin clearance versus creatinine clearance relationship is used to estimate the vancomycin clearance for this patient:

$$Cl = 0.695(CrCl) + 0.05 = 0.695[(25 \text{ mL/min})/70 \text{kg}] + 0.05 = 0.298 \text{ mL/min/kg}$$

3. *Estimate vancomycin volume of distribution.*

The average volume of distribution for vancomycin is 0.7 L/kg:

$$V = 0.7 \text{ L/kg} \cdot 70 \text{ kg} = 49 \text{ L}$$

4. *Estimate vancomycin elimination rate constant (k_e) and half-life ($t_{1/2}$).*

$$k_e = Cl/V = (0.298 \text{ mL/min/kg} \cdot 60 \text{ min/h})/(0.7 \text{ L/kg} \cdot 1000 \text{ mL/L}) = 0.0256 \text{ h}^{-1}$$
$$t_{1/2} = 0.693/k_e = 0.693/0.0256 \text{ h}^{-1} = 27 \text{ h}$$

5. *Choose desired steady-state serum concentrations.*

Patients with *S. aureus* wound infections need to be carefully assessed. This patient did not appear to be in acute distress, with a normal temperature and slightly elevated WBC. The wound was warm and red with a slight amount of purulent discharge. Because the infection was localized to the wound area, a $Css_{min} = 12 \text{ µg/mL}$ and $Css_{max} = 30 \text{ µg/mL}$ were chosen.

6. *Use intravenous bolus equations to compute dose (see Table 5-2).*

Calculate required dosage interval (τ):

$$\tau = (\ln Css_{max} - \ln Css_{min})/k_e = (\ln 30 \text{ µg/mL} - \ln 12 \text{ µg/mL})/0.0256 \text{ h}^{-1} = 36 \text{ h}$$

Dosage intervals should be rounded to clinically acceptable intervals of 8, 12, 18, 24, 36, 48, 72 hours, and multiples of 24 hours thereafter, whenever possible. In this case, the dosage interval is 36 hours.

Calculate required dose (D):

$$D = Css_{max} V(1 - e^{-k_e \tau}) = 30 \text{ mg/L} \cdot 49 \text{ L } [1 - e^{-(0.0256 \text{ h}^{-1})(36 \text{ h})}] = 884 \text{ mg}$$

Vancomycin doses should be rounded to the nearest 100-250 mg. This dose would be rounded to 1000 mg. (Note: μg/mL = mg/L, and this concentration unit was substituted for Css_{max} so that unnecessary unit conversion was not required.)

The prescribed maintenance dose would be 1000 mg every 36 hours.

7. *Compute loading dose (LD), if needed.*

Loading doses should be considered for patients with creatinine clearance values less than 60 mL/min. The administration of a loading dose in these patients will allow achievement of therapeutic concentrations quicker than if maintenance doses alone are given. However, because the pharmacokinetic parameters used to compute these initial doses are only *estimated* values and not *actual* values, the patient's own parameters may be much different than the estimated constants and steady state will not be achieved until 3-5 half-lives have passed.

$$LD = Css_{max} V = 30 \text{ mg/L} \cdot 49 \text{ L} = 1470 \text{ mg}$$

As noted, this patient has poor renal function (CrCl <60 mL/min) so a loading dose would be prescribed for this patient and given as the first dose. Vancomycin doses should be rounded to the nearest 100-250 mg. This dose would be rounded to 1500 mg. (Note: μg/mL = mg/L, and this concentration unit was substituted for Css_{max} so that unnecessary unit conversion was not required.) The first maintenance dose would be given one dosage interval (36 hours) after the loading dose was administered.

EXAMPLE 3 ▶ ▶ ▶

ZW is a 35-year-old, 150-kg (height = 5 ft 5 in) female with a *S. epidermidis* infection of a prosthetic knee joint. Her current serum creatinine is 0.7 mg/dL and is stable. Compute a vancomycin dose for this patient.

1. *Estimate creatinine clearance.*

This patient has a stable serum creatinine and is obese [$IBW_{females}$ (in kg) = 45 + 2.3(Ht − 60) = 45 + 2.3 (65 in − 60) = 57 kg]. The Salazar-Corcoran equation can be used to estimate creatinine clearance:

$$CrCl_{est(females)} = \frac{(146 - age)[(0.287 \cdot Wt) + (9.74 \cdot Ht^2)]}{(60 \cdot S_{Cr})}$$

$$CrCl_{est(females)} = \frac{(146 - 35 \text{ y})\{(0.287 \cdot 150 \text{ kg}) + [9.74 \cdot (1.65 \text{ m})^2]\}}{(60 \cdot 0.7 \text{ mg/dL})} = 184 \text{ mL/min}$$

Note: Height is converted from inches to meters: Ht = (65 in · 2.54 cm/in)/(100 cm/m) = 1.65 m.

2. *Estimate vancomycin clearance.*

The vancomycin clearance versus creatinine clearance relationship is used to estimate the vancomycin clearance for this patient. Because maintenance doses are based on total body weight (TBW), this weight factor is used to compute clearance:

$$Cl = 0.695(CrCl) + 0.05 = 0.695[(184 \text{ mL/min})/150 \text{ kg}] + 0.05 = 0.902 \text{ mL/min/kg TBW}$$

3. *Estimate vancomycin volume of distribution.*

   The average volume of distribution for vancomycin is 0.7 L/kg and computed using the patient's ideal body weight because obesity does not significantly alter this parameter:

   $$V = 0.7 \text{ L/kg} \cdot 57 \text{ kg} = 40 \text{ L}$$

4. *Estimate vancomycin elimination rate constant (k_e) and half-life ($t_{1/2}$).*

   Note that in the case of obese individuals, different weight factors are needed for vancomycin clearance and volume of distribution, so these weights are included in the equation for elimination rate constant:

   $$k_e = Cl/V = (0.902 \text{ mL/min/kg TBW} \cdot 150 \text{ kg TBW} \cdot 60 \text{ min/h})/$$
   $$(0.7 \text{ L/kg IBW} \cdot 57 \text{ kg IBW} \cdot 1000 \text{ mL/L}) = 0.205 \text{ h}^{-1}$$

   $$t_{1/2} = 0.693/k_e = 0.693/0.205 \text{ h}^{-1} = 3.4 \text{ h}$$

5. *Choose desired steady-state serum concentrations.*

   A $Css_{min} = 15 \text{ µg/mL}$ and $Css_{max} = 45 \text{ µg/mL}$ were chosen for this patient with a *S. epidermidis* prosthetic joint infection.

6. *Use intravenous bolus equations to compute dose (see Table 5-2).*

   Calculate required dosage interval (τ):

   $$\tau = (\ln Css_{max} - \ln Css_{min})/k_e = (\ln 45 \text{ µg/mL} - \ln 15 \text{ µg/mL})/0.205 \text{ h}^{-1} = 5.4 \text{ h}$$

   Dosage intervals in obese individuals should be rounded to clinically acceptable intervals of 8, 12, 18, 24, 36, 48, 72 hours, and multiples of 24 hours thereafter, whenever possible. In this case, the dosage interval would be rounded to 8 hours.

   Calculate required dose (D):

   $$D = Css_{max} V(1 - e^{-k_e\tau}) = 45 \text{ mg/L} \cdot 40 \text{ L} [1 - e^{-(0.205 \text{ h}^{-1})(8 \text{ h})}] = 1450 \text{ mg}$$

   Vancomycin doses should be rounded to the nearest 100-250 mg. This dose would be rounded to 1500 mg. (Note: µg/mL = mg/L, and this concentration unit was substituted for Css_{max} so that unnecessary unit conversion was not required.)

   The prescribed maintenance dose would be 1500 mg every 8 hours.

7. *Compute loading dose (LD), if needed.*

   Loading doses should be considered for patients with creatinine clearance values less 60 mL/min. The administration of a loading dose in these patients will allow achievement of therapeutic concentrations quicker than if maintenance doses alone are given. However, because the pharmacokinetic parameters used to compute these initial doses are only *estimated* values and not *actual* values, the patient's own parameters may be much different than the estimated constants and steady state will not be achieved until 3-5 half-lives have passed.

   $$LD = Css_{max} V = 45 \text{ mg/L} \cdot 40 \text{ L} = 1800 \text{ mg}$$

   As noted, this patient has good renal function (CrCl ≥60 mL/min) so a loading dose would not be prescribed for this patient.

EXAMPLE 4 ▶ ▶ ▶

JM is an 80-year-old, 80-kg (height = 5-ft 8-in) male with *S. viridans* endocarditis and is allergic to penicillins and cephalosporins. His current serum creatinine is 1.5 mg/dL, and it has been stable. Compute a vancomycin dose for this patient.

1. *Estimate creatinine clearance.*
   This patient has a stable serum creatinine and is not obese {IBW_{males} = 50 + 2.3(Ht − 60) = 50 + 2.3(68 in − 60) = 68 kg; % overweight = [100(80 kg − 68 kg)]/68kg = 18%}. The Cockcroft-Gault equation can be used to estimate creatinine clearance:

   $$CrCl_{est} = [(140 − age)BW]/(72 \cdot S_{Cr}) = [(140 − 80 \text{ y})80 \text{ kg}]/(72 \cdot 1.5 \text{ mg/dL})$$
   $$CrCl_{est} = 44 \text{ mL/min}$$

2. *Estimate vancomycin clearance.*
   The vancomycin clearance versus creatinine clearance relationship is used to estimate the vancomycin clearance for this patient:

   $$Cl = 0.695(CrCl) + 0.05 = 0.695[(44 \text{ mL/min})/80 \text{ kg}] + 0.05 = 0.432 \text{ mL/min/kg}$$

3. *Estimate vancomycin volume of distribution.*
   The average volume of distribution for vancomycin is 0.7 L/kg:

   $$V = 0.7 \text{ L/kg} \cdot 80 \text{ kg} = 56 \text{ L}$$

4. *Estimate vancomycin elimination rate constant (k_e) and half-life ($t_{1/2}$).*

   $$k_e = Cl/V = (0.432 \text{ mL/min/kg} \cdot 60 \text{ min/h})/(0.7 \text{ L/kg} \cdot 1000 \text{ mL/L}) = 0.0370 \text{ h}^{-1}$$
   $$t_{1/2} = 0.693/k_e = 0.693/0.0370 \text{ h}^{-1} = 18.7 \text{ h}$$

5. *Choose desired steady-state serum concentrations.*
   Steady-state vancomycin serum concentrations of Css_{min} = 10 μg/mL and Css_{max} = 30 μg/mL were chosen to treat this patient.

6. *Use intravenous bolus equations to compute dose (see Table 5-2).*
   Calculate required dosage interval (τ):

   $$τ = (\ln Css_{max} − \ln Css_{min})/k_e = (\ln 30 \text{ μg/mL} − \ln 10 \text{ μg/mL})/0.0370 \text{ h}^{-1} = 30 \text{ h}$$

   Dosage intervals should be rounded to clinically acceptable intervals of 8, 12, 18, 24, 36, 48, 72 hours, and multiples of 24 hours thereafter, whenever possible. In this case, the dosage interval would be rounded to 24 hours.
   Calculate required dose (D):

   $$D = Css_{max} V(1 − e^{-k_e τ}) = 30 \text{ mg/L} \cdot 56 \text{ L} [1 − e^{-(0.0370 \text{ h}^{-1})(24 \text{ h})}] = 988 \text{ mg}$$

   Vancomycin doses should be rounded to the nearest 100-250 mg. This dose would be rounded to 1000 mg. (Note: μg/mL = mg/L, and this concentration unit was substituted for Css_{max} so that unnecessary unit conversion was not required.)
   The prescribed maintenance dose would be 1000 mg every 24 hours.

7. *Compute loading dose (LD), if needed.*

Loading doses should be considered for patients with creatinine clearance values less than 60 mL/min. The administration of a loading dose in these patients will allow achievement of therapeutic concentrations quicker than if maintenance doses alone are given. However, because the pharmacokinetic parameters used to compute these initial doses are only *estimated* values and not *actual* values, the patient's own parameters may be much different than the estimated constants and steady state will not be achieved until 3-5 half-lives have passed.

$$LD = Css_{max} V = 30 \text{ mg/L} \cdot 56 \text{ L} = 1680 \text{ mg, round to 1500 mg}$$

As noted, this patient has poor renal function (CrCl <60 mL/min) so a loading dose would be prescribed and given as the first dose. Vancomycin doses should be rounded to the nearest 100-250 mg. (Note: μg/mL = mg/L, and this concentration unit was substituted for Css_{max} so that unnecessary unit conversion was not required.) The first maintenance dose would be given one dosage interval (24 hours) after the loading dose was administered.

Moellering Nomogram Method

Because the only two patient-specific factors that change when using the Pharmacokinetic Dosing method are patient weight and creatinine clearance, it is possible to make a simple nomogram to handle uncomplicated patients. The Moellering dosage nomogram was the first widely used approach that incorporated pharmacokinetic concepts to compute doses of vancomycin for patients with compromised renal function (Table 5-3).[75] The stated goal of the nomogram is to provide average steady-state vancomycin concentrations equal to 15 μg/mL (or 15 mg/L). In order to use the nomogram, the patient's creatinine clearance is computed and divided by their body weight so that the units for creatinine clearance are mL/min/kg. This value is converted to a vancomycin maintenance dose in terms of mg/kg/24 h. If the patient has renal impairment, a loading dose of 15 mg/kg (for obese patients >30% overweight, use IBW) is suggested. The nomogram does not provide a value for dosage interval. Because the therapeutic range for vancomycin has been moved upward since this nomogram was developed, an adjustment to the dosage rate needs to be made. To provide trough concentrations of 15-20 μg/mL, dosing values given by the nomogram can be multiplied by about 1.33-1.66.

The relationship between vancomycin clearance and creatinine clearance used in the Pharmacokinetic Dosing method is the one used to construct the Moellering nomogram. Hence, the dosage recommendations made by both these methods are generally similar although not identical because vancomycin peak and trough concentrations cannot be specified using the nomogram. A modification of the vancomycin clearance/creatinine clearance equation can be made that provides a direct calculation of the vancomycin maintenance dose.[127] Because the equation computes vancomycin clearance, it can be converted to the maintenance dose required to provide an average steady-state concentration of 20 mg/L by multiplying the equation by the concentration (MD = Css • Cl, where MD is maintenance dose) and appropriate unit conversion constants:

$$Cl \text{ (in mL/min/kg)} = 0.695(CrCl \text{ in mL/min/kg}) + 0.05$$
$$D \text{ (in mg/h/kg)} = [(20 \text{ mg/L} \cdot 60 \text{ min/h})/1000 \text{ mL/L}][0.695(CrCl \text{ in mL/min/kg}) + 0.05]$$
$$D \text{ (in mg/h/kg)} = 0.834(CrCl \text{ in mL/min/kg}) + 0.06$$

The use of this modification is straightforward. The patient's creatinine clearance is estimated using an appropriate technique (Cockcroft-Gault method[29] for normal-weight patients, Salazar-Corcoran method[128] for obese patients). The vancomycin maintenance dose is directly computed using the dosing equation and multiplied by the patient's weight to convert the answer into the units of mg/h. Guidance to the appropriate dosage interval (in hours) can be gained by dividing this dosage rate into a clinically acceptable dose such as 1000 mg, 1250 mg, or 1500 mg. To illustrate how this dosing approach is used, the same patient examples used in the previous section will be repeated for this dosage approach.

TABLE 5-3   Moellering Nomogram Vancomycin Dosage Chart

1. Compute patient's estimated creatinine clearance ($CrCl_{est}$) using Cockcroft-Gault method for normal weight or Salazar-Corcoran method for obese patients.
2. Divide $CrCl_{est}$ by patient's weight
3. Compute 24 hour maintenance dose for $CrCl_{est}$ value
4. Loading dose of 15 mg/kg should be given in patients with significant renal function impairment

Creatinine Clearance (mL/min/kg)[a]	Vancomycin Dose (mg/kg/24 h)
2	30.9
1.9	29.3
1.8	27.8
1.7	26.3
1.6	24.7
1.5	23.2
1.4	21.6
1.3	20.1
1.2	18.5
1.1	17
1.0	15.4
0.9	13.9
0.8	12.4
0.7	10.8
0.6	9.3
0.5	7.7
0.4	6.2
0.3	4.6
0.2	3.1
0.1	1.5

[a] Dose for functionally anephric patients is 1.9 mq/kq/24 h.

Adapted from Moellering et al.[75]

EXAMPLE 1 ▶ ▶ ▶

JM is a 50-year-old, 70-kg (height = 5 ft 11 in) male with an MRSA wound infection. His current serum creatinine is 0.9 mg/dL, and it has been stable over the last 5 days since admission. Compute a vancomycin dose for this patient.

1. *Estimate creatinine clearance.*

This patient has a stable serum creatinine and is not obese. The Cockcroft-Gault equation can be used to estimate creatinine clearance:

$$CrCl_{est} = [(140 - age)BW]/(72 \cdot S_{Cr}) = [(140 - 50 \text{ y})70 \text{ kg}]/(72 \cdot 0.9 \text{ mg/dL})$$
$$CrCl_{est} = 97 \text{ mL/min}$$

2. *Determine dosage interval and maintenance dose.*

The maintenance dose is calculated using the modified vancomycin dosing equation:

$$D \text{ (in mg/h/kg)} = 0.834(\text{CrCl in mL/min/kg}) + 0.06$$
$$D = 0.834[(97 \text{ mL/min})/70 \text{ kg}] + 0.06 = 1.216 \text{ mg/h/kg}$$
$$D = 1.216 \text{ mg/h/kg} \cdot 70 \text{ kg} = 85.1 \text{ mg/h}$$

Because the patient has good renal function, the typical dosage interval of 12 hours will be used:

$$D = 85.1 \text{ mg/h} \cdot 12 \text{ h} = 1021 \text{ mg}$$

Vancomycin doses should be rounded to the nearest 100-250 mg. This dose would be rounded to 1000 mg. The prescribed maintenance dose would be 1000 mg every 12 hours.

3. *Compute loading dose.*

A loading dose (LD) of 15 mg/kg is suggested by the Moellering nomogram, and this value is adjusted by 1.33:

$$LD = 15 \text{ mg/kg}(70 \text{ kg})1.33 = 1397 \text{ mg}$$

As noted, this patient has good renal function (CrCl ≥60 mL/min) so a loading dose could optionally be prescribed for this patient.

EXAMPLE 2 ▶ ▶ ▶

The same patient profile as in example 1, but serum creatinine is 3.5 mg/dL indicating renal impairment.

1. *Estimate creatinine clearance.*

This patient has a stable serum creatinine and is not obese. The Cockcroft-Gault equation can be used to estimate creatinine clearance:

$$\text{CrCl}_{est} = [(140 - \text{age})\text{BW}]/(72 \cdot \text{S}_{Cr}) = [(140 - 50 \text{ y})70 \text{ kg}]/(72 \cdot 3.5 \text{ mg/dL})$$
$$\text{CrCl}_{est} = 25 \text{ mL/min}$$

2. *Determine dosage interval and maintenance dose.*

The maintenance dose is calculated using the modified vancomycin dosing equation:

$$D \text{ (in mg/h/kg)} = 0.834(\text{CrCl in mL/min/kg}) + 0.06$$
$$D = 0.834[(25 \text{ mL/min})/70 \text{ kg}] + 0.06 = 0.358 \text{ mg/h/kg}$$
$$D = 0.358 \text{ mg/h/kg} \cdot 70 \text{ kg} = 25.1 \text{ mg/h}$$

A standard dose of 1250 mg can be used to gain an approximation for an acceptable dosage interval (τ):

$$\tau = 1250 \text{ mg}/(25.1 \text{ mg/h}) = 49.8 \text{ h}$$

Dosage intervals should be rounded to clinically acceptable intervals of 8, 12, 18, 24, 36, 48, 72 hours, and multiples of 24 hours thereafter, whenever possible. In this case, the dosage interval would be rounded to 48 hours.

$$D = 25.1 \text{ mg/h} \cdot 48 \text{ h} = 1205 \text{ mg}$$

Vancomycin doses should be rounded to the nearest 100-250 mg. This dose would be rounded to 1250 mg. The prescribed maintenance dose would be 1250 mg every 48 hours.

3. *Compute loading dose.*

A loading dose (LD) of 15 mg/kg is suggested by the Moellering nomogram, and this value is adjusted by 1.33:

$$LD = 15 \text{ mg/kg}(70 \text{ kg})1.33 = 1397 \text{ mg, rounded to } 1500 \text{ mg}$$

As noted, this patient has poor renal function (CrCl <60 mL/min) so a loading dose would be prescribed and given as the first dose. Vancomycin doses should be rounded to the nearest 100-250 mg. (Note: μg/mL = mg/L, and this concentration unit was substituted for Css_{max} so that unnecessary unit conversion was not required.) The first maintenance dose would be given one dosage interval (48 hours) after the loading dose was administered.

EXAMPLE 3 ▶ ▶ ▶

ZW is a 35-year-old, 150-kg (height = 5 ft 5 in) female with a *S. epidermidis* infection of a prosthetic knee joint. Her current serum creatinine is 0.7 mg/dL and is stable. Compute a vancomycin dose for this patient.

1. *Estimate creatinine clearance.*

This patient has a stable serum creatinine and is obese [$IBW_{females}$ (in kg) = 45 + 2.3(Ht − 60) = 45 + 2.3(65 in − 60) = 57 kg]. The Salazar-Corcoran equation can be used to estimate creatinine clearance:

$$CrCl_{est(females)} \frac{(146 - age)[(0.287 \cdot Wt) + (9.74 \cdot Ht^2)]}{(60 \cdot S_{Cr})}$$

$$CrCl_{est(females)} \frac{(146 - 35y)\{(0.287 \cdot 150kg) + [9.74 \cdot (1.65\,m)^2]\}}{(60 \cdot 0.7 \text{ mg/dL})} = 184 \text{ mL/min}$$

Note: Height is converted from inches to meters: Ht = (65 in · 2.54 cm/in)/(100 cm/m) = 1.65 m.

2. *Determine dosage interval and maintenance dose.*

The maintenance dose is calculated using the modified vancomycin dosing equation:

$$D \text{ (in mg/h/kg)} = 0.834(\text{CrCl in mL/min/kg}) + 0.06$$
$$D = 0.834[(184 \text{ mL/min})/150 \text{ kg}] + 0.06 = 1.083 \text{ mg/h/kg}$$
$$D = 1.083 \text{ mg/h/kg} \cdot 150 \text{ kg} = 162.5 \text{ mg/h}$$

Because the patient has excellent renal function and is obese, a dosage interval equal to 8 hours will be used:

$$D = 162.5 \text{ mg/h} \cdot 8 \text{ h} = 1300 \text{ mg}$$

Vancomycin doses should be rounded to the nearest 100-250 mg. This dose would be rounded to 1250 mg. The prescribed maintenance dose would be 1250 mg every 8 hours.

3. *Compute loading dose.*

A loading dose (LD) of 15 mg/kg is suggested by the Moellering nomogram. As noted, this patient has good renal function (CrCl ≥60 mL/min) so a loading dose would probably not be prescribed for this patient.

EXAMPLE 4 ▶ ▶ ▶

JM is an 80-year-old, 80-kg (height = 5 ft 8 in) male with *S. viridans* endocarditis and is allergic to penicillins and cephalosporins. His current serum creatinine is 1.5 mg/dL, and it has been stable. Compute a vancomycin dose for this patient.

1. *Estimate creatinine clearance.*

This patient has a stable serum creatinine and is not obese {IBW_{males} = 50 + 2.3(Ht − 60) = 50 + 2.3(68 in − 60) = 68 kg; % overweight = [100(80 kg − 68 kg)]/68 kg = 18%}. The Cockcroft-Gault equation can be used to estimate creatinine clearance:

$$CrCl_{est} = [(140 - age)BW]/(72 \cdot S_{Cr}) = [(140 - 80 \, y)80 \, kg]/(72 \cdot 1.5 \, mg/dL)$$
$$CrCl_{est} = 44 \, mL/min$$

2. *Determine dosage interval and maintenance dose.*

The maintenance dose is calculated using the modified vancomycin dosing equation:

$$D \, (in \, mg/h/kg) = 0.834(CrCl \, in \, mL/min/kg) + 0.06$$
$$D = 0.834[(44 \, mL/min)/80 \, kg] + 0.06 = 0.519 \, mg/h/kg$$
$$D = 0.519 \, mg/h/kg \cdot 80 \, kg = 41.5 \, mg/h$$

A standard dose of 1000 mg can be used to gain an approximation for an acceptable dosage interval (τ):

$$\tau = 1000 \, mg/(41.5 \, mg/h) = 24 \, h$$

Dosage intervals should be rounded to clinically acceptable intervals of 8, 12, 18, 24, 36, 48, 72 hours, and multiples of 24 hours thereafter, whenever possible. In this case, the dosage interval would be 24 hours.

$$D = 41.5 \, mg/h \cdot 24 \, h = 996 \, mg$$

Vancomycin doses should be rounded to the nearest 100-250 mg. This dose would be rounded to 1000 mg. The prescribed maintenance dose would be 1000 mg every 24 hours.

3. *Compute loading dose.*

A loading dose (LD) of 15 mg/kg is suggested by the Moellering nomogram, and this value is adjusted by 1.33:

$$LD = 15 \, mg/kg(80 \, kg)1.33 = 1596 \, mg$$

As noted, this patient has poor renal function (CrCl <60 mL/min) so a loading dose would be prescribed and given as the first dose. Vancomycin doses should be rounded to the nearest 100-250 mg. (Note: µg/mL = mg/L, and this concentration unit was substituted for Css_{max} so that unnecessary unit conversion was not required.) The first maintenance dose would be given one dosage interval (24 hours) after the loading dose was administered.

Matzke Nomogram Method

The Matzke dosing nomogram is a quick and efficient way to apply pharmacokinetic dosing concepts without using complicated pharmacokinetic equations (Table 5-4).[77] The nomogram has not been tested in obese subjects (>30% over ideal body weight) and should not be used in this patient population. Additionally, the authors suggest that the nomogram should not be used in patients undergoing peritoneal dialysis.

The nomogram is constructed to produce steady-state vancomycin peak and trough concentrations of 30 µg/mL and 7.5 µg/mL, respectively. A loading dose of 25 mg/kg is given as the first dose, and subsequent maintenance doses of 19 mg/kg are given according to a dosage interval that varies by the patient's creatinine clearance.

TABLE 5-4   Matzke Nomogram Vancomycin Dosage Chart

1. Compute patient's estimated creatinine clearance ($CrCl_{est}$), using Cockcroft-Gault method: $CrCl_{est} = [(140 - age)BW]/(Scr \times 72)$. Multiply by 0.85 for females.
2. Nomogram not verified in obese individuals.
3. Dosage chart designed to achieve peak serum concentrations of 30 µg/mL and trough concentrations of 7.5 µg/mL.
4. Compute loading dose of 25 mg/kg.

Compute maintenance dose of 19 mg/kg given at the dosage interval listed in the following chart for the patients $CrCl_{est}$:

$CrCl_{est}$ (mL/min)	Dosage Interval (days)
≥120	0.5
100	0.6
80	0.75
60	1.0
40	1.5
30	2.0
20	2.5
10	4.0
5	6.0
0	12.0

Adapted from Matzke et al.[77]

The dosage interval supplied by the nomogram is the time needed for 19 mg/kg of vancomycin to be eliminated from the body. By replacing the amount eliminated over the dosage interval with a maintenance dose of the same magnitude, the same peak and trough vancomycin concentration/time profile is reproduced after each dose. To illustrate how the nomogram is used, the same patient examples used in the previous section (omitting the obese patient case) will be repeated for this dosage approach. Because the nomogram uses slightly different estimates for volume of distribution and elimination rate constant as well as fixed steady-state peak and trough drug concentrations, differences in suggested doses are expected. While the Matzke nomogram has been shown to provide precise and unbiased dosage recommendations, it does supply relatively large doses so some patients may attain levels in the current therapeutic ranges.

EXAMPLE 1 ▶ ▶ ▶

JM is a 50-year-old, 70-kg (height = 5 ft 11 in) male with an MRSA wound infection. His current serum creatinine is 0.9 mg/dL, and it has been stable over the last 5 days since admission. Compute a vancomycin dose for this patient.

1. *Estimate creatinine clearance.*

   This patient has a stable serum creatinine and is not obese. The Cockcroft-Gault equation can be used to estimate creatinine clearance:

   $$CrCl_{est} = [(140 - age)BW]/(72 \cdot S_{Cr}) = [(140 - 50\ y)70\ kg]/(72 \cdot 0.9\ mg/dL) = 97\ mL/min$$

2. *Compute loading dose (see Table 5-4).*
   A loading dose (LD) of 25 mg/kg will provide a peak concentration of 30 µg/mL.

$$LD = 25 \text{ mg/kg}(70 \text{ kg}) = 1750 \text{ mg}$$

3. *Determine dosage interval and maintenance dose.*
   From the nomogram the dosage interval is 0.6 days, which would be rounded to every 12 hours. The maintenance dose would be 19 mg/kg · 70 kg = 1330 mg. Vancomycin doses should be rounded to the nearest 100-250 mg. This dose would be rounded to 1250 mg and given one dosage interval (12 hours) after the loading dose.
   The prescribed maintenance dose would be 1250 mg every 12 hours.

EXAMPLE 2 ▶ ▶ ▶

The same patient profile as in example 1, but serum creatinine is 3.5 mg/dL indicating renal impairment.

1. *Estimate creatinine clearance.*
   This patient has a stable serum creatinine and is not obese. The Cockcroft-Gault equation can be used to estimate creatinine clearance:

$$CrCl_{est} = [(140 - age)BW]/(72 \cdot S_{Cr}) = [(140 - 50 \text{ y})70 \text{ kg}]/(72 \cdot 3.5 \text{ mg/dL})$$

$$CrCl_{est} = 25 \text{ mL/min}$$

2. *Compute loading dose (see Table 5-4).*
   A loading dose (LD) of 25 mg/kg will provide a peak concentration of 30 µg/mL.

$$LD = 25 \text{ mg/kg}(70 \text{ kg}) = 1750 \text{ mg}$$

3. *Determine dosage interval and maintenance dose.*
   After rounding creatinine clearance to 30 mL/min, the nomogram suggests a dosage interval of 2 days. The maintenance dose would be 19 mg/kg · 70 kg = 1330 mg. Vancomycin doses should be rounded to the nearest 100-250 mg. This dose would be rounded to 1250 mg and given one dosage interval (2 days × 24 h/d = 48 hours) after the loading dose.
   The prescribed maintenance dose would be 1250 mg every 48 hours.

EXAMPLE 3 ▶ ▶ ▶

JM is an 80-year-old, 80-kg (height = 5 ft 8 in) male with *S. viridans* endocarditis and is allergic to penicillins and cephalosporins. His current serum creatinine is 1.5 mg/dL, and it has been stable. Compute a vancomycin dose for this patient.

1. *Estimate creatinine clearance.*
   This patient has a stable serum creatinine and is not obese {IBW$_{males}$ = 50 + 2.3(Ht − 60) = 50 + 2.3(68 in − 60) = 68 kg; % overweight = [100(80 kg − 68 kg)]/68 kg = 18%}. The Cockcroft-Gault equation can be used to estimate creatinine clearance:

$$CrCl_{est} = [(140 - age)BW]/(72 \cdot S_{Cr}) = [(140 - 80 \text{ y})80 \text{ kg}]/(72 \cdot 1.5 \text{ mg/dL})$$

$$CrCl_{est} = 44 \text{ mL/min}$$

2. *Compute loading dose (see Table 5-4).*

A loading dose (LD) of 25 mg/kg will provide a peak concentration of 30 μg/mL.

$$LD = 25 \text{ mg/kg}(80 \text{ kg}) = 2000 \text{ mg}$$

3. *Determine dosage interval and maintenance dose.*

After rounding creatinine clearance to 40 mL/min, the nomogram suggests a dosage interval of 1.5 days. The maintenance dose would be 19 mg/kg · 80 kg = 1520 mg. Vancomycin doses should be rounded to the nearest 100-250 mg. This dose would be rounded to 1500 mg and started one dosage interval (1.5 days × 24 h/d = 36 hours) after the loading dose.

The prescribed maintenance dose would be 1500 mg every 36 hours.

Rybak Nomogram Method

Similar to the other approaches suggested for the initiation of vancomycin dosing, the Ryback nomogram uses patient weight and $CrCl_{est}$ to estimate population pharmacokinetic parameters for a patient in order to derive a dose.[129] The key difference with this dosing table is that it is specifically designed to attain steady-state vancomycin trough concentrations between 15 and 20 μg/mL. The Rybak nomogram demonstrates good statistical performance in achieving the desired target concentrations (median steady-state trough concentration = 17.5 μg/mL, median percent error 14%). If desired, a loading dose of 25-30 mg/kg actual body weight can be administered as the first dose.

However, there are some notable limitations with this method. It can only be used for adult patients with weights between 50 and 110 kg and estimated creatinine clearances between 40 and 110 mL/min. Further, it has not been validated in patients with (1) a serum creatinine concentration of less than 0.6 mg/dL; (2) unstable volume of distribution or renal function; (3) organ transplant within the last 6 months; (4) surgery in the past 48 hours; (5) patients receiving vasopressors; or (6) critically ill, burn, or pediatric patients.

EXAMPLE 1 ▶ ▶ ▶

JM is a 50-year-old, 70-kg (height = 5 ft 11 in) male with an MRSA wound infection. His current serum creatinine is 0.9 mg/dL, and it has been stable over the last 5 days since admission. Compute a vancomycin dose for this patient.

1. *Estimate creatinine clearance.*

This patient has a stable serum creatinine and is not obese. The Cockcroft-Gault equation can be used to estimate creatinine clearance:

$$CrCl_{est} = [(140 - age)BW]/(72 \cdot S_{Cr}) = [(140 - 50 \text{ y})70 \text{ kg}]/(72 \cdot 0.9 \text{ mg/dL})$$
$$CrCl_{est} = 97 \text{ mL/min}$$

2. *Determine dosage interval and maintenance dose (Table 5-5).*

From the nomogram the vancomycin dosage is 1500 mg every 8 hours.

EXAMPLE 2 ▶ ▶ ▶

The same patient profile as in example 1, but serum creatinine is 2.1 mg/dL indicating renal impairment.

1. *Estimate creatinine clearance.*

This patient has a stable serum creatinine and is not obese. The Cockcroft-Gault equation can be used to estimate creatinine clearance:

$$CrCl_{est} = [(140 - age)BW]/(72 \cdot S_{Cr}) = [(140 - 50 \text{ y})70 \text{ kg}]/(72 \cdot 2.1 \text{ mg/dL})$$
$$CrCl_{est} = 42 \text{ mL/min}$$

2. *Determine dosage interval and maintenance dose (see Table 5-5).*

From the nomogram the vancomycin dosage is 750 mg every 12 hours. Because the patient's $CrCl_{est}$ is less than 60 mL/min, loading dose (LD) of 25-30 mg/kg actual body weight could be administered as the first dose: LD = 25 mg/kg • 70 kg = 1750 mg.

TABLE 5-5 Rybak Nomogram Vancomycin Dosage Chart

1. Compute patient's creatinine clearance (CrCl), using Cockcroft-Gault method: $CrCl_{est} = [(140 − age)BW]/(Scr \times 72)$. Multiply by 0.85 for females.
2. Use intersection of patient's actual weight (left column) and $CrCl_{est}$ (top row) to derive dose.
3. Dosage chart designed to achieve steady-state trough concentrations of 15–20 µg/mL.
4. A loading dose of 25-30 mg/kg (patient's actual weight) may be used as the first dose.

Weight (kg)	$CrCl_{est}$ = 40-49 mL/min	$CrCl_{est}$ = 50-59 mL/min	$CrCl_{est}$ = 60-69 mL/min	$CrCl_{est}$ = 70-79 mL/min	$CrCl_{est}$ = 80-89 mL/min	$CrCl_{est}$ = 90-99 mL/min	$CrCl_{est}$ = 100-109 mL/min
50-54	500 mg every 12 h	750 mg every 12 h	1000 mg every 12 h	750 mg every 8 h	1000 mg every 8 h	1000 mg every 8 h	1250 mg every 8 h
55-59	750 mg every 12 h	1000 mg every 12 h	1250 mg every 12 h	750 mg every 8 h	1000 mg every 8 h	1000 mg every 8 h	1250 mg every 8 h
60-64	750 mg every 12 h	1000 mg every 12 h	1250 mg every 12 h	750 mg every 8 h	1000 mg every 8 h	1250 mg every 8 h	1500 mg every 8 h
65-69	750 mg every 12 h	1000 mg every 12 h	1250 mg every 12 h	1000 mg every 8 h	1000 mg every 8 h	1250 mg every 8 h	1500 mg every 8 h
70-74	750 mg every 12 h	1250 mg every 12 h	750 mg every 8 h	1000 mg every 8 h	1250 mg every 8 h	1500 mg every 8 h	1500 mg every 8 h
75-79	1000 mg every 12 h	1250 mg every 12 h	750 mg every 8 h	1000 mg every 8 h	1250 mg every 8 h	1500 mg every 8 h	1750 mg every 8 h
80-84	1000 mg every 12 h	1250 mg every 12 h	1000 mg every 8 h	1250 mg every 8 h	1250 mg every 8 h	1500 mg every 8 h	1750 mg every 8 h
85-89	1000 mg every 12 h	1250 mg every 12 h	1000 mg every 8 h	1250 mg every 8 h	1500 mg every 8 h	1750 mg every 8 h	2000 mg every 8 h
90-94	1000 mg every 12 h	1500 mg every 12 h	1000 mg every 8 h	1250 mg every 8 h	1500 mg every 8 h	1750 mg every 8 h	2000 mg every 8 h
95-99	1250 mg every 12 h	1500 mg every 12 h	1000 mg every 8 h	1250 mg every 8 h	1500 mg every 8 h	1750 mg every 8 h	2000 mg every 8 h
100-104	1250 mg every 12 h	1500 mg every 12 h	1250 mg every 8 h	1500 mg every 8 h	1750 mg every 8 h	2000 mg every 8 h	2000 mg every 8 h
105-109	1250 mg every 12 h	1500 mg every 12 h	1250 mg every 8 h	1500 mg every 8 h	1750 mg every 8 h	2000 mg every 8 h	2250 mg every 8 h
110	1250 mg every 12 h	1500 mg every 12 h	1250 mg every 8 h	1500 mg every 8 h	1750 mg every 8 h	2000 mg every 8 h	2250 mg every 8 h

Adapted from Kullar et al.[129]

EXAMPLE 3 ▶ ▶ ▶

JM is an 80-year-old, 80-kg (height = 5 ft 8 in) male with *S. viridans* endocarditis and is allergic to penicillins and cephalosporins. His current serum creatinine is 1.5 mg/dL, and it has been stable. Compute a vancomycin dose for this patient.

1. *Estimate creatinine clearance.*
   This patient has a stable serum creatinine and is not obese {IBW_{males} = 50 + 2.3(Ht − 60) = 50 + 2.3(68 in − 60) = 68 kg; % overweight = [100(80 kg − 68 kg)]/68 kg = 18%}. The Cockcroft-Gault equation can be used to estimate creatinine clearance:

$$CrCl_{est} = [(140 - age)BW]/(72 \cdot S_{Cr}) = [(140 - 80\ y)80\ kg]/(72 \cdot 1.5\ mg/dL)$$

$$CrCl_{est} = 44\ mL/min$$

2. *Determine dosage interval and maintenance dose (see Table 5-5).*
   From the nomogram the vancomycin dosage is 1000 mg every 12 hours. Because the patient's $CrCl_{est}$ is less than 60 mL/min, a loading dose (LD) of 25-30 mg/kg actual body weight could be administered as the first dose: LD = 25 mg/kg · 80 kg = 2000 mg.

Literature-Based Recommended Dosing

Because of the large amount of variability in vancomycin pharmacokinetics, even when concurrent disease states and conditions are identified, many clinicians believe that the use of standard vancomycin doses for pediatric patients is warranted. The original computation of these doses was based on the pharmacokinetic dosing methods described in the previous section and subsequently modified based on clinical experience. In general, the expected vancomycin steady-state serum concentrations used to compute these doses were similar to those for adults. Suggested initial vancomycin doses for various pediatric patients are listed in the Effects of Disease States and Conditions on Vancomycin Pharmacokinetics and Dosing section. Doses for neonates are usually rounded to the nearest milligram. If serum creatinine values are available, estimated creatinine clearance can be computed using equations that are specific for pediatric patients [age 0-1 year, $CrCl_{est}$ (in mL/min/1.73 m^2) = (0.45 • Ht)/S_{Cr}; age 1-20 years, $CrCl_{est}$ (in mL/min/1.73 m^2) = (0.55 • Ht)/S_{Cr}, where Ht is in cm and S_{Cr} is in mg/dL].[130]

EXAMPLE 1 ▶ ▶ ▶

MM is a 3-day-old, 1015-g male premature infant (gestational age ~29 weeks) with suspected MRSA sepsis. His serum creatinine is 1.1 mg/dL. Compute an initial vancomycin dose for this patient.

1. *Compute initial dose and dosage interval.*
   From the pediatrics dosage recommendations given in earlier in this chapter, a patient in this age and renal function category should receive vancomycin 15 mg/kg every 24 hours. (Note: Grams will be converted to kilograms before the computation is made.)

$$Dose = 15\ mg/kg(1.015\ kg) = 15\ mg$$

The prescribed dose will be 15 mg every 24 hours.

USE OF VANCOMYCIN SERUM CONCENTRATIONS TO ALTER DOSAGES

Because of pharmacokinetic variability among patients, it is likely that doses calculated using patient population characteristics will not always produce vancomycin serum concentrations that are expected. Because of this, vancomycin serum concentrations are measured in most patients to ensure that therapeutic, nontoxic levels are present. However, some patients may not require serum concentration monitoring. For example, if it is expected that only a limited number of doses will be administered as is the case for surgical prophylaxis, vancomycin serum concentration monitoring may not be necessary. In addition to vancomycin concentrations, important patient parameters (fever curves, white blood cell counts, serum creatinine concentrations, etc) should be followed to confirm that the patient is responding to treatment and not developing adverse drug reactions.

When vancomycin serum concentrations are measured in patients and a dosage change is necessary, clinicians should seek to use the simplest, most straightforward method available to determine a dose that will provide safe and effective treatment. In most cases, a simple dosage ratio can be used to change vancomycin doses as these antibiotics follow *linear pharmacokinetics*. If only steady-state trough concentrations are being measured in a patient, a variant of linear pharmacokinetics can be used to perform *trough-only* dosage adjustments. The trough-only and linear pharmacokinetic methods can be combined for situations where only a dose or dosage interval alone cannot achieve the desired trough concentration.

In difficult dosage situations, both a steady-state peak and trough can be measured to assist in the dosage adjustment. Sometimes, it is not possible to simply change the dose, and the dosage interval must also be changed to achieve desired serum concentrations. In this case, it may be possible to use *pharmacokinetic concepts* to alter the vancomycin dose. In some situations, it may be necessary to compute the vancomycin pharmacokinetic parameters for the patient using the *One-Compartment Model Parameter method* and use these to calculate the best drug dose. Note that the previous two methods require both steady-state peak and trough values. Some clinicians are using individualized *area under the concentration-time curve* determinations to adjust vancomycin doses. Finally, computerized methods that incorporate expected population pharmacokinetic characteristics (*Bayesian pharmacokinetic computer programs*) can be used in difficult cases where renal function is changing, serum concentrations are obtained at suboptimal times, or the patient was not at steady state when serum concentrations were measured. If trough-only monitoring is being conducted for a patient, Bayesian computer programs can provide estimates for all vancomycin pharmacokinetic parameters even though only one serum concentration was measured. Bayesian pharmacokinetic computer programs can also be used to individualize AUC values.

Linear Pharmacokinetics Method

Because vancomycin antibiotics follow linear, dose-proportional pharmacokinetics, steady-state serum concentrations change in proportion to dose according to the following equation: $D_{new}/C_{ss,new} = D_{old}/C_{ss,old}$ or $D_{new} = (C_{ss,new}/C_{ss,old})D_{old}$, where D is the dose, Css is the steady-state peak or trough concentration, old indicates the dose that produced the steady-state concentration that the patient is currently receiving, and new denotes the dose necessary to produce the desired steady-state concentration. The advantage of this method is that it is quick and simple. The disadvantage is that steady-state concentrations are required, and it may not be possible to attain desired serum concentrations by only changing the dose.

EXAMPLE 1 ▶ ▶ ▶

JM is a 50-year-old, 70-kg (height = 5 ft 11 in) male with an MRSA pneumonia. His current serum creatinine is 0.9 mg/dL, and it has been stable over the last 5 days since admission. A vancomycin dose of 1000 mg every 12 hours was prescribed and expected to achieve steady-state peak and trough concentrations equal to 35 µg/mL and 15 µg/mL, respectively. After the third dose, steady-state peak and trough concentrations were measured and equaled 22 µg/mL and 10 µg/mL, respectively. Calculate a new vancomycin dose that would provide a steady-state trough of 15 µg/mL.

1. *Estimate creatinine clearance.*

    This patient has a stable serum creatinine and is not obese. The Cockcroft-Gault equation can be used to estimate creatinine clearance:

    $$CrCl_{est} = [(140 - age)BW]/(72 \cdot S_{Cr}) = [(140 - 50 \text{ y})70 \text{ kg}]/(72 \cdot 0.9 \text{ mg/dL})$$
    $$CrCl_{est} = 97 \text{ mL/min}$$

2. *Estimate elimination rate constant (k_e) and half-life ($t_{1/2}$).*

    The vancomycin clearance versus creatinine clearance relationship is used to estimate drug clearance for this patient:

    $$Cl = 0.695(CrCl) + 0.05 = 0.695[(97 \text{ mL/min})/70 \text{ kg}] + 0.05 = 1.013 \text{ mL/min/kg}$$

    The average volume of distribution for vancomycin is 0.7 L/kg:

    $$V = 0.7 \text{ L/kg} \cdot 70 \text{ kg} = 49 \text{ L}$$
    $$k_e = Cl/V = (1.013 \text{ mL/min/kg} \cdot 60 \text{ min/h})/(0.7 \text{ L/kg} \cdot 1000 \text{ mL/L}) = 0.0868 \text{ h}^{-1}$$
    $$t_{1/2} = 0.693/k_e = 0.693/0.0868 \text{ h}^{-1} = 8 \text{ h}$$

    Because the patient has been receiving vancomycin for ~3 estimated half-lives, it is likely that the measured serum concentrations are steady-state values.

3. *Compute new dose to achieve desired serum concentration.*

    Using linear pharmacokinetics, the new dose to attain the desired concentration should be proportional to the old dose that produced the measured concentration:

    $$D_{new} = (C_{ss,new}/C_{ss,old})D_{old} = (15 \text{ µg/mL} /10 \text{ µg/mL})1000 \text{ mg} = 1500 \text{ mg}$$

    The new suggested dose would be 1500 mg every 12 hours to be started at the next scheduled dosing time.

4. *Check steady-state peak concentration for new dosage regimen.*

    Using linear pharmacokinetics, the new steady-state concentration can be estimated and should be proportional to the old dose that produced the measured concentration:

    $$C_{ss,new} = (D_{new}/D_{old})C_{ss,old} = (1500 \text{ mg}/1000 \text{ mg}) 22 \text{ µg/mL} = 33 \text{ µg/mL}$$

    This steady-state peak concentration should be safe and effective for the infection that is being treated.

EXAMPLE 2 ▶ ▶ ▶

ZW is a 35-year-old, 150-kg (height = 5 ft 5 in) female with an enterococcal endocarditis. Her current serum creatinine is 1.1 mg/dL and is stable. A vancomycin dose of 1000 mg every 8 hours was prescribed and expected to achieve a steady-state trough concentration equal to 20 µg/mL. After the fifth dose, a steady-state trough concentration was measured and equaled 14 µg/mL. Calculate a new vancomycin dose that would provide a steady-state trough of 20 µg/mL.

1. *Estimate creatinine clearance.*

    This patient has a stable serum creatinine and is obese [$IBW_{females}$ (in kg) = 45 + 2.3(Ht − 60) = 45 + 2.3 (65 in − 60) = 57 kg]. The Salazar-Corcoran equation can be used to estimate creatinine clearance:

    $$CrCl_{est(females)} = \frac{(146 - age)[(0.287 \cdot Wt) + (9.74 \cdot Ht^2)]}{(60 \cdot S_{Cr})}$$

$$CrCl_{est(females)} = \frac{(146 - 35\ y)\{(0.287 \cdot 150\ kg) + [9.74 \cdot (1.65\ m)^2]\}}{(60 \cdot 1.1\ mg/dL)} = 117\ mL/min$$

Note: Height is converted from inches to meters: Ht = (65 in · 2.54 cm/in)/(100 cm/m) = 1.65 m.

2. *Estimate elimination rate constant (k_e) and half-life ($t_{1/2}$).*
   The vancomycin clearance versus creatinine clearance relationship is used to estimate drug clearance for this patient:

$$Cl = 0.695(CrCl) + 0.05 = 0.695[(117\ mL/min)/150\ kg] + 0.05 = 0.592\ mL/min/kg$$

The average volume of distribution for vancomycin is 0.7 L/kg IBW:

$$V = 0.7\ L/kg \cdot 57\ kg = 40\ L$$

$$k_e = Cl/V = (0.592\ mL/min/kg \cdot 150\ kg \cdot 60\ min/h)/(0.7\ L/kg \cdot 57\ kg \cdot 1000\ mL/L) = 0.134\ h^{-1}$$

$$t_{1/2} = 0.693/k_e = 0.693/0.134\ h^{-1} = 5.2\ h$$

Because the patient has been receiving vancomycin for more than 3-5 estimated half-lives, it is likely that the measured serum concentrations are steady-state values.

3. *Compute new dose to achieve desired serum concentration.*
   Using linear pharmacokinetics, the new dose to attain the desired concentration should be proportional to the old dose that produced the measured concentration:

$$D_{new} = (C_{ss,new}/C_{ss,old})D_{old} = (20\ \mu g/mL\ /\ 14\ \mu g/mL)\ 1000\ mg = 1429\ mg, \text{round to } 1500\ mg$$

The new suggested dose would be 1500 mg every 8 hours to be started at the next scheduled dosing time.

Trough-Only Method

Many clinicians adjust vancomycin doses based solely on a measurement of a steady-state trough concentration. When using this method, a typical dose of vancomycin is prescribed for the patient based on their pharmacokinetic and clinical characteristics, a steady-state trough concentration is measured, and the dosage interval is modified to attain the desired concentration. A straightforward way of accomplishing this is to use a simplified relationship between the steady-state trough concentration and the dosage interval[131]: $\tau_{new} = (C_{ss,old}/C_{ss,new})\tau_{old}$, where $C_{ss,old}$ and $C_{ss,new}$ are the original measured and new desired steady-state trough concentrations, respectively; and τ_{old} and τ_{new} are the original and new dosage intervals, respectively. New dosage intervals are rounded to clinically acceptable values (8, 12, 18, 24, 36, 48, 72 hours, and multiples of 24 hours thereafter, whenever possible), and the original dose is retained.

Because the dosage interval computation involves a simplification (eg, steady-state concentrations vary according to the inverse of the dosage interval), the actual new steady-state trough concentration should be slightly higher than that calculated if a shorter dosage interval is used or slightly lower than that calculated if a longer dosage interval is used. However, this method produces steady-state trough concentrations that are usually within 1-2 µg/mL of those computed using more sophisticated Bayesian computer methods.[131] This method can be combined with the Linear Pharmacokinetics method to adjust both the dose and dosage interval, when necessary. Combining the two methods is useful when a clinically acceptable solution cannot be achieved by changing the dose alone or the dosage interval alone.

EXAMPLE 1 ▶ ▶ ▶

UI is a 55-year-old, 78-kg (height = 6 ft 1 in) male with an MRSA pneumonia. His current serum creatinine is 1.5 mg/dL, and it has been stable over the last 3 days since admission. A vancomycin dose of 1000 mg every 24 hours was prescribed and expected to achieve a steady-state trough concentration equal to 15 μg/mL. After the second dose, the steady-state trough concentration equaled 7 μg/mL. Calculate a new vancomycin dose that would provide a steady-state trough of 15 μg/mL.

1. *Estimate creatinine clearance.*

    This patient has a stable serum creatinine and is not obese. The Cockcroft-Gault equation can be used to estimate creatinine clearance:

$$CrCl_{est} = [(140 - age)BW]/(72 \cdot S_{Cr}) = [(140 - 55\ y)78\ kg]/(72 \cdot 1.5\ mg/dL)$$

$$CrCl_{est} = 61\ mL/min$$

2. *Estimate elimination rate constant (k_e) and half-life ($t_{1/2}$).*

    The vancomycin clearance versus creatinine clearance relationship is used to estimate drug clearance for this patient:

$$Cl = 0.695(CrCl) + 0.05 = 0.695[(61\ mL/min)/78\ kg] + 0.05 = 0.594\ mL/min/kg$$

The average volume of distribution for vancomycin is 0.7 L/kg:

$$V = 0.7\ L/kg \cdot 78\ kg = 55\ L$$

$$k_e = Cl/V = (0.594\ mL/min/kg \cdot 60\ min/h)/(0.7\ L/kg \cdot 1000\ mL/L) = 0.0509\ h^{-1}$$

$$t_{1/2} = 0.693/k_e = 0.693/0.0509\ h^{-1} = 13.6\ h$$

Because the patient has been receiving vancomycin for more than 3 estimated half-lives, it is likely that the measured serum concentrations are steady-state values.

3. *Compute new dosage interval to achieve desired serum concentration.*

    The new dosage interval to attain the desired concentration should be:

$$\tau_{new} = (C_{ss,old}/C_{ss,new})\tau_{old} = (7\ \mu g/mL /15\ \mu g/mL)24\ h = 11\ h,\ round\ to\ 12\ h$$

Dosage intervals should be rounded to clinically acceptable intervals of 8, 12, 18, 24, 36, 48, 72 hours, and multiples of 24 hours thereafter, whenever possible. In this case, the dosage interval would be rounded to 12 hours. The new suggested dose would be 1000 mg every 12 hours to be started 12 hours after the last dose.

EXAMPLE 2 ▶ ▶ ▶

ZW is a 35-year-old, 150 kg (height = 5 ft 5 in), female with an enterococcal endocarditis. Her current serum creatinine is 1.1 mg/dL and is stable. A vancomycin dose of 1250 mg every 12 hours was prescribed and expected to achieve a steady-state trough concentration equal to 20 μg/mL. After the third dose, a steady-state concentration was measured and equaled 12 μg/mL. Calculate a new vancomycin dose that would provide a steady-state trough of 20 μg/mL.

1. *Estimate creatinine clearance.*

    This patient has a stable serum creatinine and is obese [$IBW_{females}$ (in kg) = 45 + 2.3(Ht − 60) = 45 + 2.3 (65 in − 60) = 57 kg]. The Salazar-Corcoran equation can be used to estimate creatinine clearance:

$$CrCl_{est(females)} = \frac{(146 - age)[(0.287 \cdot Wt) + (9.74 \cdot Ht^2)]}{(60 \cdot S_{Cr})}$$

$$CrCl_{est(females)} = \frac{(146 - 35y)\{(0.287 \cdot 150\,kg) + [9.74 \cdot (1.65\,m)^2]\}}{(60 \cdot 1.1\,mg/dL)} = 117\,mL/min$$

Note: Height is converted from inches to meters: $Ht = (65\,in \cdot 2.54\,cm/in)/(100\,cm/m) = 1.65\,m$.

2. *Estimate elimination rate constant (k_e) and half-life ($t_{1/2}$).*
The vancomycin clearance versus creatinine clearance relationship is used to estimate drug clearance for this patient:

$$Cl = 0.695(CrCl) + 0.05 = 0.695[(117\,mL/min)/150\,kg] + 0.05 = 0.592\,mL/min/kg$$

The average volume of distribution for vancomycin is 0.7 L/kg IBW:

$$V = 0.7\,L/kg \cdot 57\,kg = 40\,L$$
$$k_e = Cl/V = (0.592\,mL/min/kg \cdot 150\,kg \cdot 60\,min/h)/(0.7\,L/kg \cdot 57\,kg \cdot 1000\,mL/L) = 0.134\,h^{-1}$$
$$t_{1/2} = 0.693/k_e = 0.693/0.134\,h^{-1} = 5.2\,h$$

Because the patient has been receiving vancomycin for more than 3–5 estimated half-lives, it is likely that the measured serum concentrations are steady-state values.

3. *Compute new dosage interval to achieve desired serum concentration.*
The new dosage interval to attain the desired concentration should be:

$$\tau_{new} = (C_{ss,old}/C_{ss,new})\tau_{old} = (12\,\mu g/mL /20\,\mu g/mL)12\,h = 7\,h, \text{ round to } 8\,h$$

The new suggested dose would be 1250 mg every 8 hours to be started 8 hours after the last dose. Note that a dosage interval less than 12 hours is chosen because the patient's expected half-life is very short.

EXAMPLE 3 ▶ ▶ ▶

IK is a 75-year-old, 62-kg (height = 5 ft 9 in) male with *S. epidermidis* sepsis. His current serum creatinine is 1.3 mg/dL, and it has been stable since admission. A vancomycin dose of 1000 mg every 24 hours was prescribed and expected to achieve a steady-state trough concentration equal to 15 µg/mL. After the third dose, a steady-state concentration was measured and equaled 6 µg/mL. Calculate a new vancomycin dose that would provide a steady-state trough of 15 µg/mL.

This patient requires a large change in concentration, and it will be difficult to attain the goal by changing only the dose or only the dosage interval. Combine the Linear Pharmacokinetic and Trough-Only methods to alter both the dose and dosage interval, respectively.

1. *Estimate creatinine clearance.*
This patient has a stable serum creatinine and is not obese. The Cockcroft-Gault equation can be used to estimate creatinine clearance:

$$CrCl_{est} = [(140 - age)BW]/(72 \cdot S_{Cr}) = [(140 - 75\,y)62\,kg]/(72 \cdot 1.3\,mg/dL)$$
$$CrCl_{est} = 43\,mL/min$$

2. *Estimate vancomycin clearance.*
The vancomycin clearance versus creatinine clearance relationship is used to estimate the vancomycin clearance for this patient:

$$Cl = 0.695(CrCl) + 0.05 = 0.695[(43\,mL/min)/62\,kg] + 0.05 = 0.533\,mL/min/kg$$

3. *Estimate vancomycin volume of distribution.*

The average volume of distribution for vancomycin is 0.7 L/kg:

$$V = 0.7 \text{ L/kg} \cdot 62 \text{ kg} = 43.4 \text{ L}$$

4. *Estimate vancomycin elimination rate constant (k_e) and half-life ($t_{1/2}$).*

$$k_e = Cl/V = (0.533 \text{ mL/min/kg} \cdot 60 \text{ min/h})/(0.7 \text{ L/kg} \cdot 1000 \text{ mL/L}) = 0.0457 \text{ h}^{-1}$$

$$t_{1/2} = 0.693/k_e = 0.693/0.0457 \text{ h}^{-1} = 15.2 \text{ h}$$

Because the patient has been receiving vancomycin for more than 3-5 estimated half-lives, it is likely that the measured serum concentration is a steady-state value.

5. *Compute new dose to achieve desired serum concentration*

Using linear pharmacokinetics, a new dose to attain a portion of the desired concentration change will be computed:

$$D_{new} = (C_{ss,new}/C_{ss,old})D_{old} = (9 \text{ μg/mL} /6 \text{ μg/mL}) \, 1000 \text{ mg} = 1500 \text{ mg}$$

The new dose would be 1500 mg every 24 hours.

6. *Compute new dosage interval to achieve desired serum concentration.*

The new dosage interval to attain the desired concentration should be:

$$\tau_{new} = (C_{ss,old}/C_{ss,new})\tau_{old} = (9 \text{ μg/mL}/ 15 \text{ μg/mL}) \, 24 \text{ h} = 14.4 \text{ h, round to 12 h}$$

The new suggested dose would be 1500 mg every 12 hours to be started 12 hours after the last dose.

Pharmacokinetic Concepts Method

As implied by the name, this technique derives alternative doses by estimating actual pharmacokinetic parameters or surrogates for pharmacokinetic parameters.[132] It is a very useful way to calculate drug doses when the Linear Pharmacokinetic method is not sufficient because a dosage change that will produce a proportional change in steady-state peak and trough concentrations is not appropriate. The only requirement is a steady-state peak and trough vancomycin serum concentration pair obtained before and after a dose (Figure 5-3). The following steps are used to compute new vancomycin doses:

1. *Draw a rough sketch of the serum log concentration/time curve by hand, keeping track of the relative time between the serum concentrations (see Figure 5-3).*
2. *Because the patient is at steady state, the trough concentration can be extrapolated to the next trough value time (see Figure 5-3).*
3. *Draw the elimination curve between the steady-state peak concentration and the extrapolated trough concentration. Use this line to estimate half-life.* For example, a patient receives a vancomycin dose of 1000 mg given every 12 hours that produces a steady-state peak equal to 25 μg/mL and a steady-state trough equal to 13 μg/mL, and the dose is infused over 1 hour and the peak concentration is drawn ½ hour later (see Figure 5-3). The time between the measured steady-state peak and the extrapolated trough concentration is 10.5 hours (the 12-hour dosage interval minus the 1.5-hour combined infusion and waiting time). The definition of half-life is the time needed for serum concentrations to decrease by ½. Because the serum concentration declined by approximately ½ from the peak concentration to the trough concentration, the vancomycin half-life for this patient is approximately 10.5 hours. This information will be used to set the new dosage interval for the patient.

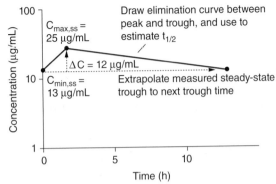

FIGURE 5-3   Graphical representation of the Pharmacokinetic Concepts method where a steady-state peak (Css_{max}) and trough (Css_{min}) concentration pair is used to individualize vancomycin therapy. Because the patient is at steady state, consecutive trough concentrations will be identical, so the trough concentration can be extrapolated to the next predose time. The change in concentration after a dose is given (ΔC) is a surrogate measure of the volume of distribution and will be used to compute the new dose for the patient.

4. *Determine the difference in concentration between the steady-state peak and trough concentrations. The difference in concentration will change proportionally with the dose size.* In the current example the patient is receiving a vancomycin dose equal to 1000 mg every 12 hours, which produced steady-state peak and trough concentrations of 25 µg/mL and 13 µg/mL, respectively. The difference between the peak and trough values is 12 µg/mL. The change in serum concentration is proportional to the dose, and this information will be used to set a new dose for the patient.

5. *Choose new steady-state peak and trough concentrations.* For the purposes of this example, the desired steady-state peak and trough concentrations will be approximately 30 µg/mL and 7 µg/mL, respectively.

6. *Determine the new dosage interval for the desired concentrations.* In this example, the patient has a desired peak concentration of 30 µg/mL. In 1 half-life, the serum concentration will decline to 15 µg/mL, and in an additional half-life the vancomycin concentration will decrease to 7.5 µg/mL (Figure 5-4). Because the approximate half-life is 10.5 hours and 2 half-lives are required for serum concentrations to decrease from the desired peak concentration to the desired trough concentration, the dosage interval should be 21 hours (10.5 hours × 2 half-lives). This value would be rounded off to the

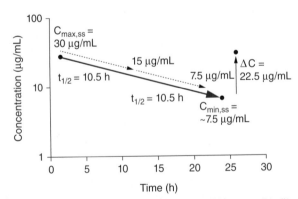

FIGURE 5-4   The Pharmacokinetic Concept method uses the estimated half-life to graphically compute the new dosage interval and the change in concentration to calculate the dose for a patient.

clinically acceptable value of 24 hours, and the actual trough concentration would be expected to be slightly lower than 7.5 µg/mL.

7. *Determine the new dose for the desired concentrations.* The desired peak concentration is 30 µg/mL, and the expected trough concentration is 7.5 µg/mL. The change in concentration between these values is 22.5 µg/mL. It is known from measured serum concentrations that administration of 1000 mg changes serum concentrations by 12 µg/mL and that the change in serum concentration between the peak and trough values is proportional to the size of the dose. Therefore, a simple ratio will be used to compute the required dose: $D_{new} = (\Delta C_{new}/\Delta C_{old})D_{old}$, where D_{new} and D_{old} are the new and old doses, respectively; ΔC_{new} is the change in concentration between the peak and trough for the new dose; and ΔC_{old} is the change in concentration between the peak and trough for the old dose. (Note: This relationship is appropriate because doses are given into a fixed, constant volume of distribution; it is not because the drug follows linear pharmacokinetics so this method will work whether the agent follows nonlinear or linear pharmacokinetics.) For this example: $D_{new} = (22.5 \text{ µg/mL} / 12 \text{ µg/mL}) 1000 \text{ mg} = 1875 \text{ mg}$, which would be rounded to 1750 mg. Vancomycin 1750 mg every 24 hours would be started 24 hours after the last dose of the previous dosage regimen.

Once this method is mastered, it can be used without the need for a calculator. The following are examples that use the Pharmacokinetic Concepts method to change vancomycin doses.

EXAMPLE 1 ▶ ▶ ▶

NE is a 50-year-old, 70-kg (height = 5 ft 10 in) male with a streptococcal (MIC = 0.25 µg/mL) wound infection of moderate severity. He is allergic to penicillins and cephalosporins. His current serum creatinine is 3.5 mg/dL, and it has been stable over the last 5 days since admission. A vancomycin dose of 800 mg every 24 hours was prescribed and expected to achieve steady-state peak and trough concentrations equal to 20 µg/mL and 5 µg/mL, respectively. After the fourth dose, steady-state peak and trough concentrations were measured and equaled 25 µg/mL and 12 µg/mL, respectively. Calculate a new vancomycin dose that would provide a steady-state peak of 20 µg/mL and a trough of 5 µg/mL.

1. *Estimate creatinine clearance.*

This patient has a stable serum creatinine and is not obese. The Cockcroft-Gault equation can be used to estimate creatinine clearance:

$$CrCl_{est} = [(140 - age)BW]/(72 \cdot S_{Cr}) = [(140 - 50 \text{ y})70 \text{ kg}]/(72 \cdot 3.5 \text{ mg/dL})$$

$$CrCl_{est} - 25 \text{ mL/min}$$

2. *Estimate elimination rate constant (k_e) and half-life ($t_{1/2}$).*

The vancomycin clearance versus creatinine clearance relationship is used to estimate drug clearance for this patient:

$$Cl = 0.695(CrCl) + 0.05 = 0.695[(25 \text{ mL/min})/70 \text{ kg}] + 0.05 = 0.298 \text{ mL/min/kg}$$

The average volume of distribution for vancomycin is 0.7 L/kg:

$$V = 0.7 \text{ L/kg} \cdot 70 \text{ kg} = 49 \text{ L}$$

$$k_e = Cl/V = (0.298 \text{ mL/min/kg} \cdot 60 \text{ min/h})/(0.7 \text{ L/kg} \cdot 1000 \text{ mL/L}) = 0.0255 \text{ h}^{-1}$$

$$t_{1/2} = 0.693/k_e = 0.693/0.0255 \text{ h}^{-1} = 27 \text{ h}$$

Because the patient has been receiving vancomycin for ~3 estimated half-lives, it is likely that the measured serum concentrations are close to steady-state values. This steady-state concentration pair can be used to compute the patient's own unique pharmacokinetic parameters that can be used to calculate individualized doses.

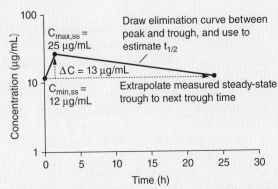

FIGURE 5-5 Graphical representation of the Pharmacokinetic Concept method where a steady-state peak (Css_{max}) and trough (Css_{min}) concentration pair is used to individualize vancomycin therapy. Because the patient is at steady state, consecutive trough concentrations will be identical, so the trough concentration can be extrapolated to the next predose time. The change in concentration after a dose is given (ΔC) is a surrogate measure of the volume of distribution and will be used to compute the new dose for the patient.

3. *Use Pharmacokinetics Concept method to compute a new dose.*
    a. *Draw a rough sketch of the serum log concentration/time curve by hand, keeping track of the relative time between the serum concentrations (Figure 5-5).*
    b. *Because the patient is at steady state, the trough concentration can be extrapolated to the next trough value time (see Figure 5–5).*
    c. *Draw the elimination curve between the steady-state peak concentration and the extrapolated trough concentration. Use this line to estimate half-life.* The patient is receiving a vancomycin dose of 800 mg given every 24 hours that produces a steady-state peak equal to 25 µg/mL and a steady-state trough equal to 12 µg/mL. The dose is infused over 1 hour and the peak concentration is drawn ½ hour later (see Figure 5-5). The time between the measured steady-state peak and the extrapolated trough concentration is 22.5 hours (the 24-hour dosage interval minus the 1.5-hour combined infusion and waiting time). The definition of half-life is the time needed for serum concentrations to decrease by ½. It would take 1 half-life for the peak serum concentration to decline from 25 to 12.5 µg/mL. The concentration of 12 µg/mL is very close to the extrapolated trough value of 12.5 µg/mL. Therefore, 1 half-life expired during the 22.5-hour time period between the peak concentration and extrapolated trough concentration, and the estimated half-life is 22.5 hours. This information will be used to set the new dosage interval for the patient.
    d. *Determine the difference in concentration between the steady-state peak and trough concentrations. The difference in concentration will change proportionally with the dose size.* In the current example, the patient is receiving a vancomycin dose equal to 800 mg every 24 hours, which produced steady-state peak and trough concentrations of 25 µg/mL and 12 µg/mL, respectively. The difference between the peak and trough values is 13 µg/mL. The change in serum concentration is proportional to the dose, and this information will be used to set a new dose for the patient.
    e. *Choose new steady-state peak and trough concentrations.* For the purposes of this example, the desired steady-state peak and trough concentrations will be 20 µg/mL and 5 µg/mL, respectively.
    f. *Determine the new dosage interval for the desired concentrations (Figure 5-6).* Using the desired concentrations, it will take 1 half-life for the peak concentration of 20 µg/mL to decrease to 10 µg/mL, and an

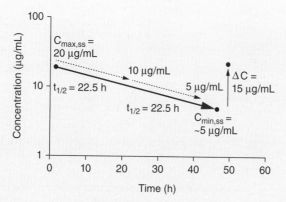

FIGURE 5-6   The Pharmacokinetic Concept method uses the estimated half-life to graphically compute the new dosage interval and the change in concentration to calculate the dose for a patient.

additional half-life for serum concentrations to decline from 10 to 5 μg/mL. Therefore, the dosage interval will need to be approximately 2 half-lives or 45 hours (22.5 hours × 2 half-live = 45 hours). This dosage interval would be rounded off to 48 hours.

g. *Determine the new dose for the desired concentrations (see Figure 5-6).* The desired peak concentration is 20 μg/mL, and the expected trough concentration is 5 μg/mL. The change in concentration between these values is 15 μg/mL. It is known from measured serum concentrations that administration of 800 mg changes serum concentrations by 13 μg/mL and that the change in serum concentration between the peak and trough values is proportional to the size of the dose. In this case: $D_{new} = (\Delta C_{new}/\Delta C_{old})D_{old} =$ (15 μg/mL / 13 μg/mL)800 mg = 923 mg, rounded to 1000 mg. Vancomycin 1000 mg every 48 hours would be started 48 hours after the last dose of the previous dosage regimen.

EXAMPLE 2 ▶▶▶

IA is a 35-year-old, 150-kg (height = 5′ 5″) female with a *S. epidermidis* (MIC = 0.5 μg/mL) wound infection. Her current serum creatinine is 1.1 mg/dL and is stable. A vancomycin dose of 2500 mg every 18 hours was prescribed and expected to achieve steady-state peak and trough concentrations equal to 30 μg/mL and 10 μg/mL, respectively. After the fifth dose, steady-state peak and trough concentrations were measured and were 40 μg/mL and 3 μg/mL, respectively. Calculate a new vancomycin dose that would provide a steady-state peak of 30 μg/mL and a steady-state trough 10 μg/mL.

1. *Estimate creatinine clearance.*

This patient has a stable serum creatinine and is obese [IBW$_{females}$ (in kg) = 45 + 2.3(Ht − 60) = 45 + 2.3 (65 in − 60) = 57 kg]) The Salazar-Corcoran equation can be used to estimate creatinine clearance:

$$CrCl_{est(females)} = \frac{(146 - age)[(0.287 \cdot Wt) + (9.74 \cdot Ht^2)]}{(60 \cdot SCr)}$$

$$CrCl_{est(females)} = \frac{(146 - 35y)\{(0.287 \cdot 150\ kg) + [9.74 \cdot (1.65\ m^2)]\}}{(60 \cdot 1.1\ mg/dL)} = 117\ mL/min$$

Note: Height is converted from inches to meters: Ht = (65 in • 2.54 cm/in)/(100 cm/m) = 1.65 m.

2. *Estimate elimination rate constant (k_e) and half-life ($t_{1/2}$).*

The vancomycin clearance versus creatinine clearance relationship is used to estimate drug clearance for this patient:

$$Cl = 0.695(CrCl) + 0.05 = 0.695[(117 \text{ mL/min})/150 \text{ kg}] + 0.05 = 0.592 \text{ mL/min/kg TBW}$$

The average volume of distribution for vancomycin is 0.7 L/kg IBW:

$$V = 0.7 \text{ L/kg} \cdot 57 \text{ kg} = 40 \text{ L}$$

$$k_e = Cl/V = (0.592 \text{ mL/min/kg TBW} \cdot 150 \text{ kg} \cdot 60 \text{ min/h})/(0.7 \text{ L/kg IBW} \cdot 57 \text{ kg} \cdot 1000 \text{ mL/L}) = 0.134 \text{ h}^{-1}$$

$$t_{1/2} = 0.693/k_e = 0.693/0.134 \text{ h}^{-1} = 5.2 \text{ h}$$

Because the patient has been receiving vancomycin for more than 5 estimated half-lives, it is likely that the measured serum concentrations are steady-state values.

3. *Use Pharmacokinetics Concept method to compute a new dose.*

  a. *Draw a rough sketch of the serum log concentration/time curve by hand, keeping track of the relative time between the serum concentrations (Figure 5-7).*

  b. *Because the patient is at steady state, the trough concentration can be extrapolated to the next trough value time (see Figure 5-7).*

  c. *Draw the elimination curve between the steady-state peak concentration and the extrapolated trough concentration. Use this line to estimate half-life.* The patient is receiving a vancomycin dose of 2500 mg given every 12 hours that produces a steady-state peak equal to 40 µg/mL and a steady-state trough equal to 3 µg/mL. The dose is infused over 1 hour and the peak concentration is drawn ½ hour later (see Figure 5-7). The time between the measured steady-state peak and the extrapolated trough concentration is 16.5 hours (the 18-hour dosage interval minus the 1.5-hour combined infusion and waiting time). The definition of half-life is the time needed for serum concentrations to decrease by ½. It would take 1 half-life for the peak serum concentration to decline from 40 to 20 µg/mL, another half-life to decrease from 20 to 10 µg/mL, an additional half-life to decrease from 10 to 5 µg/mL, and a final half-life to decrease from 5 to 2.5 µg/mL.

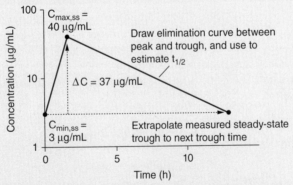

FIGURE 5-7   Graphical representation of the Pharmacokinetic Concept method where a steady-state peak (Css_{max}) and trough (Css_{min}) concentration pair is used to individualize vancomycin therapy. Because the patient is at steady state, consecutive trough concentrations will be identical, so the trough concentration can be extrapolated to the next predose time. The change in concentration after a dose is given (ΔC) is a surrogate measure of the volume of distribution and will be used to compute the new dose for the patient.

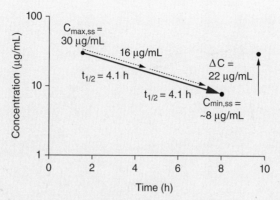

FIGURE 5-8 The Pharmacokinetic Concept method uses the estimated half-life to graphically compute the new dosage interval and the change in concentration to calculate the dose for a patient.

The concentration of 3 µg/mL is very close to the extrapolated trough value of 2.5 µg/mL. Therefore, 4 half-lives expired during the 16.5-hour time period between the peak concentration and extrapolated trough concentration, and the estimated half-life is 4.1 hours (16.5 hours/4 half-lives = 4.1 hours). This information will be used to set the new dosage interval for the patient

d. *Determine the difference in concentration between the steady-state peak and trough concentrations. The difference in concentration will change proportionally with the dose size.* In the current example the patient is receiving a vancomycin dose equal to 2500 mg every 18 hours, which produced steady-state peak and trough concentrations of 40 µg/mL and 3 µg/mL, respectively. The difference between the peak and trough values is 37 µg/mL. The change in serum concentration is proportional to the dose, and this information will be used to set a new dose for the patient.

e. *Choose new steady-state peak and trough concentrations.* For the purposes of this example, the desired steady-state peak and trough concentrations will be 30 µg/mL and 10 µg/mL, respectively.

f. *Determine the new dosage interval for the desired concentrations (Figure 5-8).* Using the desired concentrations, it will take 1 half-life for the peak concentration of 30 µg/mL to decrease to 15 µg/mL, and an additional half-life for serum concentrations to decline from 15 to 8 µg/mL. This concentration is close to the desired trough concentration of 10 µg/mL. Therefore, the dosage interval will need to be approximately 2 half-lives or 8.2 hours (4.1 hours × 2 half-live = 8.2 hours). This dosage interval would be rounded off to 8 hours.

g. *Determine the new dose for the desired concentrations (see Figure 5-8).* The desired peak concentration is 30 µg/mL, and the expected trough concentration is 8 µg/mL. The change in concentration between these values is 22 µg/mL. It is known from measured serum concentrations that administration of 2500 mg changes serum concentrations by 37 µg/mL and that the change in serum concentration between the peak and trough values is proportional to the size of the dose. In this case: $D_{new} = (\Delta C_{new}/\Delta C_{old})D_{old} = $ (22 µg/mL / 37 µg/mL)2500 mg = 1486 mg, rounded to 1500 mg. Vancomycin 1500 mg every 8 hours would be started 8 hours after the last dose of the previous dosage regimen.

One-Compartment Model Parameter Method

The One-Compartment Model Parameter method of adjusting drug doses was among the first techniques available to change doses using serum concentrations.[133] It allows the computation of an individual's own, unique pharmacokinetic constants and uses those to calculate a dose that achieves desired vancomycin concentrations. The standard One-Compartment Model Parameter method conducts a small pharmacokinetic experiment using

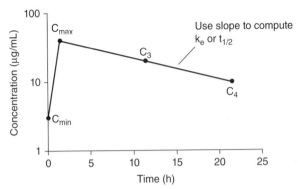

FIGURE 5-9   The One-Compartment Model Parameter method for individualization of vancomycin doses uses a trough (C_{min}), peak (C_{max}), and one to two additional postdose concentrations (C_3, C_4) to compute a patient's own, unique pharmacokinetic parameters. This version of the One-Compartment Model Parameter method does not require steady-state conditions. The peak and trough concentrations are used to calculate the volume of distribution, and the postdose concentrations (C_{max}, C_3, C_4) are used to compute half-life. Once volume of distribution and half-life have been measured, they can be used to compute the exact dose needed to achieve desired vancomycin concentrations.

three to four vancomycin serum concentrations obtained during a dosage interval and does not require steady-state conditions. The Steady-State One-Compartment Model Parameter method assumes that steady-state has been achieved and requires only a steady-state peak and trough concentration pair obtained before and after a dose. One-compartment model intravenous bolus equations are used successfully to dose drugs that are given by infusion when the infusion time is less than the drug half-life.[126]

Standard One-Compartment Model Parameter Method

The standard version of the One-Compartment Model Parameter method does not require steady-state concentrations. A trough vancomycin concentration is obtained before a dose, a peak vancomycin concentration is obtained after the dose is infused (½-1 hour after a 1-hour infusion), and one to two additional postdose serum vancomycin concentrations are obtained (Figure 5-9). Ideally, the one to two postdose concentrations should be obtained at least 1 estimated half-life from each other to minimize the influence of assay error. The postdose serum concentrations are used to calculate the vancomycin elimination rate constant and half-life (see Figure 5-9). The half-life can be computed by graphing the postdose concentrations on semilogrithmic paper, drawing the best straight line through the data points, and determining the time needed for serum concentrations to decline by one-half. Once the half-life is known, the elimination rate constant (k_e) can be computed: $k_e = 0.693/t_{1/2}$. Alternatively, the elimination rate constant can be directly calculated using the postdose serum concentrations [$k_e = (\ln C_1 - \ln C_2)/\Delta t$, where C_1 and C_2 are postdose serum concentrations and Δt is the time that expired between the times that C_1 and C_2 were obtained], and the half-life can be computed using the elimination rate constant ($t_{1/2} = 0.693/k_e$). The volume of distribution (V) is calculated using the following equation: $V = D/(C_{max} - C_{min})$ where D is the vancomycin dose, C_{max} is the peak concentration and C_{min} is the trough concentration. The elimination rate constant and volume of distribution measured in this fashion are the patient's own, unique vancomycin pharmacokinetic constants and can be used in one-compartment model intravenous bolus equations to compute the required dose to achieve any desired serum concentration.

Steady-State One-Compartment Model Parameter Method

If a steady-state peak and trough vancomycin concentration pair is available for a patient, the One-Compartment Model Parameter method can be used to compute patient pharmacokinetic parameters and vancomycin doses

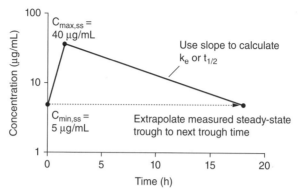

FIGURE 5-10   The steady-state version of the One-Compartment Model Parameter method uses a steady-state peak (Css$_{max}$) and trough (Css$_{min}$) concentration pair to individualize vancomycin therapy. Because the patient is at steady state, consecutive trough concentrations will be identical, so the trough concentration can be extrapolated to the next predose time. The steady-state peak and trough concentrations are used to calculate the volume of distribution and half-life. Once volume of distribution and half-life have been measured, they can be used to compute the exact dose needed to achieve desired vancomycin concentrations. This extrapolation approach can also be used to compute the steady-state AUC.

(Figure 5-10). Because the patient is at steady state, the measured trough concentration obtained before the dose was given can be extrapolated to the next dosage time and used to compute the vancomycin elimination rate constant [$k_e = (\ln Css_{max} - \ln Css_{min})/(\tau - t')$, where Css$_{max}$ and Css$_{min}$ are the steady-state peak and trough serum concentrations, respectively, and t' and τ are the infusion time and dosage interval, respectively], and the half-life can be computed using the elimination rate constant ($t_{1/2} = 0.693/k_e$). The volume of distribution (V) is calculated using the following equation: $V = D/(Css_{max} - Css_{min})$ where D is the vancomycin dose, Css$_{max}$ is the steady-state peak concentration, and Css$_{min}$ is the steady-state trough concentration. The elimination rate constant and volume of distribution measured in this way are the patient's own, unique vancomycin pharmacokinetic constants and can be used in one-compartment model intravenous bolus equations to compute the required dose to achieve any desired serum concentration. The dosage calculations are similar to those done in the initial dosage section of this chapter, except that the patient's real pharmacokinetic parameters are used in the equations instead of population pharmacokinetic estimates.

To illustrate the similarities and differences between the Pharmacokinetic Concepts and the One-Compartment Model Parameter methods, some of the same cases used in the previous section will be used as examples here.

EXAMPLE 1 ▶▶▶

NE is a 50-year-old, 70-kg (height = 5 ft 10 in) male with a streptococcal (MIC = 0.25 µg/mL) wound infection of moderate severity. He is allergic to penicillins and cephalosporins. His current serum creatinine is 3.5 mg/dL, and it has been stable over the last 5 days since admission. A vancomycin dose of 800 mg every 24 hours was prescribed and expected to achieve steady-state peak and trough concentrations equal to 20 µg/mL and 5 µg/mL, respectively. After the fourth dose, steady-state peak and trough concentrations were measured and were 25 µg/mL and 12 µg/mL, respectively. Calculate a new vancomycin dose that would provide a steady-state peak of 20 µg/mL and a trough of 5 µg/mL.

1. *Estimate creatinine clearance.*

   This patient has a stable serum creatinine and is not obese. The Cockcroft-Gault equation can be used to estimate creatinine clearance:

   $$CrCl_{est} = [(140 - age)BW]/(72 \cdot S_{Cr}) = [(140 - 50 \text{ y})70 \text{ kg}]/(72 \cdot 3.5 \text{ mg/dL})$$

   $$CrCl_{est} = 25 \text{ mL/min}$$

2. *Estimate elimination rate constant (k_e) and half-life ($t_{1/2}$).*

   The vancomycin clearance versus creatinine clearance relationship is used to estimate drug clearance for this patient:

   $$Cl = 0.695(CrCl) + 0.05 = 0.695[(25 \text{ mL/min})/70 \text{ kg}] + 0.05 = 0.298 \text{ mL/min/kg}$$

   The average volume of distribution for vancomycin is 0.7 L/kg:

   $$V = 0.7 \text{ L/kg} \cdot 70 \text{ kg} = 49 \text{ L}$$

   $$k_e = Cl/V = (0.298 \text{ mL/min/kg} \cdot 60 \text{ min/h})/(0.7 \text{ L/kg} \cdot 1000 \text{ mL/L}) = 0.0255 \text{ h}^{-1}$$

   $$t_{1/2} = 0.693/k_e = 0.693/0.0255 \text{ h}^{-1} = 27 \text{ h}$$

   Because the patient has been receiving vancomycin for ~3 estimated half-lives, it is likely that the measured serum concentrations are close to steady-state values. This steady-state concentration pair can be used to compute the patient's own unique pharmacokinetic parameters that can be used to calculate individualized doses.

3. *Use One-Compartment Model Parameter method to compute a new dose.*

   a. *Compute the patient's elimination rate constant and half-life. (Note: t′ = infusion time + waiting time of 1 hour and ½ hour, respectively.)*

   $$k_e = (\ln Css_{max} - \ln Css_{min})/(\tau - t') = (\ln 25 \text{ µg/mL} - \ln 12 \text{ µg/mL})/(24 \text{ h} - 1.5 \text{ h}) = 0.0326 \text{ h}^{-1}$$

   $$t_{1/2} = 0.693/k_e = 0.693/0.0326 \text{ h}^{-1} = 21.2 \text{ h}$$

   b. *Compute the patient's volume of distribution.*

   $$V = D/(Css_{max} - Css_{min}) = 800 \text{ mg}/(25 \text{ mg/L} - 12 \text{ mg/L}) = 61.5 \text{ L}$$

   c. *Choose new steady-state peak and trough concentrations.* For the purposes of this example, the desired steady-state peak and trough concentrations will be 20 µg/mL and 5 µg/mL, respectively.

   d. *Determine the new dosage interval for the desired concentrations.* As in the initial dosage section of this chapter, the dosage interval (τ) is computed using the following equation:

   $$\tau = (\ln Css_{max} - \ln Css_{min})/k_e = (\ln 20 \text{ µg/mL} - \ln 5 \text{ µg/mL})/0.0326 \text{ h}^{-1} = 42 \text{ h, rounded to 48 h}$$

   e. *Determine the new dose for the desired concentrations.* The dose is computed using the one-compartment model intravenous bolus equation used in the initial dosing section of this chapter:

   $$D = Css_{max} V(1 - e^{-k_e \tau}) = 20 \text{ mg/L} \cdot 61.5 \text{ L} [1 - e^{-(0.0326 \text{ h}^{-1})(48 \text{ h})}] = 974 \text{ mg, rounded to 1000 mg}$$

   A dose of vancomycin 1000 mg every 48 hours would be prescribed to begin 48 hours after the last dose of the previous regimen. This dose is identical to that derived for the patient using the Pharmacokinetic Concepts method.

EXAMPLE 2 ▶▶▶

IA is a 35-year-old, 150-kg (height = 5 ft 5 in) female with a *S. epidermidis* (MIC = 0.5 μg/mL) wound infection. Her current serum creatinine is 1.1 mg/dL and is stable. A vancomycin dose of 2500 mg every 18 hours was prescribed and expected to achieve steady-state peak and trough concentrations equal to 30 μg/mL and 10 μg/mL, respectively. After the fifth dose, steady-state peak and trough concentrations were measured and were 40 μg/mL and 3 μg/mL, respectively. Calculate a new vancomycin dose that would provide a steady-state peak of 30 μg/mL and a steady-state trough 10 μg/mL.

1. *Estimate creatinine clearance.*

   This patient has a stable serum creatinine and is obese [IBW$_{females}$ (in kg) = 45 + 2.3(Ht − 60) = 45 + 2.3 (65 in − 60) = 57 kg]. The Salazar-Corcoran equation can be used to estimate creatinine clearance:

   $$CrCl_{est(females)} = \frac{(146 - age)[(0.287 \cdot Wt) + (9.74 \cdot Ht^2)]}{(60 \cdot S_{Cr})}$$

   $$CrCl_{est(females)} = \frac{(146 - 35\ y)\{(0.287 \cdot 150\ kg) + [9.74 \cdot (1.65\ m)^2]\}}{(60 \cdot 1.1\ mg/dL)} = 117\ mL/min$$

   Note: Height is converted from inches to meters: Ht = (65 in · 2.54 cm/in)/(100 cm/m) = 1.65 m.

2. *Estimate elimination rate constant (k_e) and half-life ($t_{1/2}$).*

   The vancomycin clearance versus creatinine clearance relationship is used to estimate drug clearance for this patient:

   $$Cl = 0.695(CrCl) + 0.05 = 0.695[(117\ mL/min)/150\ kg] + 0.05 = 0.592\ mL/min/kg\ TBW$$

   The average volume of distribution for vancomycin is 0.7 L/kg IBW:

   $$V = 0.7\ L/kg \cdot 57\ kg = 40\ L$$

   $$k_e = Cl/V = (0.592\ mL/min/kg\ TBW \cdot 150\ kg \cdot 60\ min/h)/(0.7\ L/kg\ IBW \cdot 57\ kg \cdot 1000\ mL/L) = 0.134\ h^{-1}$$

   $$t_{1/2} = 0.693/k_e = 0.693/0.134\ h^{-1} = 5.2\ h$$

   Because the patient has been receiving vancomycin for more than 5 estimated half-lives, it is likely that the measured serum concentrations are steady-state values.

3. *Use One-Compartment Model Parameter method to compute a new dose.*

   a. *Compute the patient's elimination rate constant and half-life. (Note: assumed infusion time and waiting time are 1 hour and ½ hour, respectively.)*

   $$k_e = (\ln Css_{max} - \ln Css_{min})/(\tau - t') = (\ln 40\ \mu g/mL - \ln 3\ \mu g/mL)/(18\ h - 1.5\ h) = 0.157\ h^{-1}$$

   $$t_{1/2} = 0.693/k_e = 0.693/0.157\ h^{-1} = 4.4\ h$$

   b. *Compute the patient's volume of distribution.*

   $$V = D/(Css_{max} - Css_{min}) = 2500\ mg/(40\ mg/L - 3\ mg/L) = 67.6\ L$$

   c. *Choose new steady-state peak and trough concentrations.* For the purposes of this example, the desired steady-state peak and trough concentrations will be 30 μg/mL and 10 μg/mL, respectively.

   d. *Determine the new dosage interval for the desired concentrations.* As in the initial dosage section of this chapter, the dosage interval (τ) is computed using the following equation:

   $$\tau = (\ln Css_{max} - \ln Css_{min})/k_e = (\ln 30\ \mu g/mL - \ln 10\ \mu g/mL)/0.157\ h^{-1} = 7\ h, \text{rounded to } 8\ h$$

e. *Determine the new dose for the desired concentrations.* The dose is computed using the one-compartment model intravenous bolus equation used in the initial dosing section of this chapter:

$$D = Css_{max} V(1 - e^{-k_e\tau}) = 30 \text{ mg/L} \cdot 67.6 \text{ L } [1 - e^{-(0.157 \text{ h}^{-1})(8 \text{ h})}] = 1450 \text{ mg, rounded to } 1500 \text{ mg}$$

A dose of vancomycin 1500 mg every 8 hours would be prescribed to begin 8 hours after the last dose of the previous regimen. This dose is identical to that derived for the patient using the Pharmacokinetic Concepts method.

EXAMPLE 3 ▶▶▶

JH is a 24-year-old, 70-kg (height = 6 ft 0 in) male with MRSA (MIC = 0.5 µg/mL) wound infection. His current serum creatinine is 1.0 mg/dL, and it has been stable over the last 7 days since admission. A vancomycin dose of 1000 mg every 12 hours was prescribed. After the third dose, the following vancomycin serum concentrations were obtained:

Time	Vancomycin Concentration (µg/mL)
0800 H	2.0
0800–0900 H	Vancomycin 1000 mg
1000 H	18.0
1500 H	10.1
2000 H	5.7

Medication administration sheets were checked, and the previous dose was given 2 hours early (1800 H the previous day). Because of this, it is known that the patient is not at steady state. Calculate a new vancomycin dose that would provide a steady-state peak of 30 µg/mL and a trough of 10 µg/mL.

1. *Use One-Compartment Model Parameter method to compute a new dose.*

    a. *Plot serum concentration/time data (Figure 5-11). Because serum concentrations decrease in a straight line, use any two postdose concentrations to compute the patient's elimination rate constant and half-life. Compute the patient's elimination rate constant and half-life.*

$$k_e = (\ln C_{max} - \ln C_{min})/\Delta t = (\ln 18 \text{ µg/mL} - \ln 5.7 \text{ µg/mL})/(10 \text{ h}) = 0.115 \text{ h}^{-1}$$
$$t_{1/2} = 0.693/k_e = 0.693/0.115 \text{ h}^{-1} = 6 \text{ h}$$

    b. *Compute the patient's volume of distribution.*

$$V = D/(C_{max} - C_{min}) = 1000 \text{ mg}/(18 \text{ mg/L} - 2.0 \text{ mg/L}) = 62.5 \text{ L}$$

    c. *Choose new steady-state peak and trough concentrations.* For the purposes of this example, the desired steady-state peak and trough concentrations will be 30 µg/mL and 10 µg/mL, respectively.

    d. *Determine the new dosage interval for the desired concentrations.* As in the initial dosage section of this chapter, the dosage interval (τ) is computed using the following equation:

$$\tau = (\ln Css_{max} - \ln Css_{min})/k_e = (\ln 30 \text{ µg/mL} - \ln 10 \text{ µg/mL})/0.115 \text{ h}^{-1} = 10 \text{ h, rounded to } 12 \text{ h}$$

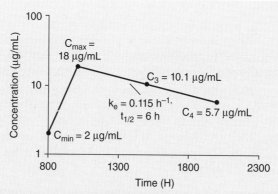

FIGURE 5-11   Graph of vancomycin serum concentrations used in One-Compartment Model Parameter method example.

e. *Determine the new dose for the desired concentrations.* The dose is computed using the one-compartment model intravenous bolus equation used in the initial dosing section of this chapter:

$$D = Css_{max} \, V(1 - e^{-k_e\tau}) = 30 \text{ mg/L} \cdot 62.5 \text{ L} \, [1 - e^{-(0.115 \text{ h}^{-1})(12 \text{ h})}] = 1403 \text{ mg, rounded to 1500 mg}$$

A dose of vancomycin 1500 mg every 12 hours would be prescribed to begin 12 hours after the last dose of the previous regimen.

AREA UNDER THE CURVE METHOD

Based on retrospective studies, the AUC_{24}/MIC ratio is a pharmacokinetic/pharmacodynamic parameter that has been established as an important index that predicts the clinical cure rate for MSSA/MRSA pneumonia.[26,27] For this particular infection and these pathogens, establishing an AUC_{24}/MIC > 400 is believed to be the best way to ensure a positive clinical outcome. Other AUC_{24}/MIC ratios may be optimal for other bacteria or other infections.[30]

Because the AUC_{24}/MIC > 400 has taken on such importance for this drug, some clinicians have begun individualizing vancomycin therapy by first determining the MIC for the infecting organism and then customizing the vancomycin dose to attain the target ratio. Because prospective clinical trials have not been done yet to establish the clinical outcomes (both therapeutic and toxic), this approach should be conducted with some caution. Because of the uncertainties surrounding the individualization of the AUC_{24}/MIC, it would be best to also keep steady-state vancomycin trough concentrations in an appropriate range when adjusting doses based on this ratio.

If a clinician wishes to customize the AUC_{24}/MIC, there are three ways this can be done: (1) estimate the AUC_{24}, using the patient's dose and an estimate of vancomycin clearance using $CrCl_{est}$, (2) compute the AUC_{24}, using a measured steady-state peak and trough pair of vancomycin concentrations, and (3) compute the AUC_{24}, using a Bayesian pharmacokinetic computer program with one or more vancomycin concentrations. It should be noted that the AUC_{24} represents the area under the concentration-time curve for an entire 24-hour dosage period. For example, if vancomycin is given every 8 hours, AUC_{24} represents three doses, but if vancomycin is given every 48 hours, AUC_{24} represents only ½ of the dosage interval. Finally, the MIC can be measured using an Etest or broth microdilution, or the MIC can be estimated using historical microbiologic data from the institution where the patient is being treated. For the purposes of the following examples, a measured MIC will be assumed.

Estimated AUC$_{24}$/MIC Ratio

In order to estimate the AUC$_{24}$, a rearrangement of a standard pharmacokinetic equation to compute drug clearance (Cl) is used: Cl = D/AUC, where D is the drug dose. The rearrangement used to compute AUC is AUC = D/Cl. In order to estimate AUC$_{24}$ from this equation, the total daily dose (mg/24 h) of vancomycin is used for the dose variable, and Cl is estimated using CrCl$_{est}$. There are several equations that relate CrCl$_{est}$ to vancomycin clearance, but for consistency the method used for this section will be the one used by the original papers that established the use of AUC$_{24}$/MIC > 400 for the treatment of pneumonia[28]: Cl = (0.79 • CrCl$_{est}$) + 15.4. Putting the AUC and vancomycin clearance equations together gives the final formula for AUC$_{24}$ (in (mg • h)/L): AUC$_{24}$ = D/{[(CrCl$_{est}$ • 0.79) + 15.4] • 0.06}, where D is the total vancomycin dose in mg for a 24-hour period, CrCl$_{est}$ is the estimated creatinine clearance in mL/min using the Cockcroft-Gault method, and 0.06 is a combined unit correction factor.[27]

EXAMPLE 1 ▶ ▶ ▶

UI is a 55-year-old, 78-kg (height = 6 ft 1 in) male with an MRSA pneumonia (MIC = 1 µg/mL). His current serum creatinine is 1.5 mg/dL, and it has been stable over the last 3 days since admission. A vancomycin dose of 1000 mg every 24 hours was prescribed and expected to achieve an AUC$_{24}$/MIC > 400. After the third dose, the steady-state trough concentration equaled 7 µg/mL. Calculate the AUC$_{24}$/MIC ratio for the patient and compute a new vancomycin dose that would provide an AUC$_{24}$/MIC > 400.

1. *Estimate creatinine clearance.*
   This patient has a stable serum creatinine and is not obese. The Cockcroft-Gault equation can be used to estimate creatinine clearance:

$$CrCl_{est} = [(140 - age)BW]/(72 • S_{Cr}) = [(140 - 55\ y)78\ kg]/(72 • 1.5\ mg/dL)$$

$$CrCl_{est} = 61\ mL/min$$

2. *Estimate AUC$_{24}$/MIC.*
   The AUC$_{24}$/MIC ratio will be estimated using the AUC$_{24}$ equation and the measured MIC:

$$AUC_{24} = D/\{[(CrCl_{est} • 0.79) + 15.4] • 0.06\} = (1000\ mg)/\{[(61\ mL/min • 0.79) + 15.4] • 0.06\} = 262.1\ (mg • h)/L$$

$$AUC_{24}/MIC = [262.1\ (mg • h)/L]/(1\ mg/L) = 262.1$$

Note: µg/mL = mg/L, so this substitution was made in the equation, and the AUC$_{24}$/MIC ratio is usually reported as a unitless value.

3. *Compute new dose based on AUC$_{24}$/MIC > 400.*
   Vancomycin follows linear pharmacokinetics, so the AUC and steady-state trough concentrations change proportionally with dose.

$$Dose_{new} = [(AUC_{24}/MIC)_{new}/(AUC_{24}/MIC)_{old}]\ Dose_{old} = (400/262.1)(1000\ mg/d)$$

$$= 1526\ mg/d,\ round\ to\ 1500\ mg/d$$

Check new expected steady-state vancomycin trough concentration for this AUC$_{24}$/MIC ratio:

$$C_{ss,new} = (D_{new}/D_{old})\ C_{ss,old} = (1500\ mg/1000\ mg)\ 7\ µg/mL = 11\ µg/mL$$

Measured AUC$_{24}$/MIC Ratio Using Steady-State Peak and Trough Concentrations

The AUC at steady state can be easily calculated using a measured steady-state vancomycin peak and trough pair around an administered dose.[133] Under steady-state conditions, the trough concentration will be the same before every dose, so can be extrapolated to the next dosing time (see Figure 5-10). The AUC during the infusion and waiting time will be computed using the linear trapezoidal rule $\{AUC_{inf} = [(Css_{min} + Css_{max})/2]\}\Delta t_{inf}$, where Css_{min} is the steady-state trough concentration, Css_{max} is the steady-state peak concentration, and Δt_{inf} is the time difference that occurred between the two concentration values during the infusion and waiting period (usually 1.5 hours for a 1-hour infusion followed by a ½-hour waiting time). The AUC after the steady-state peak concentration until the time of the next dose during the elimination phase will be computed using the log-linear trapezoidal rule $(AUC_{elim} = \{(Css_{max} - Css_{min})/[\ln (Css_{max}/Css_{min})]\}\Delta t_{elim}$, where Δt_{elim} is the time difference that occurred between the two concentration values during the elimination phase, Figure 5-10). The log-linear version of the equation is used during the elimination phase because it is a straight line when plotted on semilogarithmic paper.[133] The total AUC at steady state for a dose is calculated by taking the sum of these two partial AUC values: $AUC = AUC_{inf} + AUC_{elim}$. The AUC_{24} is then computed by multiplying the AUC for a dose by the number of doses given per day (eg, multiply by 3 for every 8-hour dosing, multiply by ½ for every 48-hour dosing, etc).

EXAMPLE 2 ▶ ▶ ▶

UI is a 55-year-old, 78-kg (height = 6 ft 1 in) male with an MRSA pneumonia (MIC = 1 µg/mL). His current serum creatinine is 1.5 mg/dL, and it has been stable over the last 3 days since admission. A vancomycin dose of 1000 mg every 24 hours was prescribed and expected to achieve an AUC_{24}/MIC > 400. After the third dose, the steady-state peak and trough concentrations equaled 25 µg/mL and 7 µg/mL, respectively. The dose was infused over 1 hour with a waiting period of ½ hour before the peak concentration was obtained. Calculate the AUC_{24}/MIC ratio for the patient and compute a new vancomycin dose that would provide an AUC_{24}/MIC > 400.

1. *Calculate AUC_{24}/MIC.*
   The AUC for a dose is: $AUC = AUC_{inf} + AUC_{elim}$ or

$$AUC = \{[(Css_{min} + Css_{max})/2]\Delta t_{inf}\} + \{(Css_{max} - Css_{min})/[\ln (Css_{max}/Css_{min})]\}\Delta t_{elim}$$
$$AUC = \{[(7\ \mu g/mL + 25\ \mu g/mL)/2]1.5\ h\} + \{(25\ \mu g/mL - 7\ \mu g/mL)/[\ln (25\ \mu g/mL / 7\ \mu g/mL)]\}$$
$$(24\ h - 1.5\ h) = 342.2\ (\mu g \cdot h)/mL = 342.2\ (mg \cdot h)/L\ (\text{Note: } \mu g/mL = mg/L)$$

Dosage interval is 24 hours, so no adjustment of AUC is needed for number of doses per day.

$$AUC_{24}/MIC = [342.2\ (\mu g \cdot h)/mL]/1\ \mu g/mL = 342.2$$

2. *Compute new dose based on AUC_{24}/MIC > 400.*
   Vancomycin follows linear pharmacokinetics, so the AUC and steady-state trough concentrations change proportionally with dose.

$$Dose_{new} = [(AUC_{24}/MIC)_{new}/(AUC_{24}/MIC)_{old}]Dose_{old} = (400/342.2)(1000\ mg/d)$$
$$= 1169\ mg/d, \text{ round to } 1250\ mg/d$$

Check new steady-state vancomycin trough concentration for this AUC_{24}/MIC ratio:

$$C_{ss,new} = (D_{new}/D_{old})C_{ss,old} = (1250\ mg/1000\ mg)\ 7\ \mu g/mL = 9\ \mu g/mL$$

Measured AUC_{24}/MIC Ratio Using Concentration(s) and Bayesian Pharmacokinetic Computer Program

Bayesian pharmacokinetic computer programs can compute pharmacokinetic values, using one or more drug concentrations, and the concentrations do not need to be at steady state (see next major section of chapter for more information). Once the program has computed vancomycin clearance, it can be used to compute AUC for the dose (AUC = D/Cl, where D is the vancomycin dose), or the program may report AUC directly. The AUC_{24} is then computed by multiplying the AUC for a dose by the number of doses given per day (eg, multiply by 3 for every 8-hour dosing, multiply by ½ for every 48-hour dosing, etc).

EXAMPLE 3 ▶ ▶ ▶

UI is a 55-year-old, 78-kg (height = 6 ft 1 in) male with an MRSA pneumonia (MIC = 1 µg/mL). His current serum creatinine is 1.5 mg/dL, and it has been stable over the last 3 days since admission. A vancomycin dose of 1000 mg every 24 hours was prescribed and expected to achieve an AUC_{24}/MIC > 400. After the third dose, the steady-state trough concentration equaled 7 µg/mL. The dose was infused over 1 hour with a waiting period of ½ hour before the peak concentration was obtained. Calculate the AUC_{24}/MIC ratio for the patient and compute a new vancomycin dose that would provide an AUC_{24}/MIC > 400.

1. *Calculate AUC_{24}/MIC, using the Bayesian pharmacokinetic computer program.*
   The pharmacokinetic parameters computed by the program are a volume of distribution of 51 L, a half-life equal to 12.7 hours, and clearance of 2.8 L/h.
   The AUC for a dose is: AUC = D/Cl = (1000 mg)/(2.8 L/h) = 357.1 (mg · h)/L
   Dosage interval is 24 hours, so no adjustment of AUC is needed for number of doses per day.

   $$AUC_{24}/MIC = [357.1 (µg · h)/mL]/1 µg/mL = 357.1$$

2. *Compute new dose based on AUC_{24}/MIC > 400.*
   Vancomycin follows linear pharmacokinetics, so the AUC and steady-state trough concentrations change proportionally with dose.

   $$Dose_{new} = [(AUC_{24}/MIC)_{new}/(AUC_{24}/MIC)_{old}]Dose_{old} = (400/357.1)(1000 mg/d)$$
   $$= 1120 mg/d, \text{ round to } 1250 mg/d$$

   Check new steady-state vancomycin trough concentration for this AUC_{24}/MIC ratio:
   The Bayesian pharmacokinetic computer program computes a steady-state vancomycin trough concentration of 9 µg/mL for the new dose.

BAYESIAN PHARMACOKINETIC COMPUTER PROGRAMS

Computer programs are available that can assist in the computation of pharmacokinetic parameters for patients.[134-139] The most reliable computer programs use a nonlinear regression algorithm that incorporates components of Bayes theorem. Nonlinear regression is a statistical technique that uses an iterative process to compute the best pharmacokinetic parameters for a concentration/time data set. Briefly, the patient's drug dosage schedule and serum concentrations are input into the computer. The computer program has a pharmacokinetic equation preprogrammed for the drug and administration method (oral, intravenous bolus, intravenous infusion, etc). Typically, a one-compartment model is used, although some programs allow the user to choose among several different equations. Using population estimates based on demographic information for the patient (age, weight, gender, renal function, etc) supplied by the user, the computer program then computes estimated serum concentrations at each time there are actual serum concentrations. Kinetic parameters are then changed by the computer program, and a new set of estimated serum concentrations are computed. The pharmacokinetic parameters that generated the estimated serum concentrations closest to the actual values are remembered by the computer program, and the process is repeated until the set of pharmacokinetic parameters that result in estimated serum concentrations that are statistically closest to the actual serum concentrations are generated. These pharmacokinetic parameters can then be used to compute improved dosing schedules for patients. Bayes theorem is used in the computer algorithm to balance the results of the computations between values based solely on the patient's serum drug concentrations and those based only on patient population parameters. Results from studies that compare various methods of dosage adjustment have consistently found that these types of computer dosing programs perform at least as well as experienced clinical pharmacokineticists and clinicians and better than inexperienced clinicians.

Some clinicians use Bayesian pharmacokinetic computer programs exclusively to alter drug doses based on serum concentrations. An advantage of this approach is that consistent dosage recommendations are made when several different practitioners are involved in therapeutic drug monitoring programs. However, because simpler dosing methods work just as well for patients with stable pharmacokinetic parameters and steady-state drug concentrations, many clinicians reserve the use of computer programs for more difficult situations. Those situations include serum concentrations that are not at steady state, serum concentrations not obtained at the specific times needed to use simpler methods, and unstable pharmacokinetic parameters. When trough-only monitoring is used during vancomycin therapy, Bayesian pharmacokinetic computer programs can be used to compute a complete patient pharmacokinetic profile that includes clearance, volume of distribution, and half-life. AUC can also be calculated, and this value can be used to compute an individual AUC_{24}/MIC ratio (please see previous section). Many Bayesian pharmacokinetic computer programs are available to users, and most should provide answers similar to the one used in the following examples. The program used to solve problems in this book is DrugCalc written by Dr Dennis Mungall.[140]

EXAMPLE 1 ▶ ▶ ▶

JM is a 50-year-old, 70-kg (height = 5 ft 10 in) male with an MRSA wound infection. His current serum creatinine is 3.5 mg/dL, and it has been stable over the last 5 days since admission. A vancomycin dose of 1000 mg every 24 hours was prescribed. After the fourth dose, steady-state peak and trough concentrations were measured and were 25 µg/mL and 12 µg/mL, respectively. Calculate a new vancomycin dose that would provide a steady-state peak of 35 µg/mL and a trough of 17 µg/mL.

1. *Enter patient demographic, drug dosing, and serum concentration/time data into the computer program.*
2. *Compute pharmacokinetic parameters for the patient using Bayesian pharmacokinetic computer program.*
   The pharmacokinetic parameters computed by the program are a volume of distribution of 66.9 L, a half-life equal to 22.6 hours, and an elimination rate constant of 0.0307 h^{-1}.
3. *Compute dose required to achieve desired vancomycin serum concentrations.*

   The one-compartment model intravenous infusion equations used by the program to compute doses indicates that a dose of 1250 mg every 24 hours will produce a steady-state peak concentration of 34.3 µg/mL and a steady-state trough concentration of 17.2 µg/mL.

EXAMPLE 2 ▶▶▶

ZW is a 35-year-old, 150-kg (height = 5 ft 5 in) female with a *S. epidermidis* infection of a prosthetic knee joint. Her current serum creatinine is 1.1 mg/dL and is stable. A vancomycin dose of 2500 mg every 18 hours was prescribed. After the fourth dose, steady-state peak and trough concentrations were measured and were 40 μg/mL and 3 μg/mL, respectively. Calculate a new vancomycin dose that would provide a steady-state peak of 40-50 μg/mL and a steady-state trough 15 μg/mL.

1. *Enter patient demographic, drug dosing, and serum concentration/time data into the computer program.*
2. *Compute pharmacokinetic parameters for the patient using Bayesian pharmacokinetic computer program.*
   The pharmacokinetic parameters computed by the program are a volume of distribution of 50.4 L, a half-life equal to 3.9 hours, and an elimination rate constant of 0.178 h^{-1}.

3. *Compute dose required to achieve desired vancomycin serum concentrations.*
   The one-compartment model intravenous infusion equations used by the program to compute doses indicates that a dose of 2500 mg every 8 hours will produce a steady-state peak concentration of 50.0 μg/mL and a steady-state trough concentration of 15.8 μg/mL.

EXAMPLE 3 ▶▶▶

KU is an 80-year-old, 65-kg (height = 5 ft 8 in) male with *S. viridans* endocarditis and is allergic to penicillins and cephalosporins. His current serum creatinine is 1.9 mg/dL, and it has been stable. A vancomycin dose of 1000 mg every 12 hours was prescribed with the expectation that it would produce steady-state peak and trough concentrations of 30 μg/mL and 10 μg/mL, respectively. After the third dose, a trough concentration was measured and equaled 17.5 μg/mL. Calculate a new vancomycin dose that would provide a steady-state peak of 30 μg/mL and a steady-state trough of 10 μg/mL.

1. *Enter patient demographic, drug dosing, and serum concentration/time data into the computer program.*
   In this patient case, it is unlikely that the patient is at steady state so the Linear Pharmacokinetics method cannot be used.
2. *Compute pharmacokinetic parameters for the patient using Bayesian pharmacokinetic computer program.*
   The pharmacokinetic parameters computed by the program are a volume of distribution of 74.8 L, a half-life equal to 33.6 hours, and an elimination rate constant of 0.0206 h^{-1}.
3. *Compute dose required to achieve desired vancomycin serum concentrations.*
   The one-compartment model intravenous infusion equations used by the program to compute doses indicates that a dose of 1250 mg every 48 hours will produce a steady-state peak concentration of 26 μg/mL and a steady-state trough concentration of 10 μg/mL.

DOSING STRATEGIES

Initial dose and dosage adjustment techniques using serum concentrations can be used in any combination as long as the limitations of each method are observed. Some dosing schemes link together logically when considered according to their basic approaches or philosophies. Dosage strategies that follow similar pathways are given in Table 5-6.

TABLE 5-6   Dosing Strategies

Dosing Approach/Philosophy	Initial Dosing	Use of Serum Concentrations to Alter Doses
Pharmacokinetic parameters/equations	Pharmacokinetic Dosing method	One-Compartment Model Parameter method
Nomogram/concepts	Moellering, Matzke, or Rybak nomogram (adults) or Literature-based recommended dosing (pediatrics)	Linear Pharmacokinetic method (≥1 concentration) Trough-only method (1 concentration) Combined Linear Pharmacokinetic/Trough-only methods (1 concentration) or Pharmacokinetic Concepts method (≥2 concentrations)
Computerized	Bayesian computer program	Bayesian computer program

PROBLEMS

The following problems are intended to emphasize the computation of initial and individualized doses using clinical pharmacokinetic techniques. Clinicians should always consult the patient's chart to confirm that antibiotic therapy is appropriate for current microbiologic cultures and sensitivities. Also, it should be confirmed that the patient is receiving other appropriate concurrent antibiotic therapy, such as aminoglycoside antibiotics, when necessary to treat the infection.

1. KI is a 75-year-old, 62-kg (5 ft 9 in) male with *S. epidermidis* sepsis. His current serum creatinine is 1.3 mg/dL, and it has been stable since admission. Compute a vancomycin dose for this patient to provide a steady-state peak concentration of 40 μg/mL and a steady-state trough concentration of 15 μg/mL.

2. Patient KI (see problem 1) was prescribed vancomycin 1000 mg every 36 hours. Steady-state vancomycin concentrations were obtained before and after the fourth dose, and the peak concentration (obtained ½ hour after a 1-hour infusion of vancomycin) was 34 μg/mL while the trough concentration (obtained immediately before dosage administration) was 2.5 μg/mL. Compute a revised vancomycin dose for this patient to provide a steady-state peak concentration of 48 μg/mL and a steady-state trough concentration of 17 μg/mL.

3. HT is a 35-year-old, 75-kg (5 ft 7 in) female with an MRSA wound infection and chronic renal failure. Her current serum creatinine is 3.7 mg/dL, and it has been stable since admission. Compute a vancomycin dose for this patient to provide a steady-state peak concentration of 45 μg/mL and a steady-state trough concentration of 15 μg/mL.

4. Patient HT (see problem 3) was prescribed vancomycin 1200 mg every 48 hours. Steady-state vancomycin concentrations were obtained before and after the fourth dose, and the peak concentration (obtained ½ hour after a 1-hour infusion of vancomycin) was 60 μg/mL while the trough concentration (obtained within ½ hour before dosage administration) was 24 μg/mL. Compute a revised vancomycin dose for this patient to provide a steady-state peak concentration of 40 μg/mL and a steady-state trough concentration of 20 μg/mL.

5. LK is a 55-year-old, 140-kg (5 ft 8 in) male with an MSSA wound infection (MIC = 0.5 μg/mL). His current serum creatinine is 0.9 mg/dL, and it has been stable since admission. Compute a vancomycin dose for this patient to provide a steady-state peak concentration of 45 μg/mL and a steady-state trough concentration of 20 μg/mL.

6. Patient LK (see problem 5) was prescribed vancomycin 1000 mg every 8 hours. Steady-state vancomycin concentrations were obtained before and after the fourth dose, and the peak concentration (obtained ½ hour after a 1-hour infusion of vancomycin) was 42 µg/mL while the trough concentration (obtained within ½ hour before dosage administration) was 18 µg/mL. Compute a revised vancomycin dose for this patient to provide a steady-state peak concentration of 40 µg/mL and a steady-state trough concentration of 10 µg/mL.

7. AF is a 45-year-old, 140-kg (5 ft 2 in) female with a *S. viridans* endocarditis who is allergic to penicillins and cephalosporins. Her current serum creatinine is 2.4 mg/dL and is stable. Compute a vancomycin dose for this patient to provide a steady-state peak concentration of 40 µg/mL, and a steady-state trough concentration of 12 µg/mL.

8. Patient AF (see problem 7) was prescribed 1300 mg every 24 hours. Steady-state vancomycin concentrations were obtained before and after the fourth dose, and the peak concentration (obtained ½ hour after a 1-hour infusion of vancomycin) was 30 µg/mL while the trough concentration (obtained within ½ hour before dosage administration) was 2.5 µg/mL. Compute a revised vancomycin dose for this patient to provide a steady-state peak concentration of 40 µg/mL and a steady-state trough concentration of 12 µg/mL.

9. DG is a 66-year-old, 65-kg (5 ft 5 in) female with an MRSA sternal osteomyelitis secondary to coronary artery bypass graft (CABG) surgery. Her current serum creatinine is 1.4 mg/dL and stable. Compute a vancomycin dose for this patient to provide a steady-state peak concentration of 50 µg/mL, and a steady-state trough concentration of 20 µg/mL.

10. Patient DG (see problem 9) was prescribed 1200 mg every 36 hours. Steady-state vancomycin concentrations were obtained before and after the fifth dose, and the peak concentration (obtained ½ hour after a 1-hour infusion of vancomycin) was 30 µg/mL while the trough concentration (obtained within ½ hour before dosage administration) was 12 µg/mL. Compute a revised vancomycin dose for this patient to provide a steady-state trough concentration of 15 µg/mL.

11. GG is a 27-year-old, 85-kg (6 ft 2 in) male trauma patient with a penicillin-resistant enterococcal pneumonia and is currently on a respirator. He sustained multiple injuries secondary to a motor vehicle accident 2 weeks ago and lost a large amount of blood at the accident site. He developed acute renal failure due to prolonged hypotension and poor perfusion of his kidneys (current postdialysis serum creatinine is 5.3 mg/dL). He is currently receiving hemodialysis on Mondays, Wednesdays, and Fridays from 0800 to 1200 H, using a low-flux dialysis filter. Recommend a vancomycin dosage regimen that will achieve peak concentrations of 40 µg/mL and trough concentrations of 20 µg/mL. The first dose of the regimen will be given immediately after hemodialysis is finished on Wednesday at 1200 H.

12. Patient GG (see problem 11) was prescribed 1600 mg loading dose on Wednesday at 1200 H, and following serum concentrations were obtained:

Date/Time	Description	Concentration (µg/mL)
Friday at 0800 H	Predialysis	20
Monday at 0800 H	Predialysis	12.1

Use these serum concentrations to compute the patient's own pharmacokinetic parameters for vancomycin and a new dosage schedule that will achieve peak concentrations of 45 µg/mL and trough concentrations of 20 µg/mL.

13. FD is a 67-year-old, 60-kg (5 ft 2 in) female with a serum creatinine equal to 1.8 mg/dL placed on vancomycin for a postsurgical brain abscess. The prescribed dose was vancomycin 900 mg every 12 hours

(infused over 1 hour), and two doses have been given at 0800 and 2000 hours. A trough concentration of 20 µg/mL was obtained at 0730 hours the next morning (½ hour before the third dose). Compute the dose to give $Css_{max} = 40$ µg/mL and $Css_{min} = 15$ µg/mL.

14. OI is a 52-year-old, 87-kg (6 ft 2 in) male with postoperative *S. epidermidis* septic arthritis. His current serum creatinine is 1.4 mg/dL and stable. Nine hours after the second dose of vancomycin 1000 mg every 12 hours, a vancomycin serum concentration equal to 20 µg/mL is measured. Compute a revised vancomycin dose for this patient to provide steady-state peak concentrations equal to 30 µg/mL and steady-state trough concentrations of 15 µg/mL.

15. HY is a 45-year-old, 65-kg (5 ft 4 in) female bone marrow transplant recipient who develops MRSA sepsis. Her current serum creatinine is 1.1 mg/dL. She is administered vancomycin 750 mg every 12 hours. A vancomycin serum concentration was obtained 5 hours after the first dose and equaled 15 µg/mL. Compute a revised vancomycin dose for this patient to provide steady-state peak concentrations equal to 40 µg/mL and steady-state trough concentrations of 20 µg/mL.

16. OF is a 9-day-old, 1550-g female premature infant (GA ~27 weeks) with a wound infection. Her serum creatinine equals 0.7 mg/dL. Compute an initial vancomycin dose for this patient.

17. Patient OF (see problem 16) was prescribed vancomycin 20 mg every 12 hours. Steady-state vancomycin concentrations were obtained, and the peak concentration was 20 µg/mL while the trough concentration was 8.6 µg/mL. Compute a revised vancomycin dose for this patient to provide a steady-state trough concentration of 15 µg/mL.

18. UL is a 7-year-old, 24-kg (3 ft 11 in) male with MRSA sepsis. His serum creatinine is 0.5 mg/dL, and it has been stable for the last 2 days. Compute an initial vancomycin dose for this patient.

19. Patient UL (see problem 18) was prescribed vancomycin 250 mg every 6 hours and was expected to achieve steady-state peak and trough concentrations equal to 38 µg/mL and 15 µg/mL, respectively. Steady-state peak and trough concentrations were measured and were 25 µg/mL and 10 µg/mL, respectively. Calculate a new vancomycin dose that would provide a steady-state trough of 15 µg/mL.

20. TK is a 75-year-old, 66-kg (5 ft 5 in) female with an MRSA pneumonia. Her current serum creatinine is 1.8 mg/dL, and it has been stable over the last 3 days since admission. A vancomycin dose of 1000 mg every 24 hours was prescribed and expected to achieve a steady-state trough concentration equal to 15 µg/mL. After the third dose, the steady-state trough concentration equaled 25 µg/mL. Calculate a new vancomycin dose that would provide a steady-state trough of 15 µg/mL.

21. VY is a 48-year-old, 170-kg (5 ft 7 in) female with septic arthritis due to MRSA. Her current serum creatinine is 1.3 mg/dL and is stable. A vancomycin dose of 1000 mg every 24 hours was prescribed and expected to achieve a steady-state trough concentration equal to 15 µg/mL. After the third dose, a steady-state concentration was measured and equaled 8 µg/mL. Calculate a new vancomycin dose that would provide a steady-state trough of 15 µg/mL.

22. NH is a 75-year-old, 62-kg (5 ft 9 in) male with MRSA bacteremia. His current serum creatinine is 1.3 mg/dL, and it has been stable since admission. A vancomycin dose of 1000 mg every 24 hours was prescribed and expected to achieve a steady-state trough concentration equal to 15 µg/mL. After the third dose, a steady-state concentration was measured and equaled 6 µg/mL. Calculate a new vancomycin dose that would provide a steady-state trough of 15 µg/mL.

23. PA is a 22-year-old, 75-kg (5 ft 11 in) male with MRSA bacteremia. His initial serum creatinine on admission was 0.8 mg/dL, but his current serum creatinine is 2.3 mg/dL, and it has been stable for the last 3 days. A vancomycin dose of 1500 mg every 8 hours was prescribed and expected to achieve a steady-state trough concentration equal to 15 µg/mL. After the sixth dose, a steady-state concentration was measured and equaled 27 µg/mL. Calculate a new vancomycin dose that would provide a steady-state trough of 15 µg/mL.

24. GA is a 55-year-old, 78-kg (6 ft 1 in) male with an MRSA endocarditis (MIC = 1 µg/mL). His current serum creatinine is 1.5 mg/dL, and it has been stable over the last 3 days since admission. A vancomycin dose of 1000 mg every 18 hours was prescribed and expected to achieve an AUC_{24}/MIC > 400. After the third dose, the steady-state trough concentration equaled 7 µg/mL. Using the estimated AUC_{24} ratio method, calculate the AUC_{24}/MIC ratio for the patient and compute a new vancomycin dose that would provide an AUC_{24}/MIC > 400.

25. RI is a 55-year-old, 78-kg (6 ft 1 in) male with an MRSA pneumonia (MIC = 1 µg/mL). His current serum creatinine is 1.5 mg/dL, and it has been stable over the last 3 days since admission. A vancomycin dose of 1000 mg every 12 hours was prescribed and expected to achieve an AUC_{24}/MIC > 400. After the third dose, the steady-state peak and trough concentrations equaled 25 µg/mL and 7 µg/mL, respectively. The dose was infused over 1 hour with a waiting period of ½ hour before the peak concentration was obtained. Use the steady-state peak and trough concentrations to calculate the AUC_{24}/MIC ratio for the patient, and compute a new vancomycin dose that would provide an AUC_{24}/MIC > 400.

26. VA is a 55-year-old, 78-kg (6 ft 1 in) male with an MRSA pneumonia (MIC = 1.5 µg/mL). His current serum creatinine is 1.5 mg/dL, and it has been stable over the last 3 days since admission. A vancomycin dose of 1000 mg every 24 hours was prescribed and expected to achieve an AUC_{24}/MIC > 400. After the third dose, the steady-state trough concentration equaled 7 µg/mL. The dose was infused over 1 hour with a waiting period of ½ hour before the peak concentration was obtained. Use a measured AUC_{24} ratio computed using concentration(s) and a Bayesian pharmacokinetic computer program to calculate the AUC_{24}/MIC ratio for the patient, and compute a new vancomycin dose that would provide an AUC_{24}/MIC > 400.

ANSWERS TO PROBLEMS

1. *Solution to Problem 1.* The initial vancomycin dose for patient KI would be calculated as follows:

Pharmacokinetic Dosing Method

1. *Estimate creatinine clearance.*
   This patient has a stable serum creatinine and is not obese. The Cockcroft-Gault equation can be used to estimate creatinine clearance:

   $$CrCl_{est} = [(140 - age)BW]/(72 \cdot S_{Cr}) = [(140 - 75 \text{ y})62 \text{ kg}]/(72 \cdot 1.3 \text{ mg/dL})$$

   $$CrCl_{est} = 43 \text{ mL/min}$$

2. *Estimate vancomycin clearance.*
   The vancomycin clearance versus creatinine clearance relationship is used to estimate the vancomycin clearance for this patient:

   $$Cl = 0.695(CrCl) + 0.05 = 0.695[(43 \text{ mL/min})/62\text{kg}] + 0.05 = 0.533 \text{ mL/min/kg}$$

3. *Estimate vancomycin volume of distribution.*
   The average volume of distribution for vancomycin is 0.7 L/kg:

   $$V = 0.7 \text{ L/kg} \cdot 62 \text{ kg} = 43.4 \text{ L}$$

4. *Estimate vancomycin elimination rate constant (k_e) and half-life $(t_{1/2})$.*

   $$k_e = Cl/V = (0.533 \text{ mL/min/kg} \cdot 60 \text{ min/h})/(0.7 \text{ L/kg} \cdot 1000 \text{ mL/L}) = 0.0457 \text{ h}^{-1}$$

   $$t_{1/2} = 0.693/k_e = 0.693/0.0457 \text{ h}^{-1} = 15.2 \text{ h}$$

5. *Choose desired steady-state serum concentrations.*

A Css_{min} = 15 µg/mL and Css_{max} = 40 µg/mL were chosen to treat this patient.

6. *Use intravenous bolus equations to compute dose (see Table 5-2).*

Calculate required dosage interval (τ):

$$\tau = (\ln Css_{max} - \ln Css_{min})/k_e = (\ln 40 \text{ µg/mL} - \ln 15 \text{ µg/mL})/0.0457 \text{ h}^{-1} = 21.5 \text{ h}$$

Dosage intervals should be rounded to clinically acceptable intervals of 8, 12, 18, 24, 36, 48, 72 hours, and multiples of 24 hours thereafter, whenever possible. In this case, the dosage interval would be rounded to 24 hours.

Calculate required dose (D):

$$D = Css_{max} V(1 - e^{-k_e\tau}) = 40 \text{ mg/L} \cdot 43.4 \text{ L } [1 - e^{-(0.0457 \text{ h}^{-1})(24 \text{ h})}] = 1156 \text{ mg}$$

Vancomycin doses should be rounded to the nearest 100-250 mg. This dose would be rounded to 1250 mg because the patient has sepsis. (Note: µg/mL = mg/L, and this concentration unit was substituted for Css_{max} so that unnecessary unit conversion was not required.)

The prescribed maintenance dose would be 1250 mg every 24 hours.

7. *Compute loading dose (LD), if needed.*

Loading doses should be considered for patients with creatinine clearance values less than 60 mL/min. The administration of a loading dose in these patients will allow achievement of therapeutic concentrations quicker than if maintenance doses alone are given. However, because the pharmacokinetic parameters used to compute these initial doses are only *estimated* values and not *actual* values, the patient's own parameters may be much different than the estimated constants and steady state will not be achieved until 3–5 half-lives have passed.

$$LD = Css_{max} V = 40 \text{ mg/L} \cdot 43.4 \text{ L} = 1736 \text{ mg}$$

As noted, this patient has poor renal function (CrCl <60 mL/min) so a loading dose would be prescribed for this patient and given as the first dose. Vancomycin doses should be rounded to the nearest 100-250 mg. This dose would be rounded to 1750 mg. (Note: µg/mL = mg/L, and this concentration unit was substituted for Css_{max} so that unnecessary unit conversion was not required.) The first maintenance dose would be given one dosage interval (24 hours) after the loading dose was administered.

Moellering Nomogram Method

1. *Estimate creatinine clearance.*

This patient has a stable serum creatinine and is not obese. The Cockcroft-Gault equation can be used to estimate creatinine clearance:

$$CrCl_{est} = [(140 - age)BW]/(72 \cdot S_{Cr}) = [(140 - 75 \text{ y})62 \text{ kg}]/(72 \cdot 1.3 \text{ mg/dL})$$
$$CrCl_{est} = 43 \text{ mL/min}$$

2. *Determine dosage interval and maintenance dose.*

The maintenance dose is calculated using the modified vancomycin dosing equation:

$$D \text{ (in mg/h/kg)} = 0.834(CrCl \text{ in mL/min/kg}) + 0.06$$
$$D = 0.834[(43 \text{ mL/min})/62 \text{ kg}] + 0.06 = 0.639 \text{ mg/h/kg}$$
$$D = 0.639 \text{ mg/h/kg} \cdot 62 \text{ kg} = 39.6 \text{ mg/h}$$

The standard dose of 1000 mg can be used to gain an approximation for an acceptable dosage interval (τ):

$$\tau = 1000 \text{ mg}/(39.6 \text{ mg/h}) = 25 \text{ h}$$

Dosage intervals should be rounded to clinically acceptable intervals of 8, 12, 18, 24, 36, 48, 72 hours, and multiples of 24 hours thereafter, whenever possible. In this case, the dosage interval would be rounded to 24 hours.

$$D = 39.6 \text{ mg/h} \cdot 24 \text{ h} = 951 \text{ mg}$$

Vancomycin doses should be rounded to the nearest 100-250 mg. This dose would be rounded to 1000 mg. The prescribed maintenance dose would be 1000 mg every 24 hours.

3. *Compute loading dose.*
   A loading dose (LD) of 15 mg/kg is suggested by the Moellering nomogram, and this value is adjusted by 1.33:

$$LD = 15 \text{ mg/kg}(62 \text{ kg})1.33 = 1237 \text{ mg, round to } 1250 \text{ mg}$$

As noted, this patient has poor renal function (CrCl <60 mL/min) so a loading dose would be prescribed and given as the first dose. Vancomycin doses should be rounded to the nearest 100–250 mg. (Note: µg/mL = mg/L, and this concentration unit was substituted for Css_{max} so that unnecessary unit conversion was not required.) The first maintenance dose would be given one dosage interval (24 hours) after the loading dose was administered.

Matzke Nomogram Method

1. *Estimate creatinine clearance.*
   This patient has a stable serum creatinine and is not obese. The Cockcroft-Gault equation can be used to estimate creatinine clearance:

$$CrCl_{est} = [(140 - \text{age})BW]/(72 \cdot S_{Cr}) = [(140 - 75 \text{ y})62 \text{ kg}]/(72 \cdot 1.3 \text{ mg/dL})$$

$$CrCl_{est} = 43 \text{ mL/min}$$

2. *Compute loading dose (see Table 5-4).*
   A loading dose (LD) of 25 mg/kg will provide a peak concentration of 30 µg/mL.

$$LD = 25 \text{ mg/kg}(62 \text{ kg}) = 1550 \text{ mg, rounded to } 1500 \text{ mg}$$

3. *Determine dosage interval and maintenance dose.*
   From the nomogram the dosage interval is 1.5 days or 36 hours. The maintenance dose would be 19 mg/kg $\cdot$ 62 kg = 1178 mg. Vancomycin doses should be rounded to the nearest 100–250 mg. This dose would be rounded to 1250 mg and given one dosage interval (36 hours) after the loading dose. The prescribed maintenance dose would be 1250 mg every 36 hours.

Rybak Nomogram Method

1. *Estimate creatinine clearance.*
   This patient has a stable serum creatinine and is not obese. The Cockcroft-Gault equation can be used to estimate creatinine clearance:

$$CrCl_{est} = [(140 - \text{age})BW]/(72 \cdot S_{Cr}) = [(140 - 75 \text{ y})62 \text{ kg}]/(72 \cdot 1.3 \text{ mg/dL})$$

$$CrCl_{est} = 43 \text{ mL/min}$$

2. *Determine dosage interval and maintenance dose (see Table 5-5).*

   From the nomogram the vancomycin dosage is 750 mg every 12 hours. Because the patient's $CrCl_{est}$ is less than 60 mL/min, loading dose (LD) of 25-30 mg/kg actual body weight could be administered as the first dose: LD = 25 mg/kg $\cdot$ 62 kg = 1550 mg, rounded to 1500 mg.

2. *Solution to Problem 2.* The revised vancomycin dose for patient KI would be calculated as follows:

Pharmacokinetics Concept Method

1. *Estimate creatinine clearance.*
   This patient has a stable serum creatinine and is not obese. The Cockcroft-Gault equation can be used to estimate creatinine clearance:

   $$CrCl_{est} = [(140 - age)BW]/(72 \cdot S_{Cr}) = [(140 - 75\ y)62\ kg]/(72 \cdot 1.3\ mg/dL)$$

   $$CrCl_{est} = 43\ mL/min$$

2. *Estimate elimination rate constant (k_e) and half-life ($t_{1/2}$).*
   The vancomycin clearance versus creatinine clearance relationship is used to estimate drug clearance for this patient:

   $$Cl = 0.695(CrCl) + 0.05 = 0.695[(43\ mL/min)/62\ kg] + 0.05 = 0.533\ mL/min/kg$$

   The average volume of distribution for vancomycin is 0.7 L/kg:

   $$V = 0.7\ L/kg \cdot 62\ kg = 43.4\ L$$
   $$k_e = Cl/V = (0.533\ mL/min/kg \cdot 60\ min/h)/(0.7\ L/kg \cdot 1000\ mL/L) = 0.0457\ h^{-1}$$
   $$t_{1/2} = 0.693/k_e = 0.693/0.0457\ h^{-1} = 15.2\ h$$

   Because the patient has been receiving vancomycin for more than 3-5 estimated half-lives, it is likely that the measured serum concentrations are close to steady-state values. This steady-state concentration pair can be used to compute the patient's own unique pharmacokinetic parameters that can be used to calculate individualized doses.

3. *Use Pharmacokinetics Concept method to compute a new dose.*
   a. *Draw a rough sketch of the serum log concentration/time curve by hand, keeping track of the relative time between the serum concentrations (Figure 5-12).*
   b. *Because the patient is at steady-state, the trough concentration can be extrapolated to the next trough value time (see Figure 5-12).*
   c. *Draw the elimination curve between the steady-state peak concentration and the extrapolated trough concentration. Use this line to estimate half-life.* The patient is receiving a vancomycin dose of 1000 mg given every 36 hours that produces a steady-state peak equal to 34 µg/mL and a steady-state trough equal to 2.5 µg/mL. The dose is infused over 1 hour and the peak concentration is drawn ½ hour later (see Figure 5-12). The time between the measured steady-state peak and the extrapolated trough

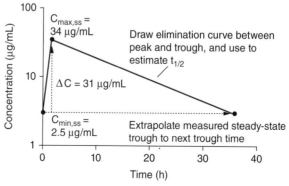

FIGURE 5-12   Solution to Problem 2 using Pharmacokinetic Concept method.

concentration is 34.5 hours (the 36-hour dosage interval minus the 1.5-hour combined infusion and waiting time). The definition of half-life is the time needed for serum concentrations to decrease by ½. It would take 1 half-life for the peak serum concentration to decline from 34 to 17 µg/mL, another half-life for concentrations to decrease from 17 to 8.5 µg/mL, an additional half-life for concentrations to drop from ~8 to 4 µg/mL, and a final half-life for the concentration to decrease to 2 µg/mL. The concentration of 2 µg/mL is very close to the extrapolated trough value of 2.5 µg/mL. Therefore, 4 half-lives expired during the 34.5-hour time period between the peak concentration and extrapolated trough concentration, and the estimated half-life is 9 hours (34.5 h/4 half-lives = ~9 hours). This information will be used to set the new dosage interval for the patient.

d. *Determine the difference in concentration between the steady-state peak and trough concentrations. The difference in concentration will change proportionally with the dose size.* In the current example the patient is receiving a vancomycin dose equal to 1000 mg every 36 hours, which produced steady-state peak and trough concentrations of 34 µg/mL and 2.5 µg/mL, respectively. The difference between the peak and trough values is 31.5 µg/mL. The change in serum concentration is proportional to the dose, and this information will be used to set a new dose for the patient.

e. *Choose new steady-state peak and trough concentrations.* For the purposes of this example, the desired steady-state peak and trough concentrations will be 48 µg/mL and 17 µg/mL, respectively.

f. *Determine the new dosage interval for the desired concentrations.* Using the desired concentrations, it will take 1 half-life for the peak concentration of 48 µg/mL to decrease to 24 µg/mL, and an additional half-life for serum concentrations to decline from 24 to 12 µg/mL. The value of 17 µg/mL is about ½ way between the final two values. Therefore, the dosage interval will need to be approximately 1.5 half-lives or 13.5 hours (9 hours × 1.5 half-live = 13.5 hours), round to 12 hours.

g. *Determine the new dose for the desired concentrations.* The desired peak concentration is 48 µg/mL, and the expected trough concentration is 17 µg/mL. The change in concentration between these values is 31 µg/mL. It is known from measured serum concentrations that administration of 1000 mg changes serum concentrations by 31.5 µg/mL and that the change in serum concentration between the peak and trough values is proportional to the size of the dose. In this case: $D_{new} = (\Delta C_{new}/\Delta C_{old})D_{old} = $ (31 µg/mL/31.5 µg/mL)1000 mg = 984 mg, rounded to 1000 mg. Vancomycin 1000 mg every 12 hours would be started 12 hours after the last dose of the previous dosage regimen.

One-Compartment Model Parameter Method

1. *Estimate creatinine clearance.*
   This patient has a stable serum creatinine and is not obese. The Cockcroft-Gault equation can be used to estimate creatinine clearance:

$$CrCl_{est} = [(140 - age)BW]/(72 \cdot S_{Cr}) = [(140 - 75 \text{ y})62 \text{ kg}]/(72 \cdot 1.3 \text{ mg/dL})$$

$$CrCl_{est} = 43 \text{ mL/min}$$

2. *Estimate elimination rate constant (k_e) and half-life ($t_{1/2}$).*
   The vancomycin clearance versus creatinine clearance relationship is used to estimate drug clearance for this patient:

$$Cl = 0.695(CrCl) + 0.05 = 0.695[(43 \text{ mL/min})/62 \text{ kg}] + 0.05 = 0.533 \text{ mL/min/kg}$$

The average volume of distribution for vancomycin is 0.7 L/kg:

$$V = 0.7 \text{ L/kg} \cdot 62 \text{ kg} = 43.4 \text{ L}$$

$$k_e = Cl/V = (0.533 \text{ mL/min/kg} \cdot 60 \text{ min/h})/(0.7 \text{ L/kg} \cdot 1000 \text{ mL/L}) = 0.0457 \text{ h}^{-1}$$

$$t_{1/2} = 0.693/k_e = 0.693/0.0457 \text{ h}^{-1} = 15.2 \text{ h}$$

Moellering Nomogram Method

1. *Estimate creatinine clearance.*
   This patient has a stable serum creatinine and is not obese. The Cockcroft-Gault equation can be used to estimate creatinine clearance:

   $$CrCl_{est} = \{[(140 - age)BW]/(72 \cdot S_{Cr})\}0.85 = \{[(140 - 35 \text{ y})75 \text{ kg}]/(72 \cdot 3.7 \text{ mg/dL})\}0.85$$
   $$CrCl_{est} = 25 \text{ mL/min}$$

2. *Determine dosage interval and maintenance dose.*
   The maintenance dose is calculated using the modified vancomycin dosing equation:

   $$D \text{ (in mg/h/kg)} = 0.834(CrCl \text{ in mL/min/kg}) + 0.06$$
   $$D = 0.834[(25 \text{ mL/min})/75 \text{ kg}] + 0.06 = 0.339 \text{ mg/h/kg}$$
   $$D = 0.339 \text{ mg/h/kg} \cdot 75 \text{ kg} = 25.5 \text{ mg/h}$$

   The standard dose of 1000 mg can be used to gain an approximation for an acceptable dosage interval (τ):

   $$\tau = 1000 \text{ mg}/(25.5 \text{ mg/h}) = 39.2 \text{ h}$$

   Dosage intervals should be rounded to clinically acceptable intervals of 8, 12, 18, 24, 36, 48, 72 hours, and multiples of 24 hours thereafter, whenever possible. In this case, the dosage interval would be rounded to 36 hours.

   $$D = 25.5 \text{ mg/h} \cdot 36 \text{ h} = 916 \text{ mg}$$

   Vancomycin doses should be rounded to the nearest 100–250 mg. This dose would be rounded to 1000 mg. The prescribed maintenance dose would be 1000 mg every 36 hours.

3. *Compute loading dose.*
   A loading dose (LD) of 15 mg/kg is suggested by the Moellering nomogram, and this value is adjusted by 1.33:

   $$LD = 15 \text{ mg/kg}(75 \text{ kg})1.33 = 1496 \text{ mg}$$

   This loading dose would be rounded off to 1500 mg and given as the first dose. The first maintenance dose would be given one dosage interval (36 hours) after the loading dose.

Matzke Nomogram Method

1. *Estimate creatinine clearance.*
   This patient has a stable serum creatinine and is not obese. The Cockcroft-Gault equation can be used to estimate creatinine clearance:

   $$CrCl_{est} = \{[(140 - age)BW]/(72 \cdot S_{Cr})\}0.85 = \{[(140 - 35 \text{ y})75 \text{ kg}]/(72 \cdot 3.7 \text{ mg/dL})\}0.85$$
   $$CrCl_{est} = 25 \text{ mL/min}$$

2. *Compute loading dose (see Table 5-4).*
   A loading dose (LD) of 25 mg/kg will provide a peak concentration of 30 μg/mL.

   $$LD = 25 \text{ mg/kg}(75 \text{ kg}) = 1875 \text{ mg, rounded to } 1750 \text{ mg}$$

3. *Determine dosage interval and maintenance dose.*
   Round the creatinine clearance value to 30 mL/min. From the nomogram the dosage interval is 2 days or 48 hours. The maintenance dose would be:

   $$19 \text{ mg/kg} \cdot 75 \text{ kg} = 1425 \text{ mg}$$

Vancomycin doses should be rounded to the nearest 100-250 mg. This dose would be rounded to 1500 mg and given one dosage interval (48 hours) after the loading dose.
The prescribed maintenance dose would be 1500 mg every 48 hours.

4. *Solution to Problem 4.* The revised vancomycin dose for patient HT would be calculated as follows:

Pharmacokinetics Concept Method

1. *Estimate creatinine clearance.*
   This patient has a stable serum creatinine and is not obese. The Cockcroft-Gault equation can be used to estimate creatinine clearance:

   $$CrCl_{est} = \{[(140 - age)BW]/(72 \cdot S_{Cr})\}0.85 = \{[(140 - 35 \text{ y})75 \text{ kg}]/(72 \cdot 3.7 \text{ mg/dL})\}0.85$$
   $$CrCl_{est} = 25 \text{ mL/min}$$

2. *Estimate elimination rate constant (k_e) and half-life ($t_{1/2}$).*
   The vancomycin clearance versus creatinine clearance relationship is used to estimate drug clearance for this patient:

   $$Cl = 0.695(CrCl) + 0.05 = 0.695[(25 \text{ mL/min})/75 \text{ kg}] + 0.05 = 0.283 \text{ mL/min/kg}$$

   The average volume of distribution for vancomycin is 0.7 L/kg:

   $$V = 0.7 \text{ L/kg} \cdot 75 \text{ kg} = 52.5 \text{ L}$$
   $$k_e = Cl/V - (0.283 \text{ mL/min/kg} \cdot 60 \text{ min/h})/(0.7 \text{ L/kg} \cdot 1000 \text{ mL/L}) = 0.0242 \text{ h}^{-1}$$
   $$t_{1/2} = 0.693/k_e = 0.693/0.0242 \text{ h}^{-1} = 28.6 \text{ h}$$

   Because the patient has been receiving vancomycin for more than 3-5 estimated half-lives, it is likely that the measured serum concentrations are close to steady-state values. This steady-state concentration pair can be used to compute the patient's own unique pharmacokinetic parameters that can be used to calculate individualized doses.

3. *Use Pharmacokinetics Concept method to compute a new dose.*
   a. *Draw a rough sketch of the serum log concentration/time curve by hand, keeping track of the relative time between the serum concentrations (Figure 5-13).*
   b. *Because the patient is at steady state, the trough concentration can be extrapolated to the next trough value time (see Figure 5-13).*
   c. *Draw the elimination curve between the steady-state peak concentration and the extrapolated trough concentration. Use this line to estimate half-life.* The patient is receiving a vancomycin dose of 1200 mg given every 48 hours that produces a steady-state peak equal to 60 µg/mL and a steady-state trough equal to 24 µg/mL. The dose is infused over 1 hour and the peak concentration is drawn ½ hour later (see Figure 5-13). The time between the measured steady-state peak and the extrapolated trough concentration is 46.5 hours (the 48-hour dosage interval minus the 1.5-hour combined infusion and waiting time). The definition of half-life is the time needed for serum concentrations to decrease by ½. It would take 1 half-life for the peak serum concentration to decline from 60 to 30 µg/mL and an additional half-life for concentrations to drop from 30 to 15 µg/mL. The concentration of 24 µg/mL is between the extrapolated values of 30 and 15 µg/mL. Therefore, ~1.5 half-lives expired during the 46.5-hour time period between the peak concentration and extrapolated trough concentration, and the estimated half-life is ~31 hours (46.5 h/1.5 half-lives = ~31 hours). This information will be used to set the new dosage interval for the patient.

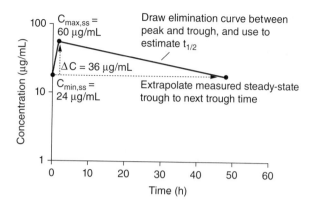

FIGURE 5-13   Solution to Problem 4 using Pharmacokinetic Concept method.

d. *Determine the difference in concentration between the steady-state peak and trough concentrations. The difference in concentration will change proportionally with the dose size.* In the current example the patient is receiving a vancomycin dose equal to 1200 mg every 48 hours, which produced steady-state peak and trough concentrations of 60 μg/mL and 24 μg/mL, respectively. The difference between the peak and trough values is 36 μg/mL. The change in serum concentration is proportional to the dose, and this information will be used to set a new dose for the patient.

e. *Choose new steady-state peak and trough concentrations.* For the purposes of this example, the desired steady-state peak and trough concentrations will be 40 μg/mL and 20 μg/mL, respectively.

f. *Determine the new dosage interval for the desired concentrations.* Using the desired concentrations, it will take 1 half-life for the peak concentration of 40 μg/mL to decrease to 20 μg/mL. Therefore, the dosage interval will need to be approximately 1 half-life or 36 hours (31 hours × 1 half-lives = 31 hours, round to 36 hours).

g. *Determine the new dose for the desired concentrations.* The desired peak concentration is 40 μg/mL, and the expected trough concentration is 20 μg/mL. The change in concentration between these values is 20 μg/mL. It is known from measured serum concentrations that administration of 1200 mg changes serum concentrations by 36 μg/mL and that the change in serum concentration between the peak and trough values is proportional to the size of the dose. In this case: $D_{new} = (\Delta C_{new}/\Delta C_{old})$ $D_{old} = (20\ \mu g/mL/36\ \mu g/mL)1200\ mg = 667\ mg$, rounded to 750 mg (dose rounded up due to MRSA infection). Vancomycin 750 mg every 36 hours would be started 36 hours after the last dose of the previous dosage regimen.

One-Compartment Model Parameter Method

1. *Estimate creatinine clearance.*
   This patient has a stable serum creatinine and is not obese. The Cockcroft-Gault equation can be used to estimate creatinine clearance:

$$CrCl_{est} = \{[(140 - age)BW]/(72 \bullet S_{Cr})\}0.85 = \{[(140 - 35\ y)75\ kg]/(72 \bullet 3.7\ mg/dL)\}0.85$$

$$CrCl_{est} = 25\ mL/min$$

2. *Estimate elimination rate constant (k_e) and half-life ($t_{1/2}$).*
The vancomycin clearance versus creatinine clearance relationship is used to estimate drug clearance for this patient:

$$Cl = 0.695(CrCl) + 0.05 = 0.695[(25 \text{ mL/min})/75 \text{ kg}] + 0.05 = 0.283 \text{ mL/min/kg}$$

The average volume of distribution for vancomycin is 0.7 L/kg:

$$V = 0.7 \text{ L/kg} \bullet 75 \text{ kg} = 52.5 \text{ L}$$

$$k_e = Cl/V = (0.283 \text{ mL/min/kg} \bullet 60 \text{ min/h})/(0.7 \text{ L/kg} \bullet 1000 \text{ mL/L}) = 0.0242 \text{ h}^{-1}$$

$$t_{1/2} = 0.693/k_e = 0.693/0.0242 \text{ h}^{-1} = 28.6 \text{ h}$$

Because the patient has been receiving vancomycin for more than 3-5 estimated half-lives, it is likely that the measured serum concentrations are close to steady-state values. This steady-state concentration pair can be used to compute the patient's own unique pharmacokinetic parameters that can be used to calculate individualized doses.

3. *Use One-Compartment Model Parameter method to compute a new dose.*
a. *Compute the patient's elimination rate constant and half-life. (Note: t' = infusion time + waiting time of 1 hour and ½ hour, respectively.)*

$$k_e = (\ln Css_{max} - \ln Css_{min})/\tau - t' = (\ln 60 \text{ μg/mL} - \ln 24 \text{ μg/mL})/(48 \text{ h} - 1.5 \text{ h}) = 0.0197 \text{ h}^{-1}$$

$$t_{1/2} = 0.693/k_e = 0.693/0.0197 \text{ h}^{-1} = 35.2 \text{ h}$$

b. *Compute the patient's volume of distribution.*

$$V = D/(Css_{max} - Css_{min}) = 1200 \text{ mg}/(60 \text{ mg/L} - 24 \text{ mg/L}) = 33.3 \text{ L}$$

c. *Choose new steady-state peak and trough concentrations.* For the purpose of this example, the desired steady-state peak and trough concentrations will be 40 μg/mL and 20 μg/mL, respectively.
d. *Determine the new dosage interval for the desired concentrations.* As in the initial dosage section of this chapter, the dosage interval (τ) is computed using the following equation:

$$\tau = (\ln Css_{max} - \ln Css_{min})/k_e = (\ln 40 \text{ μg/mL} - \ln 20 \text{ μg/mL})/0.0197 \text{ h}^{-1} = 35 \text{ h, rounded to 36 h}$$

e. *Determine the new dose for the desired concentrations.* The dose is computed using the one-compartment model intravenous bolus equation used in the initial dosing section of this chapter:

$$D = Css_{max} V(1 - e^{-k_e\tau}) = 40 \text{ mg/L} \bullet 33.3 \text{ L } [1 - e^{-(0.0197 \text{ h}^{-1})(36 \text{ h})}] = 677 \text{ mg, rounded to 750 mg}$$

A dose of vancomycin 750 mg every 36 hours would be prescribed to begin 36 hours after the last dose of the previous regimen. This dose is identical to that derived for the patient using the Pharmacokinetic Concepts method.

Bayesian Pharmacokinetic Computer Program Method

1. *Enter patient demographic, drug dosing, and serum concentration/time data into the computer program.*
2. *Compute pharmacokinetic parameters for the patient using Bayesian pharmacokinetic computer program.*
The pharmacokinetic parameters computed by the program are a volume of distribution of 35.6 L, a half-life equal to 40.4 hours, and an elimination rate constant of 0.0172 h^{-1}.
3. *Compute dose required to achieve desired vancomycin serum concentrations.*
The one-compartment model intravenous infusion equations used by the program to compute doses indicate that a dose of 750 mg every 48 hours will produce a steady-state peak concentration of

36.8 µg/mL and a steady-state trough concentration of 16.6 µg/mL. Using the Pharmacokinetic Concepts method or the One-Compartment Model Parameter method gives similar answers.

5. *Solution to Problem 5.* The initial vancomycin dose for patient LK would be calculated as follows:

Pharmacokinetic Dosing Method

1. *Estimate creatinine clearance.*
   This patient has a stable serum creatinine and is obese [IBW_{males} (in kg) = 50 + 2.3(Ht – 60) = 50 + 2.3(68 – 60) = 68.4 kg]. The Salazar-Corcoran equation can be used to estimate creatinine clearance:

   $$CrCl_{est(males)} = \frac{(137 - age)[(0.285 \bullet Wt) + (12.1 \bullet Ht^2)]}{(51 \bullet S_{Cr})}$$

   $$CrCl_{est(males)} = \frac{(137 - 55 \ y)\{(0.285 \bullet 140 \ kg) + [12.1 \bullet (1.73 \ m)^2]\}}{(51 \bullet 0.9 \ mg/dL)} = 136 \ mL/min$$

   Note: Height is converted from inches to meters: Ht = (68 in • 2.54 cm/in)/(100 cm/m) = 1.73 m.

2. *Estimate vancomycin clearance.*
   The vancomycin clearance versus creatinine clearance relationship is used to estimate the vancomycin clearance for this patient:

   Cl = 0.695(CrCl) + 0.05 = 0.695[(136 mL/min)/140 kg] + 0.05 = 0.724 mL/min/kg TBW

3. *Estimate vancomycin volume of distribution.*
   The average volume of distribution for vancomycin is 0.7 L/kg IBW:

   $$V = 0.7 \ L/kg \bullet 68.4 \ kg = 47.9 \ L$$

4. *Estimate vancomycin elimination rate constant (k_e) and half-life ($t_{1/2}$).*

   $$k_e = Cl/V = (0.724 \ mL/min/kg \ TBW \bullet 140 \ kg \bullet 60 \ min/h)/$$
   $$(0.7 \ L/kg \ IBW \bullet 68.4 \ kg \bullet 1000 \ mL/L) = 0.127 \ h^{-1}$$
   $$t_{1/2} = 0.693/k_e = 0.693/0.127 \ h^{-1} = 5.5 \ h$$

5. *Choose desired steady-state serum concentrations.*

   A Css_{min} = 20 µg/mL and Css_{max} = 45 µg/mL were chosen to treat this patient.

6. *Use intravenous bolus equations to compute dose (see Table 5-2).*
   Calculate required dosage interval (τ):

   $$\tau = (\ln Css_{max} - \ln Css_{min})/k_e = (\ln 45 \ \mu g/mL - \ln 20 \ \mu g/mL)/0.127 \ h^{-1} = 6.4 \ h$$

   Dosage intervals should be rounded to clinically acceptable intervals of 8, 12, 18, 24, 36, 48, 72 hours, and multiples of 24 hours thereafter, whenever possible. In this case, the dosage interval would be rounded to 8 hours.
   Calculate required dose (D):

   $$D = Css_{max} \ V(1 - e^{-k_e\tau}) = 45 \ mg/L \bullet 47.9 \ L \ [1 - e^{-(0.127 \ h^{-1})(8 \ h)}] = 1375 \ mg$$

   Vancomycin doses should be rounded to the nearest 100-250 mg. This dose would be rounded to 1250 mg. (Note: µg/mL = mg/L and this concentration unit was substituted for Css_{max} so that unnecessary unit conversion was not required.)
   The prescribed maintenance dose would be 1250 mg every 8 hours.

7. *Compute loading dose (LD), if needed.*
Loading doses should be considered for patients with creatinine clearance values less than 60 mL/min. The administration of a loading dose in these patients will allow achievement of therapeutic concentrations quicker than if maintenance doses alone are given. However, because the pharmacokinetic parameters used to compute these initial doses are only *estimated* values and not *actual* values, the patient's own parameters may be much different than the estimated constants and steady state will not be achieved until 3-5 half-lives have passed.

$$LD = Css_{max} V = 45 \text{ mg/L} \bullet 47.9 \text{ L} = 2155 \text{ mg}$$

As noted, this patient has good renal function (CrCl ≥60 mL/min) so a loading dose would not be necessary for this patient. (Note: μg/mL = mg/L, and this concentration unit was substituted for Css_{max} so that unnecessary unit conversion was not required.)

Moellering Nomogram Method

1. *Estimate creatinine clearance.*
This patient has a stable serum creatinine and is obese [IBW_{males} (in kg) = 50 + 2.3(Ht − 60) = 50 + 2.3(68 in − 60) = 68.4 kg]. The Salazar-Corcoran equation can be used to estimate creatinine clearance:

$$CrCl_{est(males)} = \frac{(137 - age)[(0.285 \bullet Wt) + (12.1 \bullet Ht^2)]}{(51 \bullet S_{Cr})}$$

$$CrCl_{est(males)} = \frac{(137 - 55 \text{ y})\{(0.285 \bullet 140 \text{ kg}) + [12.1 \bullet (1.73 \text{ m})^2]\}}{(51 \bullet 0.9 \text{ mg/dL})} = 136 \text{ mL/min}$$

Note: Height is converted from inches to meters: Ht = (68 in • 2.54 cm/in)/(100 cm/m) = 1.73 m.

2. *Determine dosage interval and maintenance dose.*
The maintenance dose is calculated using the modified vancomycin dosing equation:

$$D \text{ (in mg/h/kg)} = 0.834(\text{CrCl in mL/min/kg}) + 0.06$$
$$D = 0.834[(136 \text{ mL/min})/140 \text{ kg}] + 0.06 = 0.869 \text{ mg/h/kg TBW}$$
$$D = 0.869 \text{ mg/h/kg} \bullet 140 \text{ kg} = 121.6 \text{ mg/h}$$

The standard dose of 1000 mg can be used to gain an approximation for an acceptable dosage interval (τ):

$$\tau = 1000 \text{ mg/(121.6 mg/h)} = 8.2 \text{ h}$$

Dosage intervals should be rounded to clinically acceptable intervals of 8, 12, 18, 24, 36, 48, 72 hours, and multiples of 24 hours thereafter, whenever possible. In this case, the dosage interval would be rounded to 8 hours.

$$D = 121.6 \text{ mg/h} \bullet 8 \text{ h} = 973 \text{ mg}$$

Vancomycin doses should be rounded to the nearest 100-250 mg. This dose would be rounded to 1000 mg. The prescribed maintenance dose would be 1000 mg every 8 hours.

3. *Compute loading dose.*
A loading dose (LD) of 15 mg/kg IBW is suggested by the Moellering nomogram, and this value is adjusted by 1.33:

$$LD = 15 \text{ mg/kg}(68.4 \text{ kg})1.33 = 1365 \text{ mg}$$

This loading dose would be rounded off to 1500 mg and given as the first dose. The first maintenance dose would be given one dosage interval (8 hours) after the loading dose.

6. *Solution to Problem 6.* The revised vancomycin dose for patient LK would be calculated as follows:

Pharmacokinetics Concept Method

1. *Estimate creatinine clearance.*
   This patient has a stable serum creatinine and is obese (IBW_{males} (in kg) = 50 + 2.3(Ht – 60) = 50 + 2.3 (68 in – 60) = 68.4 kg). The Salazar-Corcoran equation can be used to estimate creatinine clearance:

$$CrCl_{est(males)} = \frac{(137 - age)[(0.285 \bullet Wt) + (12.1 \bullet Ht^2)]}{(51 \bullet S_{Cr})}$$

$$CrCl_{est(males)} = \frac{(137 - 55 \text{ y})\{(0.285 \bullet 140 \text{ kg}) + [12.1 \bullet (1.73 \text{ m})^2]\}}{(51 \bullet 0.9 \text{ mg/dL})} = 136 \text{ mL/min}$$

Note: Height is converted from inches to meters: Ht = (68 in • 2.54 cm/in)/(100 cm/m) = 1.73 m.

2. *Estimate elimination rate constant (k_e) and half-life ($t_{1/2}$).*
   The vancomycin clearance versus creatinine clearance relationship is used to estimate drug clearance for this patient:

$$Cl = 0.695(CrCl) + 0.05 = 0.695[(136 \text{ mL/min})/140 \text{ kg}] + 0.05 = 0.724 \text{ mL/min/kg TBW}$$

The average volume of distribution for vancomycin is 0.7 L/kg IBW:

$$V = 0.7 \text{ L/kg} \bullet 68.4 \text{ kg} = 47.9 \text{ L}$$

$$k_e = Cl/V = (0.724 \text{ mL/min/kg TBW} \bullet 140 \text{ kg} \bullet 60 \text{ min/h})/(0.7 \text{ L/kg} \bullet 68.4 \text{ kg IBW} \bullet 1000 \text{ mL/L}) = 0.127 \text{ h}^{-1}$$

$$t_{1/2} = 0.693/k_e = 0.693/0.127 \text{ h}^{-1} = 5.5 \text{ h}$$

Because the patient has been receiving vancomycin for more than 3-5 estimated half-lives, it is likely that the measured serum concentrations are close to steady-state values. This steady-state concentration pair can be used to compute the patient's own unique pharmacokinetic parameters that can be used to calculate individualized doses.

3. *Use Pharmacokinetics Concept method to compute a new dose.*
   a. *Draw a rough sketch of the serum log concentration/time curve by hand, keeping track of the relative time between the serum concentrations (Figure 5-14).*
   b. *Because the patient is at steady state, the trough concentration can be extrapolated to the next trough value time (see Figure 5-14).*
   c. *Draw the elimination curve between the steady-state peak concentration and the extrapolated trough concentration. Use this line to estimate half-life.* The patient is receiving a vancomycin dose of 1000 mg given every 8 hours that produces a steady-state peak equal to 42 μg/mL and a steady-state trough equal to 18 μg/mL. The dose is infused over 1 hour and the peak concentration is drawn ½ hour later (see Figure 5-14). The time between the measured steady-state peak and the extrapolated trough concentration is 6.5 hours (the 8-hour dosage interval minus the 1.5-hour combined infusion and waiting time). The definition of half-life is the time needed for serum concentrations to decrease by ½. It would take 1 half-life for the peak serum concentration to decline from 42 to 21 μg/mL. The concentration of 18 μg/mL is just slightly less than 21 μg/mL. Therefore, ~1.25 half-lives expired during the 6.5-hour time period between the peak concentration and extrapolated trough

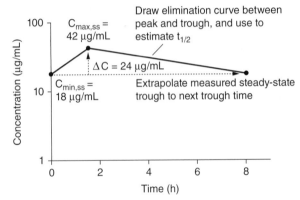

FIGURE 5-14   Solution to Problem 6 using Pharmacokinetic Concept method.

concentration, and the estimated half-life is ~5 hours (6.5 h/1.25 half-lives = ~5 hours). This information will be used to set the new dosage interval for the patient.

d. *Determine the difference in concentration between the steady-state peak and trough concentrations. The difference in concentration will change proportionally with the dose size.* In the current
example the patient is receiving a vancomycin dose equal to 1000 mg every 8 hours, which produced
steady-state peak and trough concentrations of 42 μg/mL and 18 μg/mL, respectively. The difference
between the peak and trough values is 24 μg/mL. The change in serum concentration is proportional
to the dose, and this information will be used to set a new dose for the patient.

e. *Choose new steady-state peak and trough concentrations.* For the purposes of this example, the
desired steady-state peak and trough concentrations will be 40 μg/mL and 10 μg/mL, respectively.

f. *Determine the new dosage interval for the desired concentrations.* Using the desired concentrations, it
will take 1 half-life for the peak concentration of 40 μg/mL to decrease to 20 μg/mL, and an additional
half-life for serum concentrations to decline from 20 to 10 μg/mL. Therefore, the dosage interval will
need to be approximately 2 half-lives or 12 hours (5 hours × 2 half-lives = 10 hours, round to 12 hours).

g. *Determine the new dose for the desired concentrations.* The desired peak concentration is 40 μg/
mL, and the expected trough concentration is 10 μg/mL. The change in concentration between these
values is 30 μg/mL. It is known from measured serum concentrations that administration of 1000 mg
changes serum concentrations by 24 μg/mL and that the change in serum concentration between the
peak and trough values is proportional to the size of the dose. In this case: $D_{new} = (\Delta C_{new}/\Delta C_{old})D_{old} =$
(30 μg/mL/24 μg/mL)1000 mg = 1250 mg. Vancomycin 1250 mg every 12 hours would be started
12 hours after the last dose of the previous dosage regimen.

One-Compartment Model Parameter Method

1. *Estimate creatinine clearance.*
   This patient has a stable serum creatinine and is obese [IBW_{males} (in kg) = 50 + 2.3(Ht − 60) = 50 +
   2.3(68 in − 60) = 68.4 kg]. The Salazar-Corcoran equation can be used to estimate creatinine clearance:

$$CrCl_{est(males)} = \frac{(137 - age)[(0.285 \bullet Wt) + (12.1 \bullet Ht^2)]}{(51 \bullet S_{Cr})}$$

$$CrCl_{est(males)} = \frac{(137 - 55\ y)\{(0.285 \bullet 140\ kg) + [12.1 \bullet (1.73\ m)^2]\}}{(51 \bullet 0.9\ mg/dL)} = 136\ mL/min$$

Note: Height is converted from inches to meters: Ht = (68 in • 2.54 cm/in)/(100 cm/m) = 1.73 m.

2. *Estimate elimination rate constant (k_e) and half-life ($t_{1/2}$).*
The vancomycin clearance versus creatinine clearance relationship is used to estimate drug clearance for this patient:

$$Cl = 0.695(CrCl) + 0.05 = 0.695[(136 \text{ mL/min})/140 \text{ kg}] + 0.05 = 0.724 \text{ mL/min/kg TBW}$$

The average volume of distribution for vancomycin is 0.7 L/kg IBW:

$$V = 0.7 \text{ L/kg} \bullet 68.4 \text{ kg} = 47.9 \text{ L}$$

$$k_e = Cl/V = (0.724 \text{ mL/min/kg TBW} \bullet 140 \text{ kg} \bullet 60 \text{ min/h})/(0.7 \text{ L/kg IBW} \bullet 68.4 \text{ kg} \bullet 1000 \text{ mL/L}) = 0.127 \text{ h}^{-1}$$

$$t_{1/2} = 0.693/k_e = 0.693/0.127 \text{ h}^{-1} = 5.5 \text{ h}$$

Because the patient has been receiving vancomycin for more than 3-5 estimated half-lives, it is likely that the measured serum concentrations are close to steady-state values. This steady-state concentration pair can be used to compute the patient's own unique pharmacokinetic parameters that can be used to calculate individualized doses.

3. *Use One-Compartment Model Parameter method to compute a new dose.*
   a. *Compute the patient's elimination rate constant and half-life. (Note: t' = infusion time + waiting time of 1 hour and ½ hour, respectively.)*

$$k_e = (\ln Css_{max} - \ln Css_{min})/\tau - t' = (\ln 42 \text{ μg/mL} - \ln 18 \text{ μg/mL})/(8 \text{ h} - 1.5 \text{ h}) = 0.130 \text{ h}^{-1}$$

$$t_{1/2} = 0.693/k_e = 0.693/0.130 \text{ h}^{-1} = 5.3 \text{ h}$$

   b. *Compute the patient's volume of distribution.*

$$V = D/(Css_{max} - Css_{min}) = 1000 \text{ mg}/(42 \text{ mg/L} - 18 \text{ mg/L}) = 41.7 \text{ L}$$

   c. *Choose new steady-state peak and trough concentrations.* For the purposes of this example, the desired steady-state peak and trough concentrations will be 40 μg/mL and 10 μg/mL, respectively.

   d. *Determine the new dosage interval for the desired concentrations.* As in the initial dosage section of this chapter, the dosage interval (τ) is computed using the following equation:

$$\tau = (\ln Css_{max} - \ln Css_{min})/k_e = (\ln 40 \text{ μg/mL} - \ln 10 \text{ μg/mL})/0.130 \text{ h}^{-1} = 11 \text{ h, rounded to 12 h}$$

   e. *Determine the new dose for the desired concentrations.* The dose is computed using the one-compartment model intravenous bolus equation used in the initial dosing section of this chapter:

$$D = Css_{max} V(1 - e^{-k_e \tau}) = 40 \text{ mg/L} \bullet 41.7 \text{ L } [1 - e^{-(0.130 \text{ h}^{-1})(12 \text{ h})}] = 1318 \text{ mg, rounded to 1250 mg}$$

A dose of vancomycin 1250 mg every 12 hours would be prescribed to begin 12 hours after the last dose of the previous regimen. This dose is identical to that derived for the patient using the Pharmacokinetic Concepts method.

Bayesian Pharmacokinetic Computer Program Method

1. *Enter patient demographic, drug dosing, and serum concentration/time data into the computer program.*

2. *Compute pharmacokinetic parameters for the patient using Bayesian pharmacokinetic computer program.*

The pharmacokinetic parameters computed by the program are a volume of distribution of 64.4 L, a half-life equal to 12.2 hours, and an elimination rate constant of 0.0568 h^{-1}.

3. *Compute dose required to achieve desired vancomycin serum concentrations.*

   The one-compartment model intravenous infusion equations used by the program to compute doses indicate that a dose of 1250 mg every 18 hours will produce a steady-state peak concentration of 27.8 µg/mL and a steady-state trough concentration of 10.8 µg/mL. Using the Pharmacokinetic Concepts method or the One-Compartment Model Parameter method produced the same answer of 1250 mg every 12 hours. The Bayesian computer program suggests a longer dosage interval and larger dose because of the population pharmacokinetic parameter influence for volume of distribution on the dosing algorithm. If additional concentrations are input into the program, the effect of the population parameters will diminish and eventually produce the same answer as the other two methods.

7. *Solution to Problem 7.* The initial vancomycin dose for patient AF would be calculated as follows:

Pharmacokinetic Dosing Method

1. *Estimate creatinine clearance.*
   This patient has a stable serum creatinine and is obese [IBW$_{females}$ (in kg) = 45 + 2.3(Ht − 60) = 45 + 2.3(62 in − 60) = 49.6 kg]. The Salazar-Corcoran equation can be used to estimate creatinine clearance:

$$CrCl_{est(females)} = \frac{(146 - age)[(0.287 \cdot Wt) + (9.74 \cdot Ht^2)]}{(60 \cdot S_{Cr})}$$

$$CrCl_{est(females)} = \frac{(146 - 45 \text{ y})\{(0.287 \cdot 140 \text{ kg}) + [9.74 \cdot (1.57 \text{ m})^2]\}}{(60 \cdot 2.4 \text{ mg/dL})} = 45 \text{ mL/min}$$

Note: Height is converted from inches to meters: Ht = (62 in • 2.54 cm/in)/(100 cm/m) = 1.57 m.

2. *Estimate vancomycin clearance.*
   The vancomycin clearance versus creatinine clearance relationship is used to estimate the vancomycin clearance for this patient:

   Cl = 0.695(CrCl) + 0.05 = 0.695[(45 mL/min)/140 kg] + 0.05 = 0.274 mL/min/kg TBW

3. *Estimate vancomycin volume of distribution.*
   The average volume of distribution for vancomycin is 0.7 L/kg IBW:

   V = 0.7 L/kg • 49.6 kg = 34.7 L

4. *Estimate vancomycin elimination rate constant (k_e) and half-life ($t_{1/2}$).*

   k_e = Cl/V = (0.274 mL/min/kg TBW • 140 kg • 60 min/h)/
   (0.7 L/kg IBW • 49.6 kg • 1000 mL/L) = 0.0663 h^{-1}
   $t_{1/2}$ = 0.693/k_e = 0.693/0.0663 h^{-1} = 10.5 h

5. *Choose desired steady-state serum concentrations.*

   A Css$_{min}$ = 12 µg/mL and Css$_{max}$ = 40 µg/mL were chosen to treat this patient.

6. *Use intravenous bolus equations to compute dose (see Table 5-2).*
   Calculate required dosage interval (τ):

   τ = (ln Css$_{max}$ − ln Css$_{min}$)/k_e = (ln 40 µg/mL − ln 12 µg/mL)/0.0663 h^{-1} = 18.2 h

   Dosage intervals should be rounded to clinically acceptable intervals of 8, 12, 18, 24, 36, 48, 72 hours, and multiples of 24 hours thereafter, whenever possible. In this case, the dosage interval would be rounded to 18 hours.

Calculate required dose (D):

$$D = Css_{max} \, V \, (1 - e^{-k_e\tau}) = 40 \text{ mg/L} \cdot 34.7 \text{ L} \, [1 - e^{-(0.0663 \text{ h}^{-1})(18 \text{ h})}] = 968 \text{ mg}$$

Vancomycin doses should be rounded to the nearest 100-250 mg. This dose would be rounded to 1000 mg. (Note: μg/mL = mg/L, and this concentration unit was substituted for Css_{max} so that unnecessary unit conversion was not required.)

The prescribed maintenance dose would be 1000 mg every 18 hours.

7. *Compute loading dose (LD), if needed.*

Loading doses should be considered for patients with creatinine clearance values less than 60 mL/min. The administration of a loading dose in these patients will allow achievement of therapeutic concentrations quicker than if maintenance doses alone are given. However, because the pharmacokinetic parameters used to compute these initial doses are only *estimated* values and not *actual* values, the patient's own parameters may be much different than the estimated constants and steady state will not be achieved until 3-5 half-lives have passed.

$$LD = Css_{max} \, V = 40 \text{ mg/L} \cdot 34.7 \text{ L} = 1389 \text{ mg}$$

As noted, this patient has moderate renal function (CrCl <60 mL/min) so a loading dose would be prescribed for this patient. The loading dose would be rounded to 1500 mg and given as the first dose. Maintenance doses would begin one dosage interval after the loading dose was administered. (Note: μg/mL = mg/L, and this concentration unit was substituted for Css_{max} so that unnecessary unit conversion was not required.)

Moellering Nomogram Method

1. *Estimate creatinine clearance.*

This patient has a stable serum creatinine and is obese [$IBW_{females}$ (in kg) = 45 + 2.3(Ht − 60) = 45 + 2.3 (62 in − 60) = 49.6 kg]. The Salazar-Corcoran equation can be used to estimate creatinine clearance:

$$CrCl_{est(females)} = \frac{(146 - age)[(0.287 \cdot Wt) + (9.74 \cdot Ht^2)]}{(60 \cdot S_{Cr})}$$

$$CrCl_{est(females)} = \frac{(146 - 45 \text{ y})\{(0.287 \cdot 140 \text{ kg}) + [9.74 \cdot (1.57 \text{ m})^2]\}}{(60 \cdot 2.4 \text{ mg/dL})} = 45 \text{ mL/min}$$

Note: Height is converted from inches to meters: Ht = (62 in · 2.54 cm/in)/(100 cm/m) = 1.57 m.

2. *Determine dosage interval and maintenance dose.*

The maintenance dose is calculated using the modified vancomycin dosing equation:

$$D \text{ (in mg/h/kg)} = 0.834(CrCl \text{ in mL/min/kg}) + 0.06$$
$$D = 0.834[(45 \text{ mL/min})/140 \text{ kg}] + 0.06 = 0.329 \text{ mg/h/kg TBW}$$
$$D = 0.329 \text{ mg/h/kg} \cdot 140 \text{ kg} = 46.0 \text{ mg/h}$$

The standard dose of 1000 mg can be used to gain an approximation for an acceptable dosage interval (τ):

$$\tau = 1000 \text{ mg}/(46.0 \text{ mg/h}) = 21.7 \text{ h}$$

Dosage intervals should be rounded to clinically acceptable intervals of 8, 12, 18, 24, 36, 48, 72 hours, and multiples of 24 hours thereafter, whenever possible. In this case, the dosage interval would be rounded to 24 hours.

$$D = 46.0 \text{ mg/h} \cdot 24 \text{ h} = 1105 \text{ mg}$$

Vancomycin doses should be rounded to the nearest 100-250 mg. This dose would be rounded to 1000 mg. The prescribed maintenance dose would be 1000 mg every 24 hours.

3. *Compute loading dose.*
A loading dose (LD) of 15 mg/kg IBW is suggested by the Moellering nomogram, and this value is adjusted by 1.66:

$$LD = 15 \text{ mg/kg}(49.6 \text{ kg})1.66 = 1235 \text{ mg, rounded to } 1250 \text{ mg}$$

This loading dose would be given as the first dose 1250 mg. The first maintenance dose would be given one dosage interval (24 hours) after the loading dose.

8. *Solution to Problem 8.* The revised vancomycin dose for patient AF would be calculated as follows:

Pharmacokinetics Concept Method

1. *Estimate creatinine clearance.*
This patient has a stable serum creatinine and is obese [$IBW_{females}$ (in kg) = 45 + 2.3(Ht − 60) = 45 + 2.3(62 in − 60) = 49.6 kg]. The Salazar-Corcoran equation can be used to estimate creatinine clearance:

$$CrCl_{est(females)} = \frac{(146 - \text{age})[(0.287 \bullet \text{Wt}) + (9.74 \bullet \text{Ht}^2)]}{(60 \bullet S_{Cr})}$$

$$CrCl_{est(females)} = \frac{(146 - 45 \text{ y})\{(0.287 \bullet 140 \text{ kg}) + [9.74 \bullet (1.57 \text{ m})^2]\}}{(60 \bullet 2.4 \text{ mg/dL})} = 45 \text{ mL/min}$$

Note: Height is converted from inches to meters: Ht = (62 in • 2.54 cm/in)/(100 cm/m) = 1.57 m.

2. *Estimate elimination rate constant (k_e) and half-life ($t_{1/2}$).*
The vancomycin clearance versus creatinine clearance relationship is used to estimate drug clearance for this patient:

$$Cl = 0.695(CrCl) + 0.05 = 0.695[(45 \text{ mL/min})/140 \text{ kg}] + 0.05 = 0.274 \text{ mL/min/kg TBW}$$

The average volume of distribution for vancomycin is 0.7 L/kg IBW:

$$V = 0.7 \text{ L/kg} \bullet 49.6 \text{ kg} = 34.7 \text{ L}$$

$$k_e = Cl/V = (0.274 \text{ mL/min/kg TBW} \bullet 140 \text{ kg} \bullet 60 \text{ min/h})/(0.7 \text{ L/kg} \bullet 49.6 \text{ kg} \bullet 1000 \text{ mL/L}) = 0.0663 \text{ h}^{-1}$$

$$t_{1/2} = 0.693/k_e = 0.693/0.0663 \text{ h}^{-1} = 10.5 \text{ h}$$

Because the patient has been receiving vancomycin for more than 3-5 estimated half-lives, it is likely that the measured serum concentrations are close to steady-state values. This steady-state concentration pair can be used to compute the patient's own unique pharmacokinetic parameters that can be used to calculate individualized doses.

3. *Use Pharmacokinetics Concept method to compute a new dose.*
   a. *Draw a rough sketch of the serum log concentration/time curve by hand, keeping track of the relative time between the serum concentrations (Figure 5-15).*
   b. *Because the patient is at steady state, the trough concentration can be extrapolated to the next trough value time (see Figure 5-15).*
   c. *Draw the elimination curve between the steady-state peak concentration and the extrapolated trough concentration. Use this line to estimate half-life. The patient is receiving a vancomycin*

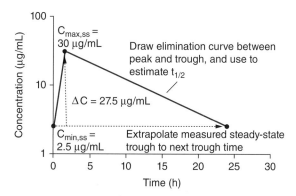

FIGURE 5-15 Solution to Problem 8 using Pharmacokinetic Concept method.

dose of 1300 mg given every 24 hours that produces a steady-state peak equal to 30 μg/mL and a steady-state trough equal to 2.5 μg/mL. The dose is infused over 1 hour and the peak concentration is drawn ½ hour later (see Figure 5-15). The time between the measured steady-state peak and the extrapolated trough concentration is 22.5 hours (the 24-hour dosage interval minus the 1.5-hour combined infusion and waiting time). The definition of half-life is the time needed for serum concentrations to decrease by ½. It would take 1 half-life for the peak serum concentration to decline from 30 to 15 μg/mL, an additional half-life for the concentration to decrease from 15 to 7.5 μg/mL, another half-life for the concentration to decline from 7.5 to 4 μg/mL, and a final half-life for the concentration to reach 2 μg/mL. The concentration of 2 μg/mL is just slightly less than 2.5 μg/mL. Therefore, 4 half-lives expired during the 22.5-hour time period between the peak concentration and extrapolated trough concentration, and the estimated half-life is ~6 hours (22.5 h/4 half-lives = ~6 hours). This information will be used to set the new dosage interval for the patient.

d. *Determine the difference in concentration between the steady-state peak and trough concentrations. The difference in concentration will change proportionally with the dose size.* In the current example the patient is receiving a vancomycin dose equal to 1300 mg every 24 hours, which produced steady-state peak and trough concentrations of 30 μg/mL and 2.5 μg/mL, respectively. The difference between the peak and trough values is 27.5 μg/mL. The change in serum concentration is proportional to the dose, and this information will be used to set a new dose for the patient.

e. *Choose new steady-state peak and trough concentrations.* For the purposes of this example, the desired steady-state peak and trough concentrations will be 40 μg/mL and 12 μg/mL, respectively.

f. *Determine the new dosage interval for the desired concentrations.* Using the desired concentrations, it will take 1 half-life for the peak concentration of 40 μg/mL to decrease to 20 μg/mL, and an additional half-life for serum concentrations to decline from 20 to 10 μg/mL. Therefore, the dosage interval will need to be approximately 2 half-lives or 12 hours (6 hours × 2 half-lives = 12 hours).

g. *Determine the new dose for the desired concentrations.* The desired peak concentration is 40 μg/mL, and the expected trough concentration is 12 μg/mL. The change in concentration between these values is 28 μg/mL. It is known from measured serum concentrations that administration of 1300 mg changes serum concentrations by 27.5 μg/mL and that the change in serum concentration between the peak and trough values is proportional to the size of the dose. In this case: $D_{new} = (\Delta C_{new}/\Delta C_{old})D_{old} = (28 \, \mu g/mL/27.5 \, \mu g/mL)1300 \, mg = 1324 \, mg$, rounded to 1250 mg. Vancomycin 1250 mg every 12 hours would be started 12 hours after the last dose of the previous dosage regimen.

One-Compartment Model Parameter Method

1. *Estimate creatinine clearance.*
   This patient has a stable serum creatinine and is obese [$IBW_{females}$ (in kg) = 45 + 2.3(Ht − 60) = 45 + 2.3 (62 in − 60) = 49.6 kg]. The Salazar-Corcoran equation can be used to estimate creatinine clearance:

   $$CrCl_{est(females)} = \frac{(146 - age)[(0.287 \bullet Wt) + (9.74 \bullet Ht^2)]}{(60 \bullet S_{Cr})}$$

   $$CrCl_{est(females)} = \frac{(146 - 45 \text{ y})\{(0.287 \bullet 140 \text{ kg}) + [9.74 \bullet (1.57 \text{ m})^2]\}}{(60 \bullet 2.4 \text{ mg/dL})} = 45 \text{ mL/min}$$

   Note: Height is converted from inches to meters: Ht = (62 in • 2.54 cm/in)/(100 cm/m) = 1.57 m.

2. *Estimate elimination rate constant (k_e) and half-life ($t_{1/2}$).*
   The vancomycin clearance versus creatinine clearance relationship is used to estimate drug clearance for this patient:

   $$Cl = 0.695(CrCl) + 0.05 = 0.695[(45 \text{ mL/min})/140 \text{ kg}] + 0.05 = 0.274 \text{ mL/min/kg TBW}$$

   The average volume of distribution for vancomycin is 0.7 L/kg IBW:

   $$V = 0.7 \text{ L/kg} \bullet 49.6 \text{ kg} = 34.7 \text{ L}$$

   $$k_e = Cl/V = (0.274 \text{ mL/min/kg TBW} \bullet 140 \text{ kg} \bullet 60 \text{ min/h})/(0.7 \text{ L/kg} \bullet 49.6 \text{ kg} \bullet 1000 \text{ mL/L}) = 0.0663 \text{ h}^{-1}$$
   $$t_{1/2} = 0.693/k_e = 0.693/0.0663 \text{ h}^{-1} = 10.5 \text{ h}$$

   Because the patient has been receiving vancomycin for more than 3-5 estimated half-lives, it is likely that the measured serum concentrations are close to steady-state values. This steady-state concentration pair can be used to compute the patient's own unique pharmacokinetic parameters that can be used to calculate individualized doses.

3. *Use One-Compartment Model Parameter method to compute a new dose.*
   a. *Compute the patient's elimination rate constant and half-life. (Note: t′ = infusion time + waiting time of 1 hour and ½ hour, respectively.)*

   $$k_e = (\ln Css_{max} - \ln Css_{min})/\tau - t' = (\ln 30 \text{ μg/mL} - \ln 2.5 \text{ μg/mL})/(24 \text{ h} - 1.5 \text{ h}) = 0.110 \text{ h}^{-1}$$
   $$t_{1/2} = 0.693/k_e = 0.693/0.110 \text{ h}^{-1} = 6.3 \text{ h}$$

   b. *Compute the patient's volume of distribution.*

   $$V = D/(Css_{max} - Css_{min}) = 1300 \text{ mg}/(30 \text{ mg/L} - 2.5 \text{ mg/L}) = 47.3 \text{ L}$$

   c. *Choose new steady-state peak and trough concentrations.* For the purposes of this example, the desired steady-state peak and trough concentrations will be 40 μg/mL and 12 μg/mL, respectively.
   d. *Determine the new dosage interval for the desired concentrations.* As in the initial dosage section of this chapter, the dosage interval (τ) is computed using the following equation:

   $$\tau = (\ln Css_{max} - \ln Css_{min})/k_e = (\ln 40 \text{ μg/mL} - \ln 12 \text{ μg/mL})/0.110 \text{ h}^{-1} = 11 \text{ h, round to 12 h}$$

   e. *Determine the new dose for the desired concentrations.* The dose is computed using the one-compartment model intravenous bolus equation used in the initial dosing section of this chapter:

   $$D = Css_{max} V(1 - e^{-k_e\tau}) = 40 \text{ mg/L} \bullet 47.3 \text{ L } [1 - e^{-(0.110 \text{ h}^{-1})(12 \text{ h})}] = 1388 \text{ mg, rounded to 1500 mg}$$

A dose of vancomycin 1500 mg every 12 hours would be prescribed to begin 12 hours after the last dose of the previous regimen (dose rounded up because patient is being treated for endocarditis).

Bayesian Pharmacokinetic Computer Program Method

1. *Enter patient demographic, drug dosing, and serum concentration/time data into the computer program.*
2. *Compute pharmacokinetic parameters for the patient using Bayesian pharmacokinetic computer program.*

   The pharmacokinetic parameters computed by the program are a volume of distribution of 39.4 L, a half-life equal to 6.3 hours, and an elimination rate constant of 0.110 h^{-1}.

3. *Compute dose required to achieve desired vancomycin serum concentrations.*

   The one-compartment model intravenous infusion equations used by the program to compute doses indicate that a dose of 1500 mg every 12 hours will produce a steady-state peak concentration of 44.2 µg/mL and a steady-state trough concentration of 14.0 µg/mL. Using the Pharmacokinetic Concepts method or the One-Compartment Model Parameter method produced the similar results.

9. *Solution to Problem 9.* The initial vancomycin dose for patient DG would be calculated as follows:

Pharmacokinetic Dosing Method

1. *Estimate creatinine clearance.*

   This patient has a stable serum creatinine and is not obese. The Cockcroft-Gault equation can be used to estimate creatinine clearance:

$$CrCl_{est} = \{[(140 - age)BW]/(72 \cdot S_{Cr})\}0.85 = \{[(140 - 66 \text{ y})65 \text{ kg}]/(72 \cdot 1.4 \text{ mg/dL})\}0.85$$

$$CrCl_{est} = 41 \text{ mL/min}$$

2. *Estimate vancomycin clearance.*

   The vancomycin clearance versus creatinine clearance relationship is used to estimate the vancomycin clearance for this patient:

$$Cl = 0.695(CrCl) + 0.05 = 0.695[(41 \text{ mL/min})/65 \text{ kg}] + 0.05 = 0.484 \text{ mL/min/kg}$$

3. *Estimate vancomycin volume of distribution.*

   The average volume of distribution for vancomycin is 0.7 L/kg:

$$V = 0.7 \text{ L/kg} \cdot 65 \text{ kg} = 45.5 \text{ L}$$

4. *Estimate vancomycin elimination rate constant (k_e) and half-life $(t_{1/2})$.*

$$k_e = Cl/V = (0.484 \text{ mL/min/kg} \cdot 60 \text{ min/h})/(0.7 \text{ L/kg} \cdot 1000 \text{ mL/L}) = 0.0415 \text{ h}^{-1}$$

$$t_{1/2} = 0.693/k_e = 0.693/0.0415 \text{ h}^{-1} = 16.7 \text{ h}$$

5. *Choose desired steady-state serum concentrations.*

   A $Css_{min} = 20$ µg/mL and $Css_{max} = 50$ µg/mL were chosen to treat this patient.

6. *Use intravenous bolus equations to compute dose (see Table 5-2).*

   Calculate required dosage interval (τ):

$$\tau = (\ln Css_{max} - \ln Css_{min})/k_e = (\ln 50 \text{ µg/mL} - \ln 20 \text{ µg/mL})/0.0415 \text{ h}^{-1} = 22.1 \text{ h}$$

Dosage intervals should be rounded to clinically acceptable intervals of 8, 12, 18, 24, 36, 48, 72 hours, and multiples of 24 hours thereafter, whenever possible. In this case, the dosage interval would be rounded to 24 hours.

Calculate required dose (D):

$$D = Css_{max} \, V(1 - e^{-k_e\tau}) = 50 \text{ mg/L} \bullet 45.5 \text{ L } [1 - e^{-(0.0415 \text{ h}^{-1})(24 \text{ h})}] = 1434 \text{ mg}$$

Vancomycin doses should be rounded to the nearest 100-250 mg. This dose would be rounded to 1500 mg. (Note: μg/mL = mg/L, and this concentration unit was substituted for Css_{max} so that unnecessary unit conversion was not required.)

The prescribed maintenance dose would be 1500 mg every 24 hours.

7. *Compute loading dose (LD), if needed.*
   Loading doses should be considered for patients with creatinine clearance values less than 60 mL/min. The administration of a loading dose in these patients will allow achievement of therapeutic concentrations quicker than if maintenance doses alone are given. However, because the pharmacokinetic parameters used to compute these initial doses are only *estimated* values and not *actual* values, the patient's own parameters may be much different than the estimated constants and steady state will not be achieved until 3-5 half-lives have passed.

$$LD = Css_{max} \, V = 50 \text{ mg/L} \bullet 45.5 \text{ L} = 2275 \text{ mg}$$

As noted, this patient has moderate renal function (CrCl <60 mL/min) so a loading dose would be prescribed for this patient and given as the first dose. Vancomycin doses should be rounded to the nearest 100-250 mg. This dose would be rounded to 2250 mg. (Note: μg/mL = mg/L, and this concentration unit was substituted for Css_{max} so that unnecessary unit conversion was not required.) The first maintenance dose would be given one dosage interval (24 hours) after the loading dose was administered.

Moellering Nomogram Method

1. *Estimate creatinine clearance.*
   This patient has a stable serum creatinine and is not obese. The Cockcroft-Gault equation can be used to estimate creatinine clearance:

$$CrCl_{est} = \{[(140 - \text{age})BW]/(72 \bullet S_{Cr})\}0.85 = \{[(140 - 66 \text{ y})65 \text{ kg}]/(72 \bullet 1.4 \text{ mg/dL})\}0.85$$
$$CrCl_{est} = 41 \text{ mL/min}$$

2. *Determine dosage interval and maintenance dose.*
   The maintenance dose is calculated using the modified vancomycin dosing equation:

$$D \text{ (in mg/h/kg)} = 0.834(CrCl \text{ in mL/min/kg}) + 0.06$$
$$D = 0.834[(41 \text{ mL/min})/65 \text{ kg}] + 0.06 = 0.586 \text{ mg/h/kg}$$
$$D = 0.586 \text{ mg/h/kg} \bullet 65 \text{ kg} = 38.1 \text{ mg/h}$$

The standard dose of 1000 mg can be used to gain an approximation for an acceptable dosage interval (τ):

$$\tau = 1000 \text{ mg}/(38.1 \text{ mg/h}) = 26.3 \text{ h}$$

Dosage intervals should be rounded to clinically acceptable intervals of 8, 12, 18, 24, 36, 48, 72 hours, and multiples of 24 hours thereafter, whenever possible. In this case, the dosage interval would be rounded to 24 hours.

$$D = 38.1 \text{ mg/h} \bullet 24 \text{ h} = 914 \text{ mg}$$

Vancomycin doses should be rounded to the nearest 100-250 mg. This dose would be rounded to 1000 mg. The prescribed maintenance dose would be 1000 mg every 24 hours.

3. *Compute loading dose.*
A loading dose (LD) of 15 mg/kg is suggested by the Moellering nomogram, and this value is adjusted by 1.5:

$$LD = 15 \text{ mg/kg}(65 \text{ kg})1.5 = 1463 \text{ mg, rounded to } 1500$$

As noted, this patient has poor renal function (CrCl <60 mL/min) so a loading dose would be prescribed and given as the first dose. Vancomycin doses should be rounded to the nearest 100-250 mg. (Note: μg/mL = mg/L, and this concentration unit was substituted for Css_{max} so that unnecessary unit conversion was not required.) The first maintenance dose would be given one dosage interval (24 hours) after the loading dose was administered.

Matzke Nomogram Method

1. *Estimate creatinine clearance.*
This patient has a stable serum creatinine and is not obese. The Cockcroft-Gault equation can be used to estimate creatinine clearance:

$$CrCl_{est} = \{[(140 - \text{age})BW]/(72 \cdot S_{Cr})\}0.85 = \{[(140 - 66 \text{ y})65 \text{ kg}]/(72 \cdot 1.4 \text{ mg/dL})\}0.85$$
$$CrCl_{est} = 41 \text{ mL/min}$$

2. *Compute loading dose (see Table 5-4).*
A loading dose (LD) of 25 mg/kg will provide a peak concentration of 30 μg/mL.

$$LD = 25 \text{ mg/kg}(65 \text{ kg}) = 1625 \text{ mg, round to } 1500 \text{ mg}$$

3. *Determine dosage interval and maintenance dose.*
From the nomogram the dosage interval is 1.5 days or 36 hours. The maintenance dose would be 19 mg/kg • 65 kg = 1235 mg. Vancomycin doses should be rounded to the nearest 100–250 mg. This dose would be rounded to 1250 mg and given one dosage interval (36 hours) after the loading dose.
The prescribed maintenance dose would be 1250 mg every 36 hours.

Rybak Nomogram Method

1. *Estimate creatinine clearance.*
This patient has a stable serum creatinine and is not obese. The Cockcroft-Gault equation can be used to estimate creatinine clearance:

$$CrCl_{est} = \{[(140 - \text{age})BW]/(72 \cdot S_{Cr})\}0.85 = \{[(140 - 66 \text{ y})65 \text{ kg}]/(72 \cdot 1.4 \text{ mg/dL})\}0.85$$
$$CrCl_{est} = 41 \text{ mL/min}$$

2. *Determine dosage interval and maintenance dose (see Table 5-5).*
From the nomogram the vancomycin dosage is 750 mg every 12 hours. Because the patient's $CrCl_{est}$ is less than 60 mL/min, loading dose (LD) of 25-30 mg/kg actual body weight could be administered as the first dose: LD = 25 mg/kg • 65 kg = 1625 mg, rounded to 1500 mg.

10. *Solution to Problem 10.* The revised vancomycin dose for patient DG would be calculated as follows:

Linear Pharmacokinetics Method

1. *Estimate creatinine clearance.*
   This patient has a stable serum creatinine and is not obese. The Cockcroft-Gault equation can be used to estimate creatinine clearance:

   $$CrCl_{est} = \{[(140 - age)BW]/(72 \cdot S_{Cr})\}0.85 = \{[(140 - 66 \text{ y})65 \text{ kg}]/(72 \cdot 1.4 \text{ mg/dL})\}0.85$$

   $$CrCl_{est} = 41 \text{ mL/min}$$

2. *Estimate elimination rate constant (k_e) and half-life ($t_{1/2}$).*
   The vancomycin clearance versus creatinine clearance relationship is used to estimate drug clearance for this patient:

   $$Cl = 0.695(CrCl) + 0.05 = 0.695[(41 \text{ mL/min})/65 \text{ kg}] + 0.05 = 0.484 \text{ mL/min/kg}$$

   The average volume of distribution for vancomycin is 0.7 L/kg:

   $$V = 0.7 \text{ L/kg} \cdot 65 \text{ kg} = 45.5 \text{ L}$$
   $$k_e = Cl/V = (0.484 \text{ mL/min/kg} \cdot 60 \text{ min/h})/(0.7 \text{ L/kg} \cdot 1000 \text{ mL/L}) = 0.0415 \text{ h}^{-1}$$
   $$t_{1/2} = 0.693/k_e = 0.693/0.0415 \text{ h}^{-1} = 16.7 \text{ h}$$

   Because the patient has been receiving vancomycin for more than 3-5 estimated half-lives, it is likely that the measured serum concentrations are steady-state values.

3. *Compute new dose to achieve desired serum concentration.*
   Using linear pharmacokinetics, the new dose to attain the desired concentration should be proportional to the old dose that produced the measured concentration:

   $$D_{new} = (C_{ss,new}/C_{ss,old})D_{old} = (15 \text{ μg/mL} / 12 \text{ μg/mL})1200 \text{ mg} = 1500 \text{ mg}$$

   The new suggested dose would be 1500 mg every 36 hours to be started at next scheduled dosing time.

4. *Check steady-state peak concentration for new dosage regimen.*
   Using linear pharmacokinetics, the new steady-state concentration can be estimated and should be proportional to the old dose that produced the measured concentration:

   $$C_{ss,new} = (D_{new}/D_{old})C_{ss,old} = (1500 \text{ mg}/1200 \text{ mg}) 30 \text{ μg/mL} = 37.5 \text{ μg/mL}$$

   This steady-state peak concentration should be safe and effective for the infection that is being treated.

11. *Solution to Problem 11.* The initial vancomycin dose for patient GG would be calculated as follows:

Pharmacokinetic Dosing Method

1. *Estimate creatinine clearance.*
   This patient is not obese. The patient is in acute renal failure and receiving hemodialysis. Because dialysis removes creatinine, the serum creatinine cannot be used to estimate creatinine clearance for the patient. Because the patient's renal function is poor enough to require dialysis, the creatinine clearance will be assumed to equal zero.

2. *Estimate vancomycin clearance.*
   The vancomycin clearance versus creatinine clearance relationship is used to estimate the vancomycin clearance for this patient:

   $$Cl = 0.695(CrCl) + 0.05 = 0.695[(0 \text{ mL/min})/85 \text{kg}] + 0.05 = 0.05 \text{ mL/min/kg}$$

3. *Estimate vancomycin volume of distribution.*
   The average volume of distribution for vancomycin is 0.7 L/kg:

   $$V = 0.7 \text{ L/kg} \bullet 85 \text{ kg} = 59.5 \text{ L}$$

4. *Estimate vancomycin elimination rate constant (k_e) and half-life ($t_{1/2}$).*

   $$k_e = Cl/V = (0.05 \text{ mL/min/kg} \bullet 60 \text{ min/h})/(0.7 \text{ L/kg} \bullet 1000 \text{ mL/L}) = 0.0043 \text{ h}^{-1}$$
   $$t_{1/2} = 0.693/k_e = 0.693/0.0043 \text{ h}^{-1} = 161 \text{ h}$$

5. *Choose desired steady-state serum concentrations.*

   A Css_{min} = 20 µg/mL and Css_{max} = 40 µg/mL were chosen to treat this patient.

6. *Use intravenous bolus equations to compute dose (see Table 5-2).*
   Calculate required dosage interval (τ):

   $$\tau = (\ln Css_{max} - \ln Css_{min})/k_e = (\ln 40 \text{ µg/mL} - \ln 20 \text{ µg/mL})/0.0043 \text{ h}^{-1} = 162 \text{ h}$$

   Dosage intervals should be rounded to clinically acceptable intervals of 8, 12, 18, 24, 36, 48, 72 hours, and multiples of 24 hours thereafter, whenever possible. In this case, the dosage interval would be rounded to 168 hours or 7 days.
   Calculate required dose (D):

   $$D = Css_{max} V(1 - e^{-k_e\tau}) = 40 \text{ mg/L} \bullet 59.5 \text{ L} [1 - e^{-(0.0043 \text{ h}^{-1})(168 \text{ h})}] = 1222 \text{ mg}$$

   Vancomycin doses should be rounded to the nearest 100-250 mg. This dose would be rounded to 1250 mg. (Note: µg/mL = mg/L, and this concentration unit was substituted for Css_{max} so that unnecessary unit conversion was not required.)
   The prescribed maintenance dose would be 1250 mg every 7 days.

7. *Compute loading dose (LD), if needed.*
   Loading doses should be considered for patients with creatinine clearance values less than 60 mL/min. The administration of a loading dose in these patients will allow achievement of therapeutic concentrations quicker than if maintenance doses alone are given. However, because the pharmacokinetic parameters used to compute these initial doses are only *estimated* values and not *actual* values, the patient's own parameters may be much different than the estimated constants and steady state will not be achieved until 3-5 half-lives have passed.

   $$LD = Css_{max} V = 40 \text{ mg/L} \bullet 59.5 \text{ L} = 2380 \text{ mg}$$

   As noted, this patient has poor renal function (CrCl <60 mL/min) so a loading dose would be prescribed for this patient and given as the first dose. Vancomycin doses should be rounded to the nearest 100-250 mg. This dose would be rounded to 2500 mg. (Note: µg/mL = mg/L, and this concentration unit was substituted for Css_{max} so that unnecessary unit conversion was not required.) The first maintenance dose would be given one dosage interval (7 days) after the loading dose was administered. In this patient case, it is possible that only one dose will need to be given if the infection resolves before a maintenance dose is due.

Moellering Nomogram Method

1. *Estimate creatinine clearance.*
   This patient is not obese. The patient is in acute renal failure and receiving hemodialysis. Because dialysis removes creatinine, the serum creatinine cannot be used to estimate creatinine clearance for

the patient. Because the patient's renal function is poor enough to require dialysis, the creatinine clearance will be assumed to equal zero.

2. *Determine dosage interval and maintenance dose.*
The maintenance dose is calculated using the nomogram suggested dose for functionally anephric patients, with value adjusted by 1.33:

$$D = 1.9 \text{ mg/kg/24 h} \bullet \text{Weight} \bullet 1.33$$
$$D = 1.9 \text{ mg/kg/24h} \bullet 85 \text{ kg} \bullet 1.33 = 214.8 \text{ mg/24 h}$$

The standard dose of 2000 mg/24 h in patients with normal renal function can be used to gain an approximation for an acceptable dosage interval (τ):

$$\tau = (2000 \text{ mg/24 h})/(214.8 \text{ mg/24 h}) = 9.3 \text{ d}$$

Dosage intervals should be rounded to clinically acceptable intervals of 8, 12, 18, 24, 36, 48, 72 hours, and multiples of 24 hours thereafter, whenever possible. In this case, the dosage interval would be rounded to 9 days.

$$D = 214.8 \text{ mg/d} \bullet 9 \text{ d} = 1933 \text{ mg}$$

Vancomycin doses should be rounded to the nearest 100-250 mg. This dose would be rounded to 2000 mg. The prescribed maintenance dose would be 2000 mg every 9 days.

3. *Compute loading dose.*
A loading dose (LD) of 15 mg/kg is suggested by the Moellering nomogram, with the value adjusted by 1.66:

$$LD = 15 \text{ mg/kg}(85 \text{ kg})1.66 = 2117 \text{ mg, round to 2250 mg}$$

This loading dose would be given as the first dose, and subsequent maintenance doses would be given every 9 days, if needed. In this patient case, it is possible that only one dose will need to be given if the infection resolves before a maintenance dose is due.

Matzke Nomogram Method

1. *Estimate creatinine clearance.*
This patient is not obese. The patient is in acute renal failure and receiving hemodialysis. Because dialysis removes creatinine, the serum creatinine cannot be used to estimate creatinine clearance for the patient. Because the patient's renal function is poor enough to require dialysis, the creatinine clearance will be assumed to equal zero.

2. *Compute loading dose (see Table 5-4).*
A loading dose (LD) of 25 mg/kg will provide a peak concentration of 30 µg/mL.

$$LD = 25 \text{ mg/kg}(85 \text{ kg}) = 2125 \text{ mg, round to 2000 mg}$$

3. *Determine dosage interval and maintenance dose.*
From the nomogram the dosage interval is 12 days. The maintenance dose would be 19 mg/kg $\bullet$ 85 kg = 1615 mg. Vancomycin doses should be rounded to the nearest 100-250 mg. This dose would be rounded to 1500 mg and given one dosage interval (12 days) after the loading dose. In this patient case, it is possible that only one dose will need to be given if the infection resolves before a maintenance dose is due. The prescribed maintenance dose would be 1500 mg every 12 days.

12. *Solution to Problem 12.* The revised vancomycin dose for patient GG would be calculated as follows:

After the first dose, this patient is not at steady state so none of the steady-state dosing methods are valid. Also, hemodialysis with a low-flux filter will not affect the elimination of the drug and is not a factor in calculating the drug dose.

One-Compartment Model Parameter Method

a. *Compute the patient's elimination rate constant and half-life. (See Table 5-2, single-dose equations. Note: t′ = infusion time + waiting time of 1 hour and ½ hour, respectively.)*

$$k_e = (\ln C_1 - \ln C_2)/\Delta t = (\ln 20\ \mu g/mL - \ln 12.1\ \mu g/mL)/(72\ h) = 0.0070\ h^{-1}$$

$$t_{1/2} = 0.693/k_e = 0.693/0.0070\ h^{-1} = 99.2\ h$$

b. *Compute the patient's volume of distribution.*

The vancomycin serum concentration needs to be extrapolated to the immediate postdose time 42.5 hours (accounting for infusion and waiting times) previous to the first measured concentration before the volume of distribution can be calculated:

$$C_{max} = C/e^{-k_e t} = (20\ \mu g/mL)/e^{-(0.0070\ h^{-1})(42.5\ h)} = 26.9\ \mu g/mL$$

$$V = D/C_{max} = 1600\ mg/(26.9\ mg/L) = 59.5\ L$$

c. *Choose new steady-state peak and trough concentrations.* For the purposes of this example, the desired steady-state peak and trough concentrations will be 45 µg/mL and 20 µg/mL, respectively.

d. *Determine the new dosage interval for the desired concentrations.* As in the initial dosage section of this chapter, the dosage interval (τ) is computed using the following equation:

$$\tau = (\ln Css_{max} - \ln Css_{min})/k_e = (\ln 45\ \mu g/mL - \ln 20\ \mu g/mL)/0.0070\ h^{-1} = 116\ h,\ \text{round to 120 h or 5 d}$$

e. *Determine the new dose for the desired concentrations.* The dose is computed using the one-compartment model intravenous bolus equation used in the initial dosing section of this chapter:

$$D = Css_{max}\ V(1 - e^{-k_e \tau}) = 45\ mg/L \cdot 59.5\ L\ [1 - e^{-(0.0070\ h^{-1})(120\ h)}] = 1522\ mg,\ \text{rounded to 1500 mg}$$

A dose of vancomycin 1500 mg every 5 days would be prescribed to begin now. In this patient case, it may not be necessary to administer another maintenance dose if the infection resolves before the next dose is due.

Bayesian Pharmacokinetic Computer Program Method

1. *Enter patient demographic, drug dosing, and serum concentration/time data into the computer program.*

2. *Compute pharmacokinetic parameters for the patient using Bayesian pharmacokinetic computer program.*

   The pharmacokinetic parameters computed by the program are a volume of distribution of 60.9 L, a half-life equal to 108 hours, and an elimination rate constant of 0.0064 h^{-1}.

3. *Compute dose required to achieve desired vancomycin serum concentrations.*
   The one-compartment model intravenous infusion equations used by the program to compute doses indicate that a dose of 1500 mg every 5 days will produce a steady-state peak concentration of 44.2 µg/mL and a steady-state trough concentration of 20.7 µg/mL.

13. *Solution to Problem 13.* The revised vancomycin dose for patient FD would be calculated as follows:

Bayesian Pharmacokinetic Computer Program Method

After the second dose, this patient is not at steady state so none of the steady-state dosing methods are valid.

1. *Enter patient demographic, drug dosing, and serum concentration/time data into the computer program.*

2. *Compute pharmacokinetic parameters for the patient using Bayesian pharmacokinetic computer program.*
   The pharmacokinetic parameters computed by the program are a volume of distribution of 63.1 L, a half-life equal to 38.1 hours, and an elimination rate constant of 0.0182 h^{-1}.

3. *Compute dose required to achieve desired vancomycin serum concentrations.*
   The one-compartment model intravenous infusion equations used by the program to compute doses indicate that a dose of 1250 mg every 48 hours will produce a steady-state peak concentration of 34 μg/mL and a steady-state trough concentration of 14 μg/mL.

14. *Solution to Problem 14.* The revised vancomycin dose for patient OI would be calculated as follows:

Bayesian Pharmacokinetic Computer Program Method

After the second dose, this patient is not at steady state so none of the steady-state dosing methods are valid.

1. *Enter patient demographic, drug dosing, and serum concentration/time data into the computer program.*

2. *Compute pharmacokinetic parameters for the patient using Bayesian pharmacokinetic computer program.*
   The pharmacokinetic parameters computed by the program are a volume of distribution of 57 L, a half-life equal to 15.3 hours, and an elimination rate constant of 0.0453 h^{-1}.

3. *Compute dose required to achieve desired vancomycin serum concentrations.*
   The one-compartment model intravenous infusion equations used by the program to compute doses indicate that a dose of 1250 mg every 18 hours will produce a steady-state peak concentration of 37 μg/mL and a steady-state trough concentration of 17 μg/mL.

15. *Solution to Problem 15.* The revised vancomycin dose for patient HY would be calculated as follows:

Bayesian Pharmacokinetic Computer Program Method

After the first dose, this patient is not at steady state so none of the steady-state dosing methods are valid.

1. *Enter patient demographic, drug dosing, and serum concentration/time data into the computer program.*

2. *Compute pharmacokinetic parameters for the patient using Bayesian pharmacokinetic computer program.*
   The pharmacokinetic parameters computed by the program are a volume of distribution of 39.2 L, a half-life equal to 13.2 hours, and an elimination rate constant of 0.0525 h^{-1}.

3. *Compute dose required to achieve desired vancomycin serum concentrations.*
   The one-compartment model intravenous infusion equations used by the program to compute doses indicate that a dose of 1250 mg every 18 hours will produce a steady-state peak concentration of 48 μg/mL and a steady-state trough concentration of 20 μg/mL.

16. *Solution to Problem 16.*

Literature-Based Recommended Dosing

1. *Compute initial dose and dosage interval.*
   From the pediatrics dosage recommendations given in earlier in this chapter, a patient in this age and renal function category should receive vancomycin 15 mg/kg every 12 hours. (*Note: Gram will be converted to kilogram before the computation is made.*)

$$Dose = 15 \text{ mg/kg}(1.550 \text{ kg}) = 23 \text{ mg}$$

   The prescribed dose will be 23 mg every 12 hours.

17. *Solution to Problem 17.*

Linear Pharmacokinetics Method

1. *Compute new dose to achieve desired serum concentration.*
   Using linear pharmacokinetics, the new dose to attain the desired concentration should be proportional to the old dose that produced the measured concentration. (*Note: The assumption that steady state was attained should be verified by checking the medication administration record.*)

$$D_{new} = (C_{ss,new}/C_{ss,old})D_{old} = (15 \text{ µg/mL}/8.6 \text{ µg/mL})20 \text{ mg} = 35 \text{ mg}$$

   The new suggested dose would be 35 mg every 12 hours to be started at next scheduled dosing time.

2. *Check steady-state peak concentration for new dosage regimen.*
   Using linear pharmacokinetics, the new steady-state concentration can be estimated and should be proportional to the old dose that produced the measured concentration:

$$C_{ss,new} = (D_{new}/D_{old})C_{ss,old} = (35 \text{ mg}/20 \text{ mg}) \ 20 \text{ µg/mL} = 35 \text{ µg/mL}$$

   This steady-state peak concentration should be safe and effective for the infection that is being treated.

18. *Solution to Problem 18.*

Literature-Based Recommended Dosing

1. *Estimate creatinine clearance.*
   This patient has a stable serum creatinine and is not obese. The pediatric CrCl equation from Chapter 3 can be used to estimate creatinine clearance. (*Note: Height is converted from inches to centimeters, 47 in • 2.54 cm/in = 119 cm.*)

$$CrCl_{est} = (0.55 \bullet Ht)/S_{Cr} = (0.55 \bullet 119 \text{ cm})/(0.5 \text{ mg/dL})$$
$$CrCl_{est} = 131 \text{ mL/min}/1.73 \text{ m}^2$$

   The patient has normal renal function, so typical initial doses can be used.

2. *Compute initial dose and dosage interval, using literature-based recommended dosing for pediatric patients.*
   The dosage recommendations for this population assume typical renal function, so it is important to verify that the assumption is valid.
   From the pediatrics dosage recommendations given earlier in this chapter, a patient in this age and weight category should receive vancomycin 45-60 mg/kg/d given as divided doses every 6-8 hours for a severe infection. Because the patient is being treated for sepsis, the highest dose and shortest dosage interval are selected.

$$Dose = 60 \text{ mg/kg/d}(24 \text{ kg}) = 1440 \text{ mg/d}$$
$$(1440 \text{ mg/d})/(4 \text{ doses/d}) = 360 \text{ mg/dose, round to 350 mg}$$

   The prescribed dose will be 350 mg every 6 hours.

19. *Solution to Problem 19.*

Linear Pharmacokinetics Method

1. *Compute new dose to achieve desired serum concentration.*
   Using linear pharmacokinetics, the new dose to attain the desired concentration should be proportional to the old dose that produced the measured concentration. (*Note: The assumption that steady state was attained should be verified by checking the medication administration record.*)

$$D_{new} = (C_{ss,new}/C_{ss,old})D_{old} = (15 \ \mu g/mL \ /10 \ \mu g/mL)250 \ mg = 375 \ mg$$

The new suggested dose would be 375 mg every 6 hours to be started at next scheduled dosing time.

2. *Check steady-state peak concentration for new dosage regimen.*
   Using linear pharmacokinetics, the new steady-state concentration can be estimated and should be proportional to the old dose that produced the measured concentration:

$$C_{ss,new} = (D_{new}/D_{old})C_{ss,old} = (375 \ mg/250 \ mg) \ 25 \ \mu g/mL = 37.5 \ \mu g/mL$$

This steady-state peak concentration should be safe and effective for the infection that is being treated.

20. *Solution to Problem 20.*

Trough-Only Method

1. *Estimate creatinine clearance.*
   This patient has a stable serum creatinine and is not obese. The Cockcroft-Gault equation can be used to estimate creatinine clearance:

$$CrCl_{est} = \{[(140 - age)BW]0.85\}/(72 \bullet S_{Cr}) = \{[(140 - 75 \ y)66 \ kg]0.85\}/(72 \bullet 1.8 \ mg/dL)$$
$$CrCl_{est} = 28 \ mL/min$$

2. *Estimate elimination rate constant (k_e) and half-life ($t_{1/2}$).*
   The vancomycin clearance versus creatinine clearance relationship is used to estimate drug clearance for this patient:

$$Cl = 0.695(CrCl) + 0.05 = 0.695[(28 \ mL/min)/66 \ kg] + 0.05 = 0.345 \ mL/min/kg$$

The average volume of distribution for vancomycin is 0.7 L/kg:

$$V = 0.7 \ L/kg \bullet 66 \ kg = 46 \ L$$

$$k_e = Cl/V = (0.345 \ mL/min/kg \bullet 60 \ min/h)/(0.7 \ L/kg \bullet 1000 \ mL/L) = 0.0296 \ h^{-1}$$
$$t_{1/2} = 0.693/k_e = 0.693/0.0296 \ h^{-1} = 23 \ h$$

Because the patient has been receiving vancomycin for more than 3 estimated half-lives, it is likely that the measured serum concentrations are steady-state values.

3. *Compute new dosage interval to achieve desired serum concentration.*
   The new dosage interval to attain the desired concentration should be:

$$\tau_{new} = (C_{ss,old}/C_{ss,new})\tau_{old} = (25 \ \mu g/mL/15 \ \mu g/mL)24 \ h = 40 \ h, \text{ round to } 36 \ h$$

Dosage intervals should be rounded to clinically acceptable intervals of 8, 12, 18, 24, 36, 48, 72 hours, and multiples of 24 hours thereafter, whenever possible. In this case, the dosage interval would be rounded to 36 hours. The new suggested dose would be 1000 mg every 36 hours to be started 36 hours after the last dose.

21. *Solution to Problem 21.*

Trough-Only method

1. *Estimate creatinine clearance.*

   This patient has a stable serum creatinine and is obese [IBW$_{females}$ (in kg) = 45 + 2.3(Ht − 60) = 45 + 2.3(67 in − 60) = 61 kg]. The Salazar-Corcoran equation can be usd to estimate creatinine clearance:

$$CrCl_{est(females)} = \frac{(146 - age)[(0.287 \bullet Wt) + (9.74 \bullet Ht^2)]}{(60 \bullet S_{Cr})}$$

$$CrCl_{est(females)} = \frac{(146 - 48\ y)\{(0.287 \bullet 170\ kg) + [9.74 \bullet (1.70\ m)^2]\}}{(60 \bullet 1.3\ mg/dL)} = 97\ mL/min$$

   Note: Height is converted from inches to meters: Ht = (67 in • 2.54 cm/in)/(100 cm/m) = 1.70 m.

2. *Estimate elimination rate constant (k_e) and half-life ($t_{1/2}$).*

   The vancomycin clearance versus creatinine clearance relationship is used to estimate drug clearance for this patient:

$$Cl = 0.695(CrCl) + 0.05 = 0.695[(97\ mL/min)/170\ kg] + 0.05 = 0.447\ mL/min/kg$$

   The average volume of distribution for vancomycin is 0.7 L/kg IBW:

$$V = 0.7\ L/kg \bullet 61\ kg = 43\ L$$

$$k_e = Cl/V = (0.447\ mL/min/kg \bullet 170\ kg \bullet 60\ min/h)/(0.7\ L/kg \bullet 61\ kg \bullet 1000\ mL/L) = 0.107\ h^{-1}$$

$$t_{1/2} = 0.693/k_e = 0.693/0.107\ h^{-1} = 6.5\ h$$

   Because the patient has been receiving vancomycin for more than 3-5 estimated half-lives, it is likely that the measured serum concentrations are steady-state values.

3. *Compute new dosage interval to achieve desired serum concentration.*

   The new dosage interval to attain the desired concentration should be:

$$\tau_{new} = (C_{ss,old}/C_{ss,new})\tau_{old} = (8\ \mu g/mL\ /\ 15\ \mu g/mL)24\ h = 12.8\ h,\ round\ to\ 12\ h$$

   The new suggested dose would be 1000 mg every 12 hours to be started 12 hours after the last dose.

22. *Solution to Problem 22.*

Combined Linear Pharmacokinetics/Trough-Only Methods

Note: This patient requires a large change in concentration, and it will be difficult to attain the goal by changing only the dose or only the dosage interval. Combine the Linear Pharmacokinetic and Trough-Only methods to alter both the dose and dosage interval, respectively.

1. *Estimate creatinine clearance.*

   This patient has a stable serum creatinine and is not obese. The Cockcroft-Gault equation can be used to estimate creatinine clearance:

$$CrCl_{est} = [(140 - age)BW]/(72 \bullet S_{Cr}) = [(140 - 75\ y)62\ kg]/(72 \bullet 1.3\ mg/dL)$$

$$CrCl_{est} = 43\ mL/min$$

2. *Estimate vancomycin clearance.*
The vancomycin clearance versus creatinine clearance relationship is used to estimate the vancomycin clearance for this patient:

$$Cl = 0.695(CrCl) + 0.05 = 0.695[(43 \text{ mL/min})/62\text{kg}] + 0.05 = 0.533 \text{ mL/min/kg}$$

3. *Estimate vancomycin volume of distribution.*
The average volume of distribution for vancomycin is 0.7 L/kg:

$$V = 0.7 \text{ L/kg} \cdot 62 \text{ kg} = 43.4 \text{ L}$$

4. *Estimate vancomycin elimination rate constant (k_e) and half-life ($t_{1/2}$).*

$$k_e = Cl/V = (0.533 \text{ mL/min/kg} \cdot 60 \text{ min/h})/(0.7 \text{ L/kg} \cdot 1000 \text{ mL/L}) = 0.0457 \text{ h}^{-1}$$

$$t_{1/2} = 0.693/k_e = 0.693/0.0457 \text{ h}^{-1} = 15.2 \text{ h}$$

Because the patient has been receiving vancomycin for more than 3-5 estimated half-lives, it is likely that the measured serum concentration is a steady-state value.

5. *Compute new dose to achieve desired serum concentration.*
Using linear pharmacokinetics, a new dose to attain a portion of the desired concentration change will be computed:

$$D_{new} = (C_{ss,new}/C_{ss,old})D_{old} = (9 \text{ μg/mL}/6 \text{ μg/mL}) \ 1000 \text{ mg} = 1500 \text{ mg}$$

The new dose would be 1500 mg.

6. *Compute new dosage interval to achieve desired serum concentration.*
The new dosage interval to attain the desired concentration should be:

$$\tau_{new} = (C_{ss,old}/C_{ss,new})\tau_{old} = (9 \text{ μg/mL}/15 \text{ μg/mL}) \ 24 \text{ h} = 14.4 \text{ h, round to } 12 \text{ h}$$

The new suggested dose would be 1500 mg every 12 hours to be started 12 hours after the last dose.

23. *Solution to Problem 23.*

Combined Linear Pharmacokinetics/Trough-Only Methods

Note: This patient requires a large change in concentration, and it will be difficult to attain the goal by changing only the dose or only the dosage interval. Combine the Linear Pharmacokinetic and Trough-Only methods to alter both the dose and dosage interval, respectively.

1. *Estimate creatinine clearance.*
This patient has a stable serum creatinine and is not obese. The Cockcroft-Gault equation can be used to estimate creatinine clearance:

$$CrCl_{est} = [(140 - age)BW]/(72 \cdot S_{Cr}) = [(140 - 22 \text{ y})75 \text{ kg}]/(72 \cdot 2.3 \text{ mg/dL})$$

$$CrCl_{est} = 53 \text{ mL/min}$$

2. *Estimate vancomycin clearance.*
The vancomycin clearance versus creatinine clearance relationship is used to estimate the vancomycin clearance for this patient:

$$Cl = 0.695(CrCl) + 0.05 = 0.695[(53 \text{ mL/min})/75\text{kg}] + 0.05 = 0.545 \text{ mL/min/kg}$$

3. *Estimate vancomycin volume of distribution.*
The average volume of distribution for vancomycin is 0.7 L/kg:

$$V = 0.7 \text{ L/kg} \bullet 75 \text{ kg} = 52.5 \text{ L}$$

4. *Estimate vancomycin elimination rate constant (k_e) and half-life ($t_{1/2}$).*

$$k_e = Cl/V = (0.545 \text{ mL/min/kg} \bullet 60 \text{ min/h})/(0.7 \text{ L/kg} \bullet 1000 \text{ mL/L}) = 0.0467 \text{ h}^{-1}$$

$$t_{1/2} = 0.693/k_e = 0.693/0.0467 \text{ h}^{-1} = 14.8 \text{ h}$$

Because the patient has been receiving vancomycin for more than 3-5 estimated half-lives, it is likely that the measured serum concentration is a steady-state value.

5. *Compute new dose to achieve desired serum concentration.*
Using linear pharmacokinetics, a new dose to attain a portion of the desired concentration change will be computed:

$$D_{new} = (C_{ss,new}/C_{ss,old})D_{old} = (20 \text{ µg/mL} /27 \text{ µg/mL}) \ 1500 \text{ mg} = 1111 \text{ mg, round to } 1000 \text{ mg}$$

The new dose would be 1000 mg.

6. *Compute new dosage interval to achieve desired serum concentration.*
The new dosage interval to attain the desired concentration should be:

$$\tau_{new} = (C_{ss,old}/C_{ss,new})\tau_{old} = (20 \text{ µg/mL} / 15 \text{ µg/mL})8 \text{ h} = 11 \text{ h, round to } 12 \text{ h}$$

The new suggested dose would be 1000 mg every 12 hours to be started 12 hours after the last dose.

24. *Solution to Problem 24.*

Estimated AUC$_{24}$ Ratio Method

1. *Estimate creatinine clearance.*
This patient has a stable serum creatinine and is not obese. The Cockcroft-Gault equation can be used to estimate creatinine clearance:

$$CrCl_{est} = [(140 - \text{age})BW]/(72 \bullet S_{Cr}) = [(140 - 55 \text{ y})78 \text{ kg}]/(72 \bullet 1.5 \text{ mg/dL})$$

$$CrCl_{est} = 61 \text{ mL/min}$$

2. *Estimate AUC$_{24}$/MIC.*
The total daily dose of vancomycin is: D = (1000 mg/18 h)24 h = 1333 mg/d.

The AUC$_{24}$/MIC ratio will be estimated using the AUC$_{24}$ equation and the measured MIC:

$$AUC_{24} = D/\{[(CrCl_{est} \bullet 0.79) + 15.4] \bullet 0.06\} = (1333 \text{ mg})/\{[(61 \text{ mL/min} \bullet 0.79)$$
$$+ 15.4] \bullet 0.06\} = 349.4 \text{ (mg} \bullet \text{h)/L}$$
$$AUC_{24}/MIC = [349.4 \text{ (mg} \bullet \text{h)/L]}/(1 \text{ mg/L}) = 349.4$$

Note: µg/mL = mg/L, so this substitution was made in the equation, and the AUC$_{24}$/MIC ratio is usually reported as a unitless value.

3. *Compute new dose based on AUC$_{24}$/MIC > 400.*
Vancomycin follows linear pharmacokinetics, so the AUC and steady-state trough concentrations change proportionally with dose.

$$Dose_{new} = [(AUC_{24}/MIC)_{new}/(AUC_{24}/MIC)_{old}]Dose_{old} = (400/349.4)(1333 \text{ mg/d})$$
$$= 1526 \text{ mg/d, round to } 1500 \text{ mg/d}$$

The new dose would be 1500 mg every 24 hours.

Check a new steady-state vancomycin trough concentration in 3-5 half-lives for this new dosage regimen to make sure that it is also consistent with treatment goals for the patient.

25. *Solution to Problem 25.*
Measured AUC_{24} using steady-state peak and trough concentrations method.

1. *Calculate AUC_{24}/MIC.*
The AUC for a dose is: $AUC = AUC_{inf} + AUC_{elim}$ or $AUC = \{[(Css_{min} + Css_{max})/2]\Delta t_{inf}\} + \{(Css_{max} - Css_{min})/[\ln (Css_{max}/Css_{min})]\}\Delta t_{elim}$

$$AUC = \{[(7 \ \mu g/mL + 25 \ \mu g/mL)/2]1.5 \ h\} + \{(25 \ \mu g/mL - 7 \ \mu g/mL)/[\ln (25 \ \mu g/mL/7 \ \mu g/mL)]\}$$
$$(12 \ h - 1.5 \ h) = 172.5 \ (\mu g \bullet h)/mL = 172.5 \ (mg \bullet h)/L \ (\text{Note: } \mu g/mL = mg/L)$$

Dosage interval is 12 hours, so an adjustment of AUC is needed for number of doses per day:

$$AUC_{24} = (2 \ doses)[172.5 \ (mg \bullet h)/L \ per \ dose] = 345.0 \ (mg \bullet h)/L$$

$$AUC_{24}/MIC = [345.0 \ (\mu g \bullet h)/mL]/ \ 1 \ \mu g/mL = 345.0$$

2. *Compute new dose based on $AUC_{24}/MIC > 400$.*
Vancomycin follows linear pharmacokinetics, so the AUC and steady-state trough concentrations change proportionally with dose.

$$Dose_{new} = [(AUC_{24}/MIC)_{new}/(AUC_{24}/MIC)_{old}]Dose_{old} = (400/345.0)(2000 \ mg/d)$$

$$= 2319 \ mg/d, \ round \ to \ 2500 \ mg/d \ or \ 1250 \ mg \ every \ 12 \ hours$$

Check new steady-state vancomycin trough concentration for this AUC_{24}/MIC ratio:

$$C_{ss,new} = (D_{new}/D_{old})C_{ss,old} = (1250 \ mg/1000 \ mg)7 \ \mu g/mL = 9 \ \mu g/mL$$

26. *Solution to Problem 26.*

Measured AUC_{24} computed using concentration(s) and a Bayesian pharmacokinetic computer program method.

1. *Calculate AUC_{24}/MIC, using the Bayesian pharmacokinetic computer program.*
The pharmacokinetic parameters computed by the program are a volume of distribution of 51 L, a half-life equal to 12.7 hours, and clearance of 2.8 L/h.

The AUC for a dose is: $AUC = D/Cl = (1000 \ mg)/(2.8 \ L/h) = 357.1 \ (mg \bullet h)/L$.

Dosage interval is 24 hours, so no adjustment of AUC is needed for number of doses per day.

$$AUC_{24}/MIC = [357.1 \ (\mu g \bullet h)/mL]/ \ 1.5 \ \mu g/mL = 238.1$$

2. *Compute new dose based on $AUC_{24}/MIC > 400$.*
Vancomycin follows linear pharmacokinetics, so the AUC and steady-state trough concentrations change proportionally with dose.

$$Dose_{new} = [(AUC_{24}/MIC)_{new}/(AUC_{24}/MIC)_{old}]Dose_{old} = (400/238.1)(1000 \ mg/d)$$

$$= 1680 \ mg/d, \ round \ to \ 1750 \ mg/d \ or \ 1750 \ mg \ every \ 24 \ hours$$

Check new steady-state vancomycin trough concentration for this AUC_{24}/MIC ratio:
The Bayesian pharmacokinetic computer program computes a steady-state vancomycin trough concentration of 12 μg/mL for the new dose.

REFERENCES

1. Ackerman BH, Vannier AM, Eudy EB. Analysis of vancomycin time-kill studies with *Staphylococcus* species by using a curve stripping program to describe the relationship between concentration and pharmacodynamic response. *Antimicrob Agents Chemother.* 1992;36(8):1766-1769.
2. Louria DB, Kaminski T, Buchman J. Vancomycin in severe staphylococcal infections. *Arch Intern Med.* 1961;107:225-240.
3. MacDougall C, Chambers HF. Protein synthesis inhibitors and miscellaneous antibacterial agents. In: Brunton L, Chabner B, Knollman B, eds. *The Pharmacological Basis of Therapeutics.* 12th ed. New York, NY: McGraw-Hill; 2011:1521-1548.
4. Kirby WMM, Perry DM, Bauer AW. Treatment of staphylococcal septicemia with vancomycin. *N Engl J Med.* 1960;262:49-55.
5. Geraci JE, Heilman FR, Nichols DR, Wellman WE, Ross GT. Some laboratory and clinical experience with a new antibiotic, vancomycin. *Antibiot Annu.* 1956-1957:90-106.
6. Gilbert DN, Chambers HF, Eliopoulos GM, Saag MS, Black D, Freedman DO, Pavia AT, Schwartz BS. *The Sanford Guide to Antimicrobial Therapy.* 44th ed. Sperryville, VA: Antimicrobial Therapy, Inc.; 2014.
7. Gump DW. Vancomycin for treatment of bacterial meningitis. *Rev Infect Dis.* 1981;3(suppl):S289-S292.
8. Young EJ, Ratner RE, Clarridge JE. Staphylococcal ventriculitis treated with vancomycin. *South Med J.* 1981;74(8):1014-1015.
9. Tenover FC, Moellering RC Jr. The rationale for revising the Clinical and Laboratory Standards Institute vancomycin minimal inhibitory concentration interpretive criteria for *Staphylococcus aureus*. *Clin Infect Dis.* May 1, 2007;44(9):1208-1215.
10. Sakoulas G, Moise-Broder PA, Schentag J, Forrest A, Moellering RC Jr, Eliopoulos GM. Relationship of MIC and bactericidal activity to efficacy of vancomycin for treatment of methicillin-resistant *Staphylococcus aureus* bacteremia. *J Clin Microbiol.* Jun 2004;42(6):2398-2402.
11. Jeffres MN, Isakow W, Doherty JA, et al. Predictors of mortality for methicillin-resistant *Staphylococcus aureus* healthcare-associated pneumonia: specific evaluation of vancomycin pharmacokinetic indices. *Chest.* Oct 2006;130(4):947-955.
12. Hidayat LK, Hsu DI, Quist R, Shriner KA, Wong-Beringer A. High-dose vancomycin therapy for methicillin-resistant *Staphylococcus aureus* infections: efficacy and toxicity. *Arch Intern Med.* Oct 23, 2006;166(19):2138-2144.
13. Lodise TP, Drusano GL, Butterfield JM, Scoville J, Gotfried M, Rodvold KA. Penetration of vancomycin into epithelial lining fluid in healthy volunteers. *Antimicrob Agents Chemother.* Dec 2011;55(12):5507-5511.
14. Lamer C, de Beco V, Soler P, et al. Analysis of vancomycin entry into pulmonary lining fluid by bronchoalveolar lavage in critically ill patients. *Antimicrob Agents Chemother.* Feb 1993;37(2):281-286.
15. Georges H, Leroy O, Alfandari S, et al. Pulmonary disposition of vancomycin in critically ill patients. *Eur J Clin Microbiol Infect Dis.* May 1997;16(5):385-388.
16. Liu C, Bayer A, Cosgrove SE, et al. Clinical practice guidelines by the Infectious Diseases Society of America for the treatment of methicillin-resistant *Staphylococcus aureus* infections in adults and children: executive summary. *Clin Infect Dis.* Feb 1, 2011;52(3):285-292.
17. Rybak MJ, Lomaestro BM, Rotschafer JC, et al. Therapeutic monitoring of vancomycin in adults summary of consensus recommendations from the American Society of Health-System Pharmacists, the Infectious Diseases Society of America, and the Society of Infectious Diseases Pharmacists. *Pharmacotherapy.* Nov 2009;29(11):1275-1279.
18. Anon. Guidelines for the management of adults with hospital-acquired, ventilator-associated, and healthcare-associated pneumonia. *Am J Respir Crit Care Med.* Feb 15, 2005;171(4):388-416.
19. Howden BP, Peleg AY, Stinear TP. The evolution of vancomycin intermediate *Staphylococcus aureus* (VISA) and heterogenous-VISA. *Infect Genet Evol.* Apr 6, 2013.
20. Moise-Broder PA, Sakoulas G, Eliopoulos GM, Schentag JJ, Forrest A, Moellering RC Jr. Accessory gene regulator group II polymorphism in methicillin-resistant *Staphylococcus aureus* is predictive of failure of vancomycin therapy. *Clin Infect Dis.* Jun 15, 2004;38(12):1700-1705.
21. Liu C, Chambers HF. *Staphylococcus aureus* with heterogeneous resistance to vancomycin: epidemiology, clinical significance, and critical assessment of diagnostic methods. *Antimicrob Agents Chemother.* Oct 2003;47(10):3040-3045.
22. Drusano GL. Antimicrobial pharmacodynamics: critical interactions of 'bug and drug'. *Nat Rev Microbiol.* Apr 2004;2(4):289-300.
23. Craig WA. Basic pharmacodynamics of antibacterials with clinical applications to the use of beta-lactams, glycopeptides, and linezolid. *Infect Dis Clin North Am.* Sep 2003;17(3):479-501.
24. Craig WA. Pharmacokinetic/pharmacodynamic parameters: rationale for antibacterial dosing of mice and men. *Clin Infect Dis.* Jan 1998;26(1):1-10; quiz 11-12.
25. Hyatt JM, McKinnon PS, Zimmer GS, Schentag JJ. The importance of pharmacokinetic/pharmacodynamic surrogate markers to outcome. Focus on antibacterial agents. *Clin Pharmacokinet.* Feb 1995;28(2):143-160.
26. Moise PA, Forrest A, Bhavnani SM, Birmingham MC, Schentag JJ. Area under the inhibitory curve and a pneumonia scoring system for predicting outcomes of vancomycin therapy for respiratory infections by *Staphylococcus aureus*. *Am J Health Syst Pharm.* Oct 15, 2000;57(suppl 2):S4-S9.
27. Moise-Broder PA, Forrest A, Birmingham MC, Schentag JJ. Pharmacodynamics of vancomycin and other antimicrobials in patients with *Staphylococcus aureus* lower respiratory tract infections. *Clin Pharmacokinet.* 2004;43(13):925-942.

28. Rodvold KA, Blum RA, Fischer JH, et al. Vancomycin pharmacokinetics in patients with various degrees of renal function. *Antimicrob Agents Chemother.* 1988;32(6):848-852.

29. Cockcroft DW, Gault MH. Prediction of creatinine clearance from serum creatinine. *Nephron.* 1976;16:31-41.

30. Brown J, Brown K, Forrest A. Vancomycin AUC24/MIC ratio in patients with complicated bacteremia and infective endocarditis due to methicillin-resistant *Staphylococcus aureus* and its association with attributable mortality during hospitalization. *Antimicrob Agents Chemother.* Feb 2012;56(2):634-638.

31. Suzuki Y, Kawasaki K, Sato Y, et al. Is peak concentration needed in therapeutic drug monitoring of vancomycin? A pharmacokinetic-pharmacodynamic analysis in patients with methicillin-resistant *Staphylococcus aureus* pneumonia. *Chemotherapy.* 2012;58(4): 308-312.

32. Kullar R, Davis SL, Levine DP, Rybak MJ. Impact of vancomycin exposure on outcomes in patients with methicillin-resistant *Staphylococcus aureus* bacteremia: support for consensus guidelines suggested targets. *Clin Infect Dis.* Apr 15, 2011;52(8):975-981.

33. Holmes NE, Turnidge JD, Munckhof WJ, et al. Vancomycin AUC/MIC ratio and 30-day mortality in patients with *Staphylococcus aureus* bacteremia. *Antimicrob Agents Chemother.* Apr 2013;57(4):1654-1663.

34. Croes S, Stolk LM. Vancomycin therapeutic guidelines: closer examination of neonatal pharmacokinetics. *Clin Infect Dis.* Nov 2011;53(9):966-967.

35. Giachetto GA, Telechea HM, Speranza N, Oyarzun M, Nanni L, Menchaca A. Vancomycin pharmacokinetic-pharmacodynamic parameters to optimize dosage administration in critically ill children. *Pediatr Crit Care Med.* Nov 2011;12(6):e250-e254.

36. Nassar L, Hadad S, Gefen A, et al. Prospective evaluation of the dosing regimen of vancomycin in children of different weight categories. *Curr Drug Saf.* Nov 1, 2012;7(5):375-381.

37. Fernandez de Gatta Mdel M, Santos Buelga D, Sanchez Navarro A, Dominguez-Gil A, Garcia MJ. Vancomycin dosage optimization in patients with malignant haematological disease by pharmacokinetic/pharmacodynamic analysis. *Clin Pharmacokinet.* 2009;48(4):273-280.

38. Revilla N, Martin-Suarez A, Perez MP, Gonzalez FM, Fernandez de Gatta Mdel M. Vancomycin dosing assessment in intensive care unit patients based on a population pharmacokinetic/pharmacodynamic simulation. *Br J Clin Pharmacol.* Aug 2010;70(2):201-212.

39. del Mar Fernandez de Gatta Garcia M, Revilla N, Calvo MV, Dominguez-Gil A, Sanchez Navarro A. Pharmacokinetic/pharmacodynamic analysis of vancomycin in ICU patients. *Intensive Care Med.* Feb 2007;33(2):279-285.

40. Frymoyer A, Hersh AL, Benet LZ, Guglielmo BJ. Current recommended dosing of vancomycin for children with invasive methicillin-resistant *Staphylococcus aureus* infections is inadequate. *Pediatr Infect Dis J.* May 2009;28(5):398-402.

41. Frymoyer A, Hersh AL, Coralic Z, Benet LZ, Joseph Guglielmo B. Prediction of vancomycin pharmacodynamics in children with invasive methicillin-resistant *Staphylococcus aureus* infections: a Monte Carlo simulation. *Clin Ther.* Mar 2010;32(3):534-542.

42. Patel N, Pai MP, Rodvold KA, Lomaestro B, Drusano GL, Lodise TP. Vancomycin: we can't get there from here. *Clin Infect Dis.* Apr 15, 2011;52(8):969-974.

43. Le J, Bradley JS, Murray W, et al. Improved vancomycin dosing in children using area under the curve exposure. *Pediatr Infect Dis J.* Apr 2013;32(4):e155-e163.

44. Thomson AH, Staatz CE, Tobin CM, Gall M, Lovering AM. Development and evaluation of vancomycin dosage guidelines designed to achieve new target concentrations. *J Antimicrob Chemother.* May 2009;63(5):1050-1057.

45. Kullar R, Davis SL, Taylor TN, Kaye KS, Rybak MJ. Effects of targeting higher vancomycin trough levels on clinical outcomes and costs in a matched patient cohort. *Pharmacotherapy.* Mar 2012;32(3):195-201.

46. Bailie GR, Neal D. Vancomycin ototoxicity and nephrotoxicity: a review. *Med Toxicol Adverse Drug Exp.* 1988;3(5):376-386.

47. Mellor JA, Kingdom J, Cafferkey M, Keane C. Vancomycin ototoxicity in patients with normal renal function. *Br J Audiol.* 1984;18(3):179-180.

48. Forouzesh A, Moise PA, Sakoulas G. Vancomycin ototoxicity: a reevaluation in an era of increasing doses. *Antimicrob Agents Chemother.* Feb 2009;53(2):483-486.

49. Zimmermann AE, Katona BG, Plaisance KI. Association of vancomycin serum concentrations with outcomes in patients with gram-positive bacteremia. *Pharmacotherapy.* 1995;15(1):85-91.

50. Welty TE, Copa AK. Impact of vancomycin therapeutic drug monitoring on patient care. *Ann Pharmacother.* 1994;28(12):1335-1339.

51. Bosso JA, Nappi J, Rudisill C, et al. Relationship between vancomycin trough concentrations and nephrotoxicity: a prospective multicenter trial. *Antimicrob Agents Chemother.* Dec 2011;55(12):5475-5479.

52. Teng CB, Rezai K, Itokazu GS, et al. Continuation of high-dose vancomycin despite nephrotoxicity. *Antimicrob Agents Chemother.* Jun 2012;56(6):3470-3471; author reply 3472.

53. Lodise TP, Lomaestro B, Graves J, Drusano GL. Larger vancomycin doses (at least four grams per day) are associated with an increased incidence of nephrotoxicity. *Antimicrob Agents Chemother.* Apr 2008;52(4):1330-1336.

54. Lodise TP, Patel N, Lomaestro BM, Rodvold KA, Drusano GL. Relationship between initial vancomycin concentration-time profile and nephrotoxicity among hospitalized patients. *Clin Infect Dis.* Aug 15, 2009;49(4):507-514.

55. van Hal SJ, Paterson DL, Lodise TP. Systematic review and meta-analysis of vancomycin-induced nephrotoxicity associated with dosing schedules that maintain troughs between 15 and 20 milligrams per liter. *Antimicrob Agents Chemother.* Feb 2013;57(2):734-744.

56. Cantu TG, Yamanaka-Yuen NA, Lietman PS. Serum vancomycin concentrations: reappraisal of their clinical value. *Clin Infect Dis.* 1994;18(4):533-543.

57. Darko W, Medicis JJ, Smith A, Guharoy R, Lehmann DE. Mississippi mud no more: cost-effectiveness of pharmacokinetic dosage adjustment of vancomycin to prevent nephrotoxicity. *Pharmacotherapy.* May 2003;23(5):643-650.

58. Murphy JE, Gillespie DE, Bateman CV. Predictability of vancomycin trough concentrations using seven approaches for estimating pharmacokinetic parameters. *Am J Health Syst Pharm.* Dec 1, 2006;63(23):2365-2370.

59. Karam CM, McKinnon PS, Neuhauser MM, Rybak MJ. Outcome assessment of minimizing vancomycin monitoring and dosing adjustments. *Pharmacotherapy.* 1999;19(3):257-266.

60. Saunders NJ. Why monitor peak vancomycin concentrations? *Lancet.* 1994;344(8939-8940):1748-1750.

61. Kirby WMM, Divelbiss CL. Vancomycin: clinical and laboratory studies. *Antibiot Annu.* 1956-1957:107-117.

62. Spitzer PG, Eliopoulos GM. Systemic absorption of enteral vancomycin in a patient with pseudomembranous colitis. *Ann Intern Med.* 1984;100(4):533-534.

63. Dudley MN, Quintiliani R, Nightingale CH, Gontarz N. Absorption of vancomycin [letter]. *Ann Intern Med.* 1984;101(1):144.

64. Thompson CM Jr, Long SS, Gilligan PH, Prebis JW. Absorption of oral vancomycin—possible associated toxicity. *Int J Pediatr Nephrol.* 1983;4(1):1-4.

65. Matzke GR, Halstenson CE, Olson PL, Collins AJ, Abraham PA. Systemic absorption of oral vancomycin in patients with renal insufficiency and antibiotic-associated colitis. *Am J Kidney Dis.* 1987;9(5):422-425.

66. Krogstad DJ, Moellering RC Jr, Greenblatt DJ. Single-dose kinetics of intravenous vancomycin. *J Clin Pharmacol.* 1980;20(41):197-201.

67. Cataldo MA, Tacconelli E, Grilli E, Pea F, Petrosillo N. Continuous versus intermittent infusion of vancomycin for the treatment of gram-positive infections: systematic review and meta-analysis. *J Antimicrob Chemother.* Jan 2011;67(1):17-24.

68. Ampe E, Delaere B, Hecq JD, Tulkens PM, Glupczynski Y. Implementation of a protocol for administration of vancomycin by continuous infusion: pharmacokinetic, pharmacodynamic and toxicological aspects. *Int J Antimicrob Agents.* May 2013;41(5):439-446.

69. Akers KS, Cota JM, Chung KK, Renz EM, Mende K, Murray CK. Serum vancomycin levels resulting from continuous or intermittent infusion in critically ill burn patients with or without continuous renal replacement therapy. *J Burn Care Res.* Nov-Dec 2012;33(6):e254-262.

70. Jeurissen A, Sluyts I, Rutsaert R. A higher dose of vancomycin in continuous infusion is needed in critically ill patients. *Int J Antimicrob Agents.* Jan 2011;37(1):75-77.

71. Payne CJ, Carmichael SJ, Stearns AT, Kingsmore DB, Byrne DS, Binning AR. Vancomycin continuous infusion as prophylaxis for vascular surgery. *Ther Drug Monit.* Dec 2009;31(6):786-788.

72. Payne CJ, Thomson AH, Stearns AT, et al. Pharmacokinetics and tissue penetration of vancomycin continuous infusion as prophylaxis for vascular surgery. *J Antimicrob Chemother.* Nov 2011;66(11):2624-2627.

73. Bauer LA, Black DJ, Lill JS. Vancomycin dosing in morbidly obese patients. *Eur J Clin Pharmacol.* 1998;54(8):621-625.

74. Blouin RA, Bauer LA, Miller DD, Record KE, Griffen WO Jr. Vancomycin pharmacokinetics in normal and morbidly obese subjects. *Antimicrob Agents Chemother.* 1982;21(4):575-580.

75. Moellering RC Jr, Krogstad DJ, Greenblatt DJ. Vancomycin therapy in patients with impaired renal function: a nomogram for dosage. *Ann Intern Med.* 1981;94(3):343-346.

76. Matzke GR, Kovarik JM, Rybak MJ, Boike SC. Evaluation of the vancomycin-clearance: creatinine-clearance relationship for predicting vancomycin dosage. *Clin Pharm.* 1985;4(3):311-315.

77. Matzke GR, McGory RW, Halstenson CE, Keane WF. Pharmacokinetics of vancomycin in patients with various degrees of renal function. *Antimicrob Agents Chemother.* 1984;25(4):433-437.

78. Dolton M, Xu H, Cheong E, et al. Vancomycin pharmacokinetics in patients with severe burn injuries. *Burns.* Jun 2010;36(4):469-476.

79. Rybak MJ, Albrecht LM, Berman JR, Warbasse LH, Svensson CK. Vancomycin pharmacokinetics in burn patients and intravenous drug abusers. *Antimicrob Agents Chemother.* 1990;34(5):792-795.

80. Buelga DS, del Mar Fernandez de Gatta M, Herrera EV, Dominguez-Gil A, Garcia MJ. Population pharmacokinetic analysis of vancomycin in patients with hematological malignancies. *Antimicrob Agents Chemother.* Dec 2005;49(12):4934-4941.

81. Al-Kofide H, Zaghloul I, Al-Naim L. Pharmacokinetics of vancomycin in adult cancer patients. *J Oncol Pharm Pract.* Dec 2010;16(4):245-250.

82. Jarkowski A 3rd, Forrest A, Sweeney RP, et al. Characterization of vancomycin pharmacokinetics in the adult acute myeloid leukemia population. *J Oncol Pharm Pract.* Mar 2011;18(1):91-96.

83. Pleasants RA, Michalets EL, Williams DM, Samuelson WM, Rehm JR, Knowles MR. Pharmacokinetics of vancomycin in adult cystic fibrosis patients. *Antimicrob Agents Chemother.* Jan 1996;40(1):186-190.

84. Vance-Bryan K, Guay DR, Gilliland SS, Rodvold KA, Rotschafer JC. Effect of obesity on vancomycin pharmacokinetic parameters as determined by using a Bayesian forecasting technique. *Antimicrob Agents Chemother.* 1993;37(3):436-440.

85. Ducharme MP, Slaughter RL, Edwards DJ. Vancomycin pharmacokinetics in a patient population: effect of age, gender, and body weight. *Ther Drug Monit.* 1994;16(5):513-518.

86. Schaad UB, McCracken GH Jr, Nelson JD. Clinical pharmacology and efficacy of vancomycin in pediatric patients. *J Pediatr.* 1980;96(1):119-126.

87. Burstein AH, Gal P, Forrest A. Evaluation of a sparse sampling strategy for determining vancomycin pharmacokinetics in preterm neonates: application of optimal sampling theory. *Ann Pharmacother.* Sep 1997;31(9):980-983.

88. Machado JK, Feferbaum R, Kobayashi CE, Sanches C, Santos SR. Vancomycin pharmacokinetics in preterm infants. *Clinics (Sao Paulo).* Aug 2007;62(4):405-410.

89. Marques-Minana MR, Saadeddin A, Peris JE. Population pharmacokinetic analysis of vancomycin in neonates. A new proposal of initial dosage guideline. *Br J Clin Pharmacol.* Nov 2010;70(5):713-720.

90. Pickering LK, Baker CJ, Kimberlin DW, Long SS. *Red book: 2012 Report of the Committee on Infectious Diseases.* 29th ed. Elk Grove Village, IL: American Academy of Pediatrics; 2012.

91. Pickering LK. *Red book: 2006 Report of the Committee on Infectious Diseases.* 27th ed. Elk Grove Village, IL: American Academy of Pediatrics; 2006.

92. Tan CC, Lee HS, Ti TY, Lee EJC. Pharmacokinetics of intravenous vancomycin in patients with end-stage renal disease. *Ther Drug Monitor.* 1990;12:29-34.

93. Decker BS, Kays MB, Chambers M, Kraus MA, Moe SM, Sowinski KM. Vancomycin pharmacokinetics and pharmacodynamics during short daily hemodialysis. *Clin J Am Soc Nephrol.* Nov 2010;5(11):1981-1987.

94. Kielstein JT, Czock D, Schopke T, et al. Pharmacokinetics and total elimination of meropenem and vancomycin in intensive care unit patients undergoing extended daily dialysis. *Crit Care Med.* Jan 2006;34(1):51-56.

95. Touchette MA, Patel RV, Anandan JV, Dumler F, Zarowitz BJ. Vancomycin removal by high-flux polysulfone hemodialysis membranes in critically ill patients with end-stage renal disease. *Am J Kidney Dis.* Sep 1995;26(3):469-474.

96. Ariano RE, Fine A, Sitar DS, Rexrode S, Zelenitsky SA. Adequacy of a vancomycin dosing regimen in patients receiving high-flux hemodialysis. *Am J Kidney Dis.* Oct 2005;46(4):681-687.

97. Scott MK, Mueller BA, Clark WR. Vancomycin mass transfer characteristics of high-flux cellulosic dialysers. *Nephrol Dial Transplant.* Dec 1997;12(12):2647-2653.

98. Foote EF, Dreitlein WB, Steward CA, Kapoian T, Walker JA, Sherman RA. Pharmacokinetics of vancomycin when administered during high flux hemodialysis. *Clin Nephrol.* Jul 1998;50(1):51-55.

99. Pollard TA, Lampasona V, Akkerman S, et al. Vancomycin redistribution: dosing recommendations following high-flux hemodialysis. *Kidney Int.* 1994;45(1):232-237.

100. Edell LS, Westby GR, Gould SR. An improved method of vancomycin administration to dialysis patients. *Clin Nephrol.* Feb 1988;29(2):86-87.

101. Kihara M, Ikeda Y, Fujita H, et al. Effects of slowly performed daytime hemodialysis (slow HD) on the pharmacokinetics of vancomycin in hemodynamically unstable patients with renal failure. *Blood Purif.* 1996;14(1):20-25.

102. Pancorbo S, Comty C. Peritoneal transport of vancomycin in 4 patients undergoing continuous ambulatory peritoneal dialysis. *Nephron.* 1982;31(1):37-39.

103. Bunke CM, Aronoff GR, Brier ME, Sloan RS, Luft FC. Vancomycin kinetics during continuous ambulatory peritoneal dialysis. *Clin Pharmacol Ther.* 1983;34(5):631-637.

104. Morse GD, Nairn DK, Walshe JJ. Once weekly intraperitoneal therapy for gram-positive peritonitis. *Am J Kidney Dis.* 1987;10(4):300-305.

105. Montanes Pauls B, Alminana MA, Casabo Alos VG. Vancomycin pharmacokinetics during continuous ambulatory peritoneal dialysis in patients with peritonitis. *Eur J Pharm Sci.* Jul 17, 2011;43(4):212-216.

106. Manley HJ, Bailie GR, Frye RF, McGoldrick MD. Intravenous vancomycin pharmacokinetics in automated peritoneal dialysis patients. *Perit Dial Int.* Jul-Aug 2001;21(4):378-385.

107. Golper TA, Marx MA. Drug dosing adjustments during continuous renal replacement therapies. *Kidney Int Suppl.* May 1998;66:S165-S168.

108. Golper TA. Update on drug sieving coefficients and dosing adjustments during continuous renal replacement therapies. *Contrib Nephrol.* 2001;(132):349-353.

109. Covajes C, Scolletta S, Penaccini L, et al. Continuous infusion of vancomycin in septic patients receiving continuous renal replacement therapy. *Int J Antimicrob Agents.* Mar 2012;41(3):261-266.

110. Joy MS, Matzke GR, Frye RF, Palevsky PM. Determinants of vancomycin clearance by continuous venovenous hemofiltration and continuous venovenous hemodialysis. *Am J Kidney Dis.* Jun 1998;31(6):1019-1027.

111. DelDot ME, Lipman J, Tett SE. Vancomycin pharmacokinetics in critically ill patients receiving continuous venovenous haemodiafiltration. *Br J Clin Pharmacol.* Sep 2004;58(3):259-268.

112. van de Vijsel LM, Walker SA, Walker SE, Yamashita S, Simor A, Hladunewich M. Initial vancomycin dosing recommendations for critically ill patients undergoing continuous venovenous hemodialysis. *Can J Hosp Pharm.* May 2010;63(3):196-206.

113. Petejova N, Martinek A, Zahalkova J, et al. Vancomycin pharmacokinetics during high-volume continuous venovenous hemofiltration in critically ill septic patients. *Biomed Pap Med Fac Univ Palacky Olomouc Czech Repub.* Nov 6, 2012.

114. Frazee EN, Kuper PJ, Schramm GE, et al. Effect of continuous venovenous hemofiltration dose on achievement of adequate vancomycin trough concentrations. *Antimicrob Agents Chemother.* Dec 2012;56(12):6181-6185.

115. Udy AA, Covajes C, Taccone FS, et al. Can population pharmacokinetic modelling guide vancomycin dosing during continuous renal replacement therapy in critically ill patients? *Int J Antimicrob Agents.* Jun 2013;41(6):564-568.

116. Paciullo CA, Harned KC, Davis GA, Connor MJ Jr, Winstead PS. Vancomycin clearance in high-volume venovenous hemofiltration. *Ann Pharmacother.* Mar 2013;47(3):e14.

117. Boereboom FT, Ververs FF, Blankestijn PJ, Savelkoul TJ, van Dijk A. Vancomycin clearance during continuous venovenous haemofiltration in critically ill patients. *Intensive Care Med.* Oct 1999;25(10):1100-1104.

118. Amaker RD, DiPiro JT, Bhatia J. Pharmacokinetics of vancomycin in critically ill infants undergoing extracorporeal membrane oxygenation. *Antimicrob Agents Chemother.* May 1996;40(5):1139-1142.

119. Mulla H, Pooboni S. Population pharmacokinetics of vancomycin in patients receiving extracorporeal membrane oxygenation. *Br J Clin Pharmacol.* Sep 2005;60(3):265-275.

120. Buck ML. Vancomycin pharmacokinetics in neonates receiving extracorporeal membrane oxygenation. *Pharmacotherapy.* Sep-Oct 1998;18(5):1082-1086.

121. Cotogni P, Passera R, Barbero C, et al. Intraoperative vancomycin pharmacokinetics in cardiac surgery with or without cardiopulmonary bypass. *Ann Pharmacother.* Apr 2013;47(4):455-463.

122. Rybak MJ, Albrecht LM, Boike SC, Chandrasekar PH. Nephrotoxicity of vancomycin, alone and with an aminoglycoside. *J Antimicrob Chemother.* 1990;25(4):679-687.

123. Farber BF, Moellering RC Jr. Retrospective study of the toxicity of preparations of vancomycin from 1974 to 1981. *Antimicrob Agents Chemother.* 1983;23(1):138-141.

124. Angaran DM, Dias VC, Arom KV, et al. The comparative influence of prophylactic antibiotics on the prothrombin response to warfarin in the postoperative prosthetic cardiac valve patient. Cefamandole, cefazolin, vancomycin. *Ann Surg.* 1987;206(2):155-161.

125. Sanchez JL, Dominguez AR, Lane JR, Anderson PO, Capparelli EV, Cornejo-Bravo JM. Population pharmacokinetics of vancomycin in adult and geriatric patients: comparison of eleven approaches. *Int J Clin Pharmacol Ther.* Aug 2010;48(8):525-533.

126. Murphy JE, Winter ME. Clinical pharmacokinetic pearls: bolus versus infusion equations. *Pharmacotherapy.* 1996;16(4):698-700.

127. Black DJ. Modification of Moellering vancomycin clearance/creatinine clearance relationship to allow direct calculation of vancomycin doses (personal communication); 1993.

128. Salazar DE, Corcoran GB. Predicting creatinine clearance and renal drug clearance in obese patients from estimated fat-free body mass. *Am J Med.* 1988;84:1053-1060.

129. Kullar R, Leonard SN, Davis SL, et al. Validation of the effectiveness of a vancomycin nomogram in achieving target trough concentrations of 15-20 mg/L suggested by the vancomycin consensus guidelines. *Pharmacotherapy.* May 2011;31(5):441-448.

130. Traub SL, Johnson CE. Comparison of methods of estimating creatinine clearance in children. *Am J Hosp Pharm.* 1980;37:195-201.

131. Bauer LA. Evaluation of a simplified method to adjust vancomycin trough concentrations. *Pharmacotherapy.* 2005;25(10):1482-1483.

132. McCormack JP, Carleton B. A simpler approach to pharmacokinetic dosage adjustments. *Pharmacotherapy.* 1997;17(6):1349-1351.

133. Shargel L, Yu A, Wu-Pong S. *Applied Biopharmaceutics and Pharmacokinetics.* 6th ed. New York, NY: McGraw-Hill; 2012.

134. Pryka RD, Rodvold KA, Garrison M, Rotschafer JC. Individualizing vancomycin dosage regimens: one- versus two-compartment Bayesian models. *Ther Drug Monit.* 1989;11(4):450-454.

135. Rodvold KA, Pryka RD, Garrison M, Rotschafer JC. Evaluation of a two-compartment Bayesian forecasting program for predicting vancomycin concentrations. *Ther Drug Monit.* 1989;11(3):269-275.

136. Rodvold KA, Rotschafer JC, Gilliland SS, Guay DR, Vance-Bryan K. Bayesian forecasting of serum vancomycin concentrations with non-steady-state sampling strategies. *Ther Drug Monit.* 1994;16(1):37-41.

137. Yamamoto T, Terakawa H, Hisaka A, Suzuki H. Bayesian estimation of pharmacokinetic parameters of vancomycin in patients with decreasing renal function. *J Pharm Sci.* Aug 2012;101(8):2968-2975.

138. Aubron C, Corallo CE, Nunn MO, Dooley MJ, Cheng AC. Evaluation of the accuracy of a pharmacokinetic dosing program in predicting serum vancomycin concentrations in critically ill patients. *Ann Pharmacother.* Oct 2011;45(10):1193-1198.

139. Nunn MO, Corallo CE, Aubron C, Poole S, Dooley MJ, Cheng AC. Vancomycin dosing: assessment of time to therapeutic concentration and predictive accuracy of pharmacokinetic modeling software. *Ann Pharmacother.* Jun 2011;45(6):757-763.

140. Wandell M, Mungall D. Computer assisted drug interpretation and drug regimen optimization. *Am Assoc Clin Chem.* 1984;6:1-11.

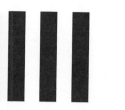

CARDIOVASCULAR AGENTS

6 Digoxin

Digoxin is the primary cardiac glycoside in clinical use. Digoxin is used for the treatment of congestive heart failure (CHF) because of its inotropic effects on the myocardium and for the treatment of atrial fibrillation because of its chronotropic effects on the electrophysiological system of the heart. The role of digoxin in the treatment of each of these disease states has changed in recent years as a better understanding of the pathophysiology of these conditions has been gained and new drug therapies have been developed.[1-5] For the treatment of chronic CHF, angiotensin I–converting enzyme inhibitors (ACE inhibitors), β-blockers, and diuretics (for patients who are fluid overloaded) are the primary pharmacotherapeutic agents. Angiotensin II receptor antagonists (ARB), aldosterone antagonists, and the combination of hydralazine and nitrates also play key roles.[6,7] For the treatment of acute or severe heart failure, agents that decrease cardiac preload (diuretics, nitrates) or afterload (vasodilators) and ACE inhibitors (decreases both preload and afterload) are used in conjunction with potent intravenously administered inotropic agents (dobutamine, milrinone, dopamine, adrenergic agonists) to balance the current cardiovascular status of the patient.[8] In either the acute or chronic heart failure situations, digoxin can be used when a mild inotropic or oral agent is needed.

If a patient presents with severe cardiovascular symptoms due to atrial fibrillation, direct-current cardioversion is a treatment option.[1,4] For the treatment of atrial fibrillation with mild or no cardiovascular symptoms, many clinicians prefer to prescribe intravenous calcium channel blockers (diltiazem or verapamil) for the control ventricular rate. If atrial fibrillation is due to excessive adrenergic tone, intravenous β-blockers can also be used. Digoxin continues to be prescribed for the control of ventricular rate in patients with atrial fibrillation with no accessory pathway and can be an excellent choice if the patient is sedentary or has heart failure or left ventricular dysfunction. It is also possible to use digoxin in combination with a β-blocker or a calcium channel blocker to treat atrial fibrillation.[1,4] Once ventricular rate is controlled, the patient's heart may spontaneously revert to normal sinus rhythm, or electrical or pharmacologic cardioversion of atrial fibrillation may be necessary.

The positive inotropic effect of digoxin is caused by binding to sodium- and potassium-activated adenosine triphosphatase, also known as Na,K-ATPase or the sodium pump.[7] Digoxin-induced inhibition of Na,K-ATPase leads to decreased transport of sodium out of myocardial cells and increased intracellular sodium concentrations that aid calcium entry and decrease calcium elimination via the sodium-calcium exchanger. The increased intracellular calcium is stored in the endoplasmic reticulum so that action potential–induced calcium release is augmented causing enhanced myocardial contractility. The chronotropic effects of digoxin are mediated via increased parasympathetic activity and vagal tone.[9]

THERAPEUTIC AND TOXIC CONCENTRATIONS

When given as oral or intravenous doses, the serum digoxin concentration/time curve follows a two-compartment model and exhibits a long and large distribution phase of 8-12 hours (Figure 6-1).[10-12] During the distribution phase, digoxin in the serum is not in equilibrium with digoxin in the tissues, so digoxin serum concentrations

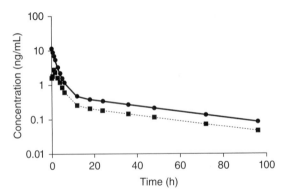

FIGURE 6-1   Digoxin serum concentrations after 250-μg doses given intravenously (circles and solid line) and orally as a tablet (squares with dashed line). After an intravenous dose, digoxin serum concentrations are very high because the entire quantity of drug is initially contained in the blood. During the distribution phase, digoxin begins to move out of the vascular system into the tissues. It is also cleared from the body during this phase. Digoxin serum concentrations decline relatively rapidly over an 8-12-hour time period until the blood and tissues are in pseudoequilibrium with each other. During the elimination phase, digoxin serum concentrations in patients with good renal function (creatinine clearance > 80 mL/min) decline with a half-life of about 36 hours. After oral tablet administration, about 70% of a digoxin dose is absorbed from the gastrointestinal tract. Maximum, or peak, concentrations occur about 1.5-2 hours after oral dosing with tablets, and the distribution phase still lasts 8-12 hours. During the elimination phase, intravenous and oral digoxin have the same terminal half-lives.

should not be measured until the distribution phase is finished. When drug distribution is complete, digoxin serum and tissue concentrations will be proportional to each other so that digoxin serum concentrations reflect concentrations at the site of action. When a digoxin serum concentration is very high but the patient is not exhibiting signs or symptoms of digitalis overdose, clinicians should consider the possibility that the blood sample for the determination of a digoxin serum concentration was obtained during the distribution phase, is too high because digoxin has not had the opportunity to diffuse out of the bloodstream into the myocardium, and is not reflective of myocardial tissue concentrations.

There is a great deal of inter- and intrapatient variability in the pharmacodynamic responses to digoxin. Clinically beneficial inotropic effects of digoxin are generally achieved at steady-state serum concentrations of 0.5-1 ng/mL.[13,14] Increasing steady-state serum concentrations to 1.2-1.5 ng/mL may provide some minor, additional inotropic effect.[13,14] Chronotropic effects usually require higher digoxin steady-state serum concentrations of 0.8-1.5 ng/mL.[15,16] Additional chronotropic effects may be observed at digoxin steady-state serum concentrations as high as 2 ng/mL. Because of pharmacodynamic variability, clinicians should consider these ranges as initial guidelines and rely heavily on patient response to monitor digoxin therapy.

Steady-state digoxin serum concentrations above 2 ng/mL are associated with an increased incidence of adverse drug reactions. At digoxin concentrations of 2.5 ng/mL or above ~50% of all patients will exhibit some form of digoxin toxicity.[17] Most digoxin side effects involve the gastrointestinal tract, central nervous system, or cardiovascular system.[18] Gastrointestinal tract–related adverse effects include anorexia, nausea, vomiting, diarrhea, abdominal pain, or constipation. Central nervous system side effects are headache, fatigue, insomnia, confusion, or vertigo. Visual disturbances can also occur and are manifested as blurred vision and changes in color vision or colored halos around objects oftentimes involving the yellow-green spectrum. As can be appreciated, most of the gastrointestinal and central nervous system side effects of digoxin are nonspecific and could be caused by many different things. Because of this, clinicians should pay close attention to any new symptoms reported by patients receiving cardiac glycosides. Cardiac side effects commonly include second- or third-degree atrioventricular block, atrioventricular dissociation, bradycardia, premature ventricular contractions, or ventricular tachycardia. Rarely, almost every cardiac arrhythmia has been reported to occur due to digoxin toxicity. If a patient develops a new arrhythmia while receiving digoxin treatment, consideration should be given to the possibility that it is digoxin induced. Also, it should be noted that relatively minor adverse effects such as nausea, headache, or changes in color vision may not occur in a patient before major cardiovascular side effects are found. In the case of life-threatening digoxin overdose, digoxin antigen-binding fragments or digoxin immune FAB (DigiFab) are portions of digoxin-specific antibodies that can be used to rapidly reverse the adverse symptoms (see Special Dosing Considerations section).

CLINICAL MONITORING PARAMETERS

In patients receiving digoxin for heart failure, the common signs and symptoms of CHF should be routinely monitored—left-sided failure: dyspnea on exertion, paroxysmal nocturnal dyspnea, orthopnea, tachypnea, cough, hemoptysis, pulmonary rales/edema, S_3 gallop, pleural effusion, Cheyne-Stokes respiration; right-sided failure: abdominal pain, anorexia, nausea, bloating, constipation, ascites, peripheral edema, jugular venous distention, hepatojugular reflux, hepatomegaly; general symptoms: fatigue, weakness, nocturia, CNS symptoms, tachycardia, pallor, digital cyanosis, cardiomegaly.[6] A very useful functional classification for heart failure patients proposed by the New York Heart Association is given in Table 6-1.

When used for the treatment of atrial fibrillation, digoxin will not stop the atrial arrhythmia but is used to decrease, or control, the ventricular rate to an acceptable value (usually <100 beats/min).[1] The patient's pulse or ventricular rate should be monitored, and an electrocardiogram can also be useful to clinicians able to interpret the output. Atrial fibrillation is characterized by 400-600 nonuniform atrial beats/min. Sinus rhythm will not be restored with the use of digoxin alone although atrial fibrillation can spontaneously remit. Depending on the symptomatology experienced by the patient, cardioversion can be attempted by using direct electrical current or by the use of an antiarrhythmic agent such as flecainide, dofetilide, propafenone, or ibutilide.[4] Adequate anticoagulation to prevent thromboembolism is needed before cardioversion if atrial fibrillation has occurred for longer than 48 hours or the duration of atrial fibrillation is unknown. Optionally, a transesophageal echocardiogram (TEE) can be performed, and if no thrombus is identified in the left atrium or left atrium appendage, cardioversion can commence after adequate anticoagulation with unfractionated heparin has been established.[4]

Patients with severe heart disease such as coronary artery disease (angina, myocardial infarction) can have increased pharmacodynamic sensitivity to cardiac glycosides, and patients receiving these drugs should be monitored closely for adverse drug effects.[17,19] Also, augmented pharmacologic responses to digitalis

TABLE 6-1   New York Heart Association (NYHA) Functional Classification for Heart Failure[6]

NYHA Heart Failure Class	Description
I	Patients with cardiac disease but without limitations of physical activity. Ordinary physical activity does not cause undue fatigue, dyspnea, or palpitation
II	Patients with cardiac disease that results in slight limitations of physical activity. Ordinary physical activity results in fatigue, palpitation, dyspnea, or angina
III	Patients with cardiac disease that results in marked limitations of physical activity. Although patients are comfortable at rest, less than ordinary activity will lead to symptoms
IV	Patients with cardiac disease that results in an inability to carry on physical activity without discomfort. Symptoms of congestive heart failure are present even at rest. With any physical activity, increased discomfort is experienced

derivatives occur with serum electrolyte disturbances such as hypokalemia, hypomagnesemia, and hypercalcemia even though steady-state digoxin serum concentrations are in the therapeutic range.[7,9] Serum potassium concentrations should be routinely monitored in patients receiving digoxin and potassium-wasting diuretics. Potassium supplementation may be necessary in some of these patients. Also, many patients receiving digoxin and diuretics will be receiving angiotensin I converting enzyme (ACE) inhibitors or angiotensin II receptor blockers (ARB) which can cause potassium retention. When receiving a combination of these drugs, it can be difficult to reasonably ascertain what the patient's serum potassium status is without measuring it.

As an adjunct to the patient's clinical response, post-distribution (8-12 hours post-dose) steady-state digoxin serum concentrations can be measured 3-5 half-lives after a stable dose is initiated. Digoxin is primarily eliminated unchanged by the kidney (~75%), so its clearance is predominately influenced by renal function.[11,12] Once stable, therapeutic steady-state digoxin serum concentrations and dosage levels have been established, serum creatinine measurements can be used to detect changes in renal function which may result in digoxin clearance and concentration alterations. Hospitalized patients with severe or acute heart failure may need to have serum creatinine determinations two or three times weekly to monitor renal function, while ambulatory patients with stable heart failure may only need yearly serum creatinine measurements.

BASIC CLINICAL PHARMACOKINETIC PARAMETERS

The primary route of digoxin elimination from the body is by the kidney via glomerular filtration and active tubular secretion of unchanged drug (~75%).[11,12] The remainder of a digoxin dose (~25%) is removed by hepatic metabolism or biliary excretion. The primary transporter involved in active tubular secretion and biliary excretion is P-glycoprotein (PGP).[20,21] Enterohepatic recirculation (reabsorption of drug from the gastrointestinal tract after elimination in the bile) of digoxin occurs.[22] Digoxin is given as an intravenous injection or orally as a tablet or solution. When given intravenously, doses should be infused over at least 5-10 minutes. Average bioavailability constants (F) for the tablet and oral solution are 0.7 and 0.8.[23-28] Digoxin is not usually administered intramuscularly due to erratic absorption and severe pain at the injection site. Plasma protein binding is ~25% for digoxin.[29,30] Usual digoxin doses for adults are 250 μg/d (range: 125-500 μg/d) in patients with good renal function (creatinine clearance ≥ 80 mL/min) and 125 μg every 2-3 days in patients with renal dysfunction (creatinine clearance ≤ 15 mL/min).

EFFECTS OF DISEASE STATES AND CONDITIONS ON DIGOXIN PHARMACOKINETICS AND DOSING

Adults with normal renal function (creatinine clearance ≥ 80 mL/min, Table 6-2) have an average digoxin half-life of 36 hours (range: 24-48 hours) and volume of distribution of 7 L/kg (range: 5-9 L/kg).[31,32] The volume of distribution is large due to the extensive tissue binding of digoxin in the body. Digoxin pharmacokinetics are not affected by obesity (>30% over ideal body weight), so volume of distribution and dosage estimates should be based on ideal body weight.[33,34]

Because digoxin is principally eliminated by the kidney, renal dysfunction is the most important disease state that effects digoxin pharmacokinetics.[12] The digoxin clearance rate decreases in proportion to creatinine clearance, and this relationship will be utilized to aid in the computation of initial doses later in the chapter (Figure 6-2). The equation that estimates digoxin clearance from creatinine clearance is: Cl = 1.303 (CrCl) + Cl_{NR}, where Cl is digoxin clearance in mL/min, CrCl is creatinine clearance in mL/min, and Cl_{NR} is digoxin clearance by nonrenal routes of elimination, which equals 40 mL/min in patients with no or mild heart failure (NYHA CHF class I or II, see Table 6-1).[12] Digoxin volume of distribution, in addition to clearance, decreases

TABLE 6-2   Disease States and Conditions That Alter Digoxin Pharmacokinetics

Disease State/ Condition	Half-Life	Volume of Distribution	Comment
Adult, normal renal function	36 hours or 1.5 days (range: 24-48 hours)	7 L/kg (range: 5-9 L/kg)	Usual dose 250 µg/d (range: 125-500 µg/d) resulting in total body stores of 8-12 µg/kg for heart failure or 13-15 µg/kg for atrial fibrillation. Digoxin is eliminated ~75% unchanged renally/~25% nonrenally
Adult, renal failure	120 hours or 5 days	4.5 L/kg $$V = \left(226 + \frac{298 \bullet CrCl}{29.1 + CrCl}\right)(Wt/70)$$ where V is digoxin volume of distribution in L/70 kg, Wt is body weight in kg (use ideal body weight if > 30% overweight) and CrCl is creatinine clearance in mL/min.	Renal failure patients have decreased digoxin clearance and volume of distribution. As a result, half-life is not as long as might be expected [$t_{1/2} = (0.693V)/Cl$]. Digoxin total body stores decrease to 6-10 µg/kg because of reduced volume of distribution
Moderate/severe heart failure	See comments	7 L/kg	Heart failure patients (NYHA Classes III-IV) have decreased cardiac output, which causes decreased liver blood flow and digoxin hepatic clearance. In patients with good renal function (creatinine clearance > 80 mL/min), the effect on digoxin total clearance is negligible. But in patients with poor renal function, (creatinine clearance < 30 mL/min) nonrenal clearance is a primary elimination pathway
Obesity (> 30% over IBW) with normal renal function	36 hours or 1.5 days	7 L/kg IBW	Digoxin does not distribute to adipose tissue, so volume of distribution calculations should be conducted with ideal body weight (IBW)
Hyperthyroidism with normal renal function	24 hours or 1 day	7 L/kg	Hyperthyroid patients are hypermetabolic and have higher digoxin renal and nonrenal clearances

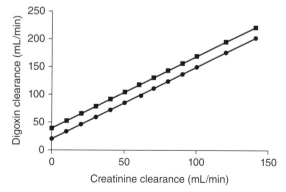

FIGURE 6-2   Digoxin clearance is proportional to creatinine clearance for patients with [circles with solid line: Cl = 1.303(CrCl) + 20] and without [squares with dashed line: Cl = 1.303(CrCl) + 40] moderate-severe (NYHA Class III or IV) heart failure. Nonrenal clearance (denoted by the y-intercept) is lower for patients with moderate-severe heart failure because reduced cardiac output results in decreased liver blood flow and digoxin hepatic clearance.

with declining renal function.[10,35] While the mechanism for this change is not as well understood, it is likely that digoxin is displaced from tissue-binding sites by an unknown substance or substances present in patients with renal dysfunction so that drug which would have been bound to tissues becomes unbound. Unbound digoxin molecules displaced from tissue-binding sites move into the blood causing the decreased volume of distribution [$\downarrow V = V_b + (f_b/\uparrow f_t) V_t$, where V is digoxin volume of distribution, V_b is blood volume, V_t is tissue volume, f_b is the unbound fraction of digoxin in the blood, and f_t is the unbound fraction of digoxin in the tissues]. The equation that estimates digoxin volume of distribution using creatinine clearance is:

$$V = \left(226 + \frac{298 \bullet CrCl}{29.1 + CrCl}\right)(Wt/70)$$

where V is digoxin volume of distribution in L/70 kg, Wt is body weight in kg (use ideal body weight if >30% overweight), and CrCl is creatinine clearance in mL/min.[35] Because digoxin volume of distribution and clearance decrease simultaneously in patients with renal failure, the average half-life for digoxin of 5 days is shorter than what might be expected if clearance alone decreased [$t_{1/2} = (0.693 \bullet V)/Cl$].

Digoxin is not significantly eliminated by hemodialysis or peritoneal dialysis.[31,32] Hemofiltration does remove digoxin with a typical sieving coefficient of 0.7.[36,37] In many cases, a sufficient amount of digoxin will not be removed to warrant an increased maintenance dose. However, due to pharmacokinetic variability, some patients may need a periodic booster dose to increase digoxin concentrations (see Special Dosing Consideration section at end of chapter).[37]

Heart failure decreases cardiac output, which in turn decreases liver blood flow. Liver blood flow is an important factor in the determination of hepatic clearance for drugs because it is the vehicle that delivers drug molecules to the liver for possible elimination. Moderate-severe heart failure (NYHA CHF class III or IV, see Table 6-1) decreases the hepatic clearance of digoxin by this mechanism.[12] When estimating digoxin clearance for the purpose of computing initial drug doses, it is necessary to decrease the nonrenal clearance (Cl_{NR}) factor to 20 mL/min in the equation to compensate for decreased hepatic clearance: $Cl = 1.303 (CrCl) + 20$, where Cl is digoxin clearance in mL/min, CrCl is creatinine clearance in mL/min, and 20 is digoxin nonrenal clearance Cl_{NR} in mL/min.

Thyroid hormone regulates basil metabolic rate, and thyroid status will influence every major organ system in the body including the heart (heart rate and cardiac output), liver (liver blood flow and microsomal drug-metabolizing enzyme function), and kidney (renal blood flow and glomerular filtration rate). Patients who are hypothyroid will have slower metabolic rates and eliminate digoxin more slowly than euthyroid patients ($t_{1/2} = 48$ hours with normal renal function).[31,32,38-40] Hyperthyroid patients have faster metabolic rates and eliminate digoxin faster than euthyroid patients ($t_{1/2} = 24$ hours with normal renal function).[31,32,38-40] Hyperthyroid patients can present with atrial fibrillation which may be treated with digoxin. Generally, these patients require higher digoxin doses to control ventricular rate because of the increase in digoxin clearance.

Similar to other drugs, digoxin clearance is lower in neonates and premature infants because renal and hepatic function are not completely developed.[41,42] Premature infants and neonates have average digoxin half-lives equal to 60 hours and 45 hours, respectively. In older babies and young children (6 months-8 years old), renal and hepatic function are fully developed and half-lives can be as short as 18 hours. Older children (≥ 12 years old) have mean digoxin half-lives ($t_{1/2} = 36$ hours) that are similar to those found in adults. Also, volume of distribution is larger in infants and children compared to adults as is found with many other drugs. Pediatric loading and maintenance doses are given in Table 6-3.

Malabsorption of oral digoxin has been reported in patients with severe diarrhea, radiation treatments to the abdomen, and gastrointestinal hypermotility.[38,43-47] In these cases, steady-state digoxin serum concentrations decrease due to poor bioavailability of the drug.

TABLE 6-3   Initial Pediatric Doses of Digoxin for Patients With Normal Renal Function (CrCl > 50 mL/min)[98]

| | Loading Dose (μg/kg)[a] | | Maintenance (μg/kg/d)[b,c] | |
Age	PO	IV/IM	PO	IV/IM
Premature	20	15	5	3-4
Full term	30	20	8-10	6-8
1 mo to <2 y	40-50	30-40	10-12	7.5-9
2-10 y	30-40	20-30	8-10	6-8
≥10 y and <100 kg	10-15	8-12	2.5-5	2-3

[a]Administer ½ dose initially, then ¼ dose at 8- to 18-hour intervals; obtain ECG after each dose to assess effect and toxicity.

[b]<10 y: Divide daily dose in half and give twice daily, ≥10 y: Give once daily.

[c]For CrCl = 10-50 mL/min give 25%-75% of daily dose every 24 hours or give total dose every 36 hours, for CrCl <10 mL/min give 10%-25% of daily dose every 24 hours or give total dose every 48 hours.

DRUG INTERACTIONS

Digoxin has an extensive list of drug interactions with other agents. Because of this, only the most common and severe drug interactions will be discussed. Inhibition of P-glycoprotein, a drug efflux pump which is found in the kidney, liver, and intestine, appears to be involved in the majority of digoxin interactions.[20,21,48] Clinicians should consult a current drug interaction reference when other medications are prescribed to patients receiving digoxin therapy.[49]

Quinidine decreases both the renal and nonrenal clearance of digoxin and also decreases the volume of distribution of digoxin.[50-55] Inhibition of P-glycoprotein may be involved in this interaction.[48] The result of this complex interaction is that concurrent quinidine therapy increases the average steady-state digoxin concentration by 30%-70%.

Verapamil, diltiazem, and bepridil inhibit digoxin clearance and increase mean digoxin steady-state concentrations by various degrees.[55-61] Of these calcium channel blockers, verapamil is the most potent inhibitor of digoxin clearance, and increases digoxin steady-state serum concentrations up to 70%. Diltiazem and bepridil therapy each increase average digoxin steady-state serum concentrations by about 30%.

Amiodarone[62-65] and propafenone[66-68] are antiarrhythmic agents that decrease digoxin clearance. In addition to this drug interaction mechanism, amiodarone also simultaneously increases digoxin oral bioavailability, and it is likely that P-glycoprotein inhibition is involved in the drug interaction between these two drugs.[69] Digoxin steady-state serum concentrations increase two-three times over baseline values with concomitant amiodarone therapy. Because amiodarone has a very long half-life (~50 hours), the onset of the drug interaction with digoxin can be very long. As serum concentrations of amiodarone slowly increase and approach steady-state values, digoxin clearance and bioavailability are simultaneously slowly changing. The insidious nature of the amiodarone–digoxin drug interaction can make it difficult to detect in patients. Propafenone therapy increases mean digoxin steady-state concentrations by 30%-60% in a dose-dependent fashion with propafenone doses of 450 mg/d causing digoxin concentration changes in the lower end of the range and propafenone doses of 900 mg/d causing digoxin concentration changes in the upper end of the range.

Cyclosporine therapy has been reported to increase average steady-state digoxin concentrations up to 50%.[70] P-glycoprotein inhibition by cyclosporine is the primary mechanism for this drug interaction.[20]

About 10% of patients receiving digoxin therapy have significant amounts of *Eubacterium lentum* in their gastrointestinal tract that metabolizes orally administered digoxin before it can be absorbed.[71,72] Erythromycin, clarithromycin, and tetracycline are antibiotics that can kill this bacteria.[73-78] Digoxin steady-state serum concentrations increase an average of 30% in these select patients when one of these three antibiotics have been prescribed. P-glycoprotein inhibition may be one of the mechanisms involved with this interaction involving macrolide antibiotics.[78]

The absorption of oral digoxin from the gastrointestinal tract is influenced by many different compounds. Aluminum-containing antacids and kaolin-pectin physically adsorb digoxin, rendering it unabsorbable.[79] These compounds should be administered no closer than 2 hours to an oral digoxin dose. Similarly, cholestyramine also reduces digoxin oral bioavailability by binding it in the gastrointestinal tract and should be given no closer than 8 hours to a digoxin oral dose.[80,81] Sulfasalazine and neomycin each decrease digoxin oral bioavailability by unknown mechanisms.[82,83] Propantheline increases oral digoxin bioavailability by prolonging gastrointestinal transit time, while metoclopramide and cisapride decreases oral digoxin bioavailability by decreasing gastrointestinal transit time.[81,84,85]

INITIAL DOSAGE DETERMINATION METHODS

Several methods to initiate digoxin therapy are available. The *Pharmacokinetic Dosing method* is the most flexible of the techniques. It allows individualized target serum concentrations to be chosen for a patient, and each pharmacokinetic parameter can be customized to reflect specific disease states and conditions present in the patient. However, it is computationally intensive.

The *Jelliffe method* is similar to the Pharmacokinetic Dosing method, except a target total body store is selected based on specific disease states and conditions present in the patient. It is also computationally intensive.

Nomograms that use the dosing concepts in the Jelliffe dosing method are available. But, in order to make calculations easier, they make simplifying assumptions. The nomograms are for adults only, and separate versions are needed for intravenous injection (Table 6-4A) and tablets (Table 6-4B) because of bioavailability

TABLE 6-4A Jelliffe Nomogram for Intravenous Digoxin (in μg) in Adult Patients With Heart Failure to Provide Total Body Stores of 10 μg/kg[99]

		Lean Body Weight						
	kg	50	60	70	80	90	100	
Corrected Ccr (mL/min per 70 kg)[a]	lb	110	132	154	176	198	220	Number of Days Before Steady-State Achieved[b]
0		75[c]	75	100	100	125	150	22
10		75	100	100	125	150	150	19
20		100	100	125	150	150	175	16
30		100	125	150	150	175	200	14
40		100	125	150	175	200	225	13
50		125	150	175	200	225	250	12
60		125	150	175	200	225	250	11
70		150	175	200	225	250	275	10
80		150	175	200	250	275	300	9
90		150	200	225	250	300	325	8
100		175	200	250	275	300	350	7

[a]Daily maintenance doses have been rounded to the nearest 25-μg increment.
[b]Ccr is creatinine clearance, corrected to 70-kg body weight or 1.73 m^2 body surface area. *For adults*, if only serum creatinine concentrations (Scr) are available, a Ccr (corrected to 70-kg body weight) may be estimated in men as (140 – age)/Scr. For women, this result should be multiplied by 0.85. *Note: This equation cannot be used for estimating creatinine clearance in infants or children.*
[c]If no loading dose administered.

TABLE 6-4B   Jelliffe Nomogram for Oral Digoxin Tablets (in μg) in Adult Patients With Heart Failure to Provide Total Body Stores of 10 μg/kg[99]

Corrected Ccr (mL/min per 70 kg)[a]	kg	Lean Body Weight						Number Of Days Before Steady-State Achieved[b]
		50	60	70	80	90	100	
	lb	110	132	154	176	198	220	
0		62.5[c]	125	125	125	187.5	187.5	22
10		125	125	125	187.5	187.5	187.5	19
20		125	125	187.5	187.5	187.5	250	16
30		125	187.5	187.5	187.5	250	250	14
40		125	187.5	187.5	250	250	250	13
50		187.5	187.5	250	250	250	250	12
60		187.5	187.5	250	250	250	375	11
70		187.5	250	250	250	250	375	10
80		187.5	250	250	250	375	375	9
90		187.5	250	250	250	375	500	8
100		250	250	250	375	375	500	7

[a]Ccr is creatinine clearance, corrected to 70-kg body weight or 1.73 m² body surface area. *For adults*, if only serum creatinine concentrations (Scr) are available, a Ccr (corrected to 70-kg body weight) may be estimated in men as (140 – age)/Scr. For women, this result should be multiplied by 0.85. *Note:* This equation cannot be used for estimating creatinine clearance in infants or children.

[b]If no loading dose administered.

differences among dosage forms. Both nomograms assume that digoxin total body stores of 10 μg/kg are adequate, so they are limited to heart failure patients requiring this dose. Another nomogram that makes other simplifying assumptions is also available for heart failure patients.[86]

Recommended initial doses for pediatric patients are given in Table 6-3.

PHARMACOKINETIC DOSING METHOD

The goal of initial dosing of digoxin is to compute the best dose possible for the patient given their set of disease states and conditions that influence digoxin pharmacokinetics and the cardiovascular disorder being treated. In order to do this, pharmacokinetic parameters for the patient will be estimated using average parameters measured in other patients with similar disease state and condition profiles. This approach is also known as the Jusko-Koup method for digoxin dosing.[12,35]

Clearance Estimate

Digoxin is predominately eliminated unchanged in the urine, and there is a good relationship between creatinine clearance and digoxin clearance (see Figure 6-2). This relationship allows the estimation of the digoxin clearance for a patient which can be used to compute an initial dose of the cardiac glycoside. Mathematically, the equation for the straight line shown in Figure 6-2 is: $Cl = 1.303 \, (CrCl) + Cl_{NR}$, where Cl is the digoxin clearance in mL/min, CrCl is creatinine clearance in mL/min, and Cl_{NR} is digoxin nonrenal clearance.[12] A digoxin nonrenal clearance value of 40 mL/min is used for patients without heart failure or who have only mild signs and symptoms of heart failure (NYHA CHF classes I or II). Patients with moderate or severe heart failure (NYHA CHF classes III or IV) have significant decreases in cardiac output which leads to a reduction in liver blood flow and digoxin hepatic clearance. In these cases, digoxin nonrenal clearance is set to equal 20 mL/min in the equation. For example, the estimated digoxin clearance for an individual with a creatinine clearance of 10 mL/min is 53 mL/min if the patient has no symptoms or mild symptoms of heart failure [Cl = 1.303 (10 mL/min) + 40 = 53 mL/min], or 33 mL/min if the patient has moderate-to-severe symptoms of heart failure [Cl = 1.303 (10 mL/min) + 20 = 33 mL/min]. Taking the patient's renal function into account when deriving initial doses of digoxin is the single most important characteristic to assess.

Volume of Distribution Estimate

The average volume of distribution for patients without disease states and conditions that change this parameter is 7 L/kg.[31,32] Because obesity does not change digoxin volume of distribution, the weight factor used in this calculation is ideal body weight (IBW) for patients that are significantly overweight (>30% over IBW).[33,34] Thus, for a 70-kg patient with good renal function, the estimated volume of distribution would be 490 L (V = 7 L/kg • 70 kg = 490 L). If a patient weighs less than their ideal body weight, actual body weight is used to estimate volume of distribution. For patients whose weight is between their ideal body weight and 30% over ideal weight, actual body weight can be used to compute estimated volume of distribution, although some clinicians prefer to use ideal body weight for these individuals. In patients who are more than 30% above their ideal body weight, volume of distribution (V) estimates should be based on ideal body weight. For an obese patient with normal renal function whose ideal body weight is 55 kg and total body weight is 95 kg, the estimated volume of distribution would be 385 L: V = 7 L/kg • IBW = 7 L/kg (55 kg) = 385 L.

For patients with renal dysfunction (creatinine clearance ≤ 30 mL/min), creatinine clearance should be used to provide an improved volume of distribution estimate (V in L) using the following formula:

$$V = \left(226 + \frac{298 \bullet \text{CrCl}}{29.1 + \text{CrCl}}\right)(\text{Wt}/70)$$

where CrCl is the patient's creatinine clearance in mL/min.[35] For example, a 70-kg patient with significant renal dysfunction (CrCl = 10 mL/min) is to receive a loading dose of digoxin and an estimate of digoxin volume of distribution is needed. The estimated volume of distribution for this patient would be 302 L:

$$V = \left(226 + \frac{298 \bullet \text{CrCl}}{29.1 + \text{CrCl}}\right)(\text{Wt}/70) = \left(226 + \frac{298 \bullet 10 \text{ mL}/\text{min}}{29.1 + 10 \text{ mL}/\text{min}}\right)(70 \text{ kg}/70) = 302 \text{ L}$$

In patients who are more than 30% above their ideal body weight, volume of distribution (V) estimates should be based on ideal body weight, so the weight factor used in the equation would be IBW.

Selection of Appropriate Pharmacokinetic Model and Equations

When given by intravenous injection or orally, digoxin follows a two-compartment pharmacokinetic model (see Figure 6-1). After the end of intravenous infusion or after peak concentration has been reached after an oral dose, serum concentrations drop over an 8–12-hour time period because of distribution of drug from blood to tissues (α or distribution phase). After distribution of digoxin is complete, drug concentrations decline more slowly, and the elimination rate constant for this segment of the concentration/time curve is the one that varies with renal function (β or elimination phase). While this model is the most correct from a strict pharmacokinetic viewpoint, it cannot easily be used clinically because of its mathematical complexity. During the elimination phase of the concentration/time curve, digoxin serum concentrations drop very slowly due to the long elimination half-life (36 hours with normal renal function, 5 days with end-stage renal disease). Because of this, a very simple pharmacokinetic equation that computes the average digoxin steady-state serum concentration

(Css in ng/mL = µg/L) is widely used and allows maintenance dosage calculation: Css = [F (D/τ)]/Cl or D/τ = (Css • Cl)/F, where F is the bioavailability fraction for the oral dosage form (F = 1 for intravenous digoxin), D is the digoxin dose in µg, τ is the dosage interval in days, and Cl is digoxin clearance in L/d.[12,35]

The equation used to calculate loading dose (LD in µg) is based on a simple one-compartment model: LD = (Css • V)/F, where Css is the desired digoxin steady-state concentration in µg/L which is equivalent to ng/mL, V is the digoxin volume of distribution, and F is the bioavailability fraction for the oral dosage form (F = 1 for intravenous digoxin). When digoxin loading doses are administered, they are usually given in divided doses separated by 4-6 hours (50% of dose at first, followed by two additional doses of 25%). A portion of the loading dose can be withheld if the patient is experiencing any digoxin adverse effects such as a low pulse rate. This technique is used to allow the assessment of clinical response before additional digoxin is given in order to avoid accidental overdosage.

Steady-State Concentration Selection

Digoxin steady-state concentrations are selected based on the cardiovascular disease being treated. For heart failure, steady-state serum concentrations of 0.5-1 ng/mL are usually effective.[13,14] For initial dosing purposes, a target digoxin concentration equal to 0.8 ng/mL is reasonable. For patients with atrial fibrillation, steady-state serum concentrations of 0.8-1.5 ng/mL are usually needed to control the ventricular rate to 100 beats/min or less.[15,32] An initial target digoxin concentration of 1.2 ng/mL is reasonable for patients with this disease state.

EXAMPLE 1 ▶▶▶

MJ is a 50-year-old, 70-kg (height = 5 ft 10 in) male with atrial fibrillation for less than 24 hours. His current serum creatinine is 0.9 mg/dL, and it has been stable over the last 5 days since admission. Compute an intravenous digoxin dose for this patient to control ventricular rate.

1. *Estimate creatinine clearance.*

This patient has a stable serum creatinine and is not obese. The Cockcroft-Gault equation can be used to estimate creatinine clearance:

$$CrCl_{est} = [(140 - age) BW]/(72 • S_{Cr}) = [(140 - 50 y) 70 kg]/(72 • 0.9 mg/dL)$$
$$CrCl_{est} = 97 mL/min$$

2. *Estimate clearance.*

The drug clearance versus creatinine clearance relationship is used to estimate the digoxin clearance for this patient (Cl_{NR} = 40 mL/min since the patient does not have moderate-severe heart failure):

$$Cl = 1.303 (CrCl) + Cl_{NR} = 1.303(97 mL/min) + 40 mL/min = 167 mL/min$$

3. *Use average steady-state concentration equation to compute digoxin maintenance dose.*

For a patient with atrial fibrillation, the desired digoxin concentration would be 0.8-1.5 ng/mL. A serum concentration equal to 1.2 ng/mL will be chosen for this patient, and intravenous digoxin will be used (F = 1). Note that for concentration units ng/mL = µg/L, and this conversion will be made before the equation is used. Also, conversion factors are needed to change milliliter units to liter (1000 mL/L) and minute units to days (1440 min/d).

$$D/τ = (Css • Cl)/F = (1.2 µg/L • 167 mL/min • 1440 min/d)/(1 • 1000 mL/L) = 288 µg/d, rounded to 250 µg/d$$

4. *Use loading dose equation to compute digoxin loading dose (if needed).*

The patient has good renal function and is nonobese. Therefore, a volume of distribution equal to 7 L/kg and actual body weight can be used to compute the digoxin loading dose. An intravenous loading dose (F = 1) could be used in this patient to achieve the desired pharmacologic effect quicker than would occur if mainte-nance doses alone were used and concentrations allowed to accumulate over 3-5 half-lives.

$$V = 7 \text{ L/kg} \bullet 70 \text{ kg} = 490 \text{ L}$$

$$LD = (Css \bullet V)/F = (1.2 \text{ μg/L} \bullet 490 \text{ L})/1 = 588 \text{ μg rounded to } 500 \text{ μg}$$

When digoxin loading doses are administered, they are usually given in divided doses separated by 4-6 hours (50% of dose at first, followed by two additional doses of 25%). In this case, an initial intravenous dose of 250 μg would be given initially, followed by two additional intravenous doses of 125 μg each. One of the loading doses could be withheld if pulse rate was less than 50-60 beats/min or other undesirable digoxin adverse effects were noted.

EXAMPLE 2 ▶▶▶

Same patient profile as in example 1, but serum creatinine is 3.5 mg/dL indicating renal impairment.

1. *Estimate creatinine clearance.*
   This patient has a stable serum creatinine and is not obese. The Cockcroft-Gault equation can be used to estimate creatinine clearance:

   $$CrCl_{est} = [(140 - \text{age}) \text{ BW}]/(72 \bullet S_{Cr}) = [(140 - 50 \text{ y}) 70 \text{ kg}]/(72 \bullet 3.5 \text{ mg/dL})$$

   $$CrCl_{est} = 25 \text{ mL/min}$$

2. *Estimate clearance.*
   The drug clearance versus creatinine clearance relationship is used to estimate the digoxin clearance for this patient ($Cl_{NR} = 40$ mL/min since the patient does not have moderate-severe heart failure):

   $$Cl = 1.303 \text{ (CrCl)} + Cl_{NR} = 1.303 \text{ (25 mL/min)} + 40 \text{ mL/min} = 73 \text{ mL/min}$$

3. *Use average steady-state concentration equation to compute digoxin maintenance dose.*
   For a patient with atrial fibrillation, the desired digoxin concentration would be 0.8-1.5 ng/mL. A serum concen-tration equal to 1.2 ng/mL will be chosen for this patient, and intravenous digoxin will be used (F = 1). Note that for concentration units ng/mL = μg/L, and this conversion will be made before the equation is used. Also, con-version factors are needed to change milliliter units to liter (1000 mL/L) and minute units to days (1440 min/d).

   $$D/\tau = (Css \bullet Cl)/F = (1.2 \text{ μg/L} \bullet 73 \text{ mL/min} \bullet 1440 \text{ min/d})/(1 \bullet 1000 \text{ mL/L}) = 125 \text{ μg/d}.$$

4. *Use loading dose equation to compute digoxin loading dose (if needed).*
   The patient has poor renal function and is nonobese. Therefore, the volume of distribution equation that adjusts the parameter estimate for renal dysfunction can be used to compute the digoxin loading dose. An intravenous loading dose (F = 1) could be given in this patient to achieve the desired pharmacologic effect quicker than would occur if maintenance doses alone were used to allow concentrations to accumulate over 3-5 half-lives.

   $$V = \left(226 + \frac{298 \bullet CrCl}{29.1 + CrCl}\right)(Wt/70) = \left(226 + \frac{298 \bullet 25 \text{ mL/min}}{29.1 + 25 \text{ mL/min}}\right)(70 \text{ kg}/70) = 364 \text{ L}$$

   $$LD = (Css \bullet V)/F = (1.2 \text{ mg/L} \bullet 364 \text{ L})/1 = 437 \text{ μg rounded to } 400 \text{ μg}$$

When digoxin loading doses are administered, they are usually given in divided doses separated by 4-6 hours (50% of dose at first, followed by two additional doses of 25%). In this case, an initial intravenous dose of 200 μg would be given initially, followed by two additional intravenous doses of 100 μg each. One of the loading doses could be withheld if the pulse rate was less than 50-60 beats/min or other undesirable digoxin adverse effects were noted.

EXAMPLE 3 ▶▶▶

Same patient profile as in example 1, but serum creatinine is 3.5 mg/dL indicating renal impairment. Additionally, the patient is being treated for NYHA Class III moderate heart failure, not atrial fibrillation. Compute an oral digoxin tablet maintenance dose for this patient.

1. *Estimate creatinine clearance.*

This patient has a stable serum creatinine and is not obese. The Cockcroft-Gault equation can be used to estimate creatinine clearance:

$$CrCl_{est} = [(140 - age)\ BW]/(72 \bullet S_{Cr}) = [(140 - 50\ y)\ 70\ kg]/(72 \bullet 3.5\ mg/dL)$$

$$CrCl_{est} = 25\ mL/min$$

2. *Estimate clearance.*

The drug clearance versus creatinine clearance relationship is used to estimate the digoxin clearance for this patient ($Cl_{NR} = 20$ mL/min since the patient has moderate heart failure):

$$Cl = 1.303\ (CrCl) + Cl_{NR} = 1.303\ (25\ mL/min) + 20\ mL/min = 53\ mL/min$$

3. *Use average steady-state concentration equation to compute digoxin maintenance dose.*

For a patient with heart failure, the desired digoxin concentration would be 0.5-1 ng/mL. A serum concentration equal to 0.8 ng/mL will be chosen for this patient, and oral digoxin will be used (F = 0.7). Note that for concentration units ng/mL = μg/L, and this conversion will be made before the equation is used. Also, conversion factors are needed to change milliliter units to liter (1000 mL/L) and minute units to days (1440 min/d).

$$D/\tau = (Css \bullet Cl)/F = (0.8\ μg/L \bullet 53\ mL/min \bullet 1440\ min/d)/(0.7 \bullet 1000\ mL/L) = 87\ μg/d,\ or\ 174\ μg\ every\ 2\ days$$
$$(87\ μg/d \bullet 2\ d = 174\ μg\ every\ 2\ days).$$

This oral tablet dose would be rounded to 125 μg every other day.

EXAMPLE 4 ▶▶▶

OI is a 65-year-old, 170-kg (height = 5 ft 5 in) female with NYHA Class III moderate heart failure. Her current serum creatinine is 4.7 mg/dL and is stable. Compute an intravenous digoxin loading and maintenance dose for this patient.

1. *Estimate creatinine clearance.*

This patient has a stable serum creatinine and is obese [$IBW_{females}$ (in kg) = 45 + 2.3 (Ht − 60) = 45 + 2.3 (65 in − 60) = 57 kg]. The Salazar and Corcoran equation can be used to estimate creatinine clearance:

$$CrCl_{est(females)} = \frac{(146 - age)[(0.287 \bullet Wt) + (9.74 \bullet Ht^2)]}{(60 \bullet S_{Cr})}$$

$$CrCl_{est(females)} = \frac{(146 - 65\ y)\{[0.287 \bullet 170\ kg] + [9.74 \bullet (1.65\ m)^2]\}}{(60 \bullet 4.7\ mg/dL)} = 22\ mL/min$$

Note: Height is converted from inches to meters: Ht = (65 in • 2.54 cm/in)/(100 cm/m) = 1.65 m.

2. *Estimate clearance.*

The drug clearance versus creatinine clearance relationship is used to estimate the digoxin clearance for this patient ($Cl_{NR} = 20$ mL/min since the patient has moderate-severe heart failure):

$$Cl = 1.303 \, (CrCl) + Cl_{NR} = 1.303 \, (22 \text{ mL/min}) + 20 \text{ mL/min} = 48 \text{ mL/min}$$

3. *Use average steady-state concentration equation to compute digoxin maintenance dose.*

For a patient with heart failure, the desired digoxin concentration would be 0.5-1 ng/mL. A serum concentration equal to 0.8 ng/mL will be chosen for this patient, and intravenous digoxin will be used (F = 1). Note that for concentration units ng/mL = µg/L, and this conversion will be made before the equation is used. Also, conversion factors are needed to change milliliter units to liter (1000 mL/L) and min units to days (1440 min/d).

$$D/\tau = (Css \bullet Cl)/F = (0.8 \text{ µg/L} \bullet 48 \text{ mL/min} \bullet 1440 \text{ min/d})/(1 \bullet 1000 \text{ mL/L}) = 56 \text{ µg/d, or } 112 \text{ µg every 2 days}$$
$$(56 \text{ µg/d} \bullet 2 \text{ d} = 112 \text{ µg every 2 days}).$$

This intravenous dose would be rounded to 125 µg every other day.

4. *Use loading dose equation to compute digoxin loading dose (if needed).*

The patient has poor renal function and is obese. Therefore, the volume of distribution equation that adjusts the parameter estimate for renal dysfunction can be used to compute the digoxin loading dose, and ideal body weight will be used as the weight factor. An intravenous loading dose (F = 1) could be given in this patient to achieve the desired pharmacologic effect quicker than would occur if maintenance doses alone were used to allow concentrations to accumulate over 3-5 half-lives.

$$V = \left(226 + \frac{298 \bullet CrCl}{29.1 + CrCl} \right)(Wt/70) = \left(226 + \frac{298 \bullet 22 \text{ mL/min}}{29.1 + 22 \text{ mL/min}} \right)(57 \text{ kg}/70) = 288 \text{ L}$$

$$LD = (Css \bullet V)/F = (0.8 \text{ µg/L} \bullet 288 \text{ L})/1 = 230 \text{ µg, rounded to } 250 \text{ µg}$$

When digoxin loading doses are administered, they are usually given in divided doses separated by 4-6 hours (50% of dose at first, followed by two additional doses of 25%). In this case, an initial intravenous dose of 125 µg would be given initially, followed by two additional intravenous doses of 62.5 µg each. One of the loading doses could be withheld if pulse rate was less than 50-60 beats/min or other undesirable digoxin adverse effects were noted.

Jelliffe Method

Another approach to derive initial doses of digoxin is to compute an appropriate loading dose which provides an amount of the drug in the body that evokes the appropriate pharmacologic response.[87,88] The amount of digoxin in the body that produces the desired effect is known at the total body stores (TBS) of digoxin. The percent of drug that is lost on a daily basis (%lost/d) is related to renal function according to the following equation: %lost/d = 14% + 0.20(CrCl), where 14% is the percent of digoxin eliminated per day by nonrenal routes and CrCl is creatinine clearance in mL/min.[88] Because the goal of therapy is to provide the total body stores of digoxin that causes the appropriate inotropic or chronotropic effect, the maintenance dose (D in µg/d) is the amount of digoxin eliminated on a daily basis: D = [TBS $\bullet$ (%lost/d)]/F, where TBS is total body stores in µg/d, %lost/d is the percent of digoxin TBS lost per day, F is the bioavailability factor for the dosage form, and 100 is a conversion factor to convert the percentage to a fraction. Combining the two equations produces the initial digoxin maintenance dose: D = {TBS $\bullet$ [14% + 0.20(CrCl)]}/(F $\bullet$100).

For patients with creatinine clearance values over 30 mL/min, digoxin total body stores of 8-12 µg/kg are usually required to cause inotropic effects while 13-15 µg/kg are generally needed to cause chronotropic effects.[89,90] Since renal disease (creatinine clearance < 30 mL/min) decreases digoxin volume of distribution, initial digoxin total body stores of 6-10 µg/kg are recommended for patients with poor renal function.[89] Because obesity does not change digoxin volume of distribution, the weight factor used in this calculation is ideal body weight (IBW) for patients that are significantly overweight (> 30% over IBW).[33,34] If a patient weighs less than their ideal body weight, actual body weight is used to calculate total body stores. For patients whose weight is between their ideal body weight and 30% over ideal weight, actual body weight can be used to compute total body stores, although some clinicians prefer to use ideal body weight for these individuals. If a loading dose is required, the total body store (TBS in µg) is calculated and used to compute the loading dose (LD in µg) after correction for dosage form bioavailability (F): LD = TBS/F.[87,88]

Nomograms that use the dosing concepts in the Jelliffe dosing method are available. But, in order to make calculations easier, they make simplifying assumptions. The nomograms are for adults only, and separate versions are needed for intravenous injection (see Table 6-4A) and tablets (see Table 6-4B) because of bioavailability differences among dosage forms. Both nomograms assume that digoxin total body stores of 10 µg/kg are adequate, so are limited to heart failure patients requiring this dose.

To contrast the Jelliffe dosage method with the Jusko-Koup dosage method, the same patient cases will be used as examples for this section.

EXAMPLE 1 ▶▶▶

MJ is a 50-year-old, 70-kg (height = 5 ft 10 in) male with atrial fibrillation for less than 24 hours. His current serum creatinine is 0.9 mg/dL, and it has been stable over the last 5 days since admission. Compute an intravenous digoxin dose for this patient to control ventricular rate.

1. *Estimate creatinine clearance.*

   This patient has a stable serum creatinine and is not obese. The Cockcroft-Gault equation can be used to estimate creatinine clearance:

   $$CrCl_{est} = [(140 - age) BW]/(72 \bullet S_{Cr}) = [(140 - 50 y) 70 kg]/(72 \bullet 0.9 mg/dL)$$
   $$CrCl_{est} = 97 mL/min$$

2. *Estimate total body store (TBS) and maintenance dose (D).*

   The patient has good renal function and is nonobese. Digoxin total body stores of 13-15 µg/kg are effective in the treatment of atrial fibrillation. A digoxin dose of 14 µg/kg is chosen for this patient.

   TBS = 14 µg/kg $\bullet$ 70 kg = 980 µg
   D = {TBS $\bullet$ [14% + 0.20(CrCl)]}/(F $\bullet$100) = {980 µg $\bullet$ [14% + 0.20(97 mL/min)]}/(1 $\bullet$100)
      = 328 µg/d, rounded to 375 µg/d

3. *Use loading dose equation to compute digoxin loading dose (if needed).*

   Digoxin total body store is used to calculate the loading dose after correcting for bioavailability:

   $$LD = TBS/F = 980 µg/1 = 980 µg, rounded to 1000 µg$$

   When digoxin loading doses are administered, they are usually given in divided doses separated by 4-6 hours (50% of dose at first, followed by two additional doses of 25%). In this case, an initial intravenous dose of 500 µg would be given initially, followed by two additional intravenous doses of 250 µg each. One of the loading doses could be withheld if pulse rate was less than 50-60 beats/min or other undesirable digoxin adverse effects were noted.

EXAMPLE 2 ▶▶▶

Same patient profile as in example 1, but serum creatinine is 3.5 mg/dL indicating renal impairment.

1. *Estimate creatinine clearance.*

   This patient has a stable serum creatinine and is not obese. The Cockcroft-Gault equation can be used to estimate creatinine clearance:

   $$CrCl_{est} = [(140 - age)\ BW]/(72 \bullet S_{Cr}) = [(140 - 50\ y)\ 70\ kg]/(72 \bullet 3.5\ mg/dL)$$

   $$CrCl_{est} = 25\ mL/min$$

2. *Estimate total body store (TBS) and maintenance dose (D).*

   The patient has poor renal function and is nonobese. Digoxin total body stores of 6-10 µg/kg are recommended for patients with renal dysfunction. A digoxin dose of 8 µg/kg is chosen for this patient.

   $$TBS = 8\ µg/kg \bullet 70\ kg = 560\ µg$$

   $$D = \{TBS \bullet [14\% + 0.20(CrCl)]\}/(F \bullet 100) = \{560\ µg \bullet [14\% + 0.20(25\ mL/min)]\}/(1 \bullet 100) = 106\ µg/d,$$
   rounded to 125 µg/d

3. *Use loading dose equation to compute digoxin loading dose (if needed).*

   Digoxin total body store is used to calculate the loading dose after correcting for bioavailability:

   $$LD = TBS/F = 560\ µg/1 = 560\ µg,\ rounded\ to\ 500\ µg$$

   When digoxin loading doses are administered, they are usually given in divided doses separated by 4-6 hours (50% of dose at first, followed by two additional doses of 25%). In this case, an initial intravenous dose of 250 µg would be given initially, followed by two additional intravenous doses of 125 µg each. One of the loading doses could be withheld if pulse rate was less than 50-60 beats/min or other undesirable digoxin adverse effects were noted.

EXAMPLE 3 ▶▶▶

Same patient profile as in example 1, but serum creatinine is 3.5 mg/dL indicating renal impairment. Additionally, the patient is being treated for NYHA Class III moderate heart failure, not atrial fibrillation. Compute an oral digoxin tablet maintenance dose for this patient.

1. *Estimate creatinine clearance.*

   This patient has a stable serum creatinine and is not obese. The Cockcroft-Gault equation can be used to estimate creatinine clearance:

   $$CrCl_{est} = [(140 - age)\ BW]/(72 \bullet S_{Cr}) = [(140 - 50\ y)\ 70\ kg]/(72 \bullet 3.5\ mg/dL)$$

   $$CrCl_{est} = 25\ mL/min$$

2. *Estimate total body store (TBS) and maintenance dose (D).*

   The patient has poor renal function and is nonobese. Digoxin total body stores of 6-10 µg/kg are recommended for patients with renal dysfunction. A digoxin dose of 8 µg/kg is chosen for this patient.

   $$TBS = 8\ µg/kg \bullet 70\ kg = 560\ µg$$

   $$D = \{TBS \bullet [14\% + 0.20(CrCl)]\}/(F \bullet 100) = \{560\ µg \bullet [14\% + 0.20(25\ mL/min)]\}/(0.7 \bullet 100) = 152\ µg/d,$$
   rounded to 125 µg/d

EXAMPLE 4 ▶▶▶

Ol is a 65-year-old, 170-kg (height = 5 ft 5 in) female with NYHA Class III moderate heart failure. Her current serum creatinine is 4.7 mg/dL and is stable. Compute an intravenous digoxin loading and maintenance dose for this patient.

1. *Estimate creatinine clearance.*

This patient has a stable serum creatinine and is obese [$IBW_{females}$ (in kg) = 45 + 2.3(Ht − 60) = 45 + 2.3(65 in − 60) = 57 kg]. The Salazar and Corcoran equation can be used to estimate creatinine clearance:

$$CrCl_{est(females)} = \frac{(146 - age)[(0.287 \bullet Wt) + (9.74 \bullet Ht^2)]}{(60 \bullet S_{Cr})}$$

$$CrCl_{est(females)} = \frac{(146 - 65\ y)\{[0.287 \bullet 170\ kg] + [9.74 \bullet (1.65\ m)^2]\}}{(60 \bullet 4.7\ mg/dL)} = 22\ mL/min$$

Note: Height is converted from inches to meters: Ht = (65 in • 2.54 cm/in)/(100 cm/m) = 1.65 m

2. *Estimate total body store (TBS) and maintenance dose (D).*

The patient has poor renal function and is obese. Digoxin total body stores of 6-10 µg/kg are recommended for patients with renal dysfunction, and ideal body weight (IBW) should be used in the computation. A digoxin dose of 8 µg/kg is chosen for this patient.

$$TBS = 8\ µg/kg \bullet 57\ kg = 456\ µg$$

D = {TBS • [14% + 0.20(CrCl)]}/(F •100) = {456 µg • [14% + 0.20(22 mL/min)]}/(1 •100) = 83 µg/d, or 166 µg every 2 days (83 µg/d • 2 days = 166 µg every 2 days)

This intravenous dose would be rounded to 150 µg every other day.

3. *Use loading dose equation to compute digoxin loading dose (if needed).*

Digoxin total body store is used to calculate the loading dose after correcting for bioavailability:

$$LD = TBS/F = 456\ µg/1 = 456\ µg, rounded\ to\ 500\ µg$$

When digoxin loading doses are administered, they are usually given in divided doses separated by 4-6 hours (50% of dose at first, followed by two additional doses of 25%). In this case, an initial intravenous dose of 250 µg would be given initially, followed by two additional intravenous doses of 125 µg each. One of the loading doses could be withheld if pulse rate was less than 50-60 beats/min or other undesirable digoxin adverse effects were noted.

USE OF DIGOXIN SERUM CONCENTRATIONS TO ALTER DOSAGES

Because of pharmacokinetic variability among patients, it is likely that doses computed using patient population characteristics will not always produce digoxin serum concentrations that are expected. Because of this, digoxin serum concentrations are measured in many patients to insure that therapeutic, nontoxic levels are present and to check for compliance to dosage regimens. However, not all patients may require serum concentration monitoring. For example, if an appropriate dose for the renal function and concurrent disease states of the patient is prescribed (e.g., 250 µg/d in a patient with a creatinine clearance of 80-100 mL/min for heart failure) and the desired clinical effect is achieved without adverse effects, digoxin serum concentration monitoring may not be necessary. Whether or not digoxin concentrations are measured, important patient parameters (dyspnea, orthopnea, tachypnea, cough, pulmonary rales/edema, S_3 gallop, etc) should be followed to confirm that the patient is responding to treatment and not developing adverse drug reactions.

When digoxin serum concentrations are measured in patients and a dosage change is necessary, clinicians should seek to use the simplest, most straightforward method available to determine a dose that will provide safe and effective treatment. In most cases, a simple dosage ratio can be used to change digoxin doses since digoxin follows *linear pharmacokinetics*. Sometimes, it is not possible to simply change the dose because of the limited number of oral dosage strengths, and the dosage interval must also be changed. Available digoxin tablet strengths are 125 μg and 250 μg while digoxin oral solution is available at a concentration of 0.05 mg/mL. In some situations, it may be necessary to compute the digoxin pharmacokinetic parameters for the patient and utilize these to calculate the best drug dose (Pharmacokinetic Parameter method).

Finally, computerized methods that incorporate expected population pharmacokinetic characteristics (*Bayesian pharmacokinetic computer programs*) can be used in difficult cases where renal function is changing, serum concentrations are obtained at suboptimal times, or the patient was not at steady-state when serum concentrations were measured. An additional benefit of this dosing method is that a complete pharmacokinetic workup (determination of clearance, volume of distribution, and half-life) can be done with one or more measured concentrations that do not have to be at steady-state.

Linear Pharmacokinetics Method

Because digoxin follows linear, dose-proportional pharmacokinetics, steady-state serum concentrations change in proportion to dose according to the following equation: $D_{new}/C_{ss,new} = D_{old}/C_{ss,old}$ or $D_{new} = (C_{ss,new}/C_{ss,old})D_{old}$. In this equation, D is the dose in μg, Css is the steady-state concentration in ng/mL, old indicates the dose that produced the steady-state concentration that the patient is currently receiving, and new denotes the dose necessary to produce the desired steady-state concentration. The advantages of this method are that it is quick and simple. The disadvantages are that steady-state concentrations are required. Also, because of a limited number of solid oral dosage strengths, it may not be possible to attain desired serum concentrations by only changing the dose. In these cases, dosage intervals are extended for patients receiving tablets so that doses can be given as multiples of 125 μg. The estimated times to achieve steady-state concentrations on a stable digoxin dosage regimen varies according to renal function and are listed in Tables 6-4A and 6-4B. An alternative to this way of estimating time to steady-state is to compute the expected digoxin half-life ($t_{1/2}$ in days) for a patient using digoxin clearance (Cl in L/d) and volume of distribution (V in L) and allow 3-5 half-lives to pass before obtaining digoxin serum concentrations: $t_{1/2} = (0.693 \cdot V)/Cl$.

EXAMPLE 1 ▶▶▶

MJ is a 50-year-old, 70-kg (height = 5 ft 10 in) male with moderate heart failure. His current serum creatinine is 0.9 mg/dL, and it has been stable over the last 6 months. A digoxin dose of 250 μg/d using oral tablets was prescribed and expected to achieve steady-state concentrations equal to 0.8 ng/mL. After a week of treatment, a steady-state digoxin concentration was measured and equaled 0.6 ng/mL. Calculate a new digoxin dose that would provide a steady-state concentration of 0.9 ng/mL.

1. *Estimate creatinine clearance.*

   This patient has a stable serum creatinine and is not obese. The Cockcroft-Gault equation can be used to estimate creatinine clearance:

   $$CrCl_{est} = [(140 - age) BW]/(72 \cdot S_{Cr}) = [(140 - 50 \text{ y}) 70 \text{ kg}]/(72 \cdot 0.9 \text{ mg/dL})$$
   $$CrCl_{est} = 97 \text{ mL/min}$$

The patient has good renal function and would be expected to have achieved steady-state after 7 days of treatment.

2. *Compute new dose to achieve the desired serum concentration.*

Using linear pharmacokinetics, the new dose to attain the desired concentration should be proportional to the old dose that produced the measured concentration:

$$D_{new} = (C_{ss,new}/C_{ss,old})\ D_{old} = (0.9\ ng/mL\ /0.6\ ng/mL)\ 250\ \mu g/d = 375\ \mu g/d$$

The new suggested dose would be 375 µg/d given as digoxin tablets to be started at the next scheduled dosing time.

EXAMPLE 2 ▶▶▶

OI is a 65-year-old, 170-kg (height = 5 ft 5 in) female with NYHA Class III heart failure. Her current serum creatinine is 4.7 mg/dL and is stable. A digoxin dose of 125 µg/d given as tablets was prescribed and expected to achieve steady-state concentrations equal to 1 ng/mL. After the 3 weeks of therapy, a steady-state digoxin concentration was measured and equaled 2.5 ng/mL. Calculate a new digoxin dose that would provide a steady-state concentration of 1.2 ng/mL.

1. *Estimate creatinine clearance.*

This patient has a stable serum creatinine and is obese [$IBW_{females}$ (in kg) = 45 + 2.3 (Ht − 60) = 45 + 2.3 (65 ft − 60) = 57 kg]. The Salazar and Corcoran equation can be used to estimate creatinine clearance:

$$CrCl_{est(females)} = \frac{(146 - age)[(0.287 \bullet Wt) + (9.74 \bullet Ht^2)]}{(60 \bullet S_{Cr})}$$

$$CrCl_{est(females)} = \frac{(146 - 65\ y)\{[0.287 \bullet 170\ kg] + [9.74 \bullet (1.65\ m)^2]\}}{(60 \bullet 4.7\ mg/dL)} = 22\ mL/min$$

Note: Height is converted from inches to meters: Ht = (65 in • 2.54 cm/in)/(100 cm/m) = 1.65 m.

This patient has poor renal function, but would be expected to be at steady-state with regard to digoxin serum concentrations after 3 weeks of treatment.

2. *Compute the new dose to achieve the desired serum concentration.*

Using linear pharmacokinetics, the new dose to attain the desired concentration should be proportional to the old dose that produced the measured concentration:

$$D_{new} = (C_{ss,new}/C_{ss,old})\ D_{old} = (1.2\ ng/mL\ /2.5\ ng/mL)\ 125\ \mu g/d = 60\ \mu g/d, \text{ or } 120\ \mu g \text{ every other day}$$

(60 µg/d • 2 days = 120 µg every 2 days)

This would be rounded to digoxin tablets 125 µg every other day.

The new suggested dose would be 125 µg every other day given as digoxin tablets to be started at next scheduled dosing time. Since the dosage interval is being changed, a day would be skipped before the next dose was given.

Pharmacokinetic Parameter Method

This method calculates the patient-specific drug clearance, and uses it to design improved dosage regimens.[31,32] Digoxin clearance can be measured using a single steady-state digoxin concentration (Css) and the following formula: Cl = [F(D/τ)]/Css, where Cl is digoxin clearance in L/d, F is the bioavailability factor for the dosage form used, τ is the dosage interval in days, and Css is the digoxin steady-state concentration in ng/mL which also equals μg/L. Although this method does allow computation of digoxin clearance, it yields exactly the same digoxin dose as that supplied using linear pharmacokinetics. As a result, most clinicians prefer to calculate the new dose directly using the Simpler Linear Pharmacokinetics method. To illustrate this point, the patient cases used to illustrate the Linear Pharmacokinetics method will be used as examples for the Pharmacokinetic Parameter method.

EXAMPLE 1 ▶▶▶

MJ is a 50-year-old, 70-kg (height = 5 ft 10 in) male with moderate heart failure. His current serum creatinine is 0.9 mg/dL, and it has been stable over the last 6 months. A digoxin dose of 250 μg/d using oral tablets was prescribed and expected to achieve steady-state concentrations equal to 0.8 ng/mL. After a week of treatment, a steady-state digoxin concentration was measured and equaled 0.6 ng/mL. Calculate a new digoxin dose that would provide a steady-state concentration of 0.9 ng/mL.

1. *Estimate creatinine clearance.*

   This patient has a stable serum creatinine and is not obese. The Cockcroft-Gault equation can be used to estimate creatinine clearance:

   $$CrCl_{est} = [(140 - age)\ BW]/(72 \bullet S_{Cr}) = [(140 - 50\ y)\ 70\ kg]/(72 \bullet 0.9\ mg/dL) = 97\ mL/min$$

   The patient has good renal function and would be expected to have achieved steady-state after 7 days of treatment.

2. *Compute drug clearance.*

   Note that digoxin concentrations in ng/mL are the same as those for μg/L. This unit substitution will be directly made to avoid conversion factors in the computation.

   $$Cl = [F\ (D/τ)]/Css = [0.7\ (250\ μg/d)]/0.6\ μg/L = 292\ L/d$$

3. *Compute the new dose to achieve the desired serum concentration.*

   The average steady-state equation is used to compute the new digoxin dose.

   $$D/τ = (Css \bullet Cl)/F = (0.9\ μg/L \bullet 292\ L/d)/0.7 = 375\ μg/d$$

   The new suggested dose would be 375 μg/d given as digoxin tablets to be started at next scheduled dosing time.

EXAMPLE 2 ▶▶▶

OI is a 65-year-old, 170-kg (height = 5 ft 5 in) female with NYHA Class III heart failure. Her current serum creatinine is 4.7 mg/dL and is stable. A digoxin dose of 125 μg/d given as tablets was prescribed and expected to achieve steady-state concentrations equal to 1 ng/mL. After the 3 weeks of therapy, a steady-state digoxin concentration was measured and equaled 2.5 ng/mL. Calculate a new digoxin dose that would provide a steady-state concentration of 1.2 ng/mL.

1. *Estimate creatinine clearance.*

This patient has a stable serum creatinine and is obese [$IBW_{females}$ (in kg) = 45 + 2.3 (Ht − 60) = 45 + 2.3 (65 in − 60) = 57 kg]. The Salazar and Corcoran equation can be used to estimate creatinine clearance:

$$CrCl_{est(females)} = \frac{(146 - age)[(0.287 \cdot Wt) + (9.74 \cdot Ht^2)]}{(60 \cdot S_{Cr})}$$

$$CrCl_{est(females)} = \frac{(146 - 65\ y)\{[0.287 \cdot 170\ kg] + [9.74 \cdot (1.65\ m)^2]\}}{(60 \cdot 4.7\ mg/dL)} = 22\ mL/min$$

Note: Height is converted from inches to meters: Ht = (65 in $\cdot$ 2.54 cm/in)/(100 cm/m) = 1.65 m.

This patient has poor renal function, but would be expected to be at steady-state with regard to digoxin serum concentrations after 3 weeks of treatment.

2. *Compute drug clearance.*

Note that digoxin concentrations in ng/mL are the same as those for µg/L. This unit substitution will be made directly to avoid conversion factors in the computation.

$$Cl = [F (D/\tau)]/Css = [0.7 (125\ µg/d)]/2.5\ µg/L = 35\ L/d$$

3. *Compute the new dose to achieve the desired serum concentration.*

The average steady-state equation is used to compute the new digoxin dose.

$$D/\tau = (Css \cdot Cl)/F = (1.2\ µg/L \cdot 35\ L/d)/0.7 = 60\ µg/d, \text{ or } 120\ µg \text{ every other day } (60\ µg/d \cdot 2\ days = 120\ µg$$
$$\text{every 2 days})$$

This would be rounded to digoxin tablets 125 µg every other day.

The new suggested dose would be 125 µg every other day given as digoxin tablets to be started at next scheduled dosing time. Since the dosage interval is being changed, a day would be skipped before the next dose was given.

BAYESIAN PHARMACOKINETIC COMPUTER PROGRAMS

Computer programs are available that can assist in the computation of pharmacokinetic parameters for patients.[91,92] The most reliable computer programs use a nonlinear regression algorithm that incorporates components of Bayes theorem. Nonlinear regression is a statistical technique that uses an iterative process to compute the best pharmacokinetic parameters for a concentration/time data set. Briefly, the patient's drug dosage schedule and serum concentrations are input into the computer. The computer program has a pharmacokinetic equation preprogrammed for the drug and administration method (oral, intravenous bolus, intravenous infusion, etc). Typically, a one-compartment model is used, although some programs allow the user to choose among several different equations. Using population estimates based on demographic information for the patient (age, weight, gender, renal function, etc) supplied by the user, the computer program then computes estimated serum concentrations at each time there are actual serum concentrations. Kinetic parameters are then changed by the computer program, and a new set of estimated serum concentrations are computed. The pharmacokinetic parameters that generated the estimated serum concentrations closest to the actual values are remembered by the computer program, and the process is repeated until the set of pharmacokinetic parameters are generated that result in estimated serum concentrations that are statistically closest to the actual serum concentrations.

These pharmacokinetic parameters can then be used to compute improved dosing schedules for patients. Bayes theorem is used in the computer algorithm to balance the results of the computations between values based solely on the patient's serum drug concentrations and those based only on patient population parameters. Results from studies that compare various methods of dosage adjustment have consistently found that these types of computer-dosing programs perform at least as well as experienced clinical pharmacokinetics and clinicians and better than inexperienced clinicians.

Some clinicians use Bayesian pharmacokinetic computer programs exclusively to alter drug doses based on serum concentrations. An advantage of this approach is that consistent dosage recommendations are made when several different practitioners are involved in therapeutic drug-monitoring programs. However, since simpler dosing methods work just as well for patients with stable pharmacokinetic parameters and steady-state drug concentrations, many clinicians reserve the use of computer programs for more difficult situations. Those situations include serum concentrations that are not at steady-state, serum concentrations not obtained at the specific times needed to employ simpler methods, and unstable pharmacokinetic parameters. Many Bayesian pharmacokinetic computer programs are available to users, and most should provide answers similar to the one used in the following examples. The program used to solve problems in this book is DrugCalc written by Dr Dennis Mungall.[93]

EXAMPLE 1 ▶▶▶

MJ is a 50-year-old, 70-kg (height = 5 ft 10 in) male with moderate heart failure. His current serum creatinine is 0.9 mg/dL, and it has been stable over the last 6 months. A digoxin dose of 250 µg/d using oral tablets was prescribed and expected to achieve steady-state concentrations equal to 0.8 ng/mL. After a week of treatment, a steady-state digoxin concentration was measured and equaled 0.6 ng/mL. Calculate a new digoxin dose that would provide a steady-state concentration of 0.9 ng/mL.

1. *Enter the patient's demographic, drug dosing, and serum concentration/time data into the computer program.*
2. *Compute pharmacokinetic parameters for the patient using Bayesian pharmacokinetic computer program.*
   The pharmacokinetic parameters computed by the program are a clearance equal to 8.8 L/h, a volume of distribution of 578 L, and a half-life equal to 46 h.
3. *Compute dose required to achieve the desired digoxin serum concentration.*
   The one-compartment model equations used by the program to compute doses indicates that a dose of 343 µg/d of digoxin tablets will produce a steady-state concentration of 0.9 ng/mL. This dose would be rounded off to 375 µg/d. Using the simpler Linear Pharmacokinetics method previously described in the chapter, the identical dose of 375 µg/d was computed.

EXAMPLE 2 ▶▶▶

OI is a 65-year-old, 170-kg (height = 5 ft 5 in) female with NYHA Class III heart failure. Her current serum creatinine is 4.7 mg/dL and is stable. A digoxin dose of 125 µg/d given as tablets was prescribed and expected to achieve steady-state concentrations equal to 1 ng/mL. After the 3 weeks of therapy, a steady-state digoxin concentration was measured and equaled 2.5 ng/mL. Calculate a new digoxin dose that would provide a steady-state concentration of 1.2 ng/mL.

1. *Enter the patient's demographic, drug dosing, and serum concentration/time data into the computer program.*
2. *Compute pharmacokinetic parameters for the patient using Bayesian pharmacokinetic computer program.*

The pharmacokinetic parameters computed by the program are a clearance equal to 1.4 L/h, a volume of distribution of 516 L, and a half-life equal to 249 h. The clearance value is slightly different than that computed using the steady-state Pharmacokinetic Parameter method (35 L/d or 1.5 L/h) because the patient probably was not at steady-state when the serum concentrations were drawn.

3. *Compute dose required to achieve the desired digoxin serum concentration.*

The one-compartment model intravenous infusion equations used by the program to compute doses indicates that a dose of 141 μg every 3 days will produce a steady-state concentration of 1.2 ng/mL. This would be rounded to 125 μg every 3 days. Using the steady-state Pharmacokinetic Parameter method previously described in the chapter, a similar dose of 125 μg every other day was computed.

EXAMPLE 3 ▶▶▶

JH is a 74-year-old, 85-kg (height = 5 ft 8 in) male with atrial fibrillation. His current serum creatinine is 1.9 mg/dL, and it has been stable over the last 7 days since admission. An intravenous digoxin loading dose of 500 μg was prescribed (given as doses of 250 μg, 125 μg, and 125 μg every 4 hours at 0800 H, 1200 H, and 1600 H, respectively). An oral maintenance dose of digoxin tablets 125 μg was given the next morning at 0800 H. Because the patient still had a rapid ventricular rate, a digoxin concentration was obtained at 1600 H and equaled 0.9 ng/mL. Recommend a stat intravenous digoxin dose to be given at 2300 H which will achieve a digoxin serum concentration of 1.5 μg and an oral maintenance dose which will provide a steady-state concentration of the same level.

1. *Enter the patient's demographic, drug dosing, and serum concentration/time data into the computer program.*

2. *Compute pharmacokinetic parameters for the patient using Bayesian pharmacokinetic computer program.*

The pharmacokinetic parameters computed by the program are a clearance equal to 4.8 L/h, a volume of distribution of 390 L, and a half-life equal to 57 h.

3. *Compute dose required to achieve the desired digoxin serum concentration.*

The stat intravenous digoxin dose will be calculated using the volume of distribution supplied by the computer program. The booster dose (BD) which will change serum concentrations by the desired amount is $BD = [V(\Delta C)]/F$, where V is the volume of distribution in L, ΔC is the necessary change in digoxin serum concentration in μg/L, and F is the bioavailability for the dosage form.

$$BD = [V(\Delta C)]/F = [390\ L\ (1.5\ \mu g/L - 0.9\ \mu g/L)]/1 = 234\ \mu g, \text{rounded to } 250\ \mu g \text{ intravenously stat}$$

The one-compartment model intravenous infusion equations used by the program to compute doses indicates that a digoxin tablet dose of 273 μg/d will produce a steady-state concentration of 1.5 ng/mL. This dose would be rounded to 250 μg/d of digoxin tablets and would be started at 0800 H the next morning.

DOSING STRATEGIES

Initial dose and dosage adjustment techniques using serum concentrations can be used in any combination as long as the limitations of each method are observed. Some dosing schemes link together logically when considered according to their basic approaches or philosophies. Dosage strategies that follow similar pathways are given in Table 6-5.

TABLE 6-5   Dosing Strategies

Dosing Approach/Philosophy	Initial Dosing	Use of Serum Concentrations to Alter Doses
Pharmacokinetic parameters/equations	Pharmacokinetic Dosing or Jelliffe method	Pharmacokinetic Parameter or Linear Pharmacokinetics method
Nomograms/Concepts	Nomograms	Linear Pharmacokinetics method
Computerized	Bayesian computer program	Bayesian computer program

SPECIAL DOSING CONSIDERATIONS

Use of Digoxin Immune FAB in Digoxin Overdoses

Digoxin immune FAB (DigiFab) are digoxin antibody molecule segments that bind and neutralize digoxin which can be used in digoxin overdose situations.[94,95] The antibody fragments are derived from antidigoxin antibodies formed in sheep. Improvements in digoxin adverse effects can be seen within 30 minutes of digoxin immune FAB administration. Digoxin serum concentrations are not useful after DigiFab has been given to a patient because pharmacologically inactive digoxin bound to the antibody segments will be measured and produce falsely high results. The elimination half-life for DigiFab is 15-20 hours in patients with normal renal function, and it is eliminated by the kidney. The half-life of DigiFab is not known in patients with impaired renal function, but is assumed to be prolonged as much as 10-fold.[96] In functionally anephric patients, the FAB fragment-digoxin complex may not be readily cleared from the body, so these patients should be closely monitored in the event digoxin dissociates from the FAB fragment and re-intoxication occurs.

Because DigiFab is a foreign protein, allergic reactions can occur including anaphylactic shock, so patient blood pressure, temperature, and other signs and symptoms of allergy (urticaria, erythema, pruritus, bronchospasm, tachycardia, angioedema, etc) should be closely monitored. Should an anaphylactic reaction occur, appropriate medical care should be initiated immediately.[97] Additionally, the electrocardiogram and serum potassium concentration should be closely followed for patients receiving this agent. Initially, patients may be hyperkalemic due to digoxin-induced displacement of intracellular potassium. However, hypokalemia can occur rapidly as the FAB fragments bind digoxin. As a result, repeated measurements of serum potassium are necessary, especially after the first few hours of DigiFab. Because the pharmacologic effects of digoxin will be lost, heart failure may worsen or a rapid ventricular rate may develop in patients treated for atrial fibrillation. Readministration of DigiFab may be necessary if digoxin adverse effects have not abated several hours after administration of the antibody fragments or if adverse effects recur. When patients do not respond to DigiFab, clinicians should consider the possibility that the patient is not digoxin toxic and seek other etiologies for the patient's clinical symptomatology.

If a digoxin serum concentration or an estimate of the number of tablets ingested is not available, 20 vials of DigiFab are usually adequate to treat most life-threatening acute overdoses in children and adults. Signs and symptoms of volume overload should be closely monitored for in young children receiving therapy with DigiFab. In less emergent situations, 10 vials may be initially given, patient response monitored, and an additional 10 vials administered, if necessary. This method of administration results in a slower response time, but it may decrease the likelihood of a febrile reaction to DigiFab. To treat chronic digoxin overdoses, six vials are usually needed for adults and older children while one vial is usually adequate for children under the weight of 20 kg.[97]

If digoxin serum concentrations are available or a reasonable estimate for the number of digoxin tablets acutely ingested is available, the DigiFab dose should be computed using one of the two approaches outlined below.[97] Most clinical assays for digoxin are optimized for concentrations ≤5 ng/mL, so some additional assay error may occur with levels above that amount. The computations assume a volume of distribution of 5 L/kg. If it is possible to calculate a DigiFab dose using both of the following methods, it is recommended that the higher dose be administered to the patient.

Chronic Overdose or Acute Overdose 8-12 Hours After Ingestion

In these cases, a post-absorption, post-distribution digoxin concentration can be used to estimate the necessary dose of DigiFab for a patient using the following formula: DigiFab dose (in vials) = (Digoxin concentration in ng/mL) (Body weight in kg)/100.

EXAMPLE ▶▶▶

HY is a 72-year-old, 80-kg male (height = 5 ft 7 in) who has accidentally been taking twice his prescribed dose of digoxin tablets. The admitting digoxin serum concentration is 4.1 ng/mL. Compute an appropriate dose of DigiFab for this patient.

DigiFab dose (in vials) = (Digoxin concentration in ng/mL)(Body weight in kg)/100 = (4.1 ng/mL • 80 kg)/ 100 = 3.3 vials, rounded up to four vials.

Acute Overdose Where Number of Tablets is Known or Can Be Estimated

For this situation, digoxin total body stores are estimated using the number of tablets ingested corrected for dosage form bioavailability: TBS = F(# dosage units)(dosage form strength), where TBS is digoxin total body stores in mg, F is the bioavailability for the dosage form. (NOTE: The suggested bioavailability constant for digoxin in the DigiFab package insert is 0.8 for tablets—which allows for variability in the fraction of the dose that was absorbed), # dosage units is the number of tablets, and dosage form strength is in mg (example: 250 μg = 0.25 mg). Each vial of DigiFab will inactivate approximately 0.5 mg of digoxin, so the dose of DigiFab (in vials) can be calculated using the following equation:

DigiFab dose = TBS/(0.5 mg/vial), where TBS is digoxin total body stores in mg.

EXAMPLE ▶▶▶

DL is a 22-year-old, 85-kg male (height = 5 ft 9 in) who took approximately 50 digoxin tablets of 0.25 mg strength about 4 hours ago. Compute an appropriate dose of DigiFab for this patient.

TBS = F(# dosage units)(dosage form strength) = 0.8 (50 tablets • 0.25 mg/tablet) = 10 mg

DigiFab dose = TBS/(0.5 mg/vial) = 10 mg/(0.5 mg/vial) = 20 vials

---

Conversion of Patient Doses Between Dosage Forms

When patients are switched between digoxin dosage forms, differences in bioavailability should be accounted for within the limits of available oral dosage forms using the following equation: $D_{IV} = D_{PO} \bullet F$, where D_{IV} is the equivalent digoxin intravenous dose in μg, D_{PO} is the equivalent digoxin oral dose, and F is the bioavailability fraction appropriate for the oral dosage form (F = 0.7 for tablets, 0.8 for oral solution). Where possible, digoxin tablet doses should be rounded to the nearest 125 μg to avoid the necessity of breaking tablets in half.

Also, it is best to avoid mixing tablet dosage strengths so that patients do not become confused with multiple prescription vials and take the wrong dose of medication. For example, if it were necessary to prescribe 375 μg/d of digoxin tablets, it would be preferable to have the patient take three 125 μg tablets daily rather than 1½ 250 μg tablets daily or a 125 μg and 250 μg tablet each day.

EXAMPLE 1 ▶▶▶

YT is a 67-year-old, 60-kg male (height = 5 ft 5 in) with atrial fibrillation receiving 200 μg of intravenous digoxin daily which produces a steady-state digoxin concentration of 1.3 ng/mL. Compute an oral tablet dose that will maintain steady-state digoxin concentrations at approximately the same level.

1. *Convert the current digoxin dose to the equivalent amount for the new dosage form/route.*

$$D_{PO} = D_{IV}/F = 200\ \mu g/0.7 = 286\ \mu g \text{ digoxin tablets, rounded to } 250\ \mu g$$

2. *Estimate change in digoxin steady-state concentration due to rounding of dose.*

The oral tablet dose of 286 μg would have produced a steady-state concentration similar to the intravenous dose of 200 μg. However, the dose had to be rounded to a dose that could be given as a tablet. The expected digoxin steady-state concentration from the rounded dose would be proportional to the ratio of the rounded dose and the actual computed dose:

$$Css_{new} = Css_{old}\ (D_{rounded}/D_{computed}) = 1.3\ ng/mL\ (250\ \mu g/286\ \mu g) = 1.1\ ng/mL$$

where Css_{new} is the new expected digoxin steady-state concentration due to tablet administration in ng/mL, Css_{old} is the measured digoxin steady-state concentration due to intravenous administration in ng/mL, $D_{rounded}$ is the oral dose rounded to account for dosage form strengths in μg, and $D_{computed}$ is the exact oral dose computed during the intravenous to oral conversion calculation in μg. However, the steady-state digoxin concentration after the dosage form change may not be exactly the value calculated due to a variety of causes. Because of interindividual variations in digoxin bioavailability, the patient's actual bioavailability constant for oral tablets may be different than the average population bioavailability constant used to convert the dose. Also, there are day-to-day intrasubject variations in the rate and extent of digoxin absorption that will affect the actual steady-state digoxin concentration obtained while taking the drug orally. Finally, other oral drug therapy that did not influence digoxin pharmacokinetics when given intravenously may alter the expected digoxin concentration.

EXAMPLE 2 ▶▶▶

KL is an 82-year-old, 45-kg female (height = 4 ft 10 in) with heart failure receiving 125 μg of oral digoxin daily as tablets which produces a steady-state digoxin concentration of 1 ng/mL. Compute an intravenous dose that will maintain steady-state digoxin concentrations at approximately the same level.

1. *Convert the current digoxin dose to the equivalent amount for the new dosage form/route.*

$$D_{IV} = D_{PO} \bullet F = 125\ \mu g \bullet 0.7 = 87.5\ \mu g \text{ digoxin tablets, rounded to } 90\ \mu g$$

2. *Estimate the change in digoxin steady-state concentration due to rounding of dose.*

The intravenous dose of 87.5 μg would have produced a steady-state concentration similar to the oral tablet dose of 125 μg. However, the dose was rounded to an amount that could be reasonably measured in a syringe. The expected digoxin steady-state concentration from the rounded dose would be proportional to the ratio of the rounded dose and the actual computed dose:

$$Css_{new} = Css_{old} (D_{rounded}/D_{computed}) = 1 \text{ ng/mL } (90 \text{ µg}/87.5 \text{ µg}) = 1 \text{ ng/mL}$$

where Css_{new} is the new expected digoxin steady-state concentration due to intravenous administration in ng/mL, Css_{old} is the measured digoxin steady-state concentration due to oral tablet administration in ng/mL, $D_{rounded}$ is the intravenous dose rounded to allow accurate dosage measurement in µg, and $D_{computed}$ is the exact intravenous dose computed during the intravenous to oral conversion calculation in µg. Since the rounded intravenous digoxin dose is so close to the exact dose needed, steady-state digoxin concentrations are not expected to change appreciably. However, the steady-state digoxin concentration after the dosage form change may not be exactly the value calculated due to a variety of causes. Because of interindividual variations in digoxin bioavailability, the patient's actual bioavailability constant for oral tablets may be different than the average population bioavailability constant used to convert the dose. Also, there are day-to-day intrasubject variations in the rate and extent of digoxin absorption that will affect the steady-state digoxin concentration obtained while taking the drug orally that will not be present when the drug is given intravenously. Finally, other oral drug therapy that influenced digoxin pharmacokinetics when given orally, but not intravenously, may alter the expected digoxin concentration.

Use of Digoxin Booster Doses to Immediately Increase Serum Concentrations

If a patient has a subtherapeutic digoxin serum concentration in an acute situation, it may be desirable to increase the digoxin concentration as quickly as possible. A rational way to increase the serum concentrations rapidly is to administer a booster dose of digoxin, a process also known as "reloading" the patient with digoxin, computed using pharmacokinetic techniques. A modified loading dose equation is used to accomplish computation of the booster dose (BD), which takes into account the current digoxin concentration present in the patient: $BD = [(C_{desired} - C_{actual}) V]/F$, where $C_{desired}$ is the desired digoxin concentration, C_{actual} is the actual current digoxin concentration for the patient, F is the bioavailability fraction of the digoxin dosage form, and V is the volume of distribution for digoxin. If the volume of distribution for digoxin is known for the patient, it can be used in the calculation. However, this value is not usually known and is assumed to equal the population average for the patient.

Concurrent with the administration of the booster dose, the maintenance dose of digoxin is usually increased. Clinicians need to recognize that the administration of a booster dose does not alter the time required to achieve steady-state conditions when a new digoxin dosage rate is prescribed. It still requires a sufficient time period to attain steady-state when the dosage rate is changed. However, usually the difference between the post-booster dose digoxin concentration and the ultimate steady-state concentration has been reduced by giving the extra dose of drug.

EXAMPLE 1 ▶ ▶ ▶

BN is a 52-year-old, 85-kg (height = 6 ft 2 in) male with atrial fibrillation who is receiving therapy with intravenous digoxin. He has normal liver and renal function. After receiving an initial loading dose of digoxin (1000 µg) and a maintenance dose of 250 µg/d of digoxin for 5 days, his digoxin concentration is measured at 0.6 ng/mL immediately after pulse rate increased to 200 beats/min. Compute a booster dose of digoxin to achieve a digoxin concentration equal to 1.5 ng/mL.

1. *Estimate the volume of distribution according to the disease states and conditions present in the patient.*

   In the case of digoxin, the population average volume of distribution equals 7 L/kg and this will be used to estimate the parameter for the patient. The patient is nonobese, so his actual body weight will be used in the computation: V = 7 L/kg • 85 kg = 595 L.

2. *Compute booster dose.*
The booster dose is computed using the following equation: BD = [(C$_{desired}$ – C$_{actual}$)V]/F = [(1.5 µg/L – 0.6 µg/L) 595 L]/1 = 536 µg, rounded to 500 µg of digoxin. (Note: ng/mL = µg/L and this concentration unit was substituted for Css in the calculations so that unnecessary unit conversion was not required). This booster dose could be split into two equal doses and given 4-6 hours apart with appropriate monitoring to avoid adverse side effects. If the maintenance dose was also increased, it will take additional time for new steady-state conditions to be achieved. Digoxin serum concentrations should be measured at this time.

PROBLEMS

The following problems are intended to emphasize the computation of initial and individualized doses using clinical pharmacokinetic techniques. Clinicians should always consult the patient's chart to confirm that other drug therapy is appropriate for current disease state signs and symptoms. Also, it should be confirmed that the patient is receiving other appropriate concurrent therapy, when necessary, to treat the cardiovascular condition.

1. UV is a 75-year-old, 62-kg (height = 5 ft 9 in) male with atrial fibrillation. His current serum creatinine is 1.3 mg/dL, and it has been stable since admission. Compute an intravenous loading and maintenance digoxin dose for this patient to provide a steady-state concentration of 1.5 ng/mL or digoxin total body store equal to 15 µg/kg.
2. Patient UV (see problem 1) was prescribed digoxin 200 µg/d intravenously, and this dose has been given for 2 weeks. A steady-state digoxin concentration was 2.4 ng/mL. Compute a revised digoxin dose for this patient to provide a steady-state concentration of 1.5 ng/mL.
3. Patient UV (see problems 1 and 2) had a dosage change to digoxin 125 µg/d intravenously which produced a steady-state concentration equal to 1.4 ng/mL. Compute an oral tablet digoxin dose for this patient that will provide about the same steady-state drug concentration as that found during intravenous therapy.
4. SD is a 35-year-old, 75-kg (height = 5 ft 7 in) female with NYHA Class IV heart failure secondary to viral cardiomyopathy. Her current serum creatinine is 3.7 mg/dL, and it has been stable since admission. Compute oral digoxin loading and maintenance doses using tablets for this patient to provide a steady-state concentration of 1 ng/mL.
5. Patient SD (see problem 4) was prescribed digoxin 187.5 µg/d orally as tablets. A steady-state digoxin concentration was obtained and equaled 0.7 ng/mL. Compute a revised digoxin dose for this patient using oral tablets to provide a steady-state concentration of 1 ng/mL.
6. Patient SD (see problems 4 and 5) had a dosage change to digoxin 250 µg/d orally as tablets which produced a steady-state concentration equal to 1.2 ng/mL. Compute an intravenous digoxin dose for this patient that will provide about the same steady-state drug concentration as that found during oral tablet therapy.
7. BN is a 55-year-old, 140-kg (height = 5 ft 8 in) male with atrial fibrillation. His current serum creatinine is 0.9 mg/dL, and it has been stable since admission. Compute an intravenous loading dose and oral tablet maintenance dose of digoxin for this patient to provide a steady-state concentration of 1.2 ng/mL.
8. Patient BN (see problem 7) was prescribed digoxin tablets 500 µg/d. A steady-state digoxin concentration was obtained and was 2.4 ng/mL. Compute a revised digoxin tablet dose for this patient to provide a steady-state concentration of 1.5 ng/mL.
9. VG is a 75-year-old, 180-kg (height = 5 ft 2 in) female with NYHA Class III heart failure. Her current serum creatinine is 6 mg/dL and is stable. Compute digoxin oral tablet loading and maintenance doses for this patient to provide a steady-state concentration of 1 ng/mL.
10. Patient VG (see problem 9) was prescribed digoxin tablets 125 µg every other day. A steady-state digoxin concentration was obtained and was 0.5 ng/mL. Compute a revised digoxin tablet dose for this patient to provide a steady-state concentration of 1 ng/mL.

11. QW is a 34-year-old, 50-kg (height = 5 ft 4 in) female with atrial fibrillation secondary to hyperthyroidism. Her current serum creatinine is 0.8 mg/dL and stable. Compute a digoxin intravenous loading dose and oral tablet maintenance dose for this patient to provide a steady-state concentration of 1.2 ng/mL.

12. RT is a 68-year-old, 88-kg (height = 5 ft 11 in) male with NYHA Class II heart failure. His current serum creatinine is 2.3 mg/dL and is stable. Digoxin therapy was initiated, and after the third oral dose of digoxin tablets 250 µg/d, a digoxin serum concentration was obtained according to the following schedule:

Time	Digoxin Dose/Concentration
Day 1/0800 H	250 µg
Day 2/0800 H	250 µg
Day 3/0800 H	250 µg
Day 4/0730 H	C = 1 ng/mL

Calculate a digoxin tablet dose that will provide a steady-state digoxin concentration equal to 0.8 ng/mL.

13. LK is a 72-year-old, 68-kg (height = 5 ft 1 in) female with NYHA Class III heart failure. Her current serum creatinine is 2.9 mg/dL and is stable. Digoxin therapy was initiated, and after an intravenous loading dose of 500 µg plus two intravenous doses of digoxin 125 µg/d, a digoxin serum concentration was obtained according to the following schedule:

Time	Digoxin Dose/Concentration
Day 1/0800 H	250 µg
Day 1/1200 H	125 µg
Day 1/1600 H	125 µg
Day 2/0800 H	125 µg
Day 3/0800 H	125 µg
Day 4/0730 H	C = 2 ng/mL

Calculate a digoxin tablet dose that will provide a steady-state digoxin concentration equal to 1 ng/mL.

14. BH is a 61-year-old, 91-kg (height = 6 ft 1 in) male with atrial fibrillation. His current serum creatinine is 1.9 mg/dL and is stable. Digoxin therapy was initiated, and after an intravenous loading dose of 1000 µg plus three oral doses of digoxin tablets 125 µg/d, a digoxin serum concentration was obtained according to the following schedule:

Time	Digoxin Dose/Concentration
Day 1/0800 H	500 µg IV
Day 1/1200 H	250 µg IV
Day 1/1600 H	250 µg IV
Day 2/0800 H	125 µg tablet
Day 3/0800 H	125 µg tablet
Day 4/0800 H	125 µg tablet
Day 5/0730 H	C = 0.9 ng/mL

Calculate a digoxin tablet dose that will provide a steady-state digoxin concentration equal to 1.5 ng/mL.

ANSWERS TO PROBLEMS

1. *Answer to problem 1.* The initial digoxin doses for patient UV would be calculated as follows:

Pharmacokinetic Dosing Method

1. *Estimate creatinine clearance.*

    This patient has a stable serum creatinine and is not obese. The Cockcroft-Gault equation can be used to estimate creatinine clearance:

$$\text{CrCl}_{est} = [(140 - \text{age}) \text{ BW}]/(72 \bullet S_{Cr}) = [(140 - 75 \text{ y}) 62 \text{ kg}]/(72 \bullet 1.3 \text{ mg/dL})$$
$$\text{CrCl}_{est} = 43 \text{ mL/min}$$

2. *Estimate clearance.*

    The drug clearance versus creatinine clearance relationship is used to estimate the digoxin clearance for this patient (Cl_{NR} = 40 mL/min since the patient does not have moderate-severe heart failure):

$$Cl = 1.303 \text{ (CrCl)} + Cl_{NR} = 1.303 \text{ (43 mL/min)} + 40 \text{ mL/min} = 96 \text{ mL/min}$$

3. *Use average steady-state concentration equation to compute digoxin maintenance dose.*

    For a patient with atrial fibrillation, the desired digoxin concentration would be 0.8-1.5 ng/mL. A serum concentration equal to 1.5 ng/mL was chosen for this patient, and intravenous digoxin will be used (F = 1). Note that for concentration units ng/mL = μg/L, and this conversion will be made before the equation is used. Also, conversion factors are needed to change milliliter units to liter (1000 mL/L) and minute units to days (1440 min/d).

$$D/\tau = (\text{Css} \bullet Cl)/F = (1.5 \text{ μg/L} \bullet 96 \text{ mL/min} \bullet 1440 \text{ min/d})/(1 \bullet 1000 \text{ mL/L}) = 208 \text{ μg/d,}$$
rounded to 200 μg/d

4. *Use loading dose equation to compute digoxin loading dose (if needed).*

    The patient has moderate renal function and is nonobese. Therefore, a volume of distribution equal to 7 L/kg and actual body weight can be used to compute the digoxin loading dose. An intravenous loading dose (F = 1) could be given in this patient to achieve the desired pharmacologic effect quicker than would occur if maintenance doses alone were used and concentrations allowed to accumulate over 3-5 half-lives.

$$V = 7 \text{ L/kg} \bullet 62 \text{ kg} = 434 \text{ L}$$
$$\text{LD} = (\text{Css} \bullet V)/F = (1.5 \text{ μg/L} \bullet 434 \text{ L})/1 = 651 \text{ μg rounded to 600 μg}$$

    When digoxin loading doses are administered, they are usually given in divided doses separated by 4-6 hours (50% of dose at first, followed by two additional doses of 25%). In this case, an initial intravenous dose of 300 μg would be given initially, followed by two additional intravenous doses of 150 μg each. One of the loading doses could be withheld if pulse rate was less than 50-60 beats/min or other undesirable digoxin adverse effects were noted.

Jelliffe Method

1. *Estimate creatinine clearance.*

    This patient has a stable serum creatinine and is not obese. The Cockcroft-Gault equation can be used to estimate creatinine clearance:

$$\text{CrCl}_{est} = [(140 - \text{age}) \text{ BW}]/(72 \bullet S_{Cr}) = [(140 - 75 \text{ y}) 62 \text{ kg}]/(72 \bullet 1.3 \text{ mg/dL}) = 43 \text{ mL/min}$$

2. *Estimate total body store (TBS) and maintenance dose (D).*

The patient has moderate renal function and is nonobese. Digoxin total body stores of 13-15 µg/kg are effective in the treatment of atrial fibrillation. A digoxin dose of 15 µg/kg was chosen for this patient.

$$TBS = 15 \text{ µg/kg} \bullet 62 \text{ kg} = 930 \text{ µg}$$

$$D = \{TBS \bullet [14\% + 0.20 \, (CrCl)]\}/(F \bullet 100) = \{930 \text{ µg} \bullet [14\% + 0.20 \, (43 \text{ mL/min})]\}/$$
$$(1 \bullet 100) = 210 \text{ µg/d, rounded to 200 µg/d}$$

3. *Use loading dose equation to compute digoxin loading dose (if needed).*

Digoxin total body store is used to calculate the loading dose after correcting for bioavailability:

$$LD = TBS/F = 930 \text{ µg/1} = 930 \text{ µg, rounded to 1000 µg}$$

When digoxin loading doses are administered, they are usually given in divided doses separated by 4-6 hours (50% of dose at first, followed by two additional doses of 25%). In this case, an initial intravenous dose of 500 µg would be given initially, followed by two additional intravenous doses of 250 µg each. One of the loading doses could be withheld if pulse rate was less than 50-60 beats/min or other undesirable digoxin adverse effects were noted.

2. *Answer to problem 2.* The revised digoxin dose for patient UV would be calculated as follows:

Linear Pharmacokinetics Method

1. *Estimate creatinine clearance.*

This patient has a stable serum creatinine and is not obese. The Cockcroft-Gault equation can be used to estimate creatinine clearance:

$$CrCl_{est} = [(140 - age) \, BW]/(72 \bullet S_{Cr}) = [(140 - 75 \text{ y}) \, 62 \text{ kg}]/(72 \bullet 1.3 \text{ mg/dL})$$
$$CrCl_{est} = 43 \text{ mL/min}$$

The patient has moderate renal function and would be expected to have achieved steady-state after 14 days of treatment.

2. *Compute new dose to achieve the desired serum concentration.*

Using linear pharmacokinetics, the new dose to attain the desired concentration should be proportional to the old dose that produced the measured concentration:

$$D_{new} = (C_{ss,new}/C_{ss,old}) \, D_{old} = (1.5 \text{ ng/mL}/2.4 \text{ ng/mL}) \, 200 \text{ µg/d} = 125 \text{ µg/d}$$

The new dose would be 125 µg/d given as intravenous digoxin to be started at next scheduled dosing time.

Pharmacokinetic Parameter Method

1. *Estimate creatinine clearance.*

This patient has a stable serum creatinine and is not obese. The Cockcroft-Gault equation can be used to estimate creatinine clearance:

$$CrCl_{est} = [(140 - age) \, BW]/(72 \bullet S_{Cr}) = [(140 - 75 \text{ y}) \, 62 \text{ kg}]/(72 \bullet 1.3 \text{ mg/dL})$$
$$CrCl_{est} = 43 \text{ mL/min}$$

The patient has good renal function and would be expected to have achieved steady-state after 14 days of treatment.

2. *Compute drug clearance.*

Note that digoxin concentrations in ng/mL are the same as those for μg/L. This unit substitution will be directly made to avoid conversion factors in the computation.

$$Cl = [F(D/\tau)]/Css = [1(200\ \mu g/d)]/2.4\ \mu g/L = 83\ L/d$$

3. *Compute new dose to achieve the desired serum concentration.*

The average steady-state equation is used to compute the new digoxin dose.

$$D/\tau = (Css \bullet Cl)/F = (1.5\ \mu g/L \bullet 83\ L/d)/1 = 125\ \mu g/d$$

The new suggested dose would be 125 μg/d given as digoxin tablets to be started at next scheduled dosing time.

3. *Answer to problem 3.* An equivalent oral dose for patient UV would be computed as follows:

1. *Convert the current digoxin dose to the equivalent amount for the new dosage form/route.*

$$D_{PO} = D_{IV}/F = 125\ \mu g/0.7 = 179\ \mu g\ \text{digoxin tablets, rounded to } 187.5\ \mu g\ (1\frac{1}{2}\ 125\ \mu g\ \text{tablets})$$

2. *Estimate the change in digoxin steady-state concentration due to rounding of dose.*

The oral tablet dose of 179 μg would have produced a steady-state concentration similar to the intravenous dose of 125 μg. However, the dose had to be rounded to a dose that could be given as tablets. The expected digoxin steady-state concentration from the rounded dose would be proportional to the ratio of the rounded dose and the actual computed dose:

$$Css_{new} = Css_{old}(D_{rounded}/D_{computed}) = 1.4\ ng/mL(187.5\ \mu g/179\ \mu g) = 1.5\ ng/mL$$

4. *Answer to problem 4.* The initial digoxin doses for patient SD would be calculated as follows:

Pharmacokinetic Dosing Method

1. *Estimate creatinine clearance.*

This patient has a stable serum creatinine and is not obese. The Cockcroft-Gault equation can be used to estimate creatinine clearance:

$$CrCl_{est} = \{[(140 - age)BW]/(72 \bullet S_{Cr})\}0.85 = \{[(140 - 35\ y)75\ kg]/(72 \bullet 3.7\ mg/dL)\}0.85$$
$$CrCl_{est} = 25\ mL/min$$

2. *Estimate clearance.*

The drug clearance versus creatinine clearance relationship is used to estimate the digoxin clearance for this patient ($Cl_{NR} = 20$ mL/min since the patient has moderate-severe heart failure):

$$Cl = 1.303\ (CrCl) + Cl_{NR} = 1.303(25\ mL/min) + 20\ mL/min = 53\ mL/min$$

3. *Use average steady-state concentration equation to compute digoxin maintenance dose.*

For a patient with heart failure, the desired digoxin concentration would be 0.5-1 ng/mL. A serum concentration equal to 1 ng/mL was chosen for this patient, and oral digoxin will be used (F = 0.7). Note that for concentration units ng/mL = μg/L, and this conversion will be made before the equation is used. Also, conversion factors are needed to change milliliter units to liter (1000 mL/L) and minute units to days (1440 min/d).

$$D/\tau = (Css \bullet Cl)/F = (1\ \mu g/L \bullet 53\ mL/min \bullet 1440\ min/d)/(0.7 \bullet 1000\ mL/L) = 108\ \mu g/d,$$
rounded to 125 μg/d

4. *Use loading dose equation to compute digoxin loading dose (if needed).*

The patient has poor renal function. Therefore, the volume of distribution equation that adjusts the parameter estimate for renal dysfunction can be used to compute the digoxin loading dose. An oral loading dose (F = 0.7) could be given in this patient to achieve the desired pharmacologic effect quicker than would occur if maintenance doses alone were used to allow concentrations to accumulate over 3-5 half-lives.

$$V = \left(226 + \frac{298 \cdot CrCl}{29.1 + CrCl}\right)(Wt/70) = \left(226 + \frac{298 \cdot 25 \text{ mL/min}}{29.1 + 25 \text{ mL/min}}\right)(75 \text{ kg}/70) = 390 \text{ L}$$

$$LD = (Css \cdot V)/F = (1 \text{ μg/L} \cdot 390 \text{ L})/0.7 = 557 \text{ μg, rounded to } 500 \text{ μg}$$

When digoxin loading doses are administered, they are usually given in divided doses separated by 4-6 hours (50% of dose at first, followed by two additional doses of 25%). In this case, an initial oral dose of 250 μg would be given initially, followed by two additional intravenous doses of 125 μg each. One of the loading doses could be withheld if pulse rate was less than 50-60 beats/min or other undesirable digoxin adverse effects were noted.

Jelliffe Method

1. *Estimate creatinine clearance.*

This patient has a stable serum creatinine and is not obese. The Cockcroft-Gault equation can be used to estimate creatinine clearance:

$$CrCl_{est} = \{[(140 - age)BW]/(72 \cdot S_{Cr})\}0.85 = \{[(140 - 35 \text{ y})75 \text{ kg}]/(72 \cdot 3.7 \text{ mg/dL})\}0.85$$

$$CrCl_{est} = 25 \text{ mL/min}$$

2. *Estimate total body store (TBS) and maintenance dose (D).*

The patient has poor renal function and is nonobese. Digoxin total body stores of 6-10 μg/kg are effective in the treatment of heart failure in patients with poor renal function. A digoxin dose of 8 μg/kg was chosen for this patient.

$$TBS = 8 \text{ μg/kg} \cdot 75 \text{ kg} = 600 \text{ μg}$$

$$D = \{TBS \cdot [14\% + 0.20(CrCl)]\}/(F \cdot 100) = \{600 \text{ μg} \cdot [14\% + 0.20(25 \text{ mL/min})]\}/$$
$$(0.7 \cdot 100) = 163 \text{ μg/d, rounded to } 187.5 \text{ μg/d}$$

3. *Use loading dose equation to compute digoxin loading dose (if needed).*

Digoxin total body store is used to calculate the loading dose after correcting for bioavailability:

$$LD = TBS/F = 600 \text{ μg}/0.7 = 857 \text{ μg, rounded to } 750 \text{ μg}$$

When digoxin loading doses are administered, they are usually given in divided doses separated by 4-6 hours (50% of dose at first, followed by two additional doses of 25%). In this case, an initial oral dose of 375 μg would be given initially, followed by two additional intravenous doses of 187.5 μg each. One of the loading doses could be withheld if pulse rate was less than 50-60 beats/min or other undesirable digoxin adverse effects were noted.

5. *Answer to problem 5.* The revised digoxin dose for patient SD would be calculated as follows:

Linear Pharmacokinetics Method

1. *Estimate creatinine clearance.*

This patient has a stable serum creatinine and is not obese. The Cockcroft-Gault equation can be used to estimate creatinine clearance:

$$CrCl_{est} = \{[(140 - age)BW]/(72 \cdot S_{Cr})\}0.85 = \{[(140 - 35 \text{ y})75 \text{ kg}]/(72 \cdot 3.7 \text{ mg/dL})\}0.85$$

$$CrCl_{est} = 25 \text{ mL/min}$$

The patient has poor renal function and would be expected to have achieved steady-state after 14 days of treatment.

2. *Compute new dose to achieve the desired serum concentration.*

Using linear pharmacokinetics, the new dose to attain the desired concentration should be proportional to the old dose that produced the measured concentration:

$$D_{new} = (C_{ss,new}/C_{ss,old})D_{old} = (1 \text{ ng/mL}/0.7 \text{ ng/mL}) \ 187.5 \ \mu g/d = 268 \ \mu g/d, \text{ rounded to } 250 \ \mu g/d$$

The new dose would be 250 μg/d given as oral digoxin tablets to be started at next scheduled dosing time.

Pharmacokinetic Parameter Method

1. *Estimate creatinine clearance.*

This patient has a stable serum creatinine and is not obese. The Cockcroft-Gault equation can be used to estimate creatinine clearance:

$$CrCl_{est} = \{[(140 - age)BW]/(72 \bullet S_{Cr})\}0.85 = \{[(140 - 35 \text{ y})75 \text{ kg}]/(72 \bullet 3.7 \text{ mg/dL})\}0.85$$
$$CrCl_{est} = 25 \text{ mL/min}$$

The patient has good renal function and would be expected to have achieved steady-state after 14 days of treatment.

2. *Compute drug clearance.*

Note that digoxin concentrations in ng/mL are the same as those for μg/L. This unit substitution will be directly made to avoid conversion factors in the computation.

$$Cl = [F(D/\tau)]/Css = [0.7(187.5 \ \mu g/d)]/0.7 \ \mu g/L = 188 \text{ L/d}$$

3. *Compute new dose to achieve the desired serum concentration.*

The average steady-state equation is used to compute the new digoxin dose.

$$D/\tau = (Css \bullet Cl)/F = (1 \ \mu g/L \bullet 188 \text{ L/d})/0.7 = 268 \ \mu g/d, \text{ rounded to } 250 \ \mu g/d$$

The new suggested dose would be 250 μg/d given as digoxin tablets to be started at next scheduled dosing time.

6. *Answer to problem 6.* An equivalent oral dose for patient SD would be computed as follows:

1. *Convert current digoxin dose to the equivalent amount for the new dosage form/route.*

$$D_{IV} = D_{PO} \bullet F = 250 \ \mu g/d \bullet 0.7 = 175 \ \mu g/d \text{ intravenous digoxin}$$

2. *Estimate change in digoxin steady-state concentration due to rounding of dose.*

This step is not necessary since the actual equivalent intravenous dose could be given without rounding.

7. *Answer to problem 7.* The initial digoxin doses for patient BN would be calculated as follows:

Pharmacokinetic Dosing Method

1. *Estimate creatinine clearance.*

This patient has a stable serum creatinine and is obese (IBW_{males} (in kg) = 50 + 2.3(Ht − 60) = 50 + 2.3(68 in − 60) = 68.4 kg). The Salazar and Corcoran equation can be used to estimate creatinine clearance:

$$CrCl_{est(males)} = \frac{(137 - age)[(0.285 \bullet Wt) + (12.1 \bullet Ht^2)]}{(51 \bullet S_{Cr})}$$

$$CrCl_{est(males)} = \frac{(137 - 55\ y)\{[0.285 \bullet 140\ kg] + [12.1 \bullet (1.73\ m)^2]\}}{(51 \bullet 0.9\ mg/dL)} = 136\ mL/min$$

Note: Height is converted from inches to meters: Ht = (68 in • 2.54 cm/in)/(100 cm/m) = 1.73 m.

2. *Estimate clearance.*

The drug clearance versus creatinine clearance relationship is used to estimate the digoxin clearance for this patient (Cl_{NR} = 40 mL/min since the patient does not have moderate-severe heart failure):

$$Cl = 1.303\ (CrCl) + Cl_{NR} = 1.303(136\ mL/min) + 40\ mL/min = 217\ mL/min$$

3. *Use average steady-state concentration equation to compute digoxin maintenance dose.*

For a patient with atrial fibrillation, the desired digoxin concentration would be 0.8-1.5 ng/mL. A serum concentration equal to 1.2 ng/mL was chosen for this patient, and oral digoxin tablets will be used (F = 0.7). Note that for concentration units ng/mL = μg/L, and this conversion will be made before the equation is used. Also, conversion factors are needed to change milliliter units to liter (1000 mL/L) and minute units to days (1440 min/d).

$$D/\tau = (Css \bullet Cl)/F = (1.2\ μg/L \bullet 217\ mL/min \bullet 1440\ min/d)/(0.7 \bullet 1000\ mL/L) = 535\ μg/d,$$
rounded to 500 μg/d

4. *Use loading dose equation to compute digoxin loading dose (if needed).*

The patient has good renal function and is obese. Therefore, a volume of distribution equal to 7 L/kg and ideal body weight can be used to compute the digoxin loading dose. An intravenous loading dose (F = 1) could be given in this patient to achieve the desired pharmacologic effect quicker than would occur if maintenance doses alone were used and concentrations allowed to accumulate over 3-5 half-lives.

$$V = 7\ L/kg \bullet 68.4\ kg = 479\ L$$
$$LD = (Css \bullet V)/F = (1.2\ μg/L \bullet 479\ L)/1 = 575\ μg\ rounded\ to\ 600\ μg$$

When digoxin loading doses are administered, they are usually given in divided doses separated by 4-6 hours (50% of dose at first, followed by two additional doses of 25%). In this case, an initial intravenous dose of 300 μg would be given initially, followed by two additional intravenous doses of 150 μg each. One of the loading doses could be withheld if pulse rate was less than 50-60 beats/min or other undesirable digoxin adverse effects were noted.

Jelliffe Method

1. *Estimate creatinine clearance.*

This patient has a stable serum creatinine and is obese [IBW_{males} (in kg) = 50 + 2.3(Ht − 60) = 50 + 2.3(68" − 60) = 68.4 kg]. The Salazar and Corcoran equation can be used to estimate creatinine clearance:

$$CrCl_{est(males)} = \frac{(137 - age)[(0.285 \bullet Wt) + (12.1 \bullet Ht^2)]}{(51 \bullet S_{Cr})}$$

$$CrCl_{est(males)} = \frac{(137 - 55\ y)\{[0.285 \bullet 140\ kg] + [12.1 \bullet (1.73\ m)^2]\}}{(51 \bullet 0.9\ mg/dL)} = 136\ mL/min$$

Note: Height is converted from inches to meters: Ht = (68 in • 2.54 cm/in)/(100 cm/m) = 1.73 m.

2. *Estimate total body store (TBS) and maintenance dose (D).*

The patient has moderate renal function and is obese. Digoxin total body stores of 13-15 µg/kg are effective in the treatment of atrial fibrillation. A digoxin dose of 14 µg/kg was chosen for this patient, and ideal body weight will be used to compute doses. Digoxin tablets will be used as the dosage form for maintenance doses.

$$TBS = 14 \ \mu g/kg \bullet 68.4 \ kg = 958 \ \mu g$$

$$D = \{TBS \bullet [14\% + 0.20(CrCl)]\}/(F \bullet 100) = \{958 \ \mu g \bullet [14\% + 0.20(136 \ mL/min)]\}/(0.7 \bullet 100) = 563 \ \mu g/d, \text{ rounded to } 500 \ \mu g/d$$

3. *Use loading dose equation to compute digoxin loading dose (if needed).*

Digoxin total body store is used to calculate the loading dose after correcting for bioavailability:

$$LD = TBS/F = 958 \ \mu g/1 = 958 \ \mu g, \text{ rounded to } 1000 \ \mu g$$

When digoxin loading doses are administered, they are usually given in divided doses separated by 4-6 hours (50% of dose at first, followed by two additional doses of 25%). In this case, an initial intravenous dose of 500 µg would be given initially, followed by two additional intravenous doses of 250 µg each. One of the loading doses could be withheld if pulse rate was less than 50-60 beats/min or other undesirable digoxin adverse effects were noted.

8. *Answer to problem 8.* The revised digoxin dose for patient BN would be calculated as follows:

Linear Pharmacokinetics Method

1. *Estimate creatinine clearance.*

This patient has a stable serum creatinine and is obese [IBW_{males} (in kg) = 50 + 2.3(Ht − 60) = 50 + 2.3(68 in − 60) = 68.4 kg]. The Salazar and Corcoran equation can be used to estimate creatinine clearance:

$$CrCl_{est(males)} = \frac{(137 - age)[(0.285 \bullet Wt) + (12.1 \bullet Ht^2)]}{(51 \bullet S_{Cr})}$$

$$CrCl_{est(males)} = \frac{(137 - 55 \ y)\{[0.285 \bullet 140 \ kg] + [12.1 \bullet (1.73 \ m)^2]\}}{(51 \bullet 0.9 \ mg/dL)} = 136 \ mL/min$$

Note: Height is converted from inches to meters: Ht = (68 in • 2.54 cm/in)/(100 cm/m) = 1.73 m.

The patient has moderate renal function and would be expected to have achieved steady-state after 7 days of treatment.

1. *Compute new dose to achieve the desired serum concentration.*

Using linear pharmacokinetics, the new dose to attain the desired concentration should be proportional to the old dose that produced the measured concentration:

$$D_{new} = (C_{ss,new}/C_{ss,old})D_{old} = (1.5 \ ng/mL/2.4 \ ng/mL) \ 500 \ \mu g/d = 313 \ \mu g/d, \text{ rounded to } 375 \ \mu g/d$$

The new dose would be 375 µg/d given as digoxin tablets to be started at next scheduled dosing time. If desired, a one daily dose could be withheld to allow the digoxin concentration to decline, and the new dose started the following day.

Pharmacokinetic Parameter Method

1. *Estimate creatinine clearance.*

This patient has a stable serum creatinine and is obese [IBW$_{males}$ (in kg) = 50 + 2.3(Ht − 60) = 50 + 2.3(68" − 60) = 68.4 kg]. The Salazar and Corcoran equation can be used to estimate creatinine clearance:

$$CrCl_{est(males)} = \frac{(137 - age)[(0.285 \bullet Wt) + (12.1 \bullet Ht^2)]}{(51 \bullet S_{Cr})}$$

$$CrCl_{est(males)} = \frac{(137 - 55\ y)\{[0.285 \bullet 140\ kg] + [12.1 \bullet (1.73\ m)^2]\}}{(51 \bullet 0.9\ mg/dL)} = 136\ mL/min$$

Note: Height is converted from inches to meters: Ht = (68 in • 2.54 cm/in)/(100 cm/m) = 1.73 m.

The patient has good renal function and would be expected to have achieved steady-state after 7 days of treatment.

2. *Compute drug clearance.*

Note that digoxin concentrations in ng/mL are the same as those for μg/L. This unit substitution will be directly made to avoid conversion factors in the computation.

$$Cl = [F(D/\tau)]/Css = [0.7(500\ \mu g/d)]/2.4\ \mu g/L = 146\ L/d$$

3. *Compute new dose to achieve the desired serum concentration.*

The average steady-state equation is used to compute the new digoxin dose.

$$D/\tau = (Css \bullet Cl)/F = (1.5\ \mu g/L \bullet 146\ L/d)/0.7 = 313\ \mu g/d, \text{ rounded to } 375\ \mu g/d$$

The new suggested dose would be 375 μg/d given as digoxin tablets to be started at next scheduled dosing time. If desired, a one daily dose could be withheld to allow the digoxin concentration to decline, and the new dose started the following day.

9. *Answer to problem 9.* The initial digoxin doses for patient VG would be calculated as follows:

Pharmacokinetic Dosing Method

1. *Estimate creatinine clearance.*

This patient has a stable serum creatinine and is obese [IBW$_{females}$ (in kg) = 45 + 2.3(Ht − 60) = 45 + 2.3(62" − 60) = 50 kg]. The Salazar and Corcoran equation can be used to estimate creatinine clearance:

$$CrCl_{est(females)} = \frac{(146 - age)[(0.287 \bullet Wt) + (9.74 \bullet Ht^2)]}{(60 \bullet S_{Cr})}$$

$$CrCl_{est(females)} = \frac{(146 - 75\ y)\{[0.287 \bullet 180\ kg] + [9.74 \bullet (1.57\ m)^2]\}}{(60 \bullet 6\ mg/dL)} = 15\ mL/min$$

Note: Height is converted from inches to meters: Ht = (62 in • 2.54 cm/in)/(100 cm/m) = 1.57 m.

The patient has poor renal function and would be expected to have achieved steady-state after ~20 days of treatment.

2. *Estimate clearance.*

The drug clearance versus creatinine clearance relationship is used to estimate the digoxin clearance for this patient ($Cl_{NR} = 20$ mL/min since the patient has moderate-severe heart failure):

$$Cl = 1.303 \, (CrCl) + Cl_{NR} = 1.303(15 \text{ mL/min}) + 20 \text{ mL/min} = 39 \text{ mL/min}$$

3. *Use average steady-state concentration equation to compute digoxin maintenance dose.*

For a patient with heart failure, the desired digoxin concentration would be 0.5-1 ng/mL. A serum concentration equal to 1 ng/mL was chosen for this patient, and oral digoxin tablets will be used (F = 0.7). Note that for concentration units ng/mL = μg/L, and this conversion will be made before the equation is used. Also, conversion factors are needed to change milliliter units to liter (1000 mL/L) and minute units to days (1440 min/d).

$$D/\tau = (Css \bullet Cl)/F = (1 \text{ μg/L} \bullet 39 \text{ mL/min} \bullet 1440 \text{ min/d})/(0.7 \bullet 1000 \text{ mL/L}) = 80 \text{ μg/d}$$

The smallest digoxin tablet size is 125 μg, so the dosage interval will have to be extended to approximate the required daily dosage rate. A dosage rate of 80 μg/d is equivalent to 160 μg given every other day (160 μg = 80 μg/d • 2 d). Since the medication is to be given as tablets, the dose would be rounded to 187.5 (1½ 125 μg tablets) every other day.

4. *Use loading dose equation to compute digoxin loading dose (if needed).*

The patient has poor renal function and is obese. Therefore, the volume of distribution equation that adjusts the parameter estimate for renal dysfunction can be used to compute the digoxin loading dose, and ideal body weight will be used as the weight factor. An oral loading dose using tablets (F = 0.7) could be given in this patient to achieve the desired pharmacologic effect quicker than would occur if maintenance doses alone were used to allow concentrations to accumulate over 3-5 half-lives.

$$V = \left(226 + \frac{298 \bullet CrCl}{29.1 + CrCl} \right)(Wt/70) = \left(226 + \frac{298 \bullet 15 \text{ mL/min}}{29.1 + 15 \text{ mL/min}} \right)(50 \text{ kg}/70) = 234 \text{ L}$$

$$LD = (Css \bullet V)/F = (1 \text{ μg/L} \bullet 234 \text{ L})/0.7 = 334 \text{ μg rounded to } 375 \text{ μg}$$

When digoxin loading doses are administered, they are usually given in divided doses separated by 4-6 hours (50% of dose at first, followed by two additional doses of 25%). In this case, an initial oral dose of 250 μg would be given, followed by two additional oral doses of 62.5 μg given 4-6 hours apart so that available tablet strengths could be used. In a nonemergent situation, three 125-μg doses separated by 4-6 hours could also be considered. The additional portions of the loading dose could be withheld if pulse rate was less than 50-60 beats/min or other undesirable digoxin adverse effects were noted.

Jelliffe Method

1. *Estimate creatinine clearance.*

This patient has a stable serum creatinine and is obese [$IBW_{females}$ (in kg) = 45 + 2.3(Ht − 60) = 45 + 2.3(62 in − 60) = 50 kg]. The Salazar and Corcoran equation can be used to estimate creatinine clearance:

$$CrCl_{est(females)} = \frac{(146 - age)[(0.287 \bullet Wt) + (9.74 \bullet Ht^2)]}{(60 \bullet S_{Cr})}$$

$$CrCl_{est(females)} = \frac{(146 - 45 \text{ y})\{[0.287 \bullet 180 \text{ kg}] + [9.74 \bullet (1.57 \text{ m})^2]\}}{(60 \bullet 6 \text{ mg/dL})} = 15 \text{ mL/min}$$

Note: Height is converted from inches to meters: Ht = (62 in • 2.54 cm/in)/(100 cm/m) = 1.57 m.

The patient has poor renal function and would be expected to have achieved steady-state after ~20 days of treatment.

2. *Estimate total body store (TBS) and maintenance dose (D).*

The patient has poor renal function and is obese. Digoxin total body stores of 6-10 µg/kg are effective in the treatment of heart failure in patients with poor renal function. A digoxin dose of 8 µg/kg was chosen for this patient, and ideal body weight will be used to compute the dose.

$$\text{TBS} = 8 \text{ µg/kg} \bullet 50 \text{ kg} = 400 \text{ µg}$$

$$D = \{\text{TBS} \bullet [14\% + 0.20(\text{CrCl})]\}/(F \bullet 100) = \{400 \text{ µg} \bullet [14\% + 0.20(15 \text{ mL/min})]\}/(0.7 \bullet 100) = 97 \text{ µg/d, rounded to } 125 \text{ µg/d}$$

3. *Use loading dose equation to compute digoxin loading dose (if needed).*

Digoxin total body store is used to calculate the loading dose after correcting for bioavailability:

$$\text{LD} = \text{TBS}/F = 400 \text{ µg}/0.7 = 571 \text{ µg, rounded to } 500 \text{ µg}$$

When digoxin loading doses are administered, they are usually given in divided doses separated by 4-6 hours (50% of dose at first, followed by two additional doses of 25%). In this case, an initial oral dose of 250 µg would be given initially, followed by two additional oral doses of 125 µg each. One of the loading doses could be withheld if pulse rate was less than 50-60 beats/min or other undesirable digoxin adverse effects were noted.

10. *Answer to problem 10.* The revised digoxin dose for patient VG would be calculated as follows:

Linear Pharmacokinetics Method

1. *Estimate creatinine clearance.*

This patient has a stable serum creatinine and is obese [$\text{IBW}_{\text{females}}$ (in kg) = 45 + 2.3(Ht − 60) = 45 + 2.3(62 in − 60) = 50 kg]. The Salazar and Corcoran equation can be used to estimate creatinine clearance:

$$\text{CrCl}_{\text{est(females)}} = \frac{(146 - \text{age})[(0.287 \bullet \text{Wt}) + (9.74 \bullet \text{Ht}^2)]}{(60 \bullet S_{\text{Cr}})}$$

$$\text{CrCl}_{\text{est(females)}} = \frac{(146 - 75 \text{ y})\{[0.287 \bullet 180 \text{ kg}] + [9.74 \bullet (1.57 \text{ m})^2]\}}{(60 \bullet 6 \text{ mg/dL})} = 15 \text{ mL/min}$$

Note: Height is converted from inches to meters: Ht = (62 in $\bullet$ 2.54 cm/in)/(100 cm/m) = 1.57 m.

The patient has poor renal function and would be expected to have achieved steady-state after ~21 days of treatment.

1. *Compute new dose to achieve the desired serum concentration.*

Using linear pharmacokinetics, the new dose to attain the desired concentration should be proportional to the old dose that produced the measured concentration:

$$D_{\text{new}} = (C_{\text{ss,new}}/C_{\text{ss,old}})D_{\text{old}} = (1 \text{ ng/mL}/0.5 \text{ ng/mL}) \, 125 \text{ µg/2d} = 250 \text{ µg/2d or } 125 \text{ µg/d}$$

The new dose would be 125 µg/d given as oral digoxin tablets to be started at next scheduled dosing time.

Pharmacokinetic Parameter Method

1. *Estimate creatinine clearance.*

    This patient has a stable serum creatinine and is obese [IBW$_{females}$ (in kg) = 45 + 2.3(Ht − 60) = 45 + 2.3(62 in − 60) = 50 kg]. The Salazar and Corcoran equation can be used to estimate creatinine clearance:

$$CrCl_{est(females)} = \frac{(146 - age)[(0.287 \bullet Wt) + (9.74 \bullet Ht^2)]}{(60 \bullet S_{Cr})}$$

$$CrCl_{est(females)} = \frac{(146 - 75\ y)\{[0.287 \bullet 180\ kg] + [9.74 \bullet (1.57\ m)^2]\}}{(60 \bullet 6\ mg/dL)} = 15\ mL/min$$

    Note: Height is converted from inches to meters: Ht = (62 in • 2.54 cm/in)/(100 cm/m) = 1.57 m. The patient has good renal function and would be expected to have achieved steady-state after ~21 days of treatment.

2. *Compute drug clearance.*

    Note that digoxin concentrations in ng/mL are the same as those for μg/L. This unit substitution will be directly made to avoid conversion factors in the computation.

$$Cl = [F(D/\tau)]/Css = [0.7(125\ \mu g/2d)]/0.5\ \mu g/L = 87.5\ L/d$$

3. *Compute new dose to achieve the desired serum concentration.*

    The average steady-state equation is used to compute the new digoxin dose.

$$D/\tau = (Css \bullet Cl)/F = (1\ \mu g/L \bullet 87.5\ L/d)/0.7 = 125\ \mu g/d$$

    The new suggested dose would be 125 μg/d given as digoxin tablets to be started at next scheduled dosing time.

11. *Answer to problem 11.* The initial digoxin doses for patient QW would be calculated as follows:

Pharmacokinetic Dosing Method

1. *Estimate creatinine clearance.*

    This patient has a stable serum creatinine and is not obese. The Cockcroft-Gault equation can be used to estimate creatinine clearance:

$$CrCl_{est} = \{[(140 - age)BW]/[72 \bullet S_{Cr}]\}0.85 = \{[(140 - 34\ y)50\ kg]/[72 \bullet 0.8\ mg/dL]\}0.85$$
$$CrCl_{est} = 78\ mL/min$$

2. *Estimate clearance.*

    The drug clearance versus creatinine clearance relationship is used to estimate the digoxin clearance for this patient (Cl$_{NR}$ = 40 mL/min since the patient does not have moderate-severe heart failure):

$$Cl = 1.303\ (CrCl) + Cl_{NR} = 1.303(78\ mL/min) + 40\ mL/min = 142\ mL/min$$

However, this patient is hyperthyroid which is a disease state known to increase digoxin metabolism and shorten half-life ($t_{1/2}$ = 1 d). Assuming a normal volume of distribution (7 L/kg) and this half-life allows the computation of the expected digoxin clearance rate for the patient:

$$V = 7 \text{ L/kg} \bullet 50 \text{ kg} = 350 \text{ L}$$

$$k_e = 0.693/t_{1/2} = 0.693/1 \text{ d} = 0.693 \text{ d}^{-1}, \text{ where } k_e \text{ is the terminal elimination rate constant}$$

$$Cl = k_e V = 0.693 \text{ d}^{-1} \bullet 350 \text{ L} = 243 \text{ L/d}$$

This clearance rate is probably more reflective of her digoxin elimination status and will be used to compute her digoxin dose.

3. *Use average steady-state concentration equation to compute digoxin maintenance dose.*

For a patient with atrial fibrillation, the desired digoxin concentration would be 0.8-1.5 ng/mL. A serum concentration equal to 1.2 ng/mL was chosen for this patient, and oral digoxin tablets will be used (F = 0.7). Note that for concentration units ng/mL = μg/L, and this conversion will be made before the equation is used. Also, conversion factors are needed to change milliliter units to liter (1000 mL/L) and minute units to days (1440 min/d).

$$D/\tau = (Css \bullet Cl)/F = (1.2 \text{ μg/L} \bullet 243 \text{ L/d})/0.7 = 417 \text{ μg/d, rounded to } 375 \text{ μg/d}$$

This is a large dose of digoxin, but hyperthyroid patients have increased digoxin clearance rates and require larger doses. If this dose were administered to the patient, she would need to be monitored several times daily for digoxin adverse effects and digoxin concentrations should be used to help guide therapy.

4. *Use loading dose equation to compute digoxin loading dose (if needed).*

$$V = 350 \text{ L from previous calculation}$$

$$LD = (Css \bullet V)/F = (1.2 \text{ μg/L} \bullet 350 \text{ L})/1 = 420 \text{ μg rounded to } 400 \text{ μg}$$

When digoxin loading doses are administered, they are usually given in divided doses separated by 4-6 hours (50% of dose at first, followed by two additional doses of 25%). In this case, an initial intravenous dose of 200 μg would be given initially, followed by two additional intravenous doses of 100 μg each. One of the loading doses could be withheld if pulse rate was less than 50-60 beats/min or other undesirable digoxin adverse effects were noted.

Jelliffe Method

1. *Estimate creatinine clearance*

This patient has a stable serum creatinine and is not obese. The Cockcroft-Gault equation can be used to estimate creatinine clearance:

$$CrCl_{est} = \{[(140 - age)BW]/[72 \bullet S_{Cr}]\}0.85 = \{[(140 - 34 \text{ y})50 \text{ kg}]/[72 \bullet 0.8 \text{ mg/dL}]\}0.85$$
$$CrCl_{est} = 78 \text{ mL/min}$$

2. *Estimate total body store (TBS) and maintenance dose (D).*

The patient has good renal function and is nonobese. Digoxin total body stores of 13-15 μg/kg are effective in the treatment of atrial fibrillation. A digoxin dose of 14 μg/kg was chosen for this patient. Digoxin tablets will be used as the dosage form for maintenance doses. Note that this dosing method does not include a way to adjust dosage requirements for disease states that cause higher than average clearance rates.

$$TBS = 14 \ \mu g/kg \bullet 50 \ kg = 700 \ \mu g$$

$$D = \{TBS \bullet [14\% + 0.20(CrCl)]\}/(F \bullet 100) = \{700 \ \mu g \bullet [14\% + 0.20(78 \ mL/min)]\}/(0.7 \bullet 100) = 296 \ \mu g/d, \ rounded \ to \ 250 \ \mu g/d$$

3. *Use loading dose equation to compute digoxin loading dose (if needed).*
   Digoxin total body store is used to calculate the loading dose after correcting for bioavailability:

$$LD = TBS/F = 700 \ \mu g/1 = 700 \ \mu g, \ rounded \ to \ 750 \ \mu g$$

When digoxin loading doses are administered, they are usually given in divided doses separated by 4-6 hours (50% of dose at first, followed by two additional doses of 25%). In this case, an initial intravenous dose of 375 μg would be given initially, followed by two additional intravenous doses of 187.5 μg each. One of the loading doses could be withheld if pulse rate was less than 50-60 beats/min or other undesirable digoxin adverse effects were noted.

12. *Answer to problem 12.* The digoxin doses for patient RT would be calculated as follows:
    1. *Enter the patient's demographic, drug-dosing, and serum concentration/time data into the computer program.*
    2. *Compute pharmacokinetic parameters for the patient using Bayesian pharmacokinetic computer program.*
       The pharmacokinetic parameters computed by the program are a clearance equal to 3 L/h, a volume of distribution of 403 L, and a half-life equal to 92 h.
    3. *Compute dose required to achieve the desired digoxin serum concentrations.*
       The one-compartment model equations used by the program to compute doses indicates that a dose of 185 μg every 2 days of digoxin tablets will produce a pre-dose steady-state concentration of 0.8 ng/mL. This dose would be rounded off to 187.5 μg (1½ 125 μg tablets) every other day.

13. *Answer to problem 13.* The digoxin doses for patient LK would be calculated as follows:
    1. *Enter the patient's demographic, drug-dosing, and serum concentration/time data into the computer program.*
    2. *Compute pharmacokinetic parameters for the patient using Bayesian pharmacokinetic computer program.*
       The pharmacokinetic parameters computed by the program are a clearance equal to 1.5 L/h, a volume of distribution of 276 L, and a half-life equal to 124 h.
    3. *Compute dose required to achieve the desired digoxin serum concentrations.*
       The one-compartment model equations used by the program to compute doses indicates that a dose of 193 μg every 3 days of digoxin tablets will produce a pre-dose steady-state concentration of 1 ng/mL. This dose would be rounded off to 187.5 μg (1½ 125-μg tablets) every third day.

14. *Answer to problem 14.* The digoxin doses for patient BH would be calculated as follows:
    1. *Enter the patient's demographic, drug-dosing, and serum concentration/time data into the computer program.*
    2. *Compute pharmacokinetic parameters for the patient using Bayesian pharmacokinetic computer program.*

The pharmacokinetic parameters computed by the program are a clearance equal to 6.5 L/h, a volume of distribution of 509 L, and a half-life equal to 54 h.

3. *Compute dose required to achieve the desired digoxin serum concentrations.*

The one-compartment model equations used by the program to compute doses indicates that a dose of 383 μg/d of digoxin tablets will produce a pre-dose steady-state concentration of 1.5 ng/mL. This dose would be rounded off to 375 μg/d.

REFERENCES

1. Sanoski CA, Bauman JL. The arrhythmias. In: DiPiro JT, Talbert RL, Yee GC, Matzke GR, Wells BG, Posey LM, eds. *Pharmacotherapy*. New York, NY: McGraw-Hill; 2011:273-309.
2. Ahmed A, Waagstein F, Pitt B, et al. Effectiveness of digoxin in reducing one-year mortality in chronic heart failure in the Digitalis Investigation Group trial. *Am J Cardiol*. Jan 1, 2009;103(1):82-87.
3. Anon. The effect of digoxin on mortality and morbidity in patients with heart failure. The Digitalis Investigation Group [see comments]. *N Engl J Med*. 1997;336(8):525-533.
4. Anderson JL, Halperin JL, Albert NM, et al. Management of patients with atrial fibrillation (Compilation of 2006 ACCF/AHA/ESC and 2011 ACCF/AHA/HRS Recommendations): a report of the American College of Cardiology/American Heart Association Task Force on Practice Guidelines. *Circulation*. 2013;127(13):1425-1443.
5. Packer M, Gheorghiade M, Young JB, et al. Withdrawal of digoxin from patients with chronic heart failure treated with angiotensin-converting-enzyme inhibitors. RADIANCE Study [see comments]. *N Engl J Med*. 1993;329(1):1-7.
6. Parker RB, Cavallari LH. Systolic heart failure. In: DiPiro JT, Talbert RL, Yee GC, Matzke GR, Wells BG, Posey LM, eds. *Pharmacotherapy*. 8th ed. New York, NY: McGraw-Hill; 2011:137-172.
7. Maron BA, Rocco TP. Pharmacotherapy of congestive heart failure. In: Brunton L, Chabner B, Knollman B, eds. *The Pharmacological Basis of Therapeutics*. 12th ed. New York, NY: McGraw-Hill; 2011:789-814.
8. Rogers JE, Lee CR. Acute decompensated heart failure. In: DiPiro JT, Talbert RL, Yee GC, Matzke GR, Wells BG, Posey LM, eds. *Pharmacotherapy*. 8th ed. New York, NY: McGraw-Hill; 2011:191-208.
9. Sampson KJ, Kass RS. Anti-arrhythmics drugs. In: Brunton L, Chabner B, Knollman B, eds. *The Pharmacological Basis of Therapeutics*. 12th ed. New York, NY: McGraw-Hill; 2011:815-848.
10. Reuning RH, Sams RA, Notari RE. Role of pharmacokinetics in drug dosage adjustment. I. Pharmacologic effect kinetics and apparent volume of distribution of digoxin. *J Clin Pharmacol New Drugs*. 1973;13(4):127-141.
11. Koup JR, Greenblatt DJ, Jusko WJ, Smith TW, Koch-Weser J. Pharmacokinetics of digoxin in normal subjects after intravenous bolus and infusion doses. *J Pharmacokinet Biopharm*. 1975;3(3):181-192.
12. Koup JR, Jusko WJ, Elwood CM, Kohli RK. Digoxin pharmacokinetics: role of renal failure in dosage regimen design. *Clin Pharmacol Ther*. 1975;18(1):9-21.
13. Slatton ML, Irani WN, Hall SA, et al. Does digoxin provide additional hemodynamic and autonomic benefit at higher doses in patients with mild to moderate heart failure and normal sinus rhythm? *J Am Coll Cardiol*. 1997;29(6):1206-1213.
14. Gheorghiade M, Hall VB, Jacobsen G, Alam M, Rosman H, Goldstein S. Effects of increasing maintenance dose of digoxin on left ventricular function and neurohormones in patients with chronic heart failure treated with diuretics and angiotensin-converting enzyme inhibitors. *Circulation*. 1995;92(7):1801-1807.
15. Beasley R, Smith DA, McHaffie DJ. Exercise heart rates at different serum digoxin concentrations in patients with atrial fibrillation. *Br Med J (Clin Res Ed)*. 1985;290(6461):9-11.
16. Aronson JK, Hardman M. ABC of monitoring drug therapy. Digoxin. *BMJ*. 1992;305(6862):1149-1152.
17. Smith TW, Haber E. Digoxin intoxication: the relationship of clinical presentation to serum digoxin concentration. *J Clin Invest*. 1970;49(12):2377-2386.
18. Chung EK. Digitalis intoxication. *Postgrad Med J*. 1972;48(557):163-179.
19. Beller GA, Smith TW, Abelmann WH, Haber E, Hood WB Jr. Digitalis intoxication. A prospective clinical study with serum level correlations. *N Engl J Med*. 1971;284(18):989-997.
20. Okamura N, Hirai M, Tanigawara Y, et al. Digoxin-cyclosporin A interaction: modulation of the multidrug transporter P-glycoprotein in the kidney. *J Pharmacol Exp Ther*. Sep 1993;266(3):1614-1619.
21. Ito S, Woodland C, Harper PA, Koren G. P-glycoprotein-mediated renal tubular secretion of digoxin: the toxicological significance of the urine-blood barrier model. *Life Sci*. 1993;53(2):PL25-PL31.
22. Norregaard-Hansen K, Klitgaard NA, Pedersen KE. The significance of the enterohepatic circulation on the metabolism of digoxin in patients with the ability of intestinal conversion of the drug. *Acta Med Scand*. 1986;220(1):89-92.

23. Johnson BF, Smith G, French J. The comparability of dosage regimens of Lanoxin tablets and Lanoxicaps. *Br J Clin Pharmacol.* 1977;4(2):209-211.

24. Johnson BF, Bye C, Jones G, Sabey GA. A completely absorbed oral preparation of digoxin. *Clin Pharmacol Ther.* 1976;19(6):746-751.

25. Kramer WG, Reuning RH. Use of area under the curve to estimate absolute bioavailability of digoxin [letter]. *J Pharm Sci.* 1978;67(1):141-142.

26. Beveridge T, Nuesch E, Ohnhaus EE. Absolute bioavailability of digoxin tablets. *Arzneimittelforschung.* 1978;28(4):701-703.

27. Ohnhaus EE, Vozeh S, Nuesch E. Absolute bioavailability of digoxin in chronic renal failure. *Clin Nephrol.* 1979;11(6):302-306.

28. Ohnhaus EE, Vozeh S, Nuesch E. Absorption of digoxin in severe right heart failure. *Eur J Clin Pharmacol.* 1979;15(2):115-120.

29. Hinderling PH. Kinetics of partitioning and binding of digoxin and its analogues in the subcompartments of blood. *J Pharm Sci.* 1984;73(8):1042-1053.

30. Storstein L. Studies on digitalis. V. The influence of impaired renal function, hemodialysis, and drug interaction on serum protein binding of digitoxin and digoxin. *Clin Pharmacol Ther.* 1976;20(1):6-14.

31. Iisalo E. Clinical pharmacokinetics of digoxin. *Clin Pharmacokinet.* 1977;2:1-16.

32. Aronson JK. Clinical pharmacokinetics of digoxin 1980. *Clin Pharmacokinet.* 1980;5(2):137-149.

33. Ewy GA, Groves BM, Ball MF, Nimmo L, Jackson B, Marcus F. Digoxin metabolism in obesity. *Circulation.* 1971;44(5):810-814.

34. Abernethy DR, Greenblatt DJ, Smith TW. Digoxin disposition in obesity: clinical pharmacokinetic investigation. *Am Heart J.* 1981;102(4):740-744.

35. Jusko WJ, Szefler SJ, Goldfarb AL. Pharmacokinetic design of digoxin dosage regimens in relation to renal function. *J Clin Pharmacol.* 1974;14(10):525-535.

36. Golper TA, Marx MA. Drug dosing adjustments during continuous renal replacement therapies. *Kidney Int Suppl.* May 1998;66:S165-S168.

37. Golper TA. Update on drug sieving coefficients and dosing adjustments during continuous renal replacement therapies. *Contrib Nephrol.* 2001;(132):349-353.

38. Ochs HR, Greenblatt DJ, Bodem G, Dengler HJ. Disease-related alterations in cardiac glycoside disposition. *Clin Pharmacokinet.* 1982;7(5):434-451.

39. Bonelli J, Haydl H, Hruby K, Kaik G. The pharmacokinetics of digoxin in patients with manifest hyperthyroidism and after normalization of thyroid function. *Int J Clin Pharmacol Biopharm.* 1978;16(7):302-306.

40. Koup JR. Distribution of digoxin in hyperthyroid patients. *Int J Clin Pharmacol Ther Toxicol.* 1980;18(5):236.

41. Nyberg L, Wettrell G. Pharmacokinetics and dosage of digoxin in neonates and infants. *Eur J Clin Pharmacol.* 1980;18(1):69-74.

42. Nyberg L, Wettrell G. Digoxin dosage schedules for neonates and infants based on pharmacokinetic considerations. *Clin Pharmacokinet.* 1978;3(6):453-461.

43. Heizer WD, Pittman AW, Hammond JE, Fitch DD, Bustrack JA, Hull JH. Absorption of digoxin from tablets and capsules in subjects with malabsorption syndromes. *DICP.* 1989;23(10):764-769.

44. Heizer WD, Smith TW, Goldfinger SE. Absorption of digoxin in patients with malabsorption syndromes. *N Engl J Med.* 1971;285(5):257-259.

45. Kolibash AJ, Kramer WG, Reuning RH, Caldwell JH. Marked decline in serum digoxin concentration during an episode of severe diarrhea. *Am Heart J.* 1977;94(6):806-807.

46. Bjornsson TD, Huang AT, Roth P, Jacob DS, Christenson R. Effects of high-dose cancer chemotherapy on the absorption of digoxin in two different formulations. *Clin Pharmacol Ther.* 1986;39(1):25-28.

47. Jusko WJ, Conti DR, Molson A, Kuritzky P, Giller J, Schultz R. Digoxin absorption from tablets and elixir. The effect of radiation-induced malabsorption. *JAMA.* 1974;230(11):1554-1555.

48. Fromm MF, Kim RB, Stein CM, Wilkinson GR, Roden DM. Inhibition of P-glycoprotein-mediated drug transport: A unifying mechanism to explain the interaction between digoxin and quinidine [see comments]. *Circulation.* 1999;99(4):552-557.

49. Hansten PD, Horn JR. *Drug Interactions Analysis and Management.* St. Louis, MO: Wolters Kluwer Health; 2014.

50. Ejvinsson G. Effect of quinidine on plasma concentrations of digoxin. *Br Med J.* 1978;1(6108):279-280.

51. Leahey EB Jr, Reiffel JA, Drusin RE, Heissenbuttel RH, Lovejoy WP, Bigger JT Jr. Interaction between quinidine and digoxin. *JAMA.* 1978;240(6):533-534.

52. Reiffel JA, Leahey EB Jr, Drusin RE, Heissenbuttel RH, Lovejoy W, Bigger JT Jr. A previously unrecognized drug interaction between quinidine and digoxin. *Clin Cardiol.* 1979;2(1):40-42.

53. Hager WD, Fenster P, Mayersohn M, et al. Digoxin-quinidine interaction Pharmacokinetic evaluation. *N Engl J Med.* 1979;300(22):1238-1241.

54. Doering W. Quinidine-digoxin interaction: pharmacokinetics, underlying mechanism and clinical implications. *N Engl J Med.* 1979;301(8):400-404.

55. Bauer LA, Horn JR, Pettit H. Mixed-effect modeling for detection and evaluation of drug interactions: digoxin-quinidine and digoxin-verapamil combinations. *Ther Drug Monit.* 1996;18(1):46-52.

56. Pedersen KE, Dorph-Pedersen A, Hvidt S, Klitgaard NA, Nielsen-Kudsk F. Digoxin-verapamil interaction. *Clin Pharmacol Ther.* 1981;30(3):311-316.

57. Klein HO, Lang R, Weiss E, et al. The influence of verapamil on serum digoxin concentration. *Circulation.* 1982;65(5):998-1003.

58. Pedersen KE, Thayssen P, Klitgaard NA, Christiansen BD, Nielsen-Kudsk F. Influence of verapamil on the inotropism and pharmacokinetics of digoxin. *Eur J Clin Pharmacol.* 1983;25(2):199-206.

59. Yoshida A, Fujita M, Kurosawa N, et al. Effects of diltiazem on plasma level and urinary excretion of digoxin in healthy subjects. *Clin Pharmacol Ther.* 1984;35(5):681-685.

60. Rameis H, Magometschnigg D, Ganzinger U. The diltiazem-digoxin interaction. *Clin Pharmacol Ther.* 1984;36(2):183-189.

61. Belz GG, Wistuba S, Matthews JH. Digoxin and bepridil: pharmacokinetic and pharmacodynamic interactions. *Clin Pharmacol Ther.* 1986;39(1):65-71.

62. Moysey JO, Jaggarao NS, Grundy EN, Chamberlain DA. Amiodarone increases plasma digoxin concentrations. *Br Med J (Clin Res Ed).* 1981;282(6260):272.

63. Maragno I, Santostasi G, Gaion RM, Paleari C. Influence of amiodarone on oral digoxin bioavailability in healthy volunteers. *Int J Clin Pharmacol Res.* 1984;4(2):149-153.

64. Nademanee K, Kannan R, Hendrickson J, Ookhtens M, Kay I, Singh BN. Amiodarone-digoxin interaction: clinical significance, time course of development, potential pharmacokinetic mechanisms and therapeutic implications. *J Am Coll Cardiol.* 1984;4(1):111-116.

65. Robinson K, Johnston A, Walker S, Mulrow JP, McKenna WJ, Holt DW. The digoxin-amiodarone interaction. *Cardiovasc Drugs Ther.* 1989;3(1):25-28.

66. Nolan PE Jr, Marcus FI, Erstad BL, Hoyer GL, Furman C, Kirsten EB. Effects of coadministration of propafenone on the pharmacokinetics of digoxin in healthy volunteer subjects. *J Clin Pharmacol.* 1989;29(1):46-52.

67. Bigot MC, Debruyne D, Bonnefoy L, Grollier G, Moulin M, Potier JC. Serum digoxin levels related to plasma propafenone levels during concomitant treatment. *J Clin Pharmacol.* 1991;31(6):521-526.

68. Calvo MV, Martin-Suarez A, Martin Luengo C, Avila C, Cascon M, Dominguez-Gil Hurle A. Interaction between digoxin and propafenone. *Ther Drug Monit.* 1989;11(1):10-15.

69. Kakumoto M, Takara K, Sakaeda T, Tanigawara Y, Kita T, Okumura K. MDR1-mediated interaction of digoxin with antiarrhythmic or antianginal drugs. *Biol Pharm Bull.* Dec 2002;25(12):1604-1607.

70. Dorian P, Strauss M, Cardella C, David T, East S, Ogilvie R. Digoxin-cyclosporine interaction: severe digitalis toxicity after cyclosporine treatment. *Clin Invest Med.* 1988;11(2):108-112.

71. Dobkin JF, Saha JR, Butler VP Jr, Neu HC, Lindenbaum J. Inactivation of digoxin by *Eubacterium lentum*, an anaerobe of the human gut flora. *Trans Assoc Am Physicians.* 1982;95:22-29.

72. Saha JR, Butler VP Jr, Neu HC, Lindenbaum J. Digoxin-inactivating bacteria: identification in human gut flora. *Science.* 1983;220(4594):325-327.

73. Lindenbaum J, Rund DG, Butler VP Jr, Tse-Eng D, Saha JR. Inactivation of digoxin by the gut flora: reversal by antibiotic therapy. *N Engl J Med.* 1981;305(14):789-794.

74. Morton MR, Cooper JW. Erythromycin-induced digoxin toxicity. *DICP.* 1989;23(9):668-670.

75. Maxwell DL, Gilmour-White SK, Hall MR. Digoxin toxicity due to interaction of digoxin with erythromycin. *BMJ.* 1989;298(6673):572.

76. Brown BA, Wallace RJ Jr, Griffith DE, Warden R. Clarithromycin-associated digoxin toxicity in the elderly. *Clin Infect Dis.* 1997;24(1):92-93.

77. Nawarskas JJ, McCarthy DM, Spinler SA. Digoxin toxicity secondary to clarithromycin therapy. *Ann Pharmacother.* 1997;31(7-8):864-866.

78. Wakasugi H, Yano I, Ito T, et al. Effect of clarithromycin on renal excretion of digoxin: interaction with P-glycoprotein. *Clin Pharmacol Ther.* 1998;64(1):123-128.

79. Allen MD, Greenblatt DJ, Harmatz JS, Smith TW. Effect of magnesium–aluminum hydroxide and kaolin–pectin on absorption of digoxin from tablets and capsules. *J Clin Pharmacol.* 1981;21(1):26-30.

80. Hall WH, Shappell SD, Doherty JE. Effect of cholestyramine on digoxin absorption and excretion in man. *Am J Cardiol.* 1977;39(2):213-216.

81. Brown DD, Schmid J, Long RA, Hull JH. A steady-state evaluation of the effects of propantheline bromide and cholestyramine on the bioavailability of digoxin when administered as tablets or capsules. *J Clin Pharmacol.* 1985;25(5):360-364.

82. Juhl RP, Summers RW, Guillory JK, Blaug SM, Cheng FH, Brown DD. Effect of sulfasalazine on digoxin bioavailability. *Clin Pharmacol Ther.* 1976;20(4):387-394.

83. Lindenbaum J, Maulitz RM, Butler VP Jr. Inhibition of digoxin absorption by neomycin. *Gastroenterology.* 1976;71(3):399-404.

84. Johnson BF, Bustrack JA, Urbach DR, Hull JH, Marwaha R. Effect of metoclopramide on digoxin absorption from tablets and capsules. *Clin Pharmacol Ther.* 1984;36(6):724-730.

85. Kirch W, Janisch HD, Santos SR, Duhrsen U, Dylewicz P, Ohnhaus EE. Effect of cisapride and metoclopramide on digoxin bioavailability. *Eur J Drug Metab Pharmacokinet.* 1986;11(4):249-250.

86. Bauman JL, DiDomenico RJ, Viana M, Fitch M. A method of determining the dose of digoxin for heart failure in the modern era. *Arch Intern Med.* Dec 11-25, 2006;166(22):2539-2545.

87. Jelliffe RW, Brooker G. A nomogram for digoxin therapy. *Am J Med.* 1974;57(1):63-68.

88. Jelliffe RW. An improved method of digoxin therapy. *Ann Intern Med.* 1968;69(4):703-717.

89. Anon. *Lanoxin(R) Prescribing Information*. Research Triangle Park, NC: GlaxoSmithKline; 2006.

90. Mutnick AH. Digoxin. In: Schumacher GE, ed. *Therapeutic Drug Monitoring*. 1st ed. Stamford, CT: Appleton & Lange; 1995:469-491.

91. Sheiner LB, Halkin H, Peck C, Rosenberg B, Melmon KL. Improved computer-assisted digoxin therapy. A method using feedback of measured serum digoxin concentrations. *Ann Intern Med*. 1975;82(5):619-627.

92. Peck CC, Sheiner LB, Martin CM, Combs DT, Melmon KL. Computer-assisted digoxin therapy. *N Engl J Med*. 1973;289(9):441-446.

93. Wandell M, Mungall D. Computer assisted drug interpretation and drug regimen optimization. *Amer Assoc Clin Chem*. 1984;6:1-11.

94. Smith TW, Butler VP Jr, Haber E, et al. Treatment of life-threatening digitalis intoxication with digoxin-specific Fab antibody fragments: experience in 26 cases. *N Engl J Med*. 1982;307(22):1357-1362.

95. Smolarz A, Roesch E, Lenz E, Neubert H, Abshagen P. Digoxin specific antibody (Fab) fragments in 34 cases of severe digitalis intoxication. *J Toxicol Clin Toxicol*. 1985;23(4-6):327-340.

96. Ujhelyi MR, Robert S. Pharmacokinetic aspects of digoxin-specific Fab therapy in the management of digitalis toxicity. *Clin Pharmacokinet*. Jun 1995;28(6):483-493.

97. Anon. *DigiFab(R) Prescribing Information*. Melville, NY: Savage Laboratories; 2009.

98. Tschudy MM, Arcara KM. *The Harriet Lane Handbook: A Manual for Pediatric House Officers*. 19th ed. Philadelphia, PA: Mosby; 2012.

99. Anon. *Lanoxin(R) Prescribing Information*. Cary, NC: Covis Pharmaceuticals; 2012.

7   Lidocaine

INTRODUCTION

Lidocaine is a local anesthetic agent that also has antiarrhythmic effects. It is classified as a type IB anti-arrhythmic agent and is a treatment for ventricular tachycardia.[1,2] For episodes of sustained ventricular tachycardia with signs or symptoms of hemodynamic instability (angina, pulmonary edema, hypotension, hemodynamic collapse), electrical cardioversion is the treatment of choice. However, for patients who are hemodynamically stable, sustained monomorphic ventricular tachycardia may be successfully treated using antiarrhythmic therapy. Lidocaine therapy is considered an alternative to procainamide, amiodarone, or sotalol treatment in this situation.[3]

Lidocaine inhibits transmembrane sodium influx into the His-Purkinje fiber conduction system thereby decreasing conduction velocity.[2] It also decreases the duration of the action potential and as a result decreases the duration of the absolute refractory period in Purkinje fibers and bundle of His. Automaticity is decreased during lidocaine therapy. The net effect of these cellular changes is that lidocaine eradicates ventricular reentrant arrhythmias by abolishing unidirectional blocks via increased conduction through diseased fibers.

THERAPEUTIC AND TOXIC CONCENTRATIONS

When given intravenously, the serum lidocaine concentration-time curve follows a two-compartment model.[4,5] This is especially apparent when initial loading doses of lidocaine are given as rapid intravenous injections over 1-5 minutes (maximum rate: 25-50 mg/min) and a distribution phase of 30-40 minutes is observed after drug administration (Figure 7-1). Unlike digoxin, the myocardium responds to the higher concentrations achieved during the distribution phase because lidocaine moves rapidly from the blood into the heart, and the onset of action for lidocaine after a loading dose is within a few minutes after completion of the intravenous injection.[1,2] Because of these factors, the heart is considered to be located in the central compartment of the two-compartment model for lidocaine.

The generally accepted therapeutic range for lidocaine is 1.5-5 µg/mL. In the upper end of the therapeutic range (>3 µg/mL) some patients will experience minor side effects including drowsiness, dizziness, paresthesias, or euphoria. Lidocaine serum concentrations above the therapeutic range can cause muscle twitching, confusion, agitation, dysarthria, psychosis, seizures, or coma. Cardiovascular adverse effects such as atrioventricular block, hypotension, and circulatory collapse have been reported at lidocaine concentrations above 6 µg/mL, but are not strongly correlated with specific serum levels. Lidocaine-induced seizures are not as difficult to treat as theophylline-induced seizures and usually respond to traditional antiseizure medication therapy. Lidocaine metabolites (MEGX and GX, see Basic Clinical Pharmacokinetic Parameter section) probably contribute to the central nervous system side effects attributed to lidocaine therapy.[6-8] Clinicians should understand that all patients with "toxic" lidocaine serum concentrations in the listed ranges will not exhibit signs or symptoms of lidocaine toxicity. Rather, lidocaine concentrations in the given ranges increase the likelihood that an adverse effect will occur.

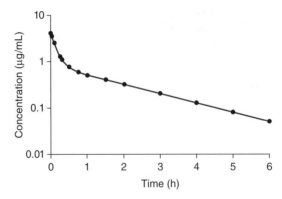

FIGURE 7-1   Lidocaine serum concentrations initially drop rapidly after an intravenous bolus as drug distributes from blood into the tissues during the distribution phase. During the distribution phase, drug leaves the blood due to tissue distribution and elimination. After 0.5-1 hour, an equilibrium is established between the blood and tissues, and serum concentrations drop more slowly since elimination is the primary process removing drug from the blood. A two-compartment model describes this type of serum concentration-time profile. The conduction system of the heart responds to the high concentrations of lidocaine present during the distribution phase, so lidocaine has a quick onset of action.

For dose adjustment purposes, lidocaine serum concentrations are best measured at steady-state after the patient has received a consistent dosage regimen for 3-5 drug half-lives. Lidocaine half-life varies from 1 to 1.5 hours in normal adults to 5 hours or more in adult patients with liver failure. If lidocaine is given as a continuous intravenous infusion, it can take a considerable amount of time (3-5 half-lives or 7.5-25 hours) for patients to achieve effective concentrations, so an intravenous loading dose is commonly administered to patients (Figure 7-2). The ideal situation is to administer an intravenous loading dose that will achieve the desired concentration immediately, then start an intravenous continuous infusion that will maintain that concentration (Figure 7-2). In order to derive this perfect situation, the lidocaine volume of distribution for the central compartment (Vc in L) would have to be known to compute the loading dose (LD in mg): LD = Css • Vc, where Css is the desired lidocaine concentration in mg/L. The volume of distribution for the central compartment of the two-compartment model is used to compute the loading dose because lidocaine distributes rapidly to the myocardium and the heart is considered to reside in the central compartment of the model. However, this pharmacokinetic parameter is rarely, if ever, known for a patient, so a loading

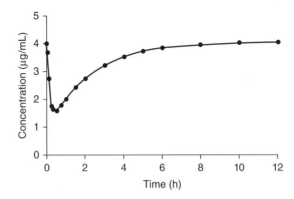

FIGURE 7-2   To maintain therapeutic lidocaine concentrations, an intravenous bolus (over 1-5 minutes) of lidocaine is followed by a continuous intravenous infusion of the drug. Even though the infusion is started right after the loading dose is given, serum concentrations due to the infusion cannot increase rapidly enough to counter the large decrease in concentrations during the distribution phase from the bolus dose. The dip in serum lidocaine concentrations below therapeutic amounts can allow previously treated arrhythmias to recur.

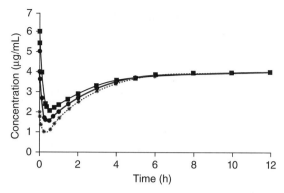

FIGURE 7-3   Because the central volume of distribution is not known at the time an intravenous loading dose of lidocaine is administered, average population parameters must be assumed and almost always result in initial lidocaine serum concentrations that are higher (dashed line with squares) or lower (dotted line with triangles) than those that were expected (solid line with circles). So, the main clinical goal of administering loading doses of lidocaine is to achieve therapeutic concentrations as soon as possible, not to attain steady-state concentrations immediately after the loading dose is given.

dose based on a population average central volume of distribution is used to calculate the amount of lidocaine needed. Since the patient's own, unique central volume of distribution will most likely be greater (resulting in too low of a loading dose) or less (resulting in too large of a loading dose) than the population average volume of distribution used to compute the loading dose, the desired steady-state lidocaine concentration will not be achieved. Because of this, it will still take 3-5 half-lives for the patient to reach steady-state conditions while receiving a constant intravenous infusion rate (Figure 7-3).

After a lidocaine-loading dose is given, serum concentrations from this dose rapidly decline due to distribution from blood to tissues, and serum concentrations due to the infusion are not able to increase rapidly enough to avoid a temporary decline or dip in lidocaine concentrations (Figure 7-2). The decline may be severe enough that ventricular arrhythmias which were initially suppressed by lidocaine may recur due to subtherapeutic antiarrhythmic concentrations. Because of this dip in concentrations due to distribution of drug after the intravenous loading dose, an additional dose (50% of original loading dose) can be given 20-30 minutes after the original loading dose. Or, several additional doses (33%-50% of original loading dose) can be given every 5-10 minutes to a total maximum of 3 mg/kg (Figure 7-4).[5] Thus, lidocaine

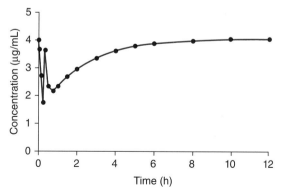

FIGURE 7-4   Since the dip in serum lidocaine concentrations below therapeutic amounts can allow previously treated arrhythmias to recur, a supplemental loading or "booster" dose is typically given 20-30 minutes after the initial loading dose. This prevents lidocaine serum concentrations from declining too far during the distribution phase of the intravenous bolus dose and before serum concentrations from the intravenous infusion have an opportunity to attain therapeutic concentrations.

intravenous loading doses do not usually achieve steady-state serum concentrations immediately, but, hopefully, they do result in therapeutic concentrations and response sooner than simply starting an intravenous infusion alone.

CLINICAL MONITORING PARAMETERS

The electrocardiogram (ECG or EKG) should be monitored to determine the response to lidocaine in patients with ventricular tachycardia. The goal of therapy is suppression of ventricular arrhythmias and avoidance of adverse drug reactions. Lidocaine therapy is often discontinued after 6-24 hours of treatment so the need for long-term antiarrhythmic drug use can be reassessed, although longer infusions may be used in patients with persistent tachyarrhythmias. For long-term therapy, electrophysiologic studies using programmed stimulation to replicate the ventricular arrhythmia or 24-hour ECG monitoring using a Holter monitor can be performed in patients while receiving a variety of antiarrhythmic agents to determine effective antiarrhythmic drug therapy. Because lidocaine is only administered parenterally, it is rarely used for more than a few days unless oral antiarrhythmic agents are ineffective.

Because lidocaine is usually given for a short duration (<24 hours), it is often not necessary to obtain serum lidocaine concentrations in patients receiving appropriate doses who currently have no ventricular arrhythmia or adverse drug effects. However, lidocaine serum concentrations should be obtained in patients who have a recurrence of ventricular tachyarrhythmias, are experiencing possible lidocaine side effects, or are receiving lidocaine doses not consistent with disease states and conditions known to alter lidocaine pharmacokinetics (see Effects of Disease States and Conditions on Lidocaine Pharmacokinetics and Dosing section). Serum concentration monitoring can aid in the decision to increase or decrease the lidocaine dose. For instance, if the ventricular arrhythmia reappears and the lidocaine serum concentration is <5 μg/mL, increasing the lidocaine dose is a therapeutic option. However, if the lidocaine serum concentration is over 5 μg/mL, it is unlikely that a dosage increase will be effective in suppressing the arrhythmia and there is an increased likelihood that drug side effects may occur. Similarly, if a possible lidocaine adverse drug reaction is noted in a patient and the lidocaine serum concentration is <3-5 μg/mL, it is possible that the observed problem may not be due to lidocaine treatment and other sources can be investigated. Patients receiving lidocaine infusions for longer than 24 hours are prone to unexpected accumulation of lidocaine concentrations in the serum and should be closely monitored for lidocaine side effects.[9-12] While receiving lidocaine, patients should be monitored for the following adverse drug effects: drowsiness, dizziness, paresthesias, euphoria, muscle twitching, confusion, agitation, dysarthria, psychosis, seizures, coma, atrioventricular block, or hypotension.

BASIC CLINICAL PHARMACOKINETIC PARAMETERS

Lidocaine is almost completely eliminated by hepatic metabolism (>95%).[4,13] Hepatic metabolism is mainly via the CYP3A enzyme system. Monoethylglycinexylidide (MEGX) is the primary metabolite resulting from lidocaine metabolism.[6-8] While a portion of MEGX is eliminated renally, most of the metabolite is further converted hepatically to glycinexylidide (GX) and other, inactive metabolites. GX is primarily eliminated by the kidney. MEGX and GX have some antiarrhythmic activity (MEGX ~80% and GX ~10%, relative to lidocaine), but have also been implicated as the cause of some adverse effects attributed to lidocaine therapy.[6-8] Because both metabolites are eliminated by the kidney, patients with renal failure should be monitored for adverse effects due to metabolite accumulation even though lidocaine serum concentrations are within the therapeutic range. The hepatic extraction ratio of lidocaine is about 70%, so lidocaine is typically classified as a high extraction ratio drug. Because of this, it is expected that liver blood flow will be the predominate factor influencing the clearance of lidocaine (Cl ≈ LBF, where Cl is lidocaine clearance and LBF is liver blood flow, both in L/min), and many disease states and conditions that alter lidocaine clearance do so via changes in liver blood flow. However, because a hepatic extraction ratio greater than 70% is the definition of a high extraction ratio agent and the extraction ratio for lidocaine is on the margin of this range, it is very possible that changes in lidocaine intrinsic clearance or plasma protein binding will change lidocaine clearance.

Lidocaine is usually given intravenously but may also be given intramuscularly.[14] After intramuscular injection, absorption is rapid and complete with maximum concentrations occurring about 1 hour after administration and 100% bioavailability as long as the patient's peripheral circulation is not compromised due to hypotension or shock. Intramuscular administration of medications can increase creatine kinase (CK) concentrations due to minor skeletal muscle trauma inflicted by the injection, and this enzyme is monitored in patients who may have had a myocardial infarction. Thus, the creatine kinase isozyme that is relatively specific to the heart (CK-MB) needs to be measured in myocardial infarction patients who have received intramuscular injections. Oral absorption of lidocaine is nearly 100%.[4] However, lidocaine is extensively metabolized by the CYP3A enzymes contained in the intestinal wall and liver resulting in a large first-pass effect and low, variable oral bioavailability (F ≈ 30%). Because roughly 70% of an oral dose is converted to metabolites, MEGX and GX concentrations are high after oral administration of lidocaine resulting in a high incidence of adverse effects.

Lidocaine can also be administered intraosseously or endotracheally. Although the optimal dose of lidocaine administered via an endotracheal tube is not known, it is typically 2-2.5 times the recommended intravenous dose.[3] Lidocaine is given through an endotracheal tube by first diluting the drug with an additional 5-10 mL of sterile water or normal saline, then injecting the entire amount into the tube.

Plasma protein binding in normal individuals is about 70%.[15-17] Of this value, approximately 30% is due to drug binding to albumin while 70% is due to lidocaine bound to α_1-acid glycoprotein (AGP).[9,11,12] AGP is classified as an acute phase reactant protein that is present in lower amounts in all individuals but is secreted in large amounts in response to certain stresses and disease states such as trauma, heart failure, and myocardial infarction. In patients with these disease states, lidocaine binding to AGP can be even larger resulting in an unbound fraction as low as 10%-15%. AGP concentrations continuously increase during the first 12-72 hours after a myocardial infarction, and, as a result, the lidocaine-unbound fraction decreases on average from about 30% to 20% during this time period. The continuous increase in protein binding due to AGP secretion causes a continuous decrease in lidocaine clearance in patients with myocardial infarction, and lidocaine concentrations can accumulate to unexpectedly high levels in patients receiving the drug for longer than 24 hours. Patients without myocardial infarction also experience accumulation of lidocaine concentrations during long-term (>24 hours) infusions due to competition for hepatic metabolism between parent drug and metabolites.[10,18] Thus, monitoring for adverse reactions in patients receiving long-term lidocaine infusions is important, and lidocaine serum concentrations can be useful adjuncts to avoid lidocaine toxicity.

The recommended dose of lidocaine is based on the concurrent disease states and conditions present in the patient that can influence lidocaine concentrations. Lidocaine pharmacokinetic parameters used to compute doses are given in the following section for specific patient profiles.

EFFECTS OF DISEASE STATES AND CONDITIONS ON LIDOCAINE PHARMACOKINETICS AND DOSING

Normal adults without the disease states and conditions given later in this section with normal liver function have an average lidocaine half-life of 1.5 hours (range: 1-2 hours), a central volume of distribution of 0.5 L/kg (Vc = 0.4-0.6 L/kg), and the volume of distribution for the entire body of 1.5 L/kg (V_{area} = 1-2 L/kg; Table 7-1).[4,10,19] Disease states and conditions that change lidocaine pharmacokinetics and dosage requirements may alter clearance, the central volume of distribution, and the volume of distribution for the

TABLE 7-1   Disease States and Conditions That Alter Lidocaine Pharmacokinetics

Disease State/ Condition	Half-Life	Central Volume of Distribution (Vc)	Volume of Distribution for Entire Body (V_{area})	Comment
Adult, normal liver function	1.5 h (range: 1-2 h)	0.5 L/kg (range: 0.4-0.6 L/kg)	1.5 L/kg (range: 1-2 L/kg)	Lidocaine has a high hepatic extraction ratio of ~70%, so liver blood flow is the primary determinate of clearance rate. Accumulation of serum lidocaine concentrations can occur with long-term (>24 h) infusions
Adult, hepatic disease (liver cirrhosis or acute hepatitis)	5 h	0.6 L/kg	2.6 L/kg	Lidocaine is metabolized >95% by hepatic microsomal enzymes (primarily CYP3A), so loss of functional liver tissue, as well as reduced liver blood flow, decreases lidocaine clearance. Pharmacokinetic parameters are highly variable in liver disease patients. Volumes of distribution are larger due to decreased α_1-acid glycoprotein and albumin drug binding in the plasma
Adult, heart failure	2 h	0.3 L/kg	1 L/kg	Decreased liver blood flow secondary to reduced cardiac output reduces lidocaine clearance. Volumes of distribution are smaller due to increased α_1-acid glycoprotein drug binding in the plasma. Heart failure results in large and variable reductions in lidocaine clearance. Cardiac status must be monitored closely in heart failure patients since lidocaine clearance changes with acute changes in cardiac output.
Adult, postmyocardial infarction (<12 h)	4 h	0.5 L/kg	1.5 L/kg	Myocardial infarction reduces cardiac output resulting in variable reductions in lidocaine clearance. These patients are especially prone to accumulation of serum lidocaine concentrations during long-term (>24 h) infusions due to secretion of α_1-acid glycoprotein
Adult, obese (>30% over ideal body weight)	According to other disease states/conditions that affect lidocaine pharmacokinetics	According to other disease states/ conditions that affect lidocaine pharmacokinetics	According to other disease states/ conditions that affect lidocaine pharmacokinetics	Lidocaine doses should be based on ideal body weight for patients who weigh more than 30% above IBW

TABLE 7-2   Child-Pugh Scores for Patients With Liver Disease[24]

Test/Symptom	Score 1 Point	Score 2 Points	Score 3 Points
Total bilirubin (mg/dL)	<2.0	2.0-3.0	>3.0
Serum albumin (g/dL)	>3.5	2.8-3.5	<2.8
Prothrombin time (seconds prolonged over control)	<4	4-6	>6
Ascites	Absent	Slight	Moderate
Hepatic encephalopathy	None	Moderate	Severe

Mild liver disease, 5-6 points; moderate liver disease, 7-9 points; severe liver disease, 10-15 points.

entire body. The volume of distribution for the central compartment of the two-compartment model is used to compute the loading dose because lidocaine distributes rapidly to the myocardium and the heart is considered to reside in the central compartment of the model. The elimination rate constant ($k = 0.693/t_{1/2}$, where $t_{1/2}$ is the half-life) and clearance ($Cl = kV_{area}$) can be computed from the aforementioned pharmacokinetic parameters.

Patients with liver cirrhosis or acute hepatitis have reduced lidocaine clearance which results in a prolonged average lidocaine half-life of 5 hours.[13,20-23] The mechanism for depressed clearance in liver disease patients is destruction of liver parenchyma, where hepatic drug-metabolizing enzymes are present, and reduction of liver blood flow. The central volume of distribution and volume of distribution for the entire body are larger in patients with liver disease because albumin and α_1-acid glycoprotein (AGP) concentrations are lower in these patients and result in reduced lidocaine plasma protein binding (average $Vc = 0.6$ L/kg, average $V_{area} = 2.6$ L/kg). However, the effect that liver disease has on lidocaine pharmacokinetics is highly variable and difficult to accurately predict, especially in patients with acute hepatitis. It is possible for a patient with liver disease to have relatively normal or grossly abnormal lidocaine clearance, volumes of distribution, and half-life. An index of liver dysfunction can be gained by applying the Child-Pugh clinical classification system to the patient (Table 7-2).[24] Child-Pugh scores are completely discussed in Chapter 3 (Drug Dosing in Special Populations: Renal and Hepatic Disease, Dialysis, Heart Failure, Obesity, and Drug Interactions), but will be briefly discussed here. The Child-Pugh score consists of five laboratory tests or clinical symptoms: serum albumin, total bilirubin, prothrombin time, ascites, and hepatic encephalopathy. Each of these areas is given a score of 1 (normal) to 3 (severely abnormal; Table 7-2), and the scores for the five areas are summed. The Child-Pugh score for a patient with normal liver function is 5 while the score for a patient with grossly abnormal serum albumin, total bilirubin, and prothrombin time values in addition to severe ascites and hepatic encephalopathy is 15. A Child-Pugh score greater than 8 is the ground for a decrease in the initial daily drug dose for lidocaine ($t_{1/2} = 5$ hours). As in any patient with or without liver dysfunction, initial doses are meant as starting points for dosage titration based on patient response and avoidance of adverse effects. Lidocaine serum concentrations and the presence of adverse drug effects should be monitored frequently in patients with liver cirrhosis.

Heart failure causes reduced lidocaine clearance because of decreased hepatic blood flow secondary to compromised cardiac output (Table 7-3).[6,13,22,25,26] Patients with cardiogenic shock experience extreme declines in lidocaine clearance due to severe decreases in cardiac output and liver blood flow. Central volume of distribution ($Vc = 0.3$ L/kg) and volume of distribution for the entire body ($V_{area} = 1$ L/kg) are decreased because heart failure patients have elevated AGP serum concentrations which lead to increased lidocaine plasma protein binding and decreased lidocaine unbound fraction. Patients with heart failure have an average lidocaine half-life equal to 2 hours (range: 1-24 hours). Half-life ($t_{1/2}$) does not change as much as expected from the change in clearance (Cl) because the volume of distribution simultaneously decreases [$t_{1/2} = (0.693 \bullet \downarrow V_{area})/\downarrow Cl$]. Obviously, the effect that heart failure has on lidocaine pharmacokinetics is highly variable and difficult to

TABLE 7-3 New York Heart Association (NYHA) Functional Classification for Heart Failure[37]

NYHA Heart Failure Class	Description
I	Patients with cardiac disease but without limitations of physical activity. Ordinary physical activity does not cause undue fatigue, dyspnea, or palpitation
II	Patients with cardiac disease that results in slight limitations of physical activity. Ordinary physical activity results in fatigue, palpitation, dyspnea, or angina
III	Patients with cardiac disease that results in marked limitations of physical activity. Although patients are comfortable at rest, less than ordinary activity will lead to symptoms
IV	Patients with cardiac disease that results in an inability to carry on physical activity without discomfort. Symptoms of congestive heart failure are present even at rest. With any physical activity, increased discomfort is experienced

accurately predict. It is possible for a patient with heart failure to have relatively normal or grossly abnormal lidocaine clearance and half-life. For heart failure patients, initial doses are meant as starting points for dosage titration based on patient response and avoidance of adverse effects. Lidocaine serum concentrations and the presence of adverse drug effects should be monitored frequently in patients with heart failure.

Patients with myocardial infarction may develop serious ventricular arrhythmias that require therapy with lidocaine. After a myocardial infarction, serum AGP concentrations increase up to 50% over a 12-72-hour time period.[9,11,12] As AGP serum concentrations increase, plasma protein binding of lidocaine decreases and the unbound fraction of lidocaine decreases from about 30% to about 20%. Although lidocaine is considered a high hepatic extraction ratio drug with liver blood flow having the major influence on lidocaine clearance, a decline in the unbound fraction of lidocaine in the plasma decreases lidocaine clearance. The reduction in lidocaine clearance is continuous as long as AGP concentrations continue to rise. A result of this phenomenon is lidocaine serum concentrations do not reach steady-state during long-term (>24 h) intravenous infusions of lidocaine in myocardial infarction patients and results of pharmacokinetic studies in this patient population differ according to when the investigation took place in relation to the myocardial damage. When studied within 12 hours of myocardial infarction, patients had decreased lidocaine clearance due to decreased cardiac output and liver blood flow, relatively normal volumes of distribution (V_c = 0.5 L/kg, V_{area} = 1.5 L/kg), and a prolonged half-life of 4 hours.[26-28] When similar myocardial infarction patients are studied after longer lidocaine infusions, the central volume of distribution and volume of distribution representing the entire body are smaller because AGP serum concentrations have had an opportunity to increase and change lidocaine plasma protein binding.[9,11,12]

Although the volume of distribution representing the entire body (V_{area}) correlates most closely with total body weight, obese patients (>30% above ideal body weight or IBW) should have central volume of distribution and clearance estimates based on ideal body weight.[19] Lidocaine pharmacokinetic parameter estimates should be based on the concurrent disease states and conditions present in the patient. If weight-based dosage recommendations are to be used, ideal body weight should be used to compute maintenance infusions (mg/kg/min) and loading doses (mg/kg) for obese individuals.

Patient age has an effect on lidocaine volumes of distribution and half-life.[25] For elderly patients over the age of 65, studies indicate that lidocaine clearance is unchanged, the volumes of distribution are slightly larger, and half-life is longer (average half-life = 2.3 hours, range: 1.7-4.5 hours) compared to younger subjects. A confounding factor found in lidocaine pharmacokinetic studies conducted in older adults is the possible accidental inclusion of subjects that have subclinical or mild cases of the disease states associated with reduced lidocaine clearance (heart failure, liver disease, etc). Additionally, most patients with serious ventricular arrhythmias studied in all of the previously mentioned studies are older and those results include any influence that age may have. Thus, in most cases elderly patients are treated with lidocaine according to the other disease states or conditions present that influence lidocaine pharmacokinetics.

Lidocaine serum concentrations accumulate in patients receiving long-term (>24 h) infusions even if the patient did not have a myocardial infarction.[10,18] Accumulation of lidocaine in these patients is due to competition for hepatic metabolism between parent drug and metabolites. Because MEGX and GX metabolites are eliminated to some extent by the kidney, patients with renal failure should be monitored for lidocaine adverse effects due to metabolite accumulation even though lidocaine serum concentrations are within the therapeutic range. Lidocaine is not appreciably removed by hemodialysis. Because lidocaine has a sieving coefficient of 0.14, continuous hemofiltration does not remove a significant amount of drug.[29,30]

DRUG INTERACTIONS

Lidocaine has serious drug interactions with β-adrenergic receptor blockers and cimetidine that decrease lidocaine clearance by 30% or more.[31] Propranolol, metoprolol, and nadolol have been reported to reduce lidocaine clearance due to the decrease in cardiac output caused by β-blocker agents. Decreased cardiac output results in reduced liver blood flow which explains the decline in lidocaine clearance caused by these drugs. Cimetidine also decreases lidocaine clearance, but the mechanism of the interaction is different. Because cimetidine does not change liver blood flow, it is believed that cimetidine decreases lidocaine clearance by inhibiting hepatic microsomal enzymes.[32,33]

Lidocaine clearance may be accelerated by concomitant use of phenobarbital or phenytoin.[31] Both of these agents are known to be hepatic drug-metabolizing enzyme inducers, and this is the probable mechanism of their drug interaction with lidocaine. It is important to remember that phenytoin has antiarrhythmic effects and is also classified as a type IB antiarrhythmic agent. Because of this, phenytoin and lidocaine may have additive pharmacologic effects that could result in a pharmacodynamic drug interaction.

INITIAL DOSAGE DETERMINATION METHODS

Several methods to initiate lidocaine therapy are available. The *pharmacokinetic dosing method* is the most flexible of the techniques. It allows individualized target serum concentrations to be chosen for a patient, and each pharmacokinetic parameter can be customized to reflect specific disease states and conditions present in the patient. *Literature-based recommended dosing* is a very commonly used method to prescribe initial doses of lidocaine. Doses are based on those that commonly produce steady-state concentrations in the lower end of the therapeutic range, although there is a wide variation in the actual concentrations for a specific patient.

Pharmacokinetic Dosing Method

The goal of initial dosing of lidocaine is to compute the best dose possible for the patient given their set of disease states and conditions that influence lidocaine pharmacokinetics and the arrhythmia being treated. In order to do this, pharmacokinetic parameters for the patient will be estimated using average parameters measured in other patients with similar disease state and condition profiles.

Half-Life and Elimination Rate Constant Estimate

Lidocaine is predominately metabolized by liver. Unfortunately, there is no good way to estimate the elimination characteristics of liver-metabolized drugs using an endogenous marker of liver function in the same manner that serum creatinine and estimated creatinine clearance are used to estimate the elimination of agents that are renally eliminated. Because of this, a patient is categorized according to the disease states and conditions that are known to change lidocaine half-life, and the half-life previously measured in these studies is used as an estimate of the current patient's half-life (Table 7-1). For example, if a patient has suffered an uncomplicated myocardial infarction, lidocaine half-life would be assumed to equal 4 hours. Alternatively, for a patient with moderate heart failure (NYHA CHF class III), lidocaine half-life would be assumed to equal 2 hours, while a patient with severe liver disease (Child-Pugh score = 12) would be assigned an estimated half-life of 5 hours. To produce the most conservative lidocaine doses in patients with multiple concurrent disease states or conditions that affect lidocaine pharmacokinetics, the disease state or condition with the longest half-life should be used to compute doses. This approach will avoid accidental overdosage as much as currently possible. Once the correct half-life is identified for the patient, it can be converted into the lidocaine elimination rate constant (k) using the following equation: $k = 0.693/t_{1/2}$.

Volume of Distribution Estimate

As with the half-life estimate, lidocaine volume of distribution values are chosen according to the disease states and conditions that are present (Table 7-1). The central volume of distribution (Vc) is used to compute loading doses because lidocaine has a rapid onset of action after administration, and the heart acts as if it is in the central compartment of the two-compartment model used to describe lidocaine pharmacokinetics. The central volume of distribution is assumed to equal 0.6 L/kg for liver disease patients, 0.3 L/kg for heart failure and cardiogenic shock patients, and 0.5 L/kg for all other patients. The volume of distribution for the entire body after distribution is complete (V_{area}) is used to help compute lidocaine clearance, and is assumed to equal 2.6 L/kg for liver disease patients, 1 L/kg for heart failure and cardiogenic shock patients, and 1.5 L/kg for all other patients. For obese patients (>30% above ideal body weight), ideal body weight is used to compute lidocaine volume of distribution. Thus, for a nonobese 80 kg patient without heart failure or liver disease, the estimated lidocaine central volume of distribution would be 40 L: Vc = 0.5 L/kg • 80 kg = 40 L. For a 150-kg obese patient with an ideal body weight of 60 kg and normal cardiac and liver function, the estimated lidocaine volume of distribution is 30 L: V = 0.5 L/kg • 60 kg = 30 L.

Selection of Appropriate Pharmacokinetic Model and Equations

When given by continuous intravenous infusion, lidocaine follows a two-compartment pharmacokinetic model (Figures 7-1, 7-2, 7-3). A simple pharmacokinetic equation that computes the lidocaine steady-state serum concentration (Css in μg/mL = mg/L) is widely used and allows dosage calculation for a continuous infusion: $Css = k_0/Cl$ or $k_0 = Css • Cl$, where k_0 is the dose of lidocaine in mg and Cl is lidocaine clearance in L/h. Clearance is computed using estimates of lidocaine elimination rate constant (k) and volume of distribution for the entire body after distribution is complete (V_{area}): $Cl = kV_{area}$. For example, if a patient has an estimated elimination rate constant equal to 0.173 h^{-1} and an estimated volume of distribution equal to 105 L, the estimated clearance would equal 18.2 L/h: Cl = 0.173 h^{-1} • 105 L = 18.2 L/h.

The equation used to calculate an intravenous loading dose (LD in mg) is based on a two-compartment model: LD = (Css • Vc), where Css is the desired lidocaine steady-state concentration in μg/mL which is equivalent to mg/L, and Vc is the lidocaine central volume of distribution. Intravenous lidocaine-loading doses should be given as an intravenous bolus no faster than 25-50 mg/min.

Steady-State Concentration Selection

The general accepted therapeutic range for lidocaine is 1.5-5 μg/mL. However, lidocaine therapy must be individualized for each patient in order to achieve optimal responses and minimal side effects.

EXAMPLE 1 ▶▶▶

LK is a 50-year-old, 75-kg (height = 5 ft 10 in) male with ventricular tachycardia who requires therapy with intravenous lidocaine. He has normal liver and cardiac function. Suggest an initial intravenous lidocaine dosage regimen designed to achieve a steady-state lidocaine concentration equal to 3 µg/mL.

1. *Estimate the half-life and elimination rate constant according to disease states and conditions present in the patient.*

   The expected lidocaine half-life ($t_{1/2}$) is 1.5 hours. The elimination rate constant is computed using the following formula: $k = 0.693/t_{1/2} = 0.693/1.5\ h = 0.462\ h^{-1}$.

2. *Estimate volume of distribution and clearance.*

   The patient is not obese, so the estimated lidocaine central volume of distribution and the volume of distribution for the entire body (V_{area}) will be based on actual body weight: $Vc = 0.5$ L/kg • 75 kg = 38 L, $V_{area} = 1.5$ L/kg • 75 kg = 113 L. Estimated lidocaine clearance is computed by taking the product of V_{area} and the elimination rate constant: $Cl = kV_{area} = 0.462\ h^{-1}$ • 113 L = 52.2 L/h.

3. *Compute dosage regimen.*

   Therapy will be started by administering an intravenous loading dose of lidocaine to the patient (note: µg/mL = mg/L and this concentration unit was substituted for Css in the calculations so that unnecessary unit conversion was not required): LD = Css • Vc = 3 mg/L • 38 L = 114 mg, rounded to 100 mg intravenously over 2-4 minutes. An additional dose equal to 50% of the loading dose can be given if arrhythmias recur 20-30 minutes after the initial loading dose.

   A lidocaine continuous intravenous infusion will be started immediately after the loading dose has been administered. (Note: µg/mL = mg/L and this concentration unit was substituted for Css in the calculations so that unnecessary unit conversion was not required.) The dosage equation for intravenous lidocaine is: $k_0 = $ Css • Cl = (3 mg/L • 52.2 L/h)/(60 min/h) = 2.6 mg/min, rounded to 2.5 mg/min.

A steady-state lidocaine serum concentration could be measured after steady-state is attained in 3-5 half-lives. Since the patient is expected to have a half-life equal to 1.5 hours, the lidocaine steady-state concentration could be obtained any time after the first 8 hours of dosing (5 half-lives = 5 • 1.5 h = 7.5 h). Lidocaine serum concentrations should also be measured if the patient experiences a return of their ventricular arrhythmia, or if the patient develops potential signs or symptoms of lidocaine toxicity.

EXAMPLE 2 ▶▶▶

OI is a 60-year-old, 85-kg (height = 6 ft 1 in) male with ventricular tachycardia who requires therapy with intravenous lidocaine. He has liver cirrhosis (Child-Pugh score = 11). Suggest an initial intravenous lidocaine dosage regimen designed to achieve a steady-state lidocaine concentration equal to 4 µg/mL.

1. *Estimate the half-life and elimination rate constant according to disease states and conditions present in the patient.*

   The expected lidocaine half-life ($t_{1/2}$) is 5 hours. The elimination rate constant is computed using the following formula: $k = 0.693/t_{1/2} = 0.693/5\ h = 0.139\ h^{-1}$.

2. *Estimate volume of distribution and clearance.*

   The patient is not obese, so the estimated lidocaine central volume of distribution and the volume of distribution for the entire body (V_{area}) will be based on actual body weight: $Vc = 0.6$ L/kg • 85 kg = 51 L, $V_{area} = 2.6$ L/kg • 85 kg = 221 L. Estimated lidocaine clearance is computed by taking the product of V_{area} and the elimination rate constant: $Cl = kV_{area} = 0.139\ h^{-1}$ • 221 L = 31 L/h.

3. *Compute dosage regimen.*

Therapy will be started by administering an intravenous loading dose of lidocaine to the patient (note: µg/mL = mg/L and this concentration unit was substituted for Css in the calculations so that unnecessary unit conversion was not required): LD = Css • Vc = 4 mg/L • 51 L = 204 mg, rounded to 200 mg intravenously over 4-8 minutes. An additional dose equal to 50% of the loading dose can be given if arrhythmias recur 20-30 minutes after the initial loading dose.

A lidocaine continuous intravenous infusion will be started immediately after the loading dose has been administered. (Note: µg/mL = mg/L and this concentration unit was substituted for Css in the calculations so that unnecessary unit conversion was not required.) The dosage equation for intravenous lidocaine is: k_0 = Css • Cl = (4 mg/L • 31 L/h)/(60 min/h) = 2.1 mg/min, rounded to 2 mg/min.

A steady-state lidocaine serum concentration could be measured after steady-state is attained in 3-5 half-lives. Since the patient is expected to have a half-life equal to 5 hours, the lidocaine steady-state concentration could be obtained any time after the first day of dosing (5 half-lives = 5 • 5 h = 25 h). Lidocaine serum concentrations should also be measured if the patient experiences a return of their ventricular arrhythmia, or if the patient develops potential signs or symptoms of lidocaine toxicity.

EXAMPLE 3 ▶▶▶

MN is a 64-year-old, 78-kg (height = 5 ft 9 in) male with ventricular tachycardia who requires therapy with intravenous lidocaine. He has moderate heart failure (NYHA CHF class III). Suggest an initial intravenous lidocaine dosage regimen designed to achieve a steady-state lidocaine concentration equal to 3 µg/mL.

1. *Estimate the half-life and elimination rate constant according to disease states and conditions present in the patient.*

The expected lidocaine half-life ($t_{1/2}$) is 2 hours. The elimination rate constant is computed using the following formula: k = $0.693/t_{1/2}$ = 0.693/2 h = 0.347 h^{-1}.

2. *Estimate volume of distribution and clearance.*

The patient is not obese, so the estimated lidocaine central volume of distribution and the volume of distribution for the entire body (V_{area}) will be based on actual body weight: Vc = 0.3 L/kg • 78 kg = 23 L, V_{area} = 1 L/kg • 78 kg = 78 L. Estimated lidocaine clearance is computed by taking the product of V_{area} and the elimination rate constant: Cl = kV_{area} = 0.347 h^{-1} • 78 L = 27 L/h.

3. *Compute dosage regimen.*

Therapy will be started by administering an intravenous loading dose of lidocaine to the patient (note: µg/mL = mg/L and this concentration unit was substituted for Css in the calculations so that unnecessary unit conversion was not required): LD = Css • Vc = 3 mg/L • 23 L = 69 mg, rounded to 75 mg intravenously over 2-3 minutes. An additional dose equal to 50% of the loading dose can be given if arrhythmias recur 20-30 minutes after the initial loading dose.

A lidocaine continuous intravenous infusion will be started immediately after the loading dose has been administered. (Note: µg/mL = mg/L and this concentration unit was substituted for Css in the calculations so that unnecessary unit conversion was not required.) The dosage equation for intravenous lidocaine is: k_0 = Css • Cl = (3 mg/L • 27 L/h)/(60 min/h) = 1.4 mg/min, rounded to 1.5 mg/min.

A steady-state lidocaine serum concentration could be measured after steady-state is attained in 3-5 half-lives. Since the patient is expected to have a half-life equal to 2 hours, the lidocaine steady-state concentration could be obtained any time after the first 10-12 hours of dosing (5 half-lives = 5 • 2 h = 10 h). Lidocaine serum concentrations should also be measured if the patient experiences a return of their ventricular arrhythmia, or if the patient develops potential signs or symptoms of lidocaine toxicity.

Literature-Based Recommended Dosing

Because of the large amount of variability in lidocaine pharmacokinetics, even when concurrent disease states and conditions are identified, many clinicians believe that the use of standard lidocaine doses for various situations is warranted.[34] The original computation of these doses were based on the pharmacokinetic dosing method described in the previous section, and subsequently modified based on clinical experience. In general, the lidocaine steady-state serum concentration expected from the lower end of the dosage range was 1.5-3 μg/mL and 3-5 μg/mL for the upper end of the dosage range. Suggested intravenous lidocaine continuous infusion maintenance doses are 1-2 mg/min for patients with liver disease or heart failure and 3-4 mg/min for all other patients. When more than one disease state or condition is present in a patient, choosing the lowest infusion rate will result in the safest, most conservative dosage recommendation. With regard to loading doses, lidocaine is given intravenously at the dose of 1-1.5 mg/kg (not to exceed 25-50 mg/min) for all patients except those with heart failure. The suggested lidocaine intravenous loading dose for heart failure patients is 0.5-0.75 mg/kg (not to exceed 25-50 mg/min), although some clinicians advocate the administration of full loading doses of lidocaine in heart failure patients. Ideal body weight is used to compute loading doses for obese patients (>30% over ideal body weight).

Pediatric doses are similar to that given to adults when adjusted for differences in body weight. Intravenous loading doses are 1 mg/kg with up to two additional doses, if needed (total dose not to exceed 3-5 mg/kg for first hour). Continuous intravenous infusions doses are 20-50 μg/kg/min. For patients with shock, heart failure, or liver disease patients, initial doses should not exceed 20 μg/kg/min.[35]

To illustrate the similarities and differences between this method of dosage calculation and the Pharmacokinetic Dosing method, the same examples used in the previous section will be used.

EXAMPLE 1 ▶▶▶

LK is a 50-year-old, 75-kg (height = 5 ft 10 in) male with ventricular tachycardia who requires therapy with intravenous lidocaine. He has normal liver and cardiac function. Suggest an initial intravenous lidocaine dosage regimen designed to achieve a steady-state lidocaine concentration equal to 3 μg/mL.

1. *Choose a lidocaine dose based on disease states and conditions present in the patient.*
   A lidocaine-loading dose of 1-1.5 mg/kg and maintenance infusion of 3-4 mg/min is suggested for a patient without heart failure or liver disease.

2. *Compute dosage regimen.*
   Because the desired concentration is in the lower end of the therapeutic range, a dose in the lower end of the suggested ranges will be used. A lidocaine-loading dose of 1 mg/kg will be administered: LD = 1 mg/kg • 75 kg = 75 mg over 1.5-3 minutes. A lidocaine maintenance infusion equal to 3 mg/min would be administered after the loading dose was given. An additional dose equal to 50% of the loading dose can be given if arrhythmias recur 20-30 minutes after the initial loading dose.

   A steady-state lidocaine serum concentration could be measured after steady-state is attained in 3-5 half-lives. Since the patient is expected to have a half-life equal to 1.5 hours, the lidocaine steady-state concentration could be obtained any time after the first 8 hours of dosing (5 half-lives = 5 • 1.5 h = 7.5 h). Lidocaine serum concentrations should also be measured if the patient experiences a return of their ventricular arrhythmia, or if the patient develops potential signs or symptoms of lidocaine toxicity.

EXAMPLE 2 ▶▶▶

OI is a 60-year-old, 85 kg (height = 6 ft 1 in) male with ventricular tachycardia who requires therapy with intravenous lidocaine. He has liver cirrhosis (Child-Pugh score = 11). Suggest an initial intravenous lidocaine dosage regimen designed to achieve a steady-state lidocaine concentration equal to 4 μg/mL.

1. *Choose the lidocaine dose based on disease states and conditions present in the patient.*
   A lidocaine-loading dose of 1-1.5 mg/kg and maintenance infusion of 1-2 mg/min is suggested for a patient with liver disease.

2. *Compute dosage regimen.*
   Because the desired concentration is in the upper end of the therapeutic range, a dose in the upper end of the suggested ranges will be used. A lidocaine loading dose of 1.5 mg/kg will be administered: LD = 1.5 mg/kg • 85 kg = 128 mg, rounded to 150 mg over 3-6 minutes. A lidocaine maintenance infusion equal to 2 mg/min would be administered after the loading dose was given. An additional dose equal to 50% of the loading dose can be given if arrhythmias recur 20-30 minutes after the initial loading dose.

   A steady-state lidocaine serum concentration could be measured after steady-state is attained in 3-5 half-lives. Since the patient is expected to have a half-life equal to 5 hours, the lidocaine steady-state concentration could be obtained any time after the first day of dosing (5 half-lives = 5 • 5 h = 25 h). Lidocaine serum concentrations should also be measured if the patient experiences a return of their ventricular arrhythmia, or if the patient develops potential signs or symptoms of lidocaine toxicity.

EXAMPLE 3 ▶▶▶

MN is a 64-year-old, 78-kg (height = 5 ft 9 in) male with ventricular tachycardia who requires therapy with intravenous lidocaine. He has moderate heart failure (NYHA CHF class III). Suggest an initial intravenous lidocaine dosage regimen designed to achieve a steady-state lidocaine concentration equal to 3 μg/mL.

1. *Choose a lidocaine dose based on disease states and conditions present in the patient.*
   A lidocaine loading dose of 0.5-0.75 mg/kg and maintenance infusion of 1-2 mg/min is suggested for a patient with heart failure.

2. *Compute dosage regimen.*
   Because the desired concentration is in the lower end of the therapeutic range, a dose in the lower end of the suggested ranges will be used. A lidocaine loading dose of 0.5 mg/kg will be administered: LD = 0.5 mg/kg • 78 kg = 39 mg, rounded to 50 mg over 1-2 minutes. A lidocaine maintenance infusion equal to 1 mg/min would be administered after the loading dose was given. An additional dose equal to 50% of the loading dose can be given if arrhythmias recur 20-30 minutes after the initial loading dose.

   A steady-state lidocaine serum concentration could be measured after steady-state is attained in 3-5 half-lives. Since the patient is expected to have a half-life equal to 2 hours, the lidocaine steady-state concentration could be obtained any time after the first 10-12 hours of dosing (5 half-lives = 5 • 2 h = 10 h). Lidocaine serum concentrations should also be measured if the patient experiences a return of their ventricular arrhythmia, or if the patient develops potential signs or symptoms of lidocaine toxicity.

USE OF LIDOCAINE SERUM CONCENTRATIONS TO ALTER DOSES

Because of the large amount of pharmacokinetic variability among patients, it is likely that doses computed using patient population characteristics will not always produce lidocaine serum concentrations that are expected or desirable. Because of pharmacokinetic variability, the narrow therapeutic index of lidocaine, and the desire to avoid lidocaine adverse side effects, measurement of lidocaine serum concentrations can be a useful adjunct for patients to insure that therapeutic, nontoxic levels are present. In addition to lidocaine serum concentrations, important patient parameters (electrocardiogram, clinical signs and symptoms of the ventricular arrhythmia, potential lidocaine side effects, etc) should be followed to confirm that the patient is responding to treatment and not developing adverse drug reactions.

When lidocaine serum concentrations are measured in patients and a dosage change is necessary, clinicians should seek to use the simplest, most straightforward method available to determine a dose that will provide safe and effective treatment. In most cases, a simple dosage ratio can be used to change lidocaine doses assuming the drug follows *linear pharmacokinetics*. Although it has been clearly demonstrated in research studies that lidocaine serum concentrations accumulate in patients during long-term (>24 hours) infusions, in the clinical setting most patients' steady-state serum concentrations change proportionally to lidocaine dose for shorter infusion times. Thus, it is assumed that linear pharmacokinetics is adequate for dosage adjustments in most patients.

Sometimes, it is useful to compute lidocaine pharmacokinetic constants for a patient and base dosage adjustments on these. In this case, it may be possible to calculate and use *pharmacokinetic parameters* to alter the lidocaine dose.

In some situations, it may be necessary to compute lidocaine clearance for the patient during a continuous infusion before steady-state conditions occur and utilize this pharmacokinetic parameter to calculate the best drug dose. Computerized methods that incorporate expected population pharmacokinetic characteristics (*Bayesian pharmacokinetic computer programs*) can be used in difficult cases where serum concentrations are obtained at suboptimal times or the patient was not at steady-state when serum concentrations were measured. An additional benefit is that a complete pharmacokinetic workup (determination of clearance, volume of distribution, and half-life) can be done with one or more measured concentrations that do not have to be at steady-state.

Linear Pharmacokinetics Method

Because lidocaine follows linear, dose-proportional pharmacokinetics in most patients during short-term infusions (<24 hours), steady-state serum concentrations change in proportion to dose according to the following equation: $D_{new}/C_{ss,new} = D_{old}/C_{ss,old}$ or $D_{new} = (C_{ss,new}/C_{ss,old})D_{old}$, where D is the dose, Css is the steady-state concentration, old indicates the dose that produced the steady-state concentration that the patient is currently receiving, and new denotes the dose necessary to produce the desired steady-state concentration. The advantages of this method are that it is quick and simple. The disadvantages are steady-state concentrations are required, and the accumulation of serum lidocaine concentrations can occur with long-term (>24 hours) infusions. When steady-state serum concentrations are higher than expected during long-term lidocaine infusions, lidocaine accumulation pharmacokinetics is a possible explanation for the observation. Because of this, suggested dosage increases greater than 75% using this method should be scrutinized by the prescribing clinician, and the risk versus benefit for the patient assessed before initiating large dosage increases (>75% over current dose).

EXAMPLE 1 ▶▶▶

LK is a 50-year-old, 75-kg (height = 5 ft 10 in) male with ventricular tachycardia who requires therapy with intravenous lidocaine. He has normal liver and cardiac function. The current steady-state lidocaine concentration equals 2.2 μg/mL at a dose of 2 mg/min. Compute a lidocaine dose that will provide a steady-state concentration of 4 μg/mL.

1. *Compute new dose to achieve the desired serum concentration.*

The patient would be expected to achieve steady-state conditions after 8 hours (5 $t_{1/2}$ = 5 • 1.5 h = 7.5 h) of therapy.

Using linear pharmacokinetics, the new dose to attain the desired concentration should be proportional to the old dose that produced the measured concentration:

$$D_{new} = (C_{ss,new}/C_{ss,old})D_{old} = (4 \text{ μg/mL} /2.2 \text{ μg/mL}) \ 2 \text{ mg/min} = 3.6 \text{ mg/min, rounded to } 3.5 \text{ mg/min}$$

The new suggested dose would be 3.5 mg/min of intravenous lidocaine to be started immediately.

A steady-state lidocaine serum concentration could be measured after steady-state is attained in 3-5 half-lives. Since the patient is expected to have a half-life equal to 1.5 hours, the lidocaine steady-state concentration could be obtained any time after the first 8 hours of dosing (5 half-lives = 5 • 1.5 h = 7.5 h). Lidocaine serum concentrations should also be measured if the patient experiences a return of their ventricular arrhythmia, or if the patient develops potential signs or symptoms of lidocaine toxicity.

EXAMPLE 2 ▶▶▶

OI is a 60-year-old, 85-kg (height = 6 ft 1 in) male with ventricular tachycardia who requires therapy with intravenous lidocaine. He has liver cirrhosis (Child-Pugh score = 11). The current steady-state lidocaine concentration equals 6.4 μg/mL at a dose of 2 mg/min. Compute a lidocaine dose that will provide a steady-state concentration of 3 μg/mL.

1. *Compute new dose to achieve the desired serum concentration.*

The patient would be expected to achieve steady-state conditions after a day (5 $t_{1/2}$ = 5 • 5 h = 25 h) of therapy.

Using linear pharmacokinetics, the new dose to attain the desired concentration should be proportional to the old dose that produced the measured concentration:

$$D_{new} = (C_{ss,new}/C_{ss,old})D_{old} = (3 \text{ μg/mL} /6.4 \text{ μg/mL}) \ 2 \text{ mg/min} = 0.9 \text{ mg/min, rounded to } 1 \text{ mg/min}$$

The new suggested dose would be 1 mg/min of intravenous lidocaine. If the patient was experiencing adverse drug effects, the infusion could be held for one estimated half-life (5 h) until the new dose was started.

A steady-state lidocaine serum concentration could be measured after steady-state is attained in 3-5 half-lives. Since the patient is expected to have a half-life equal to 5 hours, the lidocaine steady-state concentration could be obtained any time after the first day of dosing (5 half-lives = 5 • 5 h = 25 h). Lidocaine serum concentrations should also be measured if the patient experiences a return of their ventricular arrhythmia, or if the patient develops potential signs or symptoms of lidocaine toxicity.

EXAMPLE 3 ▶▶▶

MN is a 64-year-old, 78-kg (height = 5 ft 9 in) male with ventricular tachycardia who requires therapy with intravenous lidocaine. He has moderate heart failure (NYHA CHF class III). The current steady-state lidocaine concentration equals 2.2 μg/mL at a dose of 1 mg/min. Compute a lidocaine dose that will provide a steady-state concentration of 4 μg/mL.

1. *Compute new dose to achieve the desired serum concentration.*

The patient would be expected to achieve steady-state conditions after 10-12 hours ($5\,t_{1/2} = 5 \bullet 2\,h = 10\,h$) of therapy.

Using linear pharmacokinetics, the new dose to attain the desired concentration should be proportional to the old dose that produced the measured concentration:

$$D_{new} = (C_{ss,new}/C_{ss,old})D_{old} = (4\,\mu g/mL\,/2.2\,\mu g/mL)\,1\,mg/min = 1.8\,mg/min, \text{ rounded to } 2\,mg/min$$

The new suggested dose would be 2 mg/min of intravenous lidocaine to begin immediately.

A steady-state lidocaine serum concentration could be measured after steady-state is attained in 3-5 half-lives. Since the patient is expected to have a half-life equal to 2 hours, the lidocaine steady-state concentration could be obtained any time after the first 10-12 hours of dosing (5 half-lives = $5 \bullet 2\,h = 10\,h$). Lidocaine serum concentrations should also be measured if the patient experiences a return of their ventricular arrhythmia, or if the patient develops potential signs or symptoms of lidocaine toxicity.

Pharmacokinetic Parameter Method

The Pharmacokinetic Parameter method of adjusting drug doses was among the first techniques available to change doses using serum concentrations. It allows the computation of an individual's own, unique pharmacokinetic constants and uses those to calculate a dose that achieves desired lidocaine concentrations. The Pharmacokinetic Parameter method requires that steady-state has been achieved and uses only a steady-state lidocaine concentration (Css in mg/L or µg/mL). During a continuous intravenous infusion, the following equation is used to compute lidocaine clearance (Cl in L/min): $Cl = k_0/Css$, where k_0 is the dose of lidocaine in mg/min. The clearance measured using this technique is the patient's own, unique lidocaine pharmacokinetic constant and can be used in the intravenous continuous infusion equation to compute the required dose (k_0 in mg/min) to achieve any desired steady-state serum concentration (Css in mg/L or µg/mL): $k_0 = CssCl$, where Cl is lidocaine clearance in L/min. Because this method also assumes linear pharmacokinetics, lidocaine doses computed using the Pharmacokinetic Parameter method and the Linear Pharmacokinetic method should be identical.

EXAMPLE 1 ▶▶▶

LK is a 50-year-old, 75-kg (height = 5 ft 10 in) male with ventricular tachycardia who requires therapy with intravenous lidocaine. He has normal liver and cardiac function. The current steady-state lidocaine concentration equals 2.2 µg/mL at a dose of 2 mg/min. Compute a lidocaine dose that will provide a steady-state concentration of 4 µg/mL.

1. *Compute pharmacokinetic parameters.*

The patient would be expected to achieve steady-state conditions after the first 8 hours ($5\,t_{1/2} = 1.5 \bullet 5\,h = 7.5\,h$) of therapy.

Lidocaine clearance can be computed using a steady-state lidocaine concentration $Cl = k_0/Css = (2\,mg/min)/(2.2\,mg/L) = 0.91\,L/min$. (Note: µg/mL = mg/L and this concentration unit was substituted for Css in the calculations so that unnecessary unit conversion was not required.)

2. *Compute lidocaine dose.*

Lidocaine clearance is used to compute the new lidocaine infusion rate: $k_0 = Css \bullet Cl = 4\,mg/L \bullet 0.91\,L/min = 3.6\,mg/min$, round to 3.5 mg/min.

The new lidocaine infusion rate would be instituted immediately.

A steady-state lidocaine serum concentration could be measured after steady-state is attained in 3-5 half-lives. Since the patient is expected to have a half-life equal to 1.5 hours, the lidocaine steady-state concentration could be obtained any time after the first 8 hours of dosing (5 half-lives = $5 \bullet 1.5\,h = 7.5\,h$). Lidocaine serum concentrations should also be measured if the patient experiences a return of their ventricular arrhythmia, or if the patient develops potential signs or symptoms of lidocaine toxicity.

EXAMPLE 2 ▶▶▶

OI is a 60-year-old, 85-kg (height = 6 ft 1 in) male with ventricular tachycardia who requires therapy with intravenous lidocaine. He has liver cirrhosis (Child-Pugh score = 11). The current steady-state lidocaine concentration equals 6.4 μg/mL at a dose of 2 mg/min. Compute a lidocaine dose that will provide a steady-state concentration of 3 μg/mL.

1. *Compute pharmacokinetic parameters.*

   The patient would be expected to achieve steady-state conditions after a day (5 $t_{1/2}$ = 5 • 5 h = 25 h) of therapy.

   Lidocaine clearance can be computed using a steady-state lidocaine concentration Cl = k_0/Css = (2 mg/min)/(6.4 mg/L) = 0.31 L/min. (Note: μg/mL = mg/L and this concentration unit was substituted for Css in the calculations so that unnecessary unit conversion was not required.)

2. *Compute lidocaine dose.*

   Lidocaine clearance is used to compute the new lidocaine infusion rate: k_0 = Css • Cl = 3 mg/L • 0.31 L/min = 0.9 mg/min, round to 1 mg/min.

   The new suggested dose would be 1 mg/min of intravenous lidocaine. If the patient was experiencing adverse drug effects, the infusion could be held for one estimated half-life (5 h) until the new dose was started.

   A steady-state lidocaine serum concentration could be measured after steady-state is attained in 3-5 half-lives. Since the patient is expected to have a half-life equal to 5 hours, the lidocaine steady-state concentration could be obtained any time after the first day of dosing (5 half-lives = 5 • 5 h = 25 h). Lidocaine serum concentrations should also be measured if the patient experiences a return of their ventricular arrhythmia, or if the patient develops potential signs or symptoms of lidocaine toxicity.

EXAMPLE 3 ▶▶▶

MN is a 64-year-old, 78-kg (height = 5 ft 9 in) male with ventricular tachycardia who requires therapy with intravenous lidocaine. He has moderate heart failure (NYHA CHF class III). The current steady-state lidocaine concentration equals 2.2 μg/mL at a dose of 1 mg/min. Compute a lidocaine dose that will provide a steady-state concentration of 4 μg/mL.

1. *Compute pharmacokinetic parameters.*

   The patient would be expected to achieve steady-state conditions after 10-12 hours (5 $t_{1/2}$ = 5 • 2 h = 10 h) of therapy.

   Lidocaine clearance can be computed using a steady-state lidocaine concentration Cl = k_0/Css = (1 mg/min)/(2.2 mg/L) = 0.45 L/min. (Note: μg/mL = mg/L and this concentration unit was substituted for Css in the calculations so that unnecessary unit conversion was not required.)

2. *Compute lidocaine dose.*

   Lidocaine clearance is used to compute the new lidocaine infusion rate: k_0 = Css • Cl = 4 mg/L • 0.45 L/min = 1.8 mg/min, round to 2 mg/min.

   The new suggested dose would be 2 mg/min of intravenous lidocaine is to begin immediately.

   A steady-state lidocaine serum concentration could be measured after steady-state is attained in 3-5 half-lives. Since the patient is expected to have a half-life equal to 2 hours, the lidocaine steady-state concentration could be obtained any time after the first 10-12 hours of dosing (5 half-lives = 5 • 2 h = 10 h). Lidocaine serum concentrations should also be measured if the patient experiences a return of their ventricular arrhythmia, or if the patient develops potential signs or symptoms of lidocaine toxicity.

BAYESIAN PHARMACOKINETIC COMPUTER PROGRAMS

Computer programs are available that can assist in the computation of pharmacokinetic parameters for patients. The most reliable computer programs use a nonlinear regression algorithm that incorporates components of Bayes theorem. Nonlinear regression is a statistical technique that uses an iterative process to compute the best pharmacokinetic parameters for a concentration/time data set. Briefly, the patient's drug dosage schedule and serum concentrations are input into the computer. The computer program has a pharmacokinetic equation preprogrammed for the drug and administration method (oral, intravenous bolus, intravenous infusion, etc). Typically, a one-compartment model is used, although some programs allow the user to choose among several different equations. Using population estimates based on demographic information for the patient (age, weight, gender, liver function, cardiac status, etc) supplied by the user, the computer program then computes estimated serum concentrations at each time there are actual serum concentrations. Kinetic parameters are then changed by the computer program, and a new set of estimated serum concentrations are computed. The pharmacokinetic parameters that generated the estimated serum concentrations closest to the actual values are remembered by the computer program, and the process is repeated until the set of pharmacokinetic parameters that result in estimated serum concentrations that are statistically closest to the actual serum concentrations are generated. These pharmacokinetic parameters can then be used to compute improved dosing schedules for patients. Bayes theorem is used in the computer algorithm to balance the results of the computations between values based solely on the patient's serum drug concentrations and those based only on patient population parameters. Results from studies that compare various methods of dosage adjustment have consistently found that these types of computer dosing programs perform at least as well as experienced clinical pharmacokineticists and clinicians and better than inexperienced clinicians.

Some clinicians use Bayesian pharmacokinetic computer programs exclusively to alter drug doses based on serum concentrations. An advantage of this approach is that consistent dosage recommendations are made when several different practitioners are involved in therapeutic drug monitoring programs. However, since simpler dosing methods work just as well for patients with stable pharmacokinetic parameters and steady-state drug concentrations, many clinicians reserve the use of computer programs for more difficult situations. Those situations include serum concentrations that are not at steady-state, serum concentrations not obtained at the specific times needed to employ simpler methods, and unstable pharmacokinetic parameters. Many Bayesian pharmacokinetic computer programs are available to users, and most should provide answers similar to the one used in the following examples. The program used to solve problems in this book is DrugCalc written by Dr. Dennis Mungall.[36]

EXAMPLE 1 ▶▶▶

OY is a 57-year-old, 79-kg (height = 5 ft 8 in) male with ventricular tachycardia who requires therapy with intravenous lidocaine. He has normal liver (bilirubin = 0.7 mg/dL, albumin = 4.0 g/dL) and cardiac function. He received a 100-mg loading dose of lidocaine at 0800 H and a continuous intravenous infusion of lidocaine was started at 0810 H at the rate of 2 mg/min. The lidocaine serum concentration equals 2.1 μg/mL at 1030 H. Compute a lidocaine infusion rate that will provide a steady-state concentration of 4 μg/mL.

1. *Enter the patient's demographic, drug dosing, and serum concentration/time data into the computer program.*
   In this patient case, it is unlikely that the patient is at steady-state so the Linear Pharmacokinetics method cannot be used. The DrugCalc program requires lidocaine infusion rates be input in terms of mg/h. A 2-mg/min infusion rate is equivalent to 120 mg/h (k_0 = 2 mg/min • 60 min/h = 120 mg/h).

2. *Compute pharmacokinetic parameters for the patient using Bayesian pharmacokinetic computer program.*

The pharmacokinetic parameters computed by the program are a volume of distribution for the entire body (V_{area}) of 100 L, a half-life equal to 1.6 h, and a clearance equal to 43.6 L/h.

3. *Compute the dose required to achieve desired lidocaine serum concentrations.*

The continuous intravenous infusion equation used by the program to compute doses indicates that a dose of 180 mg/h or 3 mg/min ($k_0 = (180 \text{ mg/h})/(60 \text{ mg/h}) = 3$ mg/min) will produce a steady-state lidocaine concentration of 4.1 µg/mL. This infusion rate would be started immediately.

EXAMPLE 2 ▶▶▶

SL is a 71-year-old, 82 kg (height = 5 ft 10 in) male with ventricular tachycardia who requires therapy with intravenous lidocaine. He has liver cirrhosis (Child-Pugh score = 12, bilirubin = 3.2 mg/dL, albumin = 2.5 g/dL) and normal cardiac function. He received a 150 mg loading dose of lidocaine at 1300 H and a continuous intravenous infusion of lidocaine was started at 1305 H at the rate of 2 mg/min. The lidocaine serum concentration equals 5.7 µg/mL at 2300 H. Compute a lidocaine infusion rate that will provide a steady-state concentration of 4 µg/mL.

1. *Enter the patient's demographic, drug-dosing, and serum concentration/time data into the computer program.*

In this patient case, it is unlikely that the patient is at steady-state so the Linear Pharmacokinetics method cannot be used. The DrugCalc program requires lidocaine infusion rates be input in terms of mg/h. A 2-mg/min infusion rate is equivalent to 120 mg/h ($k_0 = 2$ mg/min • 60 min/h = 120 mg/h).

2. *Compute the pharmacokinetic parameters for the patient using Bayesian pharmacokinetic computer program.*

The pharmacokinetic parameters computed by the program are a volume of distribution for the entire body (V_{area}) of 142 L, a half-life equal to 6.5 h, and a clearance equal to 15 L/h.

3. *Compute the dose required to achieve desired lidocaine serum concentrations.*

The continuous intravenous infusion equation used by the program to compute doses indicates that a dose of 60 mg/h or 1 mg/min [$k_0 = (60 \text{ mg/h})/(60 \text{ mg/h}) = 1$ mg/min] will produce a steady-state lidocaine concentration of 4 µg/mL. This infusion rate could be started immediately, or if the patient was experiencing adverse drug effects, the infusion could be held for ½ to 1 half-life to allow lidocaine serum concentrations to decline and restarted at that time.

EXAMPLE 3 ▶▶▶

TR is a 75-year-old, 85-kg (height = 5 ft 8 in) male with ventricular tachycardia who requires therapy with intravenous lidocaine. He has moderate heart failure (NYHA CHF class III). He received a 75-mg loading dose of lidocaine at 0100 H and a continuous intravenous infusion of lidocaine was started at 0115 H at the rate of 1 mg/min. The lidocaine serum concentration equals 1.7 µg/mL at 0400 H. Compute a lidocaine infusion rate that will provide a steady-state concentration of 3 µg/mL.

1. *Enter the patient's demographic, drug-dosing, and serum concentration/time data into the computer program.*

In this patient case, it is unlikely that the patient is at steady-state so the Linear Pharmacokinetics method cannot be used. The DrugCalc program requires lidocaine infusion rates be input in terms of mg/h. A 1 mg/min infusion rate is equivalent to 60 mg/h ($k_0 = 1$ mg/min • 60 min/h = 60 mg/h).

2. *Compute the pharmacokinetic parameters for the patient using Bayesian pharmacokinetic computer program.*

The pharmacokinetic parameters computed by the program are a volume of distribution for the entire body (V_{area}) of 74 L, a half-life equal to 1.8 h, and a clearance equal to 29 L/h.

3. *Compute the dose required to achieve desired lidocaine serum concentrations.*
The continuous intravenous infusion equation used by the program to compute doses indicates that a dose of 90 mg/h or 1.5 mg/min [$k_0 = (90 \text{ mg/h})/(60 \text{ mg/h}) = 1.5 \text{ mg/min}$] will produce a steady-state lidocaine concentration of 3 µg/mL. This infusion rate would be started immediately.

DOSING STRATEGIES

Initial dose and dosage adjustment techniques using serum concentrations can be used in any combination as long as the limitations of each method are observed. Some dosing schemes link together logically when considered according to their basic approaches or philosophies. Dosage strategies that follow similar pathways are given in Table 7-4.

USE OF LIDOCAINE BOOSTER DOSES TO IMMEDIATELY INCREASE SERUM CONCENTRATIONS

If a patient has a subtherapeutic lidocaine serum concentration and is experiencing ventricular arrhythmias in an acute situation, it is desirable to increase the lidocaine concentration as quickly as possible. In this setting, it would not be acceptable to simply increase the maintenance dose and wait 3-5 half-lives for therapeutic serum concentrations to be established in the patient. A rational way to increase the serum concentrations rapidly is to administer a booster dose of lidocaine, a process also known as "reloading" the patient with lidocaine, computed using pharmacokinetic techniques. A modified loading dose equation is used to accomplish computation of the booster dose (BD) which takes into account the current lidocaine concentration present in the patient: $BD = (C_{desired} - C_{actual})V_c$, where $C_{desired}$ is the desired lidocaine concentration, C_{actual} is the actual current lidocaine concentration for the patient, and V_c is the central volume of distribution for lidocaine. If the central volume of distribution for lidocaine is known for the patient, it can be used in the calculation. However, this value is not usually known and is typically assumed to equal the population average appropriate for the disease states and conditions present in the patient (Table 7-1).

Concurrent with the administration of the booster dose, the maintenance dose of lidocaine is usually increased. Clinicians need to recognize that the administration of a booster dose does not alter the time required to achieve steady-state conditions when a new lidocaine dosage rate is prescribed (Figure 7-3). It still requires 3-5 half-lives to attain steady-state when the dosage rate is changed. However, usually the difference between the post-booster dose lidocaine concentration and the ultimate steady-state concentration has been reduced by giving the extra dose of drug.

TABLE 7-4   Dosing Strategies

Dosing Approach/Philosophy	Initial Dosing	Use of Serum Concentrations to Alter Doses
Pharmacokinetic parameters/equations	Pharmacokinetic Dosing method	Pharmacokinetic Parameter method
Literature-based concept	Literature-based recommended dosing	Linear Pharmacokinetic method
Computerized	Bayesian computer program	Bayesian computer program

EXAMPLE 1 ▶ ▶ ▶

BN is a 57-year-old, 50-kg (height = 5 ft 2 in) female with ventricular tachycardia who is receiving therapy with intravenous lidocaine. She has normal liver function and does not have heart failure. After receiving an initial loading dose of lidocaine (75 mg) and a maintenance infusion of lidocaine equal to 2 mg/min for 2 hours, her arrhythmia reappears and a lidocaine concentration is measured at 1.2 μg/mL. Compute a booster dose of lidocaine to achieve a lidocaine concentration equal to 4 μg/mL.

1. *Estimate volume of distribution according to disease states and conditions present in the patient.*
   In the case of lidocaine, the population average central volume of distribution equals 0.5 L/kg and this will be used to estimate the parameter for the patient. The patient is nonobese, so her actual body weight will be used in the computation: V = 0.5 L/kg • 50 kg = 25 L.

2. *Compute booster dose.*
   The booster dose is computed using the following equation: BD = $(C_{desired} - C_{actual})$ Vc = (4 mg/L – 1.2 mg/L) 25 L = 70 mg, rounded to 75 mg of lidocaine intravenously over 1.5-3 minutes. (Note: μg/mL = mg/L and this concentration unit was substituted for C in the calculations so that unnecessary unit conversion was not required.) If the maintenance dose was increased, it will take an additional 3-5 estimated half-lives for new steady-state conditions to be achieved. Lidocaine serum concentrations could be measured at this time. Lidocaine serum concentrations should also be measured if the patient experiences a return of their ventricular arrhythmia, or if the patient develops potential signs or symptoms of lidocaine toxicity.

PROBLEMS

The following problems are intended to emphasize the computation of initial and individualized doses using clinical pharmacokinetic techniques. Clinicians should always consult the patient's chart to confirm that current antiarrhythmic and other drug therapy is appropriate. Additionally, all other medications that the patient is taking, including prescription and nonprescription drugs, should be noted and checked to ascertain if a potential drug interaction with lidocaine exists.

1. VC is a 67-year-old, 72-kg (height = 6 ft 1 in) male with ventricular tachycardia who requires therapy with intravenous lidocaine. He has normal liver function and does not have heart failure. Suggest an initial lidocaine dosage regimen designed to achieve a steady-state lidocaine concentration equal to 3 μg/mL.

2. Patient VC (see problem 1) was prescribed intravenous lidocaine at a rate of 2 mg/min after receiving a loading dose. The current steady-state lidocaine concentration equals 2.5 μg/mL. Compute a new lidocaine infusion rate that will provide a steady-state concentration of 4 μg/mL.

3. EM is a 56-year-old, 81-kg (height = 5 ft 9 in) male with ventricular tachycardia who requires therapy with intravenous lidocaine. He has liver cirrhosis (Child-Pugh score = 10) and does not have heart failure. Suggest an initial lidocaine dosage regimen designed to achieve a steady-state lidocaine concentration equal to 4 μg/mL.

4. Patient EM (see problem 3) was prescribed intravenous lidocaine at the rate of 2 mg/min. The current steady-state lidocaine concentration equals 6.2 μg/mL. Compute a new intravenous lidocaine continuous infusion that will provide a steady-state concentration of 4 μg/mL.

5. OF is a 71-year-old, 60-kg (height = 5 ft 2 in) female with ventricular tachycardia who requires therapy with intravenous lidocaine. She has severe heart failure (NYHA CHF class IV) and normal liver function. Suggest an initial lidocaine dosage regimen designed to achieve a steady-state lidocaine concentration equal to 5 μg/mL.

6. Patient OF (see problem 5) was prescribed a lidocaine continuous infusion at the rate of 2 mg/min after receiving a loading dose. A steady-state lidocaine serum concentration was obtained and equaled 6.7 µg/mL. Compute a new intravenous lidocaine continuous infusion that will provide a steady-state concentration of 4 µg/mL.

7. FK is a 67-year-old, 130-kg (height = 5 ft 11 in) male with ventricular tachycardia who requires therapy with intravenous lidocaine. He has severe heart failure (NYHA CHF class IV) and normal liver function. Suggest an initial lidocaine dosage regimen designed to achieve a steady-state lidocaine concentration equal to 3 µg/mL.

8. Patient FK (see problem 7) was prescribed intravenous lidocaine. A lidocaine-loading dose of 150 mg was given at 1230 H followed by a continuous infusion of 2 mg/min starting at 1245 H. A lidocaine serum concentration was obtained at 1630 H and equaled to 6.2 µg/mL. Compute a new lidocaine dose that will provide a steady-state concentration of 4 µg/mL.

9. GP is a 76-year-old, 90-kg (height = 5 ft 11 in) male who suffered a myocardial infarction. Three hours after his heart attack, he developed ventricular tachycardia and requires therapy with intravenous lidocaine. He has a normal liver function and does not have heart failure. Suggest an initial intravenous lidocaine dosage regimen designed to achieve a steady-state lidocaine concentration equal to 4 µg/mL.

10. Patient GP (please see problem 9) was prescribed intravenous lidocaine at a rate of 2 mg/min 15 minutes after receiving a 100 mg loading dose at 1520 H. At 1930 H, the lidocaine concentration equals 1.9 µg/mL. Compute a new lidocaine infusion rate that will provide a steady-state concentration of 4 µg/mL.

11. CV is a 69-year-old, 90-kg (height 6 ft 1 in) male with ventricular tachycardia who requires therapy with intravenous lidocaine. He has liver cirrhosis (Child-Pugh score = 11, total bilirubin = 2.7 mg/dL, albumin = 2.1 g/dL) and moderate heart failure (NYHA CHF class III). At 0200 H, he received 100 mg of intravenous lidocaine as a loading dose, and a maintenance intravenous infusion of 2 mg/min was started at 0215 H. Because the patient was experiencing mental status changes, the lidocaine infusion rate was decreased to 1 mg/min at 0900 H. A lidocaine serum concentration was measured at 1000 H and equaled to 5.4 µg/mL. Suggest a lidocaine continuous infusion rate that would achieve a steady-state concentration equal to 3 µg/mL.

12. FP is a 59-year-old, 90-kg (height 5 ft 4 in) female with ventricular tachycardia who requires therapy with intravenous lidocaine. She has liver cirrhosis (Child-Pugh score = 9) and has mild heart failure (NYHA CHF class II). At 1130 H, she received 100 mg of intravenous lidocaine as a loading dose, and a maintenance intravenous infusion of 3 mg/min was started at 1200 H. Because the patient was experiencing confusion, agitation, and dysarthria, the lidocaine infusion rate was decreased to 1 mg/min at 1500 H. At 2000 H, the patient began experiencing ventricular tachycardia and an additional lidocaine booster dose of 100 mg was given while the continuous infusion was left unchanged. A lidocaine serum concentration was measured at 2200 H and equaled to 4.3 µg/mL. Suggest a lidocaine continuous infusion rate that would achieve a steady-state concentration equal to 5 µg/mL.

ANSWERS TO PROBLEMS

1. *Answer to problem 1.* The initial lidocaine dose for patient VC would be calculated as follows:

Pharmacokinetic Dosing Method

1. *Estimate half-life and elimination rate constant according to disease states and conditions present in the patient.*

   The expected lidocaine half-life ($t_{1/2}$) is 1.5 hours. The elimination rate constant is computed using the following formula: $k = 0.693/t_{1/2} = 0.693/1.5 \text{ h} = 0.462 \text{ h}^{-1}$.

2. *Estimate the volume of distribution and clearance.*

The patient is not obese, so the estimated lidocaine central volume of distribution and the volume of distribution for the entire body (V_{area}) will be based on actual body weight: $Vc = 0.5$ L/kg • 72 kg $= 36$ L, $V_{area} = 1.5$ L/kg • 72 kg $= 108$ L. Estimated lidocaine clearance is computed by taking the product of V_{area} and the elimination rate constant: $Cl = kV_{area} = 0.462$ h^{-1} • 108 L $= 50$ L/h.

3. *Compute dosage regimen.*

Therapy will be started by administering an intravenous loading dose of lidocaine to the patient (note: μg/mL = mg/L and this concentration unit was substituted for Css in the calculations so that unnecessary unit conversion was not required): LD = Css • Vc = 3 mg/L • 36 L $= 108$ mg, rounded to 100 mg intravenously over 2-4 minutes. An additional dose equal to 50% of the loading dose can be given if arrhythmias recur 20-30 minutes after the initial loading dose.

A lidocaine continuous intravenous infusion will be started immediately after the loading dose has been administered. (Note: μg/mL = mg/L and this concentration unit was substituted for Css in the calculations so that unnecessary unit conversion was not required.) The dosage equation for intravenous lidocaine is: $k_0 = $ Css • Cl $= (3$ mg/L • 50 L/h)/(60 min/h) $= 2.5$ mg/min.

A steady-state lidocaine serum concentration could be measured after steady-state is attained in 3-5 half-lives. Since the patient is expected to have a half-life equal to 1.5 hours, the lidocaine steady-state concentration could be obtained any time after the first 8 hours of dosing (5 half-lives = 5 • 1.5 h $= 7.5$ h). Lidocaine serum concentrations should also be measured if the patient experiences a return of their ventricular arrhythmia, or if the patient develops potential signs or symptoms of lidocaine toxicity.

Literature-Based Recommended Dosing

1. *Choose a lidocaine dose based on disease states and conditions present in the patient.*

A lidocaine-loading dose of 1-1.5 mg/kg and maintenance infusion of 3-4 mg/min is suggested for a patient without heart failure or liver disease.

2. *Compute dosage regimen.*

Because the desired concentration is in the lower end of the therapeutic range, a dose in the lower end of the suggested ranges will be used. A lidocaine-loading dose of 1 mg/kg will be administered: LD = 1 mg/kg • 72 kg $= 72$ mg, rounded to 75 mg over 1.5-3 minutes. A lidocaine maintenance infusion equal to 3 mg/min would be administered after the loading dose was given. An additional dose equal to 50% of the loading dose can be given if arrhythmias recur 20-30 minutes after the initial loading dose.

A steady-state lidocaine serum concentration could be measured after steady-state is attained in 3-5 half-lives. Since the patient is expected to have a half-life equal to 1.5 hours, the lidocaine steady-state concentration could be obtained any time after the first 8 hours of dosing (5 half-lives = 5 • 1.5 h $= 7.5$ h). Lidocaine serum concentrations should also be measured if the patient experiences a return of their ventricular arrhythmia, or if the patient develops potential signs or symptoms of lidocaine toxicity.

2. *Answer to problem 2.* The revised lidocaine dose for patient VC would be calculated as follows:

Linear Pharmacokinetics Method

1. *Compute new dose to achieve the desired serum concentration*

The patient would be expected to achieve steady-state conditions after 8 hours (5 $t_{1/2} = 5$ • 1.5 h $= 7.5$ h) of therapy.

Using linear pharmacokinetics, the new dose to attain the desired concentration should be proportional to the old dose that produced the measured concentration:

$$D_{new} = (C_{ss,new}/C_{ss,old})D_{old} = (4\ \mu g/mL/2.5\ \mu g/mL)\ 2\ mg/min = 3.2\ mg/min, \text{ rounded to 3 mg/min}$$

The new suggested dose would be 3 mg/min of intravenous lidocaine to be started immediately.

A steady-state lidocaine serum concentration could be measured after steady-state is attained in 3-5 half-lives. Since the patient is expected to have a half-life equal to 1.5 hours, the lidocaine steady-state concentration could be obtained any time after the first 8 hours of dosing (5 half-lives = 5 • 1.5 h = 7.5 h). Lidocaine serum concentrations should also be measured if the patient experiences a return of their ventricular arrhythmia, or if the patient develops potential signs or symptoms of lidocaine toxicity.

Pharmacokinetic Parameter Method

1. *Compute pharmacokinetic parameters.*

    The patient would be expected to achieve steady-state conditions after the first 8 hours (5 $t_{1/2}$ = 1.5 • 5 h = 7.5 h) of therapy.

    Lidocaine clearance can be computed using a steady-state lidocaine concentration $Cl = k_0/Css =$ (2 mg/min)/(2.5 mg/L) = 0.8 L/min. (Note: μg/mL = mg/L and this concentration unit was substituted for Css in the calculations so that unnecessary unit conversion was not required.)

2. *Compute lidocaine dose.*

    Lidocaine clearance is used to compute the new lidocaine infusion rate: $k_0 = Css • Cl =$ 4 mg/L • 0.8 L/min = 3.2 mg/min, round to 3 mg/min.

    The new lidocaine infusion rate would be instituted immediately.

    A steady-state lidocaine serum concentration could be measured after steady-state is attained in 3-5 half-lives. Since the patient is expected to have a half-life equal to 1.5 hours, the lidocaine steady-state concentration could be obtained any time after the first 8 hours of dosing (5 half-lives = 5 • 1.5 h = 7.5 h). Lidocaine serum concentrations should also be measured if the patient experiences a return of their ventricular arrhythmia, or if the patient develops potential signs or symptoms of lidocaine toxicity.

Computation of Booster Dose (if Needed)

1. *Use the central volume of distribution (Vc) to calculate the booster dose.*

    The booster dose is computed using the following equation (Vc population average estimate used from problem 1): $BD = (C_{desired} - C_{actual})Vc = (4\ mg/L - 2.5\ mg/L)36\ L = 54\ mg$, rounded to 50 mg of lidocaine intravenously over 1-2 minutes. (Note: μg/mL = mg/L and this concentration unit was substituted for C in the calculations so that unnecessary unit conversion was not required.) If the maintenance dose was increased, it will take an additional 3-5 estimated half-lives for new steady-state conditions to be achieved.

3. *Answer to problem 3.* The initial lidocaine dose for patient EM would be calculated as follows:

Pharmacokinetic Dosing Method

1. *Estimate half-life and elimination rate constant according to disease states and conditions present in the patient.*

    The expected lidocaine half-life ($t_{1/2}$) is 5 hours. The elimination rate constant is computed using the following formula: $k = 0.693/t_{1/2} = 0.693/5\ h = 0.139\ h^{-1}$.

2. *Estimate volume of distribution and clearance.*

The patient is not obese, so the estimated lidocaine central volume of distribution and the volume of distribution for the entire body (V_{area}) will be based on actual body weight: $Vc = 0.6$ L/kg • 81 kg = 49 L, $V_{area} = 2.6$ L/kg • 81 kg = 211 L. Estimated lidocaine clearance is computed by taking the product of V_{area} and the elimination rate constant: $Cl = kV_{area} = 0.139$ h^{-1} • 211 L = 29.3 L/h.

3. *Compute dosage regimen.*

Therapy will be started by administering an intravenous loading dose of lidocaine to the patient (note: μg/mL = mg/L and this concentration unit was substituted for Css in the calculations so that unnecessary unit conversion was not required): LD = Css • Vc = 4 mg/L • 49 L = 196 mg, rounded to 200 mg intravenously over 4-8 minutes. An additional dose equal to 50% of the loading dose can be given if arrhythmias recur 20-30 minutes after the initial loading dose.

A lidocaine continuous intravenous infusion will be started immediately after the loading dose has been administered. (Note: μg/mL = mg/L and this concentration unit was substituted for Css in the calculations so that unnecessary unit conversion was not required.) The dosage equation for intravenous lidocaine is: k_0 = Css • Cl = (4 mg/L • 29.3 L/h)/(60 min/h) = 2 mg/min.

A steady-state lidocaine serum concentration could be measured after steady-state is attained in 3-5 half-lives. Since the patient is expected to have a half-life equal to 5 hours, the lidocaine steady-state concentration could be obtained any time after the first day of dosing (5 half-lives = 5 • 5 h = 25 h). Lidocaine serum concentrations should also be measured if the patient experiences a return of their ventricular arrhythmia, or if the patient develops potential signs or symptoms of lidocaine toxicity.

Literature-Based Recommended Dosing

1. *Choose a lidocaine dose based on disease states and conditions present in the patient.*

A lidocaine-loading dose of 1-1.5 mg/kg and maintenance infusion of 1-2 mg/min is suggested for a patient with liver disease.

2. *Compute dosage regimen.*

Because the desired concentration is in the upper end of the therapeutic range, doses in the upper end of the suggested ranges will be used. A lidocaine-loading dose of 1.5 mg/kg will be administered: LD = 1.5 mg/kg • 81 kg = 122 mg, rounded to 100 mg over 2-4 minutes. A lidocaine maintenance infusion equal to 2 mg/min would be administered after the loading dose was given. An additional dose equal to 50% of the loading dose can be given if arrhythmias recur 20-30 minutes after the initial loading dose.

A steady-state lidocaine serum concentration could be measured after steady-state is attained in 3-5 half-lives. Since the patient is expected to have a half-life equal to 5 hours, the lidocaine steady-state concentration could be obtained any time after the first day of dosing (5 half-lives = 5 • 5 h = 25 h). Lidocaine serum concentrations should also be measured if the patient experiences a return of their ventricular arrhythmia, or if the patient develops potential signs or symptoms of lidocaine toxicity.

4. *Answer to problem 4.* The revised lidocaine dose for patient EM would be calculated as follows:

Linear Pharmacokinetics Method

1. *Compute new dose to achieve the desired serum concentration.*

The patient would be expected to achieve steady-state conditions after 1 day (5 $t_{1/2}$ = 5 • 5 h = 25 h) of therapy.

Using linear pharmacokinetics, the new dose to attain the desired concentration should be proportional to the old dose that produced the measured concentration:

$$D_{new} = (C_{ss,new}/C_{ss,old})D_{old} = (4\ \mu g/mL / 6.2\ \mu g/mL)\ 2\ mg/min = 1.3\ mg/min, \text{ rounded to } 1.5\ mg/min$$

The new suggested dose would be 1.5 mg/min of intravenous lidocaine to be started immediately. If the patient was experiencing lidocaine side effects, the lidocaine infusion could be held for approximately 1 half-life to allow concentrations to decline, and the new infusion would be started at that time.

A steady-state lidocaine serum concentration could be measured after steady-state is attained in 3-5 half-lives. Since the patient is expected to have a half-life equal to 5 hours, the lidocaine steady-state concentration could be obtained any time after the first day of dosing (5 half-lives = 5 • 5 h = 25 h). Lidocaine serum concentrations should also be measured if the patient experiences a return of their ventricular arrhythmia, or if the patient develops potential signs or symptoms of lidocaine toxicity.

Pharmacokinetic Parameter Method

1. *Compute pharmacokinetic parameters.*

The patient would be expected to achieve steady-state conditions after the first day (5 $t_{1/2}$ = 5 • 5 h = 25 h) of therapy.

Lidocaine clearance can be computed using a steady-state lidocaine concentration Cl = k_0/Css = (2 mg/min)/(6.2 mg/L) = 0.32 L/min. (Note: $\mu g/mL$ = mg/L and this concentration unit was substituted for Css in the calculations so that unnecessary unit conversion was not required.)

2. *Compute lidocaine dose.*

Lidocaine clearance is used to compute the new lidocaine infusion rate: k_0 = Css • Cl = 4 mg/L • 0.32 L/min = 1.3 mg/min, round to 1.5 mg/min.

The new suggested dose would be 1.5 mg/min of intravenous lidocaine to be started immediately. If the patient was experiencing lidocaine side effects, the lidocaine infusion could be held for approximately 1 half-life to allow concentrations to decline, and the new infusion would be started at that time.

A steady-state lidocaine serum concentration could be measured after steady-state is attained in 3-5 half-lives. Since the patient is expected to have a half-life equal to 5 hours, the lidocaine steady-state concentration could be obtained any time after the first day of dosing (5 half-lives = 5 • 5 h = 25 h). Lidocaine serum concentrations should also be measured if the patient experiences a return of their ventricular arrhythmia, or if the patient develops potential signs or symptoms of lidocaine toxicity.

5. *Answer to problem 5.* The initial lidocaine dose for patient OF would be calculated as follows:

Pharmacokinetic Dosing Method

1. *Estimate half-life and elimination rate constant according to disease states and conditions present in the patient.*

The expected lidocaine half-life ($t_{1/2}$) is 2 hours. The elimination rate constant is computed using the following formula: k = 0.693/$t_{1/2}$ = 0.693/2 h = 0.347 h^{-1}.

2. *Estimate volume of distribution and clearance.*

The patient is not obese, so the estimated lidocaine central volume of distribution and the volume of distribution for the entire body (V_{area}) will be based on actual body weight: Vc = 0.3 L/kg • 60 kg = 18 L, V_{area} = 1 L/kg • 60 kg = 60 L. Estimated lidocaine clearance is computed by taking the product of V_{area} and the elimination rate constant: Cl = kV_{area} = 0.347 h^{-1} • 60 L = 20.8 L/h.

3. *Compute dosage regimen.*

Therapy will be started by administering an intravenous loading dose of lidocaine to the patient (note: μg/mL = mg/L and this concentration unit was substituted for Css in the calculations so that unnecessary unit conversion was not required): LD = Css • Vc = 5 mg/L • 18 L = 90 mg, rounded to 100 mg intravenously over 2-4 minutes. An additional dose equal to 50% of the loading dose can be given if arrhythmias recur 20-30 minutes after the initial loading dose.

A lidocaine continuous intravenous infusion will be started immediately after the loading dose has been administered. (Note: μg/mL = mg/L and this concentration unit was substituted for Css in the calculations so that unnecessary unit conversion was not required.) The dosage equation for intravenous lidocaine is: k_0 = Css • Cl = (5 mg/L • 20.8 L/h)/(60 min/h) = 1.7 mg/min, rounded to 1.5 mg/min.

A steady-state lidocaine serum concentration could be measured after steady-state is attained in 3-5 half-lives. Since the patient is expected to have a half-life equal to 2 hours, the lidocaine steady-state concentration could be obtained any time after the first 10-12 hours of dosing (5 half-lives = 5 • 2 h = 10 h). Lidocaine serum concentrations should also be measured if the patient experiences a return of their ventricular arrhythmia, or if the patient develops potential signs or symptoms of lidocaine toxicity.

Literature-Based Recommended Dosing

1. *Choose a lidocaine dose based on disease states and conditions present in the patient.*

A lidocaine-loading dose of 0.5-0.75 mg/kg and maintenance infusion of 1-2 mg/min is suggested for a patient with heart failure.

2. *Compute dosage regimen.*

Because the desired concentration is in the upper end of the therapeutic range, doses in the upper end of the suggested ranges will be used. A lidocaine loading dose of 0.75 mg/kg will be administered: LD = 0.75 mg/kg • 60 kg = 45 mg, rounded to 50 mg over 1-2 minutes. A lidocaine maintenance infusion equal to 2 mg/min would be administered after the loading dose was given. An additional dose equal to 50% of the loading dose can be given if arrhythmias recur 20-30 minutes after the initial loading dose.

A steady-state lidocaine serum concentration could be measured after steady-state is attained in 3-5 half-lives. Since the patient is expected to have a half-life equal to 2 hours, the lidocaine steady-state concentration could be obtained any time after the first 10-12 hours of dosing (5 half-lives = 5 • 2 h = 10 h). Lidocaine serum concentrations should also be measured if the patient experiences a return of their ventricular arrhythmia, or if the patient develops potential signs or symptoms of lidocaine toxicity.

6. *Answer to problem 6.* The revised lidocaine dose for patient OF would be calculated as follows:

Linear Pharmacokinetics Method

1. *Compute new dose to achieve the desired serum concentration.*

The patient would be expected to achieve steady-state conditions after 10-12 hours (5 $t_{1/2}$ = 5 • 2 h = 10 h) of therapy.

Using linear pharmacokinetics, the new dose to attain the desired concentration should be proportional to the old dose that produced the measured concentration:

$$D_{new} = (C_{ss,new}/C_{ss,old})D_{old} = (4 \ \mu g/mL / 6.7 \ \mu g/mL) \ 2 \ mg/min = 1.2 \ mg/min, \text{ rounded to 1 mg/min}$$

The new suggested dose would be 1 mg/min of intravenous lidocaine to be started immediately. If the patient was experiencing lidocaine side effects, the lidocaine infusion could be held for approximately 1 half-life to allow concentrations to decline, and the new infusion would be started at that time.

A steady-state lidocaine serum concentration could be measured after steady-state is attained in 3-5 half-lives. Since the patient is expected to have a half-life equal to 2 hours, the lidocaine steady-state concentration could be obtained any time after the first 10-12 hours of dosing (5 half-lives = 5 • 2 h = 10 h). Lidocaine serum concentrations should also be measured if the patient experiences a return of their ventricular arrhythmia, or if the patient develops potential signs or symptoms of lidocaine toxicity.

Pharmacokinetic Parameter Method

1. *Compute pharmacokinetic parameters.*

The patient would be expected to achieve steady-state conditions after the first 10-12 hours ($5\,t_{1/2} = 5$ • 2 h = 10 h) of therapy.

Lidocaine clearance can be computed using a steady-state lidocaine concentration $Cl = k_0/Css =$ (2 mg/min)/(6.7 mg/L) = 0.30 L/min. (Note: $\mu g/mL = mg/L$ and this concentration unit was substituted for Css in the calculations so that unnecessary unit conversion was not required.)

2. *Compute lidocaine dose.*

Lidocaine clearance is used to compute the new lidocaine infusion rate: $k_0 = Css$ • $Cl =$ 4 mg/L • 0.30 L/min = 1.2 mg/min, round to 1 mg/min.

The new suggested dose would be 1 mg/min of intravenous lidocaine to be started immediately. If the patient was experiencing lidocaine side effects, the lidocaine infusion could be held for approximately 1 half-life to allow concentrations to decline, and the new infusion would be started at that time.

A steady-state lidocaine serum concentration could be measured after steady-state is attained in 3-5 half-lives. Since the patient is expected to have a half-life equal to 2 hours, the lidocaine steady-state concentration could be obtained any time after the first 10-12 hours of dosing (5 half-lives = 5 • 2 h = 10 h). Lidocaine serum concentrations should also be measured if the patient experiences a return of their ventricular arrhythmia, or if the patient develops potential signs or symptoms of lidocaine toxicity.

7. *Answer to problem 7.* The initial lidocaine dose for patient FK would be calculated as follows:

Pharmacokinetic Dosing Method

1. *Estimate half-life and elimination rate constant according to disease states and conditions present in the patient.*

The expected lidocaine half-life ($t_{1/2}$) is 2 hours. The elimination rate constant is computed using the following formula: $k = 0.693/t_{1/2} = 0.693/2\ h = 0.347\ h^{-1}$.

2. *Estimate volume of distribution and clearance.*

The patient is obese (>30% over ideal body weight), so the estimated lidocaine central volume of distribution (Vc) and the volume of distribution for the entire body (V_{area}) will be based on ideal body weight: IBW_{male} (in kg) = 50 kg + 2.3(Ht − 60) = 50 kg + 2.3(71 in − 60) = 75 kg, Vc = 0.3 L/kg • 75 kg = 23 L, V_{area} = 1 L/kg • 75 kg = 75 L. Estimated lidocaine clearance is computed by taking the product of V_{area} and the elimination rate constant: $Cl = kV_{area} =$ 0.347 h^{-1} • 75 L = 26 L/h.

3. *Compute dosage regimen.*

Therapy will be started by administering an intravenous loading dose of lidocaine to the patient (note: μg/mL = mg/L and this concentration unit was substituted for Css in the calculations so that unnecessary unit conversion was not required): LD = Css • Vc = 3 mg/L • 23 L = 69 mg, rounded to 75 mg intravenously over 1.5-3 minutes. An additional dose equal to 50% of the loading dose can be given if arrhythmias recur 20-30 minutes after the initial loading dose.

A lidocaine continuous intravenous infusion will be started immediately after the loading dose has been administered. (Note: μg/mL = mg/L and this concentration unit was substituted for Css in the calculations so that unnecessary unit conversion was not required.) The dosage equation for intravenous lidocaine is: k_0 = Css • Cl = (3 mg/L • 26 L/h)/(60 min/h) = 1.3 mg/min, rounded to 1.5 mg/min.

A steady-state lidocaine serum concentration could be measured after steady-state is attained in 3-5 half-lives. Since the patient is expected to have a half-life equal to 2 hours, the lidocaine steady-state concentration could be obtained any time after the first 10-12 hours of dosing (5 half-lives = 5 • 2 h = 10 h). Lidocaine serum concentrations should also be measured if the patient experiences a return of their ventricular arrhythmia, or if the patient develops potential signs or symptoms of lidocaine toxicity.

Literature-Based Recommended Dosing

1. *Choose a lidocaine dose based on disease states and conditions present in the patient.*

A lidocaine-loading dose of 0.5-0.75 mg/kg and maintenance infusion of 1-2 mg/min is suggested for a patient with heart failure. The patient is obese (>30% over ideal body weight), so lidocaine doses will be based on ideal body weight: IBW_{male} (in kg) = 50 kg + 2.3(Ht − 60) = 50 kg + 2.3(71 in − 60) = 75 kg.

2. *Compute dosage regimen.*

Because the desired concentration is in the lower end of the therapeutic range, doses in the lower end of the suggested ranges will be used. A lidocaine-loading dose of 0.5 mg/kg will be administered: LD = 0.5 mg/kg • 75 kg = 38 mg, rounded to 50 mg over 1-2 minutes. A lidocaine maintenance infusion equal to 1 mg/min would be administered after the loading dose was given. An additional dose equal to 50% of the loading dose can be given if arrhythmias recur 20-30 minutes after the initial loading dose.

A steady-state lidocaine serum concentration could be measured after steady-state is attained in 3-5 half-lives. Since the patient is expected to have a half-life equal to 2 hours, the lidocaine steady-state concentration could be obtained any time after the first 10-12 hours of dosing (5 half-lives = 5 • 2 h = 10 h). Lidocaine serum concentrations should also be measured if the patient experiences a return of their ventricular arrhythmia, or if the patient develops potential signs or symptoms of lidocaine toxicity.

8. *Answer to problem 8.* The revised lidocaine dose for patient FK would be calculated as follows:

Bayesian Pharmacokinetic Computer Programs Method

1. *Enter the patient's demographic, drug-dosing, and serum concentration/time data into the computer program.*

In this patient case, it is unlikely that the patient is at steady-state so the Linear Pharmacokinetics method cannot be used. The DrugCalc program requires lidocaine infusion rates be input in terms of mg/h. A 2-mg/min infusion rate is equivalent to 120 mg/h (k_0 = 2 mg/min • 60 min/h = 120 mg/h).

2. *Compute pharmacokinetic parameters for the patient using Bayesian pharmacokinetic computer program.*

The pharmacokinetic parameters computed by the program are a volume of distribution for the entire body (V_{area}) of 60 L, a half-life equal to 2.9 h, and a clearance equal to 14.5 L/h.

3. *Compute the dose required to achieve desired lidocaine serum concentrations.*

The continuous intravenous infusion equation used by the program to compute doses indicates that a dose of 60 mg/h or 1 mg/min [k_0 = (60 mg/h)/(60 mg/h) = 1 mg/min] will produce a steady-state lidocaine concentration of 4 µg/mL. This infusion rate could be started immediately. If the patient was experiencing lidocaine side effects, the lidocaine infusion could be held for approximately 1 half-life to allow concentrations to decline, and the new infusion would be started at that time.

9. *Answer to problem 9.* The initial lidocaine dose for patient GP would be calculated as follows:

Pharmacokinetic Dosing Method

1. *Estimate half-life and elimination rate constant according to disease states and conditions present in the patient.*

The expected lidocaine half-life ($t_{1/2}$) is 4 hours. The elimination rate constant is computed using the following formula: $k = 0.693/t_{1/2} = 0.693/4\ h = 0.173\ h^{-1}$.

2. *Estimate volume of distribution and clearance.*

The patient is not obese, so the estimated lidocaine central volume of distribution and the volume of distribution for the entire body (V_{area}) will be based on actual body weight: Vc = 0.5 L/kg • 90 kg = 45 L, V_{area} = 1.5 L/kg • 90 kg = 135 L. Estimated lidocaine clearance is computed by taking the product of V_{area} and the elimination rate constant: $Cl = kV_{area} = 0.173\ h^{-1}$ • 135 L = 23.4 L/h.

3. *Compute dosage regimen.*

Therapy will be started by administering an intravenous loading dose of lidocaine to the patient (note: µg/mL = mg/L and this concentration unit was substituted for Css in the calculations so that unnecessary unit conversion was not required): LD = Css • Vc = 4 mg/L • 45 L = 180 mg, rounded to 200 mg intravenously over 4-8 minutes. An additional dose equal to 50% of the loading dose can be given if arrhythmias recur 20-30 minutes after the initial loading dose.

A lidocaine continuous intravenous infusion will be started immediately after the loading dose has been administered. (Note: µg/mL = mg/L and this concentration unit was substituted for Css in the calculations so that unnecessary unit conversion was not required.) The dosage equation for intravenous lidocaine is: k_0 = Css • Cl = (4 mg/L • 23.4 L/h)/(60 min/h) = 1.6 mg/min, rounded to 1.5 mg/min.

A steady-state lidocaine serum concentration could be measured after steady-state is attained in 3-5 half-lives. Since the patient is expected to have a half-life equal to 4 hours, the lidocaine steady-state concentration could be obtained any time after the first day of dosing (5 half-lives = 5 • 4 h = 20 h). Lidocaine serum concentrations should also be measured if the patient experiences a return of their ventricular arrhythmia, or if the patient develops potential signs or symptoms of lidocaine toxicity.

Literature-Based Recommended Dosing

1. *Choose a lidocaine dose based on disease states and conditions present in the patient.*

A lidocaine loading dose of 1-1.5 mg/kg and maintenance infusion of 3-4 mg/min is suggested for a patient without heart failure or liver disease.

2. *Compute dosage regimen.*

Because the desired concentration is in the upper end of the therapeutic range, a dose in the upper end of the suggested ranges will be used. A lidocaine-loading dose of 1.5 mg/kg will be administered: LD = 1.5 mg/kg • 90 kg = 135 mg, rounded to 150 mg over 3-6 minutes. A lidocaine maintenance infusion equal to 3 mg/min would be administered after the loading dose was given. An additional dose equal to 50% of the loading dose can be given if arrhythmias recur 20-30 minutes after the initial loading dose.

A steady-state lidocaine serum concentration could be measured after steady-state is attained in 3-5 half-lives. Since the patient is expected to have a half-life equal to 4 hours, the lidocaine steady-state concentration could be obtained any time after the first day of dosing (5 half-lives = 5 • 4 h = 20 h). Lidocaine serum concentrations should also be measured if the patient experiences a return of their ventricular arrhythmia, or if the patient develops potential signs or symptoms of lidocaine toxicity.

10. *Answer to problem 10.* The revised lidocaine dose for patient GP would be calculated as follows:

Bayesian Pharmacokinetic Computer Programs Method

1. *Enter the patient's demographic, drug-dosing, and serum concentration/time data into the computer program.*

In this patient case, it is unlikely that the patient is at a steady-state, so the Linear Pharmacokinetics method cannot be used. The DrugCalc program requires lidocaine infusion rates be input in terms of mg/h. A 2-mg/min infusion rate is equivalent to 120 mg/h (k_0 = 2 mg/min • 60 min/h = 120 mg/h).

2. *Compute the pharmacokinetic parameters for the patient using Bayesian pharmacokinetic computer program.*

The pharmacokinetic parameters computed by the program are a volume of distribution for the entire body (V_{area}) of 118 L, a half-life equal to 1.4 h, and a clearance equal to 57 L/h.

3. *Compute the dose required to achieve desired lidocaine serum concentrations.*

The continuous intravenous infusion equation used by the program to compute doses indicates that a dose of 240 mg/h or 4 mg/min [k_0 = (240 mg/h)/(60 mg/h) = 4 mg/min] will produce a steady-state lidocaine concentration of 4.2 μg/mL. This infusion rate would be started immediately.

Computation of Booster Dose (if Needed)

1. *Use central volume of distribution (Vc) to calculate booster dose.*

The booster dose is computed using the following equation (Vc = population average estimate used from problem 9): BD = ($C_{desired}$ − C_{actual})Vc = (4.2 mg/L − 1.9 mg/L) 45 L = 104 mg, rounded to 100 mg of lidocaine intravenously over 2-4 minutes. (Note: μg/mL = mg/L and this concentration unit was substituted for C in the calculations so that unnecessary unit conversion was not required.) If the maintenance dose was increased, it will take an additional 3-5 estimated half-lives for new steady-state conditions to be achieved.

11. *Answer to problem 11.* The revised lidocaine dose for patient CV would be calculated as follows:

Bayesian Pharmacokinetic Computer Programs Method

1. *Enter the patient's demographic, drug-dosing, and serum concentration/time data into the computer program.*

In this patient case, it is unlikely that the patient is at steady-state and multiple infusion rates have been prescribed, so the Linear Pharmacokinetics method cannot be used. In addition, the patient has two disease states that change lidocaine pharmacokinetics. The DrugCalc program requires lidocaine infusion rates be input in terms of mg/h. A 2-mg/min infusion rate is equivalent to 120 mg/h (k_0 = 2 mg/min • 60 min/h = 120 mg/h), and a 1-mg/min infusion rate is equivalent to 60 mg/h (k_0 = 1 mg/min • 60 min/h = 60 mg/h).

2. *Compute pharmacokinetic parameters for the patient using Bayesian pharmacokinetic computer program.*

The pharmacokinetic parameters computed by the program are a volume of distribution for the entire body (V_{area}) of 112 L, a half-life equal to 6 h, and a clearance equal to 13 L/h.

3. *Compute dose required to achieve desired lidocaine serum concentrations.*

The continuous intravenous infusion equation used by the program to compute doses indicates that a dose of 39 mg/h or 0.7 mg/min (k_0 = (39 mg/h)/(60 mg/h) = 0.7 mg/min) will produce a steady-state lidocaine concentration of 3 μg/mL. This infusion rate could be started immediately. If the patient was experiencing lidocaine side effects, the lidocaine infusion could be held for approximately 1 half-life to allow concentrations to decline, and the new infusion would be started at that time.

12. *Answer to problem 12.* The revised lidocaine dose for patient FP would be calculated as follows:

Bayesian Pharmacokinetic Computer Programs Method

1. *Enter the patient's demographic, drug dosing, and serum concentration/time data into the computer program.*

In this patient case, it is unlikely that the patient is at steady-state and multiple infusion rates and loading doses have been prescribed, so the Linear Pharmacokinetics method cannot be used. In addition, the patient has two disease states that change lidocaine pharmacokinetics. The DrugCalc program requires lidocaine infusion rates be input in terms of mg/h. A 3-mg/min infusion rate is equivalent to 180 mg/h (k_0 = 3 mg/min • 60 min/h = 180 mg/h), and a 1-mg/min infusion rate is equivalent to 60 mg/h (k_0 = 1 mg/min • 60 min/h = 60 mg/h).

2. *Compute pharmacokinetic parameters for the patient using Bayesian pharmacokinetic computer program.*

The pharmacokinetic parameters computed by the program are a volume of distribution for the entire body (V_{area}) of 136 L, a half-life equal to 5.6 h, and a clearance equal to 17 L/h.

3. *Compute dose required to achieve desired lidocaine serum concentrations.*

The continuous intravenous infusion equation used by the program to compute doses indicates that a dose of 83 mg/h or 1.4 mg/min [k_0 = (83 mg/h)/(60 mg/h) = 1.4 mg/min], rounded to 1.5 mg/min, will produce a steady-state lidocaine concentration of 5 μg/mL. This infusion rate could be started immediately.

REFERENCES

1. Sanoski CA, Bauman JL. The arrhythmias. In: Dipiro JT, Talbert RL, Yee GC, Matzke GR, Wells BG, Posey LM, eds. *Pharmacotherapy.* New York, NY: McGraw-Hill; 2011:273-309.

2. Sampson KJ, Kass RS. Anti-arrhythmics drugs. In: Brunton L, Chabner B, Knollman B, eds. *The Pharmacological Basis of Therapeutics.* 12th ed. New York, NY: McGraw-Hill; 2011:815-848.

3. Neumar RW, Otto CW, Link MS, et al. Part 8: adult advanced cardiovascular life support: 2010 American Heart Association Guidelines for Cardiopulmonary Resuscitation and Emergency Cardiovascular Care. *Circulation.* Nov 2, 2010;122(18 suppl 3):S729-S767.

4. Boyes RN, Scott DB, Jebson PJ, Godman MJ, Julian DG. Pharmacokinetics of lidocaine in man. *Clin Pharmacol Ther.* 1971;12(1):105-116.

5. Wyman MG, Lalka D, Hammersmith L, Cannom DS, Goldreyer BN. Multiple bolus technique for lidocaine administration during the first hours of an acute myocardial infarction. *Am J Cardiol.* 1978;41(2):313-317.

6. Halkin H, Meffin P, Melmon KL, Rowland M. Influence of congestive heart failure on blood vessels of lidocaine and its active monodeethylated metabolite. *Clin Pharmacol Ther.* 1975;17(6):669-676.

7. Strong JM, Mayfield DE, Atkinson AJ Jr, Burris BC, Raymon F, Webster LT Jr. Pharmacological activity, metabolism, and pharmacokinetics of glycinexylidide. *Clin Pharmacol Ther.* 1975;17(2):184-194.

8. Narang PK, Crouthamel WG, Carliner NH, Fisher ML. Lidocaine and its active metabolites. *Clin Pharmacol Ther.* 1978;24(6):654-662.

9. Barchowsky A, Shand DG, Stargel WW, Wagner GS, Routledge PA. On the role of alpha 1-acid glycoprotein in lignocaine accumulation following myocardial infarction. *Br J Clin Pharmacol.* 1982;13(3):411-415.

10. Bauer LA, Brown T, Gibaldi M, et al. Influence of long-term infusions on lidocaine kinetics. *Clin Pharmacol Ther.* 1982;31(4):433-437.

11. Routledge PA, Stargel WW, Wagner GS, Shand DG. Increased alpha-1-acid glycoprotein and lidocaine disposition in myocardial infarction. *Ann Intern Med.* 1980;93(5):701-704.

12. Routledge PA, Shand DG, Barchowsky A, Wagner G, Stargel WW. Relationship between alpha 1-acid glycoprotein and lidocaine disposition in myocardial infarction. *Clin Pharmacol Ther.* 1981;30(2):154-157.

13. Thomson PD, Rowland M, Melmon KL. The influence of heart failure, liver disease, and renal failure on the disposition of lidocaine in man. *Am Heart J.* 1971;82(3):417-421.

14. Scott DB, Jebson PJ, Vellani CW, Julian DG. Plasma-lignocaine levels after intravenous and intramuscular injection. *Lancet.* 1970;1(7636):41.

15. Routledge PA, Stargel WW, Kitchell BB, Barchowsky A, Shand DG. Sex-related differences in the plasma protein binding of lignocaine and diazepam. *Br J Clin Pharmacol.* 1981;11(3):245-250.

16. Routledge PA, Barchowsky A, Bjornsson TD, Kitchell BB, Shand DG. Lidocaine plasma protein binding. *Clin Pharmacol Ther.* 1980;27(3):347-351.

17. McNamara PJ, Slaughter RL, Pieper JA, Wyman MG, Lalka D. Factors influencing serum protein binding of lidocaine in humans. *Anesth Analg.* 1981;60(6):395-400.

18. Suzuki T, Fujita S, Kawai R. Precursor-metabolite interaction in the metabolism of lidocaine. *J Pharm Sci.* 1984;73(1):136-138.

19. Abernethy DR, Greenblatt DJ. Lidocaine disposition in obesity. *Am J Cardiol.* 1984;53(8):1183-1186.

20. Forrest JA, Finlayson ND, Adjepon-Yamoah KK, Prescott LF. Antipyrine, paracetamol, and lignocaine elimination in chronic liver disease. *Br Med J.* 1977;1(6073):1384-1387.

21. Huet PM, Lelorier J. Effects of smoking and chronic hepatitis B on lidocaine and indocyanine green kinetics. *Clin Pharmacol Ther.* 1980;28(2):208-215.

22. Thomson PD, Melmon KL, Richardson JA, et al. Lidocaine pharmacokinetics in advanced heart failure, liver disease, and renal failure in humans. *Ann Intern Med.* 1973;78(4):499-508.

23. Williams RL, Blaschke TF, Meffin PJ, Melmon KL, Rowland M. Influence of viral hepatitis on the disposition of two compounds with high hepatic clearance: lidocaine and indocyanine green. *Clin Pharmacol Ther.* 1976;20(3):290-299.

24. Pugh RN, Murray-Lyon IM, Dawson JL, Pietroni MC, Williams R. Transection of the oesophagus for bleeding oesophageal varices. *Br J Surg.* 1973;60(8):646-649.

25. Nation RL, Triggs EJ, Selig M. Lignocaine kinetics in cardiac patients and aged subjects. *Br J Clin Pharmacol.* 1977;4(4):439-448.

26. Prescott LF, Adjepon-Yamoah KK, Talbot RG. Impaired Lignocaine metabolism in patients with myocardial infarction and cardiac failure. *Br Med J.* 1976;1(6015):939-941.

27. Bax ND, Tucker GT, Woods HF. Lignocaine and indocyanine green kinetics in patients following myocardial infarction. *Br J Clin Pharmacol.* 1980;10(4):353-361.

28. LeLorier J, Grenon D, Latour Y, et al. Pharmacokinetics of lidocaine after prolonged intravenous infusions in uncomplicated myocardial infarction. *Ann Intern Med.* 1977;87(6):700-706.

29. Golper TA, Marx MA. Drug dosing adjustments during continuous renal replacement therapies. *Kidney Int Suppl.* May 1998; 66:S165-S168.

30. Golper TA. Update on drug sieving coefficients and dosing adjustments during continuous renal replacement therapies. *Contrib Nephrol.* 2001;(132):349-353.

31. Hansten PD, Horn JR. *Drug Interactions Analysis and Management.* St. Louis, MO: Wolters Kluwer Health; 2014.

32. Bauer LA, Edwards WA, Randolph FP, Blouin RA. Cimetidine-induced decrease in lidocaine metabolism. *Am Heart J.* 1984; 108(2):413-415.

33. Bauer LA, McDonnell N, Horn JR, Zierler B, Opheim K, Strandness DE Jr. Single and multiple doses of oral cimetidine do not change liver blood flow in humans. *Clin Pharmacol Ther.* 1990;48(2):195-200.

34. Mutnick AH, Burke TG. Antiarrhythmics. In: Schumacher GE, ed. *Therapeutic Drug Monitoring.* 1st ed. Stamford, CT: Appleton & Lange; 1995:684.

35. Tschudy MM, Arcara KM. *The Harriet Lane Handbook: A Manual for Pediatric House Officers.* 19th ed. Philadelphia, PA: Mosby; 2012.

36. Wandell M, Mungall D. Computer assisted drug interpretation and drug regimen optimization. *Amer Assoc Clin Chem.* 1984;6:1-11.

37. Parker RB, Cavallari LH. Systolic heart failure. In: J.T. D, Talbert RL, Yee GC, Matzke GR, Wells BG, Posey LM, eds. *Pharmacotherapy.* New York, NY: McGraw-Hill; 2011:137-172.

8 Procainamide/*N*-acetyl Procainamide

INTRODUCTION

Procainamide is an antiarrhythmic agent that is used intravenously and orally. However, an oral dosage form is no longer available in the United States. It is classified as a type IA antiarrhythmic agent and can be used for the treatment of supraventricular or ventricular arrhythmias.[1,2] The intravenous form of procainamide is one of the drugs of choice for the treatment of hemodynamically stable monomorphic ventricular tachycardia in patients without a prolonged QT interval or heart failure.[3] Given orally, procainamide can be used for long-term suppression of ventricular arrhythmias.[4]

Procainamide can be administered orally for the long-term prevention of chronic supraventricular arrhythmias such as supraventricular tachycardia, atrial flutter, and atrial fibrillation.[4] Ventricular rate control during atrial fibrillation can be accomplished using intravenous procainamide for hemodynamically stable patients with an accessory pathway.[3,5] Procainamide is also one of the possible choices for the pharmacological cardioversion of atrial fibrillation.[5]

Procainamide inhibits transmembrane sodium influx into the conduction system of the heart thereby decreasing conduction velocity.[1,2] It also increases the duration of the action potential, increases threshold potential toward zero, and decreases the slope of phase 4 of the action potential. Automaticity is decreased during procainamide therapy. The net effect of these cellular changes is that procainamide causes increased refractoriness and decreased conduction in heart conduction tissue, which establishes a bidirectional block in reentrant pathways.

N-acetyl procainamide (NAPA) is an active metabolite of procainamide that has type III antiarrhythmic effects.[2] A common characteristic of type III antiarrhythmic agents (bretylium, amiodarone, sotalol) is prolongation of the duration of the action potential resulting in an increased absolute refractory period.

THERAPEUTIC AND TOXIC CONCENTRATIONS

When given intravenously, the serum procainamide concentration-time curve follows a two-compartment model (Figure 8-1).[6] If an intravenous loading dose is followed by a continuous infusion, serum concentrations decline rapidly at first due to distribution of the loading dose from blood to tissues (Figure 8-2).[6] When oral dosage forms are given, absorption occurs more slowly than distribution so a distribution phase is not seen (Figure 8-3).[7-11]

The generally accepted therapeutic range for procainamide is 4-10 μg/mL. Serum concentrations in the upper end of the therapeutic range (≥8 μg/mL) may result in minor side effects such as gastrointestinal disturbances (anorexia, nausea, vomiting, diarrhea), weakness, malaise, decreased mean arterial pressure (<20%), and a 10%-30% prolongation of electrocardiogram intervals (PR and QT intervals, QRS complex). Procainamide serum concentrations above 12 μg/mL can cause increased PR interval, QT interval, or QRS-complex widening (>30%) on the electrocardiogram, heart block, ventricular conduction disturbances, new ventricular arrhythmias, or cardiac arrest. Procainamide therapy is also associated with torsade de pointes.[1,2]

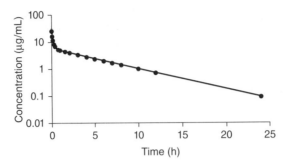

FIGURE 8-1   Procainamide serum concentrations initially drop rapidly after an intravenous bolus as drug distributes from blood into the tissues during the distribution phase. During the distribution phase, drug leaves the blood due to tissue distribution and elimination. After 20-30 minutes, an equilibrium is established between the blood and tissues, and serum concentrations drop more slowly since elimination is the primary process removing drug from the blood. A two-compartment model describes this type of serum concentration/time profile.

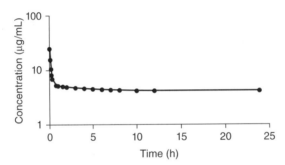

FIGURE 8-2   To maintain therapeutic procainamide concentrations, an intravenous loading dose (over 25-30 minutes) of procainamide is followed by a continuous intravenous infusion of the drug. A distribution phase is still seen due to the administration of the loading dose. Note that the administration of a loading dose may not establish steady-state conditions immediately, and the infusion needs to run 3-5 half-lives until steady-state concentrations are attained.

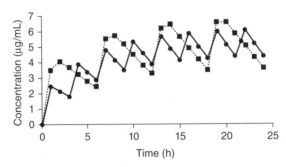

FIGURE 8-3   Serum concentration-time profile for rapid-release procainamide (solid line, given every 3 hours) or sustained-release procainamide (dashed line, given every 6 hours) oral dosage forms after multiple doses until steady-state is achieved. The curves shown would be typical for an adult with normal renal and hepatic function.

Torsade de pointes (twisting of the points) is a form of polymorphic ventricular tachycardia preceded by QT-interval prolongation. It is characterized by polymorphic QRS complexes that change in amplitude and length giving the appearance of oscillations around the electrocardiographic baseline. Torsade de pointes can develop into multiple episodes of nonsustained polymorphic ventricular tachycardia, syncope, ventricular fibrillation, or sudden cardiac death.

Nondose or concentration-related side effects to procainamide include rash, agranulocytosis, and a systemic lupus-like syndrome. Symptoms of the lupus-like syndrome include rash, photosensitivity, arthralgias, pleuritis or pericarditis, hemolytic anemia or leukopenia, and a positive antinuclear antibody (ANA) test. Patients who metabolize the drug more rapidly via N-acetyltransferase II, known as "rapid acetylators," appear to have a lower incidence of this adverse effect or at least take more time and higher doses for it to appear. While the lupus-like syndrome is usually not life threatening, it does occur in 30% to 50% of patients taking procainamide for greater than 6-12 months and requires discontinuation of the drug. Most symptoms abate within several weeks to months, but some patients have required a year or more to completely recover. Intravenous procainamide doses must be given no greater than 25-50 mg/min, as faster injection can cause profound hypotension.

An active procainamide metabolite, known as N-acetylprocainamide (NAPA) or acecainide, also possesses antiarrhythmic effects.[12-14] Based on limited clinical trials of NAPA, effective concentrations are 10-30 μg/mL. Concentration-dependent adverse effects for NAPA are similar to those given for procainamide. However, NAPA does not appear to cause a systemic lupus-like syndrome. Currently, NAPA is not commercially available in the United States and has been given orphan drug status by the U.S. Food and Drug Administration with an indication for decreasing implantable defibrillator energy requirements.[15] Some laboratories report the sum of procainamide and NAPA concentrations for a patient as the "total procainamide concentration" using the therapeutic range of 10-30 μg/mL. However, because procainamide and NAPA have different antiarrhythmic potency, serum concentrations for each agent should be considered individually. Also, many individuals feel that it is more important to maintain therapeutic procainamide concentrations in patients rather than NAPA or total procainamide levels in the suggested ranges. Clinicians should understand that all patients with "toxic" procainamide or NAPA serum concentrations in the listed ranges will not exhibit signs or symptoms of procainamide toxicity. Rather, procainamide and/or NAPA concentrations in the given ranges increase the likelihood that an adverse effect will occur.

For dose adjustment purposes, procainamide serum concentrations during oral administration are best measured as a predose or trough level at steady-state after the patient has received a consistent dosage regimen for 3-5 drug half-lives. If the drug is given as a continuous intravenous infusion, procainamide serum concentrations could be measured at steady-state after the patient has received a consistent infusion rate for 3-5 drug half-lives. Procainamide half-life varies from 2.5 to 5 hours in normal adults to 14 hours or more in adult patients with renal failure. Average NAPA half-lives are 6 hours for normal adults and 41 hours for adult patients with renal failure. If procainamide is given orally or intravenously on a stable schedule, steady-state serum concentrations for parent drug and metabolite will be achieved in about 1 day (5 • 5 h = 25 h for procainamide and 5 • 6 h = 30 h for NAPA). For a patient in renal failure, it will take 3 days for steady-state concentrations to occur for procainamide and 9 days for steady-state conditions to be established for NAPA (5 • 14 h = 70 h or ~3 days for procainamide, 5 • 41 h = 205 h or ~9 days for NAPA).

CLINICAL-MONITORING PARAMETERS

The electrocardiogram (ECG or EKG) should be monitored to determine the response to procainamide. The goal of therapy is suppression of arrhythmias and avoidance of adverse drug reactions. Electrophysiologic studies using programmed stimulation to replicate the ventricular arrhythmia or 24-hour ECG monitoring using a Holter monitor can be performed in patients while receiving a variety of antiarrhythmic agents to determine effective antiarrhythmic drug therapy.[16]

Because many procainamide therapeutic and side effects are not correlated with its serum concentration, it is often not necessary to obtain serum procainamide concentrations in patients receiving appropriate doses who currently have no arrhythmia or adverse drug effects. However, procainamide serum concentrations should be obtained in patients who have a recurrence of tachyarrhythmias, are experiencing possible procainamide side effects, or are receiving procainamide doses not consistent with disease states and conditions known to alter procainamide pharmacokinetics (see Effects of Disease States and Conditions on Procainamide Pharmacokinetics and Dosing section). Serum concentration monitoring can aid in the decision to increase or decrease the procainamide dose. For instance, if an arrhythmia reappears and the procainamide serum concentration is <10 μg/mL, increasing the procainamide dose is a therapeutic option. However, if the procainamide serum concentration is over 10-12 μg/mL, it is less likely a dosage increase will be effective in suppressing the arrhythmia and there is an increased likelihood that drug side effects may occur. Some patients have responded to procainamide serum concentrations as high as 20 μg/mL without experiencing severe adverse effects.[17] Similarly, if a possible concentration-related procainamide adverse drug reaction is noted in a patient and the procainamide serum concentration is <4 μg/mL, it is possible that the observed problem may not be due to procainamide treatment and other sources can be investigated. While receiving procainamide, patients should be monitored for the following adverse drug effects: anorexia, nausea, vomiting, diarrhea, weakness, malaise, decreased blood pressure, electrocardiogram changes (increased PR interval, QT interval, or QRS complex widening >30%), heart block, ventricular conduction disturbances, new ventricular arrhythmias, rash, agranulocytosis, and the systemic lupus-like syndrome.

BASIC CLINICAL PHARMACOKINETIC PARAMETERS

Procainamide is eliminated by both hepatic metabolism (~50%) and renal elimination of unchanged drug (~50%).[12-14,18,19] Hepatic metabolism is mainly via N-acetyltransferase II (NAT-II).[12-14] N-acetylprocainamide or NAPA is the primary active metabolite resulting from procainamide metabolism by N-acetyltransferase II. N-acetyltransferase II exhibits a bimodal genetic polymorphism that results in "slow acetylator" and "rapid acetylator" phenotypes. If the patient has normal renal function, acetylator status can be estimated using the ratio of NAPA and procainamide (PA) steady-state concentrations: acetylator ratio = NAPA/PA.[20,21] If this ratio is 1.2 or greater, it is likely the patient is a rapid acetylator. If the ratio is 0.8 or less, it is likely the patient is a slow acetylator. The Caucasian and African-American populations appear to be about evenly split between slow and rapid acetylators. Among the Japanese and Eskimo populations, 80%-90% are rapid acetylators, while only 20% or less of Egyptians and certain Jewish populations are of that phenotype. Obviously, ethnic background can play an important role in the procainamide dose required to achieve a therapeutic effect as well as the potential development of systemic lupus-like adverse effects. Metabolism of procainamide to other metabolites may be mediated by CYP2D6.[22] The ratio of procainamide renal clearance and creatinine clearance equals between 2 to 3 implying that net renal tubular secretion is taking place in the kidney.[18,19] The renal secretion probably takes place in the proximal tubule. Although there have been some reports that procainamide follows nonlinear pharmacokinetics, for the purposes of clinical drug dosing in patients, linear pharmacokinetic concepts and equations can be effectively used to compute doses and estimate serum concentrations.[23,24]

The average oral bioavailability of procainamide for both immediate-release and sustained-release dosage forms is 83%.[7-11] A lag time of 20-30 minutes occurs in some patients between oral dosage administration and the time procainamide first appears in the serum. Plasma protein binding of procainamide in normal individuals is only about 15%. The recommended dose of procainamide is based on the concurrent disease states and conditions present in the patient that can influence procainamide pharmacokinetics. Procainamide pharmacokinetic parameters used to compute doses are given in the following section for specific patient profiles.

EFFECTS OF DISEASE STATES AND CONDITIONS ON PROCAINAMIDE PHARMACOKINETICS AND DOSING

Normal adults without the disease states and conditions given later in this section and with normal liver and renal function have an average procainamide half-life of 3.3 hours (range: 2.5-4.6 hours) and a volume of distribution for the entire body of 2.7 L/kg (V = 2-3.8 L/kg; Table 8-1).[25-27] *N*-acetyltransferase II is the enzyme responsible for conversion of procainamide to NAPA. The genetic polymorphism of *N*-acetyltransferase II produces a bimodal frequency distribution for procainamide half-life and clearance that separates the population into rapid and slow acetylators (Figure 8-4). The mean procainamide half-life for rapid acetylators is 2.7 hours while for slow acetylators it is 5.2 hours. Not all studies conducted with procainamide have separated results from rapid and slow acetylators when analyzing the pharmacokinetic data. Unfortunately, it is not practical to phenotype a patient as a slow or rapid metabolizer before administration of the drug, so an average population half-life and clearance is used for the purpose of initial dosage computation. Disease states and conditions that change procainamide pharmacokinetics and dosage requirements may alter clearance and the

TABLE 8-1   Disease States and Conditions That Alter Procainamide Pharmacokinetics

Disease State/Condition	Half-Life	Volume of Distribution	Comment
Adult, normal renal and liver function	3.3 h (range: 2.6-4.6 h)	2.7 L/kg (range: 2-3.8 L/kg)	Procainamide is eliminated about 50% unchanged in the urine and about 50% metabolized. *N*-acetyltransferase II converts procainamide to an active metabolite (*N*-acetylprocainamide or NAPA). Genetically, some individuals are "rapid acetylators" and convert more procainamide to NAPA than "slow acetylators." NAPA is 85% eliminated unchanged by the kidney.
Adult, renal failure (creatinine clearance ≤10 mL/min)	13.9 h	1.7 L/kg	Because 50% of procainamide and 85% of NAPA is eliminated unchanged by the kidney, the clearance of both agents is reduced in renal failure.
Adult, liver cirrhosis	Not available	Not available	Procainamide is metabolized ~50% by hepatic enzymes (primarily *N*-acetyltransferase II). Clearance of procainamide is decreased in liver cirrhosis patients, but NAPA clearance does not substantially change. Pharmacokinetic parameters highly variable in liver disease patients.
Adult, uncompensated heart failure	5.5 h	1.6 L/kg	Decreased liver blood flow secondary to reduced cardiac output reduces procainamide clearance. Heart failure results in variable reductions in procainamide clearance.
Adult, obese (>30% over ideal body weight)	According to other disease states/conditions that affect procainamide pharmacokinetics	According to other disease states/conditions that affect procainamide pharmacokinetics	Procainamide volume of distribution should be based on ideal body weight for patients who weigh more than 30% over IBW, but clearance should be based on total body weight or TBW (0.52 L/h/kg TBW for patients with normal renal function).

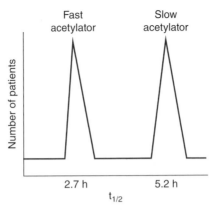

FIGURE 8-4   *N*-acetyltransferase II converts procainamide to its active metabolite, *N*-acetylprocainamide or NAPA. Patients can be phenotyped into two groups with regards to their ability to metabolize procainamide to NAPA via acetylation of the parent drug: fast acetylators convert procainamide to NAPA rapidly and have a shorter procainamide half-life, while slow acetylators convert procainamide to NAPA more slowly and have a longer procainamide half-life. This leads to a bimodal distribution of procainamide half-life for adults with normal renal function.

volume of distribution. The elimination rate constant ($k = 0.693/t_{1/2}$, where $t_{1/2}$ is the half-life) and clearance ($Cl = kV$) can be computed from the aforementioned pharmacokinetic parameters.

Because about 50% of a procainamide dose is eliminated unchanged by the kidney, renal dysfunction is the most important disease state that affects procainamide pharmacokinetics.[28-30] The procainamide clearance rate decreases as creatinine clearance decreases, but this relationship is not as helpful as it is with other drugs that are primarily renally eliminated. Digoxin, vancomycin, and the aminoglycoside antibiotics are eliminated mostly by glomerular filtration. Creatinine clearance is used as an estimate of glomerular filtration rate in patients because it is relatively easy to calculate or estimate. Since the major route of renal clearance for procainamide is via proximal tubular secretion, creatinine clearance is not as reliable a parameter to aid in the estimation of procainamide clearance. In patients with renal failure, the average procainamide half-life is 13.9 hours and volume of distribution is 1.7 L/kg.

Uncompensated heart failure reduces procainamide clearance because of decreased hepatic blood flow secondary to compromised cardiac output (Table 8-2).[27,28] Volume of distribution (V = 1.6 L/kg) is decreased in uncompensated heart failure patients as well. Because both clearance and volume of distribution simultaneously decrease, the increase in half-life is not as dramatic as might be expected, and patients with uncompensated

TABLE 8-2   New York Heart Association (NYHA) Functional Classification for Heart Failure[45]

NYHA Heart Failure Class	Description
I	Patients with cardiac disease but without limitations of physical activity. Ordinary physical activity does not cause undue fatigue, dyspnea, or palpitation.
II	Patients with cardiac disease that results in slight limitations of physical activity. Ordinary physical activity results in fatigue, palpitation, dyspnea, or angina.
III	Patients with cardiac disease that results in marked limitations of physical activity. Although patients are comfortable at rest, less than ordinary activity will lead to symptoms.
IV	Patients with cardiac disease that results in an inability to carry on physical activity without discomfort. Symptoms of congestive heart failure are present even at rest. With any physical activity, increased discomfort is experienced.

TABLE 8-3   Literature-Based Recommended Oral Procainamide Initial Dosage Ranges for Various Disease States and Conditions

Disease State/Condition	Procainamide, Oral Tablets	Procainamide, Continuous Intravenous Infusion
Adult, normal renal function (creatinine clearance >50 mL/min)	50 mg/kg/d	2-6 mg/min
Adult, renal dysfunction	Creatinine clearance = 10-50 mL/min: 25-50% dosage decrease Creatinine clearance <10 mL/min: 50%-75% dosage decrease	Creatinine clearance = 10-50 mL/min: 25%-50% dosage decrease Creatinine clearance <10 mL/min: 50%-75% dosage decrease
Adult, uncompensated heart failure	NYHA CHF class II: 25% dosage decrease NYHA CHF class III or IV: 50% dosage decrease	NYHA CHF class II: 25% dosage decrease NYHA CHF class III or IV: 50% dosage decrease
Adult, liver disease	Child/Pugh score = 8-10: 25% dosage decrease Child-Pugh score >10: 50% dosage decrease	Child/Pugh score = 8-10: 25% dosage decrease Child-Pugh score >10: 50% dosage decrease
Adult, obese (>30% over ideal body weight)	Base dose on total body weight according to other disease states/conditions	Base dose on total body weight according to other disease states/conditions

heart failure have an average procainamide half-life equal to 5.5 hours ($t_{1/2} = [0.693 \bullet \downarrow V]/\downarrow Cl$). The effect that uncompensated heart failure has on procainamide pharmacokinetics is highly variable and difficult to accurately predict. It is possible for a patient with uncompensated heart failure to have relatively normal or grossly abnormal procainamide clearance and half-life. For uncompensated heart failure patients, initial doses are meant as starting points for dosage titration based on patient response and avoidance of adverse effects. Most clinicians reduce initial procainamide doses by 25%-50% for patients with uncompensated heart failure (Table 8-3). Patients with compensated heart failure receiving appropriate treatment with good clinical response may have normal procainamide pharmacokinetics.[31] Procainamide serum concentrations and the presence of adverse drug effects should be monitored frequently in patients with heart failure.

Patients with liver cirrhosis or hepatitis have not been adequately studied with regard to procainamide pharmacokinetics. However, the majority of N-acetyltransferase II responsible for the conversion of procainamide to NAPA is thought to reside in the liver. Because of this, most clinicians recommend a decrease in initial doses for procainamide in patients with liver disease.[32] An index of liver dysfunction can be gained by applying the Child-Pugh clinical classification system to the patient (Table 8-4).[33] Child-Pugh scores are

TABLE 8-4   Child-Pugh Scores for Patients With Liver Disease[33]

Test/Symptom	Score 1 Point	Score 2 Points	Score 3 Points
Total bilirubin (mg/dL)	<2.0	2.0-3.0	>3.0
Serum albumin (g/dL)	>3.5	2.8-3.5	<2.8
Prothrombin time (seconds prolonged over control)	<4	4-6	>6
Ascites	Absent	Slight	Moderate
Hepatic encephalopathy	None	Moderate	Severe

completely discussed in Chapter 3 (Drug Dosing in Special Populations: Renal and Hepatic Disease, Dialysis, Heart Failure, Obesity, and Drug Interactions), but will be briefly discussed here. The Child-Pugh score consists of five laboratory tests or clinical symptoms: serum albumin, total bilirubin, prothrombin time, ascites, and hepatic encephalopathy. Each of these areas is given a score of 1 (normal) to 3 (severely abnormal; Table 8-4), and the scores for the five areas are summed. The Child-Pugh score for a patient with normal liver function is 5 while the score for a patient with grossly abnormal serum albumin, total bilirubin, and prothrombin time values in addition to severe ascites and hepatic encephalopathy is 15. A Child-Pugh score of 8 or more is grounds for a decrease of 25% in the initial daily drug dose for procainamide while a score greater than 10 suggests a decrease of 50% (Table 8-3). As in any patient with or without liver dysfunction, initial doses are meant as starting points for dosage titration based on patient response and avoidance of adverse effects. Procainamide serum concentrations and the presence of adverse drug effects should be monitored frequently in patients with liver cirrhosis or hepatitis.

Studies investigating the impact of obesity (30% over ideal body weight) on procainamide pharmacokinetics have found that volume of distribution correlates best with ideal body weight, but clearance correlates best with total body weight.[34] The volume of distribution for procainamide should be based on ideal body weight for obese individuals according to the other disease states and conditions present in the patient. Clearance should be based on total body weight (TBW) in obese individuals (0.52 L/h/kg TBW for normal renal failure).

Procainamide is significantly removed by hemodialysis but not by peritoneal dialysis.[35] Patients undergoing hemodialysis treatments may receive an additional dose of the usual amount taken after the procedure is finished. Because procainamide has a sieving coefficient equal to 0.86, continuous hemoperfusion removes significant amounts of the drug.[36,37] Appropriate dosage increases should be determined using serum concentration measurements of both procainamide and NAPA.

NAPA is primarily eliminated unchanged in the urine via glomerular filtration and renal tubular secretion.[18,19,25,30,38] When NAPA is given orally, 85% of the administered dose is recovered in the urine as unchanged drug. In patients with normal renal and liver function, NAPA has an average half-life of 6 hours.[13] NAPA half-life increases to 41 hours on the average in patients with renal failure.[30,38] The volume of distribution for NAPA in normal individuals is 1.4 L/kg. NAPA is significantly removed by hemodialysis but not by peritoneal dialysis.[38] In most patients with renal dysfunction, the ratio of NAPA to procainamide steady-state concentration exceeds 1, even if the patient is a slow acetylator. The reason for this is NAPA elimination is much more dependent on renal function, so NAPA concentrations accumulate more than procainamide concentrations do in patients with renal dysfunction. Thus, in patients with renal failure, NAPA may be the predominant antiarrhythmic agent present in the serum.

DRUG INTERACTIONS

Procainamide has serious drug interactions with other drugs that are capable of inhibiting its renal tubular secretion.[39-41] Cimetidine, trimethoprim, ofloxacin, levofloxacin, and ciprofloxacin are all drugs that compete for tubular secretion with procainamide and NAPA. When given with these other agents, procainamide renal clearance decreases by 30%-50% and NAPA renal clearance decreases by 10%-30%. Amiodarone increases the steady-state concentrations of procainamide and NAPA by 57% and 32%, respectively.

INITIAL DOSAGE DETERMINATION METHODS

Several methods to initiate procainamide therapy are available. The *Pharmacokinetic Dosing method* is the most flexible of the techniques. It allows individualized target serum concentrations to be chosen for a patient, and each pharmacokinetic parameter can be customized to reflect specific disease states and conditions present in the patient. *Literature-based recommended dosing* is a very commonly used method to prescribe initial doses of procainamide. Doses are based on those that commonly produce steady-state concentrations in the lower end of the therapeutic range, although there is a wide variation in the actual concentrations for a specific patient.

Pharmacokinetic Dosing Method

The goal of initial dosing of procainamide is to compute the best dose possible for the patient given their set of disease states and conditions that influence procainamide pharmacokinetics and the arrhythmia being treated. In order to do this, pharmacokinetic parameters for the patient will be estimated using average parameters measured in other patients with similar disease state and condition profiles.

Half-Life and Elimination Rate Constant Estimate

Depending on the acetylator status of the patient, procainamide is almost equally metabolized by the liver and eliminated unchanged by the kidney in patients with normal hepatic and renal function. Unfortunately, there is no good way to estimate the elimination characteristics of liver-metabolized drugs using an endogenous marker of liver function in the same manner that serum creatinine and estimated creatinine clearance are used to estimate the elimination of agents that are renally eliminated by glomerular filtration. Additionally, creatinine clearance does not accurately reflect the renal elimination of procainamide because the mechanism of elimination is active tubular secretion. Because of this, a patient is categorized according to the disease states and conditions that are known to change procainamide half-life, and the half-life previously measured in these studies is used as an estimate of the current patient's half-life (Table 8-1). For a patient with moderate heart failure (NYHA CHF class III), procainamide half-life would be assumed to equal 5.5 hours, while a patient with renal failure would be assigned an estimated half-life of 13.9 hours. To produce the most conservative procainamide doses in patients with multiple concurrent disease states or conditions that affect procainamide pharmacokinetics, the disease state or condition with the longest half-life should be used to compute doses. This approach will avoid accidental overdosage as much as currently possible. Once the correct half-life is identified for the patient, it can be converted into the procainamide elimination rate constant (k) using the following equation: $k = 0.693/t_{1/2}$.

Volume of Distribution Estimate

As with the half-life estimate, the procainamide volume of distribution is chosen according to the disease states and conditions that are present (Table 8-1). The volume of distribution is used to help compute procainamide clearance, and is assumed to equal 1.7 L/kg for renal failure patients, 1.6 L/kg for uncompensated heart failure patients, and 2.7 L/kg for all other patients. For obese patients (>30% above ideal body weight), ideal body weight is used to compute procainamide volume of distribution. Thus, for a nonobese 80-kg patient without heart failure or liver disease, the estimated procainamide volume of distribution would be 216 L: $V = 2.7$ L/kg • 80 kg = 216 L. For a 150-kg obese patient with an ideal body weight of 60 kg and normal cardiac and liver function, the estimated procainamide volume of distribution is 162 L: $V = 2.7$ L/kg • 60 kg = 162 L.

Selection of Appropriate Pharmacokinetic Model and Equations

When given orally, procainamide follows a one-compartment pharmacokinetic model (see Figure 8-3). Because procainamide has such a short half-life, most patients receive oral procainamide therapy using sustained-release dosage forms. Procainamide sustained-release dosage forms provide good bioavailability (F = 0.83), supply a continuous release of procainamide into the gastrointestinal tract, and provide a smooth procainamide serum concentration-time curve that emulates an intravenous infusion when doses are given 2-4 times daily. In the United States, two different sustained-release dosage forms have been approved that provide every 6- or 12-hour dosing. Because of this, a very simple pharmacokinetic equation that computes the average procainamide steady-state serum concentration (Css in μg/mL = mg/L) is widely used and allows maintenance dosage calculation: $Css = [F(D/\tau)]/Cl$ or $D = (Css \bullet Cl \bullet \tau)/F$, where F is the bioavailability fraction for the oral dosage form (F = 0.83 for most oral procainamide sustained-release products), D is the dose of procainamide in mg, and τ is the dosage interval in hours. Cl is procainamide clearance in L/h and is computed using estimates of procainamide elimination rate constant (k) and volume of distribution: $Cl = kV$. For example, for a patient with an estimated elimination rate constant equal to $0.210\ h^{-1}$ and an estimated volume of distribution equal to 189 L, the estimated clearance would equal 39.7 L/h: $Cl = 0.210\ h^{-1} \bullet 189\ L = 39.7\ L/h$.

When intravenous therapy is required, a similar pharmacokinetic equation that computes the procainamide steady-state serum concentration (Css in μg/mL = mg/L) is widely used and allows dosage calculation for a continuous infusion: $Css = k_0/Cl$ or $k_0 = Css \bullet Cl$, where k_0 is the dose of procainamide in mg/min, Cl is procainamide clearance in L/min and is computed using estimates of procainamide elimination rate constant (k), and volume of distribution: $Cl = kV$.

The equation used to calculate an intravenous loading dose (LD in mg) is based on a simple one-compartment model: $LD = Css \bullet V$, where Css is the desired procainamide steady-state concentration in μg/mL which is equivalent to mg/L, and V is the procainamide volume of distribution. Intravenous procainamide loading doses should be infusions no faster than 25-50 mg/min to avoid severe hypotension. Two methods are used to administer procainamide loading doses. One method administers 100 mg every 5 minutes to a maximum of 500 mg; a 10 minute waiting period to allow drug distribution to tissues is utilized if more than 500 mg is needed to abate the arrhythmia. The other method administers the loading dose as a short-term infusion at a rate of 20 mg/min over 25-30 minutes, not to exceed a total dose of 17 mg/kg.

Steady-State Concentration Selection

The generally accepted therapeutic range for procainamide is 4-10 μg/mL. If procainamide + NAPA or "total procainamide" concentrations are used, the usual therapeutic range is 10-30 μg/mL, keeping in mind that procainamide and NAPA are not equipotent antiarrhythmics. However, procainamide therapy must be individualized for each patient in order to achieve optimal responses and minimal side effects.

EXAMPLE 1 ▶▶▶

LK is a 50-year-old, 75-kg (height = 5 ft 10 in) male with ventricular tachycardia who requires therapy with oral procainamide sustained-release tablets. He has normal liver and cardiac function. Suggest an initial oral procainamide dosage regimen designed to achieve a steady-state procainamide concentration equal to 4 μg/mL.

1. *Estimate the half-life and elimination rate constant according to disease states and conditions present in the patient.*
   The expected procainamide half-life $(t_{1/2})$ for an individual with normal hepatic and renal function is 3.3 hours. The elimination rate constant is computed using the following formula: $k = 0.693/t_{1/2} = 0.693/3.3\ h = 0.210\ h^{-1}$.

2. *Estimate the volume of distribution and clearance.*
   The patient is not obese, so the estimated procainamide volume of distribution will be based on actual body weight: $V = 2.7\ L/kg \bullet 75\ kg = 203\ L$. Estimated procainamide clearance is computed by taking the product of the volume of distribution and the elimination rate constant: $Cl = kV = 0.210\ h^{-1} \bullet 203\ L = 42.6\ L/h$.

3. *Compute dosage regimen.*

Oral sustained-release procainamide tablets will be prescribed to this patient (F = 0.83). Because the patient has a rapid procainamide clearance and short half-life, the initial dosage interval (τ) will be set to 6 hours. (Note: μg/mL = mg/L and this concentration unit was substituted for Css in the calculations so that unnecessary unit conversion was not required.) The dosage equation for oral procainamide is: D = (Css • Cl • τ)/F = (4 mg/L • 42.6 L/h • 6 h)/0.83 = 1231 mg, rounded to 1250 mg every 6 hours.

　　Steady-state procainamide and NAPA serum concentrations could be measured after steady-state is attained in 3-5 half-lives. Since the patient is expected to have a half-life equal to 3.3 hours for procainamide and 6 hours for NAPA, the steady-state concentrations could be obtained any time after the first day of dosing (5 half-lives = 5 • 3.3 h = 16.5 h for procainamide, 5 half-lives = 5 • 6 h = 30 h for NAPA). Procainamide and NAPA serum concentrations should also be measured if the patient experiences a return of their arrhythmia, or if the patient develops potential signs or symptoms of procainamide toxicity.

EXAMPLE 2 ▶▶▶

OI is a 60-year-old, 85-kg (height = 6 ft 1 in) male with atrial fibrillation who requires therapy with oral procainamide. He has renal failure with an estimated creatinine clearance = 9 mL/min. Suggest an initial extended-release procainamide dosage regimen designed to achieve a steady-state procainamide concentration equal to 4 μg/mL.

1. *Estimate half-life and elimination rate constant according to disease states and conditions present in the patient.*
   Patients with severe renal disease have highly variable procainamide pharmacokinetics and dosage requirements. Renal failure decreases procainamide renal clearance, and the expected procainamide half-life ($t_{1/2}$) is 13.9 hours. The elimination rate constant is computed using the following formula: k = 0.693/$t_{1/2}$ = 0.693/13.9 h = 0.050 h^{-1}.
2. *Estimate the volume of distribution and clearance.*
   The patient is not obese, so the estimated procainamide volume of distribution will be based on actual body weight: V = 1.7 L/kg • 85 kg = 145 L. Estimated procainamide clearance is computed by taking the product of the volume of distribution and the elimination rate constant: Cl = kV = 0.050 h^{-1} • 145 L = 7.25 L/h.
3. *Compute dosage regimen.*
   Oral sustained-release procainamide tablets will be prescribed to this patient (F = 0.83). The initial dosage interval (τ) will be set to 12 hours. (Note: μg/mL = mg/L and this concentration unit was substituted for Css in the calculations so that unnecessary unit conversion was not required.) The dosage equation for oral procainamide is: D = (Css • Cl • τ)/F = (4 mg/L • 7.25 L/h • 12 h)/0.83 = 419 mg, rounded to 500 mg every 12 hours.

   　　Steady-state procainamide and NAPA serum concentrations could be measured after steady-state is attained in 3-5 half-lives. Since the patient is expected to have a half-life equal to 13.9 hours for procainamide and 41 hours for NAPA, the steady-state concentrations could be obtained any time after 3-9 days of dosing (5 half-lives = 5 • 13.9 h = 69.5 h for procainamide, 5 half-lives = 5 • 41 h = 205 h for NAPA). Procainamide and NAPA serum concentrations should also be measured if the patient experiences a return of their arrhythmia, or if the patient develops potential signs or symptoms of procainamide toxicity.

   　　To illustrate the differences and similarities between oral and intravenous procainamide dosage regimen design, the same cases will be used to compute intravenous procainamide loading doses and continuous infusions.

EXAMPLE 3 ►►►

LK is a 50-year-old, 75-kg (height = 5 ft 10 in) male with ventricular tachycardia who requires therapy with intravenous procainamide. He has normal liver and cardiac function. Suggest an intravenous procainamide dosage regimen designed to achieve a steady-state procainamide concentration equal to 4 μg/mL.

1. *Estimate half-life and elimination rate constant according to disease states and conditions present in the patient.*

   The expected procainamide half-life ($t_{1/2}$) for an individual with normal hepatic and renal function is 3.3 hours. The elimination rate constant is computed using the following formula: $k = 0.693/t_{1/2} = 0.693/3.3\,h = 0.210\,h^{-1}$.

2. *Estimate the volume of distribution and clearance.*

   The patient is not obese, so the estimated procainamide volume of distribution will be based on actual body weight: $V = 2.7\,L/kg \bullet 75\,kg = 203\,L$. Estimated procainamide clearance is computed by taking the product of the volume of distribution and the elimination rate constant: $Cl = kV = 0.210\,h^{-1} \bullet 203\,L = 42.6\,L/h$.

3. *Compute dosage regimen.*

   Therapy will be started by administering an intravenous loading dose of procainamide to the patient: $LD = Css \bullet V = 4\,mg/L \bullet 203\,L = 812\,mg$, rounded to 800 mg intravenously. Initially, a maximum dose of 600 mg over 25-30 minutes will be given, and the additional 200 mg given, if needed, at a rate of 20 mg/min. (Note: μg/mL = mg/L and this concentration unit was substituted for Css in the calculations so that unnecessary unit conversion was not required.)

   A procainamide continuous intravenous infusion will be started immediately after the loading dose has been administered. (Note: μg/mL = mg/L and this concentration unit was substituted for Css in the calculations so that unnecessary unit conversion was not required.) The dosage equation for intravenous procainamide is: $k_0 = Css \bullet Cl = (4\,mg/L \bullet 42.6\,L/h)/(60\,min/h) = 2.8\,mg/h$, rounded to 3 mg/min.

   Steady-state procainamide and NAPA serum concentrations could be measured after steady-state is attained in 3-5 half-lives. Since the patient is expected to have a half-life equal to 3.3 hours for procainamide and 6 hours for NAPA, the steady-state concentrations could be obtained any time after the first day of dosing (5 half-lives = 5 • 3.3 h = 16.5 h for procainamide, 5 half-lives = 5 • 6 h = 30 h for NAPA). Procainamide and NAPA serum concentrations should also be measured if the patient experiences a return of their arrhythmia, or if the patient develops potential signs or symptoms of procainamide toxicity.

EXAMPLE 4 ►►►

OI is a 60-year-old, 85-kg (height = 6 ft 1 in) male with atrial fibrillation who requires therapy with intravenous procainamide. He has renal failure with an estimated creatinine clearance = 9 mL/min. Suggest an initial intravenous procainamide dosage regimen designed to achieve a steady-state procainamide concentration equal to 4 μg/mL.

1. *Estimate the half-life and elimination rate constant according to disease states and conditions present in the patient.*

   Patients with severe renal disease have highly variable procainamide pharmacokinetics and dosage requirements. Renal failure decreases procainamide renal clearance, and the expected procainamide half-life ($t_{1/2}$) is 13.9 hours. The elimination rate constant is computed using the following formula: $k = 0.693/t_{1/2} = 0.693/13.9\,h = 0.050\,h^{-1}$.

2. *Estimate the volume of distribution and clearance.*

The patient is not obese, so the estimated procainamide volume of distribution will be based on actual body weight: V = 1.7 L/kg • 85 kg = 145 L. Estimated procainamide clearance is computed by taking the product of the volume of distribution and the elimination rate constant: $Cl = kV = 0.050\ h^{-1} • 145\ L = 7.25\ L/h$.

3. *Compute dosage regimen.*

Therapy will be started by administering an intravenous loading dose of procainamide to the patient: LD = Css • V = 4 mg/L • 145 L = 580 mg, rounded to 600 mg intravenously over 25-30 minutes. (Note: µg/mL = mg/L and this concentration unit was substituted for Css in the calculations so that unnecessary unit conversion was not required.)

A procainamide continuous intravenous infusion will be started immediately after the loading dose has been administered. (Note: µg/mL = mg/L and this concentration unit was substituted for Css in the calculations so that unnecessary unit conversion was not required.) The dosage equation for intravenous procainamide is: k_0 = Css • Cl = (4 mg/L • 7.25 L/h)/(60 min/h) = 0.48 mg/h, rounded to 0.5 mg/min.

Steady-state procainamide and NAPA serum concentrations could be measured after steady-state is attained in 3-5 half-lives. Since the patient is expected to have a half-life equal to 13.9 hours for procainamide and 41 hours for NAPA, the steady-state concentrations could be obtained any time after 3-9 days of dosing (5 half-lives = 5 • 13.9 h = 69.5 h for procainamide, 5 half-lives = 5 • 41 h = 205 h for NAPA). Procainamide and NAPA serum concentrations should also be measured if the patient experiences a return of their arrhythmia, or if the patient develops potential signs or symptoms of procainamide toxicity.

Literature-Based Recommended Dosing

Because of the large amount of variability in procainamide pharmacokinetics, even when concurrent disease states and conditions are identified, many clinicians believe that the use of standard procainamide doses for various situations are warranted. The original computation of these doses were based on the pharmacokinetic dosing method described in the previous section, and subsequently modified based on clinical experience. In general, the procainamide steady-state serum concentration expected from the lower end of the dosage range was 4-6 µg/mL and 6-10 µg/mL for the upper end of the dosage range. Suggested procainamide maintenance doses are given in Table 8-3. A 25%-50% reduction in initial procainamide dose is suggested for patients with moderate-severe liver disease (Child-Pugh score ≥8) or moderate-severe heart failure (NYHA class II or greater). A 25%-75% decrease is indicated with renal dysfunction. When more than one disease state or condition is present in a patient, choosing the lowest daily dose will result in the safest, most-conservative dosage recommendation.

Pediatric doses are similar to those given to adults when adjusted for differences in body weight.[42] The recommended intravenous loading dose is 2-6 mg/kg over 5 minutes (maximum dose 100 mg), repeating as necessary every 5-10 minutes to a maximum dose of 15 mg/kg (no more than 500 mg should be given within a 30-minute time period). For patients with ventricular tachycardia and poor perfusion, 15 mg/kg infused over 30-60 minutes as a single dose can be considered if cardioversion is ineffective. Intravenous maintenance infusion rates equal 20-80 µg/kg/min (maximum dose 2 g/d). Oral maintenance doses are 15-50 mg/kg/d. The dosage interval chosen should be appropriate for dosage form administered to the patient.

To illustrate the similarities and differences between this method of dosage calculation and the pharmacokinetic dosing method, the same examples used in the previous section will be used.

EXAMPLE 1 ▶▶▶

LK is a 50-year-old, 75-kg (height = 5 ft 10 in) male with ventricular tachycardia who requires therapy with oral procainamide sustained-release tablets. He has normal liver and cardiac function. Suggest an initial oral procainamide dosage regimen designed to achieve a steady-state procainamide concentration equal to 4 µg/mL.

1. *Choose procainamide dose based on disease states and conditions present in the patient.*
A procainamide maintenance dose of 50 mg/kg/d is suggested for a patient without heart failure or liver disease requiring a procainamide steady-state serum concentration in the lower end of the therapeutic range. The suggested initial dose would be 3750 mg/d (50 mg/kg/d • 75 kg = 3750 mg/d), rounded to 4000 mg/d or 1000 mg every 6 hours.

Steady-state procainamide and NAPA serum concentrations could be measured after steady-state is attained in 3-5 half-lives. Since the patient is expected to have a half-life equal to 3.3 hours for procainamide and 6 hours for NAPA, the steady-state concentrations could be obtained any time after the first day of dosing (5 half-lives = 5 • 3.3 h = 16.5 h for procainamide, 5 half-lives = 5 • 6 h = 30 h for NAPA). Procainamide and NAPA serum concentrations should also be measured if the patient experiences a return of their arrhythmia, or if the patient develops potential signs or symptoms of procainamide toxicity.

EXAMPLE 2 ▶▶▶

OI is a 60-year-old, 85-kg (height = 6 ft 1 in) male with atrial fibrillation who requires therapy with oral procainamide. He has renal failure with an estimated creatinine clearance = 9 mL/min. Suggest an initial extended-release procainamide dosage regimen designed to achieve a steady-state procainamide concentration equal to 4 µg/mL.

1. *Choose procainamide dose based on disease states and conditions present in the patient.*
A procainamide maintenance dose of 12.5 mg/kg/d (50 mg/kg/d • 0.25 = 12.5 mg/kg/d) is suggested for a patient with renal failure requiring a procainamide steady-state serum concentration in the lower end of the therapeutic range. The suggested initial dose would be 1063 mg/d (12.5 mg/kg/d • 85 kg = 1063 mg/d), rounded to 1000 mg/d or 500 mg every 12 hours.

The steady-state procainamide and NAPA serum concentrations could be measured after steady-state is attained in 3-5 half-lives. Since the patient is expected to have a half-life equal to 13.9 hours for procainamide and 41 hours for NAPA, the steady-state concentrations could be obtained any time after 3-9 days of dosing (5 half-lives = 5 • 13.9 h = 69.5 h for procainamide, 5 half-lives = 5 • 41 h = 205 h for NAPA). Procainamide and NAPA serum concentrations should also be measured if the patient experiences a return of their arrhythmia, or if the patient develops potential signs or symptoms of procainamide toxicity.

To illustrate the differences and similarities between oral and intravenous procainamide dosage regimen design, the same cases will be used to compute intravenous procainamide loading doses and continuous infusions.

EXAMPLE 3 ▶▶▶

LK is a 50-year-old, 75-kg (height = 5 ft 10 in) male with ventricular tachycardia who requires therapy with intravenous procainamide. He has normal liver and cardiac function. Suggest an intravenous procainamide dosage regimen designed to achieve a steady-state procainamide concentration equal to 4 µg/mL.

A procainamide maintenance dose of 2-4 mg/min is suggested for a patient without heart failure or liver disease requiring a procainamide steady-state serum concentration in the lower end of the therapeutic range. The suggested initial continuous infusion would be 3 mg/min. If needed, a loading dose of 500 mg infused over 25-30 minutes would also be given.

The steady-state procainamide and NAPA serum concentrations could be measured after steady-state is attained in 3-5 half-lives. Since the patient is expected to have a half-life equal to 3.3 hours for procainamide and 6 hours for NAPA, the steady-state concentrations could be obtained any time after the first day of dosing (5 half-lives = 5 • 3.3 h = 16.5 h for procainamide, 5 half-lives = 5 • 6 h = 30 h for NAPA). Procainamide and NAPA serum concentrations should also be measured if the patient experiences a return of their arrhythmia, or if the patient develops potential signs or symptoms of procainamide toxicity.

EXAMPLE 4 ▶ ▶ ▶

OI is a 60-year-old, 85-kg (height = 6 ft 1in) male with atrial fibrillation who requires therapy with intravenous procainamide. He has renal failure with an estimated creatinine clearance = 9 mL/min. Suggest an initial intravenous procainamide dosage regimen designed to achieve a steady-state procainamide concentration equal to 4 μg/mL.

1. *Choose procainamide dose based on disease states and conditions present in the patient.*
A procainamide maintenance dose of 1-2 mg/min is suggested for a patient with renal failure requiring a procainamide steady-state serum concentration in the lower end of the therapeutic range. The suggested initial dose would be 1 mg/min. If needed, a loading dose of 500 mg infused over 25-30 minutes would also be given.

The steady-state procainamide and NAPA serum concentrations could be measured after steady-state is attained in 3-5 half-lives. Since the patient is expected to have a half-life equal to 13.9 hours for procainamide and 41 hours for NAPA, the steady-state concentrations could be obtained any time after 3-9 days of dosing (5 half-lives = 5 • 13.9 h = 69.5 h for procainamide, 5 half-lives = 5 • 41 h = 205 h for NAPA). Procainamide and NAPA serum concentrations should also be measured if the patient experiences a return of their arrhythmia, or if the patient develops potential signs or symptoms of procainamide toxicity.

USE OF PROCAINAMIDE AND *N*-ACETYLPROCAINAMIDE SERUM CONCENTRATIONS TO ALTER DOSES

Because of the large amount of pharmacokinetic variability among patients, it is likely that doses computed using patient population characteristics will not always produce procainamide or NAPA serum concentrations that are expected or desirable. Because of pharmacokinetic variability, the narrow therapeutic index of procainamide, and the desire to avoid procainamide adverse side effects, measurement of procainamide and NAPA serum concentrations can be a useful adjunct for patients to insure that therapeutic, nontoxic levels are present. In addition to procainamide serum concentrations, important patient parameters (electrocardiogram, clinical signs and symptoms of the arrhythmia, potential procainamide side effects, etc) should be followed to confirm that the patient is responding to treatment and not developing adverse drug reactions.

When procainamide and NAPA serum concentrations are measured in patients and a dosage change is necessary, clinicians should seek to use the simplest, most straightforward method available to determine a dose that will provide safe and effective treatment. In most cases, a simple dosage ratio can be used to change procainamide doses, assuming the drug follows *linear pharmacokinetics*. Thus, linear pharmacokinetics is adequate for dosage adjustments in most patients.

Sometimes, it is useful to compute procainamide pharmacokinetic constants for a patient and base dosage adjustments on these parameters. In this case, it may be possible to calculate and use *pharmacokinetic parameters* to alter the procainamide dose.

In some situations, it may be necessary to compute procainamide pharmacokinetic parameters as soon as possible for the patient before steady-state conditions occur and utilize these parameters to calculate the best drug dose. Computerized methods that incorporate expected population pharmacokinetic characteristics (*Bayesian pharmacokinetic computer programs*) can be used in difficult cases where serum concentrations are obtained at suboptimal times or the patient was not at steady-state when serum concentrations were measured. An additional benefit of this method is that a complete pharmacokinetic workup (determination of clearance, volume of distribution, and half-life) can be done with one or more measured concentrations that do not have to be at steady-state.

Linear Pharmacokinetics Method

Because procainamide follows linear, dose-proportional pharmacokinetics in most patients, steady-state procainamide and NAPA serum concentrations change in proportion to dose according to the following equation: $D_{new}/C_{ss,\ new} = D_{old}/C_{ss,\ old}$ or $D_{new} = (C_{ss,\ new}/C_{ss,\ old})D_{old}$, where D is the dose, Css is the steady-state concentration, old indicates the dose that produced the steady-state concentration that the patient is currently receiving, and new denotes the dose necessary to produce the desired steady-state concentration. The advantages of this method are that it is quick and simple. The disadvantages are that steady-state concentrations are required. Because nonlinear pharmacokinetics for procainamide has been observed in some patients, suggested dosage increases greater than 75% using this method should be scrutinized by the prescribing clinician, and the risk versus benefit for the patient assessed before initiating large dosage increases (>75% over current dose).

EXAMPLE 1 ▶ ▶ ▶

LK is a 50-year-old, 75-kg (height = 5 ft 10 in) male with ventricular tachycardia who requires therapy with procainamide sustained-release tablets. He has normal liver and cardiac function. The current steady-state procainamide and NAPA concentrations equal 2.2 µg/mL and 1.5 µg/mL, respectively (total procainamide concentration = 3.7 µg/mL), at a dose of 1000 mg every 12 hours. Compute a procainamide dose that will provide a steady-state concentration of 4 µg/mL.

1. *Compute new dose to achieve desired serum concentration.*
   The patient would be expected to achieve steady-state conditions after the first day ($5\ t_{1/2} = 5 \bullet 3.3\ h = 17\ h$ for procainamide, $5\ t_{1/2} = 5 \bullet 6\ h = 30\ h$ for NAPA) of therapy.
   Using linear pharmacokinetics, the new dose to attain the desired concentration should be proportional to the old dose that produced the measured concentration. (Note: total daily dose = 1000 mg/dose • 2 dose/d = 2000 mg/d):

$$D_{new} = (C_{ss,\ new}/C_{ss,\ old})D_{old} = (4\ \mu g/mL\ /\ 2.2\ \mu g/mL)\ 2000\ mg/d = 3636\ mg/d,$$
$$\text{rounded to 4000 mg/d or 2000 mg every 12 hours}$$

   The new suggested dose would be 2000 mg every 12 hours of oral procainamide to be started immediately.

The expected NAPA steady-state serum concentration would increase in proportion to the procainamide dosage increase:

$$C_{ss, new} = (D_{new}/D_{old})C_{ss, old} = (4000 \text{ mg/d} / 2000 \text{ mg/d}) \, 1.5 \, \mu g/mL = 3 \, \mu g/mL$$

A steady-state procainamide serum concentration could be measured after steady-state is attained in 3-5 half-lives. Since the patient is expected to have a procainamide half-life equal to 3.3 hours and a NAPA half-life equal to 6 hours, procainamide and NAPA steady-state concentrations could be obtained any time after the first day of dosing (5 half-lives = 5 • 3.3 h = 17 h for procainamide, 5 half-lives = 5 • 6 h = 30 h for NAPA). Procainamide and NAPA serum concentrations should also be measured if the patient experiences a return of their arrhythmia, or if the patient develops potential signs or symptoms of procainamide toxicity.

EXAMPLE 2 ▶ ▶ ▶

OI is a 60-year-old, 85-kg (height = 6 ft 1 in) male with atrial fibrillation who requires therapy with oral procainamide sustained-release tablets. He has renal failure with an estimated creatinine clearance = 9 mL/min. The current steady-state procainamide and NAPA concentrations equal 13.1 μg/mL and 25.2 μg/mL, respectively (total procainamide concentration = 38.3 μg/mL), at a dose of 1000 mg every 12 hours. Compute a procainamide dose that will provide a steady-state concentration of 6 μg/mL.

1. *Compute new dose to achieve desired serum concentration.*

The patient would be expected to achieve steady-state conditions after the ninth day (5 $t_{1/2}$ = 5 • 13.9 h = 70 h, or 3 days for procainamide, 5 $t_{1/2}$ = 5 • 41 h = 205 h, or 9 days for NAPA) of therapy.

Using linear pharmacokinetics, the new dose to attain the desired concentration should be proportional to the old dose that produced the measured concentration. (Note: total daily dose = 1000 mg/dose • 2 dose/d = 2000 mg/d):

$$D_{new} = (C_{ss, new}/C_{ss, old})D_{old} = (6 \, \mu g/mL / 13.1 \, \mu g/mL) \, 2000 \text{ mg/d} = 916 \text{ mg/d},$$
$$\text{rounded to 1000 mg/d or 500 mg every 12 hours}$$

The new suggested dose would be 500 mg every 12 hours of oral procainamide to be started immediately. The expected NAPA steady-state serum concentration would increase in proportion to the procainamide dosage increase:

$$C_{ss, new} = (D_{new}/D_{old})C_{ss, old} = (1000 \text{ mg/d} / 2000 \text{ mg/d}) \, 25.2 \, \mu g/mL = 12.6 \, \mu g/mL$$

A steady-state procainamide serum concentration could be measured after steady-state is attained in 3-5 half-lives. Since the patient is expected to have a procainamide half-life equal to 13.9 hours and a NAPA half-life equal to 41 hours, procainamide and NAPA steady-state concentrations could be obtained any time after the ninth day of dosing (5 half-lives = 5 • 13.9 h = 70 h for procainamide, 5 half-lives = 5 • 41 h = 205 h for NAPA). Procainamide and NAPA serum concentrations should also be measured if the patient experiences a return of their arrhythmia, or if the patient develops potential signs or symptoms of procainamide toxicity.

EXAMPLE 3 ▶ ▶ ▶

MN is a 64-year-old, 78-kg (height = 5 ft 9 in) male with ventricular tachycardia who requires therapy with intravenous procainamide. He has moderate heart failure (NYHA CHF class III). The current steady-state procainamide and NAPA concentrations equal 4.5 μg/mL and 7.9 μg/mL, respectively (total procainamide concentration = 12.4 μg/mL), at a dose of 1 mg/min. Compute a procainamide dose that will provide a steady-state concentration of 8 μg/mL.

1. *Compute new dose to achieve desired serum concentration.*
   The patient would be expected to achieve steady-state conditions after the second day ($5\,t_{1/2} = 5 \bullet 5.5\,h = 28\,h$ for procainamide, $5\,t_{1/2} = 5 \bullet 6\,h = 30\,h$, for NAPA assuming normal renal function) of therapy.
   Using linear pharmacokinetics, the new dose to attain the desired concentration should be proportional to the old dose that produced the measured concentration:

   $$D_{new} = (C_{ss,\,new}/C_{ss,\,old})D_{old} = (8\,\mu g/mL\,/\,4.5\,\mu g/mL)\,1\,mg/min = 1.8\,mg/min,\ rounded\ to\ 2\,mg/min$$

   The new suggested dose would be 2 mg/min of intravenous procainamide to be started immediately.
   The expected NAPA steady-state serum concentration would increase in proportion to the procainamide dosage increase:

   $$C_{ss,\,new} = (D_{new}/D_{old})C_{ss,\,old} = (2\,mg/min\,/\,1\,mg/min)\,7.9\,\mu g/mL = 15.8\,\mu g/mL$$

   A steady-state procainamide serum concentration could be measured after steady-state is attained in 3-5 half-lives. Since the patient is expected to have a procainamide half-life equal to 5.5 hours and a NAPA half-life equal to 6 hours, procainamide and NAPA steady-state concentrations could be obtained any time after the second day of dosing (5 half-lives = 5 • 5.5 h = 28 h for procainamide, 5 half-lives = 5 • 6 h = 30 h for NAPA). Procainamide and NAPA serum concentrations should also be measured if the patient experiences a return of their arrhythmia, or if the patient develops potential signs or symptoms of procainamide toxicity.

Pharmacokinetic Parameter Method

The Pharmacokinetic Parameter method of adjusting drug doses was among the first techniques available to change doses using serum concentrations. It allows the computation of an individual's own, unique pharmacokinetic constants and uses those to calculate a dose that achieves desired procainamide concentrations. The Pharmacokinetic Parameter method requires that steady-state has been achieved and uses only a steady-state procainamide concentration (Css). During a continuous intravenous infusion, the following equation is used to compute procainamide clearance (Cl): $Cl = k_0/Css$, where k_0 is the dose of procainamide in mg/min. If the patient is receiving oral procainamide therapy, procainamide clearance (Cl) can be calculated using the following formula: $Cl = [F(D/\tau)]/Css$, where F is the bioavailability fraction for the oral dosage form (F = 0.83 for most oral procainamide products), D is the dose of procainamide in mg, Css is the steady-state procainamide concentration, and τ is the dosage interval in hours. For both oral and intravenous procainamide routes of administration, the expected NAPA steady-state serum concentration would increase in proportion to the procainamide dosage increase: $C_{ss,\,new} = (D_{new}/D_{old})C_{ss,\,old}$ where D is the dose, Css is the steady-state concentration, old indicates the dose that produced the steady-state concentration that the patient is currently receiving, and new denotes the dose necessary to produce the desired steady-state concentration. Because this method also assumes linear pharmacokinetics, procainamide doses computed using the Pharmacokinetic Parameter method and the Linear Pharmacokinetic method should be identical.

EXAMPLE 1 ▶ ▶ ▶

LK is a 50-year-old, 75-kg (height = 5 ft 10 in) male with ventricular tachycardia who requires therapy with procainamide sustained-release tablets. He has normal liver and cardiac function. The current steady-state procainamide and NAPA concentrations equal 2.2 μg/mL and 1.5 μg/mL, respectively (total procainamide concentration = 3.7 μg/mL), at a dose of 1000 mg every 12 hours. Compute a procainamide dose that will provide a steady-state concentration of 4 μg/mL.

1. *Compute pharmacokinetic parameters.*

The patient would be expected to achieve steady-state conditions after the first day (5 $t_{1/2}$ = 5 • 3.3 h = 17 h for procainamide, 5 $t_{1/2}$ = 5 • 6 h = 30 h for NAPA) of therapy.

Procainamide clearance can be computed using a steady-state procainamide concentration: Cl = [F(D/τ)] / Css = [0.83 (1000 mg/12 h)] / (2.2 mg/L) = 31.4 L/h. (Note: μg/mL = mg/L and this concentration unit was substituted for Css in the calculations so that unnecessary unit conversion was not required.)

2. *Compute procainamide dose.*

Procainamide clearance is used to compute the new dose:

D = (Css • Cl • τ)/F = (4 mg/L • 31.4 L/h • 12 h)/0.83 = 1816 mg, rounded to 2000 mg every 12 hours.

The expected NAPA steady-state serum concentration would increase in proportion to the procainamide dosage increase:

$$C_{ss,\ new} = (D_{new}/D_{old})C_{ss,\ old} = (4000\ mg/d\ /\ 2000\ mg/d)\ 1.5\ μg/mL = 3\ μg/mL$$

The new procainamide dose would be instituted immediately.

A steady-state procainamide serum concentration could be measured after steady-state is attained in 3-5 half-lives. Since the patient is expected to have a procainamide half-life equal to 3.3 hours and a NAPA half-life equal to 6 hours, procainamide and NAPA steady-state concentrations could be obtained any time after the first day of dosing (5 half-lives = 5 • 3.3 h = 17 h for procainamide, 5 half-lives = 5 • 6 h = 30 h for NAPA). Procainamide and NAPA serum concentrations should also be measured if the patient experiences a return of their arrhythmia, or if the patient develops potential signs or symptoms of procainamide toxicity.

EXAMPLE 2 ▶ ▶ ▶

OI is a 60-year-old, 85-kg (height = 6 ft 1 in) male with atrial fibrillation who requires therapy with oral procainamide sustained-release tablets. He has renal failure with an estimated creatinine clearance = 9 mL/min. The current steady-state procainamide and NAPA concentrations equal 13.1 μg/mL and 25.2 μg/mL, respectively (total procainamide concentration = 38.3 μg/mL), at a dose of 1000 mg every 12 hours. Compute a procainamide dose that will provide a steady-state concentration of 6 μg/mL.

1. *Compute pharmacokinetic parameters.*

The patient would be expected to achieve steady-state conditions after the ninth day (5 $t_{1/2}$ = 5 • 13.9 h = 70 h, or 3 days for procainamide, 5 $t_{1/2}$ = 5 • 41 h = 205 h, or 9 days for NAPA) of therapy.

Procainamide clearance can be computed using a steady-state procainamide concentration: Cl = [F(D/τ)] / Css = [0.83 (1000 mg/12 h)] / (13.1 mg/L) = 5.28 L/h. (Note: μg/mL = mg/L and this concentration unit was substituted for Css in the calculations so that unnecessary unit conversion was not required.)

2. *Compute procainamide dose.*

Procainamide clearance is used to compute the new dose:

$$D = (Css \bullet Cl \bullet \tau)/F = (6 \text{ mg/L} \bullet 5.28 \text{ L/h} \bullet 12 \text{ h})/0.83 = 458 \text{ mg, rounded to } 500 \text{ mg every } 12 \text{ hours.}$$

The expected NAPA steady-state serum concentration would change in proportion to the procainamide dosage change:

$$C_{ss, new} = (D_{new}/D_{old})C_{ss, old} = (1000 \text{ mg/d} / 2000 \text{ mg/d}) \, 25.2 \, \mu g/mL = 12.6 \, \mu g/mL$$

If the patient was experiencing side effects, the new dosage regimen would be held for one estimated half-life. Otherwise, the new procainamide dose would be instituted immediately.

A steady-state procainamide serum concentration could be measured after steady-state is attained in 3-5 half-lives. Since the patient is expected to have a procainamide half-life equal to 13.9 hours and a NAPA half-life equal to 41 hours, procainamide and NAPA steady-state concentrations could be obtained any time after the ninth day of dosing (5 half-lives = $5 \bullet 13.9 \text{ h} = 70 \text{ h}$ for procainamide, 5 half-lives = $5 \bullet 41 \text{ h} = 205 \text{ h}$ for NAPA). Procainamide and NAPA serum concentrations should also be measured if the patient experiences a return of their arrhythmia, or if the patient develops potential signs or symptoms of procainamide toxicity.

EXAMPLE 3 ▶▶▶

MN is a 64-year-old, 78-kg (height = 5 ft 9 in) male with ventricular tachycardia who requires therapy with intravenous procainamide. He has moderate heart failure (NYHA CHF class III). The current steady-state procainamide and NAPA concentrations equal 4.5 μg/mL and 7.9 μg/mL, respectively (total procainamide concentration = 12.4 μg/mL), at a dose of 1 mg/min. Compute a procainamide dose that will provide a steady-state concentration of 8 μg/mL.

1. *Compute pharmacokinetic parameters.*

The patient would be expected to achieve steady-state conditions after the second day (5 $t_{1/2} = 5 \bullet 5.5 \text{ h} = 28 \text{ h}$ for procainamide, 5 $t_{1/2} = 5 \bullet 6 \text{ h} = 30 \text{ h}$, for NAPA (assuming normal renal function) of therapy.

Procainamide clearance can be computed using a steady-state procainamide concentration: $Cl = k_0 / Css = (1 \text{ mg/min})/(4.5 \text{ mg/L}) = 0.22 \text{ L/min}$. (Note: μg/mL = mg/L and this concentration unit was substituted for Css in the calculations so that unnecessary unit conversion was not required.)

2. *Compute procainamide dose.*

Procainamide clearance is used to compute the new dose: $k_0 = Css \, Cl = 8 \text{ mg/L} \bullet 0.22 \text{ L/min} = 1.8 \text{ mg/min}$, rounded to 2 mg/min. (Note: μg/mL = mg/L and this concentration unit was substituted for Css in the calculations so that unnecessary unit conversion was not required.)

The expected NAPA steady-state serum concentration would increase in proportion to the procainamide dosage increase:

$$C_{ss, new} = (D_{new}/D_{old})C_{ss, old} = (2 \text{ mg/min} / 1 \text{ mg/min}) \, 7.9 \, \mu g/mL = 15.8 \, \mu g/mL$$

The new procainamide dose would be instituted immediately.

A steady-state procainamide serum concentration could be measured after steady-state is attained in 3-5 half-lives. Since the patient is expected to have a procainamide half-life equal to 5.5 hours and a NAPA half-life equal to 6 hours, procainamide and NAPA steady-state concentrations could be obtained any time after the second day of dosing (5 half-lives = $5 \bullet 5.5 \text{ h} = 28 \text{ h}$ for procainamide, 5 half-lives = $5 \bullet 6 \text{ h} = 30 \text{ h}$ for NAPA). Procainamide and NAPA serum concentrations should also be measured if the patient experiences a return of their arrhythmia, or if the patient develops potential signs or symptoms of procainamide toxicity.

CHIOU METHOD

For some patients, it is desirable to individualize procainamide infusion rates as rapidly as possible before steady-state is achieved.[43] Examples of these cases include patients with renal dysfunction, heart failure, or hepatic cirrhosis who have variable procainamide pharmacokinetic parameters and long procainamide half-lives. In this situation, two procainamide serum concentrations obtained at least 4-6 hours apart during a continuous infusion can be used to compute procainamide clearance and dosing rates. In addition to this requirement, the only way procainamide can be entering the patient's body must be via intravenous infusion. Thus, the last dose of sustained-release procainamide must have been administered no less than 12-16 hours before this technique is used, or some residual oral procainamide will still be absorbed from the gastrointestinal tract and cause computation errors.

The following equation is used to compute procainamide clearance (Cl) using the procainamide concentrations:

$$Cl = \frac{2k_0}{C_1 + C_2} + \frac{2V(C_1 - C_2)}{(C_1 + C_2)(t_2 - t_1)}$$

where k_0 is the infusion rate of procainamide, V is procainamide volume of distribution (chosen according to disease states and conditions present in the patient, Table 8-1), C_1 and C_2 are the first and second procainamide serum concentrations, and t_1 and t_2 are the times that C_1 and C_2 were obtained. Once procainamide clearance (Cl) is determined, it can be used to adjust the procainamide salt infusion rate (k_0) using the following relationship: $k_0 = Css \bullet Cl$.

EXAMPLE 1 ▶▶▶

JB is a 50-year-old, 60-kg (height = 5 ft 7 in) male with heart failure (NYHA CHF class III) started on a 5-mg/min procainamide infusion after being administered an intravenous loading dose. The procainamide concentration was 10.6 µg/mL at 1000 H and 14.3 µg/mL at 1400 H. What procainamide infusion rate is needed to achieve Css = 8 µg/mL?

1. *Compute procainamide clearance and dose.*

$$Cl = \frac{2k_0}{C_1 + C_2} + \frac{2V(C_1 - C_2)}{(C_1 + C_2)(t_2 - t_1)}$$

$$Cl = \frac{2(5 \text{ mg/min})}{10.6 \text{ mg/L} + 14.3 \text{ mg/L}} + \frac{2(1.6 \text{ L/kg} \bullet 60 \text{ kg})(10.6 \text{ mg/L} - 14.3 \text{ mg/L})}{(10.6 \text{ mg/L} + 14.3 \text{ mg/L}) \, 240 \text{ min}}$$

$$= 0.28 \text{ L/min}$$

(Note: µg/mL = mg/L and this concentration unit was substituted for concentrations so that unnecessary unit conversion was not required. Additionally, the time difference between t_2 and t_1, in minutes, was determined and placed directly in the calculation.)

$$k_0 = Css \bullet Cl = 8 \text{ mg/L} \bullet 0.28 \text{ L/h} = 2.2 \text{ mg/min of procainamide}$$

EXAMPLE 2 ▶▶▶

YU is a 64-year-old, 80-kg (height = 5 ft 9 in) male started on a 3-mg/min procainamide infusion after being administered an intravenous loading dose at 0900 H. The procainamide concentration was 10.3 µg/mL at 1000 H and 7.1 µg/mL at 1600 H. What procainamide infusion rate is needed to achieve Css = 10 µg/mL?

1. *Compute procainamide clearance and dose.*

$$Cl = \frac{2k_0}{C_1 + C_2} + \frac{2V(C_1 - C_2)}{(C_1 + C_2)(t_2 - t_1)}$$

$$Cl = \frac{2(3 \text{ mg / min})}{10.3 \text{ mg/L} + 7.1 \text{ mg/L}} + \frac{2(2.7 \text{ L/kg} \bullet 80 \text{ kg})(10.3 \text{ mg/L} - 7.1 \text{ mg/L})}{(10.3 \text{ mg/L} + 7.1 \text{ mg/L})360 \text{ min}}$$

$$= 0.57 \text{ L/min}$$

(Note: µg/mL = mg/L and this concentration unit was substituted for concentrations so that unnecessary unit conversion was not required. Additionally, the time difference between t_2 and t_1, in minutes, was determined and placed directly in the calculation.)

$$k_0 = Css \bullet Cl = 10 \text{ mg/L} \bullet 0.57 \text{ L/min} = 5.7 \text{ mg/min of procainamide}$$

BAYESIAN PHARMACOKINETIC COMPUTER PROGRAMS

Computer programs are available that can assist in the computation of pharmacokinetic parameters for patients. The most reliable computer programs use a nonlinear regression algorithm that incorporates components of Bayes theorem. Nonlinear regression is a statistical technique that uses an iterative process to compute the best pharmacokinetic parameters for a concentration/time data set. Briefly, the patient's drug dosage schedule and serum concentrations are input into the computer. The computer program has a pharmacokinetic equation preprogrammed for the drug and administration method (oral, intravenous bolus, intravenous infusion, etc). Typically, a one-compartment model is used, although some programs allow the user to choose among several different equations. Using population estimates based on demographic information for the patient (age, weight, gender, liver function, cardiac status, etc) supplied by the user, the computer program then computes estimated serum concentrations at each time there are actual serum concentrations. Kinetic parameters are then changed by the computer program, and a new set of estimated serum concentrations are computed. The pharmacokinetic parameters that generated the estimated serum concentrations closest to the actual values are remembered by the computer program, and the process is repeated until the set of pharmacokinetic parameters that result in estimated serum concentrations that are statistically closest to the actual serum concentrations are generated. These pharmacokinetic parameters can then be used to compute improved dosing schedules for patients. Bayes theorem is used in the computer algorithm to balance the results of the computations between values based solely on the patient's serum drug concentrations and those based only on patient population parameters. Results from studies that compare various methods of dosage adjustment have consistently found that these types of computer dosing programs perform at least as well as experienced clinical pharmacokineticists and clinicians and better than inexperienced clinicians.

Some clinicians use Bayesian pharmacokinetic computer programs exclusively to alter drug doses based on serum concentrations. An advantage of this approach is that consistent dosage recommendations are made when several different practitioners are involved in therapeutic drugmonitoring programs. However, since simpler dosing methods work just as well for patients with stable pharmacokinetic parameters and steady-state drug concentrations, many clinicians reserve the use of computer programs for more difficult situations. Those situations include serum concentrations that are not at steady-state, serum concentrations not obtained at the specific times needed to employ simpler methods, and unstable pharmacokinetic parameters. Many Bayesian pharmacokinetic computer programs are available to users, and most should provide answers similar to the one used in the following examples. The program used to solve problems in this book is DrugCalc written by Dr Dennis Mungall.[44]

EXAMPLE 1 ▶▶▶

OY is a 57-year-old, 79-kg (height = 5 ft 8 in) male with ventricular tachycardia who requires therapy with oral procainamide. He has normal liver (bilirubin = 0.7 mg/dL, albumin = 4.0 g/dL), renal (serum creatinine = 1.0 mg/dL), and cardiac function. He started taking procainamide sustained-release tablets 500 mg four times daily at 0700, 1200, 1800, and 2200 H. The procainamide serum concentration equals 2.1 µg/mL at 2130 H before the third dose is given on the first day of therapy. Compute a procainamide dose that will provide a steady-state concentration of 6 µg/mL.

1. *Enter the patient's demographic, drug dosing, and serum concentration/time data into the computer program.*
   In this patient's case, it is unlikely that the patient is at steady-state so the Linear Pharmacokinetics method cannot be used.
2. *Compute pharmacokinetic parameters for the patient using Bayesian pharmacokinetic computer program.*
   The pharmacokinetic parameters computed by the program are a volume of distribution of 152 L, a half-life equal to 3.1 hours, and a clearance equal to 33.9 L/h.
3. *Compute the dose required to achieve the desired procainamide serum concentrations.*
   The oral one-compartment model equation used by the program to compute doses indicates that 2000 mg of procainamide every 6 hours will produce a steady-state trough concentration of 6.1 µg/mL. This dose would be started immediately.

EXAMPLE 2 ▶▶▶

SL is a 71-year-old, 82-kg (height = 5 ft 10 in) male with atrial fibrillation who requires therapy with oral procainamide. He has liver cirrhosis (Child-Pugh score = 12, bilirubin = 3.2 mg/dL, albumin = 2.5 g/dL) and normal cardiac function. He began procainamide sustained-release tablets 500 mg every 12 hours at 0700 H. On the second day of therapy before the morning dose is administered, the procainamide serum concentration equals 4.5 µg/mL at 0700 H. Compute a procainamide dose that will provide a steady-state concentration of 5 µg/mL.

1. *Enter the patient's demographic, drug dosing, and serum concentration/time data into the computer program.*
   In this patient's case, it is unlikely that the patient is at steady-state so the Linear Pharmacokinetics method cannot be used.
2. *Compute pharmacokinetic parameters for the patient using Bayesian pharmacokinetic computer program.*
   The pharmacokinetic parameters computed by the program are a volume of distribution of 110 L, a half-life equal to 15.5 hours, and a clearance equal to 4.93 L/h.
3. *Compute the dose required to achieve the desired procainamide serum concentrations.*
   The oral one-compartment model equation used by the program to compute doses indicates that 250 mg of procainamide sustained-release tablets every 8 hours will produce a steady-state trough concentration of 5.5 µg/mL. This dose would be started immediately.

EXAMPLE 3 ▶ ▶ ▶

TR is a 75-year-old, 85-kg (height = 5 ft 8 in) male with atrial flutter who requires therapy wlth procain-amide sustained-release tablets. He has moderate heart failure (NYHA CHF class III). Yesterday, he was pre-scribed procainamide 500 mg four times daily, and received the first two doses at 0800 H and 1200 H. Because he felt that his arrhythmia may have returned, the patient phoned his physician who advised him to increase the dose to 1000 mg (1800 H and 2200 H). The procainamide serum concentration equals 10.7 µg/mL at 1000 H, 2 hours after the morning dose (at 0800 H, 1000 mg procainamide). Compute a procainamide sustained-release tablet dose that will provide a steady-state trough concentration of 6 µg/mL.

1. *Enter the patient's demographic, drug dosing, and serum concentration/time data into the computer program.*
   In this patient's case, it is unlikely that the patient is at steady-state so the Linear Pharmacokinetics method cannot be used.
2. *Compute pharmacokinetic parameters for the patient using Bayesian pharmacokinetic computer program.*
   The pharmacokinetic parameters computed by the program are a volume of distribution of 114 L, a half-life equal to 7.3 hours, and a clearance equal to 10.8 L/h.
3. *Compute the dose required to achieve the desired procainamide serum concentrations.*
   The oral one-compartment model equation used by the program to compute doses indicates that 500 mg of procainamide immediate-release tablets every 6 hours will produce a steady-state trough concentration of 5.9 µg/mL. This dose would be started immediately.

USE OF PROCAINAMIDE BOOSTER DOSES TO IMMEDIATELY INCREASE SERUM CONCENTRATIONS

If a patient has a subtherapeutic procainamide serum concentration in an acute situation, it may be desirable to increase the procainamide concentration as quickly as possible. In this setting, it would not be acceptable to simply increase the maintenance dose and wait 3-5 half-lives for therapeutic serum concentrations to be established in the patient. A rational way to increase the serum concentrations rapidly is to administer a booster dose of procainamide, a process also known as "reloading" the patient with procainamide, computed using pharmacokinetic techniques. A modified loading dose equation is used to accomplish computation of the booster dose (BD) which takes into account the current procainamide concentration present in the patient: $BD = (C_{desired} - C_{actual})V$, where $C_{desired}$ is the desired procainamide concentration, C_{actual} is the actual current procainamide concentration for the patient, and V is the volume of distribution for procainamide. If the volume of distribution for procainamide is known for the patient, it can be used in the calculation. However, this value is not usually known and is assumed to equal the population average for the disease states and conditions present in the patient (Table 8-1).

Concurrent with the administration of the booster dose, the maintenance dose of procainamide is usually increased. Clinicians need to recognize that the administration of a booster dose does not alter the time required to achieve steady-state conditions when a new procainamide dosage rate is prescribed. It still requires 3-5 half-lives to attain steady-state when the dosage rate is changed. However, usually the difference between the post-booster dose procainamide concentration and the ultimate steady-state concentration has been reduced by giving the extra dose of drug.

EXAMPLE 1 ▶ ▶ ▶

BN is a 42-year-old, 50-kg (height = 5 ft 2 in) female with atrial flutter, who is receiving therapy with intravenous procainamide. She has normal liver and cardiac function. After receiving an initial loading dose of procainamide (300 mg) and a maintenance infusion of procainamide equal to 4 mg/min for 16 hours, her procainamide concentration is measured at 2.1 μg/mL and her atrial rate continues to be rapid. Compute a booster dose of procainamide to achieve a procainamide concentration equal to 6 μg/mL.

1. *Estimate volume of distribution according to disease states and conditions present in the patient.*
   In the case of procainamide, the population average volume of distribution equals 2.7 L/kg and this will be used to estimate the parameter for the patient. The patient is nonobese, so her actual body weight will be used in the computation: V = 2.7 L/kg • 50 kg = 135 L.

2. *Compute booster dose.*
   The booster dose is computed using the following equation: BD = $(C_{desired} - C_{actual})V$ = (6 mg/L − 2.1 mg/L)135 L = 527 mg, rounded to 500 mg of procainamide infused over 25-30 minutes. (Note: μg/mL = mg/L and this concentration unit was substituted for Css in the calculations so that unnecessary unit conversion was not required.) If the maintenance dose was increased, it will take an additional 3-5 estimated half-lives for new steady-state conditions to be achieved. Procainamide serum concentrations can be measured at this time.

DOSING STRATEGIES

Initial dose and dosage adjustment techniques using serum concentrations can be used in any combination as long as the limitations of each method are observed. Some dosing schemes link together logically when considered according to their basic approaches or philosophies. Dosage strategies that follow similar pathways are given in Table 8-5.

CONVERSION OF PROCAINAMIDE DOSES FROM INTRAVENOUS TO ORAL ROUTE OF ADMINISTRATION

Occasionally there is a need to convert a patient stabilized on procainamide therapy from the oral route of administration to an equivalent continuous infusion or vice versa. In general, oral procainamide dosage forms, including most sustained-release tablets and capsules, have a bioavailability equal to 0.83. Assuming that equal procainamide serum concentrations are desired, this makes conversion between the intravenous [k_0 = Css • Cl] and oral [D = (Css • Cl • τ)/F] routes of administration simple since equivalent doses of drug (corrected for

TABLE 8-5   Dosing Strategies

Dosing Approach/Philosophy	Initial Dosing	Use of Serum Concentrations to Alter Doses
Pharmacokinetic parameters/equations	Pharmacokinetic Dosing method	Pharmacokinetic Parameter method
Literature-based concept	Literature-based Recommended Dosing method	Linear Pharmacokinetics method
Computerized	Bayesian computer program	Bayesian computer program

procainamide salt form) are prescribed: $k_0 = FD_{po}/(60 \text{ min/h} \cdot \tau)$ or $D_{po} = (k_0 \cdot \tau \cdot 60 \text{ min/h})/F$, where k_0 is the equivalent intravenous infusion rate for the procainamide in mg/min, D_{po} is equivalent dose of oral procainamide in mg, τ is the dosage interval in h, and F is the bioavailability fraction for oral procainamide.

EXAMPLE 1 ▶▶▶

JH is currently receiving oral sustained-release procainamide 1000 mg every 6 hours. She is responding well to therapy, has no adverse drug effects, and has a steady-state procainamide and NAPA concentrations of 8.3 µg/mL and 14.7 µg/mL, respectively. Suggest an equivalent dose of procainamide given as an intravenous infusion for this patient.

1. *Calculate equivalent intravenous dose of procainamide.*
   The equivalent intravenous procainamide dose would be: $k_0 = FD_{po}/(60 \text{ min/h} \cdot \tau) = (0.83 \cdot 1000 \text{ mg})/(60 \text{ min/h} \cdot 6 \text{ h}) = 2.3$ mg/min of procainamide as a continuous intravenous infusion.

EXAMPLE 2 ▶▶▶

LK is currently receiving a continuous infusion of procainamide at the rate of 5 mg/min. He is responding well to therapy, has no adverse drug effects, and has steady-state procainamide and NAPA concentrations of 6.2 µg/mL and 4.3 µg/mL, respectively. Suggest an equivalent dose of sustained-release oral procainamide for this patient.

1. *Calculate equivalent oral dose of procainamide.*
   The equivalent oral sustained-release procainamide dose using a 12-hour dosage interval would be: $D_{po} = (k_0 \cdot \tau \cdot 60 \text{ min/h})/F = (5 \text{ mg/min} \cdot 12 \text{ h} \cdot 60 \text{ min/h})/0.83 = 4337$ mg, rounded to 4000 mg. The patient would be prescribed procainamide sustained-release tablets 4000 mg orally every 12 hours.

PROBLEMS

The following problems are intended to emphasize the computation of initial and individualized doses using clinical pharmacokinetic techniques. Clinicians should always consult the patient's chart to confirm that current antiarrhythmic and other drug therapy is appropriate. Additionally, all other medications that the patient is taking, including prescription and nonprescription drugs, should be noted and checked to ascertain if a potential drug interaction with procainamide exists.

1. NJ is a 67-year-old, 72-kg (height = 6 ft 1 in) male with ventricular tachycardia who requires therapy with oral procainamide. He has normal renal and liver function, and does not have uncompensated heart failure. Suggest an initial oral procainamide dosage regimen designed to achieve a steady-state procainamide concentration equal to 4 µg/mL.

2. Patient NJ (see problem 1) was prescribed procainamide sustained-release tablets 1000 mg orally every 6 hours. The current steady-state procainamide and NAPA concentrations equal 4.2 µg/mL and 2.5 µg/mL, respectively (total procainamide concentration = 6.7 µg/mL). Compute a new oral procainamide dose that will provide a procainamide steady-state concentration of 6 µg/mL.

3. GF is a 56-year-old, 81-kg (height = 5 ft 9 in) male with ventricular tachycardia who requires therapy with oral procainamide. He has renal failure (estimated creatinine clearance = 10 mL/min) and normal liver function. Suggest an initial procainamide dosage regimen designed to achieve a steady-state procainamide concentration equal to 4 μg/mL.

4. Patient GF (see problem 3) was prescribed procainamide sustained-release tablets 1000 mg orally every 12 hours. The current steady-state procainamide and NAPA concentrations equal 9.5 μg/mL and 32.5 μg/mL, respectively (total procainamide concentration = 42 μg/mL). Compute a new oral procainamide dose that will provide a procainamide steady-state concentration of 6 μg/mL.

5. YU is a 71-year-old, 60-kg (height = 5 ft 2 in) female with paroxysmal atrial tachycardia who requires therapy with oral procainamide. She has severe uncompensated heart failure (NYHA CHF class IV) and normal liver function. Suggest an initial procainamide dosage regimen designed to achieve a steady-state procainamide concentration equal to 5 μg/mL.

6. Patient YU (see problem 5) was prescribed procainamide sustained-release tablets 1000 mg orally every 12 hours. The procainamide and NAPA concentrations obtained just before the third dose of this regimen equaled 11.4 μg/mL and 10.1 μg/mL, respectively (total procainamide concentration = 21.5 μg/mL). Assuming the procainamide concentration was zero before the first dose, compute a new oral procainamide dose that will provide a steady-state concentration of 8 μg/mL.

7. WE is a 54-year-old, 55-kg (height = 5 in 5 in) female with atrial fibrillation who requires therapy with oral procainamide. She has severe liver cirrhosis (Child-Pugh score = 13). Suggest an initial oral procainamide dosage regimen designed to achieve a steady-state procainamide concentration equal to 5 μg/mL.

8. Patient WE (see problem 7) was prescribed procainamide sustained-release tablets 1000 mg orally every 12 hours. The procainamide and NAPA concentrations obtained just before the third dose of this regimen equaled 9.5 μg/mL and 7.2 μg/mL, respectively (total procainamide concentration = 16.7 μg/mL). Assuming the procainamide concentration was zero before the first dose, compute a new oral procainamide dose that will provide a steady-state concentration of 7 μg/mL.

9. IO is a 62-year-old, 130-kg (height = 5 ft 11 in) male with atrial flutter who requires therapy with oral procainamide. He has normal liver and renal function. Suggest an initial procainamide sustained-release dosage regimen designed to achieve a steady-state procainamide concentration equal to 4 μg/mL.

10. Patient IO (see problem 9) was prescribed procainamide sustained-release tablets 2000 mg orally every 12 hours. After the first dose, the patient's arrhythmia returned, and his clinician advised a dosage increase to 3000 mg every 12 hours. Procainamide and NAPA serum concentrations were obtained just before the third dose (ie, after one 2000-mg and one 3000-mg dose) and equaled 2.8 μg/mL. Assuming the procainamide concentration was zero before the first dose, compute a new oral procainamide dose that will provide a steady-state concentration of 4 μg/mL.

11. LG is a 53-year-old, 69-kg (height = 5 ft 10 in) male with atrial flutter who requires therapy with intravenous procainamide. He has normal liver and cardiac function. Suggest an initial procainamide dosage regimen designed to achieve a steady-state procainamide concentration equal to 4 μg/mL.

12. Patient LG (see problem 11) was prescribed intravenous procainamide 3 mg/min. The procainamide and NAPA concentrations obtained after 24 hours of this regimen equaled 4.5 μg/mL and 2.5 μg/mL, respectively (total procainamide concentration = 7 μg/mL). Compute a new intravenous procainamide infusion and a procainamide booster dose that will provide a steady-state concentration of 8 μg/mL.

13. CV is a 69-year-old, 90-kg (height = 6 ft 1 in) male with ventricular tachycardia who requires therapy with intravenous procainamide. He has liver cirrhosis (Child-Pugh score = 11) and normal cardiac function. Suggest an initial intravenous procainamide dosage regimen designed to achieve a steady-state procainamide concentration equal to 5 μg/mL.

14. Patient CV (see problem 13) was prescribed intravenous procainamide 3 mg/min and administered a loading dose of procainamide 500 mg over 30 minutes before the continuous infusion began. A procainamide serum concentration was obtained after 12 hours of the infusion and equaled 11.2 µg/mL. Compute a new intravenous procainamide infusion that will provide a steady-state concentration of 6 µg/mL.

15. PE is a 61-year-old, 67-kg (height = 5 ft 6 in) female with atrial fibrillation who requires therapy with intravenous procainamide. She has severe heart failure (NYHA CHF class IV) and normal liver function. Suggest an initial intravenous procainamide dosage regimen designed to achieve a steady-state procainamide concentration equal to 4 µg/mL.

16. Patient PE (see problem 15) was prescribed intravenous procainamide 4 mg/min and administered a loading dose of procainamide 500 mg over 30 minutes before the continuous infusion began. Procainamide serum concentrations were obtained 4 hours and 8 hours after the infusion began and equaled 4.3 µg/mL and 8.8 µg/mL, respectively. Compute a new intravenous procainamide infusion that will provide a steady-state concentration of 6 µg/mL.

ANSWERS TO PROBLEMS

1. *Answer to problem 1.* The initial procainamide dose for patient NJ would be calculated as follows:

Pharmacokinetic Dosing Method

1. *Estimate half-life and elimination rate constant according to disease states and conditions present in the patient.*

The expected procainamide half-life ($t_{1/2}$) is 3.3 hours. The elimination rate constant is computed using the following formula: $k = 0.693/t_{1/2} = 0.693/3.3 \text{ h} = 0.210 \text{ h}^{-1}$.

2. *Estimate the volume of distribution and clearance.*

The patient is not obese, so the estimated procainamide volume of distribution will be based on actual body weight: V = 2.7 L/kg • 72 kg = 194 L. Estimated procainamide clearance is computed by taking the product of the volume of distribution and the elimination rate constant: Cl = kV = 0.210 h^{-1} • 194 L = 40.7 L/h.

3. *Compute dosage regimen.*

Oral sustained-release procainamide tablets will be prescribed to this patient (F = 0.83). Because the patient has a rapid procainamide clearance and half-life, the initial dosage interval (τ) will be set to 6 hours. (Note: µg/mL = mg/L and this concentration unit was substituted for Css in the calculations so that unnecessary unit conversion was not required.) The dosage equation for oral procainamide is: D = (Css • Cl • τ)/F = (4 mg/L • 40.7 L/h • 6 h)/0.83 = 1177 mg, rounded to 1000 mg every 6 hours.

Steady-state procainamide and NAPA serum concentrations could be measured after steady-state is attained in 3-5 half-lives. Since the patient is expected to have a half-life equal to 3.3 hours for procainamide and 6 hours for NAPA, the steady-state concentrations could be obtained any time after the first day of dosing (5 half-lives = 5 • 3.3 h = 16.5 h for procainamide, 5 half-lives = 5 • 6 h = 30 h for NAPA). Procainamide and NAPA serum concentrations should also be measured if the patient experiences a return of their arrhythmia, or if the patient develops potential signs or symptoms of procainamide toxicity.

Literature-Based Recommended Dosing

1. *Choose procainamide dose based on disease states and conditions present in the patient.*

A procainamide dose of 50 mg/kg/d is suggested by the table for an adult with normal renal and hepatic function.

2. *Compute dosage regimen.*

Oral sustained-release procainamide tablets will be prescribed to this patient every 6 hours: D = procainamide dose • Wt = 50 mg/kg/d • 72 kg = 3600 mg/d, rounded to 4000 mg/d or 1000 mg every 6 hours. This dose is identical to that suggested by the Pharmacokinetic Dosing method.

Steady-state procainamide and NAPA serum concentrations could be measured after steady-state is attained in 3-5 half-lives. Since the patient is expected to have a half-life equal to 3.3 hours for procainamide and 6 hours for NAPA, the steady-state concentrations could be obtained any time after the first day of dosing (5 half-lives = 5 • 3.3 h = 16.5 h for procainamide, 5 half-lives = 5 • 6 h = 30 h for NAPA). Procainamide and NAPA serum concentrations should also be measured if the patient experiences a return of their arrhythmia, or if the patient develops potential signs or symptoms of procainamide toxicity.

2. *Answer to problem 2.* The revised procainamide dose for patient NJ would be calculated as follows:

Linear Pharmacokinetics Method

1. *Compute new dose to achieve desired serum concentration.*

The patient would be expected to achieve steady-state conditions after the second day (5 $t_{1/2}$ = 5 • 3.3 h = 17 h for procainamide, 5 $t_{1/2}$ = 5 • 6 h = 30 h for NAPA) of therapy.

Using linear pharmacokinetics, the new dose to attain the desired concentration should be proportional to the old dose that produced the measured concentration (note: total daily dose = 1000 mg/dose • 4 doses/d = 4000 mg/d):

$$D_{new} = (C_{ss, new}/C_{ss, old})D_{old} = (6\ \mu g/mL / 4.2\ \mu g/mL)\ 4000\ mg/d = 5714\ mg/d,$$
rounded to 6000 mg/d or 1500 mg every 6 hours

The new suggested dose would be 1500 mg every 6 hours of oral procainamide to be started immediately.

The expected NAPA steady-state serum concentration would change in proportion to the procainamide dosage alteration:

$$C_{ss, new} = (D_{new}/D_{old})C_{ss, old} = (6000\ mg/d / 4000\ mg/d)\ 2.5\ \mu g/mL = 3.8\ \mu g/mL$$

A steady-state procainamide serum concentration could be measured after steady-state is attained in 3-5 half-lives. Since the patient is expected to have a procainamide half-life equal to 3.3 hours and a NAPA half-life equal to 6 hours, procainamide and NAPA steady-state concentrations could be obtained any time after the second day of dosing (5 half-lives = 5 • 3.3 h = 17 h for procainamide, 5 half-lives = 5 • 6 h = 30 h for NAPA). Procainamide and NAPA serum concentrations should also be measured if the patient experiences a return of their arrhythmia, or if the patient develops potential signs or symptoms of procainamide toxicity.

Pharmacokinetic Parameter Method

1. *Compute pharmacokinetic parameters.*

The patient would be expected to achieve steady-state conditions after the second day (5 $t_{1/2}$ = 5 • 3.3 h = 17 h for procainamide, 5 $t_{1/2}$ = 5 • 6 h = 30 h for NAPA) of therapy. Procainamide clearance can be computed using a steady-state procainamide concentration: Cl = [F(D/τ)]/ Css = [0.83 (1000 mg/6 h)]/(4.2 mg/L) = 32.9 L/h. (Note: μg/mL = mg/L and this concentration unit was substituted for Css in the calculations so that unnecessary unit conversion was not required.)

2. *Compute procainamide dose.*

Procainamide clearance is used to compute the new dose: $D = (Css \bullet Cl \bullet \tau)/F = (6 \text{ mg/L} \bullet 32.9 \text{ L/h} \bullet 6 \text{ h})/0.83 = 1427$ mg, rounded to 1500 mg every 6 hours.

The expected NAPA steady-state serum concentration would change in proportion to the procainamide dosage alteration:

$$C_{ss, new} = (D_{new}/D_{old})C_{ss, old} = (6000 \text{ mg/d}/4000 \text{ mg/d}) \ 2.5 \ \mu g/mL = 3.8 \ \mu g/mL$$

The new procainamide dose would be instituted immediately.

A steady-state procainamide serum concentration could be measured after steady-state is attained in 3-5 half-lives. Since the patient is expected to have a procainamide half-life equal to 3.3 hours and a NAPA half-life equal to 6 hours, procainamide and NAPA steady-state concentrations could be obtained any time after the second day of dosing (5 half-lives = $5 \bullet 3.3$ h = 17 h for procainamide, 5 half-lives = $5 \bullet 6$ h = 30 h for NAPA). Procainamide and NAPA serum concentrations should also be measured if the patient experiences a return of their arrhythmia, or if the patient develops potential signs or symptoms of procainamide toxicity.

3. *Answer to problem 3.* The initial procainamide dose for patient GF would be calculated as follows :

Pharmacokinetic Dosing Method

1. *Estimate half-life and elimination rate constant according to disease states and conditions present in the patient.*

The expected procainamide half-life $(t_{1/2})$ is 13.9 hours. The elimination rate constant is computed using the following formula: $k = 0.693/t_{1/2} = 0.693/13.9$ h $= 0.050$ h^{-1}.

2. *Estimate the volume of distribution and clearance.*

The patient is not obese, so the estimated procainamide volume of distribution will be based on actual body weight: $V = 1.7$ L/kg $\bullet$ 81 kg = 138 L. Estimated procainamide clearance is computed by taking the product of the volume of distribution and the elimination rate constant: $Cl = kV = 0.050$ h^{-1} $\bullet$ 138 L = 6.9 L/h.

3. *Compute dosage regimen.*

Oral sustained-release procainamide tablets will be prescribed to this patient (F = 0.83). Because the patient has a slow procainamide clearance and long half-life, the initial dosage interval (τ) will be set to 12 hours. (Note: $\mu g/mL$ = mg/L and this concentration unit was substituted for Css in the calculations so that unnecessary unit conversion was not required.) The dosage equation for oral procainamide is: $D = (Css \bullet Cl \bullet \tau)/F = (4 \text{ mg/L} \bullet 6.9 \text{ L/h} \bullet 12 \text{ h})/0.83 = 399$ mg, rounded to 500 mg every 12 hours.

Steady-state procainamide and NAPA serum concentrations could be measured after steady-state is attained in 3-5 half-lives. Since the patient is expected to have a half-life equal to 13.9 hours for procainamide and 41 hours for NAPA, the steady-state concentrations could be obtained any time after the ninth day of dosing (5 half-lives = $5 \bullet 13.9$ h = 70 h for procainamide, 5 half-lives = $5 \bullet 41$ h = 205 h for NAPA). Procainamide and NAPA serum concentrations should also be measured if the patient experiences a return of their arrhythmia, or if the patient develops potential signs or symptoms of procainamide toxicity.

Literature-Based Recommended Dosing

1. *Choose procainamide dose based on disease states and conditions present in the patient.*

A procainamide dose of 12.5 mg/kg/d (50 mg/kg/d normal dose, reduced by 75%) is suggested by the table for an adult with severe renal failure.

2. *Compute dosage regimen.*

Oral sustained-release procainamide tablets will be prescribed to this patient every 12 hours:
D = procainamide dose • Wt = 12.5 mg/kg/d • 81 kg = 1013 mg/d, rounded to 1000 mg/d or 500 mg every 12 hours. This dose is identical to that suggested by the Pharmacokinetic Dosing method.

Steady-state procainamide and NAPA serum concentrations could be measured after steady-state is attained in 3-5 half-lives. Since the patient is expected to have a half-life equal to 13.9 hours for procainamide and 41 hours for NAPA, the steady-state concentrations could be obtained any time after the ninth day of dosing (5 half-lives = 5 • 13.9 h = 70 h for procainamide, 5 half-lives = 5 • 41 h = 205 h for NAPA). Procainamide and NAPA serum concentrations should also be measured if the patient experiences a return of their arrhythmia, or if the patient develops potential signs or symptoms of procainamide toxicity.

4. *Answer to problem 4.* The revised procainamide dose for patient GF would be calculated as follows:

Linear Pharmacokinetics Method

1. *Compute new dose to achieve desired serum concentration.*

The patient would be expected to achieve steady-state conditions after the ninth day of dosing (5 half-lives = 5 • 13.9 h = 70 h for procainamide, 5 half-lives = 5 • 41 h = 205 h for NAPA).

Using linear pharmacokinetics, the new dose to attain the desired concentration should be proportional to the old dose that produced the measured concentration (note: total daily dose = 1000 mg/dose • 2 doses/d = 2000 mg/d):

$$D_{new} = (C_{ss,\ new}/C_{ss,\ old})D_{old} = (6\ \mu g/mL/9.5\ \mu g/mL)\ 2000\ mg/d = 1263\ mg/d,$$
rounded to 1500 mg/d or 750 mg every 12 hours

The new suggested dose would be 750 mg every 12 hours of oral procainamide to be started immediately if no adverse effects are present. If side effects are observed, the new dosage regimen could be held for one procainamide half-life before being instituted.

The expected NAPA steady-state serum concentration would change in proportion to the procainamide dosage alteration:

$$C_{ss,\ new} = (D_{new}/D_{old})C_{ss,\ old} = (1500\ mg/d/2000\ mg/d)\ 32.5\ \mu g/mL = 24.4\ \mu g/mL$$

Steady-state procainamide and NAPA serum concentrations could be measured after steady-state is attained in 3-5 half-lives. Since the patient is expected to have a half-life equal to 13.9 hours for procainamide and 41 hours for NAPA, the steady-state concentrations could be obtained any time after the ninth day of dosing (5 half-lives = 5 • 13.9 h = 70 h for procainamide, 5 half-lives = 5 • 41 h = 205 h for NAPA). Procainamide and NAPA serum concentrations should also be measured if the patient experiences a return of their arrhythmia, or if the patient develops potential signs or symptoms of procainamide toxicity.

Pharmacokinetic Parameter Method

1. *Compute pharmacokinetic parameters.*

The patient would be expected to achieve steady-state conditions after the ninth day of dosing (5 half-lives = 5 • 13.9 h = 70 h for procainamide, 5 half-lives = 5 • 41 h = 205 h for NAPA).

Procainamide clearance can be computed using a steady-state procainamide concentration: Cl = [F(D/τ)]/ Css = [0.83 (1000 mg/12 h)]/(9.5 mg/L) = 7.3 L/h. (Note: μg/mL = mg/L and this concentration unit was substituted for Css in the calculations so that unnecessary unit conversion was not required.)

2. *Compute procainamide dose.*

Procainamide clearance is used to compute the new dose: $D = (Css \bullet Cl \bullet \tau)/F = (6 \text{ mg/L} \bullet 7.3 \text{ L/h} \bullet 12 \text{ h})/0.83 = 633 \text{ mg}$, rounded to 750 mg every 12 hours.

The expected NAPA steady-state serum concentration would change in proportion to the procainamide dosage alteration:

$$C_{ss, new} = (D_{new}/D_{old})C_{ss, old} = (1500 \text{ mg/d}/2000 \text{ mg/d})\, 32.5 \text{ µg/mL} = 24.4 \text{ µg/mL}$$

The new suggested dose would be 750 mg every 12 hours of oral procainamide to be started immediately if no adverse effects are present. If side effects are observed, the new dosage regimen could be held for one procainamide half-life before being instituted.

Steady-state procainamide and NAPA serum concentrations could be measured after steady-state is attained in 3-5 half-lives. Since the patient is expected to have a half-life equal to 13.9 hours for procainamide and 41 hours for NAPA, the steady-state concentrations could be obtained any time after the ninth day of dosing (5 half-lives = $5 \bullet 13.9 \text{ h} = 70 \text{ h}$ for procainamide, 5 half-lives = $5 \bullet 41 \text{ h} = 205 \text{ h}$ for NAPA). Procainamide and NAPA serum concentrations should also be measured if the patient experiences a return of their arrhythmia, or if the patient develops potential signs or symptoms of procainamide toxicity.

5. *Answer to problem 5.* The initial procainamide dose for patient YU would be calculated as follows:

1. *Estimate half-life and elimination rate constant according to disease states and conditions present in the patient.*

Patients with severe uncompensated heart failure have highly variable procainamide pharmacokinetics and dosage requirements. Heart failure patients have decreased cardiac output, which leads to decreased liver blood flow, and the expected procainamide half-life ($t_{1/2}$) is 5.5 hours. The elimination rate constant is computed using the following formula: $k = 0.693/t_{1/2} = 0.693/5.5 \text{ h} = 0.126 \text{ h}^{-1}$.

2. *Estimate the volume of distribution and clearance.*

The patient is not obese, so the estimated procainamide volume of distribution will be based on actual body weight: $V = 1.6 \text{ L/kg} \bullet 60 \text{ kg} = 96 \text{ L}$. Estimated procainamide clearance is computed by taking the product of the volume of distribution and the elimination rate constant: $Cl = kV = 0.126 \text{ h}^{-1} \bullet 96 \text{ L} = 12.1 \text{ L/h}$.

3. *Compute dosage regimen.*

Oral sustained-release procainamide tablets will be prescribed to this patient ($F = 0.83$). The initial dosage interval (τ) will be set to 12 hours. (Note: µg/mL = mg/L and this concentration unit was substituted for Css in the calculations so that unnecessary unit conversion was not required.) The dosage equation for oral procainamide is: $D = (Css \bullet Cl \bullet \tau)/F = (5 \text{ mg/L} \bullet 12.1 \text{ L/h} \bullet 12 \text{ h})/0.83 = 875 \text{ mg}$, rounded to 750 mg every 12 hours.

Steady-state procainamide and NAPA serum concentrations could be measured after steady-state is attained in 3-5 half-lives. Since the patient is expected to have a half-life equal to 5.5 hours for procainamide and 6 hours for NAPA (assuming heart failure has no effect on NAPA pharmacokinetics), the steady-state concentrations could be obtained any time after the second day of dosing (5 half-lives = $5 \bullet 5.5 \text{ h} = 27.5 \text{ h}$ for procainamide, 5 half-lives = $5 \bullet 6 \text{ h} = 30 \text{ h}$ for NAPA). Procainamide and NAPA serum concentrations should also be measured if the patient experiences a return of their arrhythmia, or if the patient develops potential signs or symptoms of procainamide toxicity. Procainamide pharmacokinetic parameters can change as the patient's cardiac status changes. If heart failure improves, cardiac output will increase resulting in increased liver blood flow and procainamide clearance. Alternatively, if heart failure worsens, cardiac output will decrease further resulting in decreased liver blood flow and procainamide clearance. Thus, patients with heart failure receiving procainamide therapy must be monitored very carefully.

Literature-Based Recommended Dosing

1. *Choose procainamide dose based on disease states and conditions present in the patient.*
   A procainamide dose of 25 mg/kg/d (50 mg/kg/d normal dose, reduced by 50%) is suggested by the table for an adult with severe renal failure.

2. *Compute dosage regimen.*
   Oral sustained-release procainamide tablets will be prescribed to this patient every 12 hours: D = procainamide dose • Wt = 25 mg/kg/d • 60 kg = 1500 mg/d, 750 mg every 12 hours. This dose is identical to that suggested by the Pharmacokinetic Dosing method.
   Steady-state procainamide and NAPA serum concentrations could be measured after steady-state is attained in 3-5 half-lives. Since the patient is expected to have a half-life equal to 5.5 hours for procainamide and 6 hours for NAPA (assuming heart failure has no effect on NAPA pharmacokinetics), the steady-state concentrations could be obtained any time after the second day of dosing (5 half-lives = 5 • 5.5 h = 27.5 h for procainamide, 5 half-lives = 5 • 6 h = 30 h for NAPA). Procainamide and NAPA serum concentrations should also be measured if the patient experiences a return of their arrhythmia, or if the patient develops potential signs or symptoms of procainamide toxicity. Procainamide pharmacokinetic parameters can change as the patient's cardiac status changes. If heart failure improves, cardiac output will increase resulting in increased liver blood flow and procainamide clearance. Alternatively, if heart failure worsens, cardiac output will decrease further resulting in decreased liver blood flow and procainamide clearance. Thus, patients with heart failure receiving procainamide therapy must be monitored very carefully.

6. *Answer to problem 6.* The revised procainamide dose for patient YU would be calculated as follows:
   The patient has severe heart failure and would be expected to achieve steady-state conditions after the second day (5 $t_{1/2}$ = 5 • 5.5 h = 27.5 h) of therapy. Because the serum procainamide concentration was obtained just before the third dose, it is unlikely that steady-state has been attained. So the Linear Pharmacokinetics or Pharmacokinetic Parameter methods cannot be used.

Bayesian Pharmacokinetic Computer Programs Method

1. *Enter the patient's demographic, drug dosing, and serum concentration/time data into the computer program.*

2. *Compute pharmacokinetic parameters for the patient using Bayesian pharmacokinetic computer program.*
   The pharmacokinetic parameters computed by the program are a volume of distribution of 75 L, a half-life equal to 13.8 hours, and a clearance equal to 3.8 L/h.

3. *Compute the dose required to achieve the desired procainamide serum concentrations.*
   The one-compartment model first-order absorption equations used by the program to compute doses indicates that a dose of 500 mg every 12 hours will produce a steady-state procainamide concentration of 8 μg/mL.

7. *Answer to problem 7.* The initial procainamide dose for patient WE would be calculated as follows:

Pharmacokinetic Dosing Method

Detailed pharmacokinetic studies have not been done in patients with severe liver disease, so this method cannot be used.

Literature-Based Recommended Dosing

1. *Choose procainamide dose based on disease states and conditions present in the patient.*

   A procainamide dose of 25 mg/kg/d (50 mg/kg/d normal dose, reduced by 50%) is suggested by the table for an adult with severe liver disease.

2. *Compute dosage regimen.*

   Oral sustained-release procainamide tablets will be prescribed to this patient every 12 hours: D = procainamide dose • Wt = 25 mg/kg/d • 55 kg = 1375 mg/d, rounded to 1500 mg or 750 mg every 12 hours.

   Steady-state procainamide and NAPA serum concentrations could be measured after steady-state is attained in 3-5 half-lives. Procainamide and NAPA serum concentrations should also be measured if the patient experiences a return of their arrhythmia, or if the patient develops potential signs or symptoms of procainamide toxicity. Procainamide pharmacokinetic parameters can change as the patient's hepatic status changes. Thus, patients with heart failure receiving procainamide therapy must be monitored very carefully.

8. *Answer to problem 8.* The revised procainamide dose for patient WE would be calculated as follows:

   The patient has abnormal hepatic function and would be expected to have a prolonged half-life. Because the serum procainamide concentration was obtained before the third dose, it is unlikely that the serum concentration was obtained at steady-state. So the linear pharmacokinetics or Pharmacokinetic Parameter methods cannot be used.

Bayesian Pharmacokinetic Computer Programs Method

1. *Enter the patient's demographic, drug dosing, and serum concentration/time data into the computer program.*

2. *Compute pharmacokinetic parameters for the patient using Bayesian pharmacokinetic computer program.*

   The pharmacokinetic parameters computed by the program are a volume of distribution of 91 L, a half-life equal to 14 hours, and a clearance equal to 4.5 L/h.

3. *Compute the dose required to achieve the desired procainamide serum concentrations.*

   The one-compartment model first-order absorption equations used by the program to compute doses indicates that a dose of 500 mg every 12 hours will produce a steady-state procainamide concentration of 6.7 µg/mL.

9. *Answer to problem 9.* The initial procainamide dose for patient IO would be calculated as follows:

Pharmacokinetic Dosing Method

1. *Estimate half-life and elimination rate constant according to disease states and conditions present in the patient.*

   For an obese individual, a value of clearance is used to compute procainamide doses.

2. *Estimate the volume of distribution and clearance.*

   The patient is obese [IBW_{male} (in kg) = 50 kg + 2.3(Ht − 60) = 50 kg + 2.3(71 in − 60) = 75 kg, patient >30% over ideal body weight], so the estimated procainamide clearance will be based on total body weight and the population clearance value: Cl = 0.52 L/h/kg • 130 kg = 67.6 L/h.

3. *Compute dosage regimen.*

   Oral sustained-release procainamide tablets will be prescribed to this patient (F = 0.83). The initial dosage interval (τ) will be set to 12 hours. (Note: µg/mL = mg/L and this concentration unit was substituted for Css in the calculations so that unnecessary unit conversion was not required.) The dosage equation for oral procainamide is: $D = (Css \cdot Cl \cdot \tau)/F = (4\ mg/L \cdot 67.6\ L/h \cdot 12\ h)/0.83 = 3909\ mg$, rounded to 4000 every 12 hours.

A steady-state trough procainamide serum concentration could be measured after steady-state is attained in 3-5 half-lives. Since the patient is expected to have a half-life equal to 3.3 hours, the procainamide steady-state concentration could be obtained any time after the first day of dosing (5 half-lives = 5 • 3.3 h = 17 h). Procainamide serum concentrations should also be measured if the patient experiences an exacerbation of their arrhythmia, or if the patient develops potential signs or symptoms of procainamide toxicity.

Literature-Based Recommended Dosing

1. *Choose procainamide dose based on disease states and conditions present in the patient.*

A procainamide dose of 50 mg/kg/d is suggested by the table for an adult with normal renal and hepatic function. Because the patient is obese [IBW_{male} (in kg) = 50 kg + 2.3(Ht − 60) = 50 kg + 2.3(71 in − 60) = 75 kg, patient >30% over ideal body weight], total body weight will be used to compute doses.

2. *Compute dosage regimen.*

Oral sustained-release procainamide tablets will be prescribed to this patient. The initial dosage interval will be set to 12 hours: D = procainamide dose • Wt = 50 mg/kg/d • 130 kg = 6500 mg, rounded to 6000 or 3000 mg every 12 hours. (Note: dose rounded down to avoid possible overdosage.)

A steady-state trough procainamide serum concentration could be measured after steady-state is attained in 3-5 half-lives. Since the patient is expected to have a half-life equal to 3.3 hours, the procainamide steady-state concentration could be obtained any time after the first day of dosing (5 half-lives = 5 • 3.3 h = 17 h). Procainamide serum concentrations should also be measured if the patient experiences an exacerbation of their arrhythmia, or if the patient develops potential signs or symptoms of procainamide toxicity. Procainamide pharmacokinetic parameters can change as the patient's cardiac status changes.

10. *Answer to problem 10.* The revised procainamide dose for patient IO would be calculated as follows:

The patient has mild heart failure and would be expected to achieve steady-state conditions after the first day (5 $t_{1/2}$ = 5 • 5.5 h = 27.5 h) of therapy. Because the serum procainamide concentration was obtained on the second day of therapy, but two different doses were given on day 1, it is unlikely that the serum concentration was obtained at steady-state. So the Linear Pharmacokinetics or Pharmacokinetic Parameter methods cannot be used.

Bayesian Pharmacokinetic Computer Programs Method

1. *Enter the patient's demographic, drug dosing, and serum concentration/time data into the computer program.*

2. *Compute pharmacokinetic parameters for the patient using Bayesian pharmacokinetic computer program.*

The pharmacokinetic parameters computed by the program are a volume of distribution of 235 L, a half-life equal to 5.1 hours, and a clearance equal to 31.8 L/h.

3. *Compute the dose required to achieve the desired procainamide serum concentrations.*

The one-compartment model first-order absorption equations used by the program to compute doses indicates that a dose of 4000 mg every 12 hours will produce a steady-state procainamide concentration of 4.4 μg/mL.

A steady-state trough procainamide serum concentration could be measured after steady-state is attained in 3-5 half-lives. Since the patient is expected to have a half-life equal to 5.1 hours, the procainamide steady-state concentration could be obtained any time after the first day of dosing (5 half-lives = 5 • 5.1 h = 25.5 h). Procainamide serum concentrations should also be measured if the patient experiences an exacerbation of their arrhythmia, or if the patient develops potential signs or symptoms of procainamide toxicity.

11. *Answer to problem 11.* The initial procainamide dose for patient LG would be calculated as follows:

Pharmacokinetic Dosing Method

1. *Estimate half-life and elimination rate constant according to disease states and conditions present in the patient.*

The expected procainamide half-life ($t_{1/2}$) is 3.3 hours. The elimination rate constant is computed using the following formula: $k = 0.693/t_{1/2} = 0.693/3.3\ h = 0.210\ h^{-1}$.

2. *Estimate the volume of distribution and clearance.*

The patient is not obese, so the estimated procainamide volume of distribution will be based on actual body weight: V = 2.7 L/kg • 69 kg = 186 L. Estimated procainamide clearance is computed by taking the product of the volume of distribution and the elimination rate constant: $Cl = kV = 0.210\ h^{-1}$ • 186 L = 39.1 L/h.

3. *Compute dosage regimen.*

Therapy will be started by administering an intravenous loading dose of procainamide to the patient: LD = Css • V = 4 mg/L • 186 L = 744 mg, rounded to 750 mg. (Note: µg/mL = mg/L and this concentration unit was substituted for Css in the calculations so that unnecessary unit conversion was not required.)

A procainamide continuous intravenous infusion will be started immediately after the loading dose has been administered. (Note: µg/mL = mg/L and this concentration unit was substituted for Css in the calculations so that unnecessary unit conversion was not required.) The dosage equation for intravenous procainamide is: k_0 = Css • Cl = (4 mg/L • 39.1 L/h)/(60 min/h) = 2.6 mg/min, rounded to 3 mg/min.

A steady-state procainamide serum concentration could be measured after steady-state is attained in 3-5 half-lives. Since the patient is expected to have a half-life equal to 3.3 hours, the procainamide steady-state concentration could be obtained any time after the first day of dosing (5 half-lives = 5 • 3.3 h = 16.5 h). Procainamide serum concentrations should also be measured if the patient experiences an exacerbation of their arrhythmia, or if the patient develops potential signs or symptoms of procainamide toxicity.

Literature-Based Recommended Dosing

1. *Choose procainamide dose based on disease states and conditions present in the patient.*

A procainamide loading dose of 500 mg over 25-30 minutes would be administered followed by a continuous infusion. A procainamide dose of 2-6 mg/min is suggested by the table for an adult with normal hepatic and renal function. A dose of 3 mg/min would be expected to attain a steady-state concentration in the lower end of the therapeutic range.

A procainamide serum concentration could be measured after steady-state is attained in 3-5 half-lives. Since the patient is expected to have a half-life equal to 3.3 hours, the procainamide steady-state concentration could be obtained any time after the first day of dosing (5 half-lives = 5 • 3.3 h = 16.5 h). Procainamide serum concentrations should also be measured if the patient experiences an exacerbation of their arrhythmia, or if the patient develops potential signs or symptoms of procainamide toxicity.

12. *Answer to problem 12.* The revised procainamide dose for patient LG would be calculated as follows:

Linear Pharmacokinetics Method

1. *Compute new dose to achieve desired serum concentration.*

The patient would be expected to achieve steady-state conditions after the first day ($5 t_{1/2} = 5 \bullet 3.3$ h = 16.5 h) of therapy.

Using linear pharmacokinetics, the new infusion rate to attain the desired concentration should be proportional to the old infusion rate that produced the measured concentration:

$$D_{new} = (C_{ss, new}/C_{ss, old})D_{old} = (8 \ \mu g/mL / 4.5 \ \mu g/mL) \ 3 \ mg/min = 5.3 \ mg/min, \ rounded \ to \ 5 \ mg/min$$

The new suggested infusion rate of procainamide would be 5 mg/min.

The expected NAPA steady-state serum concentration would change in proportion to the procainamide dosage alteration:

$$C_{ss, new} = (D_{new}/D_{old})C_{ss, old} = (5 \ mg/min / 3 \ mg/min) \ 2.5 \ \mu g/mL = 4.2 \ \mu g/mL$$

A booster dose of procainamide would be computed using an estimated volume of distribution for the patient (2.7 L/kg $\bullet$ 69 kg = 186 L): $BD = (C_{desired} - C_{actual})V = (8 \ mg/L - 4.5 \ mg/L)186 \ L = 651 \ mg$, rounded to 600 mg of procainamide over 25-30 minutes. The booster dose would be given to the patient before the infusion rate was increased to the new value.

A steady-state trough procainamide serum concentration could be measured after steady-state is attained in 3-5 half-lives. Since the patient is expected to have a half-life equal to 3.3 hours, the procainamide steady-state concentration could be obtained any time after the first day of dosing (5 half-lives = 5 $\bullet$ 3.3 h = 16.5 h). Procainamide serum concentrations should also be measured if the patient experiences an exacerbation of their arrhythmia, or if the patient develops potential signs or symptoms of procainamide toxicity.

Pharmacokinetic Parameter Method

1. *Compute pharmacokinetic parameters.*

The patient would be expected to achieve steady-state conditions after the first day ($5 t_{1/2} = 5 \bullet 3.3$ h = 16.5 h) of therapy.

Procainamide clearance can be computed using a steady-state procainamide concentration $Cl = k_0/Css = (3 \ mg/min)/(4.5 \ mg/L) = 0.67 \ L/min$. (Note: $\mu g/mL = mg/L$ and this concentration unit was substituted for Css in the calculations so that unnecessary unit conversion was not required.)

2. *Compute procainamide dose.*

Procainamide clearance is used to compute the new procainamide infusion rate: $k_0 = Css \bullet Cl = 8 \ mg/L \bullet 0.67 \ L/min = 5.4 \ mg/min$, rounded to 5 mg/min.

The new suggested infusion rate would be 5 mg/min of procainamide.

The expected NAPA steady-state serum concentration would change in proportion to the procainamide dosage alteration:

$$C_{ss, new} = (D_{new}/D_{old})C_{ss, old} = (5 \ mg/min / 3 \ mg/min) \ 2.5 \ \mu g/mL = 4.2 \ \mu g/mL$$

A booster dose of procainamide would be computed using an estimated volume of distribution for the patient (2.7 L/kg $\bullet$ 69 kg = 186 L): $BD = (C_{desired} - C_{actual})V = (8 \ mg/L - 4.5 \ mg/L) \ 186 \ L = 651 \ mg$, rounded to 600 mg of procainamide over 25-30 minutes. The booster dose would be given to the patient before the infusion rate was increased to the new value.

A steady-state trough procainamide serum concentration could be measured after steady-state is attained in 3-5 half-lives. Since the patient is expected to have a half-life equal to 3.3 hours, the procainamide steady-state concentration could be obtained any time after the first day of dosing (5 half-lives = 5 • 3.3 h = 16.5 h). Procainamide serum concentrations should also be measured if the patient experiences an exacerbation of their arrhythmia, or if the patient develops potential signs or symptoms of procainamide toxicity.

13. *Answer to problem 13.* The initial procainamide dose for patient CV would be calculated as follows:

Pharmacokinetic Dosing Method

Detailed pharmacokinetic studies have not been done in patients with severe liver disease, so this method cannot be used.

Literature-Based Recommended Dosing

1. *Choose procainamide dose based on disease states and conditions present in the patient.*

A procainamide loading dose of 500 mg over 25-30 minutes would be administered followed by a continuous infusion. A procainamide dose of 1-3 mg/min (2-6 mg/min normal dose, reduced by 50%) is suggested by the table for an adult with severe liver disease. A dose in the lower end of this range should result in a procainamide steady-state concentration in the lower end of the therapeutic range. A dose of 1 mg/min would be prescribed to the patient.

Steady-state procainamide and NAPA serum concentrations could be measured after steady-state is attained in 3-5 half-lives. Procainamide and NAPA serum concentrations should also be measured if the patient experiences a return of their arrhythmia, or if the patient develops potential signs or symptoms of procainamide toxicity. Procainamide pharmacokinetic parameters can change as the patient's hepatic status changes. Thus, patients with liver failure receiving procainamide therapy must be monitored very carefully.

14. *Answer to problem 14.* The revised procainamide dose for patient CV would be calculated as follows:

The patient has liver cirrhosis and may not have achieved steady-state conditions after 12 hours of therapy. Because of this, it is unlikely that the serum concentration was obtained at steady-state even though a loading dose was given. So the Linear Pharmacokinetics or Pharmacokinetic Parameter methods cannot be used.

Bayesian Pharmacokinetic Computer Programs Method

1. *Enter the patient's demographic, drug dosing, and serum concentration/time data into the computer program.*

Note: DrugCalc requires procainamide infusion rates to be entered in the units of mg/h (3 mg/min • 60 min/h = 180 mg/h).

2. *Compute pharmacokinetic parameters for the patient using Bayesian pharmacokinetic computer program.*

The pharmacokinetic parameters computed by the program are a volume of distribution of 139 L, a half-life equal to 8.2 hours, and a clearance equal to 11.8 L/h.

3. *Compute the dose required to achieve the desired procainamide serum concentrations.*

The one-compartment model infusion equations used by the program to compute doses indicates that a procainamide infusion of 71 mg/h or 1.2 mg/min (71 mg/h / 60 min/h = 1.2 mg/min) will produce a steady-state procainamide concentration of 6 μg/mL. This dose would be started immediately if no adverse effects were noted. However, if the patient was experiencing drug side effects, the new infusion rate would be started after holding the infusion for 8 hours (~1 half-life) to allow procainamide serum concentrations to decrease by one-half.

15. *Answer to problem 15.* The initial procainamide dose for patient PE would be calculated as follows:

Pharmacokinetic Dosing Method

1. *Estimate the half-life and elimination rate constant according to disease states and conditions present in the patient.*

   Patients with severe heart failure have highly variable procainamide pharmacokinetics and dosage requirements. Heart failure patients have decreased cardiac output which leads to decreased liver blood flow, and the expected procainamide half-life ($t_{1/2}$) is 5.5 hours. The elimination rate constant is computed using the following formula: $k = 0.693/t_{1/2} = 0.693/5.5 \text{ h} = 0.126 \text{ h}^{-1}$.

2. *Estimate the volume of distribution and clearance.*

   The patient is not obese, so the estimated procainamide volume of distribution will be based on actual body weight: $V = 1.6 \text{ L/kg} \bullet 67 \text{ kg} = 107 \text{ L}$. Estimated procainamide clearance is computed by taking the product of the volume of distribution and the elimination rate constant: $Cl = kV = 0.126 \text{ h}^{-1} \bullet 107 \text{ L} = 13.5 \text{ L/h}$.

3. *Compute dosage regimen.*

   Therapy will be started by administering an intravenous loading dose of procainamide to the patient: $LD = Css \bullet V = 4 \text{ mg/L} \bullet 107 \text{ L} = 428 \text{ mg}$, rounded to 400 mg. A loading dose of 400 mg given intravenously over 25-30 minutes would be given. (Note: $\mu g/mL = mg/L$ and this concentration unit was substituted for Css in the calculations so that unnecessary unit conversion was not required.)

   A procainamide continuous intravenous infusion will be started immediately after the loading dose has been administered. (Note: $\mu g/mL = mg/L$ and this concentration unit was substituted for Css in the calculations so that unnecessary unit conversion was not required.) The dosage equation for intravenous procainamide is: $k_0 = Css \bullet Cl = (4 \text{ mg/L} \bullet 13.5 \text{ L/h})/(60 \text{ min/h}) = 0.9 \text{ mg/min}$, rounded to 1 mg/min.

   A steady-state procainamide serum concentration could be measured after steady-state is attained in 3-5 half-lives. Since the patient is expected to have a half-life equal to 5.5 hours, the procainamide steady-state concentration could be obtained any time after the second day of dosing (5 half-lives = $5 \bullet 5.5 \text{ h} = 27.5 \text{ h}$). Procainamide serum concentrations should also be measured if the patient experiences an exacerbation of their arrhythmia, or if the patient develops potential signs or symptoms of procainamide toxicity. Procainamide pharmacokinetic parameters can change as the patient's cardiac status changes. If heart failure improves, cardiac output will increase resulting in increased liver blood flow and procainamide clearance. Alternatively, if heart failure worsens, cardiac output will decrease further resulting in decreased liver blood flow and procainamide clearance. Thus, patients with heart failure that receive procainamide therapy must be monitored very carefully.

Literature-Based Recommended Dosing

1. *Choose procainamide dose based on disease states and conditions present in the patient.*

   A procainamide loading dose of 500 mg over 25-30 minutes would be administered followed by a continuous infusion. A procainamide dose of 1-3 mg/min (2-6 mg/min normal dose, reduced by 50%) is suggested by the table for an adult with severe heart failure. A dose in the lower end of this range should result in a procainamide steady-state concentration in the lower end of the therapeutic range. A dose of 1 mg/min would be prescribed to the patient.

   A steady-state procainamide serum concentration could be measured after steady-state is attained in 3-5 half-lives. Since the patient is expected to have a half-life equal to 5.5 hours, the procainamide steady-state concentration could be obtained any time after the second day of dosing (5 half-lives = 5 • 5.5 h = 27.5 h). Procainamide serum concentrations should also be measured if the patient experiences an exacerbation of their arrhythmia, or if the patient develops potential signs or symptoms of procainamide toxicity. Procainamide pharmacokinetic parameters can change as the patient's cardiac status changes. If heart failure improves, cardiac output will increase resulting in increased liver blood flow and procainamide clearance. Alternatively, if heart failure worsens, cardiac output will decrease further resulting in decreased liver blood flow and procainamide clearance. Thus, patients with heart failure that receive procainamide therapy must be monitored very carefully.

16. *Answer to problem 16.* The revised procainamide dose for patient PE would be calculated as follows:

The patient has severe heart failure and would be expected to achieve steady-state conditions after the second day (5 $t_{1/2}$ = 5 • 5.5 h = 27.5 h) of therapy. Because the serum procainamide concentrations were obtained after 4 and 8 hours of therapy, it is unlikely that the serum concentrations were obtained at steady-state even though a loading dose was given. So the Linear Pharmacokinetics or Pharmacokinetic Parameter methods cannot be used.

Chiou Method

1. *Compute procainamide clearance.*

$$Cl = \frac{2k_0}{C_1 + C_2} + \frac{2V(C_1 - C_2)}{(C_1 + C_2)(t_2 - t_1)}$$

$$Cl = \frac{2(4 \text{ mg/min})}{4.3 \text{ mg/L} + 8.8 \text{ mg/L}} + \frac{2(1.6 \text{ L/kg} \bullet 67 \text{ kg})(43 \text{ mg/L} - 8.8 \text{ mg/L})}{(4.3 \text{ mg/L} + 8.8 \text{ mg/L})240 \text{ min}}$$

$$= 0.30 \text{ L/min}$$

Note: μg/mL = mg/L and this concentration unit was substituted for concentrations so that unnecessary unit conversion was not required. Additionally, the time difference between t_2 and t_1, in minutes, was determined and placed directly in the calculation.

$$k_0 = Css \bullet Cl = 6 \text{ mg/L} \bullet 0.30 \text{ L/min} = 1.8 \text{ mg/min of procainamide}$$

Bayesian Pharmacokinetic Computer Programs Method

1. *Enter the patient's demographic, drug dosing, and serum concentration/time data into the computer program.*

In this case, the patient is not at steady-state, so the Linear Pharmacokinetics method cannot be used. DrugCalc requires procainamide continuous infusions to be entered in terms of mg/h (4 mg/min • 60 min/h = 240 mg/h).

2. *Compute pharmacokinetic parameters for the patient using Bayesian pharmacokinetic computer program.*

The pharmacokinetic parameters computed by the program are a volume of distribution of 246 L, a half-life equal to 13.9 hours, and a clearance equal to 12.3 L/h or 0.21 L/min (12.3 L/h / 60 min/h = 0.21 L/h).

3. *Compute the dose required to achieve the desired procainamide serum concentrations.*

The one-compartment model infusion equations used by the program to compute doses indicates that a procainamide infusion of 74 mg/h or 1.2 mg/min (74 mg/h / 60 min/h = 1.2 mg/min) will produce a steady-state procainamide concentration of 6 μg/mL.

REFERENCES

1. Sanoski CA, Bauman JL. The arrhythmias. In: Dipiro JT, Talbert RL, Yee GC, Matzke GR, Wells BG, Posey LM, eds. *Pharmacotherapy.* New York, NY: McGraw-Hill; 2011:273-309.
2. Sampson KJ, Kass RS. Anti-arrhythmics drugs. In: Brunton L, Chabner B, Knollman B, eds. *The Pharmacological Basis of Therapeutics.* 12th ed. New York, NY: McGraw-Hill; 2011:815-848.
3. Neumar RW, Otto CW, Link MS, et al. Part 8: adult advanced cardiovascular life support: 2010 American Heart Association Guidelines for Cardiopulmonary Resuscitation and Emergency Cardiovascular Care. *Circulation.* Nov 2, 2010;122(18 suppl 3):S729-S767.
4. Abramowicz M, Zuccotti G, Pflomm JM, eds. Drugs for cardiac arrhythmias. *Treatment Guidelines from The Medical Letter.* 2007;5(58):51-58.
5. Anderson JL, Halperin JL, Albert NM, et al. Management of patients with atrial fibrillation (Compilation of 2006 ACCF/AHA/ESC and 2011 ACCF/AHA/HRS Recommendations): a report of the American College of Cardiology/American Heart Association Task Force on Practice Guidelines. *Circulation.* 2013;127(13):1425-1443.
6. Lima JJ, Conti DR, Goldfarb AL, Golden LH, Jusko WJ. Pharmacokinetic approach to intravenous procainamide therapy. *Eur J Clin Pharmacol.* 1978;13(4):303-308.
7. Giardina EG, Fenster PE, Bigger JT Jr, Mayersohn M, Perrier D, Marcus FI. Efficacy, plasma concentrations and adverse effects of a new sustained release procainamide preparation. *Am J Cardiol.* 1980;46(5):855-862.
8. Manion CV, Lalka D, Baer DT, Meyer MB. Absorption kinetics of procainamide in humans. *J Pharm Sci.* 1977;66(7):981-984.
9. Graffner C, Johnsson G, Sjogren J. Pharmacokinetics of procainamide intravenously and orally as conventional and slow-release tablets. *Clin Pharmacol Ther.* 1975;17(4):414-423.
10. Smith TC, Kinkel AW. Plasma levels of procainamide after administration of conventional and sustained-release preparations. *Curr Ther Res.* 1980;27(2):217-228.
11. Koup JR, Abel RB, Smithers JA, Eldon MA, de Vries TM. Effect of age, gender, and race on steady state procainamide pharmacokinetics after administration of procanbid sustained-release tablets. *Ther Drug Monit.* 1998;20(1):73-77.
12. Gibson TP, Matusik J, Matusik E, Nelson HA, Wilkinson J, Briggs WA. Acetylation of procainamide in man and its relationship to isonicotinic acid hydrazide acetylation phenotype. *Clin Pharmacol Ther.* 1975;17(4):395-399.
13. Dutcher JS, Strong JM, Lucas SV, Lee WK, Atkinson AJ Jr. Procainamide and N-acetylprocainamide kinetics investigated simultaneously with stable isotope methodology. *Clin Pharmacol Ther.* 1977;22(4):447-457.
14. Lima JJ, Conti DR, Goldfarb AL, Tilstone WJ, Golden LH, Jusko WJ. Clinical pharmacokinetics of procainamide infusions in relation to acetylator phenotype. *J Pharmacokinet Biopharm.* 1979;7(1):69-85.
15. Anon. List of orphan designations and approvals. *Food and Drug Adminstration.* http://www.accessdata.fda.gov/scripts/opdlisting/oopd/OOPD_Results_2.cfm. Accessed March 25, 2014.
16. Lange RA, Hillis LD. Cardiovascular testing. In: Dipiro JT, Talbert RL, Yee GC, Matzke GR, Wells BG, Posey LM, eds. *Pharmacotherapy.* New York, NY: McGraw-Hill; 2011:55-81.
17. Myerburg RJ, Kessler KM, Kiem I, et al. Relationship between plasma levels of procainamide, suppression of premature ventricular complexes and prevention of recurrent ventricular tachycardia. *Circulation.* 1981;64(2):280-290.
18. Galeazzi RL, Sheiner LB, Lockwood T, Benet LZ. The renal elimination of procainamide. *Clin Pharmacol Ther.* 1976;19(1):55-62.
19. Reidenberg MM, Camacho M, Kluger J, Drayer DE. Aging and renal clearance of procainamide and acetylprocainamide. *Clin Pharmacol Ther.* 1980;28(6):732-735.
20. Lima JJ, Jusko WJ. Determination of procainamide acctylator status. *Clin Pharmacol Ther.* 1978;23(1):25-29.
21. Reidenberg MM, Drayer DE, Levy M, Warner H. Polymorphic acetylation procainamide in man. *Clin Pharmacol Ther.* 1975;17(6):722-730.
22. Lessard E, Fortin A, Belanger PM, Beaune P, Hamelin BA, Turgeon J. Role of CYP2D6 in the N-hydroxylation of procainamide. *Pharmacogenetics.* 1997;7(5):381-390.
23. Tilstone WJ, Lawson DH. Capacity-limited elimination of procainamide in man. *Res Commun Chem Pathol Pharmacol.* 1978;21(2):343-346.
24. Coyle JD, Boudoulas H, Mackichan JJ, Lima JJ. Concentration-dependent clearance of procainamide in normal subjects. *Biopharm Drug Dispos.* 1985;6(2):159-165.
25. Giardina EG, Dreyfuss J, Bigger JT Jr, Shaw JM, Schreiber EC. Metabolism of procainamide in normal and cardiac subjects. *Clin Pharmacol Ther.* 1976;19(3):339-351.
26. Koch-Weser J. Pharmacokinetic of procainamide in man. *Ann N Y Acad Sci.* 1971;179:370-382.
27. Koch-Weser J, Klein SW. Procainamide dosage schedules, plasma concentrations, and clinical effects. *JAMA.* 1971;215(9):1454-1460.
28. Bauer LA, Black D, Gensler A, Sprinkle J. Influence of age, renal function and heart failure on procainamide clearance and N-acetylprocainamide serum concentrations. *Int J Clin Pharmacol Ther Toxicol.* 1989;27(5):213-216.
29. Gibson TP, Lowenthal DT, Nelson HA, Briggs WA. Elimination of procainamide in end stage renal failure. *Clin Pharmacol Ther.* 1975;17(3):321-329.

30. Gibson TP, Atkinson AJ Jr, Matusik E, Nelson LD, Briggs WA. Kinetics of procainamide and *N*-acetylprocainamide in renal failure. *Kidney Int.* 1977;12(6):422-429.

31. Tisdale JE, Rudis MI, Padhi ID, et al. Disposition of procainamide in patients with chronic congestive heart failure receiving medical therapy. *J Clin Pharmacol.* 1996;36(1):35-41.

32. Mutnick AH, Burke TG. Antiarrhythmics. In: Schumacher GE, ed. *Therapeutic Drug Monitoring.* 1st ed. Stamford, CT: Appleton & Lange; 1995:684.

33. Pugh RN, Murray-Lyon IM, Dawson JL, Pietroni MC, Williams R. Transection of the oesophagus for bleeding oesophageal varices. *Br J Surg.* 1973;60(8):646-649.

34. Christoff PB, Conti DR, Naylor C, Jusko WJ. Procainamide disposition in obesity. *Drug Intell Clin Pharm.* 1983;17(7-8):516-522.

35. Atkinson AJ Jr, Krumlovsky FA, Huang CM, del Greco F. Hemodialysis for severe procainamide toxicity: clinical and pharmacokinetic observations. *Clin Pharmacol Ther.* 1976;20(5):585-592.

36. Golper TA, Marx MA. Drug dosing adjustments during continuous renal replacement therapies. *Kidney Int Suppl.* May 1998;66:S165-168.

37. Golper TA. Update on drug sieving coefficients and dosing adjustments during continuous renal replacement therapies. *Contrib Nephrol.* 2001;132:349-353.

38. Gibson TP, Matusik EJ, Briggs WA. *N*-Acetylprocainamide levels in patients with end-stage renal failure. *Clin Pharmacol Ther.* 1976;19(2):206-212.

39. Bauer LA, Black D, Gensler A. Procainamide-cimetidine drug interaction in elderly male patients. *J Am Geriatr Soc.* 1990;38(4):467-469.

40. Bauer LA, Black DJ, Lill JS, Garrison J, Raisys VA, Hooton TM. Levofloxacin and ciprofloxacin decrease procainamide and *N*-acetylprocainamide renal clearances. *Antimicrob Agents Chemother.* Apr 2005;49(4):1649-1651.

41. Hansten PD, Horn JR. *Drug Interactions Analysis and Management.* St. Louis, MO: Wolters Kluwer Health; 2014.

42. Tschudy MM, Arcara KM. *The Harriet Lane Handbook: A Manual for Pediatric House Officers.* 19th ed. Philadelphia, PA: Mosby; 2012.

43. Chiou WL, Gadalla MA, Peng GW. Method for the rapid estimation of the total body drug clearance and adjustment of dosage regimens in patients during a constant-rate intravenous infusion. *J Pharmacokinet Biopharm.* 1978;6(2):135-151.

44. Wandell M, Mungall D. Computer assisted drug interpretation and drug regimen optimization. *Amer Assoc Clin Chem.* 1984;6:1-11.

45. Parker RB, Cavallari LH. Systolic heart failure. In: Dipiro JT, Talbert RL, Yee GC, Matzke GR, Wells BG, Posey LM, eds. *Pharmacotherapy.* New York, NY: McGraw-Hill; 2011:137-172.

9 Quinidine

INTRODUCTION

Quinidine was one of the first agents used for its antiarrhythmic effects. It is classified as a type IA antiarrhythmic agent and can be used for the treatment of supraventricular or ventricular arrhythmias.[1] After ventricular rate has been controlled, quinidine therapy can be used to chemically convert atrial fibrillation to normal sinus rhythm for a patient.[2] Because of its side effect profile, quinidine is considered by many clinicians to be a second-line antiarrhythmic choice. Quinidine inhibits transmembrane sodium influx into the conduction system of the heart, thereby decreasing conduction velocity.[1,3] It also increases the duration of the action potential, increases threshold potential toward zero, and decreases the slope of phase 4 of the action potential. Automaticity is decreased during quinidine therapy. The net effect of these cellular changes is that quinidine causes increased refractoriness and decreased conduction in heart conduction tissue which establishes a bidirectional block in reentrant pathways.

THERAPEUTIC AND TOXIC CONCENTRATIONS

When given intravenously, the serum quinidine concentration-time curve follows a two-compartment model.[4-7] However, due to marked hypotension and tachycardia when given intravenously to some patients, the oral route of administration is far more common. When oral quinidine is given as a rapidly absorbed dosage form such as quinidine sulfate tablets, a similar distribution phase is also observed with a duration of 20-30 minutes.[4,5,8,9] If extended-release oral dosage forms are given, absorption occurs more slowly than distribution so a distribution phase is not seen (Figure 9-1).[10-14]

The generally accepted therapeutic range for quinidine is 2-6 µg/mL. Quinidine serum concentrations above the therapeutic range can cause increased QT interval or QRS complex widening (>35%-50%) on the electrocardiogram, cinchonism, hypotension, high-degree atrioventricular block, and ventricular arrhythmias. Cinchonism is a collection of symptoms that includes tinnitus, blurred vision, lightheadedness, tremor, giddiness, and altered hearing which decreases in severity with lower quinidine concentrations. Gastrointestinal adverse effects such as anorexia, nausea, vomiting, and diarrhea are the most common side effects of quinidine therapy, can occur after both oral and intravenous quinidine routes of administration, but are not strongly correlated with specific serum levels. Quinidine therapy is also associated with syncope and torsade de pointes. Quinidine syncope occurs when ventricular tachycardia, ventricular fibrillation, or a prolongation of QT intervals occurs in a non–dose-dependent manner. Torsade de pointes (twisting of the points) is a form of polymorphic ventricular tachycardia preceded by QT interval prolongation. It is characterized by polymorphic QRS complexes that change in amplitude and length, giving the appearance of oscillations around the electrocardiographic baseline. Torsade de pointes can develop into multiple episodes of nonsustained polymorphic ventricular tachycardia, syncope, ventricular fibrillation, or sudden cardiac death. Hypersensitivity reactions to quinidine include rash, drug fever, thrombocytopenia, hemolytic anemia, asthma, respiratory depression, a systemic lupus-like syndrome, hepatitis, and anaphylactic shock.

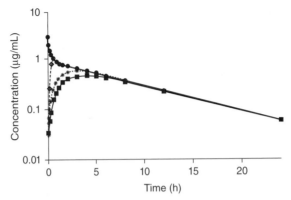

FIGURE 9-1   Quinidine serum concentrations after an intravenous dose (circles with solid line) and three different oral tablets (doses normalized to provide 200 mg of quinidine base systemically). After an intravenous dose, quinidine serum concentrations decline according to a two-compartment model, which demonstrates a distribution phase that lasts for 20-30 minutes postinjection. Immediate-release quinidine tablets (diamonds with dashed line) are rapidly absorbed and also show a distinct distribution phase. Extended-release quinidine gluconate (stars with dotted line) and quinidine sulfate (squares with solid line) have slower absorption profiles, so the drug has an opportunity to distribute to tissues while absorption is occurring. Because of this, no distribution phase is observed for these dosage forms.

Quinidine metabolites (3-hydroxyquinidine, 2′-quinidinone, quinidine-*N*-oxide, *O*-desmethylquinidine) have antiarrhythmic effects in animal models.[15-18] Of these compounds, 3-hydroxyquinidine is the most potent (60%-80% compared to the parent drug) and achieves high enough serum concentrations in humans that its antiarrhythmic effects probably contribute to the clinical effects observed during quinidine treatment. Dihydroquinidine is an impurity contained in commercially available quinidine products that also has antiarrhythmic effects.[19-21] Most products contain less than 10% of the labeled quinidine amount as dihydroquinidine. Clinicians should understand that all patients with "toxic" quinidine serum concentrations in the listed ranges will not exhibit signs or symptoms of quinidine toxicity. Rather, quinidine concentrations in the given ranges increase the likelihood that an adverse effect will occur.

For dose-adjustment purposes, quinidine serum concentrations are best measured as a predose or trough level at steady-state after the patient has received a consistent dosage regimen for 3-5 drug half-lives. Quinidine half-life varies from 6-8 hours in normal adults to 9-10 hours or more in adult patients with liver failure. If quinidine is given orally or intravenously on a stable schedule, steady-state serum concentrations will be achieved in about 2 days (5 • 8 h = 40 h).

CLINICAL MONITORING PARAMETERS

The electrocardiogram (ECG or EKG) should be monitored to determine the response to quinidine. The goal of therapy is suppression of arrhythmias and avoidance of adverse drug reactions. Electrophysiologic studies using programmed stimulation to replicate the ventricular arrhythmia or 24-hour ECG monitoring using a Holter monitor can be performed in patients while receiving a variety of antiarrhythmic agents to determine effective antiarrhythmic drug therapy.[22]

Because many quinidine therapeutic and side effects are not correlated with its serum concentration, it is often not necessary to obtain serum quinidine concentrations in patients receiving appropriate doses who currently have no arrhythmia or adverse drug effects. However, quinidine serum concentrations should be obtained in patients who have a recurrence of tachyarrhythmias, are experiencing possible quinidine side effects, or are receiving quinidine doses not consistent with disease states and conditions known to alter quinidine pharmacokinetics (see Effects of Disease States and Conditions on Quinidine Pharmacokinetics and Dosing section). Serum concentration monitoring can aid in the decision to increase or decrease the quinidine dose. For instance, if an arrhythmia reappears and the quinidine serum concentration is <6 μg/mL, increasing the quinidine dose is a therapeutic option. However, if the quinidine serum concentration is over 6 μg/mL, it is unlikely that a dosage increase will be effective in suppressing the arrhythmia and there is an increased likelihood that drug side effects may occur. Similarly, if a possible concentration-related quinidine adverse drug reaction is noted in a patient and the quinidine serum concentration is <2 μg/mL, it is possible that the observed problem may not be due to quinidine treatment and other sources can be investigated. While receiving quinidine, patients should be monitored for the following adverse drug effects: anorexia, nausea, vomiting, diarrhea, cinchonism, syncope, increased QT interval or QRS complex widening (>35%-50%) on the electrocardiogram, hypotension, high-degree atrioventricular block, ventricular arrhythmias, and hypersensitivity reactions (rash, drug fever, thrombocytopenia, hemolytic anemia, asthma, respiratory depression, a lupus-like syndrome, hepatitis, anaphylactic shock).

BASIC CLINICAL PHARMACOKINETIC PARAMETERS

Quinidine is almost completely eliminated by hepatic metabolism (~80%).[5,8] Hepatic metabolism is mainly via the CYP3A enzyme system. 3-Hydroxyquinidine is the primary active metabolite resulting from quinidine metabolism while dihydroquinidine is an active compound that is found as an impurity in most quinidine dosage forms. The hepatic extraction ratio of quinidine is about 30%, so quinidine is typically classified as an intermediate extraction ratio drug. Because of this, it is expected that liver blood flow, unbound fraction of drug in the blood, and intrinsic clearance will all be important factors influencing the clearance of quinidine. After oral administration, quinidine is subject to moderate first-pass metabolism by CYP3A contained in the liver and intestinal wall. Quinidine is also a substrate for P-glycoprotein. Approximately 20% of a quinidine dose is eliminated unchanged in the urine. Although there have been some reports that quinidine follows nonlinear pharmacokinetics, for the purposes of clinical drug dosing in patients, linear pharmacokinetic concepts and equations can be effectively used to compute doses and estimate serum concentrations.[23]

Two salt forms of quinidine are available. Quinidine sulfate contains 83% quinidine base, and quinidine gluconate contains 62% quinidine base. The gluconate salt is available for intravenous injection and oral use. Quinidine sulfate is available only for oral use. The oral bioavailability of both quinidine-based drugs is moderate and generally equals 70% reflecting first-pass metabolism in the intestinal wall and liver.[4,8] Although quinidine injection can be given intramuscularly, this route of administration may lead to erratic absorption and serum concentrations.[7]

Plasma protein binding of quinidine in normal individuals is about 80%-90%.[24-26] The drug binds to both albumin and α_1-acid glycoprotein (AGP). AGP is classified as an acute-phase reactant protein that is present in lower amounts in all individuals but is secreted in large amounts in response to certain stresses and disease states such as trauma, heart failure, and myocardial infarction. In patients with these disease states, quinidine binding to AGP can be even larger resulting in an unbound fraction as low as 8%.

The recommended dose of quinidine is based on the concurrent disease states and conditions present in the patient that can influence quinidine pharmacokinetics. Quinidine pharmacokinetic parameters used to compute doses are given in the following section for specific patient profiles.

EFFECTS OF DISEASE STATES AND CONDITIONS ON QUINIDINE PHARMACOKINETICS AND DOSING

Normal adults without the disease states and conditions given later in this section and with normal liver function have an average quinidine half-life of 7 hours (range: 6-8 hours) and a volume of distribution for the entire body of 2.4 L/kg (V = 2-3 L/kg; Table 9-1).[4-7,10,27-29] Disease states and conditions that change quinidine pharmacokinetics and dosage requirements may alter clearance and the volume of distribution. The elimination rate constant (k = $0.693/t_{1/2}$, where $t_{1/2}$ is the half-life) and clearance (Cl = kV) can be computed from the aforementioned pharmacokinetic parameters.

Patients with liver cirrhosis have increased quinidine clearance and volume of distribution which results in a prolonged average quinidine half-life of 9 hours.[30,31] Clearance and volume of distribution are larger in patients with liver disease because albumin and α_1-acid glycoprotein (AGP) concentrations are lower in these

TABLE 9-1   Disease States and Conditions That Alter Quinidine Pharmacokinetics

Disease State/ Condition	Half-Life	Volume of Distribution	Comment
Adult, normal liver function	7 h (range: 6-8 h)	2.4 L/kg (range: 2-3 L/kg)	Quinidine has a moderate hepatic extraction ratio of ~30%, so liver blood flow, unbound fraction of drug in the blood, and intrinsic clearance are all important factors in clearance rate. ~20% of quinidine is eliminated unchanged in urine
Adult, liver cirrhosis	9 h	3.8 L/kg	Quinidine is metabolized ~80% by hepatic microsomal enzymes (primarily CYP3A) and is a substrate for P-glycoprotein. Clearance of total drug increased in cirrhosis patients, but intrinsic clearance is decreased. Pharmacokinetic parameters highly variable in liver disease patients. Volume of distribution is larger due to decreased α_1-acid glycoprotein and albumin production by liver which decreases drug binding in the plasma
Adult, heart failure	7 h	1.7 L/kg	Decreased liver blood flow secondary to reduced cardiac output reduces quinidine clearance. Volume of distribution is smaller due to increased α_1-acid glycoprotein drug binding in the plasma. Heart failure results in large and variable reductions in quinidine clearance. Cardiac status must be monitored closely in heart failure patients since quinidine clearance changes with acute changes in cardiac output
Adult, obese (>30% over ideal body weight)	According to other disease states/conditions that affect quinidine pharmacokinetics	According to other disease states/conditions that affect quinidine pharmacokinetics	Quinidine doses should be based on ideal body weight for patients who weigh more that 30% over IBW

TABLE 9-2   Child-Pugh Scores for Patients With Liver Disease[32]

Test/Symptom	Score 1 Point	Score 2 Points	Score 3 Points
Total bilirubin (mg/dL)	<2.0	2.0-3.0	>3.0
Serum albumin (g/dL)	>3.5	2.8-3.5	<2.8
Prothrombin time (seconds prolonged over control)	<4	4-6	>6
Ascites	Absent	Slight	Moderate
Hepatic encephalopathy	None	Moderate	Severe

Mild liver disease, 5-6 points; moderate liver disease, 7-9 points; severe liver disease, 10-15 points.

patients and result in reduced quinidine plasma protein binding (average V = 3.8 L/kg). The increased unbound fraction in the plasma allows more quinidine to enter the liver parenchyma where hepatic drug-metabolizing enzymes are present and leads to increased drug clearance. Decreased plasma protein binding also leads to higher unbound levels for a given total quinidine serum concentration. For example, a quinidine total serum concentration of 3 μg/mL would yield an unbound concentration of 0.3 μg/mL in a patient with normal plasma protein binding (3 μg/mL • 0.1 unbound fraction = 0.3 μg/mL), but an unbound concentration of 0.6 μg/mL in a cirrhosis patient with decreased plasma protein binding (3 μg/mL • 0.2 unbound fraction = 0.6 μg/mL). The significance of this difference in unbound concentrations has not been assessed in cirrhosis patients, but clinicians should bear it in mind when monitoring quinidine levels as only total serum concentrations are available from laboratories. The exact effect that liver disease has on quinidine pharmacokinetics is highly variable and difficult to accurately predict. It is possible for a patient with liver disease to have relatively normal or grossly abnormal quinidine clearance, volume of distribution, and half-life. An index of liver dysfunction can be gained by applying the Child-Pugh clinical classification system to the patient (Table 9-2).[32] Child-Pugh scores are completely discussed in Chapter 3 (Drug Dosing in Special Populations: Renal and Hepatic Disease, Dialysis, Heart Failure, Obesity, and Drug Interactions), but will be briefly discussed here. The Child-Pugh score consists of five laboratory tests or clinical symptoms: serum albumin, total bilirubin, prothrombin time, ascites, and hepatic encephalopathy. Each of these areas is given a score of 1 (normal) to 3 (severely abnormal; see Table 9-2), and the scores for the five areas are summed. The Child-Pugh score for a patient with normal liver function is 5 while the score for a patient with grossly abnormal serum albumin, total bilirubin, and prothrombin time values in addition to severe ascites and hepatic encephalopathy is 15. A Child-Pugh score greater than 8 is grounds for a decrease of 25%-50% in the initial daily drug dose for quinidine. As in any patient with or without liver dysfunction, initial doses are meant as starting points for dosage titration based on patient response and avoidance of adverse effects. Quinidine serum concentrations and the presence of adverse drug effects should be monitored frequently in patients with liver cirrhosis.

Heart failure reduces quinidine clearance because of decreased hepatic blood flow secondary to compromised cardiac output (Table 9-3).[8,9,33,34] Volume of distribution (V = 1.7 L/kg) is decreased because heart failure patients have elevated AGP serum concentrations which leads to increased quinidine plasma protein binding and decreased quinidine unbound fraction. Because both clearance and volume of distribution simultaneously decrease, patients with heart failure have an average quinidine half-life equal to 7 hours which is similar to a normal individual [$t_{1/2} = (0.693 • \downarrow V)/\downarrow Cl$]. Increased plasma protein binding also leads to lower unbound levels for a given total quinidine serum concentration. For example, a quinidine total serum concentration of 3 μg/mL would yield an unbound concentration of 0.3 μg/mL in a patient with normal plasma protein binding (3 μg/mL • 0.1 unbound fraction = 0.3 μg/mL), but an unbound concentration of 0.15 μg/mL in a heart failure patient with increased plasma protein binding (3 μg/mL • 0.05 unbound fraction = 0.15 μg/mL).

TABLE 9-3   New York Heart Association (NYHA) Functional Classification for Heart Failure[43]

NYHA Heart Failure Class	Description
I	Patients with cardiac disease but without limitations of physical activity. Ordinary physical activity does not cause undue fatigue, dyspnea, or palpitation
II	Patients with cardiac disease that results in slight limitations of physical activity. Ordinary physical activity results in fatigue, palpitation, dyspnea, or angina
III	Patients with cardiac disease that results in marked limitations of physical activity. Although patients are comfortable at rest, less than ordinary activity will lead to symptoms
IV	Patients with cardiac disease that results in an inability to carry on physical activity without discomfort. Symptoms of congestive heart failure are present even at rest. With any physical activity, increased discomfort is experienced

The clinical significance of this difference in unbound concentrations has not been assessed in heart failure patients. Obviously, the effect that heart failure has on quinidine pharmacokinetics is highly variable and difficult to accurately predict. It is possible for a patient with heart failure to have relatively normal or grossly abnormal quinidine clearance and half-life. For heart failure patients, initial doses are meant as starting points for dosage titration based on patient response and avoidance of adverse effects. Quinidine serum concentrations and the presence of adverse drug effects should be monitored frequently in patients with heart failure.

Patients with myocardial infarction may develop serious arrhythmias that require therapy with quinidine. After a myocardial infarction, serum AGP concentrations increase up to 50% over a 12-72-hour time period. As AGP serum concentrations increase, plasma protein binding of quinidine increases and the unbound fraction of quinidine decreases. Because quinidine is considered a moderate hepatic extraction ratio drug, a decline in the unbound fraction of quinidine in the plasma decreases quinidine clearance.

Patient age has an effect on quinidine clearance and half-life.[16,35] For elderly patients over the age of 65, studies indicate that quinidine clearance is reduced, the volume of distribution is unchanged, and half-life is longer (average half-life = 10 hours) compared to younger subjects. A confounding factor found in quinidine pharmacokinetic studies conducted in older adults is the possible accidental inclusion of subjects that have subclinical or mild cases of the disease states associated with reduced quinidine clearance (heart failure, liver disease, etc). Additionally, most patients with serious arrhythmias studied in all of the previously mentioned investigations are older and those results include any influence of age. Thus, in most cases elderly patients are treated with quinidine according to the other disease states or conditions present that influence quinidine pharmacokinetics.

Because detailed studies have not been conducted in obese patients, ideal body weight should be used to compute initial doses of quinidine to avoid accidental overdose in overweight individuals (>30% above ideal body weight or IBW). Since only 20% of a quinidine dose is eliminated unchanged by the kidney, dosage adjustments for renal failure patients are usually not required.[15,34] Quinidine is not appreciably removed by hemodialysis or peritoneal dialysis.[36,37]

DRUG INTERACTIONS

Quinidine has serious interactions with other drugs that are capable of inhibiting the CYP3A enzyme system.[38] Because this isozyme is present in the intestinal wall and liver, quinidine serum concentrations may increase due to decreased clearance, decreased first-pass metabolism, or a combination of both. P-glycoprotein is also inhibited by quinidine, so drug transport may be decreased and cause drug interactions. Erythromycin, keto-conazole, and verapamil have been reported to increase quinidine serum concentrations or area under the concentration-time curve (AUC) by greater than 30%-50%. Other macrolide antibiotics (such as clarithromycin) or azole antifungals (such as fluconazole, miconazole, and itraconazole) that inhibit CYP3A probably cause similar drug interactions with quinidine. Cimetidine and amiodarone also have been reported to cause increases in quinidine concentrations or AUC of a similar magnitude. Drugs that induce CYP3A (phenytoin, phenobarbital, rifampin, rifabutin) decrease quinidine serum concentrations by increasing quinidine clearance and first-pass metabolism. It is important to remember that phenytoin has antiarrhythmic effects and is also classified as a type IB antiarrhythmic agent. Because of this, phenytoin and quinidine may have additive pharmacologic effects that could result in a pharmacodynamic drug interaction.

Although it is not a substrate for the enzyme, quinidine is a potent inhibitor of the CYP2D6 enzyme system.[38-41] As little as 50 mg of quinidine can effectively turn an "extensive metabolizer" into a "poor metabolizer" for this isozyme. Because poor metabolizers of CYP2D6 substrates have little to none of this enzyme in their liver, the administration of quinidine does not result in a drug interaction in these individuals. Quinidine can markedly decrease the clearance β-adrenergic receptor blockers eliminated via CYP2D6 by 30% or more. Propranolol, metoprolol, and timolol have decreased clearance due to quinidine coadministration. Tricyclic antidepressants (nortriptyline, imipramine, and desipramine), haloperidol, and dextromethorphan also have increased serum concentrations when given with quinidine. Codeine is a prodrug with no analgesic effect that relies on conversion to morphine via the CYP2D6 enzyme system to decrease pain. When quinidine is given concomitantly with codeine, the conversion from codeine to morphine does not take place, and patients do not experience analgesia. A similar drug interaction may occur with dihydrocodeine and hydrocodone. Although it may not be reported in the literature for a specific compound, clinicians should consider that a drug interaction is possible between quinidine and any CYP2D6 substrate.

Quinidine increases digoxin serum concentrations 30%-50% by decreasing digoxin renal and nonrenal clearance as well as digoxin volume of distribution.[38] The probable mechanisms of this drug interaction are inhibition of digoxin renal and hepatic P-glycoprotein (PGP) elimination and tissue-binding displacement of digoxin by quinidine. Antacids can increase urinary pH leading to increased renal tubular reabsorption of unionized quinidine and decreased quinidine renal clearance. Kaolin-pectin administration results in physical adsorption of quinidine in the gastrointestinal tract and decreased quinidine oral absorption. The pharmacologic effects of warfarin and neuromuscular blockers have been enhanced when given with quinidine.

INITIAL DOSAGE DETERMINATION METHODS

Several methods to initiate quinidine therapy are available. The *Pharmacokinetic Dosing method* is the most flexible of the techniques. It allows individualized target serum concentrations to be chosen for a patient, and each pharmacokinetic parameter can be customized to reflect specific disease states and conditions present in the patient. *Literature-based Recommended Dosing* is a very commonly used method to prescribe initial doses of quinidine. Doses are based on those that commonly produce steady-state concentrations in the lower end of the therapeutic range, although there is a wide variation in the actual concentrations for a specific patient.

Pharmacokinetic Dosing Method

The goal of initial dosing of quinidine is to compute the best dose possible for the patient, given their set of disease states and conditions that influence quinidine pharmacokinetics and the arrhythmia being treated. In order to do this, pharmacokinetic parameters for the patient will be estimated using average parameters measured in other patients with similar disease state and condition profiles.

Half-Life and Elimination Rate Constant Estimate

Quinidine is predominately metabolized by liver. Unfortunately, there is no good way to estimate the elimination characteristics of liver-metabolized drugs using an endogenous marker of liver function in the same manner that serum creatinine and estimated creatinine clearance are used to estimate the elimination of agents that are renally eliminated. Because of this, a patient is categorized according to the disease states and conditions that are known to change quinidine half-life, and the half-life previously measured in these studies is used as an estimate of the current patient's half-life (see Table 9-1). For a patient with moderate heart failure (NYHA CHF class III), quinidine half-life would be assumed to equal 7 hours, while a patient with severe liver disease (Child-Pugh score = 12) would be assigned an estimated half-life of 9 hours. To produce the most conservative quinidine doses in patients with multiple concurrent disease states or conditions that affect quinidine pharmacokinetics, the disease state or condition with the longest half-life should be used to compute doses. This approach will avoid accidental overdosage as much as currently possible. Once the correct half-life is identified for the patient, it can be converted into the quinidine elimination rate constant (k) using the following equation: $k = 0.693/t_{1/2}$.

Volume of Distribution Estimate

As with the half-life estimate, the quinidine volume of distribution is chosen according to the disease states and conditions that are present (see Table 9-1). The volume of distribution is used to help compute quinidine clearance, and is assumed to equal 3.8 L/kg for liver disease patients, 1.7 L/kg for heart failure patients, and 2.4 L/kg for all other patients. For obese patients (>30% above ideal body weight), ideal body weight is used to compute quinidine volume of distribution. Thus, for a nonobese 80-kg patient without heart failure or liver disease, the estimated quinidine volume of distribution would be 192 L: V = 2.4 L/kg • 80 kg = 192 L. For a 150-kg obese patient with an ideal body weight of 60 kg and normal cardiac and liver function, the estimated quinidine volume of distribution is 144 L: V = 2.4 L/kg • 60 kg = 144 L.

Selection of Appropriate Pharmacokinetic Model and Equations

When given orally, quinidine follows a one- or two-compartment pharmacokinetic model (see Figure 9-1). When oral therapy is required, most clinicians utilize a sustained-release dosage form that has good bioavailability (F = 0.7), supplies a continuous release of quinidine into the gastrointestinal tract, and provides a smooth quinidine serum concentration-time curve that emulates an intravenous infusion when given every 8-12 hours. Because of this, a very simple pharmacokinetic equation that computes the average quinidine steady-state serum concentration (Css in μg/mL = mg/L) is widely used and allows maintenance dosage calculation: Css = [F • S (D/τ)]/Cl or D = (Css • Cl • τ)/(F • S), where F is the bioavailability fraction for the oral dosage form (F = 0.7 for most oral quinidine products), S is the fraction of the quinidine salt form that is active quinidine (S = 0.83 for sulfate: immediate-release tablets = 200, 300 mg, extended-release tablets = 300 mg; S = 0.62 for gluconate: extended-release tablets = 324 mg), D is the dose of quinidine salt in mg, and τ is the dosage interval in hours. Cl is quinidine clearance in L/h and is computed using estimates of quinidine elimination rate constant (k) and volume of distribution: Cl = kV. For example, for a patient with an estimated elimination rate constant equal to 0.099 h^{-1} and an estimated volume of distribution equal to 168 L, the estimated clearance would equal 16.6 L/h: Cl = 0.099h^{-1} • 168 L = 16.6 L/h.

Steady-State Concentration Selection

The general accepted therapeutic range for quinidine is 2-6 μg/mL. However, quinidine therapy must be individualized for each patient in order to achieve optimal responses and minimal side effects.

EXAMPLE 1 ▶▶▶

LK is a 50-year-old, 75-kg (height = 5 ft 10 in) male with ventricular tachycardia who requires therapy with oral quinidine gluconate. He has normal liver and cardiac function. Suggest an initial oral quinidine dosage regimen designed to achieve a steady-state quinidine concentration equal to 3 μg/mL.

1. *Estimate half-life and elimination rate constant according to disease states and conditions present in the patient.*
   The expected quinidine half-life ($t_{1/2}$) is 7 hours. The elimination rate constant is computed using the following formula: $k = 0.693/t_{1/2} = 0.693/7\ h = 0.099\ h^{-1}$.

2. *Estimate the volume of distribution and clearance.*
   The patient is not obese, so the estimated quinidine volume of distribution will be based on actual body weight: V = 2.4 L/kg • 75 kg = 180 L. Estimated quinidine clearance is computed by taking the product of V and the elimination rate constant: $Cl = kV = 0.099\ h^{-1}$ • 180 L = 17.8 L/h.

3. *Compute dosage regimen.*
   Oral extended-release quinidine gluconate tablets will be prescribed to this patient (F = 0.7, S = 0.62). The initial dosage interval (τ) will be set to 8 hours. (Note: μg/mL = mg/L and this concentration unit was substituted for Css in the calculations so that unnecessary unit conversion was not required). The dosage equation for oral quinidine is: D = (Css • Cl • τ)/(F • S) = (3 mg/L • 17.8 L/h • 8 h)/(0.7 • 0.62) = 984 mg, rounded to 972 mg every 8 hours.
   A steady-state quinidine serum concentration could be measured after steady-state is attained in 3-5 half-lives. Since the patient is expected to have a half-life equal to 7 hours, the quinidine steady-state concentration could be obtained any time after the second day of dosing (5 half-lives = 5 • 7 h = 35 h). Quinidine serum concentrations should also be measured if the patient experiences a return of their arrhythmia, or if the patient develops potential signs or symptoms of quinidine toxicity.

EXAMPLE 2 ▶▶▶

OI is a 60-year-old, 85-kg (height = 6 ft 1 in) male with atrial fibrillation who requires therapy with oral quinidine sulfate. He has liver cirrhosis (Child-Pugh score = 11). Suggest an initial extended-release quinidine sulfate dosage regimen designed to achieve a steady-state quinidine concentration equal to 2 μg/mL.

1. *Estimate half-life and elimination rate constant according to disease states and conditions present in the patient.*
   The expected quinidine half-life ($t_{1/2}$) is 9 hours. The elimination rate constant is computed using the following formula: $k = 0.693/t_{1/2} = 0.693/9\ h = 0.077\ h^{-1}$.

2. *Estimate the volume of distribution and clearance.*
   The patient is not obese, so the estimated quinidine volume of distribution will be based on actual body weight: Vc = 3.8 L/kg • 85 kg = 323 L. Estimated quinidine clearance is computed by taking the product of V and the elimination rate constant: $Cl = kV = 0.077\ h^{-1}$ • 323 L = 24.9 L/h.

3. *Compute dosage regimen.*
   Oral extended-release quinidine sulfate tablets will be prescribed to this patient (F = 0.7, S = 0.83). The initial dosage interval (τ) will be set to 8 hours. (Note: μg/mL = mg/L and this concentration unit was substituted for Css in the calculations so that unnecessary unit conversion was not required). The dosage equation for oral quinidine is: D = (Css • Cl • τ)/(F • S) = (2 mg/L • 24.9 L/h • 8 h)/(0.7 • 0.83) = 686 mg, rounded to 600 mg every 8 hours.
   A steady-state quinidine serum concentration could be measured after steady-state is attained in 3-5 half-lives. Since the patient is expected to have a half-life equal to 9 hours, the quinidine steady-state concentration could be obtained any time after the second day of dosing (5 half-lives = 5 • 9 h = 45 h). Quinidine serum concentrations should also be measured if the patient experiences a return of their arrhythmia, or if the patient develops potential signs or symptoms of quinidine toxicity.

EXAMPLE 3 ▶ ▶ ▶

MN is a 64-year-old, 78-kg (height = 5 ft 9 in) male with ventricular tachycardia who requires therapy with oral quinidine. He has moderate heart failure (NYHA CHF class III). Suggest an initial extended-release quinidine gluconate dosage regimen designed to achieve a steady-state quinidine concentration equal to 3 μg/mL.

1. *Estimate half-life and elimination rate constant according to disease states and conditions present in the patient.*
   The expected quinidine half-life ($t_{1/2}$) is 7 hours. The elimination rate constant is computed using the following formula: $k = 0.693/t_{1/2} = 0.693/7 \text{ h} = 0.099 \text{ h}^{-1}$.
2. *Estimate the volume of distribution and clearance.*
   The patient is not obese, so the estimated quinidine volume of distribution will be based on actual body weight: V = 1.7 L/kg • 78 kg = 133 L. Estimated quinidine clearance is computed by taking the product of V and the elimination rate constant: $Cl = kV = 0.099 \text{ h}^{-1}$ • 133 L = 13.2 L/h.
3. *Compute dosage regimen.*
   Oral extended-release quinidine gluconate tablets will be prescribed to this patient (F = 0.7, S = 0.62). The initial dosage interval (τ) will be set to 12 hours. (Note: μg/mL = mg/L and this concentration unit was substituted for Css in the calculations so that unnecessary unit conversion was not required.) The dosage equation for oral quinidine is: D = (Css • Cl • τ)/(F • S) = (3 mg/L • 13.2 L/h • 8 h)/(0.7 • 0.62) = 730 mg, rounded to 648 mg every 8 hours.

   A steady-state quinidine serum concentration could be measured after steady-state is attained in 3-5 half-lives. Since the patient is expected to have a half-life equal to 7 hours, the quinidine steady-state concentration could be obtained any time after the second day of dosing (5 half-lives = 5 • 7 h = 35 h). Quinidine serum concentrations should also be measured if the patient experiences a return of their arrhythmia, or if the patient develops potential signs or symptoms of quinidine toxicity.

Literature-Based Recommended Dosing

Because of the large amount of variability in quinidine pharmacokinetics, even when concurrent disease states and conditions are identified, many clinicians believe that the use of standard quinidine doses for various situations are warranted. The original computation of these doses were based on the Pharmacokinetic Dosing method described in the previous section, and subsequently modified based on clinical experience. In general, the quinidine steady-state serum concentration expected from the lower end of the dosage range was 2-4 μg/mL and 4-6 μg/mL for the upper end of the dosage range. Suggested quinidine maintenance doses for adults and children are given in Table 9-4. A 25%-50% reduction in initial quinidine dose is suggested for patients with moderate-severe liver disease (Child-Pugh score ≥8) or moderate-severe heart failure (NYHA class II or greater). When more than one disease state or condition is present in a patient, choosing the lowest daily dose will result in the safest, most conservative dosage recommendation.

To illustrate the similarities and differences between this method of dosage calculation and the Pharmacokinetic Dosing method, the same examples used in the previous section will be used.

EXAMPLE 1 ▶ ▶ ▶

LK is a 50-year-old, 75-kg (height = 5 ft 10 in) male with ventricular tachycardia who requires therapy with oral quinidine gluconate. He has normal liver and cardiac function. Suggest an initial oral quinidine dosage regimen designed to achieve a steady-state quinidine concentration equal to 3 μg/mL.

1. *Choose quinidine dose based on disease states and conditions present in the patient.*

A quinidine gluconate maintenance dose of 628 mg every 12 hours (1256 mg/d) is suggested for a patient without heart failure or liver disease requiring a quinidine steady-state serum concentration in the lower end of the therapeutic range.

A steady-state quinidine serum concentration could be measured after steady-state is attained in 3-5 half-lives. Since the patient is expected to have a half-life equal to 7 hours, the quinidine steady-state concentration could be obtained any time after the second day of dosing (5 half-lives = 5 • 7 h = 35 h). Quinidine serum concentrations should also be measured if the patient experiences a return of their arrhythmia, or if the patient develops potential signs or symptoms of quinidine toxicity.

EXAMPLE 2 ▶▶▶

OI is a 60-year-old, 85-kg (height = 6 ft 1 in) male with atrial fibrillation who requires therapy with oral quinidine sulfate. He has liver cirrhosis (Child-Pugh score = 11). Suggest an initial immediate-release quinidine sulfate dosage regimen designed to achieve a steady-state quinidine concentration equal to 2 µg/mL.

1. *Choose quinidine dose based on disease states and conditions present in the patient.*
   A quinidine sulfate maintenance dose of 100 mg every 6 hours (400 mg/d) is suggested for a patient with liver disease requiring a quinidine steady-state serum concentration in the lower end of the therapeutic range.

   A steady-state quinidine serum concentration could be measured after steady-state is attained in 3-5 half-lives. Since the patient is expected to have a half-life equal to 9 hours, the quinidine steady-state concentration could be obtained any time after the second day of dosing (5 half-lives = 5 • 9 h = 45 h). Quinidine serum concentrations should also be measured if the patient experiences a return of their arrhythmia, or if the patient develops potential signs or symptoms of quinidine toxicity.

TABLE 9-4   Literature-Based Recommended Oral Quinidine Initial Dosage Ranges for Various Disease States and Conditions

Disease State/ Condition	Quinidine Sulfate, Immediate-Release Tablets	Quinidine Sulfate, Extended-Release Tablets	Quinidine Gluconate Extended-Release Tablets
Adult, normal liver function	200-300 mg every 6-8 h	600 mg every 8-12 h	324-648 mg every 8-12 h
Adult, liver cirrhosis or heart failure	100-200 mg every 6-8 h	300 mg every 8-12 h	324 mg every 8-12 h
Children, normal liver function[a]	15-60 mg/kg/d given every 6 h	—	—

[a]For intravenous use, the dose of quinidine gluconate injection is 2-10 mg/kg/dose administered every 3-6 h, as needed. A 2-mg/kg test dose of oral quinidine sulfate or injectable quinidine gluconate (IM) is recommended to determine if an idiosyncratic adverse effect will occur (maximum test dose is 200 mg).[44]

EXAMPLE 3 ▶▶▶

MN is a 64-year-old, 78-kg (height = 5 ft 9 in) male with ventricular tachycardia who requires therapy with oral quinidine. He has moderate heart failure (NYHA CHF class III). Suggest an initial extended-release quinidine gluconate dosage regimen designed to achieve a steady-state quinidine concentration equal to 3 μg/mL.

1. *Choose quinidine dose based on disease states and conditions present in the patient.*

A quinidine gluconate maintenance dose of 324 mg every 12 hours (648 mg/d) is suggested for a patient with heart failure requiring a quinidine steady-state serum concentration in the lower end of the therapeutic range.

A steady-state quinidine serum concentration could be measured after steady state is attained in 3-5 half-lives. Since the patient is expected to have a half-life equal to 7 hours, the quinidine steady-state concentration could be obtained any time after the second day of dosing (5 half-lives = 5 • 7 h = 35 h). Quinidine serum concentrations should also be measured if the patient experiences a return of their arrhythmia, or if the patient develops potential signs or symptoms of quinidine toxicity.

USE OF QUINIDINE SERUM CONCENTRATIONS TO ALTER DOSES

Because of the large amount of pharmacokinetic variability among patients, it is likely that doses computed using patient population characteristics will not always produce quinidine serum concentrations that are expected or desirable. Because of pharmacokinetic variability, the narrow therapeutic index of quinidine, and the desire to avoid quinidine adverse side effects, measurement of quinidine serum concentrations can be a useful adjunct for patients to insure that therapeutic, nontoxic levels are present. In addition to quinidine serum concentrations, important patient parameters (electrocardiogram, clinical signs and symptoms of the arrhythmia, potential quinidine side effects, etc) should be followed to confirm that the patient is responding to treatment and not developing adverse drug reactions.

When quinidine serum concentrations are measured in patients and a dosage change is necessary, clinicians should seek to use the simplest, most straightforward method available to determine a dose that will provide safe and effective treatment. In most cases, a simple dosage ratio can be used to change quinidine doses assuming the drug follows *linear pharmacokinetics*. Thus, assuming linear pharmacokinetics is adequate for dosage adjustments in most patients.

Sometimes, it is useful to compute quinidine pharmacokinetic constants for a patient and base dosage adjustments on these parameters. In this case, it may be possible to calculate and use *pharmacokinetic parameters* to alter the quinidine dose.

In some situations, it may be necessary to compute quinidine pharmacokinetic parameters as soon as possible for the patient before steady-state conditions occur and utilize these parameters to calculate the best drug dose. Computerized methods that incorporate expected population pharmacokinetic characteristics (*Bayesian pharmacokinetic computer programs*) can be used in difficult cases where serum concentrations are obtained at suboptimal times or the patient was not at a steady state when serum concentrations were measured. An additional benefit of this method is that a complete pharmacokinetic workup (determination of clearance, volume of distribution, and half-life) can be done with one or more measured concentrations that do not have to be at a steady state.

Linear Pharmacokinetics Method

Because quinidine follows linear, dose-proportional pharmacokinetics in most patients, steady-state serum concentrations change in proportion to dose according to the following equation: $D_{new}/C_{ss, new} = D_{old}/C_{ss, old}$ or

$D_{new} = (C_{ss, new}/C_{ss, old})D_{old}$, where D is the dose, Css is the steady-state concentration, old indicates the dose that produced the steady-state concentration that the patient is currently receiving, and new denotes the dose necessary to produce the desired steady-state concentration. The advantages of this method are that it is quick and simple. The disadvantages are that steady-state concentrations are required. Because nonlinear pharmacokinetics for quinidine has been observed in some patients, suggested dosage increases greater than 75% using this method should be scrutinized by the prescribing clinician, and the risk versus benefit for the patient assessed before initiating large dosage increases (>75% over current dose).

EXAMPLE 1 ▶▶▶

LK is a 50-year-old, 75-kg (height = 5 ft 10 in) male with ventricular tachycardia who requires therapy with quinidine gluconate. He has normal liver and cardiac function. The current steady-state quinidine concentration equals 2.2 µg/mL at a dose of 324 mg every 8 hours. Compute a quinidine dose that will provide a steady-state concentration of 4 µg/mL.

1. *Compute new dose to achieve desired serum concentration.*

The patient would be expected to achieve steady-state conditions after the second day (5 $t_{1/2}$ = 5 • 7 h = 35 h) of therapy.

Using linear pharmacokinetics, the new dose to attain the desired concentration should be proportional to the old dose that produced the measured concentration (note: total daily dose = 324 mg/dose • 3 dose/d = 972 mg/d):

$$D_{new} = (C_{ss, new}/C_{ss, old})\,D_{old} = (4\,\mu g/mL / 2.2\,\mu g/mL)\,972\,mg/d = 1767\,mg/d,$$
rounded to 1944 mg/d or 648 mg every 8 hours

The new suggested dose would be 648 mg every 8 hours of oral quinidine gluconate to be started immediately.

A steady-state quinidine serum concentration could be measured after steady state is attained in 3-5 half-lives. Since the patient is expected to have a half-life equal to 7 hours, the quinidine steady-state concentration could be obtained any time after the day of dosing (5 half-lives = 5 • 7 h = 35 h). Quinidine serum concentrations should also be measured if the patient experiences a return of their arrhythmia, or if the patient develops potential signs or symptoms of quinidine toxicity.

EXAMPLE 2 ▶▶▶

OI is a 60-year-old, 85-kg (height = 6 ft 1 in) male with atrial fibrillation who requires therapy with oral quinidine sulfate extended-release tablets. He has liver cirrhosis (Child-Pugh score = 11). The current steady-state quinidine concentration equals 7.4 µg/mL at a dose of 600 mg every 12 hours. Compute a quinidine dose that will provide a steady-state concentration of 3 µg/mL.

1. *Compute new dose to achieve the desired serum concentration.*

The patient would be expected to achieve steady-state conditions after 2 days (5 $t_{1/2}$ = 5 • 9 h = 45 h) of therapy.

Using linear pharmacokinetics, the new dose to attain the desired concentration should be proportional to the old dose that produced the measured concentration (note: total daily dose = 600 mg/dose • 2 dose/d = 1200 mg/d):

$$D_{new} = (C_{ss, new}/C_{ss, old})\,D_{old} = (3\,\mu g/mL / 7.4\,\mu g/mL)\,1200\,mg/d = 486\,mg/d, \text{ rounded to } 600\,mg/d$$

The new suggested dose would be 300 mg every 12 hours of quinidine sulfate extended-release tablets. If the patient was experiencing adverse drug effects, the new dosage regimen could be held for 1-2 estimated half-lives ($t_{1/2} = 9$ h).

A steady-state quinidine serum concentration could be measured after steady state is attained in 3-5 half-lives. Since the patient is expected to have a half-life equal to 9 hours, the quinidine steady-state concentration could be obtained any time after the second day of dosing (5 half-lives = 5 • 9 h = 45 h). Quinidine serum concentrations should also be measured if the patient experiences a return of their arrhythmia, or if the patient develops potential signs or symptoms of quinidine toxicity.

EXAMPLE 3 ▶▶▶

MN is a 64-year-old, 78-kg (height = 5 ft 9 in) male with ventricular tachycardia who requires therapy with oral quinidine sulfate immediate-release tablets. He has moderate heart failure (NYHA CHF class III). The current steady-state quinidine concentration equals 2.2 µg/mL at a dose of 100 mg every 6 hours. Compute a quinidine dose that will provide a steady-state concentration of 4 µg/mL.

1. *Compute new dose to achieve desired serum concentration.*

The patient would be expected to achieve steady-state conditions after 2 days (5 $t_{1/2}$ = 5 • 7 h = 35 h) of therapy.

Using linear pharmacokinetics, the new dose to attain the desired concentration should be proportional to the old dose that produced the measured concentration. (Note: total daily dose = 100 mg/dose • 4 doses/d = 400 mg/d):

$$D_{new} = (C_{ss,\,new}/C_{ss,\,old})\, D_{old} = (4\ \mu g/mL\, /\, 2.2\ \mu g/mL)\ 400\ mg/d = 727\ mg/d,$$
$$\text{rounded to 800 mg/d or 200 mg every 6 hours}$$

The new suggested dose would be 200 mg every 6 hours of quinidine sulfate immediate-release tablets to begin immediately.

A steady-state quinidine serum concentration could be measured after steady-state is attained in 3-5 half-lives. Since the patient is expected to have a half-life equal to 7 hours, the quinidine steady-state concentration could be obtained any time after the second day of dosing (5 half-lives = 5 • 7 h = 35 h). Quinidine serum concentrations should also be measured if the patient experiences a return of their arrhythmia, or if the patient develops potential signs or symptoms of quinidine toxicity.

Pharmacokinetic Parameter Method

The Pharmacokinetic Parameter method of adjusting drug doses was among the first techniques available to change doses using serum concentrations. It allows the computation of an individual's own, unique pharmacokinetic constants and uses those to calculate a dose that achieves desired quinidine concentrations. The Pharmacokinetic Parameter method requires that steady state has been achieved and uses only a steady-state quinidine concentration (Css). If the patient is receiving oral quinidine therapy, quinidine clearance (Cl) can be calculated using the following formula: Cl = [F • S (D/τ)]/ Css, where F is the bioavailability fraction for the oral dosage form (F = 0.7 for most oral quinidine products), S is the fraction of the quinidine salt form that is active quinidine (S = 0.83 for quinidine sulfate, S = 0.62 for quinidine gluconate), D is the dose of quinidine salt in mg, Css is the steady-state quinidine concentration, and τ is the dosage interval in hours. Because this method also assumes linear pharmacokinetics, quinidine doses computed using the Pharmacokinetic Parameter method and the Linear Pharmacokinetic method should be identical.

EXAMPLE 1 ▶▶▶

LK is a 50-year-old, 75-kg (height = 5 ft 10 in) male with ventricular tachycardia who requires therapy with quinidine gluconate. He has normal liver and cardiac function. The current steady-state quinidine concentration equals 2.2 µg/mL at a dose of 324 mg every 8 hours. Compute a quinidine dose that will provide a steady-state concentration of 4 µg/mL.

1. *Compute pharmacokinetic parameters.*

   The patient would be expected to achieve steady-state conditions after the second day (5 $t_{1/2}$ = 5 • 7 h = 35 h) of therapy.

   Quinidine clearance can be computed using a steady-state quinidine concentration: Cl = [F • S (D/τ)] / Css = [0.7 • 0.62 (324 mg/8 h)] / (2.2 mg/L) = 7.99 L/h. (Note: µg/mL = mg/L and this concentration unit was substituted for Css in the calculations so that unnecessary unit conversion was not required.)

2. *Compute quinidine dose.*

   Quinidine clearance is used to compute the new dose: D = (Css • Cl • τ)/(F • S) = (4 mg/L • 7.99 L/h • 8h)/ (0.7 • 0.62) = 589 mg, rounded to 648 mg every 8 hours.

   The new quinidine dose would be instituted immediately.

   A steady-state quinidine serum concentration could be measured after steady state is attained in 3-5 half-lives. Since the patient is expected to have a half-life equal to 7 hours, the quinidine steady-state concentration could be obtained any time after the second day of dosing (5 half-lives = 5 • 7 h = 35 h). Quinidine serum concentrations should also be measured if the patient experiences a return of their arrhythmia, or if the patient develops potential signs or symptoms of quinidine toxicity.

EXAMPLE 2 ▶▶▶

OI is a 60-year-old, 85-kg (height = 6 ft 1 in) male with atrial fibrillation who requires therapy with oral quinidine sulfate extended-release tablets. He has liver cirrhosis (Child-Pugh score = 11). The current steady-state quinidine concentration equals 7.4 µg/mL at a dose of 600 mg every 12 hours. Compute a quinidine dose that will provide a steady-state concentration of 3 µg/mL.

1. *Compute pharmacokinetic parameters.*

   The patient would be expected to achieve steady-state conditions after the second day (5 $t_{1/2}$ = 5 • 9 h = 45 h) of therapy.

   Quinidine clearance can be computed using a steady-state quinidine concentration: Cl = [F • S (D/τ)] / Css = [0.7 • 0.83 (600 mg/12 h)] / (7.4 mg/L) = 3.93 L/h. (Note: µg/mL = mg/L and this concentration unit was substituted for Css in the calculations so that unnecessary unit conversion was not required.)

2. *Compute quinidine dose.*

   Quinidine clearance is used to compute the new dose: D = (Css • Cl • τ)/(F • S) = (3 mg/L • 3.93 L/h • 12 h)/ (0.7 • 0.83) = 244 mg, rounded to 300 mg every 12 hours.

   The new quinidine dose would be instituted immediately.

   A steady-state quinidine serum concentration could be measured after steady-state is attained in 3-5 half-lives. Since the patient is expected to have a half-life equal to 9 hours, the quinidine steady-state concentration could be obtained any time after the second day of dosing (5 half-lives = 5 • 9 h = 45 h). Quinidine serum concentrations should also be measured if the patient experiences a return of their arrhythmia, or if the patient develops potential signs or symptoms of quinidine toxicity.

EXAMPLE 3 ▶ ▶ ▶

MN is a 64-year-old, 78-kg (height = 5 ft 9 in) male with ventricular tachycardia who requires therapy with oral quinidine sulfate immediate-release tablets. He has moderate heart failure (NYHA CHF class III). The current steady-state quinidine concentration equals 2.2 μg/mL at a dose of 100 mg every 6 hours. Compute a quinidine dose that will provide a steady-state concentration of 4 μg/mL.

1. *Compute pharmacokinetic parameters.*

The patient would be expected to achieve steady-state conditions after the second day (5 $t_{1/2}$ = 5 • 7 h = 35 h) of therapy.

Quinidine clearance can be computed using a steady-state quinidine concentration: Cl = [F • S (D/τ)] / Css = [0.7 • 0.83 (100 mg/6 h)] / (2.2 mg/L) = 4.40 L/h. (Note: μg/mL = mg/L and this concentration unit was substituted for Css in the calculations so that unnecessary unit conversion was not required.)

2. *Compute quinidine dose.*

Quinidine clearance is used to compute the new dose: D = (Css • Cl • τ)/(F • S) = (4 mg/L • 4.40 L/h • 6 h)/(0.7 • 0.83) = 182 mg, rounded to 200 mg every 6 hours.

The new quinidine dose would be instituted immediately.

A steady-state quinidine serum concentration could be measured after steady-state is attained in 3-5 half-lives. Since the patient is expected to have a half-life equal to 7 hours, the quinidine steady-state concentration could be obtained any time after the second day of dosing (5 half-lives = 5 • 7 h = 35 h). Quinidine serum concentrations should also be measured if the patient experiences a return of their arrhythmia, or if the patient develops potential signs or symptoms of quinidine toxicity.

Bayesian Pharmacokinetic Computer Programs

Computer programs are available that can assist in the computation of pharmacokinetic parameters for patients. The most reliable computer programs use a nonlinear regression algorithm that incorporates components of Bayes theorem. Nonlinear regression is a statistical technique that uses an iterative process to compute the best pharmacokinetic parameters for a concentration/time data set. Briefly, the patient's drug dosage schedule and serum concentrations are input into the computer. The computer program has a pharmacokinetic equation pre-programmed for the drug and administration method (oral, intravenous bolus, intravenous infusion, etc). Typically, a one-compartment model is used, although some programs allow the user to choose among several different equations. Using population estimates based on demographic information for the patient (age, weight, gender, liver function, cardiac status, etc) supplied by the user, the computer program then computes estimated serum concentrations at each time there are actual serum concentrations. Kinetic parameters are then changed by the computer program, and a new set of estimated serum concentrations are computed. The pharmacokinetic parameters that generated the estimated serum concentrations closest to the actual values are remembered by the computer program, and the process is repeated until the set of pharmacokinetic parameters that result in esti-mated serum concentrations that are statistically closest to the actual serum concentrations are generated. These pharmacokinetic parameters can then be used to compute improved dosing schedules for patients. Bayes theorem is used in the computer algorithm to balance the results of the computations between values based solely on the patient's serum drug concentrations and those based only on patient population parameters. Results from studies that compare various methods of dosage adjustment have consistently found that these types of computer dosing programs perform at least as well as experienced clinical pharmacokineticists and clinicians and better than inexperienced clinicians.

Some clinicians use Bayesian pharmacokinetic computer programs exclusively to alter drug doses based on serum concentrations. An advantage of this approach is that consistent dosage recommendations are made when several different practitioners are involved in therapeutic drug-monitoring programs. However, since simpler dosing methods work just as well for patients with stable pharmacokinetic parameters and steady-state drug concentrations, many clinicians reserve the use of computer programs for more difficult situations. Those situations include serum concentrations that are not at steady state, serum concentrations not obtained at the specific times needed to employ simpler methods, and unstable pharmacokinetic parameters. Many Bayesian pharmacokinetic computer programs are available to users, and most should provide answers similar to the one used in the following examples. The program used to solve problems in this book is DrugCalc written by Dr Dennis Mungall.[42]

EXAMPLE 1 ▶▶▶

OY is a 57-year-old, 79-kg (height = 5 ft 8 in) male with ventricular tachycardia who requires therapy with oral quinidine gluconate. He has normal liver (bilirubin = 0.7 mg/dL, albumin = 4.0 g/dL) and cardiac function. He started taking quinidine gluconate 648 mg every 12 hours at 0800 H. The quinidine serum concentration equals 2.1 µg/mL at 0730 H before the morning dose is given on the second day of therapy. Compute a quinidine gluconate dose that will provide a steady-state concentration of 4 µg/mL.

1. *Enter the patient's demographic, drug-dosing, and serum concentration/time data into the computer program.*
   In this patient's case, it is unlikely that the patient is at steady state so the Linear Pharmacokinetics method cannot be used. The DrugCalc program requires quinidine salt doses be input in terms of quinidine base. A 648 mg of quinidine gluconate is equivalent to 400 mg of quinidine base (400 mg quinidine base = 648 mg quinidine gluconate • 0.62).

2. *Compute pharmacokinetic parameters for the patient using Bayesian pharmacokinetic computer program.*
   The pharmacokinetic parameters computed by the program are a volume of distribution of 181 L, a half-life equal to 15.2 h, and a clearance equal to 8.21 L/h.

3. *Compute the dose required to achieve desired quinidine serum concentrations.*
   The oral one-compartment model equation used by the program to compute doses indicates that 972 mg of quinidine gluconate every 12 hours will produce a steady-state trough concentration of 4.7 µg/mL. (Note: DrugCalc uses salt form A and sustained-action options for quinidine gluconate.) This dose would be started immediately.

EXAMPLE 2 ▶▶▶

SL is a 71-year-old, 82-kg (height = 5 ft 10 in) male with atrial fibrillation who requires therapy with oral quinidine. He has liver cirrhosis (Child-Pugh score = 12, bilirubin = 3.2 mg/dL, albumin = 2.5 g/dL) and normal cardiac function. He began quinidine sulfate extended-release tablets 600 mg every 12 hours at 0700 H. On the second day of therapy before the morning dose is administered, the quinidine serum concentration equals 4.5 µg/mL at 0700 H. Compute a quinidine sulfate dose that will provide a steady-state concentration of 4 µg/mL.

1. *Enter the patient's demographic, drug-dosing, and serum concentration/time data into the computer program.*
   In this patient's case, it is unlikely that the patient is at steady state so the Linear Pharmacokinetics method cannot be used. The DrugCalc program requires quinidine salt doses be input in terms of quinidine base. A 600 mg of quinidine sulfate is equivalent to 500 mg of quinidine base (500 mg quinidine base = 600 mg quinidine sulfate • 0.83).

2. *Compute pharmacokinetic parameters for the patient using Bayesian pharmacokinetic computer program.*
   The pharmacokinetic parameters computed by the program are a volume of distribution of 161 L, a half-life equal to 21.4 h, and a clearance equal to 5.24 L/h.
3. *Compute the dose required to achieve the desired quinidine serum concentrations.*
   The oral one-compartment model equation used by the program to compute doses indicates that 300 mg of quinidine sulfate extended-release tablets every 12 hours will produce a steady-state trough concentration of 4.1 µg/mL. (Note: DrugCalc uses salt form B and sustained-action options for quinidine sulfate extended-release tablets.) This dose would be started immediately.

EXAMPLE 3 ▶▶▶

TR is a 75-year-old, 85-kg (height = 5 ft 8 in) male with atrial flutter who requires therapy with quinidine sulfate immediate-release tablets. He has moderate heart failure (NYHA CHF class III). Yesterday, he was prescribed quinidine sulfate 200 mg four times daily, and received the first two doses at 0800 H and 1200 H. Because he felt that his arrhythmia may have returned, the patient phoned his physician who advised him to increase the dose to 400 mg (1800 H and 2200 H). The quinidine serum concentration equals 4.7 µg/mL at 1000 H, 2 hours after the morning dose (at 0800 H, 400 mg quinidine sulfate). Compute a quinidine sulfate dose that will provide a steady-state trough concentration of 4 µg/mL.

1. *Enter the patient's demographic, drug-dosing, and serum concentration/time data into the computer program.*
   In this patient's case, it is unlikely that the patient is at steady-state so the Linear Pharmacokinetics method cannot be used. The DrugCalc program requires quinidine salt doses be input in terms of quinidine base. A 200 mg of quinidine sulfate is equivalent to 165 mg of quinidine base while 400 mg of quinidine sulfate is equivalent to 330 mg of quinidine base (165 mg quinidine base = 200 mg quinidine sulfate • 0.83, 330 mg quinidine base = 400 mg quinidine sulfate • 0.83).
2. *Compute pharmacokinetic parameters for the patient using Bayesian pharmacokinetic computer program.*
   The pharmacokinetic parameters computed by the program are a volume of distribution of 126 L, a half-life equal to 11.6 h, and a clearance equal to 7.53 L/h.
3. *Compute the dose required to achieve the desired quinidine serum concentrations.*
   The oral one-compartment model equation used by the program to compute doses indicates that 300 mg of quinidine sulfate immediate-release tablets every 6 hours will produce a steady-state trough concentration of 4.2 µg/mL. (Note: DrugCalc uses salt form B and oral options for quinidine sulfate immediate-release tablets.) This dose would be started immediately.

DOSING STRATEGIES

Initial dose and dosage adjustment techniques using serum concentrations can be used in any combination as long as the limitations of each method are observed. Some dosing schemes link together logically when considered according to their basic approaches or philosophies. Dosage strategies that follow similar pathways are given in Table 9-5.

TABLE 9-5   Dosing Strategies

Dosing Approach/Philosophy	Initial Dosing	Use of Serum Concentrations to Alter Doses
Pharmacokinetic parameters/equations	Pharmacokinetic Dosing method	Pharmacokinetic Parameter method
Literature-based concepts	Literature-based recommended dosing	Linear Pharmacokinetics method
Computerized	Bayesian computer programs	Bayesian computer programs

CONVERSION OF QUINIDINE DOSES FROM ONE SALT FORM TO ANOTHER

Occasionally there is a need to convert a patient stabilized on quinidine therapy from one salt form to an equivalent amount of quinidine base using another salt form. In general, oral quinidine dosage forms, including most sustained-release tablets, have a bioavailability equal to 0.7. Assuming that equal quinidine serum concentrations are desired, this makes conversion between the two salt forms simple since equivalent doses of drug are prescribed: $D_{new} = (D_{old} \bullet S_{old})/S_{new}$, where D_{new} is the equivalent quinidine base dose for the new quinidine salt dosage form in mg/d, D_{old} is the dose of oral quinidine salt old dosage form in mg/d, and S_{old} and S_{new} are the fraction of the old and new quinidine salt dosage forms that is active quinidine.

EXAMPLE 1 ▶▶▶

JH is currently receiving oral extended-release quinidine sulfate 600 mg every 12 hours. She is responding well to therapy, has no adverse drug effects, and has a steady-state quinidine concentration of 4.7 µg/mL. Suggest an equivalent dose of extended-release quinidine gluconate given every 8 hours for this patient.

1. *Calculate equivalent oral dose of quinidine.*
   The patient is currently receiving 600 mg every 12 hours or 1200 mg/d (600 mg/dose • 2 doses/d = 1200 mg/d) of quinidine sulfate. The equivalent quinidine gluconate dose would be: $D_{new} = (D_{old} \bullet S_{old})/S_{new} = $ (1200 mg/d • 0.83)/0.62 = 1606 mg/d, rounded to 1620 mg/d of quinidine gluconate, or 648 mg at 0700 H, 324 mg at 1500 H, and 648 mg at 2300 H.

EXAMPLE 2 ▶▶▶

LK is currently receiving oral extended-release quinidine gluconate 648 mg every 12 hours. He is responding well to therapy, has no adverse drug effects, and has a steady-state quinidine concentration of 3.3 µg/mL. Suggest an equivalent dose of immediate-release oral quinidine sulfate for this patient.

1. *Calculate equivalent oral dose of quinidine.*
   The patient is currently receiving 648 mg every 12 hours or 1296 mg/d (648 mg/dose • 2 doses/d = 1296 mg/d) of quinidine gluconate. The equivalent quinidine sulfate dose would be: $D_{new} = (D_{old} \bullet S_{old})/S_{new} = $ (1296 mg/d • 0.62)/0.83 = 968 mg/d, rounded to 800 mg/d of quinidine sulfate, or 200 mg every 6 hours.

PROBLEMS

The following problems are intended to emphasize the computation of initial and individualized doses using clinical pharmacokinetic techniques. Clinicians should always consult the patient's chart to confirm that current antiarrhythmic and other drug therapy is appropriate. Additionally, all other medications that the patient is taking, including prescription and nonprescription drugs, should be noted and checked to ascertain if a potential drug interaction with quinidine exists.

1. VC is a 67-year-old, 72-kg (height = 6 ft 1 in) male with ventricular tachycardia who requires therapy with oral quinidine. He has normal liver function and does not have heart failure. Suggest an initial extended-release quinidine gluconate dosage regimen designed to achieve a steady-state quinidine concentration equal to 3 μg/mL.

2. Patient VC (see problem 1) was prescribed oral quinidine gluconate 648 mg every 12 hours. The current steady-state quinidine concentration equals 2.5 μg/mL. Compute a new quinidine gluconate dose that will provide a steady-state concentration of 4 μg/mL.

3. EM is a 56-year-old, 81-kg (height 5 ft 9 in) male with ventricular tachycardia who requires therapy with oral quinidine. He has liver cirrhosis (Child-Pugh score = 10) and does not have heart failure. Suggest an initial quinidine gluconate extended-release tablet dosage regimen designed to achieve a steady-state quinidine concentration equal to 2 μg/mL.

4. Patient EM (see problem 3) was prescribed oral quinidine gluconate extended-release tablets 648 mg every 8 hours. The current steady-state quinidine concentration equals 5.1 μg/mL, and the patient is experiencing symptoms that could be adverse effects related to quinidine therapy. Compute a new quinidine gluconate dose that will provide a steady-state concentration of 3 μg/mL.

5. OF is a 71-year-old, 60-kg (height = 5 ft 2 in) female with paroxysmal atrial tachycardia who requires therapy with oral quinidine. She has severe heart failure (NYHA CHF class IV) and normal liver function. Suggest an initial quinidine sulfate extended-release dosage regimen designed to achieve a steady-state quinidine concentration equal to 4 μg/mL.

6. Patient OF (see problem 5) was prescribed quinidine sulfate extended-release tablets 600 mg orally every 12 hours. A steady-state quinidine serum concentration was obtained and equaled 6.7 μg/mL. Compute a new quinidine sulfate dose that will provide a steady-state concentration of 4 μg/mL.

7. FK is a 67-year-old, 130-kg (height = 5 ft 11 in) male with ventricular tachycardia who requires therapy with oral quinidine. He has severe heart failure (NYHA CHF class IV) and normal liver function. Suggest an initial quinidine sulfate immediate-release dosage regimen designed to achieve a steady-state quinidine concentration equal to 3 μg/mL.

8. Patient FK (see problem 7) was prescribed oral quinidine. Immediate-release quinidine sulfate tablets 300 mg every 8 hours were prescribed starting at 0700 H. A quinidine serum concentration was obtained just before the third dose at 2300 H and equaled 1.7 μg/mL. Compute a new dose that will provide a steady-state concentration of 4 μg/mL.

9. CV is a 69-year-old, 90-kg (height = 6 ft 1 in) male with ventricular tachycardia who requires therapy with quinidine. He has liver cirrhosis (Child-Pugh score = 11, total bilirubin = 2.7 mg/dL, albumin = 2.1 g/dL) and moderate heart failure (NYHA CHF class III). At 0200 H, he received 500 mg of intravenous quinidine gluconate over 2 hours as a loading dose. At 0800 H, quinidine gluconate 648 mg orally every 12 hours was started. A quinidine serum concentration was measured before the third dose at 0800 H the next day and equaled 5.4 μg/mL. Suggest an oral quinidine gluconate dosage regimen that would achieve a steady-state trough concentration equal to 4 μg/mL.

10. FP is a 59-year-old, 90-kg (height = 5 ft 4 in) female with atrial fibrillation who requires therapy with oral quinidine. She has liver cirrhosis (Child-Pugh score = 9) and has mild heart failure

(NYHA CHF class II). She received 600 mg of quinidine sulfate sustained-release every 12 hours at 0600 H and 1800 H for nine doses. Because the patient was experiencing anorexia, nausea, vomiting, and 40% widening of the ORS complex, the quinidine doses were held after the ninth dose. A quinidine serum concentration was measured at 0800 H the next morning and equaled 7.1 µg/mL. Suggest a quinidine sulfate immediate-release tablet dose that would achieve a steady-state trough concentration equal to 4 µg/mL.

ANSWERS TO PROBLEMS

1. *Answer to problem 1.* The initial quinidine dose for patient VC would be calculated as follows:

Pharmacokinetic Dosing Method

1. *Estimate half-life and elimination rate constant according to disease states and conditions present in the patient.*

The expected quinidine half-life $(t_{1/2})$ is 7 hours. The elimination rate constant is computed using the following formula: $k = 0.693/t_{1/2} = 0.693/7 \text{ h} = 0.099 \text{ h}^{-1}$.

2. *Estimate the volume of distribution and clearance.*

The patient is not obese, so the estimated quinidine volume of distribution will be based on actual body weight: $V = 2.4 \text{ L/kg} \bullet 72 \text{ kg} = 173 \text{ L}$. Estimated quinidine clearance is computed by taking the product of V and the elimination rate constant: $Cl = kV = 0.099 \text{ h}^{-1} \bullet 173 \text{ L} = 17.1 \text{ L/h}$.

3. *Compute dosage regimen.*

Oral extended-release quinidine gluconate tablets will be prescribed to this patient (F = 0.7, S = 0.62). The initial dosage interval (τ) will be set to 8 hours. (Note: µg/mL = mg/L and this concentration unit was substituted for Css in the calculations so that unnecessary unit conversion was not required.) The dosage equation for oral quinidine is: $D = (Css \bullet Cl \bullet \tau)/(F \bullet S) = (3 \text{ mg/L} \bullet 17.1 \text{ L/h} \bullet 8 \text{ h})/(0.7 \bullet 0.62) = 945 \text{ mg}$, rounded to 972 mg every 8 hours.

A steady-state quinidine serum concentration could be measured after steady state is attained in 3-5 half-lives. Since the patient is expected to have a half-life equal to 7 hours, the quinidine steady-state concentration could be obtained any time after the second day of dosing (5 half-lives = 5 $\bullet$ 7 h = 35 h). Quinidine serum concentrations should also be measured if the patient experiences a return of their arrhythmia, or if the patient develops potential signs or symptoms of quinidine toxicity.

Literature-Based Recommended Dosing

1. *Choose quinidine dose based on disease states and conditions present in the patient.*

A quinidine gluconate maintenance dose of 324 mg every 12 hours (648 mg/d) is suggested for a patient without heart failure or liver disease requiring a quinidine steady-state serum concentration in the lower end of the therapeutic range.

A steady-state quinidine serum concentration could be measured after steady state is attained in 3-5 half-lives. Since the patient is expected to have a half-life equal to 7 hours, the quinidine steady-state concentration could be obtained any time after the second day of dosing (5 half-lives = 5 $\bullet$ 7 h = 35 h). Quinidine serum concentrations should also be measured if the patient experiences a return of their arrhythmia, or if the patient develops potential signs or symptoms of quinidine toxicity.

2. *Answer to problem 2.* The revised quinidine dose for patient VC would be calculated as follows:

Linear Pharmacokinetics Method

1. *Compute new dose to achieve the desired serum concentration.*

The patient would be expected to achieve steady-state conditions after 2 days ($5\ t_{1/2} = 5 \bullet 7\ h = 35\ h$) of therapy.

Using linear pharmacokinetics, the new dose to attain the desired concentration should be proportional to the old dose that produced the measured concentration (note: total daily dose is 1296 mg/d = 648 mg/d $\bullet$ 2 doses/d):

$$D_{new} = (C_{ss,\ new}/C_{ss,\ old})\ D_{old} = (4\ \mu g/mL\ /\ 2.5\ \mu g/mL)\ 1296\ mg/d = 2074\ mg/d,$$
rounded to 1944 mg/d or 648 mg every 8 hours

The new suggested dose would be 648 mg every 8 hours of quinidine gluconate to be started immediately.

A steady-state quinidine serum concentration could be measured after steady state is attained in 3-5 half-lives. Since the patient is expected to have a half-life equal to 7 hours, the quinidine steady-state concentration could be obtained any time after the 2 days of dosing (5 half-lives = $5 \bullet 7\ h = 35\ h$). Quinidine serum concentrations should also be measured if the patient experiences a return of their arrhythmia, or if the patient develops potential signs or symptoms of quinidine toxicity.

Pharmacokinetic Parameter Method

1. *Compute pharmacokinetic parameters.*

The patient would be expected to achieve steady-state conditions after the second day ($5\ t_{1/2} = 5 \bullet 7\ h = 35\ h$) of therapy.

Quinidine clearance can be computed using a steady-state quinidine concentration: $Cl = [F \bullet S\ (D/\tau)]/Css = [0.7 \bullet 0.62\ (648\ mg/12\ h)]/(2.5\ mg/L) = 9.37\ L/h$. (Note: $\mu g/mL = mg/L$ and this concentration unit was substituted for Css in the calculations so that unnecessary unit conversion was not required.)

2. *Compute quinidine dose.*

Quinidine clearance is used to compute the new dose: $D = (Css \bullet Cl \bullet \tau)/(F \bullet S) = (4\ mg/L \bullet 9.37\ L/h \bullet 8h)/(0.7 \bullet 0.62) = 691\ mg$, rounded to 648 mg every 8 hours.

The new quinidine dose would be instituted immediately.

A steady-state quinidine serum concentration could be measured after steady state is attained in 3-5 half-lives. Since the patient is expected to have a half-life equal to 7 hours, the quinidine steady-state concentration could be obtained any time after the second day of dosing (5 half-lives = $5 \bullet 7\ h = 35\ h$). Quinidine serum concentrations should also be measured if the patient experiences a return of their arrhythmia, or if the patient develops potential signs or symptoms of quinidine toxicity.

3. *Answer to problem 3.* The initial quinidine dose for patient EM would be calculated as follows:

Pharmacokinetic Dosing Method

1. *Estimate half-life and elimination rate constant according to disease states and conditions present in the patient.*

The expected quinidine half-life ($t_{1/2}$) is 9 hours. The elimination rate constant is computed using the following formula: $k = 0.693/t_{1/2} = 0.693/9\ h = 0.077\ h^{-1}$.

2. *Estimate the volume of distribution and clearance.*

The patient is not obese, so the estimated quinidine volume of distribution will be based on actual body weight: V = 3.8 L/kg • 81 kg = 308 L. Estimated quinidine clearance is computed by taking the product of V and the elimination rate constant: Cl = kV = 0.077 h^{-1} • 308 L = 23.7 L/h.

3. *Compute dosage regimen.*

Oral extended-release quinidine gluconate tablets will be prescribed to this patient (F = 0.7, S = 0.62). The initial dosage interval (τ) will be set to 8 hours. (Note: μg/mL = mg/L and this concentration unit was substituted for Css in the calculations so that unnecessary unit conversion was not required.) The dosage equation for oral quinidine is: D = (Css • Cl • τ)/(F • S) = (2 mg/L • 23.7 L/h • 8 h)/(0.7 • 0.62) = 873 mg, rounded to 972 mg every 8 hours.

A steady-state quinidine serum concentration could be measured after steady state is attained in 3-5 half-lives. Since the patient is expected to have a half-life equal to 9 hours, the quinidine steady-state concentration could be obtained any time after the second day of dosing (5 half-lives = 5 • 9 h = 45 h). Quinidine serum concentrations should also be measured if the patient experiences a return of their arrhythmia, or if the patient develops potential signs or symptoms of quinidine toxicity.

Literature-Based Recommended Dosing

1. *Choose quinidine dose based on disease states and conditions present in the patient.*

A quinidine gluconate maintenance dose of 324 mg every 12 hours (648 mg/d) is suggested for a patient with liver disease requiring a quinidine steady-state serum concentration in the lower end of the therapeutic range.

A steady-state quinidine serum concentration could be measured after steady state is attained in 3-5 half-lives. Since the patient is expected to have a half-life equal to 9 hours, the quinidine steady-state concentration could be obtained any time after the second day of dosing (5 half-lives = 5 • 9 h = 45 h). Quinidine serum concentrations should also be measured if the patient experiences a return of their arrhythmia, or if the patient develops potential signs or symptoms of quinidine toxicity.

4. *Answer to problem 4.* The revised quinidine dose for patient EM would be calculated as follows:

Linear Pharmacokinetics Method

1. *Compute new dose to achieve desired serum concentration.*

The patient would be expected to achieve steady-state conditions after 2 days (5 t$_{1/2}$ = 5 • 9 h = 45 h) of therapy.

Using linear pharmacokinetics, the new dose to attain the desired concentration should be proportional to the old dose that produced the measured concentration (note: total daily dose is 1944 mg/d = 648 mg/d • 3 doses/d):

$$D_{new} = (C_{ss,\ new}/C_{ss,\ old})\ D_{old} = (3\ \mu g/mL\ /\ 5.1\ \mu g/mL)\ 1944\ mg/d = 1144\ mg/d,$$
rounded to 1296 mg/d or 648 mg every 12 hours

The new suggested dose would be 648 mg every 12 hours of quinidine gluconate to be started in 1-2 half-lives (9-18 hours) to allow time for possible side effects to subside.

A steady-state quinidine serum concentration could be measured after steady-state is attained in 3-5 half-lives. Since the patient is expected to have a half-life equal to 9 hours, the quinidine steady-state concentration could be obtained any time after the 2 days of dosing (5 half-lives = 5 • 9 h = 45 h). Quinidine serum concentrations should also be measured if the patient experiences a return of their arrhythmia, or if the patient develops potential signs or symptoms of quinidine toxicity.

Pharmacokinetic Parameter Method

1. *Compute pharmacokinetic parameters.*

The patient would be expected to achieve steady-state conditions after the second day (5 $t_{1/2}$ = 5 • 9 h = 45 h) of therapy.

Quinidine clearance can be computed using a steady-state quinidine concentration: Cl = [F • S (D/τ)]/Css = [0.7 • 0.62 (648 mg/8 h)]/(5.1 mg/L) = 6.89 L/h. (Note: µg/mL = mg/L and this concentration unit was substituted for Css in the calculations so that unnecessary unit conversion was not required.)

2. *Compute quinidine dose.*

Quinidine clearance is used to compute the new dose: D = (Css • Cl • τ)/(F • S) = (3 mg/L • 6.89 L/h • 12 h)/(0.7 • 0.62) = 572 mg, rounded to 648 mg every 12 hours.

The new suggested dose would be 648 mg every 12 hours of quinidine gluconate to be started in 1-2 half-lives (9-18 hours) to allow time for possible side effects to subside.

A steady-state quinidine serum concentration could be measured after steady state is attained in 3-5 half-lives. Since the patient is expected to have a half-life equal to 9 hours, the quinidine steady-state concentration could be obtained any time after the 2 days of dosing (5 half-lives = 5 • 9 h = 45 h). Quinidine serum concentrations should also be measured if the patient experiences a return of their arrhythmia, or if the patient develops potential signs or symptoms of quinidine toxicity.

5. *Answer to problem 5.* The initial quinidine dose for patient OF would be calculated as follows:

Pharmacokinetic Dosing Method

1. *Estimate half-life and elimination rate constant according to disease states and conditions present in the patient.*

The expected quinidine half-life ($t_{1/2}$) is 7 hours. The elimination rate constant is computed using the following formula: k = 0.693/$t_{1/2}$ = 0.693/7 h = 0.099 h^{-1}.

2. *Estimate the volume of distribution and clearance.*

The patient is not obese, so the estimated quinidine volume of distribution will be based on actual body weight: V = 1.7 L/kg • 60 kg = 102 L. Estimated quinidine clearance is computed by taking the product of V and the elimination rate constant: Cl = kV = 0.099 h^{-1} • 102 L = 10.1 L/h.

3. *Compute dosage regimen.*

Oral extended-release quinidine sulfate tablets will be prescribed to this patient (F = 0.7, S = 0.83). The initial dosage interval (τ) will be set to 12 hours. (Note: µg/mL = mg/L and this concentration unit was substituted for Css in the calculations so that unnecessary unit conversion was not required.) The dosage equation for oral quinidine is: D = (Css • Cl • τ)/(F • S) = (4 mg/L • 10.1 L/h • 12 h)/(0.7 • 0.83) = 834 mg, rounded to 900 mg every 12 hours.

A steady-state quinidine serum concentration could be measured after steady state is attained in 3-5 half-lives. Since the patient is expected to have a half-life equal to 7 hours, the quinidine steady-state concentration could be obtained any time after the second day of dosing (5 half-lives = 5 • 7 h = 35 h). Quinidine serum concentrations should also be measured if the patient experiences a return of their arrhythmia, or if the patient develops potential signs or symptoms of quinidine toxicity.

Literature-Based Recommended Dosing

1. *Choose quinidine dose based on disease states and conditions present in the patient.*

A extended-release quinidine sulfate maintenance dose of 300 mg every 8 hours (900 mg/d) is suggested for a patient with heart failure requiring a quinidine steady-state serum concentration in the upper end of the therapeutic range.

A steady-state quinidine serum concentration could be measured after steady state is attained in 3-5 half-lives. Since the patient is expected to have a half-life equal to 7 hours, the quinidine steady-state concentration could be obtained any time after the second day of dosing (5 half-lives = 5 • 7 h = 35 h). Quinidine serum concentrations should also be measured if the patient experiences a return of their arrhythmia, or if the patient develops potential signs or symptoms of quinidine toxicity.

6. *Answer to problem 6.* The revised quinidine dose for patient OF would be calculated as follows:

Linear Pharmacokinetics Method

1. *Compute new dose to achieve the desired serum concentration.*

The patient would be expected to achieve steady-state conditions after 2 days (5 $t_{1/2}$ = 5 • 7 h = 35 h) of therapy.

Using linear pharmacokinetics, the new dose to attain the desired concentration should be proportional to the old dose that produced the measured concentration (note: total daily dose is 1200 mg/d = 600 mg/dose • 2 doses/d):

$$D_{new} = (C_{ss, new}/C_{ss, old}) \, D_{old} = (4 \text{ μg/mL} / 6.7 \text{ μg/mL}) \, 1200 \text{ mg/d} = 716 \text{ mg/d},$$
$$\text{rounded to 600 mg/d or 300 mg every 12 hours}$$

The new suggested dose would be 300 mg every 12 hours of quinidine sulfate extended-release tablets to be started in 1-2 half-lives (7-14 hours) to allow time for serum concentrations to decline.

A steady-state quinidine serum concentration could be measured after steady state is attained in 3-5 half-lives. Since the patient is expected to have a half-life equal to 7 hours, the quinidine steady-state concentration could be obtained any time after the 2 days of dosing (5 half-lives = 5 • 7 h = 35 h). Quinidine serum concentrations should also be measured if the patient experiences a return of their arrhythmia, or if the patient develops potential signs or symptoms of quinidine toxicity.

Pharmacokinetic Parameter Method

1. *Compute pharmacokinetic parameters.*

The patient would be expected to achieve steady-state conditions after the second day (5 $t_{1/2}$ = 5 • 7 h = 35 h) of therapy.

Quinidine clearance can be computed using a steady-state quinidine concentration: Cl = [F • S (D/τ)] / Css = [0.7 • 0.83 (600 mg/12 h)] / (6.7 mg/L) = 4.34 L/h. (Note: μg/mL = mg/L and this concentration unit was substituted for Css in the calculations so that unnecessary unit conversion was not required.)

2. *Compute quinidine dose.*

Quinidine clearance is used to compute the new dose: D = (Css • Cl • τ)/(F • S) = (4 mg/L • 4.34 L/h • 12 h)/(0.7 • 0.83) = 359 mg, rounded to 300 mg every 12 hours.

The new suggested dose would be 300 mg every 12 hours of quinidine sulfate extended-release tablets to be started in 1-2 half-lives (7-14 hours) to allow time for possible side effects to subside.

A steady-state quinidine serum concentration could be measured after steady state is attained in 3-5 half-lives. Since the patient is expected to have a half-life equal to 7 hours, the quinidine steady-state concentration could be obtained any time after the 2 days of dosing (5 half-lives = 5 • 7 h = 35 h). Quinidine serum concentrations should also be measured if the patient experiences a return of their arrhythmia, or if the patient develops potential signs or symptoms of quinidine toxicity.

7. *Answer to problem 7.* The initial quinidine dose for patient FK would be calculated as follows:

Pharmacokinetic Dosing Method

1. *Estimate half-life and elimination rate constant according to disease states and conditions present in the patient.*

    The expected quinidine half-life ($t_{1/2}$) is 7 hours. The elimination rate constant is computed using the following formula: $k = 0.693/t_{1/2} = 0.693/7\ h = 0.099\ h^{-1}$.

2. *Estimate the volume of distribution and clearance.*

    The patient is obese (>30% over ideal body weight), so the estimated quinidine volume of distribution will be based on ideal body weight: IBW_{male} (in kg) = 50 kg + 2.3(Ht − 60) = 50 kg + 2.3 (71 in − 60) = 75 kg, V = 1.7 L/kg • 75 kg = 128 L. Estimated quinidine clearance is computed by taking the product of V and the elimination rate constant: $Cl = kV = 0.099\ h^{-1}$ • 128 L = 12.7 L/h.

3. *Compute dosage regimen.*

    Oral immediate-release quinidine sulfate tablets will be prescribed to this patient (F = 0.7, S = 0.83). The initial dosage interval (τ) will be set to 6 hours. (Note: μg/mL = mg/L and this concentration unit was substituted for Css in the calculations so that unnecessary unit conversion was not required.) The dosage equation for oral quinidine is: D = (Css • Cl • τ)/(F • S) = (3 mg/L • 12.7 L/h • 6 h)/ (0.7 • 0.83) = 393 mg, rounded to 400 mg every 6 hours.

    A steady-state quinidine serum concentration could be measured after steady state is attained in 3-5 half-lives. Since the patient is expected to have a half-life equal to 7 hours, the quinidine steady-state concentration could be obtained any time after the second day of dosing (5 half-lives = 5 • 7 h = 35 h). Quinidine serum concentrations should also be measured if the patient experiences a return of their arrhythmia, or if the patient develops potential signs or symptoms of quinidine toxicity.

Literature-Based Recommended Dosing

1. *Choose quinidine dose based on disease states and conditions present in the patient.*

    A quinidine sulfate maintenance dose of 100 mg every 6 hours (400 mg/d) is suggested for a patient with heart failure requiring a quinidine steady-state serum concentration in the upper end of the therapeutic range.

    A steady-state quinidine serum concentration could be measured after steady state is attained in 3-5 half-lives. Since the patient is expected to have a half-life equal to 7 hours, the quinidine steady-state concentration could be obtained any time after the second day of dosing (5 half-lives = 5 • 7 h = 35 h). Quinidine serum concentrations should also be measured if the patient experiences a return of their arrhythmia, or if the patient develops potential signs or symptoms of quinidine toxicity.

8. *Answer to problem 8.* The revised quinidine dose for patient FK would be calculated as follows:

Bayesian Pharmacokinetic Computer Program Method

1. *Enter the patient's demographic, drug-dosing, and serum concentration/time data into the computer program.*

    In this patient's case, it is unlikely that the patient is at steady state so the linear pharmacokinetics method cannot be used. The DrugCalc program requires quinidine salt doses be input in terms of quinidine base. A 300-mg dose of quinidine sulfate is equivalent to 250 mg of quinidine base (250 mg quinidine base = 300 mg quinidine sulfate • 0.83).

2. *Compute the pharmacokinetic parameters for the patient using Bayesian pharmacokinetic computer program.*

The pharmacokinetic parameters computed by the program are a volume of distribution of 171 L, a half-life equal to 16.1 h, and a clearance equal to 7.36 L/h.

3. *Compute the dose required to achieve the desired quinidine serum concentrations.*

The oral one-compartment model equation used by the program to compute doses indicates that 300 mg of quinidine sulfate immediate-release tablets every 6 hours will produce a steady-state trough concentration of 4.7 μg/mL. (Note: DrugCalc uses salt form B and oral options for quinidine sulfate immediate-release tablets.) This dose would be started immediately.

9. *Answer to problem 9.* The revised quinidine dose for patient CV would be calculated as follows:

Bayesian Pharmacokinetic Computer Program Method

1. *Enter the patient's demographic, drug-dosing, and serum concentration/time data into the computer program.*

In this patient's case, it is unlikely that the patient is at steady state so the Linear Pharmacokinetics method cannot be used. The DrugCalc program requires quinidine salt doses be input in terms of quinidine base. A 500-mg dose of quinidine gluconate is equivalent to 300 mg of quinidine base while a 648-mg dose of quinidine gluconate is equal to 400 mg of quinidine base (300 mg quinidine base = 500 mg quinidine gluconate • 0.62, 400 mg quinidine base = 648 mg quinidine gluconate • 0.62).

2. *Compute pharmacokinetic parameters for the patient using Bayesian pharmacokinetic computer program.*

The pharmacokinetic parameters computed by the program are a volume of distribution of 130 L, a half-life equal to 23.6 h, and a clearance equal to 3.83 L/h.

3. *Compute the dose required to achieve the desired quinidine serum concentrations.*

The oral one-compartment model equation used by the program to compute doses indicates that 324 mg of quinidine gluconate extended-release tablets every 12 hours will produce a steady-state trough concentration of 4.2 μg/mL. (Note: DrugCalc uses salt form B and sustained-release options for quinidine gluconate extended-release tablets.) This dose could be held for 1 half-life (1 day) if adverse drug effects were occurring or started immediately.

10. *Answer to problem 10.* The revised quinidine dose for patient FP would be calculated as follows:

Bayesian Pharmacokinetic Computer Program Method

1. *Enter the patient's demographic, drug-dosing, and serum concentration/time data into the computer program.*

In this patient's case, it is unlikely that the patient is at steady state so the Linear Pharmacokinetics method cannot be used. The DrugCalc program requires quinidine salt doses be input in terms of quinidine base. A 600-mg dose of quinidine sulfate is equivalent to 500 mg of quinidine base (500 mg quinidine base = 600 mg quinidine sulfate • 0.83).

2. *Compute the pharmacokinetic parameters for the patient using Bayesian pharmacokinetic computer program.*

The pharmacokinetic parameters computed by the program are a volume of distribution of 238 L, a half-life equal to 51.3 h, and a clearance equal to 3.21 L/h.

3. *Compute the dose required to achieve the desired quinidine serum concentrations.*

The oral one-compartment model equation used by the program to compute doses indicates that 200 mg of quinidine sulfate immediate-release tablets every 12 hours will produce a steady-state trough concentration of 3.6 μg/mL. (Note: DrugCalc uses salt form B and oral options for quinidine sulfate immediate-release tablets.) This dose could be held for 1 half-life (2 days) if adverse drug effects continued to occur or started immediately.

REFERENCES

1. Sampson KJ, Kass RS. Anti-arrhythmics drugs. In: Brunton L, Chabner B, Knollman B, eds. *The Pharmacological Basis of Therapeutics.* 12th ed. New York, NY: McGraw-Hill; 2011:815-848.
2. Anderson JL, Halperin JL, Albert NM, et al. Management of patients with atrial fibrillation (Compilation of 2006 ACCF/AHA/ESC and 2011 ACCF/AHA/HRS Recommendations): a report of the American College of Cardiology/American Heart Association Task Force on Practice Guidelines. *Circulation.* 2013;127(13):1425-1443.
3. Sanoski CA, Bauman JL. The arrhythmias. In: DiPirio JT, Talbert RL, Yee GC, Matzke GR, Wells BG, Posey LM, eds. *Pharmacotherapy.* New York, NY: McGraw-Hill; 2011:273-309.
4. Ueda CT, Williamson BJ, Dzindzio BS. Absolute quinidine bioavailability. *Clin Pharmacol Ther.* 1976;20(3):260-265.
5. Ueda CT, Hirschfeld DS, Scheinman MM, Rowland M, Williamson BJ, Dzindzio BS. Disposition kinetics of quinidine. *Clin Pharmacol Ther.* 1976;19(1):30-36.
6. Woo E, Greenblatt DJ. A reevaluation of intravenous quinidine. *Am Heart J.* 1978;96(6):829-832.
7. Greenblatt DJ, Pfeifer HJ, Ochs HR, et al. Pharmacokinetics of quinidine in humans after intravenous, intramuscular and oral administration. *J Pharmacol Exp Ther.* 1977;202(2):365-378.
8. Ueda CT, Dzindzio BS. Quinidine kinetics in congestive heart failure. *Clin Pharmacol Ther.* 1978;23(2):158-164.
9. Ueda CT, Dzindzio BS. Bioavailability of quinidine in congestive heart failure. *Br J Clin Pharmacol.* 1981;11(6):571-577.
10. Covinsky JO, Russo J Jr, Kelly KL, Cashman J, Amick EN, Mason WD. Relative bioavailability of quinidine gluconate and quinidine sulfate in healthy volunteers. *J Clin Pharmacol.* 1979;19(5-6):261-269.
11. Gibson DL, Smith GH, Koup JR, Stewart DK. Relative bioavailability of a standard and a sustained-release quinidine tablet. *Clin Pharm.* 1982;1(4):366-368.
12. McGilveray IJ, Midha KK, Rowe M, Beaudoin N, Charette C. Bioavailability of 11 quinidine formulations and pharmacokinetic variation in humans. *J Pharm Sci.* 1981;70(5):524-529.
13. Ochs HR, Greenblatt DJ, Woo E, Franke K, Pfeifer HJ, Smith TW. Single and multiple dose pharmacokinetics of oral quinidine sulfate and gluconate. *Am J Cardiol.* 1978;41(4):770-777.
14. Woo E, Greenblatt DJ, Ochs HR. Short- and long-acting oral quinidine preparations: clinical implications of pharmacokinetic differences. *Angiology.* 1978;29(3):243-250.
15. Drayer DE, Lowenthal DT, Restivo KM, Schwartz A, Cook CE, Reidenberg MM. Steady-state serum levels of quinidine and active metabolites in cardiac patients with varying degrees of renal function. *Clin Pharmacol Ther.* 1978;24(1):31-39.
16. Drayer DE, Hughes M, Lorenzo B, Reidenberg MM. Prevalence of high (3S)-3-hydroxyquinidine/quinidine ratios in serum, and clearance of quinidine in cardiac patients with age. *Clin Pharmacol Ther.* 1980;27(1):72-75.
17. Holford NH, Coates PE, Guentert TW, Riegelman S, Sheiner LB. The effect of quinidine and its metabolites on the electrocardiogram and systolic time intervals: concentration–effect relationships. *Br J Clin Pharmacol.* 1981;11(2):187-195.
18. Rakhit A, Holford NH, Guentert TW, Maloney K, Riegelman S. Pharmacokinetics of quinidine and three of its metabolites in man. *J Pharmacokinet Biopharm.* 1984;12(1):1-21.
19. Ueda CT, Dzindzio BS. Pharmacokinetics of dihydroquinidine in congestive heart failure patients after intravenous quinidine administration. *Eur J Clin Pharmacol.* 1979;16(2):101-105.
20. Ueda CT, Williamson BJ, Dzindzio BS. Disposition kinetics of dihydroquinidine following quinidine administration. *Res Commun Chem Pathol Pharmacol.* 1976;14(2):215-225.
21. Narang PK, Crouthamel WG. Dihydroquinidine contamination of quinidine raw materials and dosage forms: rapid estimation by high-performance liquid chromatography. *J Pharm Sci.* 1979;68(7):917-919.
22. Lange RA, Hillis LD. Cardiovascular testing. In: Dipiro JT, Talbert RL, Yee GC, Matzke GR, Wells BG, Posey LM, eds. *Pharmacotherapy.* New York, NY: McGraw-Hill; 2011:55-81.
23. Russo J Jr, Russo ME, Smith RA, Pershing LK. Assessment of quinidine gluconate for nonlinear kinetics following chronic dosing. *J Clin Pharmacol.* 1982;22(5-6):264-270.
24. Chen BH, Taylor EH, Ackerman BH, Olsen K, Pappas AA. Effect of pH on free quinidine [letter]. *Drug Intell Clin Pharm.* 1988;22(10):826.
25. Mihaly GW, Cheng MS, Klein MB. Difference in the binding of quinine and quinidine to plasma proteins. *Br J Clin Pharmacol.* 1987;24:769-774.
26. Woo E, Greenblatt DJ. Pharmacokinetic and clinical implications of quinidine protein binding. *J Pharm Sci.* 1979;68(4):466-470.
27. Carliner NH, Crouthamel WG, Fisher ML, et al. Quinidine therapy in hospitalized patients with ventricular arrhythmias. *Am Heart J.* 1979;98(6):708-715.
28. Conrad KA, Molk BL, Chidsey CA. Pharmacokinetic studies of quinidine in patients with arrhythmias. *Circulation.* 1977;55(1):1-7.
29. Guentert TW, Holford NH, Coates PE, Upton RA, Riegelman S. Quinidine pharmacokinetics in man: choice of a disposition model and absolute bioavailability studies. *J Pharmacokinet Biopharm.* 1979;7(4):315-330.

30. Kessler KM, Humphries WC Jr, Black M, Spann JF. Quinidine pharmacokinetics in patients with cirrhosis or receiving propranolol. *Am Heart J.* 1978;96(5):627-635.
31. Powell JR, Okada R, Conrad KA, Guentert TW, Riegelman S. Altered quinidine disposition in a patient with chronic active hepatitis. *Postgrad Med J.* 1982;58(676):82-84.
32. Pugh RN, Murray-Lyon IM, Dawson JL, Pietroni MC, Williams R. Transection of the oesophagus for bleeding oesophageal varices. *Br J Surg.* 1973;60(8):646-649.
33. Crouthamel WG. The effect of congestive heart failure on quinidine pharmacokinetics. *Am Heart J.* 1975;90(3):335-339.
34. Kessler KM, Lowenthal DT, Warner H, Gibson T, Briggs W, Reidenberg MM. Quinidine elimination in patients with congestive heart failure or poor renal function. *N Engl J Med.* 1974;290(13):706-709.
35. Ochs HR, Greenblatt DJ, Woo E, Smith TW. Reduced quinidine clearance in elderly persons. *Am J Cardiol.* 1978;42(3):481-485.
36. Hall K, Meatherall B, Krahn J, Penner B, Rabson JL. Clearance of quinidine during peritoneal dialysis. *Am Heart J.* 1982;104(3): 646-647.
37. Chin TW, Pancorbo S, Comty C. Quinidine pharmacokinetics in continuous ambulatory peritoneal dialysis. *Clin Exp Dial Apheresis.* 1981;5(4):391-397.
38. Hansten PD, Horn JR. *Drug Interactions Analysis and Management.* St. Louis, MO: Wolters Kluwer Health; 2014.
39. Muralidharan G, Cooper JK, Hawes EM, Korchinski ED, Midha KK. Quinidine inhibits the 7-hydroxylation of chlorpromazine in extensive metabolisers of debrisoquine. *Eur J Clin Pharmacol.* 1996;50(1-2):121-128.
40. von Moltke LL, Greenblatt DJ, Cotreau-Bibbo MM, Duan SX, Harmatz JS, Shader RI. Inhibition of desipramine hydroxylation in vitro by serotonin-reuptake-inhibitor antidepressants, and by quinidine and ketoconazole: a model system to predict drug interactions in vivo. *J Pharmacol Exp Ther.* 1994;268(3):1278-1283.
41. von Moltke LL, Greenblatt DJ, Duan SX, Daily JP, Harmatz JS, Shader RI. Inhibition of desipramine hydroxylation (Cytochrome P450-2D6) in vitro by quinidine and by viral protease inhibitors: relation to drug interactions in vivo. *J Pharm Sci.* 1998;87(10):1184-1189.
42. Wandell M, Mungall D. Computer assisted drug interpretation and drug regimen optimization. *Amer Assoc Clin Chem.* 1984;6:1-11.
43. Parker RB, Cavallari LH. Systolic heart failure. In: DiPirio JT, Talbert RL, Yee GC, Matzke GR, Wells BG, Posey LM, eds. *Pharmacotherapy.* New York, NY: McGraw-Hill; 2011:137-172.
44. Tschudy MM, Arcara KM. *The Harriet Lane Handbook: A Manual for Pediatric House Officers.* 19th ed. Philadelphia, PA: Mosby; 2012.

IV ANTICONVULSANTS

10 Phenytoin/Fosphenytoin

INTRODUCTION

Phenytoin is a hydantoin compound related to the barbiturates that are used for the treatment of seizures. It is an effective anticonvulsant for the chronic treatment of tonic-clonic (grand mal) or partial seizures and the acute treatment of generalized status epilepticus (Table 10-1).[1-4] After generalized status epilepticus has been controlled with intravenous benzodiazepine therapy and supportive measures have been instituted, phenytoin therapy is often immediately instituted with the administration of intravenous phenytoin or fosphenytoin. Orally administered phenytoin is used chronically to provide prophylaxis against tonic-clonic or partial seizures. Phenytoin is a type 1B antiarrhythmic and is also used in the treatment of trigeminal neuralgia.

The antiseizure activity of phenytoin is related to its ability to inhibit the repetitive firing of action potentials caused by prolonged depolarization of neurons.[7,8] Additionally, phenytoin stops the spread of abnormal discharges from epileptic foci thereby decreasing the spread of seizure activity throughout the brain.

TABLE 10-1 International Classification of Epileptic Seizures With Recommended Therapies

| Major Class | Subset of Class | Drug Treatment for Selected Seizure Type | | | |
		2004 AAN/AES	2013 Medical Letter	2012 NICE	2013 ILAE[a]
Partial seizures (beginning locally)	1. Simple partial seizures (without impaired consciousness) a. with motor symptoms b. with somatosensory or special sensory symptoms c. with autonomic symptoms d. with psychological symptoms	Carbamazepine Phenytoin Valproate Phenobarbital Lamotrigine Gabapentin Oxcarbazepine Topiramate	Lamotrigine Carbamazepine Levetiracetam Oxcarbazepine *Alternatives:* Topiramate Valproate Gabapentin Zonisamide Phenytoin Pregabalin Lacosamide Ezogabine	Carbamazepine Lamotrigine Levetiracetam Oxcarbazepine Valproate *Adjunctive:* Carbamazepine Clobazam Gabapentin Lamotrigine Levetiracetam Oxcarbazepine Valproate Topiramate	*Adults:* Carbamazepine Levetiracetam Phenytoin Zonisamide Valproate *Children:* Oxcarbazepine Carbamazepine Phenobarbital Phenytoin Topiramate Valproate Vigabatrin *Elderly:* Gabapentin Lamotrigine Carbamazepine

(Continued)

TABLE 10-1   International Classification of Epileptic Seizures With Recommended Therapies (*Continued*)

Major Class	Subset of Class	Drug Treatment for Selected Seizure Type			
		2004 AAN/AES	2013 Medical Letter	2012 NICE	2013 ILAE[a]
	2. Complex partial seizures (with impaired consciousness) a. simple partial onset followed by impaired consciousness b. impaired consciousness at onset	Carbamazepine Phenytoin Valproate Phenobarbital Lamotrigine Gabapentin Oxcarbazepine Topiramate	Lamotrigine Carbamazepine Levetiracetam Oxcarbazepine *Alternatives:* Topiramate Valproate Gabapentin Zonisamide Phenytoin Pregabalin Lacosamide Ezogabine	Carbamazepine Lamotrigine Levetiracetam Oxcarbazepine Valproate *Adjunctive:* Carbamazepine Clobazam Gabapentin Lamotrigine Levetiracetam Oxcarbazepine Valproate Topiramate	*Adults:* Carbamazepine Levetiracetam Phenytoin Zonisamide Valproate *Children:* Oxcarbazepine Carbamazepine Phenobarbital Phenytoin Topiramate Valproate Vigabatrin *Elderly:* Gabapentin Lamotrigine Carbamazepine
	3. Partial seizures evolving into secondary generalized seizures	Carbamazepine Phenytoin Valproate Phenobarbital Lamotrigine Gabapentin Oxcarbazepine Topiramate	Lamotrigine Carbamazepine Levetiracetam Oxcarbazepine *Alternatives:* Topiramate Valproate Gabapentin Zonisamide Phenytoin Pregabalin Lacosamide Ezogabine	Carbamazepine Lamotrigine Levetiracetam Oxcarbazepine Valproate *Adjunctive:* Carbamazepine Clobazam Gabapentin Lamotrigine Levetiracetam Oxcarbazepine Valproate Topiramate	*Adults:* Carbamazepine Levetiracetam Phenytoin Zonisamide Valproate *Children:* Oxcarbazepine Carbamazepine Phenobarbital Phenytoin Topiramate Valproate Vigabatrin *Elderly:* Gabapentin Lamotrigine Carbamazepine
Generalized seizures (convulsive or nonconvulsive)	1. Absence seizures[b] (typical or atypical; also known as petite mal seizures)	*Children:*[c] Ethosuximide Valproate Lamotrigine	Ethosuximide Valproate *Alternatives:* Lamotrigine Clonazepam Zonisamide Levetiracetam	Ethosuximide Lamotrigine Valproate *Adjunctive:* Ethosuximide Lamotrigine Valproate	*Children:* Ethosuximide Valproate Lamotrigine

(*Continued*)

TABLE 10-1 **International Classification of Epileptic Seizures With Recommended Therapies** (*Continued*)

Major Class	Subset of Class	Drug Treatment for Selected Seizure Type			
		2004 AAN/AES	2013 Medical Letter	2012 NICE	2013 ILAE[a]
	2. Tonic-clonic seizures (also known as grand mal seizures)	Carbamazepine Phenytoin Valproate Phenobarbital Lamotrigine Oxcarbazepine Topiramate	Valproate Lamotrigine Levetiracetam *Alternatives:* Topiramate Zonisamide Phenytoin	Carbamazepine Lamotrigine Oxcarbazepine Valproate *Adjunctive:* Clobazam Lamotrigine Levetiracetam Valproate Topiramate	*Adults:* Carbamazepine Lamotrigine Oxcarbazepine Phenobarbital Phenytoin Topiramate Valproate Gabapentin Levetiracetam Vigabatrin *Children:* Carbamazepine Phenobarbital Phenytoin Topiramate Valproate Oxcarbazepine

[a]Only two highest available levels of evidence listed.
[b]Recent literature suggests either ethosuximide or valproic acid is a superior initial therapy compared to lamotrigine for absence seizures.[5,6]
[c]Lamotrigine added to previous recommendation per expert panel.
Abbreviations: ANN, American Academy of Neurology; AES, American Epilepsy Society; ILAE, International League Against Epilepsy; NICE, UK National Institute for Clinical Excellence.

Posttetanic potentiation at synaptic junctions are blocked which alters synaptic transmission. At the cellular level, the mechanism of action for phenytoin appears related to its ability to prolong the inactivation of voltage-activated sodium ion channels and reduction of the ability of neurons to fire at high frequencies.

THERAPEUTIC AND TOXIC CONCENTRATIONS

The usual therapeutic range for total (unbound + bound) phenytoin serum concentrations when the drug is used in the treatment of seizures is 10-20 μg/mL. Since phenytoin is highly bound (~90%) to albumin, it is prone to plasma protein–binding displacement due to a large variety of factors. Because of this, unbound or "free" phenytoin concentrations are widely available. Although there is clinical data to support the therapeutic range for total phenytoin concentrations, the suggested therapeutic range for unbound phenytoin concentrations is based on the usual unbound fraction (10%) of phenytoin in individuals with normal plasma protein binding. Thus, the generally accepted therapeutic range for unbound phenytoin concentrations is 1-2 μg/mL, which is simply 10% of the lower and upper bounds for the total concentration range, respectively.

In the upper end of the therapeutic range (>15 μg/mL) some patients will experience minor central nervous system depression side effects such as drowsiness or fatigue.[7,8] At total phenytoin concentrations above 20 μg/mL, nystagmus may occur and can be especially prominent upon lateral gaze. When total concentrations exceed 30 μg/mL, ataxia, slurred speech, and/or incoordination similar to ethanol intoxication can be observed.

If total phenytoin concentrations are above 40 µg/mL, mental status changes, including decreased mentation, severe confusion or lethargy, and coma are possible. Drug-induced seizure activity has been observed at concentrations over 50-60 µg/mL. Because phenytoin follows nonlinear or saturable metabolism pharmacokinetics, it is possible to attain excessive drug concentrations much easier than for other compounds that follow linear pharmacokinetics. Clinicians should understand that all patients with "toxic" phenytoin serum concentrations in the listed ranges will not exhibit signs or symptoms of phenytoin toxicity. Rather, phenytoin concentrations in the ranges given increase the likelihood that an adverse drug effect will occur.

CLINICAL USEFULNESS OF UNBOUND PHENYTOIN CONCENTRATIONS

Unbound phenytoin concentrations are an extremely useful monitoring tool when used correctly. The relationship between total concentration (C), unbound or "free" concentration (C_f), and unbound or "free" fraction (f_B) is: $C_f = f_B C$. For routine therapeutic drug monitoring purposes, total phenytoin serum concentrations are still the mainstream way to gauge therapy with the anticonvulsant. In most patients without known or identifiable plasma protein–binding abnormalities, the unbound fraction of phenytoin will be normal (~10%) and unbound drug concentration measurement is unnecessary. At present, unbound drug concentrations are 50%-100% more expensive than total concentrations, take longer to conduct by the laboratory and have results returned to clinicians, and are not available at all laboratories. Generally, unbound phenytoin serum concentration monitoring should be restricted to those patients with known reasons to have altered drug plasma protein binding. Exceptions to this approach are patients with an augmented or excessive pharmacologic response compared to their total phenytoin concentration. For example, if a patient has a satisfactory anticonvulsant response to a low total phenytoin concentration, one possible reason would be abnormal plasma protein binding (20%) for some unidentified reason, so that even though the total concentration was low (5 µg/mL), a therapeutic unbound concentration was present in the patient ($C_f = f_B C = 0.2 \bullet 5$ µg/mL = 1 µg/mL). Conversely, if a patient has a possible phenytoin-related adverse drug reaction and the total phenytoin concentration is within the therapeutic range, a possible reason could be abnormal protein binding (20%) for an unidentified reason, so that even though the total concentration appeared to be appropriate (15 µg/mL), a toxic unbound concentration was present in the patient ($C_f = f_B C = 0.2 \bullet 15$ µg/mL = 3 µg/mL).

Unbound phenytoin serum concentrations should be measured in patients with factors known to alter phenytoin plasma protein binding. These factors fall into three broad categories: (1) lack of binding protein where there are insufficient plasma concentrations of albumin, (2) displacement of phenytoin from albumin-binding sites by endogenous compounds, and (3) displacement of phenytoin from albumin-binding sites by exogenous compounds (Table 10-2).[9-27] When multiple factors that decrease phenytoin plasma protein binding are present in a patient, the free fraction can be as high as 30%-40%.[28]

TABLE 10-2   Disease States and Conditions That Alter Phenytoin Plasma Protein Binding

Insufficient Albumin Concentration (Hypoalbuminemia)	Displacement By Endogenous Compounds	Displacement By Exogenous Compounds
Liver disease	Hyperbilirubinemia	Drug interactions
Nephrotic syndrome	Jaundice	Warfarin
Pregnancy	Liver disease	Valproic acid
Cystic fibrosis	Renal dysfunction	Aspirin (>2 g/d)
Burns		NSAIDs with high albumin binding
Trauma		
Malnourishment		
Elderly		

Low albumin concentrations, known as hypoalbuminemia, can be found in patients with liver disease or the nephrotic syndrome, pregnant women, cystic fibrosis patients, burn patients, trauma patients, malnourished individuals, and the elderly. Albumin concentrations below 3 g/dL are associated with high phenytoin-unbound fractions in the plasma. Patients with albumin concentrations between 2.5 and 3 g/dL typically have phenytoin-unbound fractions of 15%-20%, while patients with albumin concentrations between 2.0 and 2.5 g/dL often have unbound phenytoin fractions greater than 20%. Albumin is manufactured by the liver so patients with hepatic disease may have difficulty synthesizing the protein. Patients with nephrotic syndrome waste albumin by eliminating it in the urine. Malnourished patients can be so nutritionally deprived that albumin production is impeded. Malnourishment is the reason for hypoalbuminemia in some elderly patients, although there is a general downtrend in albumin concentrations in older patients. While recovering from their injuries, burn and trauma patients can become hypermetabolic and albumin concentrations decrease if enough calories are not supplied during this phase of their disease state. Albumin concentrations may decline during pregnancy as maternal reserves are shifted to the developing fetus and are especially prevalent during the third trimester.

Displacement of phenytoin from plasma protein–binding sites by endogenous substances can occur in patients with hepatic or renal dysfunction. The mechanism is competition for albumin plasma protein–binding sites between the exogenous substances and phenytoin. Bilirubin (a byproduct of heme metabolism) is broken down by the liver, so patients with hepatic disease can have excessive bilirubin concentrations. Total bilirubin concentrations in excess of 2 mg/dL are associated with abnormal phenytoin plasma protein binding. End-stage renal disease patients (creatinine clearance <10-15 mL/min) with uremia (blood urea nitrogen concentrations >80-100 mg/dL) accumulate unidentified compound(s) in their blood that displace phenytoin from plasma protein–binding sites. Abnormal phenytoin binding persists in these patients even when dialysis procedures are instituted.

Phenytoin plasma protein–binding displacement can also occur due to exogenously administered compounds such as drugs. In this case, the mechanism is competition for albumin-binding sites between phenytoin and other agents. Other drugs that are highly bound to albumin and cause plasma protein–binding displacement drug interactions with phenytoin include warfarin, valproic acid, aspirin (>2 g/d), and some highly bound nonsteroidal anti-inflammatory agents.

Once the free fraction (f_B) has been determined for a patient with altered phenytoin plasma protein binding ($f_B = C_f/C$, where C is the total concentration and C_f is the unbound concentration), it is often not necessary to obtain additional unbound drug concentrations. If the situations that caused altered plasma protein binding are stable (albumin or bilirubin concentration, hepatic or renal function, other drug doses, etc), total phenytoin concentrations can be converted to concurrent unbound values and used for therapeutic drug-monitoring purposes. For example, an end-stage renal failure patient is receiving phenytoin therapy as well as valproic acid and warfarin. The concurrently measured total and unbound phenytoin concentrations are 5 μg/mL and 1.5 μg/mL, respectively, yielding an unbound fraction of 30% ($f_B = C_f/C$ = 1.5 μg/mL / 5 μg/mL = 0.30). The next day, a total phenytoin concentration is measured and equals 6 μg/mL. The estimated unbound concentration using this information would be 1.8 μg/mL: $C_f = f_B C$ = 0.30 • 6 μg/mL = 1.8 μg/mL. Of course, if the disease state status or drug therapy changes, a new unbound phenytoin fraction will be present and need to be remeasured using an unbound/total phenytoin concentration pair.

When unbound phenytoin concentrations are unavailable, several methods have been suggested to estimate the value or a surrogate measure of the value. The most common surrogate is an estimation of the equivalent total phenytoin concentration that would provide the same unbound phenytoin concentration if the patient had a normal unbound fraction value of 10%. These calculations "normalize" the total phenytoin concentration so that it can be compared to the usual phenytoin therapeutic range of 10-20 μg/mL and used for dosage adjustment purposes. The equation for hypoalbuminemia is: $C_{NormalBinding} = C/(X • Alb + 0.1)$, where $C_{NormalBinding}$ is the normalized total phenytoin concentration in μg/mL, C is the actual measured phenytoin concentration in μg/mL, X is a constant equal to 0.2 if protein-binding measurements were conducted at 37°C or 0.25 if conducted at 25°C, and Alb is the albumin concentration in g/dL.[29,30] If the patient has end-stage renal disease (creatinine clearance <10-15 mL/min), the same equation is used with a different constant value (X = 0.1).[29] (Note: in most experimental laboratories, protein binding is determined at normal body temperature [37°C], in most clinical laboratories, protein binding is determined at room temperature [25°C]). Because these methods assume that the normal unbound fraction of phenytoin is 10%, the estimated unbound phenytoin concentration ($C_{f_{EST}}$) is computed using the following formula: $(C_{f_{EST}}) = 0.1\ C_{NormalBinding}$. A different approach is taken by the equations used for patients with concurrent valproic acid administration. In this case, the unbound phenytoin concentration ($C_{f_{EST}}$) is estimated using simultaneously measured total phenytoin (PHT in µg/mL) and valproic acid (VPA in µg/mL) concentrations: $C_{f_{EST}} = (0.095 + 0.001 \bullet VPA)PHT$.[31,32] This value is compared to the usual therapeutic range for unbound phenytoin concentrations (1-2 µg/mL) and used for dosage adjustment purposes. It should be noted that these equations only provide estimates of their respective concentrations, and actual unbound phenytoin concentrations should be measured whenever possible in patients with suspected abnormal phenytoin plasma protein binding.

EXAMPLE 1 ▶▶▶

JM is an epileptic patient being treated with phenytoin. He has hypoalbuminemia (albumin = 2.2 g/dL) and normal renal function (creatinine clearance = 90 mL/min). His total phenytoin concentration is 7.5 µg/mL. Assuming that any unbound concentrations performed by the clinical laboratory will be conducted at 25°C, compute an estimated normalized phenytoin concentration for this patient.

1. *Choose the appropriate equation to estimate normalized total phenytoin concentration at the appropriate temperature.*

$$C_{NormalBinding} = C/(0.25 \bullet Alb + 0.1) = (7.5\ \mu g/mL)/(0.25 \bullet 2.2\ g/dL + 0.1) = 11.5\ \mu g/mL$$

$$C_{f_{EST}} = 0.1\ C_{NormalBinding} = 0.1 \bullet 11.5\ \mu g/mL = 1.2\ \mu g/mL$$

This patient's estimated normalized total phenytoin concentration is expected to provide an unbound concentration equivalent to a total phenytoin concentration of 11.5 µg/mL for a patient with normal drug protein binding ($C_{f_{EST}} = 1.2\ \mu g/mL$). Because the estimated total value is within the therapeutic range of 10-20 µg/mL, it is likely that the patient has an unbound phenytoin concentration within the therapeutic range. If possible, this should be confirmed by obtaining an actual, measured unbound phenytoin concentration.

EXAMPLE 2 ▶▶▶

LM is an epileptic patient being treated with phenytoin. He has hypoalbuminemia (albumin = 2.2 g/dL) and poor renal function (creatinine clearance = 10 mL/min). His total phenytoin concentration is 7.5 µg/mL. Compute an estimated normalized phenytoin concentration for this patient.

1. *Choose appropriate equation to estimate normalized total phenytoin concentration.*

$$C_{NormalBinding} = C/(0.1 \bullet Alb + 0.1) = (7.5\ \mu g/mL)/(0.1 \bullet 2.2\ g/dL + 0.1) = 23.4\ \mu g/mL$$

$$C_{f_{EST}} = 0.1\ C_{NormalBinding} = 0.1 \bullet 23.4\ \mu g/mL = 2.3\ \mu g/mL$$

This patient's estimated normalized total phenytoin concentration is expected to provide an unbound concentration equivalent to a total phenytoin concentration of 23.4 µg/mL for a patient with normal drug protein binding ($C_{f_{EST}} = 2.3\ \mu g/mL$). Because the estimated total value is above the therapeutic range of 10-20 µg/mL, it is likely that the patient has an unbound phenytoin concentration above the therapeutic range. If possible, this should be confirmed by obtaining an actual, measured unbound phenytoin concentration.

EXAMPLE 3 ▶▶▶

PM is an epileptic patient being treated with phenytoin and valproic acid. He has a normal albumin concentration (albumin = 4.2 g/dL) and normal renal function (creatinine clearance = 90 mL/min). His steady-state total phenytoin and valproic acid concentrations are 7.5 μg/mL and 100 μg/mL, respectively. Compute an estimated unbound phenytoin concentration for this patient.

1. *Choose appropriate equation to estimate unbound phenytoin concentration.*

$$C_{f_{EST}} = (0.095 + 0.001 \bullet VPA)PHT = (0.095 + 0.001 \bullet 100 \text{ μg/mL})7.5 \text{ μg/mL} = 1.5 \text{ μg/mL}$$

This patient's estimated unbound phenytoin concentration is expected to be within the therapeutic range for unbound concentrations. If possible, this should be confirmed by obtaining an actual, measured unbound phenytoin concentration.

CLINICAL MONITORING PARAMETERS

The goal of therapy with anticonvulsants is to reduce seizure frequency and maximize quality of life with a minimum of adverse drug effects.[7] While it is desirable to entirely abolish all seizure episodes, it may not be possible to accomplish this in many patients. Patients should be monitored for concentration-related side effects (drowsiness, fatigue, nystagmus, ataxia, slurred speech, incoordination, mental status changes, decreased mentation, confusion, lethargy, coma) as well as adverse reactions associated with long-term use (behavioral changes, cerebellar syndrome, connective tissue changes, coarse facies, skin thickening, folate deficiency, gingival hyperplasia, lymphadenopathy, hirsutism, osteomalacia). Idiosyncratic side effects include skin rash, Stevens-Johnson syndrome, bone marrow suppression, systemic lupus-like reactions, and hepatitis.

Phenytoin serum concentrations should be measured in most patients. Because epilepsy is an episodic disease state, patients do not experience seizures on a continuous basis. Thus, during dosage titration, it is difficult to tell if the patient is responding to drug therapy or simply is not experiencing any abnormal central nervous system discharges at that time. Phenytoin serum concentrations are also valuable tools to avoid adverse drug effects. Patients are more likely to accept drug therapy if adverse reactions are held to the absolute minimum. Because phenytoin follows nonlinear or saturable pharmacokinetics, it is fairly easy to attain toxic concentrations with modest changes in drug dose.

BASIC CLINICAL PHARMACOKINETIC PARAMETERS

Phenytoin is primarily eliminated by hepatic metabolism (>95%). Hepatic metabolism is mainly via the CYP2C9 enzyme system with a smaller amount metabolized by CYP2C19. About 5% of a phenytoin dose is recovered in the urine as unchanged drug. Phenytoin follows Michaelis-Menten or saturable pharmacokinetics.[33-35] This is the type of nonlinear pharmacokinetics that occurs when the number of drug molecules overwhelms or saturates the enzyme's ability to metabolize the drug. When this occurs, steady-state drug serum concentrations increase in a disproportionate manner after a dosage increase (Figure 10-1). In this case, the rate of drug removal is described by the classic Michaelis-Menten relationship that is used for all enzyme systems: rate of metabolism = $(V_{max} \bullet C)/(K_m + C)$, where V_{max} is the maximum rate of metabolism in mg/d, C is the phenytoin concentration in mg/L or μg/mL, and K_m is the substrate concentration in mg/L or μg/mL where the rate of metabolism = $V_{max}/2$.

The clinical implication of Michaelis-Menten pharmacokinetics is that the clearance of phenytoin is not a constant as it is with linear pharmacokinetics, but is concentration or dose dependent. As the dose or

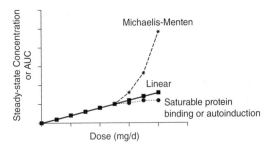

FIGURE 10-1   If a drug follows linear pharmacokinetics, Css or AUC increases proportionally with dose resulting in a straight line on the plot. Nonlinear pharmacokinetics occurs when the Css or AUC versus dose plot results in something other than a straight line. If a drug follows Michaelis-Menten pharmacokinetics (eg, phenytoin, aspirin), as steady-state drug concentrations approach K_m serum concentrations increase more than expected due to dose increases. If a drug follows nonlinear protein binding (eg, valproic acid, disopyramide) or demonstrates autoinduction (eg, carbamazepine), total steady-state drug concentrations increase less than expected as dose increases.

concentration of phenytoin increases, the clearance rate (Cl) decreases as the enzyme approaches saturable conditions: $Cl = V_{max}/(K_m + C)$. This is the reason concentrations increase disproportionately after a phenytoin dosage increase. For example, phenytoin follows saturable pharmacokinetics with average Michaelis-Menten constants of $V_{max} = 500$ mg/d and $K_m = 4$ mg/L. The therapeutic range of phenytoin is 10-20 μg/mL. As the steady-state concentration of phenytoin increases from 10 μg/mL to 20 μg/mL, clearance decreases from 36 L/d to 21 L/d: $Cl = V_{max}/(K_m + C)$; Cl = (500 mg/d)/(4 mg/L + 10 mg/L) = 36 L/d; Cl = (500 mg/d)/(4 mg/L + 20 mg/L) = 21 L/d (note: μg/mL = mg/L and this substitution was directly made to avoid unnecessary unit conversion). Unfortunately, there is so much interpatient variability in Michaelis-Menten pharmacokinetic parameters for phenytoin (typically $V_{max} = 100$-1000 mg/d and $K_m = 1$-15 μg/mL) that dosing the drug is extremely difficult.

Phenytoin volume of distribution (V = 0.7 L/kg) is unaffected by saturable metabolism and is still determined by the physiological volume of blood (V_B) and tissues (V_T) as well as the unbound concentration of drug in the blood (f_B) and tissues (f_T): $V = V_B + (f_B/f_T)V_T$. Also, half-life ($t_{1/2}$) is still related to clearance and volume of distribution using the same equation as for linear pharmacokinetics: $t_{1/2} = (0.693 \bullet V)/Cl$. However, since clearance is dose or concentration dependent, half-life also changes with phenytoin dosage or concentration changes. As doses or concentrations increase for a drug that follows Michaelis-Menten pharmacokinetics, clearance decreases and half-life becomes longer for the drug: $\uparrow t_{1/2} = (0.693 \bullet V)/\downarrow Cl$. Using the above example for clearance and the volume of distribution for a 70-kg person (V = 0.7 L/kg $\bullet$ 70 kg $\approx$ 50 L), half-life changes from 1 day [$t_{1/2} = (0.693 \bullet V)/Cl = (0.693 \bullet 50$ L)/36 L/d = 1 d] to 1.7 days [$t_{1/2} = (0.693 \bullet 50$ L)/ 21 L/d = 1.7 d] as phenytoin serum concentrations increase from 10 μg/mL to 20 μg/mL. The clinical implication of this finding is that the time to steady-state (3-5 $t_{1/2}$) is longer as the dose or concentration is increased for phenytoin. On average, the time to steady-state serum concentrations is approximately 5 days at a dosage rate of 300 mg/d and 15 days at a dosage rate of 400 mg/d.[34]

Under steady-state conditions, the rate of drug administration equals the rate of drug removal.[36] Therefore, the Michaelis-Menten equation can be used to compute the maintenance dose (MD in mg/d) required to achieve a target steady-state phenytoin serum concentration (Css in μg/mL or mg/L):

$$MD = \frac{V_{max} \bullet Css}{K_m + Css}$$

Or, solved for Css:

$$Css = \frac{K_m \bullet MD}{V_{max} - MD}$$

When phenytoin steady-state concentrations are far below the K_m value for a patient, this equation simplifies to: $MD = (V_{max}/K_m)Css$ or, since V_{max}/K_m is a constant, $MD = Cl \bullet Css$. Therefore, when $K_m \gg Css$, phenytoin follows linear pharmacokinetics. When phenytoin steady-state concentrations are far above the K_m value for a patient, the rate of metabolism becomes a constant equal to V_{max}. Under these conditions, only a fixed amount of phenytoin is metabolized per day because the enzyme system is completely saturated and cannot increase its metabolic capacity. This situation is also known as zero-order pharmacokinetics. First-order pharmacokinetics is another name for linear pharmacokinetics.

For parenteral use, phenytoin is available in two different dosage forms. Phenytoin sodium, the sodium salt of phenytoin, contains 92% phenytoin by weight. Even though it is a salt of phenytoin, the drug is still relatively insoluble in water. To facilitate dissolution, ethanol and propylene glycol are added to the vehicle, and the pH of the solution is adjusted to between 10 and 12. When given intramuscularly, phenytoin sodium injections are very painful.[37] Some of the drug probably precipitates in the muscle injection site and this results in prolonged absorption of drug over several days. When given intravenously, injection rates should not exceed 50 mg/min to avoid hypotension. Even at lower infusion rates, profound hypotension can result in patients with unstable blood pressure or shock. Phenytoin sodium injection can be given by slow intravenous push of undiluted drug, or added to normal saline at a concentration of 10 mg/mL or less and infused <50 mg/min. When added to normal saline, the drug should be given as soon as possible after being mixed to avoid precipitation, and a 0.22-μm inline filter should be used to remove any drug crystals before they reach the patient.

To avoid many of the problems associated with phenytoin sodium injection, a water-soluble phosphate ester prodrug of phenytoin, fosphenytoin, has been developed. Conversion of fosphenytoin to phenytoin is rapid, with a fosphenytoin half-life of approximately 15 minutes.[38] To avoid confusion, fosphenytoin is prescribed in terms of phenytoin sodium equivalents (PE). Thus, 100 mg PE of fosphenytoin is equivalent to 100 mg of phenytoin sodium. Hypotension during intravenous administration of fosphenytoin is much less of a problem than with phenytoin sodium. The maximal intravenous infusion rate is 150 mg PE/min. Transient pruritus and paresthesia are associated with this route of administration. Intramuscular absorption is rapid with a peak concentration that occurs about 30 minutes after injection, and bioavailability via this route of administration is 100%. However, fosphenytoin is much more expensive that phenytoin sodium injection, and this has limited its widespread use. Because of this, most clinicians have reserved fosphenytoin use to patients requiring intramuscular phenytoin or to patients with unstable or low blood pressure requiring intravenous phenytoin therapy.

For oral use, capsules contain phenytoin sodium (92% phenytoin, by weight) while tablets and suspension contain phenytoin. Phenytoin sodium capsules are labeled as extended phenytoin sodium capsules or prompt phenytoin capsules. Extended phenytoin capsules release phenytoin slowly from the gastrointestinal tract into the systemic circulation. The extended-release characteristics of this dosage form are due to the slow dissolution of the drug in gastric juices and not the result of extended-release dosage form technology. Prompt phenytoin sodium capsules are absorbed fairly quickly from the gastrointestinal tract because they contain microcrystalline phenytoin sodium, which dissolves quicker in gastric juices. As a result of their sustained-release properties, phenytoin doses given as extended phenytoin sodium capsules can be given every once or twice daily, but prompt phenytoin sodium capsules must be given multiple times daily. Extended phenytoin sodium capsules are available in 30-mg, 100-mg, 200-mg, and 300-mg strengths. Because phenytoin follows nonlinear pharmacokinetics, even subtle differences in bioavailability may alter steady-state serum concentrations.[39,40] Any time therapy is changed from one brand of phenytoin to another, clinicians should carefully monitor patients for any changes in seizure frequency, adverse effects, and steady-state concentration.

Phenytoin tablets (50 mg, chewable) and suspension (125 mg/5 mL) for oral use are available as the acid form of the drug. Both the tablet and suspension dosage forms are absorbed more rapidly than extended phenytoin sodium capsules, and once daily dosing with these may not be possible in some patients. The suspension is thick, and the drug is difficult to disperse evenly throughout the liquid. If not shaken well before dispensing a dose, the drug can flocculate out into the bottom of the bottle. When this occurs, phenytoin concentrations near the top of the bottle will be less than average, and doses given when the bottle is ⅔ or more full will contain less phenytoin. Conversely, phenytoin concentrations near the bottom of the bottle will be greater than average, and doses given when the bottle is ⅓ or less full will contain more phenytoin. This problem can be avoided to a large extent if the dispensing pharmacist shakes the bottle very well (several minutes) before giving to the patient.

For most drugs, the 8% difference in dose between dosage forms containing phenytoin (suspension and tablets, 100 mg = 100 mg phenytoin) and phenytoin sodium (capsules and injection, 100 mg = 92 mg phenytoin) would be trivial and could easily be ignored. However, because phenytoin follows nonlinear pharmacokinetics, an 8% difference in dose can result in major changes in phenytoin serum concentrations. For example, if a patient is stabilized on a dose of intravenous phenytoin sodium 300 mg/d (300 mg/d phenytoin sodium × 0.92 = 276 mg phenytoin) with a steady-state concentration of 17 µg/mL, switching the patient to phenytoin suspension 300 mg/d could result in steady-state phenytoin concentrations exceeding 20 µg/mL (15%-30% increase or more) and result in toxicity. Conversely, if a different patient is stabilized on a dose of phenytoin suspension 300 mg/d with a steady-state concentration of 12 µg/mL, switching the patient to intravenous phenytoin sodium 300 mg/d (300 mg/d phenytoin sodium × 0.92 = 276 mg phenytoin) could result in steady-state phenytoin concentrations below 10 µg/mL (15%-30% decrease or more) and result in loss of efficacy. Usually, phenytoin doses are not fine-tuned to the point of directly accounting for the difference in phenytoin content (ie, 276 mg of phenytoin suspension would not be prescribed for the patient receiving 300 mg of phenytoin sodium injection). Rather, clinicians are aware that when phenytoin dosage forms are changed, phenytoin content may change and anticipate that the drug concentration may increase or decrease because of this. Because of this, most individuals recheck phenytoin serum concentrations after a dosage form change is instituted.

The oral bioavailability of phenytoin is very good for capsule, tablet, and suspension dosage forms and approximates 100%.[41-44] At larger amounts, there is some dose dependency on absorption characteristics.[45] Single oral doses of 800 mg or more produce longer times for maximal concentrations to occur (T_{max}) and decreased bioavailability. Since larger oral doses also produce a higher incidence of gastrointestinal side effects (primarily nausea and vomiting due to local irritation), it is prudent to break maintenance doses larger than 800 mg/d into multiple doses. If oral phenytoin loading doses are given, a common total dose is 1000 mg given as 400 mg, 300 mg, and 300 mg separated by 2- to 6-hour time intervals. Enteral feedings given by nasogastric tube interfere with phenytoin absorption.[46-49] Possible mechanisms include decreased gastrointestinal transit time which reduces absorption contact time, binding of phenytoin to proteins contained in the feedings, and adherence of phenytoin to the lumen of the feeding tube. The solution to this problem is to stop the feedings, when possible, for 1-2 hours before and after phenytoin administration, and increase the oral phenytoin dose.[48] It is not unusual for phenytoin oral dosage requirements to double or triple while the patient receives concurrent nasogastric feedings (eg, usual dose of 300-400 mg/d increasing to 600-1200 mg/d while receiving nasogastric feedings). Of course, intravenous or intramuscular phenytoin or fosphenytoin doses could also be substituted while nasogastric feedings were being administered. Although poorly documented, phenytoin oral malabsorption may also occur in patients with severe diarrhea, malabsorption syndromes, or gastric resection.

The typical recommended loading dose for phenytoin is 15-20 mg/kg resulting in 1000 mg for most adult patients. Usual initial maintenance doses are 5-10 mg/kg/d for children (6 months to 16 years old) and 4-6 mg/kg/d for adults. For adults, the most prescribed dose is 300-400 mg/d of phenytoin. Because of an increased incidence of adverse effects in older patients (>65 years old), many clinicians prescribe a maximum of 200 mg/d as an initial dose for these individuals.[50,51]

IMPACT OF ALTERED PLASMA PROTEIN BINDING ON PHENYTOIN PHARMACOKINETICS

The pharmacokinetic alterations that occur with altered plasma protein binding result in complex changes for total and unbound steady-state phenytoin concentrations and drug response. As previously discussed (see Chapter 3, Drug Dosing in Special Populations: Renal and Hepatic Disease, Dialysis, Heart Failure, Obesity, and Drug Interactions), hepatic drug metabolism is described by the following equation:

$$Cl_H = \frac{LBF \bullet (f_B \bullet Cl'_{int})}{LBF + (f_B \bullet Cl'_{int})}$$

where LBF is liver blood flow, f_B is the fraction of unbound drug in the blood, and Cl'_{int} is intrinsic clearance. For drugs such as phenytoin with a low hepatic extraction ratio ($\leq 30\%$), the numeric value of liver blood flow is much greater than the product of unbound fraction of drug in the blood and the intrinsic clearance of the compound ($LBF >> f_B \bullet Cl'_{int}$), and the sum in the denominator of the hepatic clearance equation is almost equal to liver blood flow [$LBF \approx LBF + (f_B \bullet Cl'_{int})$]. When this substitution is made into the hepatic clearance equation, hepatic clearance is equal to the product of free fraction in the blood and the intrinsic clearance of the drug for a drug with a low hepatic extraction ratio:

$$Cl_H = \frac{LBF \bullet (f_B \bullet Cl'_{int})}{LBF} = f_B \bullet Cl'_{int}$$

In order to illustrate the differences that may occur in steady-state drug concentrations and pharmacologic effects for patients with altered phenytoin plasma protein binding, a graphical technique will be used (Figure 10-2A). The example assumes that phenytoin is being given to a patient as a continuous intravenous infusion, and that all physiologic, pharmacokinetic, and drug effect parameters (shown on the y-axis) are initially stable. However, the same changes occur for average total and unbound steady-state concentrations when the drug is given on a continuous dosage schedule (every 8, 12, 24, etc hours) or orally. On the x-axis, an arrow indicates that phenytoin plasma protein binding decreases and unbound fraction increases in the patient; an assumption made for this illustration is that any changes in the parameters are instantaneous. An increase in the parameter is denoted as an uptick in the line while a decrease in the parameter is shown as a downtick in the line.

For a drug with a low hepatic extraction ratio, plasma protein–binding displacement drug interactions cause major pharmacokinetic alterations but are not clinically significant because the pharmacologic effect of the drug does not change (Figure 10-2A). Because the clearance of the drug is dependent on the fraction of unbound drug in the blood and intrinsic clearance for a low hepatic extraction ratio agent, a decrease in plasma protein binding and increase in unbound fraction will increase clearance ($\uparrow Cl = \uparrow f_B Cl'_{int}$) and volume of distribution [$\uparrow V = V_B + (\uparrow f_B/f_T)V_T$]. Since half-life depends on clearance and volume of distribution, it is likely

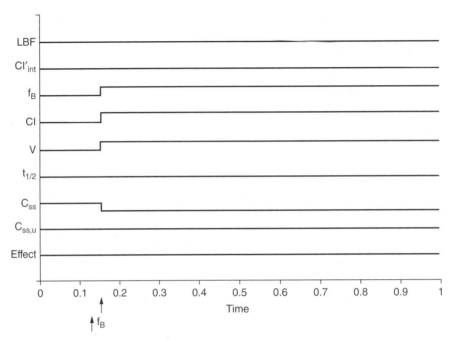

FIGURE 10-2A   Schematic representation of physiologic (LBF = liver blood flow, Cl'_{int} = intrinsic or unbound clearance, f_B = unbound fraction of drug in blood/plasma), pharmacokinetic (Cl = clearance; V = volume of distribution; $t_{1/2}$ = half-life; Css = total steady-state drug concentration; Css, u = unbound steady-state drug concentration), and pharmacodynamic (Effect = pharmacodynamic effect) changes that occur with decreased protein binding of phenytoin (arrow denotes ↑f_B).

that because both increase, half-life will not substantially change [$t_{1/2} = (0.693 \bullet ↑V)/↑Cl$]. However, it is possible that if either clearance or volume of distribution changes disproportionately, half-life will change. The total steady-state concentration will decline because of the increase in clearance ($↓Css = k_0/↑Cl$, where k_0 is the infusion rate of drug). But, the unbound steady-state concentration will remain unaltered because the free fraction of drug in the blood is higher than it was before the increase in unbound fraction occurred (Css, u = ↑f_B↓Css). The pharmacologic effect of the drug does not change because the free concentration of drug in the blood is unchanged. This can be an unexpected outcome for the decrease in plasma protein binding, especially because the total steady-state concentration of the drug decreased. Clinicians need to be on the outlook for situations like this because the total drug concentration (bound + unbound) can be misleading and cause an unwarranted increase in drug dosage. Unbound drug concentrations should be used to convince clinicians that a drug dosage increase is not needed even though total concentrations decline as a result of this interaction.

EFFECTS OF DISEASE STATES AND CONDITIONS ON PHARMACOKINETICS AND DOSING

Measurement of V_{max} and K_m for phenytoin is very difficult to accomplish for research or clinical purposes. Because of this, the effects of disease states and conditions on these parameters are largely unknown. By necessity, this discussion must be done in qualitative terms for phenytoin. Adults without the disease states and conditions given later in this section, with normal liver and renal function as well as normal plasma protein binding (~90%), have an average phenytoin V_{max} of 7 mg/kg/d (range: 1.5-14 mg/kg/d) and K_m of 4 μg/mL (range: 1-15 µg/mL).[35] Michaelis-Menten parameters for younger children (6 months-6 years) are V_{max} = 12 mg/kg/d and K_m = 6 µg/mL while for older children (7-16 years) V_{max} = 9 mg/kg/d and K_m = 6 µg/mL.[52-58] The most difficult and frustrating aspect of phenytoin dosage determination is the 10-15-fold variation in Michaelis-Menten pharmacokinetic parameters which creates a huge amount of variability in dose requirements. An individualized dosage regimen for each patient prescribed phenytoin must be determined to accomplish therapeutic goals. Unfortunately, measurement of V_{max} and K_m for phenytoin is very difficult to accomplish for research or clinical purposes. Because of this, the effects of disease states and conditions on these parameters are largely unknown. By necessity, this discussion must be done in qualitative terms for phenytoin.

Patients with liver cirrhosis or acute hepatitis have reduced phenytoin clearance because of destruction of liver parenchyma. This loss of functional hepatic cells reduces the amount of CYP2C9 and CYP2C19 available to metabolize the drug and decreases V_{max}. The volume of distribution is larger because of reduced plasma protein binding. Protein binding is reduced and unbound fraction is increased due to hypoalbuminemia and/ or hyperbilirubinemia (especially albumin ≤3 g/dL and/or total bilirubin ≥2 mg/dL). However, the effects that liver disease have on phenytoin pharmacokinetics are highly variable and difficult to accurately predict. It is possible for a patient with liver disease to have relatively normal or grossly abnormal phenytoin clearance and volume of distribution. For example, a liver disease patient who has relatively normal albumin and bilirubin concentrations can have a normal volume of distribution for phenytoin. An index of liver dysfunction can be gained by applying the Child-Pugh clinical classification system to the patient (Table 10-3).[59] Child-Pugh scores are completely discussed in Chapter 3 (Drug Dosing in Special Populations: Renal and Hepatic Disease, Dialysis, Heart Failure, Obesity, and Drug Interactions), but will be briefly discussed here. The Child-Pugh score consists of five laboratory tests or clinical symptoms: serum albumin, total bilirubin, prothrombin time, ascites, and hepatic encephalopathy. Each of these areas is given a score of 1 (normal) to 3 (severely abnormal; see Table 10-3), and the scores for the five areas are summed. The Child-Pugh score for a patient with normal liver function is 5 while the score for a patient with grossly abnormal serum albumin, total bilirubin, and prothrombin time values in addition to severe ascites and hepatic encephalopathy is 15. A Child-Pugh score greater than 8 is grounds for a decrease of 25%-50% in the initial daily drug dose for phenytoin. As in any patient with or without liver dysfunction, initial doses are meant as starting points for dosage titration based on patient response and avoidance of adverse effects. Phenytoin serum concentrations and the presence of adverse drug effects should be monitored frequently in patients with liver cirrhosis.

Other patients are also prone to hypoalbuminemia, including patients with the nephrotic syndrome, cystic fibrosis patients, and malnourished individuals. Unbound phenytoin concentration monitoring should be considered in these patients especially when albumin concentrations are ≤3 g/dL. High bilirubin concentrations can also be found in patients with biliary tract obstruction or hemolysis. Unbound phenytoin

TABLE 10-3 Child-Pugh Scores for Patients With Liver Disease[59]

Test/Symptom	Score 1 Point	Score 2 Points	Score 3 Points
Total bilirubin (mg/dL)	<2.0	2.0-3.0	>3.0
Serum albumin (g/dL)	>3.5	2.8-3.5	<2.8
Prothrombin time (seconds prolonged over control)	<4	4-6	>6
Ascites	Absent	Slight	Moderate
Hepatic encephalopathy	None	Moderate	Severe

Mild liver disease, 5-6 points; moderate liver disease, 7-9 points; severe liver disease, 10-15 points.

concentration monitoring should be considered in these patients especially when total bilirubin concentrations are ≥2 mg/dL.

Trauma and burn patients have an increased ability to metabolize phenytoin beginning 3-7 days after their initial injury.[60,61] At this time, these patients become hypermetabolic in order to repair damaged tissue, and the V_{max} for phenytoin increases due to this general increase in metabolic rate. If caloric needs are not met during this phase of recovery for trauma patients, many become hypoalbuminemic, and phenytoin plasma protein binding decreases resulting in an increased unbound fraction. Phenytoin dosage requirements are increased while trauma patients are in their hypermetabolic phase, and unbound concentration monitoring is indicated when patients have low albumin concentrations (especially for albumin levels ≤3 g/dL).

Pregnant women taking phenytoin have increased dosage requirements, particularly during the third trimester (>26 weeks).[9,10,62-66] There are several reasons for this change, including malabsorption of drug resulting in decreased bioavailability, increased metabolism of phenytoin, and decreased protein binding due to low albumin concentrations. Aggressive drug serum concentration monitoring, including the measurement of unbound phenytoin concentrations if the patient is hypoalbuminemic, is necessary to avoid seizures and subsequent harm to the unborn fetus. An additional concern when administering phenytoin to pregnant patients is the development of fetal hydantoin syndrome by the baby.

Elderly individuals over the age of 65 years have a decreased capacity to metabolize phenytoin, possibly due to age-related losses of liver parenchyma resulting in decreased amounts of CYP2C9 and CYP2C19.[50,51] Older patients also may have hypoalbuminemia with resulting decreases in plasma protein binding and increases in unbound fraction.[26,27] Many elderly patients also seem to have an increased propensity for central nervous system side effects due to phenytoin, and because of these pharmacokinetic and pharmacodynamic changes, clinicians tend to prescribe lower initial phenytoin doses for older patients (~200 mg/d).

End-stage renal disease patients with creatinine clearances <10-15 mL/min have an unidentified substance in their blood that displaces phenytoin from its plasma protein–binding sites.[19-23,25] This unknown compound is not removed by dialysis.[24] In addition to this, these patients tend to have hypoalbuminemia which increases the unbound fraction of phenytoin even further. Unbound phenytoin serum concentration monitoring is very helpful in determining dosage requirements for renal failure patients. Other patients are also prone to hypoalbuminemia, including patients with the nephrotic syndrome, cystic fibrosis patients, and malnourished individuals. High bilirubin concentrations can also be found in patients with biliary tract obstruction or hemolysis. Unbound phenytoin concentration monitoring should be considered in these patients especially when albumin concentrations are ≤3 g/dL or total bilirubin concentrations are ≥2 mg/dL.

Hemodialysis does not remove enough phenytoin that supplemental postdialysis doses are necessary.[66] The typical sieving coefficient during hemoperfusion for phenytoin is 0.45, so in some cases supplemental phenytoin doses could be needed.[68,69] Because of pharmacokinetic variability, check phenytoin concentrations in patients receiving hemoperfusion.

The ratio between simultaneous breast milk and plasma areas under the curve averaged 0.13.[70] The mean ratio between breast milk and plasma concentration determined at various times during a dosage interval is 0.28.[71]

DRUG INTERACTIONS

Because phenytoin is so highly liver metabolized by CYP2C9 and CYP2C19, it is prone to drug interactions that inhibit hepatic microsomal enzymes.[72,73] Cimetidine, valproic acid, amiodarone, chloramphenicol, isoniazid, disulfiram, and omeprazole have been reported to inhibit phenytoin metabolism and increase phenytoin serum concentrations. Phenytoin is also a broad-based hepatic enzyme inducer affecting most cytochrome P-450 systems. Drugs with narrow therapeutic ranges that can have their metabolism increased by concurrent phenytoin administration include carbamazepine, phenobarbital, cyclosporin, tacrolimus, and warfarin. When phenytoin therapy is added to the medication regimen for a patient, a comprehensive review for drug interactions should be conducted. Valproic acid, aspirin (>2 g/d), some highly protein-bound nonsteroidal anti-inflammatory drugs, and warfarin can displace phenytoin from plasma protein–binding sites necessitating monitoring of unbound phenytoin concentrations.

The drug interaction between valproic acid and phenytoin deserves special examination because of its complexity and because these two agents are regularly used together for the treatment of seizures.[11-14] The drug interaction involves the plasma protein–binding displacement and intrinsic clearance inhibition of phenytoin by valproic acid. What makes this interaction so difficult to detect and understand is that these two changes do not occur simultaneously, so the impression left by the drug interaction depends on when in time it is observed in a patient. For example, a patient is stabilized on phenytoin therapy (Figure 10-2B), but because adequate control of seizures has not been attained, valproic acid is added to the regimen. As valproic acid concentrations accumulate, the first interaction observed is phenytoin plasma protein binding as the two drugs compete for binding sites on albumin. The result of this portion of the drug interaction is an increase in phenytoin unbound fraction and a decrease in phenytoin total serum concentration, but the unbound phenytoin serum concentration remains the same. As valproic acid serum concentrations achieve steady-state conditions, the higher concentrations of the drug bathe the hepatic microsomal enzyme system and inhibit the intrinsic clearance of phenytoin. This portion of the interaction decreases intrinsic clearance and hepatic clearance for

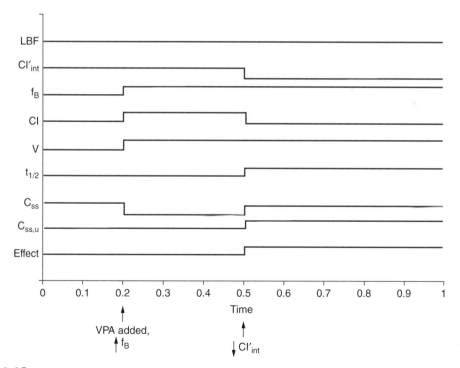

FIGURE 10-2B Schematic representation of the effect of initiating valproic acid (VPA) treatment in an individual stabilized on phenytoin therapy (see Figure 10-2A legend for symbol definition). Initially, valproic acid decreases phenytoin plasma protein binding via competitive displacement for binding sites on albumin (arrow denotes $\uparrow f_B$). As valproic acid concentrations increase, the hepatic enzyme inhibition component of the drug interaction comes into play (arrow denotes $\downarrow Cl'_{int}$). The net result is total phenytoin concentrations are largely unchanged from baseline, but unbound phenytoin concentrations and pharmacologic effect increase.

phenytoin, so both unbound and total phenytoin concentrations increase. When phenytoin concentrations finally equilibrate and reach steady-state under the new plasma protein binding and intrinsic clearance conditions imposed by concurrent valproic acid therapy, the total concentration of phenytoin is often times at about the same level as before the drug interaction occurred, but unbound phenytoin concentrations are much higher. If only total phenytoin concentrations are measured at this point in time, clinicians will be under the impression that total concentrations did not change and no drug interaction occurred. However, if unbound phenytoin concentrations are simultaneously measured, it will be found that these concentrations have risen and that the phenytoin unbound fraction is twice or more ($\geq 20\%$) of the baseline amount. In this situation, the patient may have unbound phenytoin concentrations that are toxic and a decrease in phenytoin dosage may be in order.

INITIAL DOSAGE DETERMINATION METHODS

Several methods to initiate phenytoin therapy are available. The *Pharmacokinetic Dosing method* is the most flexible of the techniques. It allows individualized target serum concentrations to be chosen for a patient, and each pharmacokinetic parameter can be customized to reflect specific disease states and conditions present in the patient. Unfortunately, specific values for Michaelis-Menten pharmacokinetic variables are not known for many disease states and conditions because they are difficult to measure. Even when values are available, there is 10-15-fold variation for each parameter. Also, it is computationally intensive. *Literature-based recommended dosing* is a very commonly used method to prescribe initial doses of phenytoin. Doses are based on those that commonly produce steady-state concentrations in the lower end of the therapeutic range, although there is a wide variation in the actual concentrations for a specific patient.

Pharmacokinetic Dosing Method

The goal of initial dosing with phenytoin is to compute the best dose possible for the patient given their set of disease states and conditions that influence phenytoin pharmacokinetics. The optimal way to accomplish this goal is to use average parameters measured in other patients with similar disease state and condition profiles as estimates of pharmacokinetic constants for the patient currently being treated with the drug. Unfortunately, because of the difficulty in computing Michaelis-Menten parameters, accurate estimates of V_{max} and K_m are not available for many important patient populations. Even if average-population Michaelis-Menten constants are available, the 10-15-fold variation in these parameters means that initial doses derived from these parameters will not be successful in achieving desired goals for all patients. Phenytoin serum concentration monitoring, including unbound concentration measurement if altered plasma protein binding is suspected, is an important component of therapy for this drug. If the patient has significant hepatic dysfunction (Child-Pugh score ≥ 8), maintenance doses computed using this method should be decreased by 25%-50% depending on how aggressive therapy is required to be for the individual.

Michaelis-Menten Parameter Estimates

Normal adults with normal liver and renal function as well as normal plasma protein binding have an average phenytoin V_{max} of 7 mg/kg/d and K_m of 4 μg/mL. Michaelis-Menten parameters for younger children (6 months-6 years) are V_{max} = 12 mg/kg/d and K_m = 6 μg/mL while for older children (7-16 years) V_{max} = 9 mg/kg/d and K_m = 6 μg/mL. These are the only parameters required to estimate a maintenance dose for phenytoin.

Volume of Distribution Estimate

The volume of distribution for patients with normal phenytoin plasma protein binding is estimated at 0.7 L/kg for adults. For obese individuals 30% or more above their ideal body weight, the volume of distribution can be estimated using the following equation: V = 0.7 L/kg [IBW + 1.33(TBW − IBW)], where IBW is ideal body weight in kg [$IBW_{females}$ (in kg) = 45 + 2.3(Ht − 60) or IBW_{males} (in kg) = 50 + 2.3(Ht − 60)], Ht is height in inches, and TBW is total body weight in kg.[74] This parameter is used to estimate the loading dose (LD in mg) for phenytoin, if one is indicated: LD = Css • V, where Css is the desired total phenytoin concentration in mg/L (note: mg/L = µg/mL and this conversion was directly made to avoid unnecessary unit conversion) and V is volume of distribution in L. For example, the volume of distribution for a 70-kg, nonobese patient would equal 49 L (V = 0.7 L/kg • 70 kg = 49 L). The loading dose to achieve a total phenytoin concentration of 15 µg/mL is 750 mg [LD = Css • V = 15 mg/L • 49 L = 735 mg, rounded to 750 mg (note: mg/L = µg/mL and this conversion was directly made to avoid unnecessary unit conversion)]. For an obese individual with a total body weight of 150 kg and an ideal body weight of 70 kg, the volume of distribution would equal 123 L: V = 0.7 L/kg [IBW + 1.33(TBW − IBW)] = 0.7 L/kg [70 kg + 1.33(150 kg − 70 kg)] = 123 L.

Selection of Appropriate Pharmacokinetic Model and Equations

When given by short-term intravenous infusion or orally, phenytoin follows a one-compartment pharmacokinetic model. When oral therapy is required, most clinicians utilize an extended phenytoin capsule dosage form that has good bioavailability (F = 1), supplies a continuous release of phenytoin into the gastrointestinal tract, and provides a smooth phenytoin serum concentration-time curve that emulates an intravenous infusion after once or twice daily dosing. Because of this, the Michaelis-Menten pharmacokinetic equation that computes the average phenytoin steady-state serum concentration (Css in µg/mL = mg/L) is widely used and allows maintenance dosage calculation:

$$MD = \frac{V_{max} \bullet Css}{S(K_m + Css)}$$

Or, solved for Css:

$$Css = \frac{K_m \bullet (S \bullet MD)}{V_{max} - (S \bullet MD)}$$

where V_{max} is the maximum rate of metabolism in mg/d, S is the fraction of the phenytoin salt form that is active phenytoin (0.92 for phenytoin sodium injection and capsules; 0.92 for fosphenytoin because doses are prescribed as a phenytoin sodium equivalent or PE, 1.0 for phenytoin acid suspensions and tablets), MD is the maintenance dose of the phenytoin salt contained in the dosage form in mg/d, Css is the phenytoin concentration in mg/L (which equals µg/mL), and K_m is the substrate concentration in mg/L (which equals µg/mL) where the rate of metabolism = $V_{max}/2$.

The equation used to calculate loading doses (LD in mg) is based on a simple one-compartment model: LD = (Css • V)/S, where Css is the desired phenytoin steady-state concentration in µg/mL which is equivalent to mg/L, V is the phenytoin volume of distribution, and S is the fraction of the phenytoin salt form that is active (0.92 for phenytoin sodium injection and capsules; 0.92 for fosphenytoin because doses are prescribed as a phenytoin sodium equivalent or PE, 1.0 for phenytoin acid suspensions and tablets). Intravenous phenytoin sodium doses should be short-term infusions given no greater than 50 mg/min, and intravenous fosphenytoin doses should be short-term infusions given no greater than 150 mg/min PE.

Steady-State Concentration Selection

The general accepted therapeutic ranges for total and unbound phenytoin concentrations are 10-20 µg/mL and 1-2 µg/mL, respectively, for the treatment seizures. As previously discussed, unbound concentrations represent the portion of phenytoin that is in equilibrium with the central nervous system and should most accurately reflect drug concentration at the site of action. Thus, for patients with altered phenytoin plasma protein binding, it is more important to have the unbound concentration within its therapeutic range than the total concentration. To establish that the unbound fraction (f_B) is altered for a patient, phenytoin total and unbound concentrations should be simultaneously measured from the same blood sample: $f_B = C_f/C$, where C is the total phenytoin concentration in µg/mL and C_f is the unbound, or "free," phenytoin concentration in µg/mL. As long as the disease states or conditions that caused altered phenytoin plasma protein binding is stable, a previously measured unbound fraction can be used to convert newly measured total phenytoin concentrations to their unbound equivalent ($C_f = f_B C$). Phenytoin therapy must be individualized for each patient in order to achieve optimal responses and minimal side effects.

EXAMPLE 1 ▶▶▶

TD is a 50-year-old, 75-kg (height = 5 ft 10 in) male with simple partial seizures who requires therapy with oral phenytoin. He has normal liver and renal function. Suggest an initial phenytoin dosage regimen designed to achieve a steady-state phenytoin concentration equal to 12 µg/mL.

1. *Estimate Michaelis-Menten constants according to disease states and conditions present in the patient.*

   The V_{max} for a nonobese adult patient with normal liver and renal function is 7 mg/kg/d. For a 75-kg patient, $V_{max} = 525$ mg/d: $V_{max} = 7$ mg/kg/d • 75 kg = 525 mg/d. For this individual, $K_m = 4$ mg/L.

2. *Compute dosage regimen.*

   Oral extended phenytoin sodium capsules will be prescribed to this patient (F = 1, S = 0.92). The initial dosage interval (τ) will be set to 24 hours. (Note: µg/mL = mg/L and this concentration unit was substituted for Css in the calculations so that unnecessary unit conversion was not required.) The dosage equation for phenytoin is:

   $$MD = \frac{V_{max} \bullet Css}{S(K_m + Css)} = \frac{525 \text{ mg/d} \bullet 12 \text{ mg/L}}{0.92(4 \text{ mg/L} + 12 \text{ mg/L})} = 428 \text{ mg/d, rounded to 400 mg/d}$$

   A steady-state trough total phenytoin serum concentration should be measured after steady-state is attained in 7-14 days. Phenytoin serum concentrations should also be measured if the patient experiences an exacerbation of their epilepsy, or if the patient develops potential signs or symptoms of phenytoin toxicity.

EXAMPLE 2 ▶▶▶

UO is a 10-year-old, 40-kg male with simple partial seizures who requires therapy with oral phenytoin. He has normal liver and renal function. Suggest an initial phenytoin dosage regimen designed to achieve a steady-state phenytoin concentration equal to 12 µg/mL.

1. *Estimate Michaelis-Menten constants according to disease states and conditions present in the patient.*

   The V_{max} for a 7-16-year-old adolescent patient with normal liver and renal function is 9 mg/kg/d. For a 40-kg patient, $V_{max} = 360$ mg/d: $V_{max} = 9$ mg/kg/d • 40 kg = 360 mg/d. For this individual, $K_m = 6$ mg/L.

2. *Compute dosage regimen.*

   Oral phenytoin suspension will be prescribed to this patient (F = 1, S = 1). The initial dosage interval (τ) will be set to 12 hours. (Note: µg/mL = mg/L and this concentration unit was substituted for Css in the calculations so that unnecessary unit conversion was not required.) The dosage equation for phenytoin is:

   $$MD = \frac{V_{max} \bullet Css}{S(K_m + Css)} = \frac{360 \text{ mg/d} \bullet 12 \text{ mg/L}}{1.0(6 \text{ mg/L} + 12 \text{ mg/L})} = 240 \text{ mg/d, rounded to 250 mg/d}$$

Phenytoin suspension 125 mg every 12 hours would be prescribed for the patient. A steady-state trough total phenytoin serum concentration should be measured after steady-state is attained in 7-14 days. Phenytoin serum concentrations should also be measured if the patient experiences an exacerbation of their epilepsy, or if the patient develops potential signs or symptoms of phenytoin toxicity.

To illustrate the differences and similarities between oral and intravenous phenytoin dosage regimen design, the same cases will be used to compute intravenous phenytoin or fosphenytoin loading and maintenance doses.

EXAMPLE 3 ▶▶▶

TD is a 50-year-old, 75-kg (height = 5 ft 10 in) male with simple partial seizures who requires therapy with intravenous phenytoin sodium. He has normal liver and renal function. Suggest an initial phenytoin dosage regimen designed to achieve a steady-state phenytoin concentration equal to 12 µg/mL.

1. *Estimate Michaelis-Menten and volume of distribution constants according to disease states and conditions present in the patient.*

   The V_{max} for a nonobese adult patient with normal liver and renal function is 7 mg/kg/d. For a 75-kg patient, $V_{max} = 525$ mg/d: $V_{max} = 7$ mg/kg/d • 75 kg = 525 mg/d. For this individual, $K_m = 4$ mg/L. The volume of distribution for this patient would equal 53 L: V = 0.7 L/kg • 75 kg = 53 L.

2. *Compute dosage regimen.*

   Intravenous phenytoin sodium will be prescribed to this patient (F = 1, S = 0.92). If a loading dose is needed it would be computed using the following equation: LD = (V • Css)/S = (53 L • 12 mg/L)/0.92 = 691 mg, rounded to 700 mg given at a maximal rate of 50 mg/min. (Note: µg/mL = mg/L and this concentration unit was substituted for Css in the calculations so that unnecessary unit conversion was not required.)

   For the maintenance dose, the initial dosage interval (τ) will be set to 12 hours. The dosage equation for phenytoin is:

$$MD = \frac{V_{max} \cdot Css}{S(K_m + Css)} = \frac{525 \text{ mg/d} \cdot 12 \text{ mg/L}}{0.92(4 \text{ mg/L} + 12 \text{ mg/L})} = 428 \text{ mg/d, rounded to 400 mg/d}$$

The patient would be prescribed 200 mg of phenytoin sodium injection every 12 hours using an infusion rate no greater than 50 mg/min. A steady-state trough total phenytoin serum concentration should be measured after steady-state is attained in 7-14 days. Phenytoin serum concentrations should also be measured if the patient experiences an exacerbation of their epilepsy, or if the patient develops potential signs or symptoms of phenytoin toxicity.

EXAMPLE 4 ▶▶▶

UO is a 10-year-old, 40-kg male with simple partial seizures who requires therapy with intravenous fosphenytoin. He has normal liver and renal function. Suggest an initial phenytoin dosage regimen designed to achieve a steady-state phenytoin concentration equal to 12 µg/mL.

1. *Estimate Michaelis-Menten and volume of distribution constants according to disease states and conditions present in the patient.*

The V_{max} for a 7-16-year-old adolescent patient with normal liver and renal function is 9 mg/kg/d. For a 40-kg patient, V_{max} = 360 mg/d: V_{max} = 9 mg/kg/d • 40 kg = 360 mg/d. For this individual, K_m = 6 mg/L. The volume of distribution for this patient would equal 28 L: V = 0.7 L/kg • 40 kg = 28 L.

2. *Compute dosage regimen.*

Intravenous fosphenytoin will be prescribed, in phenytoin sodium equivalents or PE, to this patient (F = 1, S = 0.92). If a loading dose is needed, it would be computed using the following equation: LD = (V • Css)/S = (28 L • 12 mg/L)/0.92 = 365 mg, rounded to 350 mg given at a maximal rate of 150 mg/min PE. (Note: µg/mL = mg/L and this concentration unit was substituted for Css in the calculations so that unnecessary unit conversion was not required.) The dosage equation for phenytoin is:

$$MD = \frac{V_{max} \bullet Css}{S(K_m + Css)} = \frac{360 \text{ mg/d} \bullet 12 \text{ mg/L}}{0.92(6 \text{ mg/L} + 12 \text{ mg/L})} = 261 \text{ mg/d, rounded to } 250 \text{ mg/d}$$

Intravenous fosphenytoin 125 mg PE every 12 hours given no greater than 150 mg/min PE would be prescribed for the patient. A steady-state trough total phenytoin serum concentration should be measured after steady-state is attained in 7-14 days. Phenytoin serum concentrations should also be measured if the patient experiences an exacerbation of their epilepsy, or if the patient develops potential signs or symptoms of phenytoin toxicity.

LITERATURE-BASED RECOMMENDED DOSING

Because of the large amount of variability in phenytoin pharmacokinetics, even when concurrent disease states and conditions are identified, many clinicians believe that the use of standard phenytoin doses for various situations are warranted. The original computations of these doses were based on the Pharmacokinetic Dosing methods described in the previous section, and subsequently modified based on clinical experience. In general, the expected phenytoin steady-state serum concentrations used to compute these doses was 10-15 µg/mL. Suggested phenytoin maintenance doses are 4-6 mg/kg/d for adults and 5-10 mg/kg/d for children (6 months-16 years old). Phenytoin-loading doses are 15-20 mg/kg. For obese individuals (>30% over ideal body weight), adjusted body weight (ABW) should be used to compute loading doses: ABW (in kg) = IBW + 1.33(TBW − IBW), where IBW is ideal body weight in kg [IBW$_{females}$ (in kg) = 45 + 2.3(Ht − 60) or IBW$_{males}$ (in kg) = 50 + 2.3(Ht − 60)], Ht is height in inches, and TBW is total body weight in kg.[74] Although clearance probably is increased in obese individuals, precise information regarding the best weight factor is lacking for maintenance dose computation, so most clinicians use ideal body weight to calculate this dose. If the patient has significant hepatic dysfunction (Child-Pugh score ≥8), maintenance doses prescribed using this method should be decreased by 25%-50% depending on how aggressive therapy is required to be for the individual. Doses of phenytoin, phenytoin sodium, or fosphenytoin (in PE or phenytoin sodium equivalents) are computed using these dosage rates since dosage amounts will be rounded to clinically acceptable amounts.

To illustrate the similarities and differences between this method of dosage calculation and the Pharmacokinetic Dosing method, the same examples used in the previous section will be used.

EXAMPLE 1 ▶▶▶

TD is a 50-year-old, 75-kg (height = 5 ft 10 in) male with simple partial seizures who requires therapy with oral phenytoin. He has normal liver and renal function. Suggest an initial phenytoin dosage regimen designed to achieve a steady-state phenytoin concentration equal to 12 μg/mL.

1. *Estimate phenytoin dose according to disease states and conditions present in the patient.*

The suggested initial dosage rate for extended phenytoin sodium capsules in an adult patient is 4-6 mg/kg/d. Using a rate of 5 mg/kg/d, the initial dose would be 400 mg/d: 5 mg/kg/d • 75 kg = 375 mg/d, rounded to 400 mg/d. Using a dosage interval of 24 hours, the prescribed dose would be 400 mg of extended phenytoin sodium capsules daily.

A steady-state trough total phenytoin serum concentration should be measured after steady-state is attained in 7-14 days. Phenytoin serum concentrations should also be measured if the patient experiences an exacerbation of their epilepsy, or if the patient develops potential signs or symptoms of phenytoin toxicity.

EXAMPLE 2 ▶▶▶

UO is a 10-year-old, 40-kg male with simple partial seizures who requires therapy with oral phenytoin. He has normal liver and renal function. Suggest an initial phenytoin dosage regimen designed to achieve a steady-state phenytoin concentration equal to 12 μg/mL.

1. *Estimate phenytoin dose according to disease states and conditions present in the patient.*

The suggested initial dosage rate for phenytoin suspension in an adolescent patient is 5-10 mg/kg/d. Using a rate of 6 mg/kg/d, the initial dose would be 250 mg/d: 6 mg/kg/d • 40 kg = 240 mg/d, rounded to 250 mg/d. Using a dosage interval of 12 hours, the prescribed dose would be 125 mg of phenytoin suspension every 12 hours.

A steady-state trough total phenytoin serum concentration should be measured after steady-state is attained in 7-14 days. Phenytoin serum concentrations should also be measured if the patient experiences an exacerbation of their epilepsy, or if the patient develops potential signs or symptoms of phenytoin toxicity.

To illustrate the differences and similarities between oral and intravenous phenytoin dosage regimen design, the same cases will be used to compute intravenous phenytoin or fosphenytoin loading and maintenance doses.

EXAMPLE 3 ▶▶▶

TD is a 50-year-old, 75-kg (height = 5 ft 10 in) male with simple partial seizures who requires therapy with intravenous phenytoin sodium. He has normal liver and renal function. Suggest an initial phenytoin dosage regimen designed to achieve a steady-state phenytoin concentration equal to 12 μg/mL.

1. *Estimate phenytoin dose according to disease states and conditions present in the patient.*

The suggested initial dosage rate for phenytoin sodium injection in an adult patient is 4-6 mg/kg/d. Using a rate of 5 mg/kg/d, the initial dose would be 400 mg/d: 5 mg/kg/d • 75 kg = 375 mg/d, rounded to 400 mg/d. Using a dosage interval of 12 hours, the prescribed dose would be 200 mg of phenytoin sodium injection every 12 hours. If loading dose administration was necessary, the suggested amount is 15-20 mg/kg. Using 15 mg/kg, the suggested loading dose would be 1250 mg of phenytoin sodium injection given no faster than 50 mg/min: 15 mg/kg • 75 kg = 1125 mg, rounded to 1250 mg.

A steady-state trough total phenytoin serum concentration should be measured after steady-state is attained in 7-14 days. Phenytoin serum concentrations should also be measured if the patient experiences an exacerbation of their epilepsy, or if the patient develops potential signs or symptoms of phenytoin toxicity.

EXAMPLE 4 ▶▶▶

UO is a 10-year-old, 40-kg male with simple partial seizures who requires therapy with intravenous fosphenytoin. He has normal liver and renal function. Suggest an initial phenytoin dosage regimen designed to achieve a steady-state phenytoin concentration equal to 12 µg/mL.

1. *Estimate phenytoin dose according to disease states and conditions present in the patient.*
   The suggested initial dosage rate for fosphenytoin injection in an adolescent patient is 5-10 mg/kg/d PE. Using a rate of 6 mg/kg/d, the initial dose would be 250 mg/d PE: 6 mg/kg/d • 40 kg = 240 mg/d, rounded to 250 mg/d. Using a dosage interval of 12 hours, the prescribed dose would be 125 mg of fosphenytoin injection every 12 hours. If loading dose administration was necessary, the suggested amount is 15-20 mg/kg PE. Using 15 mg/kg, the suggested loading dose would be 600 mg PE of fosphenytoin injection given no faster than 150 mg/min PE: 15 mg/kg • 40 kg = 600 mg.

   A steady-state trough total phenytoin serum concentration should be measured after steady-state is attained in 7-14 days. Phenytoin serum concentrations should also be measured if the patient experiences an exacerbation of their epilepsy, or if the patient develops potential signs or symptoms of phenytoin toxicity.

USE OF PHENYTOIN SERUM CONCENTRATIONS TO ALTER DOSES

Because of the large amount of pharmacokinetic variability among patients, it is likely that doses computed using patient population characteristics will not always produce phenytoin serum concentrations that are expected or desirable. Because of pharmacokinetic variability, the Michaelis-Menten pharmacokinetics followed by the drug, the narrow therapeutic index of phenytoin, and the desire to avoid adverse side effects of phenytoin, measurement of phenytoin serum concentrations is conducted for almost all patients to insure that therapeutic, nontoxic levels are present. In addition to phenytoin serum concentrations, important patient parameters (seizure frequency, potential phenytoin side effects, etc) should be followed to confirm that the patient is responding to treatment and not developing adverse drug reactions.

When phenytoin serum concentrations are measured in patients and a dosage change is necessary, clinicians should seek to use the simplest, most straightforward method available to determine a dose that will provide safe and effective treatment. A variety of methods are used to estimate new maintenance doses or Michaelis-Menten parameters when one steady-state phenytoin serum concentration is available. Based on typical Michaelis-Menten parameters, it is possible to adjust phenytoin doses with one or more steady-state concentrations using the *Empiric Dosing method*. This is a widely used technique to adjust doses by experienced clinicians. The *Graves-Cloyd method* allows adjustment of phenytoin doses using one steady-state concentration. Because it uses a power function, it is computationally intensive. The *Vozeh-Sheiner method* utilizes a specialized graph and Bayesian pharmacokinetic concepts to individualize phenytoin doses using a single steady-state concentration. Because of this, a copy of the graph paper with population orbits must be available, and plotting the data is time consuming.

Sometimes, it is useful to compute phenytoin pharmacokinetic constants for a patient and base dosage adjustments on these. If two or more steady-state phenytoin serum concentrations are available from two or more daily dosage rates, it may be possible to calculate and use *pharmacokinetic parameters* to alter the phenytoin dose. Two graphical methods allow the computation of V_{max} and K_m for patients receiving phenytoin, but they are cumbersome and time consuming. The *Mullen method* uses the same specialized graph as the Vozeh-Sheiner method, but computes the patients own Michaelis-Menten parameters instead of Bayesian pharmacokinetic estimates. The *Ludden method* uses standard graph paper to plot the concentration-time data, and V_{max} and K_m are computed from the intercept and slope of the resulting line.

Finally, computerized methods that incorporate expected population pharmacokinetic characteristics (*Bayesian pharmacokinetic computer programs*) can be used in difficult cases where serum concentrations are obtained at suboptimal times or the patient was not at steady-state when serum concentrations were measured. An additional benefit of this method is that a complete pharmacokinetic workup (V_{max}, K_m, V) can be done with one or more measured concentrations.

So that results from the different methods can be compared, the same cases are used to compute adjusted doses for phenytoin.

Single Total Phenytoin Steady-State Serum Concentration Methods

Empiric Dosing Method

Based on the knowledge of population Michaelis-Menten pharmacokinetic parameters, it is possible to suggest empiric dosage increases for phenytoin when one steady-state serum concentration is available (Table 10-4).[75] The lower end of the suggested dosage range for each category tends to produce more conservative increases in steady-state concentration while the upper end of the suggested dosage range tends to produce more aggressive increases. These dosage changes are based on outpatients where avoiding adverse drug reactions is paramount. For hospitalized patients or patients requiring aggressive treatment, larger empiric dosage adjustments may be needed. When dosage increases >100 mg/d are recommended, phenytoin concentrations and patient response should be carefully monitored.

Wherever possible, clinicians should avoid using more than one solid dosage form strength (ie, mixing 30 and 100 mg extended phenytoin capsules, etc) for a patient. An effective way to increase the phenytoin dose for an individual that requires an increase in dose of 50 mg/d when using the 100-mg extended phenytoin sodium capsule dosage form is to increase the dose by 100 mg every other day. For example, if a dosage increase of 50 mg/d is desired for an individual receiving 300 mg/d of extended phenytoin sodium capsule, a dosage increase of 300 mg/d alternating with 400 mg/d is possible if the patient is able to comply with a more complex dosage schedule. Dosage aids such as calendars, prefilled dosage cassettes, or memory-aiding schemes (400 mg/d on even days, 300 mg/d on odd days) are all useful in different patient situations. Alternate daily dosages are possible because of the extended-release characteristics of extended phenytoin capsules and the long half-life of phenytoin.

TABLE 10-4   Empiric Phenytoin Dosage Increases Based On a Single Total Steady-State Concentration

Measured Phenytoin Total Serum Concentration (μg/mL)	Suggested Dosage Increase[a]
<7	100 mg/d or more
7-12	50-100 mg/d
>12	30-50 mg/d

[a]Higher dosage used if more aggressive therapy desired, lower dosage used if less aggressive therapy desired.
Modified from Mauro, et al.[75]

EXAMPLE 1 ▶▶▶

TD is a 50-year-old, 75-kg (height = 5 ft 10 in) male with simple partial seizures who requires therapy with oral phenytoin. He has normal liver and renal function. The patient was prescribed 400 mg/d of extended phenytoin sodium capsules for 1 month, and the steady-state phenytoin total concentration equals 6.2 µg/mL. The patient is assessed to be compliant with his dosage regimen. Suggest an initial phenytoin dosage regimen designed to achieve a steady-state phenytoin concentration within the therapeutic range.

1. *Use Table 10-4 to suggest new phenytoin dose.*

   The table suggests a dosage increase of ≥100 mg/d for this patient. The dose would be increased to 500 mg/d.

   A steady-state trough total phenytoin serum concentration should be measured after steady-state is attained in 7-14 days. Phenytoin serum concentrations should also be measured if the patient experiences an exacerbation of their epilepsy, or if the patient develops potential signs or symptoms of phenytoin toxicity.

EXAMPLE 2 ▶▶▶

GF is a 35-year-old, 55-kg female with tonic-clonic seizures who requires therapy with oral phenytoin. She has normal liver and renal function. The patient was prescribed 300 mg/d of extended phenytoin sodium capsules for 1 month, and the steady-state phenytoin total concentration equals 10.7 µg/mL. The patient is assessed to be compliant with her dosage regimen. Suggest an initial phenytoin dosage regimen designed to achieve a steady-state phenytoin concentration within the middle of the therapeutic range.

1. *Use Table 10-4 to suggest new phenytoin dose.*

   The table suggests a dosage increase of 50-100 mg/d for this patient. The dose would be increased to 300 mg/d alternating with 400 mg/d.

   A steady-state trough total phenytoin serum concentration should be measured after steady-state is attained in 7-14 days. Phenytoin serum concentrations should also be measured if the patient experiences an exacerbation of their epilepsy, or if the patient develops potential signs or symptoms of phenytoin toxicity.

Pseudolinear Pharmacokinetics Method

A simple, easy way to approximate new total serum concentrations after a dosage adjustment with phenytoin is to temporarily assume linear pharmacokinetics, then add 15%-33% for a dosage increase or subtract 15%-33% for a dosage decrease to account for Michaelis-Menten pharmacokinetics: $Css_{new} = (D_{new}/D_{old})Css_{old}$, where Css_{new} is the expected steady-state concentration from the new phenytoin dose in µg/mL, Css_{old} is the measured steady-state concentration from the old phenytoin dose in µg/mL, D_{new} is the new phenytoin dose to be prescribed in mg/d, and D_{old} is the currently prescribed phenytoin dose in mg/d.[76] *Note:* This method is only intended to provide a rough approximation of the resulting phenytoin steady-state concentration after an appropriate dosage adjustment, such as that suggested by the Mauro dosage chart, has been made. The Pseudolinear Pharmacokinetics method should never be used to compute a new dose based on measured and desired phenytoin concentrations.

EXAMPLE 3 ▶▶▶

TD is a 50-year-old, 75-kg (height = 5 ft 10 in) male with simple partial seizures who requires therapy with oral phenytoin. He has normal liver and renal function. The patient was prescribed 400 mg/d of extended phenytoin sodium capsules for 1 month, and the steady-state phenytoin total concentration equals 6.2 μg/mL. The patient is assessed to be compliant with his dosage regimen. Suggest an initial phenytoin dosage regimen designed to achieve a steady-state phenytoin concentration within the therapeutic range.

1. *Use pseudolinear pharmacokinetics to predict new concentration for a dosage increase, then compute 15%-33% factor to account for Michaelis-Menten pharmacokinetics.*

   Since the patient is receiving extended phenytoin sodium capsules, a convenient dosage change would be 100 mg/d and an increase to 500 mg/d is suggested. Using pseudolinear pharmacokinetics, the resulting total steady-state phenytoin serum concentration would be estimated as: $Css_{new} = (D_{new}/D_{old})Css_{old} = (500$ mg/d / 400 mg/d)6.2 μg/mL = 7.8 μg/mL. Because of Michaelis-Menten pharmacokinetics, the serum concentration would be expected to increase 15%, or 1.15 times, to 33%, or 1.33 times, greater than that predicted by linear pharmacokinetics: Css = 7.8 μg/mL • 1.15 = 9.0 μg/mL and Css = 7.8 μg/mL • 1.33 = 10.4 μg/mL. Thus, a dosage increase of 100 mg/d would be expected to yield a total phenytoin steady-state serum concentration between 9 and 11 μg/mL.

   A steady-state trough total phenytoin serum concentration should be measured after steady-state is attained in 7-14 days. Phenytoin serum concentrations should also be measured if the patient experiences an exacerbation of their epilepsy, or if the patient develops potential signs or symptoms of phenytoin toxicity.

EXAMPLE 4 ▶▶▶

GF is a 35-year-old, 55-kg female with tonic-clonic seizures who requires therapy with oral phenytoin. She has normal liver and renal function. The patient was prescribed 300 mg/d of extended phenytoin sodium capsules for 1 month, and the steady-state phenytoin total concentration equals 10.7 μg/mL. The patient is assessed to be compliant with her dosage regimen. Suggest an initial phenytoin dosage regimen designed to achieve a steady-state phenytoin concentration within the middle of the therapeutic range.

1. *Use pseudolinear pharmacokinetics to predict new concentration for a dosage increase, then compute 15%-33% factor to account for Michaelis-Menten pharmacokinetics.*

   Since the patient is receiving extended phenytoin sodium capsules, a convenient dosage change would be 100 mg/d and an increase to 400 mg/d is suggested. Using pseudolinear pharmacokinetics, the resulting total steady-state phenytoin serum concentration would be estimated as: $Css_{new} = (D_{new}/D_{old})Css_{old} = (400$ mg/d / 300 mg/d)10.7 μg/mL = 14.3 μg/mL. Because of Michaelis-Menten pharmacokinetics, the serum concentration would be expected to increase 15%, or 1.15 times, to 33%, or 1.33 times, greater than that predicted by linear pharmacokinetics: Css = 14.3 μg/mL • 1.15 = 16.4 μg/mL and Css = 14.3 μg/mL • 1.33 = 19.0 μg/mL. Thus, a dosage increase of 100 mg/d would be expected to yield a total phenytoin steady-state serum concentration between 16 and 19 μg/mL.

   A steady-state trough total phenytoin serum concentration should be measured after steady-state is attained in 7-14 days. Phenytoin serum concentrations should also be measured if the patient experiences an exacerbation of their epilepsy, or if the patient develops potential signs or symptoms of phenytoin toxicity.

Graves-Cloyd Method

This dosage adjustment method uses a steady-state phenytoin serum concentration to compute the patient's own phenytoin clearance rate (D_{old}/Css_{old}, where D_{old} is the administered phenytoin dose in mg/d and Css_{old} is the resulting measured total phenytoin steady-state concentration in µg/mL) at the dosage being given, then uses the measured concentration and desired concentration (Css_{new} in µg/mL) to estimate a new dose (D_{new} in mg/d) for the patient:[77] $D_{new} = (D_{old}/Css_{old}) \bullet Css_{new}^{0.199} \bullet Css_{old}^{0.804}$.

EXAMPLE 5 ▶▶▶

TD is a 50-year-old, 75-kg (height = 5 ft 10 in) male with simple partial seizures who requires therapy with oral phenytoin. He has normal liver and renal function. The patient was prescribed 400 mg/d of extended phenytoin sodium capsules for 1 month, and the steady-state phenytoin total concentration equals 6.2 µg/mL. The patient is assessed to be compliant with his dosage regimen. Suggest an initial phenytoin dosage regimen designed to achieve a steady-state phenytoin concentration within the therapeutic range.

1. *Use Graves-Cloyd method to estimate a new phenytoin dose for desired steady-state concentration.*

   Phenytoin sodium 400 mg equals 368 mg of phenytoin (400 mg • 0.92 = 368 mg). A new total phenytoin steady-state serum concentration equal to 10 µg/mL is chosen for the patient: $D_{new} = (D_{old}/Css_{old}) \bullet Css_{new}^{0.199} \bullet Css_{old}^{0.804}$ = (368 mg/d / 6.2 mg/L) • (10 mg/L)$^{0.199}$ • (6.2 mg/L)$^{0.804}$ = 407 mg/d. This is equivalent to 442 mg/d of phenytoin sodium (407 mg/0.92 = 442 mg) rounded to 450 mg/d, or 400 mg/d on even days alternating with 500 mg/d on odd days.

   A steady-state trough total phenytoin serum concentration should be measured after steady-state is attained in 7-14 days. Phenytoin serum concentrations should also be measured if the patient experiences an exacerbation of their epilepsy, or if the patient develops potential signs or symptoms of phenytoin toxicity.

EXAMPLE 6 ▶▶▶

GF is a 35-year-old, 55-kg female with tonic-clonic seizures who requires therapy with oral phenytoin. She has normal liver and renal function. The patient was prescribed 300 mg/d of extended phenytoin sodium capsules for 1 month, and the steady-state phenytoin total concentration equals 10.7 µg/mL. The patient is assessed to be compliant with her dosage regimen. Suggest an initial phenytoin dosage regimen designed to achieve a steady-state phenytoin concentration of 18 µg/mL.

1. *Use Graves-Cloyd method to estimate a new phenytoin dose for desired steady-state concentration.*

   Phenytoin sodium 300 mg equals 276 mg of phenytoin (300 mg • 0.92 = 276 mg). A new total phenytoin steady-state serum concentration equal to 18 µg/mL is chosen for the patient: $D_{new} = (D_{old}/Css_{old}) \bullet Css_{new}^{0.199} \bullet Css_{old}^{0.804}$ = (276 mg/d / 10.7 mg/L) • (18 mg/L)$^{0.199}$ • (10.7 mg/L)$^{0.804}$ = 308 mg/d. This is equivalent to 335 mg/d of phenytoin sodium (308 mg/0.92 = 335 mg) rounded to 350 mg/d, or 300 mg/d on odd days alternating with 400 mg/d on even days.

   A steady-state trough total phenytoin serum concentration should be measured after steady-state is attained in 7-14 days. Phenytoin serum concentrations should also be measured if the patient experiences an exacerbation of their epilepsy, or if the patient develops potential signs or symptoms of phenytoin toxicity.

Vozeh-Sheiner or Orbit Graph Method

A graphical method that employs population Michaelis-Menten information using Bayes theorem can also be used to adjust phenytoin doses using a single steady-state total concentration.[78] This method employs a series of orbs encompassing 50%, 75%, 85%, etc of the population parameter combinations for V_{max} and K_m on the plot suggested by Mullen for use with multiple steady-state/dosage pairs (Figure 10-3). The use of the population's parameter orbs allows the plot to be used with one phenytoin steady-state concentration/dose pair.

The graph is divided into two sectors. On the left side of the x-axis, a steady-state total phenytoin concentration is plotted. On the y-axis, the phenytoin dosage rate (in mg/kg/d of phenytoin; S = 0.92 for phenytoin sodium and fosphenytoin PE dosage forms) is plotted. A straight line is drawn between these two points, extended into the right sector, and through the orbs contained in the right sector. If the line intersects more than one orb, the innermost orb is selected, and the midpoint of the line contained within that orb is found and marked with a point. The midpoint within the orb and the desired steady-state phenytoin total concentration (on the left portion of the x-axis) are connected by a straight line. The intersection of this line with the y-axis is the new phenytoin dose required to achieve the new phenytoin concentration. If needed, the phenytoin dose is converted to phenytoin sodium or fosphenytoin amounts. If a line parallel to the y-axis is drawn down to the x-axis from the midpoint of the line contained within the orb, an estimate of K_m (in µg/mL) is obtained. Similarly, if a line parallel to the x-axis is drawn to the left to the y-axis from the midpoint of the line contained within the orb, an estimate of V_{max} (in mg/kg/d) is obtained.

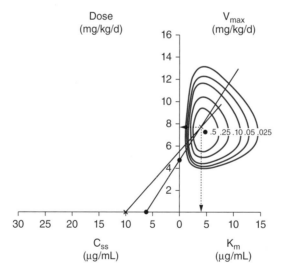

FIGURE 10-3   Vozeh-Sheiner or Orbit Graph employing Bayesian feedback used to estimate Michaelis-Menten parameters and phenytoin dose using one steady-state dose/concentration pair (example 7 data shown). The orbs represent 50%, 75%, 85%, etc of the population parameter combinations for V_{max} and K_m. The drug dose is converted into a phenytoin amount (in mg/kg/d) and plotted on the y-axis (circle, 4.9 mg/kg/d). The concurrent steady-state phenytoin serum concentration is plotted on the left portion of the x-axis (circle, 6.2 µg/mL), and the two points are joined with a straight line across the orbs. If the line intersects more than one orb, the innermost orb is selected, and the midpoint of the line contained within that orb is found and marked (x mark within orbs). The new desired steady-state concentration is identified on the left portion of the x-axis (x mark on x-axis, 10 µg/mL), and the two x marks are connected by a straight line. The required phenytoin dose is identified at the intersection of the drawn line and the y-axis (5.5 mg/kg/d). If necessary, the dose would be converted to phenytoin sodium or fosphenytoin amounts. Estimates of V_{max} (7.9 mg/kg/d) and K_m (4 µg/mL) are obtained by extrapolating parallel lines to the y- and x-axes, respectively.

EXAMPLE 7 ▶▶▶

TD is a 50-year-old, 75-kg (height = 5 ft 10 in) male with simple partial seizures who requires therapy with oral phenytoin. He has normal liver and renal function. The patient was prescribed 400 mg/d of extended phenytoin sodium capsules for 1 month, and the steady-state phenytoin total concentration equals 6.2 µg/mL. The patient is assessed to be compliant with his dosage regimen. Suggest an initial phenytoin dosage regimen designed to achieve a steady-state phenytoin concentration within the therapeutic range.

1. *Use Vozeh-Sheiner method to estimate a new phenytoin dose for desired steady-state concentration.*
   A new total phenytoin steady-state serum concentration equal to 10 µg/mL is chosen for the patient. Using the orbit graph, the serum concentration/dose information is plotted (note: phenytoin dose = 0.92 • phenytoin sodium dose = 0.92 • 400 mg/d = 368 mg/d; 368 mg/d / 75 kg = 4.9 mg/kg/d; see Figure 10-3). According to the graph, a dose of 5.5 mg/kg/d of phenytoin is required to achieve a steady-state concentration equal to 10 µg/mL. This equals an extended phenytoin sodium capsule dose of 450 mg/d, administered by alternating 400 mg/d on even days and 500 mg/d on odd days: (5.5 mg/kg/d • 75 kg)/0.92 = 448 mg/d, rounded to 450 mg/d.
   A steady-state trough total phenytoin serum concentration should be measured after steady-state is attained in 7-14 days. Phenytoin serum concentrations should also be measured if the patient experiences an exacerbation of their epilepsy, or if the patient develops potential signs or symptoms of phenytoin toxicity.

EXAMPLE 8 ▶▶▶

GF is a 35-year-old, 55-kg female with tonic-clonic seizures who requires therapy with oral phenytoin. She has normal liver and renal function. The patient was prescribed 300 mg/d of extended phenytoin sodium capsules for 1 month, and the steady-state phenytoin total concentration equals 10.7 µg/mL. The patient is assessed to be compliant with her dosage regimen. Suggest an initial phenytoin dosage regimen designed to achieve a steady-state phenytoin concentration of 18 µg/mL.

1. *Use Vozeh-Sheiner method to estimate a new phenytoin dose for desired steady-state concentration.*
   A new total phenytoin steady-state serum concentration equal to 18 µg/mL is chosen for the patient. Using the orbit graph, the serum concentration/dose information is plotted (note: phenytoin dose = 0.92 • phenytoin sodium dose = 0.92 • 300 mg/d = 276 mg/d; 276 mg/d / 55 kg = 5.0 mg/kg/d; see Figure 10-4). According to the graph, a dose of 5.7 mg/kg/d of phenytoin is required to achieve a steady-state concentration equal to 18 µg/mL. This equals an extended phenytoin sodium capsule dose of 350 mg/d, administered by alternating 300 mg/d on even days and 400 mg/d on odd days: (5.7 mg/kg/d • 55 kg)/0.92 = 341 mg/d, rounded to 350 mg/d.
   A steady-state trough total phenytoin serum concentration should be measured after steady-state is attained in 7-14 days. Phenytoin serum concentrations should also be measured if the patient experiences an exacerbation of their epilepsy, or if the patient develops potential signs or symptoms of phenytoin toxicity.

Two or More Phenytoin Steady-State Serum Concentrations at Two or More Dosage Levels Methods

In order to utilize each of the dosage schemes in this section, at least two phenytoin steady-state serum concentrations at different dosage rates are needed. This requirement can be difficult to achieve.

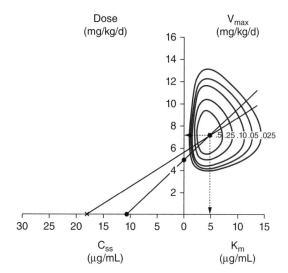

FIGURE 10-4   Vozeh-Sheiner or Orbit Graph employing Bayesian feedback used to estimate Michaelis-Menten parameters and phenytoin dose using one steady-state dose/concentration pair. The graph shows the solution for example 8.

Empiric Dosing Method

Based on the knowledge of population Michaelis-Menten pharmacokinetic parameters, it is possible to suggest empiric dosage increases for phenytoin with two or more steady-state serum concentrations at two or more dosage levels.[76] For instance, if a patient has a steady-state phenytoin concentration equal to 11.2 μg/mL on 300 mg/d of phenytoin sodium and 25.3 μg/mL on 400 mg/d of phenytoin sodium, it is obvious that a dose of 350 mg/d of phenytoin sodium will probably produce a steady-state phenytoin serum concentration in the mid-to-upper end of the therapeutic range. Similarly, if a patient has a steady-state phenytoin concentration equal to 11.2 μg/mL on 300 mg/d of phenytoin sodium and 15.0 μg/mL on 400 mg/d of phenytoin sodium, it is apparent that a dose of 450 mg/d of phenytoin sodium will probably produce a steady-state phenytoin serum concentration in the upper end of the therapeutic range. In the latter situation, Table 10-4 can be useful to suggest dosage increases.

EXAMPLE 1 ▶▶▶

TD is a 50-year-old, 75-kg (height = 5 ft 10 in) male with simple partial seizures who requires therapy with oral phenytoin. He has normal liver and renal function. The patient was prescribed 400 mg/d of extended phenytoin sodium capsules for 1 month, and the steady-state phenytoin total concentration equals 6.2 μg/mL. The dosage was increased to 500 mg/d of extended phenytoin sodium capsules for another month, the steady-state phenytoin total concentration equals 22.0 μg/mL, and the patient has some lateral-gaze nystagmus. The patient is assessed to be compliant with his dosage regimen. Suggest a new phenytoin dosage regimen designed to achieve a steady-state phenytoin concentration within the mid-to-upper end of the therapeutic range.

1. *Empirically suggest new phenytoin dose.*

The next logical dose to prescribe is phenytoin sodium 450 mg/d to be taken by the patient as 400 mg/d on even days and 500 mg/d on odd days.

A steady-state trough total phenytoin serum concentration should be measured after steady-state is attained in 7-14 days. Phenytoin serum concentrations should also be measured if the patient experiences an exacerbation of their epilepsy, or if the patient develops potential signs or symptoms of phenytoin toxicity.

EXAMPLE 2 ▶▶▶

GF is a 35-year-old, 55-kg female with tonic-clonic seizures who requires therapy with oral phenytoin. She has normal liver and renal function. The patient was prescribed 300 mg/d of extended phenytoin sodium capsules for 1 month, and the steady-state phenytoin total concentration equals 10.7 µg/mL. At that time, the dose was increased to 350 mg/d of extended phenytoin sodium capsules for an additional month, and the resulting steady-state concentration was 15.8 µg/mL. The patient is assessed to be compliant with her dosage regimen. Suggest a new phenytoin dosage regimen increase designed to achieve a steady-state phenytoin concentration within the upper end of the therapeutic range.

1. *Empirically suggest new phenytoin dose.*
   The next logical dose to prescribe is phenytoin sodium 400 mg/d (see Table 10-4).
      A steady-state trough total phenytoin serum concentration should be measured after steady-state is attained in 7-14 days. Phenytoin serum concentrations should also be measured if the patient experiences an exacerbation of their epilepsy, or if the patient develops potential signs or symptoms of phenytoin toxicity.

Mullen Method

This dosage approach uses the same dose/concentration plot as that described for the Vozeh-Sheiner or Orbit Graph method, but the population orbs denoting the Bayesian distribution of V_{max} and K_m parameters are omitted.[79,80] As before, the graph is divided into two sectors. On the left side of the x-axis, a steady-state total phenytoin concentration is plotted. On the y-axis, the phenytoin dosage rate (in mg/kg/d of phenytoin; S = 0.92 for phenytoin sodium and fosphenytoin PE dosage forms) is plotted. A straight line is drawn between these two points and extended into the right sector. This process is repeated for all steady-state dose/concentrations pairs that are available. The intersection of these lines in the right sector provides the Michaelis-Menten constant values for the patient. If a line parallel to the y-axis is drawn down to the x-axis from the intersection point, K_m (in µg/mL) is obtained. Similarly, if a line parallel to the x-axis is drawn to the left to the y-axis from the intersection point, an estimate of V_{max} (in mg/kg/d) is obtained. To compute the new phenytoin dose, the intersection point and the desired steady-state phenytoin total concentration (on the left portion of the x-axis) are connected by a straight line. The intersection of this line with the y-axis is the new phenytoin dose required to achieve the new phenytoin concentration. If needed, the phenytoin dose is converted to phenytoin sodium or fosphenytoin amounts.

EXAMPLE 3 ▶▶▶

TD is a 50–year-old, 75-kg (height = 5 ft 10 in) male with simple partial seizures who requires therapy with oral phenytoin. He has normal liver and renal function. The patient was prescribed 400 mg/d of extended phenytoin sodium capsules for 1 month, and the steady-state phenytoin total concentration equals 6.2 µg/mL. The dosage was increased to 500 mg/d of extended phenytoin sodium capsules for another month, the steady state phenytoin total concentration equals 22.0 µg/mL, and the patient has some lateral-gaze nystagmus. The patient is assessed to be compliant with his dosage regimen. Suggest a new phenytoin dosage regimen designed to achieve a steady-state phenytoin concentration within the therapeutic range.

1. *Use Mullen method to estimate a new phenytoin dose for desired steady-state concentration.*
   Using the graph, the serum concentration/dose information is plotted (note: phenytoin dose = 0.92 • phenytoin sodium dose = 0.92 • 400 mg/d = 368 mg/d, 368 mg/d / 75 kg = 4.9 mg/kg/d; phenytoin dose = 0.92 • phenytoin sodium dose = 0.92 • 500 mg/d = 460 mg/d, 460 mg/d / 75 kg = 6.1 mg/kg/d; see Figure 10-5).

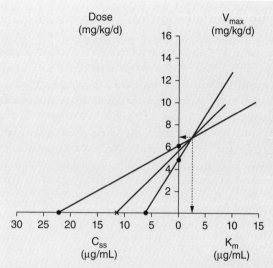

FIGURE 10-5 Mullen graph used to compute Michaelis-Menten parameters and phenytoin dose using two or more steady-state dose/concentration pairs (example 3 data shown). The first dose and concentration are plotted as circles on the y- (4.9 mg/kg/d) and x-axes (6.2 μg/mL), respectively, and joined by a straight line. This process is repeated for the second dose/concentration pair (6.1 mg/kg/d, 22 μg/mL) plus any others that are available. The intersection of the lines in the right sector of the graph is used to compute a new dose by drawing a straight line between the intersection and the new desired steady-state concentration on the left portion of the x-axis (x on x-axis, 11.5 μg/mL). The required dose is the intersection of this new line with the y-axis (5.5 mg/kg/d). Estimates of V_{max} (6.8 mg/kg/d) and K_m (2.2 μg/mL) are obtained by extrapolating parallel lines to the y- and x-axes, respectively.

According to the graph, a dose of 5.5 mg/kg/d of phenytoin is required to achieve a steady-state concentration equal to 11.5 μg/mL. This equals an extended phenytoin sodium capsule dose of 450 mg/d, administered by alternating 400 mg/d on even days and 500 mg/d on odd days: (5.5 mg/kg/d • 75 kg)/0.92 = 448 mg/d, rounded to 450 mg/d. V_{max} = 6.8 mg/kg/d and K_m = 2.2 μg/mL for this patient.

A steady-state trough total phenytoin serum concentration should be measured after steady-state is attained in 7-14 days. Phenytoin serum concentrations should also be measured if the patient experiences an exacerbation of their epilepsy, or if the patient develops potential signs or symptoms of phenytoin toxicity.

EXAMPLE 4 ▶▶▶

GF is a 35-year-old, 55-kg female with tonic-clonic seizures who requires therapy with oral phenytoin. She has normal liver and renal function. The patient was prescribed 300 mg/d of extended phenytoin sodium capsules for 1 month, and the steady-state phenytoin total concentration equals 10.7 μg/mL. At that time, the dose was increased to 350 mg/d of extended phenytoin sodium capsules for an additional month, and the resulting steady-state concentration was 15.8 μg/mL. The patient is assessed to be compliant with her dosage regimen. Suggest a new phenytoin dosage regimen increase designed to achieve a steady-state phenytoin concentration within the upper end of the therapeutic range.

1. *Use Mullen method to estimate a new phenytoin dose for desired steady-state concentration.*

   Using the graph, the serum concentration/dose information is plotted (note: phenytoin dose = 0.92 • phenytoin sodium dose = 0.92 • 300 mg/d = 276 mg/d, 276 mg/d/55 kg = 5 mg/kg/d; phenytoin dose = 0.92 • phenytoin sodium dose = 0.92 • 350 mg/d = 322 mg/d, 322 mg/d/55 kg = 5.9 mg/kg/d; Figure 10-6). According to the graph, a dose of 6.7 mg/kg/d of phenytoin is required to achieve a steady-state concentration equal to 22 μg/mL. This equals an extended phenytoin sodium capsule dose of 400 mg/d: (6.7 mg/kg/d • 55 kg)/0.92 = 401 mg/d, rounded to 400 mg/d. V_{max} = 9.4 mg/kg/d and K_m = 9.5 μg/mL for this patient.

   A steady-state trough total phenytoin serum concentration should be measured after steady-state is attained in 7-14 days. Phenytoin serum concentrations should also be measured if the patient experiences an exacerbation of their epilepsy, or if the patient develops potential signs or symptoms of phenytoin toxicity.

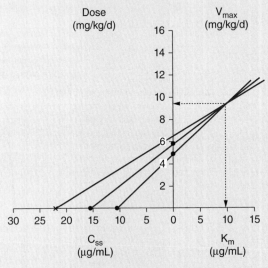

FIGURE 10-6   Mullen graph used to estimate Michaelis-Menten parameters and phenytoin dose using two or more steady-state dose/concentration pairs. The graph shows the solution for example 4.

Ludden Method

This method involves the arrangement of the Michaelis-Menten equation so that two or more maintenance doses (MD, in mg/d of phenytoin) and steady-state concentrations (Css in mg/L = μg/mL) can be used to obtain graphical solutions for V_{max} and K_m: MD = $-K_m$(MD/Css) + V_{max}.[36] When maintenance dose is plotted on the y-axis and MD/Css is plotted on the x-axis of Cartesian graph paper, a straight line with a y-intercept of V_{max} and a slope equal to $-K_m$ is found. If three or more dose/concentration pairs are available, it is best to actually plot the data so the best straight line can be drawn through the points. However, if only two dose/concentration pairs are available, a direct mathematical solution can be used. The slope for a simple linear equation is the quotient of the change in the y-axis values (Δy) and the change in the x-axis values (Δx): slope = $\Delta y/\Delta x$. Applying this to the above rearrangement of the Michaels-Menten equation, $-K_m$ = (MD$_1$ − MD$_2$)/[(MD$_1$/Css$_1$) − (MD$_2$/Css$_2$)], where the subscript 1 indicates the higher dose and 2 indicates the lower dose. Once this has been accomplished, V_{max} can be solved for in the rearranged Michaels-Menten equation: V_{max} = MD + K_m(MD/Css). The Michaels-Menten equation can be used to compute steady-state concentrations for a given dose or vice versa.

EXAMPLE 5 ▶▶▶

TD is a 50-year-old, 75-kg (height = 5 ft 10 in) male with simple partial seizures who requires therapy with oral phenytoin. He has normal liver and renal function. The patient was prescribed 400 mg/d of extended phenytoin sodium capsules for 1 month, and the steady-state phenytoin total concentration equals 6.2 μg/mL. The dosage was increased to 500 mg/d of extended phenytoin sodium capsules for another month, the steady state phenytoin total concentration equals 22.0 μg/mL, and the patient has some lateral-gaze nystagmus. The patient is assessed to be compliant with his dosage regimen. Suggest a new phenytoin dosage regimen designed to achieve a steady-state phenytoin concentration within the therapeutic range.

1. *Use Ludden method to estimate V_{max} and K_m.*

Using the graph, the serum concentration/dose information is plotted (note: phenytoin dose = 0.92 • phenytoin sodium dose = 0.92 • 400 mg/d = 368 mg/d, 368 mg/d / 75 kg = 4.9 mg/kg/d; phenytoin dose = 0.92 • phenytoin sodium dose = 0.92 • 500 mg/d = 460 mg/d, 460 mg/d / 75 kg = 6.1 mg/kg/d; see Figure 10-7). According to the graph, $V_{max} = 510$ mg/d and $K_m = 2.4$ mg/L.

Because only two doses/steady-state concentrations pairs are available, a direct mathematical solution can also be conducted: $-K_m = (MD_1 - MD_2)/[(MD_1/Css_1) - (MD_2/Css_2)] = (460$ mg/d $- 368$ mg/d)/[(460 mg/d / 22 mg/L) − (368 mg/d / 6.2 mg/L)] = −2.4 mg/L, $K_m = 2.4$ mg/L; $V_{max} = MD + K_m(MD/Css) = 368$ mg/d + 2.4(368 mg/d / 6.2 mg/L) = 510 mg/d.

2. *Use Michaelis-Menten equation to compute a new phenytoin dose for desired steady-state concentration.*

According to the Michaelis-Menten equation, a dose equal to 450 mg of phenytoin sodium is required to achieve a steady-state concentration equal to 10.4 μg/mL:

$$Css = \frac{K_m \bullet (S \bullet MD)}{V_{max} - (S \bullet MD)} = \frac{2.4 \text{ mg/L} \bullet (0.92 \bullet 450 \text{ mg/d})}{510 \text{ mg/d} - (0.92 \bullet 450 \text{ mg/d})} = 10.4 \text{ mg/L}$$

This dose would be administered by alternating 400 mg/d on even days and 500 mg/d on odd days.

A steady-state trough total phenytoin serum concentration should be measured after steady-state is attained in 7-14 days. Phenytoin serum concentrations should also be measured if the patient experiences an exacerbation of their epilepsy, or if the patient develops potential signs or symptoms of phenytoin toxicity.

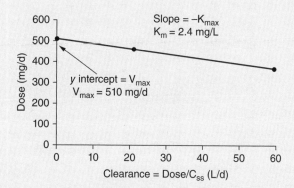

FIGURE 10-7 Ludden graph used to compute Michaelis-Menten parameters and phenytoin dose using two or more steady-state dose/concentration pairs (example 5 data shown). Dose is plotted on the y-axis while clearance (Dose/Css) is plotted on the x-axis for each data pair. The best straight line is drawn through the points. Slope equals $-K_m$, and V_{max} is the y-intercept. These values are then used to compute the required maintenance dose (MD) for any desired steady-state serum concentration: $MD = (V_{max} \times Css)/[S(K_m + Css)]$.

EXAMPLE 6 ▶▶▶

GF is a 35-year-old, 55-kg female with tonic-clonic seizures who requires therapy with oral phenytoin. She has normal liver and renal function. The patient was prescribed 300 mg/d of extended phenytoin sodium capsules for 1 month, and the steady-state phenytoin total concentration equals 10.7 µg/mL. At that time, the dose was increased to 350 mg/d of extended phenytoin sodium capsules for an additional month, and the resulting steady-state concentration was 15.8 µg/mL. The patient is assessed to be compliant with her dosage regimen. Suggest a new phenytoin dosage regimen increase designed to achieve a steady-state phenytoin concentration within the upper end of the therapeutic range.

1. *Use Ludden method to estimate V_{max} and K_m.*
   Using the graph, the serum concentration/dose information is plotted (note: phenytoin dose = 0.92 • phenytoin sodium dose = 0.92 • 300 mg/d = 276 mg/d, phenytoin dose = 0.92 • phenytoin sodium dose = 0.92 • 350 mg/d = 322 mg/d; see Figure 10-8). According to the graph, V_{max} = 495 mg/d and K_m = 8.5 mg/L.
   Because only two doses/steady-state concentrations pairs are available, a direct mathematical solution can also be conducted: $-K_m = (MD_1 - MD_2)/[(MD_1/Css_1) - (MD_2/Css_2)]$ = (322 mg/d − 276 mg/d)/[(322 mg/d / 15.8 mg/L) − (276 mg/d / 10.7 mg/L)] = −8.5 mg/L, K_m = 8.5 mg/L; V_{max} = MD + K_m(MD/Css) = 322 mg/d + 8.5 mg/L(322 mg/d / 15.8 mg/L) = 495 mg/d.

2. *Use Michaelis-Menten equation to compute a new phenytoin dose for desired steady-state concentration.*
   According to the Michaelis-Menten equation, a dose equal to 400 mg of phenytoin sodium is required to achieve a steady-state concentration equal to 24.6 µg/mL:

$$Css = \frac{K_m \bullet (S \bullet MD)}{V_{max} - (S \bullet MD)} = \frac{8.5 \text{ mg/L} \bullet (0.92 \bullet 400 \text{ mg/d})}{495 \text{ mg/d} - (0.92 \bullet 400 \text{ mg/d})} = 24.6 \text{ mg/L}$$

A steady-state trough total phenytoin serum concentration should be measured after steady-state is attained in 7-14 days. Phenytoin serum concentrations should also be measured if the patient experiences an exacerbation of their epilepsy, or if the patient develops potential signs or symptoms of phenytoin toxicity.

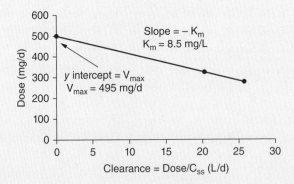

FIGURE 10-8 Ludden graph used to compute Michaelis-Menten parameters and phenytoin dose using two or more steady-state dose/concentration pairs. The graph shows the solution for example 6.

BAYESIAN PHARMACOKINETIC COMPUTER PROGRAMS

Computer programs are available that can assist in the computation of pharmacokinetic parameters for patients. The most reliable computer programs use a nonlinear regression algorithm that incorporates components of Bayes theorem. Nonlinear regression is a statistical technique that uses an iterative process to compute the best pharmacokinetic parameters for a concentration/time data set. Briefly, the patient's drug dosage schedule and serum concentrations are input into the computer. The computer program has a pharmacokinetic equation pre-programmed for the drug and administration method (oral, intravenous bolus, intravenous infusion, etc). Typically, a one-compartment model is used, although some programs allow the user to choose among several different equations. Using population estimates based on demographic information for the patient (age, weight, gender, liver function, cardiac status, etc) supplied by the user, the computer program then computes estimated serum concentrations at each time there are actual serum concentrations. Kinetic parameters are then changed by the computer program, and a new set of estimated serum concentrations are computed. The pharmacokinetic parameters that generated the estimated serum concentrations closest to the actual values are remembered by the computer program, and the process is repeated until the set of pharmacokinetic parameters that result in estimated serum concentrations that are statistically closest to the actual serum concentrations are generated. These pharmacokinetic parameters can then be used to compute improved dosing schedules for patients. Bayes theorem is used in the computer algorithm to balance the results of the computations between values based solely on the patient's serum drug concentrations and those based only on patient population parameters. Results from studies that compare various methods of dosage adjustment have consistently found that these types of computer-dosing programs perform at least as well as experienced clinical pharmacokineticists and clinicians and better than inexperienced clinicians.

Some clinicians use Bayesian pharmacokinetic computer programs exclusively to alter drug doses based on serum concentrations. An advantage of this approach is that consistent dosage recommendations are made when several different practitioners are involved in therapeutic drug-monitoring programs. However, since simpler dosing methods work just as well for patients with stable pharmacokinetic parameters and steady-state drug concentrations, many clinicians reserve the use of computer programs for more difficult situations. Those situations include serum concentrations that are not at steady-state, serum concentrations not obtained at the specific times needed to employ simpler methods, and unstable pharmacokinetic parameters. When only a limited number of phenytoin concentrations are available, Bayesian pharmacokinetic computer programs can be used to compute a complete patient pharmacokinetic profile that includes V_{max}, K_m, and volume of distribution. These are distinct advantages compared to the other methods used to adjust phenytoin dose based on one steady-state serum concentration. Many Bayesian pharmacokinetic computer programs are available to users, and most should provide answers similar to the one used in the following examples. The program used to solve problems in this book is DrugCalc written by Dr Dennis Mungall.[81]

EXAMPLE 1 ▶▶▶

TD is a 50-year-old, 75-kg (height = 5 ft 10 in) male with simple partial seizures who requires therapy with oral phenytoin. He has normal liver and renal function (total bilirubin = 0.5 mg/dL, albumin = 4.0 g/dL, serum creatinine = 0.9 mg/dL). The patient was prescribed 400 mg/d of extended phenytoin sodium capsules for 1 month, and the steady-state phenytoin total concentration equals 6.2 µg/mL. The patient is assessed to be compliant with his dosage regimen. Suggest an initial phenytoin dosage regimen designed to achieve a steady-state phenytoin concentration within the therapeutic range.

1. *Enter the patient's demographic, drug-dosing, and serum concentration/time data into the computer program.*
   DrugCalc requires doses to be entered in terms of phenytoin. A 400-mg dose of phenytoin sodium is equal to 368 mg of phenytoin (400 mg phenytoin sodium • 0.92 = 368 mg phenytoin). Extended phenytoin sodium capsules are input as a slow release dosage form.
2. *Compute pharmacokinetic parameters for the patient using Bayesian pharmacokinetic computer program.*
   The pharmacokinetic parameters computed by the program are a volume of distribution of 53 L, a V_{max} equal to 506 mg/d, and a K_m equal to 4.3 mg/L.
3. *Compute the dose required to achieve desired phenytoin serum concentrations.*
   The one-compartment model Michaelis-Menten equations used by the program to compute doses indicates that a dose of 414 mg/d of phenytoin will produce a total steady-state concentration of 12.1 µg/mL. This is equivalent to 450 mg/d of phenytoin sodium (414 mg/d phenytoin / 0.92 = 450 mg/d phenytoin sodium). Extended phenytoin sodium capsules would be prescribed as 400 mg/d on even days alternating with 500 mg/d on odd days.

   A steady-state trough total phenytoin serum concentration should be measured after steady-state is attained in 7-14 days. Phenytoin serum concentrations should also be measured if the patient experiences an exacerbation of their epilepsy, or if the patient develops potential signs or symptoms of phenytoin toxicity.

EXAMPLE 2 ▶ ▶ ▶

GF is a 35-year-old, 55-kg, 5 ft 4 in tall female with tonic-clonic seizures who requires therapy with oral phenytoin. She has normal liver and renal function (total bilirubin = 0.6 mg/dL, albumin = 4.6 g/dL, serum creatinine = 0.6 mg/dL). The patient was prescribed 300 mg/d of extended phenytoin sodium capsules for 1 month, and the steady-state phenytoin total concentration equals 10.7 µg/mL. The patient is assessed to be compliant with her dosage regimen. Suggest an initial phenytoin dosage regimen designed to achieve a steady-state phenytoin concentration of 18 µg/mL.

1. *Enter the patient's demographic, drug-dosing, and serum concentration/time data into the computer program.*
   DrugCalc requires doses to be entered in terms of phenytoin. A 300-mg dose of phenytoin sodium is equal to 276 mg of phenytoin (300 mg phenytoin sodium • 0.92 = 276 mg phenytoin). Extended phenytoin sodium capsules are input as a slow release dosage form.
2. *Compute pharmacokinetic parameters for the patient using Bayesian pharmacokinetic computer program.*
   The pharmacokinetic parameters computed by the program are a volume of distribution of 34 L, a V_{max} equal to 354 mg/d, and a K_m equal to 5.8 mg/L.
3. *Compute the dose required to achieve the desired phenytoin serum concentrations.*
   The one-compartment model Michaelis-Menten equations used by the program to compute doses indicates that a dose of 304 mg/d of phenytoin will produce a total steady-state concentration of 19.6 µg/mL. This is equivalent to 330 mg/d of phenytoin sodium (304 mg/d phenytoin/0.92 = 330 mg/d phenytoin sodium). Extended phenytoin sodium capsules would be prescribed as 330 mg/d (three 100-mg capsules + one 30-mg capsule).

   A steady-state trough total phenytoin serum concentration should be measured after steady-state is attained in 7-14 days. Phenytoin serum concentrations should also be measured if the patient experiences an exacerbation of their epilepsy, or if the patient develops potential signs or symptoms of phenytoin toxicity.

EXAMPLE 3 ▶▶▶

TY is a 27-year-old, 60-kg, 5 ft 6 in female with complex partial seizures who requires therapy with oral phenytoin. She has normal liver and renal function (total bilirubin = 0.8 mg/dL, albumin = 5.1 g/dL, serum creatinine = 0.4 mg/dL). The patient was prescribed 300 mg/d of extended phenytoin sodium capsules for 1 month, and the steady-state phenytoin total concentration equals 8.7 μg/mL. At that time, the dose was increased to 400 mg/d of extended phenytoin sodium capsules for an additional month, and the resulting steady-state concentration was 13.2 μg/mL. The patient is assessed to be compliant with her dosage regimen. Suggest a new phenytoin dosage regimen increase designed to achieve a steady-state phenytoin concentration within the upper end of the therapeutic range.

1. *Enter the patient's demographic, drug-dosing, and serum concentration/time data into the computer program.*
   DrugCalc requires doses to be entered in terms of phenytoin. A 300-mg dose of phenytoin sodium is equal to 276 mg of phenytoin (300 mg phenytoin sodium • 0.92 = 276 mg phenytoin) while a 400-mg dose of phenytoin sodium equals 368 mg of phenytoin (400 mg phenytoin sodium • 0.92 = 368 mg phenytoin). Extended phenytoin sodium capsules are input as a slow release dosage form.

2. *Compute pharmacokinetic parameters for the patient using Bayesian pharmacokinetic computer program.*
   The pharmacokinetic parameters computed by the program are a volume of distribution of 43 L, a V_{max} equal to 586 mg/d, and a K_m equal to 13.2 mg/L.

3. *Compute the dose required to achieve the desired phenytoin serum concentrations.*
   The one-compartment model Michaelis-Menten equations used by the program to compute doses indicates that a dose of 396 mg/d of phenytoin will produce a total steady-state concentration of 20.4 μg/mL. This is equivalent to 430 mg/d of phenytoin sodium (396 mg/d phenytoin/0.92 = 430 mg/d phenytoin sodium). Extended phenytoin sodium capsules would be prescribed as 430 mg/d (four 100-mg capsules + one 30-mg capsule).

   A steady-state trough total phenytoin serum concentration should be measured after steady-state is attained in 7-14 days. Phenytoin serum concentrations should also be measured if the patient experiences an exacerbation of their epilepsy, or if the patient develops potential signs or symptoms of phenytoin toxicity.

DOSING STRATEGIES

Initial dose and dosage adjustment techniques using serum concentrations can be used in any combination as long as the limitations of each method are observed. Some dosing schemes link together logically when considered according to their basic approaches or philosophies. Dosage strategies that follow similar pathways are given in Table 10-5.

USE OF PHENYTOIN BOOSTER DOSES TO IMMEDIATELY INCREASE SERUM CONCENTRATIONS

If a patient has a subtherapeutic phenytoin serum concentration in an acute situation, it may be desirable to increase the phenytoin concentration as quickly as possible. In this setting, it would not be acceptable to simply increase the maintenance dose and wait for therapeutic steady-state serum concentrations to be established in the patient. A rational way to increase the serum concentrations rapidly is to administer a booster dose of phenytoin, a process also known as "reloading" the patient with phenytoin, computed using pharmacokinetic techniques. A modified loading dose equation is used to accomplish computation of the

TABLE 10-5 Dosing Strategies

Dosing Approach/Philosophy	Initial Dosing	Use of Serum Concentrations to Alter Doses
Pharmacokinetic parameters/equations	Pharmacokinetic Dosing method	Vozeh-Sheiner method (one concentration/dose pair) or Mullen method (≥2 concentration/dose pairs) or Ludden method (≥2 concentration/dose pairs)
Literature-based/concept	Literature-based Recommended Dosing	Empiric Dosing method
Mathematical	—[a]	Graves-Cloyd method (one concentration/dose pair)
Computerized	Bayesian computer program	Bayesian computer program

[a]Any initial dosing method appropriate for the patient.

booster dose (BD) which takes into account the current phenytoin concentration present in the patient: $BD = [(C_{desired} - C_{actual})V]/S$, where $C_{desired}$ is the desired phenytoin concentration, C_{actual} is the actual current phenytoin concentration for the patient, S is the fraction of the phenytoin salt form that is active phenytoin (0.92 for phenytoin sodium injection and capsules; 0.92 for fosphenytoin because doses are prescribed as a phenytoin sodium equivalent or PE, 1.0 for phenytoin acid suspensions and tablets), and V is the volume of distribution for phenytoin. If the volume of distribution for phenytoin is known for the patient, it can be used in the calculation. However, this value is not usually known and is assumed to equal the population average of 0.7 L/kg. For obese individuals, 30% or more above their ideal body weight, the volume of distribution can be estimated using the following equation: $V = 0.7$ L/kg [IBW + 1.33(TBW − IBW)], where IBW is ideal body weight in kg [$IBW_{females}$ (in kg) = 45 + 2.3(Ht − 60) or IBW_{males} (in kg) = 50 + 2.3(Ht − 60)], Ht is height in inches, and TBW is total body weight in kg.

Concurrent with the administration of the booster dose, the maintenance dose of phenytoin is usually increased. Clinicians need to recognize that the administration of a booster dose does not alter the time required to achieve steady-state conditions when a new phenytoin dosage rate is prescribed. It still requires a sufficient time period to attain steady-state when the dosage rate is changed. However, usually the difference between the post-booster dose phenytoin concentration and the ultimate steady-state concentration has been reduced by giving the extra dose of drug.

EXAMPLE 1 ▶▶▶

BN is a 22-year-old, 85-kg (height = 6 ft 2 in) male with complex partial seizures who is receiving therapy with intravenous phenytoin sodium. He has normal liver and renal function. After receiving an initial loading dose of phenytoin sodium (1000 mg) and a maintenance dose of 300 mg/d of phenytoin sodium for 5 days, his phenytoin concentration is measured at 5.6 μg/mL immediately after seizure activity was observed. Compute a booster dose of phenytoin to achieve a phenytoin concentration equal to 15 μg/mL.

1. *Estimate the volume of distribution according to disease states and conditions present in the patient.*
   In the case of phenytoin, the population average volume of distribution equals 0.7 L/kg and this will be used to estimate the parameter for the patient. The patient is nonobese, so his actual body weight will be used in the computation: V = 0.7 L/kg • 85 kg = 60 L.

2. *Compute booster dose.*

The booster dose is computed using the following equation: BD = [($C_{desired}$ − C_{actual})V]/S = [(15 mg/L − 5.6 mg/L)60 L]/0.92 = 613 mg, rounded to 600 mg of phenytoin sodium infused no faster than 50 mg/min. (Note: μg/mL = mg/L and this concentration unit was substituted for Css in the calculations so that unnecessary unit conversion was not required.) If the maintenance dose was increased, it will take additional time for new steady-state conditions to be achieved. Phenytoin serum concentrations should be measured at this time.

PROBLEMS

The following problems are intended to emphasize the computation of initial and individualized doses using clinical pharmacokinetic techniques. Clinicians should always consult the patient's chart to confirm that current anticonvulsant therapy is appropriate. Additionally, all other medications that the patient is taking, including prescription and nonprescription drugs, should be noted and checked to ascertain if a potential drug interaction with phenytoin exists.

1. DF is a 23-year-old, 85-kg (height = 6 ft 1 in) male with tonic-clonic seizures who requires therapy with oral phenytoin. He has normal liver and renal function (bilirubin = 1.0 mg/dL, albumin = 4.9 g/dL, serum creatinine = 0.7 mg/dL). Suggest an initial extended phenytoin sodium capsule dosage regimen designed to achieve a steady-state phenytoin concentration equal to 10 μg/mL.

2. Patient DF (see problem 1) was prescribed extended phenytoin sodium capsules 500 mg/d orally. The current steady-state phenytoin concentration equals 23.5 μg/mL. Compute a new oral phenytoin dose that will provide a steady-state concentration of 15 μg/mL.

3. TR is a 56-year-old, 70-kg (height = 5 ft 9 in) male with complex partial seizures who requires therapy with oral phenytoin. He has normal liver and renal function (bilirubin = 0.8 mg/dL, albumin = 4.4 g/dL, serum creatinine = 0.9 mg/dL). Suggest an initial phenytoin suspension dosage regimen designed to achieve a steady-state phenytoin concentration equal to 15 μg/mL.

4. Patient TR (see problem 3) was prescribed phenytoin suspension 200 mg orally every 12 hours. The current steady-state phenytoin concentration equals 8 μg/mL. Compute a new oral phenytoin dose that will provide a steady-state concentration of 15 μg/mL.

5. PL is a 64-year-old, 60-kg (height = 5 ft 2 in) female with simple partial seizures who requires therapy with intravenous fosphenytoin. She has normal liver and renal function (bilirubin = 0.8 mg/dL, albumin = 3.6 g/dL, serum creatinine = 1.2 mg/dL). Suggest an initial intravenous fosphenytoin regimen designed to achieve a steady-state phenytoin concentration equal to 12 μg/mL.

6. Patient PL (see problem 5) was prescribed intravenous fosphenytoin injection 200 mg/d PE. A phenytoin serum concentration was obtained just before the fourth dose of this regimen and equaled 4.1 μg/mL. Assuming the phenytoin concentration was zero before the first dose, compute a new intravenous fosphenytoin injection that will provide a steady-state concentration of 12 μg/mL.

7. MN is a 24-year-old, 55-kg (height = 5 ft 5 in) female with complex partial seizures who requires therapy with intravenous phenytoin sodium. She has normal liver and renal function (bilirubin = 0.8 mg/dL, albumin = 3.6 g/dL, serum creatinine = 1.2 mg/dL). Suggest an initial intravenous phenytoin sodium dosage regimen designed to achieve a steady-state phenytoin concentration equal to 12 μg/mL.

8. Patient MN (see problem 7) was prescribed intravenous phenytoin sodium injection 300 mg/d. A phenytoin serum concentration was obtained at steady-state and equaled 6.4 µg/mL. The dose was increased to intravenous phenytoin sodium injection 400 mg/d and the measured steady-state concentration equaled 10.7 µg/mL. Compute a new intravenous phenytoin sodium injection dose that will provide a steady-state concentration of 15 µg/mL.

9. SA is a 62-year-old, 130-kg (height = 5 ft 11 in) male with complex partial seizures who requires therapy with oral phenytoin. He has normal liver and renal function (bilirubin = 0.6 mg/dL, albumin = 3.9 g/dL, serum creatinine = 1.0 mg/dL). Suggest an initial extended phenytoin sodium capsule dosage regimen designed to achieve a steady-state concentration equal to 10 µg/mL.

10. Patient SA (see problem 9) was prescribed extended phenytoin sodium capsules 200 mg orally every 12 hours. A phenytoin serum concentration was obtained at steady-state and equaled 6.2 µg/mL. The dose was increased to extended phenytoin sodium capsules 300 mg orally every 12 hours, and the measured steady-state concentration equaled 25.7 µg/mL. Compute a new oral phenytoin dose that will provide a steady-state concentration of 15 µg/mL.

11. VG is an epileptic patient being treated with phenytoin. He has hypoalbuminemia (albumin = 2.4 g/dL) and normal renal function (creatinine clearance = 90 mL/min). His total phenytoin concentration is 8.9 µg/mL. Assuming that any unbound concentrations performed by the clinical laboratory will be conducted at 25°C, compute an estimated normalized phenytoin concentration for this patient.

12. DE is an epileptic patient being treated with phenytoin. He has hypoalbuminemia (albumin = 2.0 g/dL) and poor renal function (creatinine clearance = 10 mL/min). His total phenytoin concentration is 8.1 µg/mL. Compute an estimated normalized phenytoin concentration for this patient.

13. KL is an epileptic patient being treated with phenytoin and valproic acid. He has a normal albumin concentration (albumin = 4.0 g/dL) and normal renal function (creatinine clearance = 95 mL/min). His steady-state total phenytoin and valproic acid concentrations are 6 µg/mL and 90 µg/mL, respectively. Compute an estimated unbound phenytoin concentration for this patient.

14. YS is a 9-year-old, 35-kg female with complex partial seizures who requires therapy with oral phenytoin. She has normal liver and renal function. Suggest an initial phenytoin dosage regimen designed to achieve a steady-state phenytoin concentration equal to 12 µg/mL.

15. Patient YS (see problem 14) was prescribed phenytoin suspension 150 mg orally every 12 hours. The current steady-state phenytoin concentration equals 23 µg/mL. Compute a new oral phenytoin dose that will provide a steady-state concentration of 15 µg/mL.

ANSWERS TO PROBLEMS

1. *Answer to problem 1.* The initial phenytoin dose for patient DF would be calculated as follows:

Pharmacokinetic Dosing Method

1. *Estimate Michaelis-Menten constants according to disease states and conditions present in the patient.*

    The V_{max} for a nonobese adult patient with normal liver and renal function is 7 mg/kg/d. For an 85-kg patient, V_{max} = 595 mg/d: V_{max} = 7 mg/kg/d • 85 kg = 595 mg/d. For this individual, K_m = 4 mg/L.

2. *Compute dosage regimen.*

Oral phenytoin sodium capsules will be prescribed to this patient (F = 1, S = 0.92). The initial dosage interval (τ) will be set to 24 hours. (Note: μg/mL = mg/L and this concentration unit was substituted for Css in the calculations so that unnecessary unit conversion was not required.) The dosage equation for phenytoin is:

$$MD = \frac{V_{max} \bullet Css}{S(K_m + Css)} = \frac{595 \text{ mg/d} \bullet 10 \text{ mg/L}}{0.92(4 \text{ mg/L} + 10 \text{ mg/L})} = 462 \text{ mg/d, rounded to } 500 \text{ mg/d}$$

A steady-state trough total phenytoin serum concentration should be measured after steady-state is attained in 7-14 days. Phenytoin serum concentrations should also be measured if the patient experiences an exacerbation of their epilepsy, or if the patient develops potential signs or symptoms of phenytoin toxicity.

Literature-Based Dosing Method

1. *Estimate phenytoin dose according to disease states and conditions present in the patient.*

The suggested initial dosage rate for extended phenytoin sodium capsules in an adult patient is 4-6 mg/kg/d. Using a rate of 5 mg/kg/d, the initial dose would be 400 mg/d: 5 mg/kg/d • 85 kg = 425 mg/d, rounded to 400 mg/d. Using a dosage interval of 24 hours, the prescribed dose would be 400 mg of extended phenytoin sodium capsules daily.

A steady-state trough total phenytoin serum concentration should be measured after steady-state is attained in 7-14 days. Phenytoin serum concentrations should also be measured if the patient experiences an exacerbation of their epilepsy, or if the patient develops potential signs or symptoms of phenytoin toxicity.

2. *Answer to problem 2.* The revised phenytoin dose of patient DF would be calculated as follows:

Empiric Dosing Method

1. *Suggest new phenytoin dose.*

Since the patient is receiving extended phenytoin sodium capsules, a convenient dosage change would be 100 mg/d and a decrease to 400 mg/d is suggested.

A steady-state trough total phenytoin serum concentration should be measured after steady-state is attained in 7-14 days. Phenytoin serum concentrations should also be measured if the patient experiences an exacerbation of their epilepsy, or if the patient develops potential signs or symptoms of phenytoin toxicity.

Pseudolinear Pharmacokinetics Method

1. *Use pseudolinear pharmacokinetics to predict new concentration for a dosage decrease, then compute 15%-33% factor to account for Michaelis-Menten pharmacokinetics.*

Since the patient is receiving extended phenytoin sodium capsules, a convenient dosage change would be 100 mg/d and a decrease to 400 mg/d is suggested. Using pseudolinear pharmacokinetics, the resulting total steady-state phenytoin serum concentration would equal: $Css_{new} = (D_{new}/D_{old})Css_{old} =$ (400 mg/d / 500 mg/d)23.5 μg/mL = 18.8 μg/mL. Because of Michaelis-Menten pharmacokinetics, the serum concentration would be expected to decrease 15%, or 0.85 times, to 33%, or 0.67 times, greater than that predicted by linear pharmacokinetics: Css = 18.8 μg/mL • 0.85 = 16 μg/mL and Css = 18.8 μg/mL • 0.67 = 12.6 μg/mL. Thus, a dosage decrease of 100 mg/d would be expected to yield a total phenytoin steady-state serum concentration between 12 and 16 μg/mL.

A steady-state trough total phenytoin serum concentration should be measured after steady-state is attained in 7-14 days. Phenytoin serum concentrations should also be measured if the patient experiences an exacerbation of their epilepsy, or if the patient develops potential signs or symptoms of phenytoin toxicity.

Graves-Cloyd Method

1. *Use Graves-Cloyd method to estimate a new phenytoin dose for desired steady-state concentration.*
   A new total phenytoin steady-state serum concentration equal to 15 µg/mL is chosen for the patient (460 mg phenytoin = 500 mg phenytoin sodium • 0.92): $D_{new} = (D_{old}/Css_{old}) \cdot Css_{new}^{0.199} \cdot Css_{old}^{0.804}$ = (460 mg/d/23.5 mg/L) • (15 mg/L)$^{0.199}$ • (23.5 mg/L)$^{0.804}$ = 425 mg/d of phenytoin acid, which equals 462 mg of phenytoin sodium (462 mg phenytoin sodium = 425 mg phenytoin/0.92). This dose would be rounded to 450 mg/d, or 400 mg/d on even days alternating with 500 mg/d on odd days.
   A steady-state trough total phenytoin serum concentration should be measured after steady-state is attained in 7-14 days. Phenytoin serum concentrations should also be measured if the patient experiences an exacerbation of their epilepsy, or if the patient develops potential signs or symptoms of phenytoin toxicity.

Vozeh-Sheiner Method

1. *Use Vozeh-Sheiner method to estimate a new phenytoin dose for desired steady-state concentration.*
   A new total phenytoin steady-state serum concentration equal to 15 µg/mL is chosen for the patient. Using the orbit graph, the serum concentration/dose information is plotted (note: phenytoin dose = 0.92 • phenytoin sodium dose = 0.92 • 500 mg/d = 460 mg/d; 460 mg/d/85 kg = 5.4 mg/kg/d; see Figure 10-9). According to the graph, a dose of 4.9 mg/kg/d of phenytoin is required to achieve a steady-state concentration equal to 15 µg/mL. This equals an extended phenytoin sodium capsule dose of 450 mg/d, administered by alternating 400 mg/d on even days and 500 mg/d on odd days: (4.9 mg/kg/d • 85 kg)/0.92 = 453 mg/d, rounded to 450 mg/d.

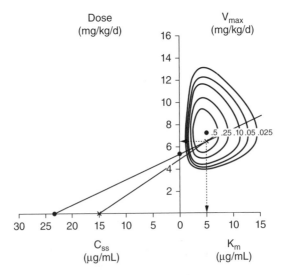

FIGURE 10-9   Solution to problem 2 using Vozeh-Sheiner or Orbit Graph.

A steady-state trough total phenytoin serum concentration should be measured after steady-state is attained in 7-14 days. Phenytoin serum concentrations should also be measured if the patient experiences an exacerbation of their epilepsy, or if the patient develops potential signs or symptoms of phenytoin toxicity.

3. *Answer to problem 3.* The initial phenytoin dose for patient TR would be calculated as follows:

Pharmacokinetic Dosing Method

1. *Estimate Michaelis-Menten constants according to disease states and conditions present in the patient.*

The V_{max} for a nonobese adult patient with normal liver and renal function is 7 mg/kg/d. For a 70-kg patient, V_{max} = 490 mg/d: V_{max} = 7 mg/kg/d • 70 kg = 490 mg/d. For this individual, K_m = 4 mg/L.

2. *Compute dosage regimen.*

Oral phenytoin suspension will be prescribed to this patient (F = 1, S = 1). The initial dosage interval (τ) will be set to 12 hours. (Note: µg/mL = mg/L and this concentration unit was substituted for Css in the calculations so that unnecessary unit conversion was not required.) The dosage equation for phenytoin is:

$$MD = \frac{V_{max} \bullet Css}{S(K_m + Css)} = \frac{490 \text{ mg/d} \bullet 15 \text{ mg/L}}{1(4 \text{ mg/L} + 15 \text{ mg/L})} = 387 \text{ mg/d, rounded to 400 mg/d}$$

A dose of phenytoin suspension 200 mg every 12 hours would be prescribed. A steady-state trough total phenytoin serum concentration should be measured after steady-state is attained in 7-14 days. Phenytoin serum concentrations should also be measured if the patient experiences an exacerbation of their epilepsy, or if the patient develops potential signs or symptoms of phenytoin toxicity.

Literature-Based Dosing Method

1. *Estimate phenytoin dose according to disease states and conditions present in the patient.*

The suggested initial dosage rate for extended phenytoin sodium capsules in an adult patient is 4-6 mg/kg/d. Using a rate of 5 mg/kg/d, the initial dose would be 400 mg/d: 5 mg/kg/d • 70 kg = 350 mg/d, rounded to 400 mg/d. Using a dosage interval of 12 hours, the prescribed dose would be 200 mg of phenytoin suspension every 12 hours.

A steady-state trough total phenytoin serum concentration should be measured after steady-state is attained in 7-14 days. Phenytoin serum concentrations should also be measured if the patient experiences an exacerbation of their epilepsy, or if the patient develops potential signs or symptoms of phenytoin toxicity.

4. *Answer to problem 4.* The revised phenytoin dose of patient TR would be calculated as follows:

Empiric Dosing Method

1. *Suggest new phenytoin dose.*

Since the patient is receiving phenytoin suspension, a convenient dosage change would be 100 mg/d and an increase to 500 mg/d or 250 mg every 12 hours is suggested (see Table 10-4).

A steady-state trough total phenytoin serum concentration should be measured after steady-state is attained in 7-14 days. Phenytoin serum concentrations should also be measured if the patient experiences an exacerbation of their epilepsy, or if the patient develops potential signs or symptoms of phenytoin toxicity.

Pseudolinear Pharmacokinetics Method

1. *Use pseudolinear pharmacokinetics to predict new concentration for a dosage increase, then compute 15%-33% factor to account for Michaelis-Menten pharmacokinetics.*

    Since the patient is receiving phenytoin suspension, a convenient dosage change would be 100 mg/d and an increase to 500 mg/d is suggested. Using pseudolinear pharmacokinetics, the resulting total steady-state phenytoin serum concentration would equal: $Css_{new} = (D_{new}/D_{old})Css_{old} = (500 \text{ mg/d} / 400 \text{ mg/d})8 \text{ µg/mL} = 10 \text{ µg/mL}$. Because of Michaelis-Menten pharmacokinetics, the serum concentration would be expected to increase 15%, or 1.15 times, to 33%, or 1.33 times, greater than that predicted by linear pharmacokinetics: $Css = 10 \text{ µg/mL} \bullet 1.15 = 11.5 \text{ µg/mL}$ and $Css = 10 \text{ µg/mL} \bullet 1.33 = 13.3 \text{ µg/mL}$. Thus, a dosage increase of 100 mg/d would be expected to yield a total phenytoin steady-state serum concentration between 11 and 13 µg/mL.

    A steady-state trough total phenytoin serum concentration should be measured after steady-state is attained in 7-14 days. Phenytoin serum concentrations should also be measured if the patient experiences an exacerbation of their epilepsy, or if the patient develops potential signs or symptoms of phenytoin toxicity.

Graves-Cloyd Method

1. *Use Graves-Cloyd method to estimate a new phenytoin dose for desired steady-state concentration.*

    A new total phenytoin steady-state serum concentration equal to 15 µg/mL is chosen for the patient: $D_{new} = (D_{old}/Css_{old}) \bullet Css_{new}^{0.199} \bullet Css_{old}^{0.804} = (400 \text{ mg/d} / 8 \text{ mg/L}) \bullet (15 \text{ mg/L})^{0.199} \bullet (8 \text{ mg/L})^{0.804} = 456 \text{ mg/d}$, rounded to 450 mg/d, or 225 mg every 12 hours.

    A steady-state trough total phenytoin serum concentration should be measured after steady state is attained in 7-14 days. Phenytoin serum concentrations should also be measured if the patient experiences an exacerbation of their epilepsy, or if the patient develops potential signs or symptoms of phenytoin toxicity.

Vozeh-Sheiner Method

1. *Use Vozeh-Sheiner method to estimate a new phenytoin dose for desired steady-state concentration.*

    A new total phenytoin steady-state serum concentration equal to 15 µg/mL is chosen for the patient. Using the orbit graph, the serum concentration/dose information is plotted (note: 400 mg/d / 70 kg = 5.7 mg/kg/d; see Figure 10-10). According to the graph, a dose of 6.6 mg/kg/d of phenytoin is required to achieve a steady-state concentration equal to 15 µg/mL. This equals a phenytoin suspension dose of 450 mg/d, administered as 225 mg every 12 hours: 6.6 mg/kg/d $\bullet$ 70 kg = 462 mg/d, rounded to 450 mg/d.

    A steady-state trough total phenytoin serum concentration should be measured after steady-state is attained in 7-14 days. Phenytoin serum concentrations should also be measured if the patient experiences an exacerbation of their epilepsy, or if the patient develops potential signs or symptoms of phenytoin toxicity.

5. *Answer to problem 5.* The initial phenytoin dose for patient PL would be calculated as follows:

Pharmacokinetic Dosing Method

1. *Estimate Michaelis-Menten constants and volume of distribution according to disease states and conditions present in the patient.*

    The V_{max} for a nonobese adult patient with normal liver and renal function is 7 mg/kg/d. For a 60-kg patient, $V_{max} = 420 \text{ mg/d}$: $V_{max} = 7 \text{ mg/kg/d} \bullet 60 \text{ kg} = 420 \text{ mg/d}$. For this individual, $K_m = 4 \text{ mg/L}$. The volume of distribution for this patient would equal 42 L: $V = 0.7 \text{ L/kg} \bullet 60 \text{ kg} = 42 \text{ L}$.

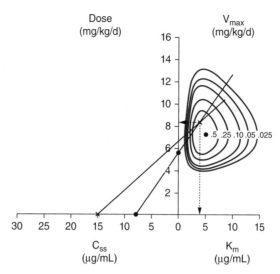

FIGURE 10-10   Solution to problem 4 using Vozeh-Sheiner or Orbit Graph.

2. *Compute dosage regimen.*

Fosphenytoin will be given to this patient, which is prescribed in phenytoin sodium equivalents or PE (F = 1, S = 0.92). The initial dosage interval (τ) will be set to 12 hours. (Note: µg/mL = mg/L and this concentration unit was substituted for Css in the calculations so that unnecessary unit conversion was not required.) The dosage equation for phenytoin is:

$$MD = \frac{V_{max} \bullet Css}{S(K_m + Css)} = \frac{420 \text{ mg/d} \bullet 12 \text{ mg/L}}{0.92(4 \text{ mg/L} + 12 \text{ mg/L})} = 342 \text{ mg/d, rounded to 350 mg}$$

$$LD = (V \bullet Css)/S = (42 \text{ L} \bullet 12 \text{ mg/L}) / 0.92 = 548 \text{ mg, rounded to 550 mg}$$

The maintenance dose would be given as 175 mg every 12 hours. Maintenance and loading dose infusion rates should not exceed 150 mg/min PE. A steady-state trough total phenytoin serum concentration should be measured after steady-state is attained in 7-14 days. Phenytoin serum concentrations should also be measured if the patient experiences an exacerbation of their epilepsy, or if the patient develops potential signs or symptoms of phenytoin toxicity.

Literature-Based Dosing Method

1. *Estimate phenytoin dose according to disease states and conditions present in the patient.*

The suggested initial dosage rate for fosphenytoin injection in an adult patient is 4-6 mg/kg/d PE. Using a rate of 5 mg/kg/d, the initial dose would be 300 mg/d or 150 mg every 12 hours: 5 mg/kg/d • 60 kg = 300 mg/d. Suggested loading doses for fosphenytoin is 15-20 mg/kg PE. Using a dose of 18 mg/kg PE, the loading dose would be 1000 mg PE: 18 mg/kg PE • 60 kg = 1080 mg PE, rounded to 1000 mg PE. Maintenance and loading dose infusion rates should not exceed 150 mg/min PE.

A steady-state trough total phenytoin serum concentration should be measured after steady-state is attained in 7-14 days. Phenytoin serum concentrations should also be measured if the patient experiences an exacerbation of their epilepsy, or if the patient develops potential signs or symptoms of phenytoin toxicity.

6. *Answer to problem 6.* The revised phenytoin dose of patient PL would be calculated as follows:

Bayesian Pharmacokinetic Computer Method

Because the patient has only received three doses of fosphenytoin, it is very unlikely that the measured serum concentration is a steady-state concentration. Thus, methods that require a single steady-state serum concentration should not be used.

1. *Enter the patient's demographic, drug-dosing, and serum concentration/time data into the computer program.*

    DrugCalc requires doses to be entered in terms of phenytoin. A 200-mg/d PE dose of fosphenytoin is equal to 184 mg of phenytoin (200 mg PE fosphenytoin • 0.92 = 184 mg phenytoin). This dose was entered into the program along with a dose length time of 1.

2. *Compute pharmacokinetic parameters for the patient using Bayesian pharmacokinetic computer program.*

    The pharmacokinetic parameters computed by the program are a volume of distribution of 47 L, a V_{max} equal to 299 mg/d, and a K_m equal to 6.0 mg/L.

3. *Compute the dose required to achieve the desired phenytoin serum concentrations.*

    The one-compartment model Michaelis-Menten equations used by the program to compute doses indicates that a dose of 200 mg/d of phenytoin will produce a total steady-state concentration of 12 µg/mL. This is equivalent to 217 mg/d of phenytoin sodium (200 mg/d phenytoin/0.92 = 217 mg/d PE fosphenytoin), and this dose would be rounded to 200 mg/d PE. Fosphenytoin would be prescribed as 200 mg/d PE at an infusion rate no greater than 150 mg/min PE.

    A steady-state trough total phenytoin serum concentration should be measured after steady-state is attained in 7-14 days. Phenytoin serum concentrations should also be measured if the patient experiences an exacerbation of their epilepsy, or if the patient develops potential signs or symptoms of phenytoin toxicity.

7. *Answer to problem 7.* The initial phenytoin dose for patient MN would be calculated as follows:

Pharmacokinetic Dosing Method

1. *Estimate Michaelis-Menten constants and volume of distribution according to disease states and conditions present in the patient.*

    The V_{max} for a nonobese adult patient with normal liver and renal function is 7 mg/kg/d. For a 55-kg patient, V_{max} = 385 mg/d: V_{max} = 7 mg/kg/d • 55 kg = 385 mg/d. For this individual, K_m = 4 mg/L. The volume of distribution for this patient would equal 39 L: V = 0.7 L/kg • 55 kg = 39 L.

2. *Compute dosage regimen.*

    Phenytoin sodium injection will be given to this patient (F = 1, S = 0.92). The initial dosage interval (τ) will be set to 12 hours. (Note: µg/mL = mg/L and this concentration unit was substituted for Css in the calculations so that unnecessary unit conversion was not required.) The dosage equation for phenytoin is:

$$MD = \frac{V_{max} \bullet Css}{S(K_m + Css)} = \frac{385 \text{ mg/d} \bullet 12 \text{ mg/L}}{0.92(4 \text{ mg/L} + 12 \text{ mg/L})} = 314 \text{ mg/d, rounded to 300 mg/d}$$

$$LD = (V \bullet Css)/S = (39 \text{ L} \bullet 12 \text{ mg/L}) / 0.92 = 509 \text{ mg, rounded to 500 mg}$$

The maintenance dose would be given as 150 mg every 12 hours. Maintenance and loading dose infusion rates should not exceed 50 mg/min. A steady-state trough total phenytoin serum concentration should be measured after steady-state is attained in 7-14 days. Phenytoin serum concentrations should also be measured if the patient experiences an exacerbation of their epilepsy, or if the patient develops potential signs or symptoms of phenytoin toxicity.

Literature-Based Dosing Method

1. *Estimate phenytoin dose according to disease states and conditions present in the patient.*

The suggested initial dosage rate for fosphenytoin injection in an adult patient is 4-6 mg/kg/d PE. Using a rate of 5 mg/kg/d, the initial dose would be 300 mg/d or 150 mg every 12 hours: 5 mg/kg/d • 55 kg = 275 mg/d, rounded to 300 mg/d. The suggested loading dose for phenytoin sodium injection is 15-20 mg/kg. Using a dose of 18 mg/kg, the loading dose would be 1000 mg: 18 mg/kg • 55 kg = 990 mg PE, rounded to 1000 mg PE. Maintenance and loading dose infusion rates should not exceed 50 mg/min.

A steady-state trough total phenytoin serum concentration should be measured after steady-state is attained in 7-14 days. Phenytoin serum concentrations should also be measured if the patient experiences an exacerbation of their epilepsy, or if the patient develops potential signs or symptoms of phenytoin toxicity.

8. *Answer to problem 8.* The revised phenytoin dose of patient MN would be calculated as follows:

Empiric Dosing Method

1. *Empirically suggest new phenytoin dose.*

The next logical dose to prescribe is phenytoin sodium 500 mg/d (see Table 10-4).

A steady-state trough total phenytoin serum concentration should be measured after steady-state is attained in 7-14 days. Phenytoin serum concentrations should also be measured if the patient experiences an exacerbation of their epilepsy, or if the patient develops potential signs or symptoms of phenytoin toxicity.

Mullen Method

1. *Use Mullen method to estimate a new phenytoin dose for the desired steady-state concentration.*

Using the graph, the serum concentration/dose information is plotted (note: phenytoin dose = 0.92 • phenytoin sodium dose = 0.92 • 300 mg/d = 276 mg/d, 276 mg/d / 55 kg = 5 mg/kg/d; phenytoin dose = 0.92 • phenytoin sodium dose = 0.92 • 400 mg/d = 368 mg/d, 368 mg/d / 55 kg = 6.7 mg/kg/d; see Figure 10-11). According to the graph, a dose of 7.7 mg/kg/d of phenytoin is

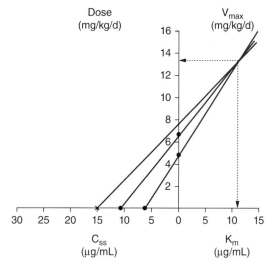

FIGURE 10-11   Solution to problem 8 using Mullen graph.

required to achieve a steady-state concentration equal to 15 µg/mL. This equals a phenytoin sodium injection dose of 450 mg/d or 225 mg every 12 hours: (7.7 mg/kg/d • 55 kg)/0.92 = 460 mg/d, rounded to 450 mg/d. The dose would be given as 225 mg every 12 hours. V_{max} = 13.4 mg/kg/d and K_m = 10.6 µg/mL for this patient.

A steady-state trough total phenytoin serum concentration should be measured after steady state is attained in 7-14 days. Phenytoin serum concentrations should also be measured if the patient experiences an exacerbation of their epilepsy, or if the patient develops potential signs or symptoms of phenytoin toxicity.

Ludden Method

1. *Use Ludden method to estimate V_{max} and K_m.*

    Using the graph, the serum concentration/dose information is plotted (note: phenytoin dose = 0.92 • phenytoin sodium dose = 0.92 • 300 mg/d = 276 mg/d, 276 mg/d/55 kg = 5 mg/kg/d; phenytoin dose = 0.92 • phenytoin sodium dose = 0.92 • 400 mg/d = 368 mg/d, 368 mg/d/55 kg = 6.7 mg/kg/d; see Figure 10-12). According to the graph, V_{max} = 729 mg/d and K_m = 10.5 mg/L.

    Because only two dose/steady-state concentration pairs are available, a direct mathematical solution can also be conducted: $-K_m = (MD_1 - MD_2)/[(MD_1/Css_1) - (MD_2/Css_2)] = (368 \text{ mg/d} - 276 \text{ mg/d})/[(368 \text{ mg/d}/10.7 \text{ mg/L}) - (276 \text{ mg/d}/6.4 \text{ mg/L})] = -10.5 \text{ mg/L}$, K_m = 10.5 mg/L; $V_{max} = MD + K_m(MD/Css) = 368 \text{ mg/d} + 10.5 \text{ mg/L}(368 \text{ mg/d}/10.7 \text{ mg/L}) = 729 \text{ mg/d}$.

2. *Use Michaelis-Menten equation to compute a new phenytoin dose for desired steady-state concentration.*

    According to the Michaelis-Menten equation, a dose equal to 450 mg of phenytoin sodium is required to achieve a steady-state concentration equal to 10.4 µg/mL:

$$MD = \frac{V_{max} \bullet Css}{S(K_m + Css)} = \frac{729 \text{ mg/d} \bullet 15 \text{ mg/L}}{0.92(10.5 \text{ mg/L} + 15 \text{ mg/L})} = 466 \text{ mg/d, rounded to 450 mg/d}$$

This dose would be administered by giving 225 mg every 12 hours.

A steady-state trough total phenytoin serum concentration should be measured after steady-state is attained in 7-14 days. Phenytoin serum concentrations should also be measured if the patient experiences an exacerbation of their epilepsy, or if the patient develops potential signs or symptoms of phenytoin toxicity.

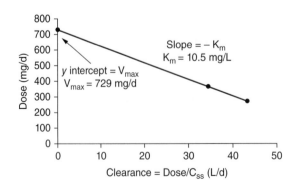

FIGURE 10-12   Solution to problem 8 using Ludden graph.

Bayesian Pharmacokinetic Computer Method

1. *Enter the patient's demographic, drug-dosing, and serum concentration/time data into the computer program.*

   DrugCalc requires doses to be entered in terms of phenytoin. (Phenytoin dose = 0.92 • phenytoin sodium dose = 0.92 • 300 mg/d = 276 mg/d; phenytoin dose = 0.92 • phenytoin sodium dose = 0.92 • 400 mg/d = 368 mg/d.) These doses were entered into the program along with a dose length time of 1 d.

2. *Compute pharmacokinetic parameters for the patient using Bayesian pharmacokinetic computer program.*

   The pharmacokinetic parameters computed by the program are a volume of distribution of 49 L, a V_{max} equal to 633 mg/d, and a K_m equal to 10.8 mg/L.

3. *Compute the dose required to achieve the desired phenytoin serum concentrations.*

   The one-compartment model Michaelis-Menten equations used by the program to compute doses indicates that a dose of 414 mg/d of phenytoin will produce a total steady-state concentration of 20.3 µg/mL. This is equivalent to 450 mg/d of phenytoin sodium (414 mg/d phenytoin/0.92 = 450 mg/d phenytoin sodium), and this dose would be given as 225 mg every 12 hours.

   A steady-state trough total phenytoin serum concentration should be measured after steady-state is attained in 7-14 days. Phenytoin serum concentrations should also be measured if the patient experiences an exacerbation of their epilepsy, or if the patient develops potential signs or symptoms of phenytoin toxicity.

9. *Answer to problem 9.* The initial phenytoin dose for patient SA would be calculated as follows:

Pharmacokinetic Dosing Method

1. *Estimate Michaelis-Menten constants and volume of distribution according to disease states and conditions present in the patient.*

   The V_{max} for an adult patient with normal liver and renal function is 7 mg/kg/d. In obese individuals, it is unclear whether to use ideal body weight (IBW) or total body weight (TBW) for maintenance dose calculation. Currently, most clinicians use ideal body weight since it produces the most conservative dosage recommendation: $IBW_{males} = 50 + 2.3(Ht - 60) = 50 + 2.3(71\ in - 60) = 75\ kg$. For a 75-kg patient, $V_{max} = 525$ mg/d: $V_{max} = 7$ mg/kg/d • 75 kg = 525 mg/d. For this individual, $K_m = 4$ mg/L.

2. *Compute dosage regimen.*

   Extended phenytoin sodium capsules will be given to this patient (F = 1, S = 0.92). The initial dosage interval (τ) will be set to 24 hours. (Note: µg/mL = mg/L and this concentration unit was substituted for Css in the calculations so that unnecessary unit conversion was not required.) The dosage equation for phenytoin is:

$$MD = \frac{V_{max} \bullet Css}{S(K_m + Css)} = \frac{525\ mg/d \bullet 10\ mg/L}{0.92(4\ mg/L + 10\ mg/L)} = 408\ mg/d,\ \text{rounded to 400 mg/d}$$

   The maintenance dose would be given as 400 mg/d. A steady-state trough total phenytoin serum concentration should be measured after steady-state is attained in 7-14 days. Phenytoin serum concentrations should also be measured if the patient experiences an exacerbation of their epilepsy, or if the patient develops potential signs or symptoms of phenytoin toxicity.

Literature-Based Dosing Method

1. *Estimate phenytoin dose according to disease states and conditions present in the patient.*

      The suggested initial dosage rate for phenytoin sodium injection in an adult patient is 4-6 mg/kg/d. In obese individuals, it is unclear whether to use ideal body weight (IBW) or total body weight (TBW) for dose calculation. Currently, most clinicians use ideal body weight since it produces the most conservative dosage recommendation: $IBW_{males} = 50 + 2.3(Ht - 60) = 50 + 2.3(71\ in - 60) = 75$ kg. Using a rate of 5 mg/kg/d, the initial dose would be 400 mg/d or 200 mg every 12 hours: 5 mg/kg/d • 75 kg = 375 mg/d, rounded to 400 mg/d.

      A steady-state trough total phenytoin serum concentration should be measured after steady-state is attained in 7-14 days. Phenytoin serum concentrations should also be measured if the patient experiences an exacerbation of their epilepsy, or if the patient develops potential signs or symptoms of phenytoin toxicity.

10. *Answer to problem 10.* The revised phenytoin dose of patient SA would be calculated as follows:

Empiric Dosing Method

1. *Empirically suggest new phenytoin dose.*

      The next logical dose to prescribe is phenytoin sodium 200 mg every morning plus 300 mg every evening.

      A steady-state trough total phenytoin serum concentration should be measured after steady-state is attained in 7-14 days. Phenytoin serum concentrations should also be measured if the patient experiences an exacerbation of their epilepsy, or if the patient develops potential signs or symptoms of phenytoin toxicity.

Mullen Method

1. *Use Mullen method to estimate a new phenytoin dose for the desired steady-state concentration.*

      Using the graph, the serum concentration/dose information is plotted (note: phenytoin dose = 0.92 • phenytoin sodium dose = 0.92 • 600 mg/d = 552 mg/d, 552 mg/d/75 kg IBW = 7.4 mg/kg/d; phenytoin dose = 0.92 • phenytoin sodium dose = 0.92 • 400 mg/d = 368 mg/d, 368 mg/d/75 kg IBW = 4.9 mg/kg/d; see Figure 10-13). According to the graph, a dose of 6.7 mg/kg/d of phenytoin

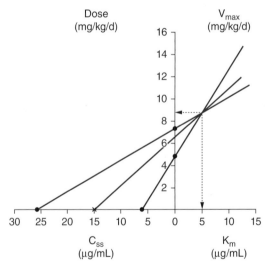

FIGURE 10-13   Solution to problem 10 using Mullen graph.

is required to achieve a steady-state concentration equal to 15 µg/mL. This equals an extended phenytoin sodium capsule dose of 500 mg/d or 200 mg every morning plus 300 mg every evening: (6.7 mg/kg/d • 75 kg)/0.92 = 546 mg/d, rounded to 500 mg/d. V_{max} = 8.8 mg/kg/d and K_m = 5 µg/mL for this patient.

A steady-state trough total phenytoin serum concentration should be measured after steady-state is attained in 7-14 days. Phenytoin serum concentrations should also be measured if the patient experiences an exacerbation of their epilepsy, or if the patient develops potential signs or symptoms of phenytoin toxicity.

Ludden Method

1. *Use Ludden method to estimate V_{max} and K_m.*

   Using the graph, the serum concentration/dose information is plotted (note: phenytoin dose = 0.92 • phenytoin sodium dose = 0.92 • 600 mg/d = 552 mg/d, 552 mg/d/75 kg IBW = 7.4 mg/kg/d; phenytoin dose = 0.92 • phenytoin sodium dose = 0.92 • 400 mg/d = 368 mg/d, 368 mg/d/75 kg IBW = 4.9 mg/kg/d; see Figure 10-14). According to the graph, V_{max} = 659 mg/d and K_m = 4.9 mg/L.

   Because only two doses/steady-state concentrations pairs are available, a direct mathematical solution can also be conducted: $-K_m = (MD_1 - MD_2)/[(MD_1/Css_1) - (MD_2/Css_2)] = (552$ mg/d $- 368$ mg/d$)/[(552$ mg/d/25.7 mg/L$) - (368$ mg/d/6.2 mg/L$)] = -4.9$ mg/L, $K_m = 4.9$ mg/L; $V_{max} = MD + K_m(MD/Css) = 368$ mg/d $+ 4.9$ mg/L $(368$ mg/d/6.2 mg/L$) = 659$ mg/d.

2. *Use Michaelis-Menten equation to compute a new phenytoin dose for the desired steady-state concentration.*

   According to the Michaelis-Menten equation, a dose equal to 500 mg of phenytoin sodium is required to achieve a steady-state concentration equal to 15 µg/mL:

$$MD = \frac{V_{max} \bullet Css}{S(K_m + Css)} = \frac{659 \text{ mg/d} \bullet 15 \text{ mg/L}}{0.92(4.9 \text{ mg/L} + 15 \text{ mg/L})} = 540 \text{ mg/d, rounded to 500 mg/d}$$

This dose would administered by giving 200 mg every morning plus 300 mg every evening.

A steady-state trough total phenytoin serum concentration should be measured after steady-state is attained in 7-14 days. Phenytoin serum concentrations should also be measured if the patient experiences an exacerbation of their epilepsy, or if the patient develops potential signs or symptoms of phenytoin toxicity.

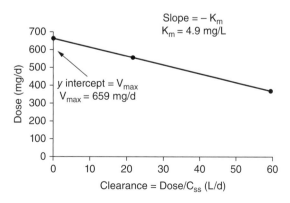

FIGURE 10-14   Solution to problem 10 using Ludden graph.

Bayesian Pharmacokinetic Computer Method

1. *Enter the patient's demographic, drug-dosing, and serum concentration/time data into the computer program.*

    DrugCalc requires doses to be entered in terms of phenytoin (phenytoin dose = 0.92 • phenytoin sodium dose = 0.92 • 600 mg/d = 552 mg/d; phenytoin dose = 0.92 • phenytoin sodium dose = 0.92 • 400 mg/d = 368 mg/d).

2. *Compute pharmacokinetic parameters for the patient using Bayesian pharmacokinetic computer program.*

    The pharmacokinetic parameters computed by the program are a volume of distribution of 90 L, a V_{max} equal to 510 mg/d, and a K_m equal to 4.3 mg/L.

3. *Compute the dose required to achieve the desired phenytoin serum concentrations.*

    The one-compartment model Michaelis-Menten equations used by the program to compute doses indicates that a dose of 440 mg/d of phenytoin will produce a total steady-state concentration of 15 µg/mL. This is equivalent to 478 mg/d of phenytoin sodium (440 mg/d phenytoin/0.92 = 478 mg/d phenytoin sodium), and this dose would be rounded to 500 mg/d given as 200 mg in the morning plus 300 mg in the evening.

    A steady-state trough total phenytoin serum concentration should be measured after steady-state is attained in 7-14 days. Phenytoin serum concentrations should also be measured if the patient experiences an exacerbation of their epilepsy, or if the patient develops potential signs or symptoms of phenytoin toxicity.

11. *Answer to problem 11.* For patient VG:

    1. *Choose appropriate equation to estimate normalized total phenytoin concentration at the appropriate temperature.*

$$C_{NormalBinding} = C/(0.25 • Alb + 0.1) = (8.9 \text{ µg/mL})/(0.25 • 2.4 \text{ g/dL} + 0.1) = 12.7 \text{ µg/mL}$$

$$C_{f_{EST}} = 0.1 \ C_{NormalBinding} = 0.1 • 12.7 \text{ µg/mL} = 1.3 \text{ µg/mL}$$

    This patient's estimated normalized total phenytoin concentration is expected to provide an unbound concentration equivalent to a total phenytoin concentration of 12.7 µg/mL for a patient with normal drug protein binding ($C_{f_{EST}}$ = 1.3 µg/mL). Because the estimated total value is within the therapeutic range of 10-20 µg/mL, it is likely that the patient has an unbound phenytoin concentration within the therapeutic range. If possible, this should be confirmed by obtaining an actual, measured unbound phenytoin concentration.

12. *Answer to problem 12.* For patient DE:

    1. *Choose appropriate equation to estimate normalized total phenytoin concentration.*

$$C_{NormalBinding} = C/(0.1 • Alb + 0.1) = (8.1 \text{ µg/mL})/(0.1 • 2.0 \text{ g/dL} + 0.1) = 27 \text{ µg/mL}$$

$$C_{f_{EST}} = 0.1 \ C_{NormalBinding} = 0.1 • 27 \text{ µg/mL} = 2.7 \text{ µg/mL}$$

    This patient's estimated normalized total phenytoin concentration is expected to provide an unbound concentration equivalent to a total phenytoin concentration of 27 µg/mL for a patient with normal drug protein binding ($C_{f_{EST}}$ = 2.7 µg/mL). Because the estimated total value is above the therapeutic range of 10-20 µg/mL, it is likely that the patient has an unbound phenytoin concentration above the therapeutic range. If possible, this should be confirmed by obtaining an actual, measured unbound phenytoin concentration.

13. *Answer to problem 13.* For patient KL:

1. *Choose appropriate equation to estimate unbound phenytoin concentration.*

$$C_{f_{EST}} = (0.095 + 0.001 \bullet VPA)PHT = (0.095 + 0.001 \bullet 90 \text{ μg/mL})6 \text{ μg/mL} = 1.1 \text{ μg/mL}$$

This patient's estimated unbound phenytoin concentration is expected to be within the therapeutic range for unbound concentrations. If possible, this should be confirmed by obtaining an actual, measured unbound phenytoin concentration.

14. *Answer to problem 14.* For patient YS:

Pharmacokinetic Dosing Method

1. *Estimate Michaelis-Menten constants according to disease states and conditions present in the patient.*

The V_{max} for a 7-16-year-old adolescent patient with normal liver and renal function is 9 mg/kg/d. For a 35-kg patient, V_{max} = 315 mg/d: V_{max} = 9 mg/kg/d $\bullet$ 35 kg = 315 mg/d. For this individual, K_m = 6 mg/L.

2. *Compute dosage regimen.*

Oral phenytoin suspension will be prescribed to this patient (F = 1, S = 1). The initial dosage interval (τ) will be set to 12 hours. (Note: μg/mL = mg/L and this concentration unit was substituted for Css in the calculations so that unnecessary unit conversion was not required.) The dosage equation for phenytoin is:

$$MD = \frac{V_{max} \bullet Css}{S(K_m + Css)} = \frac{315 \text{ mg/d} \bullet 12 \text{ mg/L}}{1.0(6 \text{ mg/L} + 12 \text{ mg/L})} = 210 \text{ mg/d, rounded to 200 mg/d}$$

Phenytoin suspension 100 mg every 12 hours would be prescribed for the patient. A steady-state trough total phenytoin serum concentration should be measured after steady-state is attained in 7-14 days. Phenytoin serum concentrations should also be measured if the patient experiences an exacerbation of their epilepsy, or if the patient develops potential signs or symptoms of phenytoin toxicity.

Literature-Based Recommended Dosing

1. *Estimate phenytoin dose according to disease states and conditions present in the patient.*

The suggested initial dosage rate for phenytoin suspension in an adolescent patient is 5-10 mg/kg/d. Using a rate of 6 mg/kg/d, the initial dose would be 200 mg/d: 6 mg/kg/d $\bullet$ 35 kg = 210 mg/d, rounded to 200 mg/d. Using a dosage interval of 12 hours, the prescribed dose would be 100 mg of phenytoin suspension every 12 hours.

A steady-state trough total phenytoin serum concentration should be measured after steady-state is attained in 7-14 days. Phenytoin serum concentrations should also be measured if the patient experiences an exacerbation of their epilepsy, or if the patient develops potential signs or symptoms of phenytoin toxicity.

15. *Answer to problem 15.* The revised phenytoin dose of patient YS would be calculated as follows:

Empiric Dosing Method

1. *Suggest new phenytoin dose.*

Since the patient is receiving phenytoin suspension, a convenient dosage change would be 50 mg/d and a decrease to 250 mg/d or 125 mg every 12 hours is empirically suggested.

A steady-state trough total phenytoin serum concentration should be measured after steady-state is attained in 7-14 days. Phenytoin serum concentrations should also be measured if the patient experiences an exacerbation of their epilepsy, or if the patient develops potential signs or symptoms of phenytoin toxicity.

Pseudolinear Pharmacokinetics Method

1. *Use pseudolinear pharmacokinetics to predict new concentration for a dosage decrease, then compute 15%-33% factor to account for Michaelis-Menten pharmacokinetics.*

    Since the patient is receiving phenytoin suspension, a convenient dosage change would be 50 mg/d and a decrease to 250 mg/d is suggested. Using pseudolinear pharmacokinetics, the resulting total steady-state phenytoin serum concentration would equal: $Css_{new} = (D_{new}/D_{old})Css_{old} =$ (250 mg/d / 300 mg/d)23 µg/mL = 19 µg/mL. Because of Michaelis-Menten pharmacokinetics, the serum concentration would be expected to decrease 15%, or 0.85 times, to 33%, or 0.67 times, more than that predicted by linear pharmacokinetics: Css = 19 µg/mL • 0.85 = 16.2 µg/mL and Css = 19 µg/mL • 0.67 = 12.7 µg/mL. Thus, a dosage decrease of 50 mg/d would be expected to yield a total phenytoin steady-state serum concentration between 13 and 16 µg/mL.

    A steady-state trough total phenytoin serum concentration should be measured after steady-state is attained in 7-14 days. Phenytoin serum concentrations should also be measured if the patient experiences an exacerbation of their epilepsy, or if the patient develops potential signs or symptoms of phenytoin toxicity.

REFERENCES

1. Abramowicz M, Zuccotti G, Pflomm JM, eds. Drugs for epilepsy. *Treatment Guidelines from The Medical Letter.* 2013;11(126):9-18.
2. Anon. The epilepsies: the diagnosis and management of the epilepsies in adults and children in primary and secondary care. *UK National Institute for Health and Care Excellence.* http://www.nice.org.uk/nicemedia/live/13635/57779/57779.pdf. April 1, 2014.
3. French JA, Kanner AM, Bautista J, et al. Efficacy and tolerability of the new antiepileptic drugs I: treatment of new onset epilepsy: report of the Therapeutics and Technology Assessment Subcommittee and Quality Standards Subcommittee of the American Academy of Neurology and the American Epilepsy Society. *Neurology.* Apr 27, 2004;62(8):1252-1260.
4. Glauser T, Ben-Menachem E, Bourgeois B, et al. Updated ILAE evidence review of antiepileptic drug efficacy and effectiveness as initial monotherapy for epileptic seizures and syndromes. *Epilepsia.* Mar 2013;54(3):551-563.
5. Glauser TA, Cnaan A, Shinnar S, et al. Ethosuximide, valproic acid, and lamotrigine in childhood absence epilepsy. *N Engl J Med.* Mar 4, 2010;362(9):790-799.
6. Glauser TA, Cnaan A, Shinnar S, et al. Ethosuximide, valproic acid, and lamotrigine in childhood absence epilepsy: initial monotherapy outcomes at 12 months. *Epilepsia.* Jan 2013;54(1):141-155.
7. Rogers SJ, Cavazos JE. Epilepsy. In: DiPiro JT, Talbert RL, Yee GC, Matzke GR, Wells BG, Posey LM, eds. *Pharmacotherapy.* 8th ed. New York, NY: McGraw-Hill; 2011:979-1005.
8. McNamara JO. Pharmacotherapy of the epilepsies. In: Brunton L, Chabner B, Knollman B, eds. *The Pharmacological Basis of Therapeutics.* 12th ed. New York, NY: McGraw-Hill; 2011:583-608.
9. Chen SS, Perucca E, Lee JN, Richens A. Serum protein binding and free concentration of phenytoin and phenobarbitone in pregnancy. *Br J Clin Pharmacol.* 1982;13(4):547-552.
10. Knott C, Williams CP, Reynolds F. Phenytoin kinetics during pregnancy and the puerperium. *Br J Obstet Gynaecol.* 1986;93(10): 1030-1037.
11. Perucca E, Hebdige S, Frigo GM, Gatti G, Lecchini S, Crema A. Interaction between phenytoin and valproic acid: plasma protein binding and metabolic effects. *Clin Pharmacol Ther.* 1980;28(6):779-789.
12. Pisani FD, Di Perri RG. Intravenous valproate: effects on plasma and saliva phenytoin levels. *Neurology.* 1981;31(4):467-470.
13. Riva R, Albani F, Contin M, et al. Time-dependent interaction between phenytoin and valproic acid. *Neurology.* 1985;35(4):510-515.
14. Frigo GM, Lecchini S, Gatti G, Perucca E, Crema A. Modification of phenytoin clearance by valproic acid in normal subjects. *Br J Clin Pharmacol.* 1979;8(6):553-556.

15. Paxton JW. Effects of aspirin on salivary and serum phenytoin kinetics in healthy subjects. *Clin Pharmacol Ther.* 1980;27(2):170-178.

16. Leonard RF, Knott PJ, Rankin GO, Robinson DS, Melnick DE. Phenytoin-salicylate interaction. *Clin Pharmacol Ther.* 1981;29(1): 56-60.

17. Fraser DG, Ludden TM, Evens RP, Sutherland EW 3rd. Displacement of phenytoin from plasma binding sites by salicylate. *Clin Pharmacol Ther.* 1980;27(2):165-169.

18. Olanow CW, Finn AL, Prussak C. The effects of salicylate on the pharmacokinetics of phenytoin. *Neurology.* 1981;31(3):341-342.

19. Mabuchi H, Nakahashi H. A major inhibitor of phenytoin binding to serum protein in uremia. *Nephron.* 1988;48(4):310-314.

20. Dasgupta A, Malik S. Fast atom bombardment mass spectrometric determination of the molecular weight range of uremic compounds that displace phenytoin from protein binding: absence of midmolecular uremic toxins. *Am J Nephrol.* 1994;14(3):162-168.

21. Odar-Cederlof I, Borga O. Kinetics of diphenylhydantoin in uraemic patients: consequences of decreased plasma protein binding. *Eur J Clin Pharmacol.* 1974;7:31-37.

22. Odar-Cederlof I, Borga O. Impaired plasma protein binding of phenytoin in uremia and displacement effect of salicylic acid. *Clin Pharmacol Ther.* 1976;20(1):36-47.

23. Odar-Cederlof I. Plasma protein binding of phenytoin and warfarin in patients undergoing renal transplantation. *Clin Pharmacokin.* 1977;2:147-153.

24. Dodson WE, Loney LC. Hemodialysis reduces the unbound phenytoin in plasma. *J Pediatr.* 1982;101(3):465-468.

25. Kinniburgh DW, Boyd ND. Isolation of peptides from uremic plasma that inhibit phenytoin binding to normal plasma proteins. *Clin Pharmacol Ther.* 1981;30(2):276-280.

26. Peterson GM, McLean S, Aldous S, Von Witt RJ, Millingen KS. Plasma protein binding of phenytoin in 100 epileptic patients. *Br J Clin Pharmacol.* 1982;14(2):298-300.

27. Patterson M, Heazelwood R, Smithurst B, Eadie MJ. Plasma protein binding of phenytoin in the aged: in vivo studies. *Br J Clin Pharmacol.* 1982;13(3):423-425.

28. Bauer LA. Use of mixed-effect modeling to determine the influence of albumin, bilirubin, valproic acid, warfarin, and aspirin on phenytoin unbound fraction and pharmacokinetics. *J Amer Pharm Assoc.* 2004;44:236-237.

29. Winter ME, Tozer TN. Phenytoin. In: Evans WE, Schentag JJ, Jusko WJ, eds. *Applied Pharmacokinetics.* 3rd ed. Vancouver, WA: Applied Therapeutics; 1992:25.21-44.

30. Anderson GD, Pak C, Doane KW, et al. Revised Winter-Tozer equation for normalized phenytoin concentrations in trauma and elderly patients with hypoalbuminemia. *Ann Pharmacother.* 1997;31(3):279-284.

31. Haidukewych D, Rodin EA, Zielinski JJ. Derivation and evaluation of an equation for prediction of free phenytoin concentration in patients co-medicated with valproic acid. *Ther Drug Monit.* 1989;11(2):134-139.

32. Kerrick JM, Wolff DL, Graves NM. Predicting unbound phenytoin concentrations in patients receiving valproic acid: a comparison of two prediction methods. *Ann Pharmacother.* 1995;29(5):470-474.

33. Aarons L, Ahmed IA, Deleu D. Estimation of population pharmacokinetic parameters of free-phenytoin in adult epileptic patients. *Arch Med Res.* Jan-Feb 2005;36(1):49-53.

34. Allen JP, Ludden TM, Burrow SR, Clementi WA, Stavchansky SA. Phenytoin cumulation kinetics. *Clin Pharmacol Ther.* 1979;26(4):445-448.

35. Grasela TH, Sheiner LB, Rambeck B, et al. Steady-state pharmacokinetics of phenytoin from routinely collected patient data. *Clin Pharmacokin.* 1983;8:355-364.

36. Ludden TM, Allen JP, Valutsky WA, et al. Individualization of phenytoin dosage regimens. *Clin Pharmacol Ther.* 1977;21(3):287-293.

37. Perrier D, Rapp R, Young B, et al. Maintenance of therapeutic phenytoin plasma levels via intramuscular administration. *Ann Intern Med.* 1976;85(3):318-321.

38. Tanaka J, Kasai H, Shimizu K, Shimasaki S, Kumagai Y. Population pharmacokinetics of phenytoin after intravenous administration of fosphenytoin sodium in pediatric patients, adult patients, and healthy volunteers. *Eur J Clin Pharmacol.* Mar 2013;69(3): 489-497.

39. Kinikar SA, Delate T, Menaker-Wiener CM, Bentley WH. Clinical outcomes associated with brand-to-generic phenytoin interchange. *Ann Pharmacother.* May 2012;46(5):650-658.

40. Burkhardt RT, Leppik IE, Blesi K, Scott S, Gapany SR, Cloyd JC. Lower phenytoin serum levels in persons switched from brand to generic phenytoin. *Neurology.* Oct 26, 2004;63(8):1494-1496.

41. Jusko WJ, Koup JR, Alvan G. Nonlinear assessment of phenytoin bioavailability. *J Pharmacokinet Biopharm.* 1976;4(4):327-336.

42. Gugler R, Manion CV, Azarnoff DL. Phenytoin: pharmacokinetics and bioavailability. *Clin Pharmacol Ther.* 1976;19(2):135-142.

43. Smith TC, Kinkel A. Absorption and metabolism of phenytoin from tablets and capsules. *Clin Pharmacol Ther.* 1976;20(6):738-742.

44. Chakrabarti S, Belpaire F, Moerman E. Effect of formulation on dissolution and bioavailability of phenytoin tablets. *Pharmazie.* 1980;35(10):627-629.

45. Jung D, Powell JR, Walson P, Perrier D. Effect of dose on phenytoin absorption. *Clin Pharmacol Ther.* 1980;28(4):479-485.

46. Fleisher D, Sheth N, Kou JH. Phenytoin interaction with enteral feedings administered through nasogastric tubes. *JPEN J Parenter Enteral Nutr.* 1990;14(5):513-516.

47. Cacek AT, DeVito JM, Koonce JR. In vitro evaluation of nasogastric administration methods for phenytoin. *Am J Hosp Pharm.* 1986;43(3):689-692.

48. Bauer LA. Interference of oral phenytoin absorption by continuous nasogastric feedings. *Neurology.* 1982;32(5):570-572.

49. Ozuna J, Friel P. Effect of enteral tube feeding on serum phenytoin levels. *J Neurosurg Nurs.* 1984;16(6):289-291.

50. Bach B, Molholm Hansen J, Kampmann JP, Rasmussen SN, Skovsted L. Disposition of antipyrine and phenytoin correlated with age and liver volume in man. *Clin Pharmacokin.* 1981;6:389-396.

51. Bauer LA, Blouin RA. Age and phenytoin kinetics in adult epileptics. *Clin Pharmacol Ther.* 1982;31(3):301-304.

52. Blain PG, Mucklow JC, Bacon CJ, Rawlins MD. Pharmacokinetics of phenytoin in children. *Br J Clin Pharmacol.* 1981;12(5):659-661.

53. Chiba K, Ishizaki T, Miura H, Minagawa K. Apparent Michaelis-Menten kinetic parameters of phenytoin in pediatric patients. *Pediatr Pharmacol.* 1980;1(2):171-180.

54. Chiba K, Ishizaki T, Miura H, Minagawa K. Michaelis-Menten pharmacokinetics of diphenylhydantoin and application in the pediatric age patient. *J Pediatr.* 1980;96(3 Pt 1):479-484.

55. Dodson WE. Nonlinear kinetics of phenytoin in children. *Neurology.* 1982;32(1):42-48.

56. Leff RD, Fischer LJ, Roberts RJ. Phenytoin metabolism in infants following intravenous and oral administration. *Dev Pharmacol Ther.* 1986;9(4):217-223.

57. Bauer LA, Blouin RA. Phenytoin Michaelis-Menten pharmacokinetics in Caucasian paediatric patients. *Clin Pharmacokinet.* 1983;8(6):545-549.

58. Lee FX, Kong ST, Chan DW, Chan E, Tan WW, Ho PC. Developing a nomogram for dose individualization of phenytoin in Asian pediatric patients derived from population pharmacokinetic modeling of saturable pharmacokinetic profiles of the drug. *Ther Drug Monit.* Feb 2013;35(1):54-62.

59. Pugh RN, Murray-Lyon IM, Dawson JL, Pietroni MC, Williams R. Transection of the oesophagus for bleeding oesophageal varices. *Br J Surg.* 1973;60(8):646-649.

60. Bauer LA, Edwards WA, Dellinger EP, Raisys VA, Brennan C. Importance of unbound phenytoin serum levels in head trauma patients. *J Trauma.* 1983;23(12):1058-1060.

61. Boucher BA, Rodman JH, Jaresko GS, Rasmussen SN, Watridge CB, Fabian TC. Phenytoin pharmacokinetics in critically ill trauma patients. *Clin Pharmacol Ther.* 1988;44(6):675-683.

62. Chiba K, Ishizaki T, Tabuchi T, Wagatsuma T, Nakazawa Y. Antipyrine disposition in relation to lowered anticonvulsant plasma level during pregnancy. *Obstet Gynecol.* 1982;60(5):620-626.

63. Dickinson RG, Hooper WD, Wood B, Lander CM, Eadie MJ. The effect of pregnancy in humans on the pharmacokinetics of stable isotope labelled phenytoin. *Br J Clin Pharmacol.* 1989;28(1):17-27.

64. Lander CM, Smith MT, Chalk JB, et al. Bioavailability and pharmacokinetics of phenytoin during pregnancy. *Eur J Clin Pharmacol.* 1984;27(1):105-110.

65. Kochenour NK, Emery MG, Sawchuk RJ. Phenytoin metabolism in pregnancy. *Obstet Gynecol.* 1980;56(5):577-582.

66. Landon MJ, Kirkley M. Metabolism of diphenylhydantoin (phenytoin) during pregnancy. *Br J Obstet Gynaecol.* 1979;86(2):125-132.

67. Brier ME, Aronoff GR. *Drug Prescribing in Renal Failure.* 5th ed. Philadelphia, PA: American College of Physicians; 2007.

68. Golper TA, Marx MA. Drug dosing adjustments during continuous renal replacement therapies. *Kidney Int Suppl.* May 1998; 66:S165-S168.

69. Golper TA. Update on drug sieving coefficients and dosing adjustments during continuous renal replacement therapies. *Contrib Nephrol.* 2001;132:349-353.

70. Steen B, Rane A, Lonnerholm G, Falk O, Elwin CE, Sjoqvist F. Phenytoin excretion in human breast milk and plasma levels in nursed infants. *Ther Drug Monit.* 1982;4(4):331-334.

71. Shimoyama R, Ohkubo T, Sugawara K, et al. Monitoring of phenytoin in human breast milk, maternal plasma and cord blood plasma by solid-phase extraction and liquid chromatography. *J Pharm Biomed Anal.* Aug 1998;17(4-5):863-869.

72. Hansten PD, Horn JR. *Drug Interactions Analysis and Management.* St. Louis, MO: Wolters Kluwer Health; 2014.

73. Hansten PD, Horn JR. *The Top 100 Drug Interactions.* Freeland, WA: H&H Publications; 2014.

74. Abernethy DR, Greenblatt DJ. Phenytoin disposition in obesity. Determination of loading dose. *Arch Neurol.* 1985;42(5):468-471.

75. Mauro LS, Mauro VF, Bachmann KA, Higgins JT. Accuracy of two equations in determining normalized phenytoin concentrations. *DICP.* 1989;23(1):64-68.

76. Bauer LA. Clinical pharmacokinetics and pharmacodynamics. In: DiPiro JT, Talbert RL, Yee GC, Matzke GR, Wells BG, Posey LM, eds. *Pharmacotherapy.* 9th ed. New York, NY: McGraw-Hill; 2014.

77. Graves N, Cloyd J, Leppik I. Phenytoin dosage predictions using population clearances. *Ann Pharmacother.* 1982;16:473-478.

78. Vozeh S, Muir KT, Sheiner LB, Follath F. Predicting individual phenytoin dosage. *J Pharmacokinet Biopharm.* 1981;9(2):131-146.

79. Mullen PW. Optimal phenytoin therapy: a new technique for individualizing dosage. *Clin Pharmacol Ther.* 1978;23(2):228-232.

80. Mullen PW, Foster RW. Comparative evaluation of six techniques for determining the Michaelis-Menten parameters relating phenytoin dose and steady-state serum concentrations. *J Pharm Pharmacol.* 1979;31(2):100-104.

81. Wandell M, Mungall D. Computer assisted drug interpretation and drug regimen optimization. *Amer Assoc Clin Chem.* 1984;6:1-11.

11 Carbamazepine

INTRODUCTION

Carbamazepine is an iminostilbene derivative related to the tricyclic antidepressants that is used in the treatment of tonic-clonic (grand mal), partial, or secondarily generalized seizures (Table 11-1).[1-4] Although methods have been suggested to treat acute seizures with carbamazepine, lack of an intravenous dosage form has limited its use in this area. Thus, the drug is used primarily as a prophylactic agent in the chronic therapy of epilepsy. Carbamazepine is also a useful agent to treat trigeminal neuralgia and bipolar affective disorders.[7-9]

The antiseizure activity of carbamazepine is related to its ability to decrease transmission in the nucleus ventralis anterior section of the thalamus, an area of the brain thought to be involved with the generalization and propagation of epileptic discharges.[7,10] Although the exact cellular mechanism of action is unclear, inhibition of voltage-gated sodium channels appears to be involved. Additionally, carbamazepine depresses posttetanic potentiation and may prevent increases in cyclic adenosine monophosphate (cAMP).

THERAPEUTIC AND TOXIC CONCENTRATIONS

The accepted therapeutic range for carbamazepine is 4-12 μg/mL when the drug is used for the treatment of seizures. Carbamazepine plasma protein binding is quite variable among individuals because it is bound to both albumin and α_1-acid glycoprotein (AGP). In patients with normal concentrations of these proteins, plasma protein binding is 75%-80% resulting in a free fraction of drug of 20%-25%.[11-14] AGP is classified as an acute-phase reactant protein that is present in lower amounts in all individuals but is secreted in large amounts in response to certain stresses and disease states such as trauma, heart failure, and myocardial infarction. In patients with these disease states, carbamazepine binding to AGP can be even larger resulting in an unbound fraction as low as 10%-15%.

Little prospective work has been done to establish the therapeutic range for unbound carbamazepine serum concentrations or the clinical situations where unbound carbamazepine serum concentration measurement is useful. As an initial guide, 25% of the total carbamazepine therapeutic range as been used to establish a preliminary desirable range for unbound carbamazepine serum concentrations of 1-3 μg/mL. Although carbamazepine is highly plasma protein bound, it is harder to displace this agent to the extent that a clinically important change in protein binding takes place. Generally speaking, a doubling in unbound fraction in the plasma is required to produce such an alteration. In comparison, phenytoin is 90% protein bound under usual circumstances resulting in an unbound fraction in the plasma of 10%. It is relatively easy to change the protein binding of phenytoin from 90% to 80%, under a variety of disease states or conditions, which increases the unbound fraction in the plasma from 10% to 20%. However, it is very difficult to change the protein binding of carbamazepine from 80% to 60% to achieve the same doubling of unbound fraction in the plasma (20%-40%). As a result of this, the use of unbound carbamazepine serum concentrations are currently limited

TABLE 11-1 International Classification of Epileptic Seizures With Recommended Therapies

Major Class	Subset of Class	Drug Treatment for Selected Seizure Type			
		2004 AAN/AES	**2013 Medical Letter**	**2012 NICE**	**2013 ILAE**[a]
Partial seizures (beginning locally)	1. Simple partial seizures (without impaired consciousness) a. with motor symptoms b. with somatosensory or special sensory symptoms c. with autonomic symptoms d. with psychological symptoms	Carbamazepine Phenytoin Valproate Phenobarbital Lamotrigine Gabapentin Oxcarbazepine Topiramate	Lamotrigine Carbamazepine Levetiracetam Oxcarbazepine *Alternatives:* Topiramate Valproate Gabapentin Zonisamide Phenytoin Pregabalin Lacosamide Ezogabine	Carbamazepine Lamotrigine Levetiracetam Oxcarbazepine Valproate *Adjunctive:* Carbamazepine Clobazam Gabapentin Lamotrigine Levetiracetam Oxcarbazepine Valproate Topiramate	*Adults:* Carbamazepine Levetiracetam Phenytoin Zonisamide Valproate *Children:* Oxcarbazepine Carbamazepine Phenobarbital Phenytoin Topiramate Valproate Vigabatrin *Elderly:* Gabapentin Lamotrigine Carbamazepine
	2. Complex partial seizures (with impaired consciousness) a. simple partial onset followed by impaired consciousness b. impaired consciousness at onset	Carbamazepine Phenytoin Valproate Phenobarbital Lamotrigine Gabapentin Oxcarbazepine Topiramate	Lamotrigine Carbamazepine Levetiracetam Oxcarbazepine *Alternatives:* Topiramate Valproate Gabapentin Zonisamide Phenytoin Pregabalin Lacosamide Ezogabine	Carbamazepine Lamotrigine Levetiracetam Oxcarbazepine Valproate *Adjunctive:* Carbamazepine Clobazam Gabapentin Lamotrigine Levetiracetam Oxcarbazepine Valproate Topiramate	*Adults:* Carbamazepine Levetiracetam Phenytoin Zonisamide Valproate *Children:* Oxcarbazepine Carbamazepine Phenobarbital Phenytoin Topiramate Valproate Vigabatrin *Elderly:* Gabapentin Lamotrigine Carbamazepine
	3. Partial seizures evolving into secondary generalized seizures	Carbamazepine Phenytoin Valproate Phenobarbital Lamotrigine Gabapentin Oxcarbazepine Topiramate	Lamotrigine Carbamazepine Levetiracetam Oxcarbazepine *Alternatives:* Topiramate Valproate Gabapentin Zonisamide Phenytoin Pregabalin Lacosamide Ezogabine	Carbamazepine Lamotrigine Levetiracetam Oxcarbazepine Valproate *Adjunctive:* Carbamazepine Clobazam Gabapentin Lamotrigine Levetiracetam Oxcarbazepine Valproate Topiramate	*Adults:* Carbamazepine Levetiracetam Phenytoin Zonisamide Valproate *Children:* Oxcarbazepine Carbamazepine Phenobarbital Phenytoin Topiramate Valproate Vigabatrin *Elderly:* Gabapentin Lamotrigine Carbamazepine

(Continued)

TABLE 11-1   International Classification of Epileptic Seizures With Recommended Therapies (*Continued*)

Major Class	Subset of Class	Drug Treatment for Selected Seizure Type			
		2004 AAN/AES	**2013 Medical Letter**	**2012 NICE**	**2013 ILAE**[a]
Generalized seizures (convulsive or nonconvulsive)	1. Absence seizures[b] (typical or atypical; also known as petite mal seizures)	*Children:*[c] Ethosuximide Valproate Lamotrigine	Ethosuximide Valproate *Alternatives:* Lamotrigine Clonazepam Zonisamide Levetiracetam	Ethosuximide Lamotrigine Valproate *Adjunctive:* Ethosuximide Lamotrigine Valproate	*Children:* Ethosuximide Valproate Lamotrigine
	2. Tonic-clonic seizures (also known as grand mal seizures)	Carbamazepine Phenytoin Valproate Phenobarbital Lamotrigine Oxcarbazepine Topiramate	Valproate Lamotrigine Levetiracetam *Alternatives:* Topiramate Zonisamide Phenytoin	Carbamazepine Lamotrigine Oxcarbazepine Valproate *Adjunctive:* Clobazam Lamotrigine Levetiracetam Valproate Topiramate	*Adults:* Carbamazepine Lamotrigine Oxcarbazepine Phenobarbital Phenytoin Topiramate Valproate Gabapentin Levetiracetam Vigabatrin *Children:* Carbamazepine Phenobarbital Phenytoin Topiramate Valproate Oxcarbazepine

[a]Only two highest available levels of evidence listed.

[b]Recent literature suggests either ethosuximide or valproic acid is a superior initial therapy compared to lamotrigine for absence seizures.[5,6]

[c]Lamotrigine added to previous recommendation per expert panel.

Abbreviations: ANN, American Academy of Neurology; AES, American Epilepsy Society; ILAE, International League Against Epilepsy; NICE, UK National Institute for Clinical Excellence.

to those patients that have total concentrations within the therapeutic range but experience adverse effects usually seen at higher concentrations, or those patients that have total concentrations below the therapeutic range but have a therapeutic response usually observed at higher concentrations.

Carbamazepine-10, 11-epoxide is an active metabolite of carbamazepine that contributes to both the therapeutic and toxic effects of the drug, and can be measured in serum samples at a limited number of epilepsy centers.[15-21] The concentration of the epoxide is often related to the presence or absence of other inhibitors or inducers of hepatic drug-metabolizing enzymes. Epoxide concentrations tend to be higher in patients taking enzyme inducers and lower in patients taking enzyme inhibitors. The percent of epoxide to parent drug in chronically treated patients averages about 12% for carbamazepine monotherapy, 14% when carbamazepine is taken with phenobarbital, 18% when carbamazepine is taken with phenytoin, and about 25% when carbamazepine is taken with both phenytoin and phenobarbital. Currently, the therapeutic range of carbamazepine-10, 11-epoxide is not known although a suggested range of 0.4-4 µg/mL is used by several research centers.

In the upper end of the therapeutic range (>8 μg/mL) some patients will begin to experience the concentration-related adverse effects of carbamazepine treatment: nausea, vomiting, lethargy, dizziness, drowsiness, headache, blurred vision, diplopia, unsteadiness, ataxia, incoordination. Because carbamazepine induces its own hepatic metabolism, these adverse effects can also be seen early during dosage titration periods soon after dosage increases are made. To improve patient acceptance, it is important to initiate and titrate carbamazepine doses at a slow rate to minimize side effects. Clinicians should understand that all patients with "toxic" carbamazepine serum concentrations in the listed ranges will not exhibit signs or symptoms of carbamazepine toxicity. Rather, carbamazepine concentrations in the ranges given increase the likelihood that an adverse drug effect will occur.

CLINICAL MONITORING PARAMETERS

The goal of therapy with anticonvulsants is to reduce seizure frequency and maximize quality of life with a minimum of adverse drug effects. While it is desirable to entirely abolish all seizure episodes, it may not be possible to accomplish this in many patients. Patients should be monitored for concentration-related side effects (nausea, vomiting, lethargy, dizziness, drowsiness, headache, blurred vision, diplopia, unsteadiness, ataxia, incoordination). Because carbamazepine has antidiuretic effects associated with reduced levels of antidiuretic hormone, some patients may develop hyponatremia during chronic therapy with carbamazepine, and serum sodium concentrations can be periodically measured.

Hematologic adverse effects can be divided into two types. The first is a leukopenia that occurs in many patients and requires no therapeutic intervention. The typical clinical picture is an individual with a normal white blood cell count who develops a transient decrease in this index. In a few patients, a decreased, stable white blood cell count of 3000 cells/mm^2 or less may persist and does not appear to cause any deleterious effects. The second hematologic effect is severe and usually requires discontinuation of the drug. Thrombocytopenia, leukopenia (trend downward in white blood cell count with <2500 cells/mm^2 or absolute neutrophil count <1000 cells/mm^2), or anemia are in this category. Rarely, aplastic anemia and agranulocytosis has been reported during carbamazepine treatment. Drug-induced hepatitis due to carbamazepine therapy has also been reported. The severe hematologic and hepatic adverse effects tend to occur early in treatment. Because of this, many clinicians measure a complete blood cell count and liver function tests monthly for the first 3-6 months after a patient first begins carbamazepine treatment, and repeat these tests every 3-6 months for the first year. Other idiosyncratic side effects include skin rash, Stevens-Johnson syndrome, and systemic lupus-like reactions.

Carbamazepine serum concentrations should be measured in most patients. Because epilepsy is an episodic disease state, patients do not experience seizures on a continuous basis. Thus, during dosage titration it is difficult to tell if the patient is responding to drug therapy or simply is not experiencing any abnormal central nervous system discharges at that time. Carbamazepine serum concentrations are also valuable tools to avoid adverse drug effects. Patients are more likely to accept drug therapy if adverse reactions are held to the absolute minimum. Because carbamazepine induces its own hepatic metabolism, it is fairly easy to attain toxic concentrations with modest increases in drug dose before maximal enzyme induction has occurred.

BASIC CLINICAL PHARMACOKINETIC PARAMETERS

Carbamazepine is primarily eliminated by hepatic metabolism (>99%) mainly via the CYP3A4 enzyme system.[22,23] Altogether 33 metabolites have been identified with carbamazepine-10, 11-epoxide being the major species. The epoxide metabolite is active and probably contributes to both the therapeutic and toxic side effects observed during therapy. Carbamazepine is a potent inducer of hepatic drug-metabolizing enzymes,

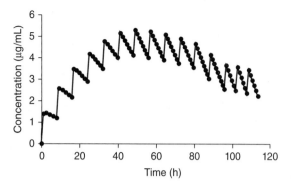

FIGURE 11-1 Carbamazepine induces its own metabolism via the hepatic microsomal enzyme system CYP3A4 system. This process is known as autoinduction. When dosing is initiated, serum concentrations increase according to the baseline clearance and half-life. After a few doses of carbamazepine, enough autoinduction has occurred that clearance increases, half-life decreases, and drug accumulation slows down. With additional exposure of liver tissue to carbamazepine, clearance continues to increase and half-life continues to shorten. As a result of these pharmacokinetic changes, carbamazepine concentrations decline and ultimately stabilize in accord with the new clearance and half-life values. Maximal autoinduction usually occurs 2-3 weeks after dosing commenced. Because of the autoinduction phenomenon, the ultimate desired maintenance dose cannot be started with the first dose. Additional autoinduction occurs with subsequent increases in dose.

and induces it's own metabolism, a process known as autoinduction (Figures 11-1, 11-2).[24-28] As a result, patients cannot initially be placed on the dose of carbamazepine that will ultimately result in a safe and effective outcome. At first, patients are started on ¼-⅓ of the desired maintenance dose. This exposes hepatic drug-metabolizing enzymes to carbamazepine and begins the induction process. The dose is increased by a similar amount every 2-3 weeks until the total desired daily dose is ultimately given. This gradual exposure of carbamazepine allows liver enzyme induction and carbamazepine clearance increases to occur over a 6-12 week time period. Therapeutic effect and steady-state carbamazepine serum concentrations can be assessed 2-3 weeks after the final dosage increase. Autoinduction continues to occur in patients who are stabilized on a carbamazepine dose but require a dosage increase. It appears that a 2-3 week time period is also needed under chronic dosing conditions for maximal autoinduction to occur after a dosage increase. The effects of autoinduction are reversible even when doses are held for as few as 6 days.[29]

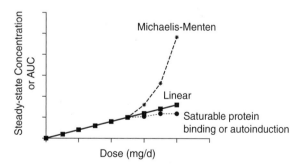

FIGURE 11-2 If a drug follows linear pharmacokinetics, Css or AUC increases proportionally with dose resulting in a straight line on the plot. Nonlinear pharmacokinetics occurs when the Css or AUC versus dose plot results in something other than a straight line. If a drug follows Michaelis-Menten pharmacokinetics (eg, phenytoin, aspirin), as steady-state drug concentrations approach K_m serum concentrations increase more than expected due to dose increases. If a drug follows nonlinear protein binding (eg, valproic acid, disopyramide) or demonstrates autoinduction (eg, carbamazepine), total steady-state drug concentrations increase less than expected as dose increases.

An injectable form of carbamazepine is not available for clinical use. For oral use, the drug is available as immediate-release tablets (chewable: 100 mg, regular: 200 mg), extended-release tablets (100, 200, 400 mg), extended-release capsules (100, 200, 300 mg), and suspension (100 mg/5 mL). The rapid release dosage forms are erratically absorbed from the gastrointestinal tract resulting in peak concentrations between 2 and 24 hours after a single dose of tablets (average 6 hours). During multiple dose studies after maximal autoinduction has taken place, peak concentrations occur about 3 hours after tablet administration. Peak concentrations after multiple doses of the extended-release dosage forms are observed 3 to 12 hours after administration. Rectal administration of an extemporaneously compounded carbamazepine retention enema results in similar serum concentrations as that produced by a comparable immediate-release tablet.[30,31]

The absolute oral bioavailability of commercially available carbamazepine dosage forms for adult epileptics determined using an experimental intravenous injection for comparison is 78%.[32] The relative oral bioavailability of other dosage forms (chewable tablet, suspension, extended-release tablets, and extended-release capsules) compared to the immediate-release tablet approaches 100%. If a patient is receiving a stable dose of carbamazepine on one dosage form, the same total daily dose of another dosage form can typically be substituted without adjustment. However, some bioequivalence problems have been reported for generic carbamazepine products.[33-35]

Usual initial maintenance doses are 10-20 mg/kg/d for children under 6 years of age, 200 mg/d for children 6-12 years old, and 400 mg/d for adults. Twice daily dosing is initially used until autoinduction takes place. Dosage increases to allow for autoinduction are made every 2-3 weeks depending on response and adverse effects. Most adults will require 800-1200 mg/d of carbamazepine while older children will require 400-800 mg/d. Although some minor side effects occur, single loading doses of 8 mg/kg have been given to adults as suspension or immediate-release tablets in order to achieve therapeutic concentrations within 2-4 hours after administration.[36]

EFFECTS OF DISEASE STATES AND CONDITIONS ON PHARMACOKINETICS AND DOSING

After single doses of carbamazepine, the oral clearance (Cl/F) is 11-26 mL/h/kg and half-life is 35 hours for adults.[37-39] During multiple dosing after maximal autoinduction has taken place, oral clearance equals 50-100 mg/h/kg and half-life equals 5-27 hours. In children 6-12 years old, oral clearance and half-life equal 50-200 mL/h/kg and 3-15 hours, respectively, during chronic dosing. Clearance rates can be higher and half-lives shorter in patients receiving other hepatic drug-metabolizing enzyme inducers (phenytoin, phenobarbital, rifampin).[40-42] Carbamazepine volume of distribution using immediate-release tablets (V/F) is 1-2 L/kg. The volume of distribution (V) using an experimental intravenous form of the drug is 1.1 L/kg.[32]

Patients with liver cirrhosis or acute hepatitis have reduced carbamazepine clearance because of destruction of liver parenchyma. This loss of functional hepatic cells reduces the amount of CYP3A4 available to metabolize the drug and decreases clearance. The volume of distribution may be larger because of reduced plasma protein binding. Protein binding may be reduced and unbound fraction maybe increased due to hypoalbuminemia and/or hyperbilirubinemia (especially albumin ≤ 3 g/dL and/or total bilirubin ≥ 2 mg/dL). However, the effects that liver disease has on carbamazepine pharmacokinetics are highly variable and difficult to accurately predict. It is possible for a patient with liver disease to have relatively normal or grossly abnormal carbamazepine clearance and volume of distribution. For example, a liver disease patient who has relatively normal albumin and bilirubin concentrations can have a normal volume of distribution for carbamazepine. An index of liver dysfunction can be gained by applying the Child-Pugh clinical classification system to the patient (Table 11-2).[43] Child-Pugh scores are completely discussed in Chapter 3 (Drug Dosing in Special Populations: Renal and Hepatic Disease, Dialysis, Heart Failure, Obesity, and Drug Interactions), but will be briefly discussed here. The Child-Pugh score consists of five laboratory tests or clinical symptoms: serum albumin, total bilirubin, prothrombin time, ascites, and hepatic encephalopathy. Each of these areas is given a score of 1 (normal) to 3 (severely abnormal;

TABLE 11-2   Child-Pugh Scores for Patients With Liver Disease

Test/Symptom	Score 1 Point	Score 2 Points	Score 3 Points
Total bilirubin (mg/dL)	<2.0	2.0-3.0	>3.0
Serum albumin (g/dL)	>3.5	2.8-3.5	<2.8
Prothrombin time (seconds prolonged over control)	<4	4-6	>6
Ascites	Absent	Slight	Moderate
Hepatic encephalopathy	None	Moderate	Severe

Mild liver disease, 5-6 points; moderate liver disease, 7-9 points; severe liver disease, 10-15 points.

see Table 11-2), and the scores for the five areas are summed. The Child-Pugh score for a patient with normal liver function is 5 while the score for a patient with grossly abnormal serum albumin, total bilirubin, and pro-thrombin time values in addition to severe ascites and hepatic encephalopathy is 15. A Child-Pugh score greater than 8 is grounds for a decrease of 25%-50% in the initial daily drug dose for carbamazepine. As in any patient with or without liver dysfunction, initial doses are meant as starting points for dosage titration based on patient response and avoidance of adverse effects. Carbamazepine serum concentrations and the presence of adverse drug effects should be monitored frequently in patients with liver cirrhosis.

Elderly and younger epileptic patients have similar carbamazepine clearances.[14,32] However, older patients may be more sensitive to the central nervous system adverse effects of carbamazepine, and a lower starting dose of 100 mg/d is often used in elderly patients to avoid these problems. Compared to men, women have ~26% higher clearance rates for carbamazepine.[32] Carbamazepine clearance is ~19% lower in African American patients compared to Caucasian patients.[14,32] During the third trimester of pregnancy, oral clearance of carbamazepine may decrease and require dosage adjustment. Doses of carbamazepine do not require adjustment for patients with renal failure, and the drug is not removed by dialysis.[44,45] Breast milk concentrations of carbamazepine are about 60% of concurrent serum concentrations.

DRUG INTERACTIONS

Carbamazepine is a potent inducer of hepatic drug-metabolizing enzyme systems and P-glycoprotein.[46] The CYP1A2, CYP2C9, and CYP3A4 enzyme systems are all induced by carbamazepine, and drug substrates for other enzyme systems also have known drug interactions with carbamazepine. Other antiepileptic drugs that have their clearance rates increased and steady-state concentrations decreased by carbamazepine-related enzyme induction include felbamate, lamotrigine, phenytoin, primidone, tiagabine, topiramate, and valproic acid. Carbamazepine therapy also increases the clearance and decreases steady-state concentrations of many other drugs including oral contraceptives, calcium channel blockers, tricyclic antidepressants, cyclosporine, tacrolimus, theophylline, and warfarin. Generally, when carbamazepine is added to a patient's drug regimen, loss of therapeutic effect due to one of the other drugs must be considered as a possible drug interaction with carbamazepine.

Carbamazepine is a substrate for CYP3A4, and other drugs can affect carbamazepine clearance and steady-state serum concentrations.[46] Phenytoin and phenobarbital can increase carbamazepine clearance and decrease carbamazepine steady-state serum concentrations. Cimetidine, macrolide antibiotics, azole antifungals, fluox-etine, fluvoxamine, nefazodone, cyclosporine, diltiazem, verapamil, indinavir, and ritonavir are examples of drugs that decrease carbamazepine clearance and increase carbamazepine steady-state concentrations. Administration of single doses of carbamazepine with grapefruit juice increases both area under the serum con-centration versus time curve (AUC) and maximal serum concentration (C_{max}) of carbamazepine by about 40%.

INITIAL DOSAGE DETERMINATION METHODS

Because of the large amount of variability in carbamazepine pharmacokinetics, even when concurrent disease states and conditions are identified, most clinicians believe that the use of standard carbamazepine doses for various situations is warranted. The original computation of these doses were based on the Pharmacokinetic Dosing methods, and subsequently modified based on clinical experience. In general, the expected carbamazepine steady-state serum concentrations used to compute these doses was 6-8 µg/mL. Usual initial maintenance doses are 10-20 mg/kg/d for children under 6 years of age, 200 mg/d for children 6-12 years old and 400 mg/d for adults. Twice daily dosing is initially used until autoinduction takes place. Dosage increases to allow for autoinduction are made every 2-3 weeks depending on response and adverse effects. Most adults will require 800-1200 mg/d of carbamazepine while older children will require 400-800 mg/d. If the patient has significant hepatic dysfunction (Child-Pugh score ≥8), maintenance doses prescribed using this method should be decreased by 25%-50% depending on how aggressive therapy is required to be for the individual.

EXAMPLE 1 ▶▶▶

KL is a 51-year-old, 75-kg (height = 5 ft 10 in) male with simple partial seizures who requires therapy with oral carbamazepine. He has normal liver function. Suggest an initial carbamazepine dosage regimen designed to achieve a steady-state carbamazepine concentration equal to 6-8 µg/mL.

1. *Estimate carbamazepine dose according to disease states and conditions present in the patient.*

    The suggested initial dosage rate for immediate-release carbamazepine tablets in an adult patient is 200 mg twice daily (400 mg/d). This dose would be titrated upward in 200-mg increments every 2-3 weeks while monitoring for adverse and therapeutic effects. The goal of therapy includes maximal suppression of seizures, avoidance of side effects, and a target drug range of 800-1200 mg/d.

    A steady-state trough total carbamazepine serum concentration should be measured after steady-state is achieved in 2-3 weeks at the highest dosage rate attained. Carbamazepine serum concentrations should also be measured if the patient experiences an exacerbation of their epilepsy, or if the patient develops potential signs or symptoms of carbamazepine toxicity.

EXAMPLE 2 ▶▶▶

UO is a 10-year-old, 40-kg male with simple partial seizures who requires therapy with oral carbamazepine. He has normal liver function. Suggest an initial carbamazepine dosage regimen designed to achieve a steady-state carbamazepine concentration equal to 6-8 µg/mL.

1. *Estimate carbamazepine dose according to disease states and conditions present in the patient.*

    The suggested initial dosage rate for immediate-release carbamazepine tablets for a child in this age range is 100 mg twice daily (200 mg/d). This dose would be titrated upward in 100-mg increments every 2-3 weeks while monitoring for adverse and therapeutic effects. The goal of therapy includes maximal suppression of seizures, avoidance of side effects, and a target drug range of 400-800 mg/d.

    A steady-state trough total carbamazepine serum concentration should be measured after steady-state is achieved in 2-3 weeks at the highest dosage rate attained. Carbamazepine serum concentrations should also be measured if the patient experiences an exacerbation of their epilepsy, or if the patient develops potential signs or symptoms of carbamazepine toxicity.

USE OF CARBAMAZEPINE SERUM CONCENTRATIONS TO ALTER DOSES

Because of the large amount of pharmacokinetic variability among patients, it is likely that doses computed using patient population characteristics will not always produce carbamazepine serum concentrations that are expected or desirable. Because of pharmacokinetic variability, the autoinduction pharmacokinetics followed by the drug, the narrow therapeutic index of carbamazepine, and the desire to avoid adverse side effects of carbamazepine, measurement of carbamazepine serum concentrations is conducted for almost all patients to insure that therapeutic, nontoxic levels are present. In addition to carbamazepine serum concentrations, important patient parameters (seizure frequency, potential carbamazepine side effects, etc) should be followed to confirm that the patient is responding to treatment and not developing adverse drug reactions. When carbamazepine serum concentrations are measured in patients and a dosage change is necessary, clinicians should seek to use the simplest, most straightforward method available to determine a dose that will provide safe and effective treatment.

Pseudolinear Pharmacokinetics Method

A simple, easy way to approximate new total serum concentrations after a dosage adjustment with carbamazepine is to temporarily assume linear pharmacokinetics, then subtract 10%-20% for a dosage increase or add 10%-20% for a dosage decrease to account for autoinduction pharmacokinetics: $Css_{new} = (D_{new}/D_{old})Css_{old}$, where Css_{new} is the expected steady-state concentration from the new carbamazepine dose in $\mu g/mL$, Css_{old} is the measured steady-state concentration from the old carbamazepine dose in $\mu g/mL$, D_{new} is the new carbamazepine dose to be prescribed in mg/d, and D_{old} is the currently prescribed carbamazepine dose in mg/d.

Note: This method is only intended to provide a rough approximation of the resulting carbamazepine steady-state concentration after an appropriate dosage adjustment, such as 100-200 mg/d, has been made. The Pseudolinear Pharmacokinetics method should never be used to compute a new dose based on measured and desired carbamazepine concentrations.

EXAMPLE 1 ▶▶▶

KL is a 51-year-old, 75-kg (height = 5 ft 10 in) male with simple partial seizures who requires therapy with oral carbamazepine. He has normal liver function. After dosage titration, the patient was prescribed 200 mg of carbamazepine tablets in the morning, 200 mg in the afternoon, and 400 mg at bedtime (800 mg/d) for 1 month, and the steady-state carbamazepine total concentration equals 3.8 µg/mL. The patient is assessed to be compliant with his dosage regimen. Suggest a carbamazepine dosage regimen designed to achieve a steady-state carbamazepine concentration within the therapeutic range.

1. *Use pseudolinear pharmacokinetics to predict new concentration for a dosage increase, then compute 10%-20% factor to account for autoinduction pharmacokinetics.*

   Since the patient is receiving carbamazepine tablets, a convenient dosage change would be 200 mg/d and an increase to 1000 mg/d (400 mg in the morning and bedtime, 200 mg in the afternoon) is suggested. Using pseudolinear pharmacokinetics, the resulting total steady-state carbamazepine serum concentration would equal: $Css_{new} = (D_{new}/D_{old})Css_{old} = (1000 \text{ mg/d} / 800 \text{ mg/d})3.8 \text{ µg/mL} = 4.8 \text{ µg/mL}$. Because of autoinduction pharmacokinetics, the serum concentration would be expected to increase 10% less, or 0.90 times, to 20%, or 0.80 times, less than that predicted by linear pharmacokinetics: Css = 4.8 µg/mL • 0.90 = 4.3 µg/mL and Css = 4.8 µg/mL • 0.80 = 3.8 µg/mL. Thus, a dosage increase of 200 mg/d would be expected to yield a total carbamazepine steady-state serum concentration between 3.8 and 4.3 µg/mL.

   A steady-state trough total carbamazepine serum concentration should be measured after steady-state is attained in 2-3 weeks. Carbamazepine serum concentrations should also be measured if the patient experiences an exacerbation of their epilepsy, or if the patient develops potential signs or symptoms of carbamazepine toxicity.

EXAMPLE 2 ▶▶▶

UO is a 10-year-old, 40-kg male with simple partial seizures who requires therapy with oral carbamazepine. He has normal liver function. After dosage titration, the patient was prescribed 200 mg of carbamazepine tablets three times daily (600 mg/d) for 1 month, and the steady-state carbamazepine total concentration equals 5.1 µg/mL. The patient is assessed to be compliant with his dosage regimen. Suggest a carbamazepine dosage regimen designed to achieve a steady-state carbamazepine concentration within the middle of the therapeutic range.

1. *Use pseudolinear pharmacokinetics to predict new concentration for a dosage increase, then compute 10%-20% factor to account for autoinduction pharmacokinetics.*

   Since the patient is receiving carbamazepine tablets, a convenient dosage change would be 200 mg/d and an increase to 800 mg/d (300 mg in the morning and bedtime, 200 mg in the afternoon) is suggested. Using pseudolinear pharmacokinetics, the resulting total steady-state carbamazepine serum concentration would equal: $Css_{new} = (D_{new}/D_{old})Css_{old} = (800\ mg/d\ /\ 600\ mg/d)\ 5.1\ \mu g/mL = 6.8\ \mu g/mL$. Because of autoinduction pharmacokinetics, the serum concentration would be expected to increase 10% less, or 0.90 times, to 20%, or 0.80 times, less than that predicted by linear pharmacokinetics: $Css = 6.8\ \mu g/mL \bullet 0.90 = 6.1\ \mu g/mL$ and $Css = 6.8\ \mu g/mL \bullet 0.80 = 5.4\ \mu g/mL$. Thus, a dosage increase of 200 mg/d would be expected to yield a total carbamazepine steady-state serum concentration between 5.4 and 6.1 µg/mL.

   A steady-state trough total carbamazepine serum concentration should be measured after steady-state is attained in 2-3 weeks. Carbamazepine serum concentrations should also be measured if the patient experiences an exacerbation of their epilepsy, or if the patient develops potential signs or symptoms of carbamazepine toxicity.

BAYESIAN PHARMACOKINETIC COMPUTER PROGRAMS

Computer programs are available that can assist in the computation of pharmacokinetic parameters for patients.[47] The most reliable computer programs use a nonlinear regression algorithm that incorporates components of Bayes theorem. Nonlinear regression is a statistical technique that uses an iterative process to compute the best pharmacokinetic parameters for a concentration/time data set. Unfortunately, these types of computer programs have not been able to give acceptable solutions unless four or more carbamazepine concentrations are available. This is due to the complexity of the autoinduction pharmacokinetics that carbamazepine follows under chronic dosing conditions. Because of the large number of concentrations needed, this dosage adjustment approach cannot be recommended at this time.

PROBLEMS

The following problems are intended to emphasize the computation of initial and individualized doses using clinical pharmacokinetic techniques. Clinicians should always consult the patient's chart to confirm that current anticonvulsant therapy is appropriate. Additionally, all other medications that the patient is taking, including prescription and nonprescription drugs, should be noted and checked to ascertain if a potential drug interaction with carbamazepine exists.

1. TY is a 47-year-old, 85-kg (height = 6 ft 1 in) male with tonic-clonic seizures who requires therapy with oral carbamazepine. He has normal liver function. Suggest an initial carbamazepine dosage regimen designed to achieve a steady-state carbamazepine concentration equal to 6-8 µg/mL.

2. Patient TY (see problem 1) was prescribed 400 mg every 12 hours of extended-release carbamazepine tablets for 1 month after dosage titration, and the steady-state carbamazepine total concentration equals 4.5 µg/mL. The patient is assessed to be compliant with his dosage regimen. Suggest a carbamazepine dosage regimen designed to achieve a steady-state carbamazepine concentration within the middle portion of the therapeutic range.

3. IU is a 9-year-old, 35-kg female with simple partial seizures who requires therapy with oral carbamazepine. She has normal liver function. Suggest an initial carbamazepine dosage regimen designed to achieve a steady-state carbamazepine concentration equal to 6-8 µg/mL.

4. Patient IU (see problem 3) was prescribed 150 mg of carbamazepine suspension three times daily (450 mg/d) for 1 month after dosage titration, and the steady-state carbamazepine total concentration equals 4.9 µg/mL. The patient is assessed to be compliant with her dosage regimen. Suggest a carbamazepine dosage regimen designed to achieve a steady-state carbamazepine concentration within the middle of the therapeutic range.

5. LK is a 4-year-old, 22-kg male with complex partial seizures who requires therapy with carbamazepine suspension. He has normal liver function. Suggest an initial carbamazepine dosage regimen designed to achieve a steady-state carbamazepine concentration equal to 6-8 µg/mL.

6. Patient LK (see problem 5) was prescribed 100 mg of carbamazepine suspension three times daily (300 mg/d) for 1 month after dosage titration, and the steady-state carbamazepine total concentration equals 6.1 µg/mL. The patient is assessed to be compliant with her dosage regimen. Suggest a carbamazepine dosage regimen designed to achieve a steady-state carbamazepine concentration within the upper end of the therapeutic range.

ANSWERS TO PROBLEMS

1. *Answer to problem 1.*
   1. *Estimate carbamazepine dose according to disease states and conditions present in the patient.*
      The suggested initial dosage rate for immediate-release carbamazepine tablets in an adult patient is 200 mg twice daily (400 mg/d). This dose would be titrated upward in 200-mg increments every 2-3 weeks while monitoring for adverse and therapeutic effects. The goal of therapy includes maximal suppression of seizures, avoidance of side effects, and a target drug range of 800-1200 mg/d.
      A steady-state trough total carbamazepine serum concentration should be measured after steady-state is achieved in 2-3 weeks at the highest dosage rate attained. Carbamazepine serum concentrations should also be measured if the patient experiences an exacerbation of their epilepsy, or if the patient develops potential signs or symptoms of carbamazepine toxicity.

2. *Answer to problem 2.*
   1. *Use pseudolinear pharmacokinetics to predict new concentration for a dosage increase, then compute 10%-20% factor to account for autoinduction pharmacokinetics.*
      Since the patient is receiving extended-release carbamazepine tablets, a convenient dosage change would be 400 mg/d and an increase to 1200 mg/d (600 mg every 12 hours) is suggested. Using pseudolinear pharmacokinetics, the resulting total steady-state carbamazepine serum concentration would equal: $Css_{new} = (D_{new}/D_{old})Css_{old} = (1200 \text{ mg/d} / 800 \text{ mg/d}) \, 4.5 \text{ µg/mL} = 6.8 \text{ µg/mL}$. Because of autoinduction pharmacokinetics, the serum concentration would be expected to increase 10% less, or 0.90 times, to 20%, or 0.80 times, less than that predicted by linear pharmacokinetics: $Css = 6.8 \text{ µg/mL} \bullet 0.90 = 6.1 \text{ µg/mL}$ and $Css = 6.8 \text{ µg/mL} \bullet 0.80 = 5.4 \text{ µg/mL}$. Thus, a dosage increase of 400 mg/d would be expected to yield a total carbamazepine steady-state serum concentration between 5.4 and 6.1 µg/mL.

A steady-state trough total carbamazepine serum concentration should be measured after steady-state is attained in 2-3 weeks. Carbamazepine serum concentrations should also be measured if the patient experiences an exacerbation of their epilepsy, or if the patient develops potential signs or symptoms of carbamazepine toxicity.

3. *Answer to problem 3.*
  1. *Estimate carbamazepine dose according to disease states and conditions present in the patient.*
     The suggested initial dosage rate for carbamazepine suspension in a child in this age range is 100 mg twice daily (200 mg/d). This dose would be titrated upward in 100-mg increments every 2-3 weeks while monitoring for adverse and therapeutic effects. The goal of therapy includes maximal suppression of seizures, avoidance of side effects, and a target drug range of 400-800 mg/d.
     A steady-state trough total carbamazepine serum concentration should be measured after steady-state is achieved in 2-3 weeks at the highest dosage rate attained. Carbamazepine serum concentrations should also be measured if the patient experiences an exacerbation of their epilepsy, or if the patient develops potential signs or symptoms of carbamazepine toxicity.

4. *Answer to problem 4.*
  1. *Use pseudolinear pharmacokinetics to predict new concentration for a dosage increase, then compute 10%-20% factor to account for autoinduction pharmacokinetics.*
     Since the patient is receiving carbamazepine suspension, a convenient dosage change would be 150 mg/d and an increase to 600 mg/d (200 mg three times daily) is suggested. Using pseudolinear pharmacokinetics, the resulting total steady-state carbamazepine serum concentration would equal: $Css_{new} = (D_{new}/D_{old})Css_{old} = (600 \text{ mg/d} / 450 \text{ mg/d})4.9 \text{ µg/mL} = 6.5 \text{ µg/mL}$. Because of autoinduction pharmacokinetics, the serum concentration would be expected to increase 10% less, or 0.90 times, to 20%, or 0.80 times, less than that predicted by linear pharmacokinetics: $Css = 6.5 \text{ µg/mL} \bullet 0.90 = 5.9 \text{ µg/mL}$ and $Css = 6.5 \text{ µg/mL} \bullet 0.80 = 5.2 \text{ µg/mL}$. Thus, a dosage increase of 150 mg/d would be expected to yield a total carbamazepine steady-state serum concentration between 5.2 and 5.9 µg/mL.
     A steady-state trough total carbamazepine serum concentration should be measured after steady-state is attained in 2-3 weeks. Carbamazepine serum concentrations should also be measured if the patient experiences an exacerbation of their epilepsy, or if the patient develops potential signs or symptoms of carbamazepine toxicity.

5. *Answer to problem 5.*
  1. *Estimate carbamazepine dose according to disease states and conditions present in the patient.*
     The suggested initial dosage rate for carbamazepine suspension in a child in this age range is 10-20 mg/kg/d. Using a dose of 15 mg/kg/d, the target maintenance dose equals 300 mg/d (15 mg/kg/d • 22 kg = 330 mg/d, rounded to 300 mg/d). The starting dose would be ¼-⅓ of the target maintenance dose or 100 mg/d given as 50 mg twice daily. This dose would be titrated upward in 100 mg/d increments every 2-3 weeks while monitoring for adverse and therapeutic effects. The goal of therapy includes maximal suppression of seizures, avoidance of side effects, and a target drug range of 300 mg/d given as 100 mg three times daily.
     A steady-state trough total carbamazepine serum concentration should be measured after steady-state is achieved in 2-3 weeks at the highest dosage rate attained. Carbamazepine serum concentrations should also be measured if the patient experiences an exacerbation of their epilepsy, or if the patient develops potential signs or symptoms of carbamazepine toxicity.

6. *Answer to problem 6.*
  1. *Use pseudolinear pharmacokinetics to predict new concentration for a dosage increase, then compute 10%-20% factor to account for autoinduction pharmacokinetics.*

Since the patient is receiving carbamazepine suspension, a convenient dosage change would be 150 mg/d and an increase to 450 mg/d (150 mg three times daily) is suggested. Using pseudolinear pharmacokinetics, the resulting total steady-state carbamazepine serum concentration would equal: $Css_{new} = (D_{new}/D_{old})Css_{old} = (450 \text{ mg/d} / 300 \text{ mg/d})6.1 \text{ μg/mL} = 9.2 \text{ μg/mL}$. Because of autoinduction pharmacokinetics, the serum concentration would be expected to increase 10% less, or 0.90 times, to 20%, or 0.80 times, less than that predicted by linear pharmacokinetics: $Css = 9.2 \text{ μg/mL} \bullet 0.90 = 8.3 \text{ μg/mL}$ and $Css = 9.2 \text{ μg/mL} \bullet 0.80 = 7.4 \text{ μg/mL}$. Thus, a dosage increase of 150 mg/d would be expected to yield a total carbamazepine steady-state serum concentration between 7.4 and 8.3 μg/mL.

A steady-state trough total carbamazepine serum concentration should be measured after steady-state is attained in 2-3 weeks. Carbamazepine serum concentrations should also be measured if the patient experiences an exacerbation of their epilepsy, or if the patient develops potential signs or symptoms of carbamazepine toxicity.

REFERENCES

1. Abramowicz M, Zuccotti G, Pflomm JM, eds. Drugs for epilepsy. *Treatment Guidelines from The Medical Letter*. 2013;11(126):9-18.
2. Anon. The epilepsies: the diagnosis and management of the epilepsies in adults and children in primary and secondary care. *UK National Institute for Health and Care Excellence*. http://www.nice.org.uk/nicemedia/live/13635/57779/57779.pdf. Accessed April 2, 2014.
3. French JA, Kanner AM, Bautista J, et al. Efficacy and tolerability of the new antiepileptic drugs I: treatment of new onset epilepsy: report of the Therapeutics and Technology Assessment Subcommittee and Quality Standards Subcommittee of the American Academy of Neurology and the American Epilepsy Society. *Neurology*. Apr 27 2004;62(8):1252-1260.
4. Glauser T, Ben-Menachem E, Bourgeois B, et al. Updated ILAE evidence review of antiepileptic drug efficacy and effectiveness as initial monotherapy for epileptic seizures and syndromes. *Epilepsia*. Mar 2013;54(3):551-563.
5. Glauser TA, Cnaan A, Shinnar S, et al. Ethosuximide, valproic acid, and lamotrigine in childhood absence epilepsy. *N Engl J Med*. Mar 4 2010;362(9):790-799.
6. Glauser TA, Cnaan A, Shinnar S, et al. Ethosuximide, valproic acid, and lamotrigine in childhood absence epilepsy: initial monotherapy outcomes at 12 months. *Epilepsia*. Jan 2013;54(1):141-155.
7. McNamara JO. Pharmacotherapy of the epilepsies. In: Brunton L, Chabner B, Knollman B, eds. *The Pharmacological Basis of Therapeutics*. 12th ed. New York, NY: McGraw-Hill; 2011:583-608.
8. Abramowicz M, Zuccotti G, Pflomm JM, eds. Drugs for depression and bipolar disorder. *Treatment Guidelines from The Medical Letter*. 2010;8(93):35-42.
9. Drayton SJ. Bipolar disorders. In: DiPiro JT, Talbert RL, Yee GC, Matzke GR, Wells BG, Poscy LM, eds. *Pharmacotherapy*. 8th ed. New York, NY: McGraw-Hill; 2011:1191-1208.
10. Rogers SJ, Cavazos JE. Epilepsy. In: DiPiro JT, Talbert RL, Yee GC, Matzke GR, Wells BG, Posey LM, eds. *Pharmacotherapy*. 8th ed. New York, NY: McGraw-Hill; 2011:979-1005.
11. Hooper WD, Dubetz DK, Bochner F, et al. Plasma protein binding of carbamazepine. *Clin Pharmacol Ther*. 1975;17(4):433-440.
12. Lawless LM, DeMonaco HJ, Muido LR. Protein binding of carbamazepine in epileptic patients. *Neurology*. 1982;32(4):415-418.
13. Paxton JW, Donald RA. Concentrations and kinetics of carbamazepine in whole saliva, parotid saliva, serum ultrafiltrate, and serum. *Clin Pharmacol Ther*. 1980;28(5):695-702.
14. Ahmed GF, Brundage RC, Marino SE, et al. Population pharmacokinetics of unbound and total drug concentrations following intravenously administered carbamazepine in elderly and younger adult patients with epilepsy. *J Clin Pharmacol*. Mar 2013;53(3):276-284.
15. Rane A, Hojer B, Wilson JT. Kinetics of carbamazepine and its 10, 11-epoxide metabolite in children. *Clin Pharmacol Ther*. 1976;19(3):276-283.
16. McKauge L, Tyrer JH, Eadie MJ. Factors influencing simultaneous concentrations of carbamazepine and its epoxide in plasma. *Ther Drug Monit*. 1981;3(1):63-70.
17. Brodie MJ, Forrest G, Rapeport WG. Carbamazepine 10, 11 epoxide concentrations in epileptics on carbamazepine alone and in combination with other anticonvulsants. *Br J Clin Pharmacol*. 1983;16(6):747-749.
18. Eichelbaum M, Bertilsson L, Lund L, Palmer L, Sjoqvist F. Plasma levels of carbamazepine and carbamazepine-10, 11-epoxide during treatment of epilepsy. *Eur J Clin Pharmacol*. 1976;09(5-6):417-421.

19. MacKichan JJ, Duffner PK, Cohen ME. Salivary concentrations and plasma protein binding of carbamazepine and carbamazepine 10, 11-epoxide in epileptic patients. *Br J Clin Pharmacol.* 1981;12(1):31-37.

20. Hundt HK, Aucamp AK, Muller FO, Potgieter MA. Carbamazepine and its major metabolites in plasma: a summary of eight years of therapeutic drug monitoring. *Ther Drug Monit.* 1983;5(4):427-435.

21. Elyas AA, Patsalos PN, Agbato OA, Brett EM, Lascelles PT. Factors influencing simultaneous concentrations of total and free carbamazepine and carbamazepine-10, 11-epoxide in serum of children with epilepsy. *Ther Drug Monit.* 1986;8(3):288-292.

22. Bertilsson L, Tybring G, Widen J, Chang M, Tomson T. Carbamazepine treatment induces the CYP3A4 catalysed sulphoxidation of omeprazole, but has no or less effect on hydroxylation via CYP2C19. *Br J Clin Pharmacol.* 1997;44(2):186-189.

23. Kerr BM, Thummel KE, Wurden CJ, et al. Human liver carbamazepine metabolism. Role of CYP3A4 and CYP2C8 in 10, 11-epoxide formation. *Biochem Pharmacol.* 1994;47(11):1969-1979.

24. Perucca E, Bittencourt P, Richens A. Effect of dose increments on serum carbamazepine concentration in epileptic patients. *Clin Pharmacokinet.* 1980;5(6):576-582.

25. McNamara PJ, Colburn WA, Gibaldi M. Time course of carbamazepine self-induction. *J Pharmacokinet Biopharm.* 1979;7(1):63-68.

26. Eichelbaum M, Kothe KW, Hoffmann F, von Unruh GE. Use of stable labelled carbamazepine to study its kinetics during chronic carbamazepine treatment. *Eur J Clin Pharmacol.* 1982;23(3):241-244.

27. Pitlick WH, Levy RH, Tropin AS, Green JR. Pharmacokinetic model to describe self-induced decreases in steady-state concentrations of carbamazepine. *J Pharm Sci.* 1976;65(3):462-463.

28. Bertilsson L, Hojer B, Tybring G, Osterloh J, Rane A. Autoinduction of carbamazepine metabolism in children examined by a stable isotope technique. *Clin Pharmacol Ther.* 1980;27(1):83-88.

29. Schaffler L, Bourgeois BF, Luders HO. Rapid reversibility of autoinduction of carbamazepine metabolism after temporary discontinuation. *Epilepsia.* 1994;35(1):195-198.

30. Graves NM, Kriel RL, Jones-Saete C, Cloyd JC. Relative bioavailability of rectally administered carbamazepine suspension in humans. *Epilepsia.* 1985;26(5):429-433.

31. Neuvonen PJ, Tokola O. Bioavailability of rectally administered carbamazepine mixture. *Br J Clin Pharmacol.* 1987;24(6):839-841.

32. Marino SE, Birnbaum AK, Leppik IE, et al. Steady-state carbamazepine pharmacokinetics following oral and stable-labeled intravenous administration in epilepsy patients: effects of race and sex. *Clin Pharmacol Ther.* Mar 2012;91(3):483-488.

33. Hartley R, Aleksandrowicz J, Ng PC, McLain B, Bowmer CJ, Forsythe WI. Breakthrough seizures with generic carbamazepine: a consequence of poorer bioavailability? *Br J Clin Pract.* 1990;44(7):270-273.

34. Meyer MC, Straughn AB, Mhatre RM, Shah VP, Williams RL, Lesko LJ. The relative bioavailability and in vivo-in vitro correlations for four marketed carbamazepine tablets. *Pharm Res.* 1998;15(11):1787-1791.

35. Olling M, Mensinga TT, Barends DM, Groen C, Lake OA, Meulenbelt J. Bioavailability of carbamazepine from four different products and the occurrence of side effects. *Biopharm Drug Dispos.* 1999;20(1):19-28.

36. Cohen H, Howland MA, Luciano DJ, et al. Feasibility and pharmacokinetics of carbamazepine oral loading doses. *Am J Health Syst Pharm.* 1998;55(11):1134-1140.

37. Cotter LM, Eadie MJ, Hooper WD, Lander CM, Smith GA, Tyrer JH. The pharmacokinetics of carbamazepine. *Eur J Clin Pharmacol.* 1977;12(6):451-456.

38. Levy RH, Pitlick WH, Troupin AS, Green JR, Neal JM. Pharmacokinetics of carbamazepine in normal man. *Clin Pharmacol Ther.* 1975;17(6):657-668.

39. Rawlins MD, Collste P, Bertilsson L, Palmer L. Distribution and elimination kinetics of carbamazepine in man. *Eur J Clin Pharmacol.* 1975;8(2):91-96.

40. Monaco F, Riccio A, Benna P, et al. Further observations on carbamazepine plasma levels in epileptic patients. Relationships with therapeutic and side effects. *Neurology.* 1976;26(10):936-973.

41. Battino D, Bossi L, Croci D, et al. Carbamazepine plasma levels in children and adults: influence of age, dose, and associated therapy. *Ther Drug Monit.* 1980;2(4):315-322.

42. Eichelbaum M, Kothe KW, Hoffman F, von Unruh GE. Kinetics and metabolism of carbamazepine during combined antiepileptic drug therapy. *Clin Pharmacol Ther.* 1979;26(3):366-371.

43. Pugh RN, Murray-Lyon IM, Dawson JL, Pietroni MC, Williams R. Transection of the oesophagus for bleeding oesophageal varices. *Br J Surg.* 1973;60(8):646-649.

44. Lee CS, Wang LH, Marbury TC, Bruni J, Perchalski RJ. Hemodialysis clearance and total body elimination of carbamazepine during chronic hemodialysis. *Clin Toxicol.* 1980;17(3):429-438.

45. Kandrotas RJ, Oles KS, Gal P, Love JM. Carbamazepine clearance in hemodialysis and hemoperfusion. *Dicp.* 1989;23(2):137-140.

46. Hansten PD, Horn JR. *The Top 100 Drug Interactions.* Freeland, WA, USA: H&H Publications; 2014.

47. Wandell M, Mungall D. Computer assisted drug interpretation and drug regimen optimization. *Amer Assoc Clin Chem.* 1984;6:1-11.

12 Valproic Acid

INTRODUCTION

Valproic acid is an agent that is chemically related to free fatty acids and is used in the treatment of generalized, partial, and absence (petit mal) seizures.[1-4] As such, it has the widest spectrum of activity compared to the other currently available antiepileptic drugs (Table 12-1). Available in intravenous, as well as oral, form, valproic acid can be used for the acute treatment and chronic prophylaxis of seizures.[5,6] Valproic acid is also a useful agent for the treatment of bipolar affective disorders and the prevention of migraine headaches.[7,8]

Although the precise mechanism of action for valproic acid is unknown, its antiepileptic effect is thought to be due to its ability to increase concentrations of the neuroinhibitor γ-aminobutyric acid (GABA), to potentate the postsynaptic response to GABA, or to exert a direct effect on cellular membranes.[11,12]

THERAPEUTIC AND TOXIC CONCENTRATIONS

The generally accepted therapeutic range for total valproic acid steady-state concentrations is 50-100 μg/mL, although some clinicians suggest drug concentrations as high as 175 μg/mL with appropriate monitoring of serum concentrations and possible adverse effects. Valproic acid is highly protein bound to albumin with typical values of 90%-95%.[13,14] Plasma protein binding of valproic acid is saturable within the therapeutic range which results in less protein binding and higher unbound fraction of drug at higher concentrations. The concentration-dependent protein binding of valproic acid causes the drug to follow nonlinear pharmacokinetics (Figure 12-1). This type of nonlinear pharmacokinetics is fundamentally different than that observed during phenytoin administration. Phenytoin hepatic metabolism becomes saturated which causes Michaelis-Menten pharmacokinetics to take place. As a result, when phenytoin doses are increased total and unbound steady-state concentrations increase more than a proportional amount (eg, when the dose is doubled, serum concentrations may increase 3-5-fold or more). In the case of valproic acid, when the dose is increased total drug steady-state concentration increases less than expected, but unbound steady-state drug concentration increases in a proportional fashion (eg, when the dose is doubled, total serum concentration increases 1.6-1.9 times but unbound steady-state serum concentration doubles; Figure 12-2). The pharmacokinetic rational for these changes is explained fully in the Basic Clinical Pharmacokinetic Parameters section found later in this chapter.

Insufficient prospective work has been done to establish the therapeutic range for unbound valproic acid steady-state serum concentrations. As an initial guide, 5% of the lower end and 10% of the upper end of the total concentration therapeutic range is used to construct the preliminary unbound steady-state concentration therapeutic range for valproic acid of 2.5-10 μg/mL. The percent used for each case is the average unbound fraction of drug at the appropriate concentration.

More information is available that identifies the clinical situations where unbound valproic acid serum concentration measurement is useful. As is the case with phenytoin, measurement of unbound valproic acid

TABLE 12-1   International Classification of Epileptic Seizures With Recommended Therapies

Major Class	Subset of Class	Drug Treatment for Selected Seizure Type			
		2004 AAN/AES	**2013 Medical Letter**	**2012 NICE**	**2013 ILAE[a]**
Partial seizures (beginning locally)	1. Simple partial seizures (without impaired consciousness) a. with motor symptoms b. with somato-sensory or special sensory symptoms c. with autonomic symptoms d. with psychological symptoms	Carbamazepine Phenytoin Valproate Phenobarbital Lamotrigine Gabapentin Oxcarbazepine Topiramate	Lamotrigine Carbamazepine Levetiracetam Oxcarbazepine *Alternatives:* Topiramate Valproate Gabapentin Zonisamide Phenytoin Pregabalin Lacosamide Ezogabine	Carbamazepine Lamotrigine Levetiracetam Oxcarbazepine Valproate *Adjunctive:* Carbamazepine Clobazam Gabapentin Lamotrigine Levetiracetam Oxcarbazepine Valproate Topiramate	*Adults:* Carbamazepine Levetiracetam Phenytoin Zonisamide Valproate *Children:* Oxcarbazepine Carbamazepine Phenobarbital Phenytoin Topiramate Valproate Vigabatrin *Elderly:* Gabapentin Lamotrigine Carbamazepine
	2. Complex partial seizures (with impaired consciousness) a. simple partial onset followed by impaired consciousness b. impaired consciousness at onset	Carbamazepine Phenytoin Valproate Phenobarbital Lamotrigine Gabapentin Oxcarbazepine Topiramate	Lamotrigine Carbamazepine Levetiracetam Oxcarbazepine *Alternatives:* Topiramate Valproate Gabapentin Zonisamide Phenytoin Pregabalin Lacosamide Ezogabine	Carbamazepine Lamotrigine Levetiracetam Oxcarbazepine Valproate *Adjunctive:* Carbamazepine Clobazam Gabapentin Lamotrigine Levetiracetam Oxcarbazepine Valproate Topiramate	*Adults:* Carbamazepine Levetiracetam Phenytoin Zonisamide Valproate *Children:* Oxcarbazepine Carbamazepine Phenobarbital Phenytoin Topiramate Valproate Vigabatrin *Elderly:* Gabapentin Lamotrigine Carbamazepine
	3. Partial seizures evolving into secondary generalized seizures	Carbamazepine Phenytoin Valproate Phenobarbital Lamotrigine Gabapentin Oxcarbazepine Topiramate	Lamotrigine Carbamazepine Levetiracetam Oxcarbazepine *Alternatives:* Topiramate Valproate Gabapentin Zonisamide Phenytoin Pregabalin Lacosamide Ezogabine	Carbamazepine Lamotrigine Levetiracetam Oxcarbazepine Valproate *Adjunctive:* Carbamazepine Clobazam Gabapentin Lamotrigine Levetiracetam Oxcarbazepine Valproate Topiramate	*Adults:* Carbamazepine Levetiracetam Phenytoin Zonisamide Valproate *Children:* Oxcarbazepine Carbamazepine Phenobarbital Phenytoin Topiramate Valproate Vigabatrin *Elderly:* Gabapentin Lamotrigine Carbamazepine

(Continued)

TABLE 12-1   International Classification of Epileptic Seizures With Recommended Therapies (Continued)

Major Class	Subset of Class	Drug Treatment for Selected Seizure Type			
		2004 AAN/AES	**2013 Medical Letter**	**2012 NICE**	**2013 ILAE[a]**
Generalized seizures (convulsive or nonconvulsive)	1. Absence seizures[b] (typical or atypical; also known as petite mal seizures)	*Children:[c]* Ethosuximide Valproate Lamotrigine	Ethosuximide Valproate *Alternatives:* Lamotrigine Clonazepam Zonisamide Levetiracetam	Ethosuximide Lamotrigine Valproate *Adjunctive:* Ethosuximide Lamotrigine Valproate	*Children:* Ethosuximide Valproate Lamotrigine
	2. Tonic-clonic seizures (also known as grand mal seizures)	Carbamazepine Phenytoin Valproate Phenobarbital Lamotrigine Oxcarbazepine Topiramate	Valproate Lamotrigine Levetiracetam *Alternatives:* Topiramate Zonisamide Phenytoin	Carbamazepine Lamotrigine Oxcarbazepine Valproate *Adjunctive:* Clobazam Lamotrigine Levetiracetam Valproate Topiramate	*Adults:* Carbamazepine Lamotrigine Oxcarbazepine Phenobarbital Phenytoin Topiramate Valproate Gabapentin Levetiracetam Vigabatrin *Children:* Carbamazepine Phenobarbital Phenytoin Topiramate Valproate Oxcarbazepine

[a]Only two highest available levels of evidence listed.

[b]Recent literature suggests either ethosuximide or valproic acid is superior initial therapy compared to lamotrigine for absence seizures.[9,10]

[c]Lamotrigine added to previous recommendation per expert panel.

Abbreviations: ANN, American Academy of Neurology; AES, American Epilepsy Society; ILAE, International League Against Epilepsy; NICE, UK National Institute for Clinical Excellence.

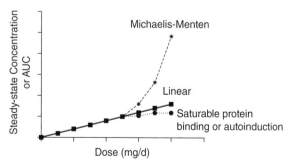

FIGURE 12-1   If a drug follows linear pharmacokinetics, Css or AUC increases proportionally with dose resulting in a straight line on the plot. Nonlinear pharmacokinetics occurs when the Css or AUC versus dose plot results in something other than a straight line. If a drug follows Michaelis-Menten pharmacokinetics (eg phenytoin, aspirin), as steady-state drug concentrations approach Km, serum concentrations increase more than expected due to dose increases. If a drug follows nonlinear protein binding (eg, valproic acid, disopyramide) or autoinduction (eg, carbamazepine), total steady-state drug concentrations increase less than expected as dose increases.

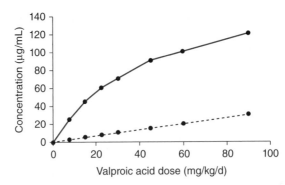

FIGURE 12-2   Although total valproic acid concentrations increase in a nonlinear fashion with dosage increases (solid line), unbound, or "free" valproic acid concentrations increase in a linear fashion with dosage increases (dashed line). Valproic acid is a low-extraction ratio drug, and its unbound serum concentrations are only a function of intrinsic clearance (Cl'_{int}): $Css, u = (D/\tau)/Cl'_{int}$, where D is valproic acid dose in mg, τ is the dosage interval in h, and Css, u is the unbound steady-state valproic acid concentration.

serum concentrations should be considered in patients with factors known to alter valproic acid plasma protein binding.[14-18] These factors fall into three broad categories: (1) lack of binding protein where there are insufficient plasma concentrations of albumin, (2) displacement of valproic acid from albumin-binding sites by endogenous compounds, and (3) displacement of valproic acid from albumin-binding sites by exogenous compounds (Table 12-2).

Low albumin concentrations, known as hypoalbuminemia, can be found in patients with liver disease or the nephrotic syndrome, pregnant women, cystic fibrosis patients, burn patients, trauma patients, malnourished individuals, and the elderly. Albumin concentrations below 3 g/dL are associated with high valproic acid unbound fractions in the plasma. Albumin is manufactured by the liver so patients with hepatic disease may have difficulty synthesizing the protein. Patients with nephrotic syndrome waste albumin by eliminating it in the urine. Malnourished patients can be so nutritionally deprived that albumin production is impeded. Malnourishment is the reason for hypoalbuminemia in some elderly patients, although there is a general downtrend in albumin concentrations in older patients. However, the unbound fraction of valproic acid is higher in elderly patients even if albumin concentrations are within the normal range. While recovering from their injuries, burn and trauma patients can become hypermetabolic and albumin concentrations decrease if enough calories are not supplied during this phase of their disease state. Albumin concentrations may decline during

TABLE 12-2   Disease States and Conditions That Alter Valproic Acid Plasma Protein Binding

Insufficient Albumin Concentration (Hypoalbuminemia)	Displacement by Endogenous Compounds	Displacement by Exogenous Compounds
Liver disease	Hyperbilirubinemia	Drug interactions
Nephrotic syndrome	Jaundice	Warfarin
Pregnancy	Liver disease	Phenytoin
Cystic fibrosis	Renal dysfunction	Aspirin (>2 g/d)
Burns		NSAIDs with high albumin binding
Trauma		
Malnourishment		
Elderly		

pregnancy as maternal reserves are shifted to the developing fetus and are especially prevalent during the third trimester.

Displacement of valproic acid from plasma protein–binding sites by endogenous substances can occur in patients with hepatic or renal dysfunction. The mechanism is competition for albumin plasma protein–binding sites between the exogenous substances and valproic acid. Bilirubin (a byproduct of heme metabolism) is broken down by the liver, so patients with hepatic disease can have excessive bilirubin concentrations. Total bilirubin concentrations in excess of 2 mg/dL are associated with abnormal valproic acid plasma protein binding. End-stage renal disease patients (creatinine clearance <10-15 mL/min) with uremia (blood urea nitrogen concentrations >80-100 mg/dL) accumulate unidentified compound(s) in their blood that displace valproic acid from plasma protein–binding sites. Abnormal valproic acid binding persists in these patients even when dialysis procedures are instituted.

Valproic acid plasma protein–binding displacement can also occur due to exogenously administered compounds such as drugs. In this case, the mechanism is competition for albumin-binding sites between valproic acid and other agents. Other drugs that are highly bound to albumin and cause plasma protein–binding displacement drug interactions with valproic acid include warfarin, phenytoin, aspirin (>2 g/d), and some highly bound nonsteroidal anti-inflammatory agents.

In the upper end of the therapeutic range (>75 μg/mL) some patients will begin to experience the concentration-dependent adverse effects of valproic acid therapy: ataxia, sedation, lethargy, and tiredness. In many individuals, these side effects dissipate with continued dosing, and slow dosage titration may assist in minimizing these adverse reactions in newly treated patients. Other concentration-related side effects of valproic acid therapy include tremor at concentrations >100 μg/mL, and stupor or coma at concentrations >175 μg/mL. Additionally, valproic acid–associated thrombocytopenia can usually be limited by a decrease in drug dose.

CLINICAL MONITORING PARAMETERS

The goal of therapy with anticonvulsants is to reduce seizure frequency and maximize quality of life with a minimum of adverse drug effects. While it is desirable to entirely abolish all seizure episodes, it may not be possible to accomplish this in many patients. Patients should be monitored for concentration-related side effects (ataxia, sedation, lethargy, tiredness, tremor, stupor, coma, thrombocytopenia) as well as gastrointestinal upset associated with local irritation of gastric mucosa (nausea, vomiting, anorexia).[12] Elevated liver function tests, increased serum ammonia, alopecia, and weight gain have been reported during chronic valproic acid treatment. Serious, but rare, idiosyncratic side effects include hepatotoxicity, pancreatitis, pitting edema, systemic lupus-like reactions, and leukopenia with bone marrow changes.

Valproic acid serum concentrations should be measured in most patients. Because epilepsy is an episodic disease state, patients do not experience seizures on a continuous basis. Thus, during dosage titration it is difficult to tell if the patient is responding to drug therapy or simply is not experiencing any abnormal central nervous system discharges at that time. Valproic acid serum concentrations are also valuable tools to avoid adverse drug effects. Patients are more likely to accept drug therapy if adverse reactions are held to the absolute minimum.

BASIC CLINICAL PHARMACOKINETIC PARAMETERS

Valproic acid is primarily eliminated by hepatic metabolism (>95%). Hepatic metabolism is via glucuronidation, β-oxidation, and α-hydroxylation. When measured using *in vitro* techniques, glucuronidation is mediated by UGT1A3, UGT1A4, UGT1A6, UGT1A8, UGT1A9, UGT1A10, UGT2B7, and UGT2B15, with UGT1A6 and UGT2B7 responsible for the majority of the reactions.[19-22] Over 10 metabolites have been identified for valproic acid, and the 4-en-valproic acid metabolite may be associated with the drug's propensity to cause hepatotoxicity. About 1%-5% of a valproic acid dose is recovered in the urine as unchanged drug. Valproic acid follows nonlinear pharmacokinetics due to saturable, or concentration-dependent, plasma protein binding. This is the type of nonlinear pharmacokinetics that occurs when the number of drug molecules overwhelms or saturates albumin's ability to bind the drug in the plasma. When this occurs, total steady-state drug serum concentrations increase in a disproportionate manner after a dosage increase, but unbound steady-state drug serum concentrations increase in a proportional fashion (see Figure 12-2). Valproic acid is eliminated almost completely by hepatic metabolism, and it is a low-hepatic extraction ratio drug. In this case the hepatic clearance rate is described by the classic relationship that is used to describe hepatic clearance: $Cl_H = [LBF \bullet (f_B Cl'_{int})]/(LBF + f_B Cl'_{int})$, where LBF is liver blood flow, f_B is the unbound fraction of drug in the blood, and Cl'_{int} is the intrinsic ability of the enzyme system to metabolize the drug. Since valproic acid has a low hepatic extraction ratio, this expression for hepatic clearance simplifies to $Cl_H = f_B Cl'_{int}$.

The clinical implication of concentration-dependent plasma protein–binding pharmacokinetics is that the clearance of valproic acid is not a constant as it is with linear pharmacokinetics, but is concentration or dose dependent. As the dose or concentration of valproic acid increases, the clearance rate (Cl) increases because more unbound drug is available to hepatic enzymes for metabolism: $\uparrow Cl_H = \uparrow f_B Cl'_{int}$. This is the reason total steady-state concentrations increase disproportionately after a valproic acid dosage increase: $\uparrow Css = [F(\Uparrow D/\tau)]/\uparrow Cl_H$, where F is valproic acid bioavailability, D is valproic acid dose, τ is the dosage interval, and Cl_H is hepatic clearance. When valproic acid dose is increased, the unbound fraction increases and causes an increase in hepatic clearance. Because both dose and hepatic clearance simultaneously increase, total valproic acid concentrations increase, but by a smaller than expected amount. For example, valproic acid follows concentration-dependent plasma protein–binding pharmacokinetics with average unbound fractions of 5% in the lower end of the therapeutic range (50 µg/mL) and 10% in the upper end of the therapeutic range (100 µg/mL). When the dose is increased and steady-state concentration of valproic acid increases from 50 µg/mL to 100 µg/mL, the unbound fraction increases by a factor of 2 from 5% to 10% and hepatic clearance of total drug will double within the therapeutic range: $2Cl_H = 2f_B Cl'_{int}$. Unfortunately, there is so much interpatient variability in concentration-dependent plasma protein–binding parameters for valproic acid that predicting changes in unbound fraction and hepatic clearance is extremely difficult. However, since unbound steady-state concentrations are only influenced by intrinsic clearance, unbound concentrations increase in a proportional amount to dose: $Css,u = [F(D/\tau)]/Cl'_{int}$.

Valproic acid volume of distribution (V = 0.15-0.2 L/kg) is also effected by concentration-dependent plasma protein binding and is determined by the physiological volume of blood (V_B) and tissues (V_T) as well as the unbound fraction of drug in the blood (f_B) and tissues (f_T): $V = V_B + (f_B/f_T)V_T$. As valproic acid concentrations increase, unbound fraction of drug in the blood increases which causes an increase in the volume of distribution for the drug: $\uparrow V = V_B + (\uparrow f_B/f_T)V_T$. Half-life ($t_{1/2}$) is related to clearance and volume of distribution using the same equation as for linear pharmacokinetics: $t_{1/2} = (0.693 \bullet V)/Cl$. However, since clearance and volume of distribution are a function of dose- or concentration-dependent plasma protein binding for valproic acid, half-life also changes with drug dosage or concentration changes. As doses or concentrations increase for a drug that follows concentration-dependent plasma protein–binding pharmacokinetics, clearance and volume of distribution simultaneously increase, and half-life changes are variable depending on the relative changes in clearance and volume of distribution: $\leftrightarrow t_{1/2} = (0.693 \bullet \uparrow V)/\uparrow Cl$. Using the average clearance and the volume of distribution for an adult (V = 0.15 L/kg, Cl = 10 mL/h/kg or 0.010 L/h/kg), half-life remains at 10 h [$t_{1/2} = (0.693 \bullet V)/Cl$] = [0.693 • 0.15 L/kg]/0.010 L/h/kg = 10 h. Clearance and volume of distribution increase to 0.30 L/kg and 0.020 L/h/kg, respectively, due to decreased protein binding: $t_{1/2}$ = [0.693 • 0.30 L]/0.020 L/h/kg = 10 h as valproic acid serum concentrations increase from 50 µg/mL to 100 µg/mL. The clinical implication of this finding is that the time to steady-state (3-5 $t_{1/2}$) is variable as the dose or concentration is increased for valproic acid. On average, valproic acid half-life is 12-18 hours in adult patients with total concentrations within the therapeutic range.

Valproic acid is available as three different entities, and all of them are prescribed as valproic acid equivalents: valproic acid, sodium valproate (the sodium salt of valproic acid), and divalproex sodium (a stable coordination compound consisting of a 1:1 ratio of valproic acid and sodium valproate). For parenteral use, valproic acid is available as a 100 mg/mL solution. When given intravenously, it should be diluted in at least 50 mL of intravenous solution, and given over 1 hour (injection rates should not exceed 20 mg/min). For oral use, a syrup (50 mg/mL), soft capsule (250 mg), enteric coated capsules (125, 250, and 500 mg), extended-release tablets (250 mg and 500 mg) and sprinkle capsule (125 mg, used to sprinkle into foods) are available. The enteric-coated capsules are not extended-release products, but only delay the absorption of drug after ingestion. As a result, there are less gastrointestinal side effects with the enteric-coated product.

The oral bioavailability of valproic acid is very good for all dosage forms and ranges from 90% for the extended-release tablets to 100% for the other oral dosage forms. Extended-release tablets produce an AUC that is about 10% less than other oral dosage forms, and drug serum concentrations should be measured for patients converted between extended-release and other oral dosage forms.[23,24] If a patient is stabilized on an oral valproic acid product, and it is necessary to switch the patient to intravenous drug, the same total daily dose of injectable valproic acid can be given to the individual. Usually, valproic acid doses are not fine tuned to the point of directly accounting for the difference in valproic acid bioavailability. Rather, clinicians are aware that when valproic acid dosage forms are changed, the serum concentration versus time profile may change. Because of this, most individuals recheck valproic acid steady-state serum concentrations after a dosage form change is instituted.

The typical maintenance dose for valproic acid is 15 mg/kg/d resulting in 1000 mg or 500 mg twice daily for most adult patients. However, because age and coadministration of other antiepileptic drugs that are enzyme inducers (eg, carbamazepine, phenytoin, phenobarbital) effect valproic acid pharmacokinetics, many clinicians recommend the administration of 7.5 mg/kg/d for adults or 10 mg/kg/d for children under 12 years of age receiving monotherapy and 15 mg/kg/d for adults or 20 mg/kg/d for children under 12 years old receiving other drugs that are enzyme inducers.[25]

EFFECTS OF DISEASE STATES AND CONDITIONS ON PHARMACOKINETICS AND DOSING

For valproic acid, oral clearance (Cl/F) is 7-12 mL/h/kg and half-life is 12-18 hours for adults.[26] In children 6-12 years old, oral clearance and half-life equal 10-20 mL/h/kg and 6-8 hours, respectively.[27] Clearance rates can be higher and half-lives shorter in patients receiving other hepatic drug-metabolizing enzyme inducers (phenytoin, phenobarbital, carbamazepine). For adults receiving other antiepileptic drugs that are enzyme inducers, valproic acid clearance for adults is 15-18 mL/h/kg and half-lives range from 4 to 12 hours. Similarly, if children receive therapy with other antiepileptic drugs that are enzyme inducers, clearance is 20-30 mL/h/kg and half-life is 4-6 h.[28,29] Valproic acid volume of distribution (V/F) is 0.15-0.2 L/kg.[26,30]

Patients with liver cirrhosis or acute hepatitis have reduced valproic acid clearance because of destruction of liver parenchyma.[31] This loss of functional hepatic cells reduces the amount of enzymes available to metabolize the drug and decreases clearance. Valproic acid clearance in patients with liver disease is 3-4 mL/h/kg. The volume of distribution may be larger because of reduced plasma protein binding (free fraction ≈ 29%). Protein binding may be reduced and unbound fraction maybe increased due to hypoalbuminemia and/or hyperbilirubinemia (especially albumin ≤3 g/dL and/or total bilirubin ≥2 mg/dL). Average half-life for valproic acid in patients with liver disease is 25 hours. However, the effects that liver disease has on valproic acid pharmacokinetics are highly variable and difficult to accurately predict. It is possible for a patient with liver disease to have relatively normal or grossly abnormal valproic acid clearance and volume of distribution. For example, a liver disease patient who has relatively normal albumin and bilirubin concentrations can have

TABLE 12-3   Child-Pugh Scores for Patients With Liver Disease

Test/Symptom	Score 1 Point	Score 2 Points	Score 3 Points
Total Bilirubin (mg/dL)	<2.0	2.0-3.0	>3.0
Serum albumin (g/dL)	>3.5	2.8-3.5	<2.8
Prothrombin time (seconds prolonged over control)	<4	4-6	>6
Ascites	Absent	Slight	Moderate
Hepatic encephalopathy	None	Moderate	Severe

Mild liver disease, 5-6 points; moderate liver disease, 7-9 points; severe liver disease, 10-15 points.

a normal volume of distribution for valproic acid. An index of liver dysfunction can be gained by applying the Child-Pugh clinical classification system to the patient (Table 12-3).[32] Child-Pugh scores are completely discussed in Chapter 3 (Drug Dosing in Special Populations: Renal and Hepatic Disease, Dialysis, Heart Failure, Obesity, and Drug Interactions), but will be briefly discussed here. The Child-Pugh score consists of five laboratory tests or clinical symptoms: serum albumin, total bilirubin, prothrombin time, ascites, and hepatic encephalopathy. Each of these areas is given a score of 1 (normal) to 3 (severely abnormal; see Table 12-3), and the scores for the five areas are summed. The Child-Pugh score for a patient with normal liver function is 5 while the score for a patient with grossly abnormal serum albumin, total bilirubin, and prothrombin time values in addition to severe ascites and hepatic encephalopathy is 15. A Child-Pugh score greater than 8 is grounds for a decrease of 25%-50% in the initial daily drug dose for valproic acid. As in any patient with or without liver dysfunction, initial doses are meant as starting points for dosage titration based on patient response and avoidance of adverse effects. Since the drug has been associated with hepatic damage, valproic acid therapy should be avoided in patients with liver disease whenever possible. Valproic acid serum concentrations and the presence of adverse drug effects should be monitored frequently in patients with liver cirrhosis.

Elderly patients have lower valproic acid oral clearance rates and higher unbound fractions than younger adults, so lower initial doses may be used in older individuals.[14] For patients between 65 and 99 years old, there does not appear to be a further decline in valproic acid clearance as age advances.[33] During the third trimester of pregnancy, oral clearance of valproic acid may decrease and require dosage adjustment.[34] Valproic acid serum concentrations exhibit some diurnal variation in patients, so the time that steady-state serum concentrations are obtained should be noted when comparing multiple values.[14,35] Doses of valproic acid do not require adjustment for patients with renal failure, and the drug is not removed by dialysis.[36] Breast milk concentrations of valproic acid are about 10% of concurrent serum concentrations.

DRUG INTERACTIONS

Valproic acid is a potent inhibitor of hepatic drug-metabolizing enzyme systems and glucuronidation.[37-40] Other antiepileptic drugs that have their clearance rates decreased and steady-state concentrations increased by valproic acid–related enzyme inhibition include clonazepam, carbamazepine, phenytoin, primidone, lamotrigine, and ethosuximide. Valproic acid therapy also decreases the clearance and increases steady-state concentrations of other drugs including zidovudine, amitriptyline, and nortriptyline. As a general rule, when valproic acid is added to a patient's drug regimen, an adverse effect due to one of the other drugs must be considered as a possible drug interaction with valproic acid.

Additionally, other drugs can affect valproic acid clearance and steady-state serum concentrations.[40] Phenytoin, lamotrigine, rifampin, and carbamazepine can increase valproic acid clearance and decrease valproic acid steady-state serum concentrations. Cimetidine, chlorpromazine, and felbamate are examples of drugs that decrease valproic acid clearance and increase valproic acid steady-state concentrations. Carbapenem antibiotics decrease valproic acid concentrations to the extent that of loss of seizure control has occurred in some epileptic patients. Because valproic acid is highly protein bound, plasma protein–binding drug interactions can occur with other drugs that are highly bound to albumin.[40] Aspirin, warfarin, and phenytoin all have plasma protein–binding drug interactions with valproic acid, and these drugs have higher unbound fractions when given concurrently with valproic acid. The drug interaction between valproic acid and phenytoin deserves special examination because of its complexity and because these two agents are regularly used together for the treatment of seizures.[41-44] The drug interaction involves the plasma protein–binding displacement and intrinsic clearance inhibition of phenytoin by valproic acid. What makes this interaction so difficult to detect and understand is that these two changes do not occur simultaneously, so the impression left by the drug interaction depends on when in time it is observed in a patient. For example, a patient is stabilized on phenytoin therapy (Figure 12-3), but because adequate control of seizures has not been attained, valproic acid is added to the regimen. As valproic acid concentrations accumulate, the first interaction observed is phenytoin plasma protein binding as the two drugs compete for binding sites on albumin. The result of this portion of the drug interaction is an increase in

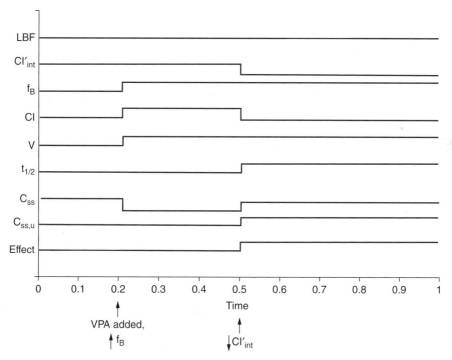

FIGURE 12-3 Schematic representation of the effect on physiologic (LBF = liver blood flow, Cl'_{int} = intrinsic or unbound clearance, f_B = unbound fraction of drug in blood/plasma), pharmacokinetic (Cl = clearance; V = volume of distribution; $t_{1/2}$ = half-life; Css = total steady-state drug concentration; Css, u = unbound steady-state drug concentration), and pharmacodynamic (Effect = pharmacodynamic effect) parameters that occur when initiating valproic acid (VPA) treatment in an individual stabilized on phenytoin therapy. Initially, valproic acid decreases phenytoin plasma-protein binding via competitive displacement for binding sites on albumin (arrow denotes ↑f_B). As valproic acid concentrations increase, the hepatic enzyme inhibition component of the drug interaction comes into play (arrow denotes ↓ Cl'_{int}). The net result is total phenytoin concentrations are largely unchanged from baseline, but unbound phenytoin concentrations and pharmacologic effect increase.

phenytoin-unbound fraction and a decrease in phenytoin total serum concentration, but the unbound phenytoin serum concentration remains the same. As valproic acid serum concentrations achieve steady-state conditions, the higher concentrations of the drug bathe the hepatic microsomal enzyme system and inhibit the intrinsic clearance of phenytoin. This portion of the interaction decreases intrinsic clearance and hepatic clearance for phenytoin, so both unbound and total phenytoin concentrations increase. When phenytoin concentrations finally equilibrate and reach steady-state under the new plasma protein binding and intrinsic clearance conditions imposed by concurrent valproic acid therapy, the total concentration of phenytoin is oftentimes at about the same level as before the drug interaction occurred, but unbound phenytoin concentrations are much higher. If only total phenytoin concentrations are measured at this point in time, clinicians will be under the impression that total concentrations did not change and no drug interaction occurred. However, if unbound phenytoin concentrations are simultaneously measured, it will be found that these concentrations have risen and that the phenytoin-unbound fraction is twice or more ($\geq 20\%$) of the baseline amount. In this situation, the patient may have unbound phenytoin concentrations that are toxic and a decrease in phenytoin dosage may be in order.

INITIAL DOSAGE DETERMINATION METHODS

Several methods to initiate valproic acid therapy are available. The *Pharmacokinetic Dosing method* is the most flexible of the techniques. It allows individualized target serum concentrations to be chosen for a patient, and each pharmacokinetic parameter can be customized to reflect specific disease states and conditions present in the patient. *Literature-based Recommended dosing* is a very commonly used method to prescribe initial doses of valproic acid. Doses are based on those that commonly produce steady-state concentrations in the lower end of the therapeutic range, although there is a wide variation in the actual concentrations for a specific patient.

Pharmacokinetic Dosing Method

The goal of initial dosing of valproic acid is to compute the best dose possible for the patient given their set of disease states and conditions that influence valproic acid pharmacokinetics and the epileptic disorder being treated. In order to do this, pharmacokinetic parameters for the patient will be estimated using average parameters measured in other patients with similar disease state and condition profiles.

Clearance Estimate

Valproic acid is predominately metabolized by liver. Unfortunately, there is no good way to estimate the elimination characteristics of liver-metabolized drugs using an endogenous marker of liver function in the same manner that serum creatinine and estimated creatinine clearance are used to estimate the elimination of agents that are renally eliminated. Because of this, a patient is categorized according to the disease states and conditions that are known to change valproic acid clearance, and the clearance previously measured in these studies is used as an estimate of the current patient's clearance. For example, for a 70-kg adult patient with liver cirrhosis or acute hepatitis, valproic acid clearance would be assumed to equal 3-4 mL/h/kg: 70 kg • 3.5 mL/h/kg = 245 mL/h or 0.245 L/h. To produce the most conservative valproic acid doses in patients with multiple concurrent disease states or conditions that affect valproic acid pharmacokinetics, the disease state or condition with the smallest clearance should be used to compute doses. This approach will avoid accidental overdosage as much as currently possible.

Volume of Distribution Estimate

Valproic acid volume of distribution is assumed to equal 0.15 L/kg for adults and 0.2 L/kg for children under 12 years of age. Thus, for an 80-kg adult patient, the estimated valproic volume of distribution would be 12 L: V = 0.15 L/kg • 80 kg = 12 L. Patients with cirrhosis or renal failure may have larger volumes of distribution due to decreased plasma protein binding.

Half-Life and Elimination Rate Constant Estimate

Once the correct clearance and volume of distribution estimates are identified for the patient, they can be converted into the valproic acid half-life ($t_{1/2}$) and elimination rate constant (k) estimates using the following equations: $t_{1/2} = (0.693 \bullet V)/Cl$, $k = 0.693/t_{1/2} = Cl/V$.

Selection of Appropriate Pharmacokinetic Model and Equations

When given by intravenous injection or orally, valproic acid follows a one-compartment pharmacokinetic model. When oral therapy is required, valproic acid has good bioavailability (F = 1), and every 8-12 hour dosing provides a relatively smooth serum concentration-time curve that emulates an intravenous infusion. Because of this, a very simple pharmacokinetic equation that computes the average valproic acid steady-state serum concentration (Css in µg/mL = mg/L) is widely used and allows maintenance dosage calculation: Css = [F(D/τ)]/Cl or D = (Css • Cl • τ)/F, where F is the bioavailability fraction for the oral dosage form (F = 1 for oral rapid-release products, F = 0.9 for oral extended-release tablets), D is the dose of valproic acid in mg, and τ is the dosage interval in hours. Cl is valproic acid clearance in L/h. When intravenous therapy is required, the same pharmacokinetic equation is widely used: Css = (D/τ)/Cl or D = Css • Cl • τ, where D is the dose of valproic acid in mg, and τ is the dosage interval in hours. Cl is valproic acid clearance in L/h.

The equation used to calculate an intravenous loading dose (LD in mg) is based on a simple one-compartment model: LD = Css • V, where Css is the desired valproic acid steady-state concentration in µg/mL which is equivalent to mg/L, and V is the valproic acid volume of distribution. Intravenous valproic acid doses should be infusions over at least 60 minutes (≤20 mg/minute).

EXAMPLE 1 ▶▶▶

KL is a 51-year-old, 75-kg (height = 5 ft 10 in) male with tonic-clonic seizures who requires therapy with oral valproic acid. He has normal liver function and takes no medications that induce hepatic enzymes. Suggest an initial valproic acid dosage regimen designed to achieve a steady-state valproic acid concentration equal to 50 µg/mL.

1. *Estimate clearance and volume of distribution according to disease states and conditions present in the patient.*
   The clearance rate for an adult patient not taking other drugs that induce hepatic drug metabolism is 7-12 mL/h/kg. Using a value of 10 mL/h/kg, the estimated clearance would equal 0.75 L/h: Cl = 75 kg • 10 mL/h/kg = 750 mL/h or 0.75 L/h. Using 0.15 L/kg, the estimated volume of distribution would be 11 L: 75 kg • 0.15 L/kg = 11 L.

2. *Estimate half-life and elimination rate constant.*
   Once the correct clearance and volume of distribution estimates are identified for the patient, they can be converted into the valproic acid half-life ($t_{1/2}$) and elimination rate constant (k) estimates using the following equations: $t_{1/2} = (0.693 \bullet V)/Cl = (0.693 \bullet 11 \text{ L})/0.75 \text{ L/h} = 10 \text{ h}$, $k = 0.693/t_{1/2} = 0.693/10 \text{ h} = 0.069 \text{ h}^{-1}$.

3. *Compute dosage regimen.*
   Oral enteric-coated divalproex sodium tablets will be prescribed to this patient (F = 1). (Note: µg/mL = mg/L and this concentration unit was substituted for Css in the calculations so that unnecessary unit conversion was not required.) The dosage equation for oral valproic acid is: D = (Css • Cl • τ)/F = (50 mg/L• 0.75 L/h • 12 h)/1 = 450 mg, rounded to 500 every 12 hours.

   A steady-state trough valproic acid serum concentration should be measured after steady-state is attained in 3-5 half-lives. Since the patient is expected to have a half-life equal to 10 hours, the valproic acid steady-state concentration could be obtained any time after the second day of dosing (5 half-lives = 5 • 10 h = 50 h). Valproic acid serum concentrations should also be measured if the patient experiences an exacerbation of their epilepsy, or if the patient develops potential signs or symptoms of valproic acid toxicity.

EXAMPLE 2 ▶▶▶

UO is a 10-year-old, 40-kg male with absence seizures who requires therapy with oral valproic acid. He has normal liver function and currently takes carbamazepine. Suggest an initial valproic acid dosage regimen designed to achieve a steady-state valproic acid concentration equal to 50 μg/mL.

1. *Estimate clearance and volume of distribution according to disease states and conditions present in the patient.*
   The clearance rate for a child who takes other drugs that induce hepatic drug metabolism is 20-30 mL/h/kg. Using a value of 25 mL/h/kg, the estimated clearance would equal 1 L/h: Cl = 40 kg • 25 mL/h/kg = 1000 mL/h or 1 L/h. Using 0.2 L/kg, the estimated volume of distribution would be 8 L: 40 kg • 0.2 L/kg = 8 L.

2. *Estimate half-life and elimination rate constant.*
   Once the correct clearance and volume of distribution estimates are identified for the patient, they can be converted into the valproic acid half-life ($t_{1/2}$) and elimination rate constant (k) estimates using the following equations: $t_{1/2} = (0.693 • V)/Cl = (0.693 • 8 L)/1 L/h = 6 h$, $k = 0.693/t_{1/2} = 0.693/6 h = 0.116 h^{-1}$.

3. *Compute dosage regimen.*
   Oral valproic acid syrup will be prescribed to this patient (F = 1). (Note: μg/mL = mg/L and this concentration unit was substituted for Css in the calculations so that unnecessary unit conversion was not required.) The dosage equation for oral valproic acid is: $D = (Css • Cl • τ)/F = (50 mg/L • 1 L/h • 8 h)/1 = 400 mg$, or 400 mg every 8 h.

   A steady-state trough valproic acid serum concentration should be measured after steady-state is attained in 3-5 half-lives. Since the patient is expected to have a half-life equal to 6 hours, the valproic acid steady-state concentration could be obtained any time after the first day of dosing (5 half-lives = 5 • 6 h = 30 h). Valproic acid serum concentrations should also be measured if the patient experiences an exacerbation of their epilepsy, or if the patient develops potential signs or symptoms of valproic acid toxicity.

EXAMPLE 3 ▶▶▶

HU is a 25-year-old, 85-kg (height = 6 ft 2 in) male with tonic-clonic seizures who requires therapy with intravenous valproic acid. He has normal liver function and takes no medications that induce hepatic enzymes. Suggest an initial valproic acid dosage regimen designed to achieve a steady-state valproic acid concentration equal to 75 μg/mL.

1. *Estimate clearance and volume of distribution according to disease states and conditions present in the patient.*
   The clearance rate for an adult patient not taking other drugs that induce hepatic drug metabolism is 7-12 mL/h/kg. Using a value of 10 mL/h/kg, the estimated clearance would equal 0.85 L/h: Cl = 85 kg • 10 mL/h/kg = 850 mL/h or 0.85 L/h. Using 0.15 L/kg, the estimated volume of distribution would be 13 L: 85 kg • 0.15 L/kg = 13 L.

2. *Estimate half-life and elimination rate constant.*
   Once the correct clearance and volume of distribution estimates are identified for the patient, they can be converted into the valproic acid half-life ($t_{1/2}$) and elimination rate constant (k) estimates using the following equations: $t_{1/2} = (0.693 • V)/Cl = (0.693 • 13 L)/0.85 L/h = 11 h$, $k = 0.693/t_{1/2} = 0.693/11 h = 0.063 h^{-1}$.

3. *Compute dosage regimen.*
   Valproic acid injection will be prescribed to this patient (F = 1). (Note: μg/mL = mg/L and this concentration unit was substituted for Css in the calculations so that unnecessary unit conversion was not required.) The maintenance dosage equation for valproic acid is: $D = (Css • Cl • τ)/F = (75 mg/L • 0.85 L/h • 8 h)/1 = 510 mg$, rounded to 500 every 8 hours. The loading dose equation for valproic acid is: $LD = Css • V = 75 mg/L • 13 L = 975 mg$, rounded to 1000 mg. Intravenous doses should be given over 1 h (≤20 mg/min).

   A steady-state trough valproic acid serum concentration should be measured after steady-state is attained in 3-5 half-lives. Since the patient is expected to have a half-life equal to 11 hours, the valproic acid steady-state concentration could be obtained any time after the second day of dosing (5 half-lives = 5 • 11 h = 55 h). Valproic acid serum concentrations should also be measured if the patient experiences an exacerbation of their epilepsy, or if the patient develops potential signs or symptoms of valproic acid toxicity.

Literature-Based Recommended Dosing

Because of the large amount of variability in valproic acid pharmacokinetics, even when concurrent disease states and conditions are identified, most clinicians believe that the use of standard valproic acid doses for various situations is warranted. The original computation of these doses were based on the Pharmacokinetic Dosing methods and subsequently modified based on clinical experience. In general, the expected valproic acid steady-state serum concentrations used to compute these doses was 50 µg/mL. Usual initial maintenance doses for pediatric patients are 10 mg/kg/d if the child is not taking a hepatic enzyme inducer (phenytoin, phenobarbital, carbamazepine, rifampin) or 20 mg/kg/d if the child is taking a hepatic enzyme inducer. For adults, initial maintenance doses are 7.5 mg/kg/d if the patient is not taking hepatic enzyme inducers or 15 mg/kg/d if a hepatic enzyme inducer is concurrently administered. Two or three divided daily doses are initially used for these total doses. To avoid gastrointestinal side effects, doses over 1500 mg given at one time should be avoided. Dosage increases of 5-10 mg/kg/d are made every 1-2 weeks depending on response and adverse effects. Most adults will require 1500-3000 mg/d of valproic acid. If the patient has significant hepatic dysfunction (Child-Pugh score ≥8), maintenance doses prescribed using this method should be decreased by 25%-50% depending on how aggressive therapy is required to be for the individual.

To illustrate the similarities and differences between this method of dosage calculation and the Pharmacokinetic Dosing method, the same examples used in the previous section will be used.

EXAMPLE 4 ▶▶▶

KL is a 51-year-old, 75 kg (height = 5 ft 10 in) male with tonic-clonic seizures who requires therapy with oral valproic acid. He has normal liver function and takes no medications that induce hepatic enzymes. Suggest an initial valproic acid dosage regimen for this patient.

1. *Estimate valproic acid dose according to disease states and conditions present in the patient.*

   Oral enteric-coated divalproex sodium tablets will be prescribed to this patient. The suggested initial maintenance dosage rate for valproic acid in an adult patient not taking enzyme inducers is 7.5 mg/kg/d: 75 kg • 7.5 mg/kg/d = 563 mg/d or 250 mg every 12 hours. This dose would be titrated upward in 5-10 mg/kg/d increments every 1-2 weeks while monitoring for adverse and therapeutic effects. The goals of therapy include maximal suppression of seizures and avoidance of side effects.

   A steady-state trough total valproic acid serum concentration should be measured after steady-state is attained in 1-2 weeks. Valproic acid serum concentrations should also be measured if the patient experiences an exacerbation of their epilepsy, or if the patient develops potential signs or symptoms of valproic acid toxicity.

EXAMPLE 5 ▶▶▶

UO is a 10-year-old, 40-kg male with absence seizures who requires therapy with oral valproic acid. He has normal liver function and currently takes carbamazepine. Suggest an initial valproic acid dosage regimen for this patient.

1. *Estimate valproic acid dose according to disease states and conditions present in the patient.*

   Oral valproic acid syrup will be prescribed to this patient. The suggested initial maintenance dosage rate for valproic acid for a child taking enzyme inducers is 20 mg/kg/d: 40 kg • 20 mg/kg/d = 800 mg/d or 250 mg every 8 hours. This dose would be titrated upward in 5-10 mg/kg/d increments every 1-2 weeks while monitoring for adverse and therapeutic effects. The goals of therapy include maximal suppression of seizures and avoidance of side effects.

   A steady-state trough total valproic acid serum concentration should be measured after steady-state is attained in 1-2 weeks. Valproic acid serum concentrations should also be measured if the patient experiences an exacerbation of their epilepsy, or if the patient develops potential signs or symptoms of valproic acid toxicity.

EXAMPLE 6 ▶ ▶ ▶

HU is a 25-year-old, 85-kg (height = 6 ft 2 in) male with tonic-clonic seizures who requires therapy with intravenous valproic acid. He has normal liver function and takes no medications that induce hepatic enzymes. Suggest an initial valproic acid dosage regimen for this patient.

1. *Estimate valproic acid dose according to disease states and conditions present in the patient.*

   Intravenous valproic acid injection will be prescribed to this patient. The suggested initial maintenance dosage rate for an adult patient not taking enzyme inducers is 7.5 mg/kg/d: 85 kg • 7.5 mg/kg/d = 638 mg/d, rounded to 750 mg/d or 250 mg every 12 hours. This dose would be titrated upward in 5-10 mg/kg/d increments every 1-2 weeks while monitoring for adverse and therapeutic effects. If needed, a loading dose of 7.5 mg/kg could be given as the first dose: 85 kg • 7.5 mg/kg = 638 mg, rounded to 750 mg. Intravenous doses should be administered over 1 hour (≤20 mg/min). The goals of therapy include maximal suppression of seizures and avoidance of side effects.

   A steady-state trough total valproic acid serum concentration should be measured after steady-state is attained in 1-2 weeks. Valproic acid serum concentrations should also be measured if the patient experiences an exacerbation of their epilepsy, or if the patient develops potential signs or symptoms of valproic acid toxicity.

USE OF VALPROIC ACID SERUM CONCENTRATIONS TO ALTER DOSES

Because of the large amount of pharmacokinetic variability among patients, it is likely that doses computed using patient population characteristics will not always produce valproic acid serum concentrations that are expected or desirable. Because of pharmacokinetic variability, the nonlinear pharmacokinetics followed by the drug due to concentration-dependent plasma protein binding, the narrow therapeutic index of valproic acid, and the desire to avoid adverse side effects of valproic acid, measurement of valproic acid serum concentrations is conducted for most patients to ensure that therapeutic, nontoxic levels are present.

In addition to valproic acid serum concentrations, important patient parameters (seizure frequency, potential valproic acid side effects, etc) should be followed to confirm that the patient is responding to treatment and not developing adverse drug reactions. When valproic acid serum concentrations are measured in patients and a dosage change is necessary, clinicians should seek to use the simplest, most straightforward method available to determine a dose that will provide safe and effective treatment. In most cases, a simple dosage ratio can be used to change valproic acid doses by temporarily assuming valproic acid follows linear pharmacokinetics (*Pseudolinear Pharmacokinetics method*). An empiric adjustment is made in the estimated steady-state concentrations to adjust for nonlinear, concentration-dependent plasma protein binding. In some situations, it may be necessary or desirable to compute the valproic acid *pharmacokinetic parameters* for the patient and utilize these to calculate the best drug dose. Computerized methods that incorporate expected population pharmacokinetic characteristics (*Bayesian pharmacokinetic computer programs*) can be used in difficult cases where renal function is changing, serum concentrations are obtained at suboptimal times, or the patient was not at steady-state when serum concentrations were measured. An additional benefit of this method is that a complete pharmacokinetic workup (determination of clearance, volume of distribution, and half-life) can be done with one or more measured concentrations that do not have to be at steady-state.

Pseudolinear Pharmacokinetics Method

A simple, easy way to approximate new total serum concentrations after a dosage adjustment with valproic acid is to temporarily assume linear pharmacokinetics, then subtract 10%-20% for a dosage increase or add 10%-20% for a dosage decrease to account for nonlinear, concentration-dependent plasma protein binding pharmacokinetics: $D_{new} = (Css_{new}/Css_{old}) D_{old}$, where Css_{new} is the expected steady-state concentration from the new valproic acid dose in µg/mL, Css_{old} is the measured steady-state concentration from the old valproic acid dose in µg/mL, D_{new} is the new valproic acid dose to be prescribed in mg/d, and D_{old} is the currently prescribed valproic acid dose in mg/d. *Note:* This method is only intended to provide a rough approximation of the resulting valproic acid total steady-state concentration after an appropriate dosage adjustment has been made. Of course, as expected, unbound steady-state concentrations increase or decrease in a linear fashion with dose.

EXAMPLE 7 ▶▶▶

KL is a 51-year-old, 75-kg (height = 5 ft 10 in) male with tonic-clonic seizures who requires therapy with oral valproic acid. After dosage titration, the patient was prescribed 500 mg every 12 hours of enteric-coated divalproex sodium tablets (1000 mg/d) for 1 month, and the steady-state valproic acid total concentration equals 38 µg/mL. The patient is assessed to be compliant with his dosage regimen. Suggest a valproic acid dosage regimen designed to achieve a steady-state valproic acid concentration of 80 µg/mL.

1. *Use pseudolinear pharmacokinetics to predict new concentration for a dosage increase, then compute 10%-20% factor to account for nonlinear, concentration-dependent plasma protein–binding pharmacokinetics.*

   Using pseudolinear pharmacokinetics, the resulting total steady-state valproic acid serum concentration would equal: $D_{new} = (Css_{new}/Css_{old}) D_{old} = (80 \,µg/mL / 38 \,µg/mL) 1000 \,mg/d = 2105 \,mg/d$, rounded to 2000 mg/d or 1000 mg every 12 hours. Because of nonlinear, concentration-dependent protein-binding pharmacokinetics, the total steady-state serum concentration would be expected to be 10% less, or 0.90 times, to 20% less, or 0.80 times, than that predicted by linear pharmacokinetics: $Css = 80 \,µg/mL \bullet 0.90 = 72 \,µg/mL$ and $Css = 80 \,µg/mL \bullet 0.80 = 64 \,µg/mL$. Thus, a dosage rate of 2000 mg/d would be expected to yield a total valproic acid steady-state serum concentration between 64 and 72 µg/mL.

   A steady-state trough total valproic acid serum concentration should be measured after steady-state is attained in 1-2 weeks. Valproic acid serum concentrations should also be measured if the patient experiences an exacerbation of their epilepsy, or if the patient develops potential signs or symptoms of valproic acid toxicity.

EXAMPLE 8 ▶▶▶

UO is a 10-year-old, 40-kg male with absence seizures who requires therapy with oral valproic acid. He has normal liver function. After dosage titration, the patient was prescribed 400 mg three times daily (1200 mg/d) of valproic acid syrup for 1 month, and the steady-state valproic acid total concentration equals 130 µg/mL. The patient is assessed to be compliant with his dosage regimen. Suggest a valproic acid dosage regimen designed to achieve a steady-state valproic acid concentration of 75 µg/mL.

1. *Use pseudolinear pharmacokinetics to predict new concentration for a dosage decrease, then compute 10%-20% factor to account for nonlinear, concentration-dependent plasma protein binding pharmacokinetics.*

   Using pseudolinear pharmacokinetics, the resulting total steady-state valproic acid serum concentration would equal: $D_{new} = (Css_{new}/Css_{old}) D_{old} = (75 \,µg/mL / 130 \,µg/mL) 1200 \,mg/d = 692 \,mg/d$, rounded to 750 mg/d or 250 mg every 8 hours. Because of nonlinear, concentration-dependent protein-binding pharmacokinetics, the total steady-state serum concentration would be expected to be 10% greater, or 1.10 times, to 20% greater, or 1.2 times, than that predicted by linear pharmacokinetics: $Css = 75 \,µg/mL \bullet 1.10 = 83 \,µg/mL$ and $Css = 75 \,µg/mL \bullet 1.20 = 90 \,µg/mL$. Thus, a dosage rate of 750 mg/d would be expected to yield a total valproic acid steady-state serum concentration between 83 and 90 µg/mL.

   A steady-state trough total valproic acid serum concentration should be measured after steady-state is attained in 1-2 weeks. Valproic acid serum concentrations should also be measured if the patient experiences an exacerbation of their epilepsy, or if the patient develops potential signs or symptoms of valproic acid toxicity.

PHARMACOKINETIC PARAMETER METHOD

The Pharmacokinetic Parameter method of adjusting drug doses was among the first techniques available to change doses using serum concentrations. It allows the computation of an individual's own, unique pharmacokinetic constants and uses those to calculate a dose that achieves desired valproic acid concentrations. The Pharmacokinetic Parameter method requires that steady-state has been achieved and uses only a steady-state valproic acid concentration (Css). During an intravenous dosing, the following equation is used to compute valproic acid clearance (Cl): $Cl = (D/\tau)/Css$, where D is the dose of valproic acid in mg, Css is the steady-state valproic acid concentration in mg/L, and τ is the dosage interval in hours. If the patient is receiving oral valproic acid therapy, valproic acid clearance (Cl) can be calculated using the following formula: $Cl = [F(D/\tau)]/Css$, where F is the bioavailability fraction for the oral dosage form (F = 1 for oral valproic acid products), D is the dose of valproic acid in mg, Css is the steady-state valproic acid concentration in mg/L, and τ is the dosage interval in hours.

Occasionally, valproic acid serum concentrations are obtained before and after an intravenous dose. Assuming a one-compartment model, the volume of distribution (V) is calculated using the following equation: $V = D/(C_{postdose} - C_{predose})$ where D is the dose of valproic acid in mg, $C_{postdose}$ is the postloading dose concentration in mg/L, and $C_{predose}$ is the concentration before the loading dose was administered in mg/L. ($C_{predose}$ should be obtained within 30 minutes of dosage administration; $C_{postdose}$ should be obtained 30-60 minutes after the end of infusion to avoid the distribution phase.) If the predose concentration was also a steady-state concentration, valproic acid clearance can also be computed. If both clearance (Cl) and volume of distribution (V) have been measured using these techniques, the half-life [$t_{1/2} = (0.693 \bullet V)/Cl$] and elimination rate constant ($k = 0.693/t_{1/2} = Cl/V$) can be computed. The clearance, volume of distribution, elimination rate constant, and half-life measured using these techniques are the patient's own, unique valproic acid pharmacokinetic constants and can be used in one-compartment model equations to compute the required dose to achieve any desired serum concentration. Because this method also assumes linear pharmacokinetics, valproic acid doses computed using the Pharmacokinetic Parameter method and the Pseudolinear Pharmacokinetic method should be identical. As with the previous method, to account for nonlinear, concentration-dependent plasma protein–binding pharmacokinetics, 10%-20% for a dosage increase can be subtracted or 10%-20% for a dosage decrease can be added to the expected steady-state serum concentration.

To illustrate the similarities and differences between this method of dosage calculation and the Pharmacokinetic Parameter method, the same examples used in the previous section will be used.

EXAMPLE 9 ▶▶▶

KL is a 51-year-old, 75-kg (height = 5 ft 10 in) male with tonic-clonic seizures who requires therapy with oral valproic acid. After dosage titration, the patient was prescribed 500 mg every 12 hours of enteric-coated divalproex sodium tablets (1000 mg/d) for 1 month, and the steady-state valproic acid total concentration equals 38 μg/mL. The patient is assessed to be compliant with his dosage regimen. Suggest a valproic acid dosage regimen designed to achieve a steady-state valproic acid concentration of 80 μg/mL.

1. *Compute pharmacokinetic parameters.*

The patient would be expected to achieve steady-state conditions after 2-3 days of therapy.

Valproic acid clearance can be computed using a steady-state valproic acid concentration: Cl = [F(D/τ)]/Css = [1(500 mg/12 h)]/(38 mg/L) = 1.1 L/h. (Note: μg/mL = mg/L and this concentration unit was substituted for Css in the calculations so that unnecessary unit conversion was not required.)

2. *Compute valproic acid dose.*

Valproic acid clearance is used to compute the new dose: D = (Css • Cl • τ)/F = (80 mg/L• 1.1 L/h • 12 h)/1 = 1056 mg, rounded to 1000 mg every 12 hours.

Because of nonlinear, concentration-dependent protein-binding pharmacokinetics, the total steady-state serum concentration would be expected to be 10% less, or 0.90 times, to 20% less, or 0.80 times, than that predicted by linear pharmacokinetics: Css = 80 μg/mL • 0.90 = 72 μg/mL and Css = 80 μg/mL • 0.80 = 64 μg/mL. Thus, a dosage rate of 2000 mg/d would be expected to yield a total valproic acid steady-state serum concentration between 64 and 72 μg/mL.

A steady-state trough total valproic acid serum concentration should be measured after steady-state is attained in 1-2 weeks. Valproic acid serum concentrations should also be measured if the patient experiences an exacerbation of their epilepsy, or if the patient develops potential signs or symptoms of valproic acid toxicity.

EXAMPLE 10 ▶▶▶

UO is a 10-year-old, 40-kg male with absence seizures who requires therapy with oral valproic acid. He has normal liver function. After dosage titration, the patient was prescribed 400 mg three times daily (1200 mg/d) of valproic acid syrup for 1 month, and the steady-state valproic acid total concentration equals 130 μg/mL. The patient is assessed to be compliant with his dosage regimen. Suggest a valproic acid dosage regimen designed to achieve a steady-state valproic acid concentration of 75 μg/mL.

1. *Compute pharmacokinetic parameters.*

The patient would be expected to achieve steady-state conditions after 2-3 days of therapy.

Valproic acid clearance can be computed using a steady-state valproic acid concentration: Cl = [F(D/τ)]/Css = [1(400 mg/8 h)]/(130 mg/L) = 0.38 L/h. (Note: μg/mL = mg/L and this concentration unit was substituted for Css in the calculations so that unnecessary unit conversion was not required.)

2. *Compute valproic acid dose.*

Valproic acid clearance is used to compute the new dose: D = (Css • Cl • τ)/F = (75 mg/L • 0.38 L/h • 8 h)/1 = 228 mg, rounded to 250 mg every 8 hours.

Because of nonlinear, concentration-dependent protein-binding pharmacokinetics, the total steady-state serum concentration would be expected to be 10% more, or 1.10 times, to 20%, or 1.20 times, more than that predicted by linear pharmacokinetics: Css = 75 μg/mL • 1.10 = 83 μg/mL and Css = 75 μg/mL • 1.2 = 90 μg/mL. Thus, a dosage rate of 750 mg/d would be expected to yield a total valproic acid steady-state serum concentration between 83 and 90 μg/mL.

A steady-state trough total valproic acid serum concentration should be measured after steady-state is attained in 1-2 weeks. Valproic acid serum concentrations should also be measured if the patient experiences an exacerbation of their epilepsy, or if the patient develops potential signs or symptoms of valproic acid toxicity.

EXAMPLE 11 ▶▶▶

PP is a 59-year-old, 65-kg (height = 5 ft 8 in) male with tonic-clonic seizures who is receiving valproic acid injection 500 mg every 8 hours. The current steady-state valproic acid concentration (obtained 30 minutes before "booster" dose administration) equals 40 μg/mL. Compute a valproic acid maintenance dose that will provide a steady-state concentration of 75 μg/mL. Additionally, in an attempt to boost valproic acid concentrations as soon as possible, an additional, single valproic acid "booster" dose of 500 mg over 60 minutes was given before the maintenance dosage rate was increased. The valproic acid total serum concentration 30 minutes after the additional dose was 105 μg/mL.

1. *Compute pharmacokinetic parameters.*

The patient would be expected to achieve steady-state conditions after 2-3 days of therapy.

Valproic acid clearance can be computed using a steady-state valproic acid concentration: $Cl = [F(D/\tau)]/Css =$ [1(500 mg/ 8 h)]/(40 mg/L) = 1.6 L/h. (Note: μg/mL = mg/L and this concentration unit was substituted for Css in the calculations so that unnecessary unit conversion was not required.)

Valproic acid volume of distribution can be computed using the prebolus dose (Css = 40 μg/mL) and postbolus dose concentrations: $V = D/(C_{postdose} - C_{predose}) = 500$ mg/(105 mg/L − 40 mg/L) = 8 L. (Note: μg/mL = mg/L and this concentration unit was substituted for Css in the calculations so that unnecessary unit conversion was not required.)

Valproic acid half-life $(t_{1/2})$ and elimination rate constant (k) can also be computed: $t_{1/2} = (0.693 \bullet V)/Cl =$ (0.693 • 8 L)/(1.6 L/h) = 3.5 h; $k = Cl/V = (1.6$ L/h)/(8 L) = 0.20 h^{-1}.

2. *Compute valproic acid dose.*

Valproic acid clearance is used to compute the new valproic acid maintenance dose: $D = (Css \bullet Cl \bullet \tau) =$ (75 mg/L • 1.6 L/h • 8 h) = 960 mg, rounded to 1000 mg every 8 hours.

Because of nonlinear, concentration-dependent protein-binding pharmacokinetics, the total steady-state serum concentration would be expected to be 10% less, or 0.90 times, to 20% less, or 0.80 times, than that predicted by linear pharmacokinetics: Css = 75 μg/mL • 0.90 = 68 μg/mL and Css = 75 μg/mL • 0.80 = 60 μg/mL. Thus, a dosage rate of 3000 mg/d would be expected to yield a total valproic acid steady-state serum concentration between 60 and 68 μg/mL.

The new valproic acid maintenance dose would be instituted one dosage interval after the additional "booster" dose was given.

A valproic acid serum concentration should be measured after steady-state is attained in 3-5 half-lives. Since the patient has a half-life equal to 3.5 hours, the valproic acid steady-state concentration could be obtained after 1 day of continuous dosing (5 half-lives = 5 • 3.5 h = 17.5 h). Valproic acid serum concentrations should also be measured if the patient experiences an exacerbation of their epilepsy, or if the patient develops potential signs or symptoms of valproic acid toxicity.

BAYESIAN PHARMACOKINETIC COMPUTER PROGRAMS

Computer programs are available that can assist in the computation of pharmacokinetic parameters for patients. The most reliable computer programs use a nonlinear regression algorithm that incorporates components of Bayes theorem.[45] Nonlinear regression is a statistical technique that uses an iterative process to compute the best pharmacokinetic parameters for a concentration/time data set. Briefly, the patient's drug dosage schedule and serum concentrations are input into the computer. The computer program has a pharmacokinetic equation preprogrammed for the drug and administration method (oral, intravenous bolus, intravenous infusion, etc). Typically, a one-compartment model is used, although some programs allow the user to choose among several different equations. Using population estimates based on demographic information for the patient (age, weight, gender, liver function, cardiac status, etc) supplied by the user, the computer program then computes estimated serum concentrations at each time there are actual serum concentrations. The computer program then changes the kinetic parameters, and computes a new set of estimated serum concentrations. The computer program remembers the pharmacokinetic parameters that generated the estimated serum concentrations closest to the actual values. This process is repeated until the set of pharmacokinetic parameters that result in estimated serum concentrations that are statistically closest to the actual serum concentrations are generated. These pharmacokinetic parameters can then be used to compute improved dosing schedules for patients. Bayes theorem is used in the computer algorithm to balance the results of the computations between values based solely on the patient's serum drug concentrations and those based only on patient population parameters. Results from studies that compare various methods of dosage adjustment have consistently found that these types of computer-dosing programs perform at least as well as experienced clinical pharmacokineticists and clinicians and better than inexperienced clinicians.

Some clinicians use Bayesian pharmacokinetic computer programs exclusively to alter drug doses based on serum concentrations. An advantage of this approach is that consistent dosage recommendations are made when several different practitioners are involved in therapeutic drug-monitoring programs. However, since simpler dosing methods work just as well for patients with stable pharmacokinetic parameters and steady-state drug concentrations, many clinicians reserve the use of computer programs for more difficult situations. Those situations include serum concentrations that are not at steady-state, serum concentrations not obtained at the specific times needed to employ simpler methods, and unstable pharmacokinetic parameters. Many Bayesian pharmacokinetic computer programs are available to users, and most should provide answers similar to the one used in the following examples. The program used to solve problems in this book is DrugCalc written by Dr Dennis Mungall.[45]

EXAMPLE 12 ▶▶▶

LK is a 50-year-old, 75 kg (height = 5 ft 10 in) male with complex partial seizures who is receiving 500 mg every 8 hours of oral enteric-coated valproic acid tablets. He has normal liver (bilirubin = 0.7 mg/dL, albumin = 4.0 g/dL) function, and also takes 1200 mg/d of carbamazepine. The current steady-state valproic acid concentration equals 31 µg/mL. Compute a valproic acid dose that will provide a steady-state concentration of 70 µg/mL.

1. *Enter the patient's demographic, drug-dosing, and serum concentration/time data into the computer program.*

2. *Compute pharmacokinetic parameters for the patient using Bayesian pharmacokinetic computer program.*
   The pharmacokinetic parameters computed by the program are a volume of distribution of 8.6 L, a half-life equal to 5.2 h, and a clearance equal to 1.13 L/h.

3. *Compute dose required to achieve desired valproic acid serum concentrations.*
   The one-compartment model first-order absorption equations used by the program to compute doses indicates that a dose of 1000 mg every 8 hours will produce a steady-state valproic acid concentration of 68 µg/mL.

EXAMPLE 13 ▶▶▶

HJ is a 62-year-old, 87-kg (height = 6 ft 1 in) male with tonic-clonic seizures who was given a new prescription of 500 mg every 12 hours of an oral valproic acid capsules. He has liver cirrhosis (Child-Pugh score = 12, bilirubin = 3.2 mg/dL, albumin = 2.5 g/dL). The trough valproic acid concentration before the seventh dose equals 72 μg/mL, and he is experiencing some minor adverse effects (sedation, lethargy, tiredness). Compute a valproic acid dose that will provide a total steady-state concentration of 50 μg/mL.

1. *Enter the patient's demographic, drug-dosing, and serum concentration/time data into the computer program.*

   In this patient case, it is unlikely that the patient is at steady-state so the Linear Pharmacokinetics method cannot be used.

2. *Compute pharmacokinetic parameters for the patient using Bayesian pharmacokinetic computer program.*

   The pharmacokinetic parameters computed by the program are a volume of distribution of 12.5 L, a half-life equal to 19 h, and a clearance equal to 0.46 L/h.

3. *Compute dose required to achieve desired valproic acid serum concentrations.*

   The one-compartment first-order absorption equations used by the program to compute doses indicates that a dose of 750 mg every 24 hours will produce a steady-state concentration of 46 μg/mL.

EXAMPLE 14 ▶▶▶

JB is a 50-year-old, 60-kg (height = 5 ft 7 in) male with tonic-clonic seizures was started on valproic acid 500 mg every 8 hours intravenously after being administered an intravenous loading dose of valproic acid 750 mg at 0800 H over 60 minutes. The valproic acid concentration was 30 μg/mL before the third maintenance dose. What valproic acid dose is needed to achieve Css = 75 μg/mL?

1. *Enter the patient's demographic, drug-dosing, and serum concentration/time data into the computer program.*

   In this patient case, it is unlikely that the patient is at steady-state so the Linear Pharmacokinetics method cannot be used. Valproic acid doses will be input as intravenous bolus doses.

2. *Compute pharmacokinetic parameters for the patient using Bayesian pharmacokinetic computer program.*

   The pharmacokinetic parameters computed by the program are a volume of distribution of 8.9 L, a half-life equal to 15 h, and clearance equal to 0.42 L/h.

3. *Compute dose required to achieve the desired valproic acid serum concentrations.*

   The one-compartment model intravenous bolus equations used by the program to compute doses indicates that a dose of valproic acid 300 mg every 8 hours will produce a steady-state concentration of 75 μg/mL.

DOSING STRATEGIES

Initial dose and dosage adjustment techniques using serum concentrations can be used in any combination as long as the limitations of each method are observed. Some dosing schemes link together logically when considered according to their basic approaches or philosophies. Dosage strategies that follow similar pathways are given in Table 12-4.

TABLE 12-4   Dosing Strategies

Dosing Approach/Philosophy	Initial Dosing	Use of Serum Concentrations to Alter Doses
Pharmacokinetic parameters/equations	Pharmacokinetic Dosing method	Pharmacokinetic Parameter method
Literature-based concepts	Literature-based recommended dosing	Empiric dosing changes with Pseudolinear Pharmacokinetic method
Computerized	Bayesian computer programs	Bayesian computer programs

PROBLEMS

The following problems are intended to emphasize the computation of initial and individualized doses using clinical pharmacokinetic techniques. Clinicians should always consult the patient's chart to confirm that current anticonvulsant therapy is appropriate. Additionally, all other medications that the patient is taking, including prescription and nonprescription drugs, should be noted and checked to ascertain if a potential drug interaction with valproic acid exists.

1. CD is a 42-year-old, 85-kg (height = 6 ft 1 in) male with tonic-clonic seizures who requires therapy with oral valproic acid. He has normal liver function. Suggest an initial valproic acid dosage regimen designed to achieve a steady-state valproic acid concentration equal to 50 µg/mL.

2. Patient CD (see problem 1) was prescribed 750 mg every 12 hours of enteric-coated divalproex sodium tablets for 1 month, and the steady-state valproic acid total concentration equals 40 µg/mL. The patient is assessed to be compliant with his dosage regimen. Suggest a valproic acid dosage regimen designed to achieve a steady-state valproic acid concentration of 75 µg/mL.

3. BP is a 9-year-old, 35-kg female (height = 4 ft 6 in) with absence seizures who requires therapy with oral valproic acid. She has normal liver function. Suggest an initial valproic acid dosage regimen designed to achieve a steady-state valproic acid concentration equal to 75 µg/mL.

4. Patient BP (see problem 3) was prescribed 150 mg three times daily (450 mg/d) of valproic acid syrup for 2 weeks, and the steady-state valproic acid total concentration equals 55 µg/mL. The patient is assessed to be compliant with her dosage regimen. Suggest a valproic acid dosage regimen designed to achieve a steady-state valproic acid concentration equal to 90 µg/mL.

5. PH is a 4-year-old, 22-kg male (height = 40 in) with tonic-clonic seizures who requires therapy with valproic acid syrup. He has normal liver function and is also treated with carbamazepine. Suggest an initial valproic acid dosage regimen designed to achieve a steady-state valproic acid concentration equal to 50 µg/mL.

6. Patient PH (see problem 5) was prescribed 100 mg three times daily (300 mg/d) of valproic acid syrup for 1 week, and the steady-state valproic acid total concentration equals 40 µg/mL. The patient is assessed to be compliant with his dosage regimen. Suggest a valproic acid dosage regimen designed to achieve a steady-state valproic acid concentration of 60 µg/mL.

7. FL is a 29-year-old, 75-kg (height = 5 ft 11 in) male with tonic-clonic seizures who requires therapy with oral valproic acid. He has normal liver function and is also receiving phenytoin therapy. Suggest an initial valproic acid dosage regimen designed to achieve a steady-state valproic acid concentration equal to 50 µg/mL.

8. Patient FL (see problem 7) was prescribed 750 mg every 8 hours of enteric-coated divalproex sodium tablets for 2 weeks, and the steady-state valproic acid total concentration equals 55 µg/mL. The patient

is assessed to be compliant with his dosage regimen. Suggest a valproic acid dosage regimen designed to achieve a steady-state valproic acid concentration of 90 μg/mL.

9. WE is a 55-year-old, 68-kg (height = 5 ft 8 in) male with complex partial seizures who is receiving 500 mg every 8 hours of an oral enteric-coated divalproex sodium tablets. He has normal liver (bilirubin = 0.7 mg/dL, albumin = 4.0 g/dL) function, and also takes 800 mg/d of carbamazepine. The total valproic acid concentration equals 22 μg/mL before the fourth dose. Compute a valproic acid dose that will provide a steady-state concentration of 50 μg/mL.

10. YF is a 5-year-old, 20-kg (height = 42 in) female with tonic-clonic seizures who was given a new prescription of 250 mg every 12 hours of oral valproic acid capsules. She has normal liver function and is receiving no enzyme inducers. The trough valproic acid concentration before the third dose equals 42 μg/mL. Compute a valproic acid dose that will provide a total steady-state concentration of 75 μg/mL.

ANSWERS TO PROBLEMS

1. *Answer to problem 1.*

Pharmacokinetic Dosing Method

1. *Estimate clearance and volume of distribution according to disease states and conditions present in the patient.*

    The clearance rate for an adult patient not taking other drugs that induce hepatic drug metabolism is 7-12 mL/h/kg. Using a value of 10 mL/h/kg, the estimated clearance would equal 0.85 L/h: Cl = 85 kg • 10 mL/h/kg = 850 mL/h or 0.85 L/h. Using 0.15 L/kg, the estimated volume of distribution would be 13 L: 85 kg • 0.15 L/kg = 13 L.

2. *Estimate half-life and elimination rate constant.*

    Once the correct clearance and volume of distribution estimates are identified for the patient, they can be converted into the valproic acid half-life $(t_{1/2})$ and elimination rate constant (k) estimates using the following equations: $t_{1/2} = (0.693 • V)/Cl = (0.693 • 13 L)/0.85 L/h = 11 h$, $k = 0.693/t_{1/2} = 0.693/11 h = 0.063 h^{-1}$.

3. *Compute dosage regimen.*

    Oral enteric-coated divalproex sodium tablets will be prescribed to this patient (F = 1). (Note: μg/mL = mg/L and this concentration unit was substituted for Css in the calculations so that unnecessary unit conversion was not required.) The dosage equation for oral valproic acid is: D = (Css • Cl • τ)/F = (50 mg/L • 0.85 L/h • 12 h)/1 = 510 mg, rounded to 500 every 12 hours.

    A steady-state trough valproic acid serum concentration should be measured after steady-state is attained in 3-5 half-lives. Since the patient is expected to have a half-life equal to 11 hours, the valproic acid steady-state concentration could be obtained any time after the second day of dosing (5 half-lives = 5 • 11 h = 55 h). Valproic acid serum concentrations should also be measured if the patient experiences an exacerbation of their epilepsy, or if the patient develops potential signs or symptoms of valproic acid toxicity.

Literature-Based Recommended Dosing

1. *Estimate valproic acid dose according to disease states and conditions present in the patient.*

    Oral enteric-coated divalproex sodium tablets will be prescribed to this patient. The suggested initial maintenance dosage rate for valproic acid in an adult patient not taking enzyme inducers is 7.5 mg/kg/d: 85 kg • 7.5 mg/kg/d = 638 mg/d, rounded to 750 mg or 250 mg every 8 hours.

This dose would be titrated upward in 5-10 mg/kg/d increments every 1-2 weeks while monitoring for adverse and therapeutic effects. The goals of therapy include maximal suppression of seizures and avoidance of side effects.

A steady-state trough total valproic acid serum concentration should be measured after steady-state is attained in 1-2 weeks. Valproic acid serum concentrations should also be measured if the patient experiences an exacerbation of their epilepsy, or if the patient develops potential signs or symptoms of valproic acid toxicity.

2. *Answer to problem 2.*

Pseudolinear Pharmacokinetics Method

1. *Use pseudolinear pharmacokinetics to predict new concentration for a dosage increase, then compute 10%-20% factor to account for nonlinear, concentration-dependent plasma protein–binding pharmacokinetics.*

Using pseudolinear pharmacokinetics, the resulting total steady-state valproic acid serum concentration would equal : $D_{new} = (Css_{new}/Css_{old}) D_{old} = (75\ \mu g/mL\ /\ 40\ \mu g/mL)\ 1500\ mg/d = 2813\ mg/d$, rounded to 3000 mg/d or 1000 mg every 8 hours. Because of nonlinear, concentration-dependent protein-binding pharmacokinetics, the total steady-state serum concentration would be expected to be 10% less, or 0.90 times, to 20% less, or 0.80 times, than that predicted by linear pharmacokinetics: $Css = 75\ \mu g/mL \bullet 0.90 = 68\ \mu g/mL$ and $Css = 75\ \mu g/mL \bullet 0.80 = 60\ \mu g/mL$. Thus, a dosage rate of 3000 mg/d would be expected to yield a total valproic acid steady-state serum concentration between 60 and 68 μg/mL.

A steady-state trough total valproic acid serum concentration should be measured after steady-state is attained in 1-2 weeks. Valproic acid serum concentrations should also be measured if the patient experiences an exacerbation of their epilepsy, or if the patient develops potential signs or symptoms of valproic acid toxicity.

Pharmacokinetic Parameter Method

1. *Compute pharmacokinetic parameters.*

The patient would be expected to achieve steady-state conditions after 2-3 days of therapy.

Valproic acid clearance can be computed using a steady-state valproic acid concentration: $Cl = [F(D/\tau)]/Css = [1(750\ mg/12\ h)]/(40\ mg/L) = 1.6\ L/h$. (Note: μg/mL = mg/L and this concentration unit was substituted for Css in the calculations so that unnecessary unit conversion was not required.)

2. *Compute valproic acid dose.*

Valproic acid clearance is used to compute the new dose: $D = (Css \bullet Cl \bullet \tau)/F = (75\ mg/L \bullet 1.6\ L/h \bullet 8\ h)/1 = 960\ mg$, rounded to 1000 mg every 8 hours. (Note: Dosage interval was changed to every 8 hours to avoid large single doses and gastrointestinal upset.)

Because of nonlinear, concentration-dependent protein-binding pharmacokinetics, the total steady-state serum concentration would be expected to be 10% less, or 0.90 times, to 20% less, or 0.80 times, than that predicted by linear pharmacokinetics: $Css = 75\ \mu g/mL \bullet 0.90 = 68\ \mu g/mL$ and $Css = 75\ \mu g/mL \bullet 0.80 = 60\ \mu g/mL$. Thus, a dosage rate of 3000 mg/d would be expected to yield a total valproic acid steady-state serum concentration between 60 and 68 μg/mL.

A steady-state trough total valproic acid serum concentration should be measured after steady-state is attained in 1-2 weeks. Valproic acid serum concentrations should also be measured if the patient experiences an exacerbation of their epilepsy, or if the patient develops potential signs or symptoms of valproic acid toxicity.

Bayesian Pharmacokinetic Computer Programs

1. *Enter the patient's demographic, drug-dosing, and serum concentration/time data into the computer program.*

2. *Compute pharmacokinetic parameters for the patient using Bayesian pharmacokinetic computer program.*

    The pharmacokinetic parameters computed by the program are a volume of distribution of 10.7 L, a half-life equal to 8.1 h, and a clearance equal to 0.91 L/h.

3. *Compute dose required to achieve the desired valproic acid serum concentrations.*

    The one-compartment model first-order absorption equations used by the program to compute doses indicates that a dose of 750 mg every 8 hours will produce a steady-state valproic acid concentration of 78 µg/mL.

3. *Answer to problem 3.*

Pharmacokinetic Dosing Method

1. *Estimate clearance and volume of distribution according to the disease states and conditions present in the patient.*

    The clearance rate for a pediatric patient not taking other drugs that induce hepatic drug metabolism is 10-20 mL/h/kg. Using a value of 15 mL/h/kg, the estimated clearance would equal 0.53 L/h: $Cl = 35$ kg • 15 mL/h/kg = 525 mL/h or 0.53 L/h. Using 0.2 L/kg, the estimated volume of distribution would be 7 L: 35 kg • 0.2 L/kg = 7 L.

2. *Estimate half-life and elimination rate constant.*

    Once the correct clearance and volume of distribution estimates are identified for the patient, they can be converted into the valproic acid half-life ($t_{1/2}$) and elimination rate constant (k) estimates using the following equations: $t_{1/2} = (0.693 • V)/Cl = (0.693 • 7$ L)/0.53 L/h = 9 h, $k = 0.693/t_{1/2} = 0.693/9$ h $= 0.077$ h^{-1}.

3. *Compute dosage regimen.*

    Oral valproic acid syrup will be prescribed to this patient (F = 1). (Note: µg/mL = mg/L and this concentration unit was substituted for Css in the calculations so that unnecessary unit conversion was not required.) The dosage equation for oral valproic acid is: $D = (Css • Cl • \tau)/F = (75$ mg/L • 0.53 L/h • 8 h)/1 = 318 mg, rounded to 300 every 8 hours.

    A steady-state trough valproic acid serum concentration should be measured after steady-state is attained in 3-5 half-lives. Since the patient is expected to have a half-life equal to 9 hours, the valproic acid steady-state concentration could be obtained any time after the second day of dosing (5 half-lives = 5 • 9 h = 45 h). Valproic acid serum concentrations should also be measured if the patient experiences an exacerbation of their seizures, or if the patient develops potential signs or symptoms of valproic acid toxicity.

Literature-Based Recommended Dosing

1. *Estimate valproic acid dose according to disease states and conditions present in the patient.*

    Oral valproic acid syrup will be prescribed to this patient. The suggested initial maintenance dosage rate for valproic acid in an adult patient not taking enzyme inducers is 10 mg/kg/d: 35 kg • 10 mg/kg/d = 350 mg/d, rounded to 400 mg or 200 mg every 12 hours. This dose would be titrated upward in 5-10 mg/kg/d increments every 1-2 weeks while monitoring for adverse and therapeutic effects. The goals of therapy include maximal suppression of seizures and avoidance of side effects.

A steady-state trough total valproic acid serum concentration should be measured after steady-state is attained in 1-2 weeks. Valproic acid serum concentrations should also be measured if the patient experiences an exacerbation of their epilepsy, or if the patient develops potential signs or symptoms of valproic acid toxicity.

4. *Answer to problem 4.*

Pseudolinear Pharmacokinetics Method

1. *Use pseudolinear pharmacokinetics to predict new concentration for a dosage increase, then compute 10%-20% factor to account for nonlinear, concentration-dependent plasma protein–binding pharmacokinetics.*

Using pseudolinear pharmacokinetics, the resulting total steady-state valproic acid serum concentration would equal: $D_{new} = (Css_{new}/Css_{old}) D_{old} = (90 \text{ μg/mL} / 55 \text{ μg/mL}) 450 \text{ mg/d} = 736$ mg/d, rounded to 750 mg/d or 250 mg every 8 hours. Because of nonlinear, concentration-dependent protein-binding pharmacokinetics, the total steady-state serum concentration would be expected to be 10% less, or 0.90 times, to 20% less, or 0.80 times, than that predicted by linear pharmacokinetics: $Css = 90 \text{ μg/mL} \bullet 0.90 = 81 \text{ μg/mL}$ and $Css = 90 \text{ μg/mL} \bullet 0.80 = 72 \text{ μg/mL}$. Thus, a dosage rate of 750 mg/d would be expected to yield a total valproic acid steady-state serum concentration between 72 and 81 μg/mL.

A steady-state trough total valproic acid serum concentration should be measured after steady-state is attained in 1-2 weeks. Valproic acid serum concentrations should also be measured if the patient experiences an exacerbation of their epilepsy, or if the patient develops potential signs or symptoms of valproic acid toxicity.

Pharmacokinetic Parameter Method

1. *Compute pharmacokinetic parameters.*

The patient would be expected to achieve steady-state conditions after 2-3 days of therapy.

Valproic acid clearance can be computed using a steady-state valproic acid concentration: $Cl = [F(D/\tau)]/Css = [1(150 \text{ mg/8 h})]/(55 \text{ mg/L}) = 0.34 \text{ L/h}$. (Note: μg/mL = mg/L and this concentration unit was substituted for Css in the calculations so that unnecessary unit conversion was not required.)

2. *Compute valproic acid dose.*

Valproic acid clearance is used to compute the new dose: $D = (Css \bullet Cl \bullet \tau)/F = (90 \text{ mg/L} \bullet 0.34 \text{ L/h} \bullet 8 \text{ h})/1 = 245 \text{ mg}$, rounded to 250 mg every 8 hours.

Because of nonlinear, concentration-dependent protein-binding pharmacokinetics, the total steady-state serum concentration would be expected to be 10% less, or 0.90 times, to 20% less, or 0.80 times, than that predicted by linear pharmacokinetics: $Css = 90 \text{ μg/mL} \bullet 0.90 = 81 \text{ μg/mL}$ and $Css = 90 \text{ μg/mL} \bullet 0.80 = 72 \text{ μg/mL}$. Thus, a dosage rate of 750 mg/d would be expected to yield a total valproic acid steady-state serum concentration between 72 and 81 μg/mL.

A steady-state trough total valproic acid serum concentration should be measured after steady-state is attained in 1-2 weeks. Valproic acid serum concentrations should also be measured if the patient experiences an exacerbation of their epilepsy, or if the patient develops potential signs or symptoms of valproic acid toxicity.

Bayesian Pharmacokinetic Computer Programs

1. *Enter the patient's demographic, drug-dosing, and serum concentration/time data into the computer program.*

2. *Compute pharmacokinetic parameters for the patient using Bayesian pharmacokinetic computer program.*

   The pharmacokinetic parameters computed by the program are a volume of distribution of 2 L, a half-life equal to 6.4 h, and a clearance equal to 0.21 L/h.

3. *Compute dose required to achieve desired valproic acid serum concentrations.*

   The one-compartment model first-order absorption equations used by the program to compute doses indicates that a dose of 250 mg every 8 hours will produce a steady-state valproic acid concentration of 100 μg/mL.

5. *Answer to problem 5.*

Pharmacokinetic Dosing Method

1. *Estimate clearance and volume of distribution according to disease states and conditions present in the patient.*

   The clearance rate for a pediatric patient that takes other drugs that induce hepatic drug metabolism is 20-30 mL/h/kg. Using a value of 25 mL/h/kg, the estimated clearance would equal 0.55 L/h: Cl = 22 kg • 25 mL/h/kg = 550 mL/h or 0.55 L/h. Using 0.2 L/kg, the estimated volume of distribution would be 4.4 L: 22 kg • 0.2 L/kg = 4.4 L.

2. *Estimate half-life and elimination rate constant.*

   Once the correct clearance and volume of distribution estimates are identified for the patient, they can be converted into the valproic acid half-life ($t_{1/2}$) and elimination rate constant (k) estimates using the following equations: $t_{1/2} = (0.693 • V)/Cl = (0.693 • 4.4 L)/0.55 L/h = 5.5 h$, $k = 0.693/t_{1/2} = 0.693/5.5 h = 0.126 h^{-1}$.

3. *Compute dosage regimen.*

   Oral valproic acid syrup will be prescribed to this patient (F = 1). (Note: μg/mL = mg/L and this concentration unit was substituted for Css in the calculations so that unnecessary unit conversion was not required.) The dosage equation for oral valproic acid is: D = (Css • Cl • τ)/F = (50 mg/L • 0.55 L/h • 8 h)/1 = 220 mg, rounded to 250 mg every 8 hours.

   A steady-state trough valproic acid serum concentration should be measured after steady-state is attained in 3-5 half-lives. Since the patient is expected to have a half-life equal to 5.5 hours, the valproic acid steady-state concentration could be obtained any time after the first day of dosing (5 half-lives = 5 • 5.5 h = 28 h). Valproic acid serum concentrations should also be measured if the patient experiences an exacerbation of their seizures, or if the patient develops potential signs or symptoms of valproic acid toxicity.

Literature-Based Recommended Dosing

1. *Estimate valproic acid dose according to disease states and conditions present in the patient.*

   Oral valproic acid syrup will be prescribed to this patient. The suggested initial maintenance dosage rate for valproic acid in an adult patient not taking enzyme inducers is 20 mg/kg/d: 22 kg • 20 mg/kg/d = 440 mg/d, rounded to 400 mg or 200 mg every 12 hours. This dose would be titrated upward in 5-10 mg/kg/d increments every 1-2 weeks while monitoring for adverse and therapeutic effects. The goals of therapy include maximal suppression of seizures and avoidance of side effects.

   A steady-state trough total valproic acid serum concentration should be measured after steady-state is attained in 1-2 weeks. Valproic acid serum concentrations should also be measured if the patient experiences an exacerbation of their epilepsy, or if the patient develops potential signs or symptoms of valproic acid toxicity.

6. *Answer to problem 6.*

Pseudolinear Pharmacokinetics Method

1. *Use pseudolinear pharmacokinetics to predict new concentration for a dosage increase, then compute 10%-20% factor to account for nonlinear, concentration-dependent plasma protein–binding pharmacokinetics.*

Using pseudolinear pharmacokinetics, the resulting total steady-state valproic acid serum concentration would equal: $D_{new} = (Css_{new}/Css_{old}) D_{old} = (60\ \mu g/mL\ /\ 40\ \mu g/mL)\ 300\ mg/d = 450\ mg/d$, 150 mg every 8 hours. Because of nonlinear, concentration-dependent protein-binding pharmacokinetics, the total steady-state serum concentration would be expected to be 10% less, or 0.90 times, to 20% less, or 0.80 times, than that predicted by linear pharmacokinetics: $Css = 60\ \mu g/mL \bullet 0.90 = 54\ \mu g/mL$ and $Css = 60\ \mu g/mL \bullet 0.80 = 48\ \mu g/mL$. Thus, a dosage rate of 450 mg/d would be expected to yield a total valproic acid steady-state serum concentration between 48 and 54 μg/mL.

A steady-state trough total valproic acid serum concentration should be measured after steady-state is attained in 1-2 weeks. Valproic acid serum concentrations should also be measured if the patient experiences an exacerbation of their epilepsy, or if the patient develops potential signs or symptoms of valproic acid toxicity.

Pharmacokinetic Parameter Method

1. *Compute pharmacokinetic parameters.*

The patient would be expected to achieve steady-state conditions after 2-3 days of therapy.

Valproic acid clearance can be computed using a steady-state valproic acid concentration: $Cl = [F(D/\tau)]/Css = [1(100\ mg/8\ h)]/(40\ mg/L) = 0.31\ L/h$. (Note: μg/mL = mg/L and this concentration unit was substituted for Css in the calculations so that unnecessary unit conversion was not required.)

2. *Compute valproic acid dose.*

Valproic acid clearance is used to compute the new dose: $D = (Css \bullet Cl \bullet \tau)/F = (60\ mg/L \bullet 0.31\ L/h \bullet 8\ h)/1 = 149\ mg$, rounded to 150 mg every 8 hours.

Because of nonlinear, concentration-dependent protein-binding pharmacokinetics, the total steady-state serum concentration would be expected to be 10% less, or 0.90 times, to 20% less, or 0.80 times, than that predicted by linear pharmacokinetics: $Css = 60\ \mu g/mL \bullet 0.90 = 54\ \mu g/mL$ and $Css = 60\ \mu g/mL \bullet 0.80 = 48\ \mu g/mL$. Thus, a dosage rate of 450 mg/d would be expected to yield a total valproic acid steady-state serum concentration between 48 and 54 μg/mL.

A steady-state trough total valproic acid serum concentration should be measured after steady-state is attained in 1-2 weeks. Valproic acid serum concentrations should also be measured if the patient experiences an exacerbation of their epilepsy, or if the patient develops potential signs or symptoms of valproic acid toxicity.

Bayesian Pharmacokinetic Computer Programs

1. *Enter the patient's demographic, drug-dosing, and serum concentration/time data into the computer program.*

2. *Compute pharmacokinetic parameters for the patient using Bayesian pharmacokinetic computer program.*

The pharmacokinetic parameters computed by the program are a volume of distribution of 2.9 L, a half-life equal to 8.9 h, and a clearance equal to 0.23 L/h.

3. *Compute dose required to achieve the desired valproic acid serum concentrations.*

The one-compartment model first-order absorption equations used by the program to compute doses indicates that a dose of 150 mg every 8 hours will produce a steady-state valproic acid concentration of 64 μg/mL.

7. *Answer to problem 7.*

Pharmacokinetic Dosing Method

1. *Estimate clearance and volume of distribution according to disease states and conditions present in the patient.*

    The clearance rate for an adult patient taking other drugs that induce hepatic drug metabolism is 15-18 mL/h/kg. Using a value of 16 mL/h/kg, the estimated clearance would equal 1.2 L/h: Cl = 75 kg • 16 mL/h/kg = 1200 mL/h or 1.2 L/h. Using 0.15 L/kg, the estimated volume of distribution would be 11 L: 75 kg • 0.15 L/kg = 11 L.

2. *Estimate half-life and elimination rate constant.*

    Once the correct clearance and volume of distribution estimates are identified for the patient, they can be converted into the valproic acid half-life ($t_{1/2}$) and elimination rate constant (k) estimates using the following equations: $t_{1/2}$ = (0.693 • V)/Cl = (0.693 • 11 L)/1.2 L/h = 6 h, k = $0.693/t_{1/2}$ = 0.693/6 h = 0.116 h^{-1}.

3. *Compute dosage regimen.*

    Oral enteric-coated divalproex sodium tablets will be prescribed to this patient (F = 1). (Note: μg/mL = mg/L and this concentration unit was substituted for Css in the calculations so that unnecessary unit conversion was not required.) The dosage equation for oral valproic acid is: D = (Css • Cl • τ)/F = (50 mg/L• 1.2 L/h • 8 h)/1 = 480 mg, rounded to 500 every 8 hours.

    A steady-state trough valproic acid serum concentration should be measured after steady-state is attained in 3-5 half-lives. Since the patient is expected to have a half-life equal to 6 hours, the valproic acid steady-state concentration could be obtained any time after the second day of dosing (5 half-lives = 5 • 6 h = 30 h). Valproic acid serum concentrations should also be measured if the patient experiences an exacerbation of their epilepsy, or if the patient develops potential signs or symptoms of valproic acid toxicity.

Literature-Based Recommended Dosing

1. *Estimate valproic acid dose according to disease states and conditions present in the patient.*

    Oral enteric-coated divalproex sodium tablets will be prescribed to this patient. The suggested initial maintenance dosage rate for valproic acid in an adult patient taking enzyme inducers is 15 mg/kg/d: 75 kg • 15 mg/kg/d = 1125 mg/d, rounded to 1000 mg or 500 mg every 12 hours. This dose would be titrated upward in 5-10 mg/kg/d increments every 1-2 weeks while monitoring for adverse and therapeutic effects. The goals of therapy include maximal suppression of seizures and avoidance of side effects.

    A steady-state trough total valproic acid serum concentration should be measured after steady-state is attained in 1-2 weeks. Valproic acid serum concentrations should also be measured if the patient experiences an exacerbation of their epilepsy, or if the patient develops potential signs or symptoms of valproic acid toxicity.

8. *Answer to problem 8.*

Pseudolinear Pharmacokinetics Method

1. *Use pseudolinear pharmacokinetics to predict new concentration for a dosage increase, then compute 10%-20% factor to account for nonlinear, concentration-dependent plasma protein–binding pharmacokinetics.*

    Using pseudolinear pharmacokinetics, the resulting total steady-state valproic acid serum concentration would equal: D_{new} = (Css_{new}/Css_{old}) D_{old} = (90 μg/mL / 55 μg/mL) 2250 mg/d = 3682 mg/d, rounded to 3750 mg/d or 1250 mg every 8 hours. Because of nonlinear, concentration-dependent protein-binding pharmacokinetics, the total steady-state serum concentration would be expected to be 10% less, or 0.90 times, to 20% less, or 0.80 times, than that predicted by linear pharmacokinetics: Css = 90 µg/mL • 0.90 = 81 µg/mL and Css = 90 µg/mL • 0.80 = 72 µg/mL. Thus, a dosage rate of 3750 mg/d would be expected to yield a total valproic acid steady-state serum concentration between 72 and 81 µg/mL.

A steady-state trough total valproic acid serum concentration should be measured after steady-state is attained in 1-2 weeks. Valproic acid serum concentrations should also be measured if the patient experiences an exacerbation of their epilepsy, or if the patient develops potential signs or symptoms of valproic acid toxicity.

Pharmacokinetic Parameter Method

1. *Compute pharmacokinetic parameters.*

The patient would be expected to achieve steady-state conditions after 2-3 days of therapy.

Valproic acid clearance can be computed using a steady-state valproic acid concentration: Cl = [F(D/τ)]/Css = [1(750 mg/8 h)]/(55 mg/L) = 1.7 L/h. (Note: µg/mL = mg/L and this concentration unit was substituted for Css in the calculations so that unnecessary unit conversion was not required.)

2. *Compute valproic acid dose.*

Valproic acid clearance is used to compute the new dose: D = (Css • Cl • τ)/F = (90 mg/L• 1.7 L/h • 8 h)/1 = 1224 mg, rounded to 1250 mg every 8 hours.

Because of nonlinear, concentration-dependent protein-binding pharmacokinetics, the total steady-state serum concentration would be expected to be 10% less, or 0.90 times, to 20% less, or 0.80 times, than that predicted by linear pharmacokinetics: Css = 90 µg/mL • 0.90 = 81 µg/mL and Css = 90 µg/mL • 0.80 = 72 µg/mL. Thus, a dosage rate of 3750 mg/d would be expected to yield a total valproic acid steady-state serum concentration between 72 and 81 µg/mL.

A steady-state trough total valproic acid serum concentration should be measured after steady-state is attained in 1-2 weeks. Valproic acid serum concentrations should also be measured if the patient experiences an exacerbation of their epilepsy, or if the patient develops potential signs or symptoms of valproic acid toxicity.

Bayesian Pharmacokinetic Computer Programs

1. *Enter the patient's demographic, drug-dosing, and serum concentration/time data into the computer program.*

2. *Compute pharmacokinetic parameters for the patient using Bayesian pharmacokinetic computer program.*

The pharmacokinetic parameters computed by the program are a volume of distribution of 9 L, a half-life equal to 6.1 h, and a clearance equal to 1 L/h.

3. *Compute dose required to achieve the desired valproic acid serum concentrations.*

The one-compartment model first-order absorption equations used by the program to compute doses indicates that a dose of 1000 mg every 8 hours will produce a steady-state valproic acid concentration of 82 µg/mL.

9. *Answer to problem 9.*

Bayesian Pharmacokinetic Computer Programs

1. *Enter the patient's demographic, drug-dosing, and serum concentration/time data into the computer program.*

2. *Compute pharmacokinetic parameters for the patient using Bayesian pharmacokinetic computer program.*

The pharmacokinetic parameters computed by the program are a volume of distribution of 6.8 L, a half-life equal to 3.9 h, and a clearance equal to 1.2 L/h.

3. *Compute the dose required to achieve the desired valproic acid serum concentrations.*

The one-compartment model first-order absorption equations used by the program to compute doses indicates that a dose of 1000 mg every 8 hours will produce a steady-state valproic acid concentration of 50 μg/mL.

10. *Answer to problem 10.*

Bayesian Pharmacokinetic Computer Programs

1. *Enter the patient's demographic, drug-dosing, and serum concentration/time data into the computer program.*

2. *Compute pharmacokinetic parameters for the patient using Bayesian pharmacokinetic computer program.*

The pharmacokinetic parameters computed by the program are a volume of distribution of 4.3 L, a half-life equal to 9.2 h, and a clearance equal to 0.32 L/h.

3. *Compute dose required to achieve the desired valproic acid serum concentrations.*

The one-compartment model first-order absorption equations used by the program to compute doses indicates that a dose of 250 mg every 8 hours will produce a steady-state valproic acid concentration of 70 μg/mL. (Note: Dosage interval was decreased to avoid excessive doses and gastrointestinal side effects.)

REFERENCES

1. Abramowicz M, Zuccotti G, Pflomm JM, eds. Drugs for epilepsy. *Treatment Guidelines From The Medical Letter.* 2013;11(126):9-18.
2. Anon. The epilepsies: the diagnosis and management of the epilepsies in adults and children in primary and secondary care. *UK National Institute for Health and Care Excellence.* http://www.nice.org.uk/nicemedia/live/13635/57779/57779.pdf. Accessed April 2, 2014.
3. French JA, Kanner AM, Bautista J, et al. Efficacy and tolerability of the new antiepileptic drugs I: treatment of new onset epilepsy: report of the Therapeutics and Technology Assessment Subcommittee and Quality Standards Subcommittee of the American Academy of Neurology and the American Epilepsy Society. *Neurology.* Apr 27 2004;62(8):1252-1260.
4. Glauser T, Ben-Menachem E, Bourgeois B, et al. Updated ILAE evidence review of antiepileptic drug efficacy and effectiveness as initial monotherapy for epileptic seizures and syndromes. *Epilepsia.* Mar 2013;54(3):551-563.
5. Naritoku DK, Mueed S. Intravenous loading of valproate for epilepsy. *Clin Neuropharmacol.* Mar-Apr 1999;22(2):102-106.
6. Alehan FK, Morton LD, Pellock JM. Treatment of absence status with intravenous valproate. *Neurology.* Mar 10 1999;52(4):889-890.
7. Abramowicz M, Zuccotti G, Pflomm JM, eds. Drugs for depression and bipolar disorder. *Treatment Guidelines From The Medical Letter.* 2010;8(93):35-42.
8. Drayton SJ. Bipolar disorders. In: DiPiro JT, Talbert RL, Yee GC, Matzke GR, Wells BG, Posey LM, eds. *Pharmacotherapy.* 8th ed. New York, NY: McGraw-Hill; 2011:1191-1208.
9. Glauser TA, Cnaan A, Shinnar S, et al. Ethosuximide, valproic acid, and lamotrigine in childhood absence epilepsy. *N Engl J Med.* Mar 4 2010;362(9):790-799.
10. Glauser TA, Cnaan A, Shinnar S, et al. Ethosuximide, valproic acid, and lamotrigine in childhood absence epilepsy: initial monotherapy outcomes at 12 months. *Epilepsia.* Jan 2013;54(1):141-155.
11. McNamara JO. Pharmacotherapy of the epilepsies. In: Brunton L, Chabner B, Knollman B, eds. *The Pharmacological Basis of Therapeutics.* 12th ed. New York, NY: McGraw-Hill; 2011:583-608.
12. Rogers SJ, Cavazos JE. Epilepsy. In: DiPiro JT, Talbert RL, Yee GC, Matzke GR, Wells BG, Posey LM, eds. *Pharmacotherapy.* 8th ed. New York, NY: McGraw-Hill; 2011:979-1005.
13. Kodama Y, Koike Y, Kimoto H, et al. Binding parameters of valproic acid to serum protein in healthy adults at steady state. *Ther Drug Monit.* 1992;14(1):55-60.

14. Bauer LA, Davis R, Wilensky A, Raisys V, Levy RH. Valproic acid clearance: unbound fraction and diurnal variation in young and elderly adults. *Clin Pharmacol Ther.* 1985;37(6):697-700.

15. Urien S, Albengres E, Tillement JP. Serum protein binding of valproic acid in healthy subjects and in patients with liver disease. *Int J Clin Pharmacol Ther Toxicol.* 1981;19(7):319-325.

16. Brewster D, Muir NC. Valproate plasma protein binding in the uremic condition. *Clin Pharmacol Ther.* 1980;27(1):76-82.

17. Bruni J, Wang LH, Marbury TC, Lee CS, Wilder BJ. Protein binding of valproic acid in uremic patients. *Neurology.* 1980;30(5):557-559.

18. Gugler R, Mueller G. Plasma protein binding of valproic acid in healthy subjects and in patients with renal disease. *Br J Clin Pharmacol.* 1978;5(5):441-446.

19. Chatzistefanidis D, Georgiou I, Kyritsis AP, Markoula S. Functional impact and prevalence of polymorphisms involved in the hepatic glucuronidation of valproic acid. *Pharmacogenomics.* Jul 2012;13(9):1055-1071.

20. Argikar UA, Remmel RP. Effect of aging on glucuronidation of valproic acid in human liver microsomes and the role of UDP-glucuronosyltransferase UGT1A4, UGT1A8, and UGT1A10. *Drug Metab Dispos.* Jan 2009;37(1):229-236.

21. Ghodke-Puranik Y, Thorn CF, Lamba JK, et al. Valproic acid pathway: pharmacokinetics and pharmacodynamics. *Pharmacogenet Genomics.* Apr 2013;23(4):236-241.

22. Ethell BT, Anderson GD, Burchell B. The effect of valproic acid on drug and steroid glucuronidation by expressed human UDP-glucuronosyltransferases. *Biochem Pharmacol.* May 1 2003;65(9):1441-1449.

23. Dutta S, Zhang Y. Bioavailability of divalproex extended-release formulation relative to the divalproex delayed-release formulation. *Biopharm Drug Dispos.* Nov 2004;25(8):345-352.

24. Dutta S, Reed RC. Distinct absorption characteristics of oral formulations of valproic acid/divalproex available in the United States. *Epilepsy Res.* Mar 2007;73(3):275-283.

25. Garnett WR. Antiepileptics. In: Schumacher GE, ed. *Therapeutic Drug Monitoring.* Stamford, CT: Appleton & Lange; 1995:345-395.

26. Zaccara G, Messori A, Moroni F. Clinical pharmacokinetics of valproic acid—1988. *Clin Pharmacokinet.* 1988;15(6):367-389.

27. Hall K, Otten N, Johnston B, Irvine-Meek J, Leroux M, Seshia S. A multivariable analysis of factors governing the steady-state pharmacokinetics of valproic acid in 52 young epileptics. *J Clin Pharmacol.* 1985;25(4):261-268.

28. Cloyd JC, Kriel RL, Fischer JH. Valproic acid pharmacokinetics in children. II. Discontinuation of concomitant antiepileptic drug therapy. *Neurology.* 1985;35(11):1623-1627.

29. Chiba K, Suganuma T, Ishizaki T, et al. Comparison of steady-state pharmacokinetics of valproic acid in children between monotherapy and multiple antiepileptic drug treatment. *J Pediatr.* 1985;106(4):653-658.

30. Gugler R, von Unruh GE. Clinical pharmacokinetics of valproic acid. *Clin Pharmacokinet.* 1980;5(1):67-83.

31. Klotz U, Rapp T, Muller WA. Disposition of valproic acid in patients with liver disease. *Eur J Clin Pharmacol.* 1978;13(1):55-60.

32. Pugh RN, Murray-Lyon IM, Dawson JL, Pietroni MC, Williams R. Transection of the oesophagus for bleeding oesophageal varices. *Br J Surg.* 1973;60(8):646-649.

33. Birnbaum AK, Ahn JE, Brundage RC, Hardie NA, Conway JM, Leppik IE. Population pharmacokinetics of valproic acid concentrations in elderly nursing home residents. *Ther Drug Monit.* Oct 2007;29(5):571-575.

34. Omtzigt JG, Nau H, Los FJ, Pijpers L, Lindhout D. The disposition of valproate and its metabolites in the late first trimester and early second trimester of pregnancy in maternal serum, urine, and amniotic fluid: effect of dose, co-medication, and the presence of spina bifida. *Eur J Clin Pharmacol.* 1992;43(4):381-388.

35. Bauer LA, Davis R, Wilensky A, Raisys V, Levy RH. Diurnal variation in valproic acid clearance. *Clin Pharmacol Ther.* 1984;35(4):505-509.

36. Kandrotas RJ, Love JM, Gal P, Oles KS. The effect of hemodialysis and hemoperfusion on serum valproic acid concentration. *Neurology.* 1990;40(9):1456-1458.

37. Bauer LA, Harris C, Wilensky AJ, Raisys VA, Levy RH. Ethosuximide kinetics: possible interaction with valproic acid. *Clin Pharmacol Ther.* 1982;31(6):741-745.

38. Trapnell CB, Klecker RW, Jamis-Dow C, Collins JM. Glucuronidation of 3′-azido-3′-deoxythymidine (zidovudine) by human liver microsomes: relevance to clinical pharmacokinetic interactions with atovaquone, fluconazole, methadone, and valproic acid. *Antimicrob Agents Chemother.* 1998;42(7):1592-1596.

39. Hansten PD, Horn JR. *The Top 100 Drug Interactions.* Freeland, WA: H&H Publications; 2014.

40. Hansten PD, Horn JR. *Drug Interactions Analysis and Management.* St. Louis, MO: Wolters Kluwer; 2014.

41. Pisani FD, Di Perri RG. Intravenous valproate: effects on plasma and saliva phenytoin levels. *Neurology.* 1981;31(4):467-470.

42. Perucca E, Hebdige S, Frigo GM, Gatti G, Lecchini S, Crema A. Interaction between phenytoin and valproic acid: plasma protein binding and metabolic effects. *Clin Pharmacol Ther.* 1980;28(6):779-789.

43. Riva R, Albani F, Contin M, et al. Time-dependent interaction between phenytoin and valproic acid. *Neurology.* 1985;35(4):510-515.

44. Frigo GM, Lecchini S, Gatti G, Perucca E, Crema A. Modification of phenytoin clearance by valproic acid in normal subjects. *Br J Clin Pharmacol.* 1979;8(6):553-556.

45. Wandell M, Mungall D. Computer assisted drug interpretation and drug regimen optimization. *Amer Assoc Clin Chem.* 1984;6:1-11.

13

Phenobarbital/Primidone

INTRODUCTION

Phenobarbital is a barbiturate and primidone is a deoxybarbiturate effective in the treatment of generalized tonic-clonic and partial seizures (Table 13-1).[1-4] Phenobarbital is available as a separate agent, but is also an active metabolite produced via hepatic metabolism during primidone treatment. Because of this, and because they share a similar antiseizure spectrum, these two drugs are considered together in this chapter. The probable mechanism of action for phenobarbital is elevation of seizure threshold by interacting with γ-aminobutyric acid$_A$ (GABA$_A$) postsynaptic receptors which potentates synaptic inhibition.[5,6] While the exact mechanism of action is not known for the antiepileptic effect of primidone, a portion of its antiseizure activity is due to its active metabolites phenobarbital and phenylethylmalonamide (PEMA).[6,7]

THERAPEUTIC AND TOXIC CONCENTRATIONS

The therapeutic range for phenobarbital and primidone are defined by most laboratories as 15-40 µg/mL and 5-12 µg/mL, respectively. When primidone is given, sufficient doses are usually administered to produce therapeutic concentrations of both phenobarbital and primidone. At present, concentrations of the other possible active metabolite of primidone, phenylethylmalonamide (PEMA) are not routinely measured. While animal experiments indicate that primidone has inherent antiseizure activity, some clinicians believe that phenobarbital is the predominate species responsible for the therapeutic effect of primidone in humans.[7,10] Because phenobarbital and PEMA are produced via hepatic metabolism of primidone, it is very difficult to study the antiepileptic activity of primidone alone in patients.

The most common concentration-related adverse effects of phenobarbital involve the central nervous system: ataxia, headache, unsteadiness, sedation, confusion, and lethargy.[6,11] Other concentration-related side effects are nausea, and in children, irritability and hyperactivity. At phenobarbital concentrations >60 µg/mL, stupor and coma have been reported. During long-term treatment with phenobarbital, changes in behavior, porphyria, decreased cognitive function, and osteomalacia can occur. For primidone, concentration-related side effects include nausea, vomiting, diplopia, dizziness, sedation, unsteadiness, and ataxia.[6,11] Generally, slow dosage titration, administration of smaller doses and more frequent dosing of the drug produce relief from these side effects. Long-term treatment with primidone is associated with behavioral changes, decreased cognitive function, and disorders of the connective tissue. Obviously, some of the adverse effects noted during treatment with primidone may, in fact, be due to phenobarbital. Idiosyncratic side effects that are independent of concentration for both drugs include skin rashes and blood dyscrasias.

TABLE 13-1   International Classification of Epileptic Seizures With Recommended Therapies

Major Class	Subset of Class	Drug Treatment for Selected Seizure Type			
		2004 AAN/AES	**2013 Medical Letter**	**2012 NICE**	**2013 ILAE**[a]
Partial seizures (beginning locally)	1. Simple partial seizures (without impaired consciousness) a. with motor symptoms b. with somato-sensory or special sensory symptoms c. with auto-nomic symptoms d. with psy-chological symptoms	Carbamazepine Phenytoin Valproate Phenobarbital Lamotrigine Gabapentin Oxcarbazepine Topiramate	Lamotrigine Carbamazepine Levetiracetam Oxcarbazepine *Alternatives:* Topiramate Valproate Gabapentin Zonisamide Phenytoin Pregabalin Lacosamide Ezogabine	Carbamazepine Lamotrigine Levetiracetam Oxcarbazepine Valproate *Adjunctive:* Carbamazepine Clobazam Gabapentin Lamotrigine Levetiracetam Oxcarbazepine Valproate Topiramate	*Adults:* Carbamazepine Levetiracetam Phenytoin Zonisamide Valproate *Children:* Oxcarbazepine Carbamazepine Phenobarbital Phenytoin Topiramate Valproate Vigabatrin *Elderly:* Gabapentin Lamotrigine Carbamazepine
	2. Complex partial seizures (with impaired consciousness) a. simple partial onset followed by impaired consciousness b. impaired consciousness at onset	Carbamazepine Phenytoin Valproate Phenobarbital Lamotrigine Gabapentin Oxcarbazepine Topiramate	Lamotrigine Carbamazepine Levetiracetam Oxcarbazepine *Alternatives:* Topiramate Valproate Gabapentin Zonisamide Phenytoin Pregabalin Lacosamide Ezogabine	Carbamazepine Lamotrigine Levetiracetam Oxcarbazepine Valproate *Adjunctive:* Carbamazepine Clobazam Gabapentin Lamotrigine Levetiracetam Oxcarbazepine Valproate Topiramate	*Adults:* Carbamazepine Levetiracetam Phenytoin Zonisamide Valproate *Children:* Oxcarbazepine Carbamazepine Phenobarbital Phenytoin Topiramate Valproate Vigabatrin *Elderly:* Gabapentin Lamotrigine Carbamazepine
	3. Partial seizures evolving into secondary gener-alized seizures	Carbamazepine Phenytoin Valproate Phenobarbital Lamotrigine Gabapentin Oxcarbazepine Topiramate	Lamotrigine Carbamazepine Levetiracetam Oxcarbazepine *Alternatives:* Topiramate Valproate Gabapentin Zonisamide Phenytoin Pregabalin Lacosamide Ezogabine	Carbamazepine Lamotrigine Levetiracetam Oxcarbazepine Valproate *Adjunctive:* Carbamazepine Clobazam Gabapentin Lamotrigine Levetiracetam Oxcarbazepine Valproate Topiramate	*Adults:* Carbamazepine Levetiracetam Phenytoin Zonisamide Valproate *Children:* Oxcarbazepine Carbamazepine Phenobarbital Phenytoin Topiramate Valproate Vigabatrin *Elderly:* Gabapentin Lamotrigine Carbamazepine

(Continued)

TABLE 13-1 **International Classification of Epileptic Seizures With Recommended Therapies (*Continued*)**

Major Class	Subset of Class	Drug Treatment for Selected Seizure Type			
		2004 AAN/AES	**2013 Medical Letter**	**2012 NICE**	**2013 ILAE[a]**
Generalized seizures (convulsive or nonconvulsive)	1. Absence seizures[b] (typical or atypical; also known as petite mal seizures)	*Children:[c]* Ethosuximide Valproate Lamotrigine	Ethosuximide Valproate *Alternatives:* Lamotrigine Clonazepam Zonisamide Levetiracetam	Ethosuximide Lamotrigine Valproate *Adjunctive:* Ethosuximide Lamotrigine Valproate	*Children:* Ethosuximide Valproate Lamotrigine
	2. Tonic-clonic seizures (also known as grand mal seizures)	Carbamazepine Phenytoin Valproate Phenobarbital Lamotrigine Oxcarbazepine Topiramate	Valproate Lamotrigine Levetiracetam *Alternatives:* Topiramate Zonisamide Phenytoin	Carbamazepine Lamotrigine Oxcarbazepine Valproate *Adjunctive:* Clobazam Lamotrigine Levetiracetam Valproate Topiramate	*Adults:* Carbamazepine Lamotrigine Oxcarbazepine Phenobarbital Phenytoin Topiramate Valproate Gabapentin Levetiracetam Vigabatrin *Children:* Carbamazepine Phenobarbital Phenytoin Topiramate Valproate Oxcarbazepine

[a]Only two highest available levels of evidence listed.
[b]Recent literature suggests either ethosuximide or valproic acid is a superior initial therapy compared to lamotrigine for absence seizures.[8,9]
[c]Lamotrigine added to previous recommendation per expert panel.
Abbreviations: ANN, American Academy of Neurology; AES, American Epilepsy Society; NICE, UK National Institute for Clinical Excellence; ILAE, International League Against Epilepsy.

CLINICAL MONITORING PARAMETERS

The goal of therapy with anticonvulsants is to reduce seizure frequency and maximize quality of life with a minimum of adverse drug effects. While it is desirable to entirely abolish all seizure episodes, it may not be possible to accomplish this in many patients. Patients should be monitored for concentration-related side effects (diplopia, ataxia, dizziness, headache, unsteadiness, sedation, confusion, lethargy) as well as gastrointestinal upset (nausea, vomiting) when receiving these drugs. Serious, but rare, idiosyncratic side effects include connective tissue disorders, blood dyscrasias, and skin rashes.

Phenobarbital serum concentrations, or primidone plus phenobarbital serum concentrations for those patients receiving primidone therapy, should be measured in most patients. Because epilepsy is an episodic disease state, patients do not experience seizures on a continuous basis. Thus, during dosage titration it is difficult to tell if the patient is responding to drug therapy or simply is not experiencing any abnormal central nervous system discharges at that time. Serum concentrations are also valuable tools to avoid adverse drug effects. Patients are more likely to accept drug therapy if adverse reactions are held to the absolute minimum.

BASIC CLINICAL PHARMACOKINETIC PARAMETERS

Phenobarbital is eliminated primarily by hepatic metabolism (65%-70%) via CYP2C9 and CYP2C19 to inactive metabolites.[12,13] About 30%-35% of a phenobarbital dose is recovered as unchanged drug in the urine. Renal excretion of unchanged phenobarbital is pH dependent with alkaline urine increasing renal clearance. Phenobarbital is about 50% bound to plasma proteins. The absolute bioavailability of oral phenobarbital in humans approaches 100%.[14] Phenobarbital is available in tablet (15, 16, 30, 60, 100 mg), solution (20 mg/5 mL), elixir (20 mg/5 mL), and injectable (65 mg/mL and 130 mg/mL for intravenous or intramuscular use) forms. The typical maintenance dose for phenobarbital is 2.5-5 mg/kg/d for neonates, 3-4.5 mg/kg/d for pediatric patients (<10 years old), and 1.5-2 mg/kg/d for older patients.[6,11] For the acute treatment of status epilepticus, intravenous phenobarbital doses of 15-20 mg/kg are used.

Primidone is eliminated by hepatic metabolism (40%-60%) and renal excretion of unchanged drug (40%-60%).[12] In adults, approximately 15%-20% of a primidone dose is converted by the liver into phenobarbital. Phenylethylmalonamide (PEMA) is another active metabolite of primidone.[15,16] When starting treatment with primidone, PEMA concentrations are detectable after the first dose, but phenobarbital concentrations may not be measurable for 5-7 days (Figure 13-1). Primidone does not significantly bind to plasma proteins in humans. Because an intravenous form of the drug is not commercially available, the absolute bioavailability of primidone in humans is not known. Primidone is available as 50-mg and 250-mg tablets. Usual maintenance doses for primidone are 12-20 mg/kg/d for neonates, 12-23 mg/kg/d for pediatric patients (<15 years old), and 10-25 mg/kg/d for older patients.

EFFECTS OF DISEASE STATES AND CONDITIONS ON PHARMACOKINETICS AND DOSING

Phenobarbital clearance rate (Cl) for older children (≥12 years old) and adults is 4 mL/h/kg, and for children is 8 mL/h/kg.[11,14,17] Phenobarbital volume of distribution (V) equals 0.7 L/kg, and its half-life averages 120 hours in neonates (0-4 weeks old), 60 hours in children (≥2 months old), and 100 hours in adults. Although only limited studies in patients with hepatic disease are available, a 50% increase in half-life is seen in adults with liver cirrhosis or acute viral hepatitis.[18] Based on this information, patients with liver cirrhosis or acute

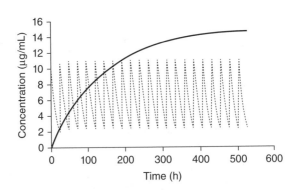

FIGURE 13-1   Primidone and phenobarbital concentrations after administration of primidone. Primidone concentrations fluctuate over the dosage interval with half-lives of 8-15 hours, but phenobarbital concentrations accumulate slowly with an average half-life of 100 h in adults as primidone is converted to phenobarbital. Because of this, primidone concentrations achieve steady-state conditions long before phenobarbital concentrations reach steady-state. In order to measure steady-state serum concentrations of both drugs, one must wait at least 3-4 weeks after a primidone dosage change.

TABLE 13-2   Child-Pugh Scores for Patients With Liver Disease

Test/Symptom	Score 1 Point	Score 2 Points	Score 3 Points
Total bilirubin (mg/dL)	<2.0	2.0-3.0	>3.0
Serum albumin (g/dL)	>3.5	2.8-3.5	<2.8
Prothrombin time (seconds prolonged over control)	<4	4-6	>6
Ascites	Absent	Slight	Moderate
Hepatic encephalopathy	None	Moderate	Severe

Mild liver disease, 5-6 points; moderate liver disease, 7-9 points; severe liver disease, 10-15 points.

hepatitis may have reduced phenobarbital clearance because of destruction of liver parenchyma. This loss of functional hepatic cells reduces the amount of enzymes available to metabolize the drug and decreases clearance. An index of liver dysfunction can be gained by applying the Child-Pugh clinical classification system to the patient (Table 13-2).[19] Child-Pugh scores are completely discussed in Chapter 3 (Drug Dosing in Special Populations: Renal and Hepatic Disease, Dialysis, Heart Failure, Obesity, and Drug Interactions), but will be briefly discussed here. The Child-Pugh score consists of five laboratory tests or clinical symptoms: serum albumin, total bilirubin, prothrombin time, ascites, and hepatic encephalopathy. Each of these areas is given a score of 1 (normal) to 3 (severely abnormal; see Table 13-2), and the scores for the five areas are summed. The Child-Pugh score for a patient with normal liver function is 5 while the score for a patient with grossly abnormal serum albumin, total bilirubin, and prothrombin time values in addition to severe ascites and hepatic encephalopathy is 15. A Child-Pugh score greater than 8 is grounds for a decrease of 25%-50% in the initial daily drug dose for phenobarbital. As in any patient with or without liver dysfunction, initial doses are meant as starting points for dosage titration based on patient response and avoidance of adverse effects. Phenobarbital serum concentrations and the presence of adverse drug effects should be monitored frequently in patients with liver cirrhosis.

Similarly, because phenobarbital is also eliminated by the kidney, patients with renal dysfunction (creatinine clearance <30 mL/min) receiving phenobarbital should be closely monitored. Phenobarbital is significantly removed (~30% of total body amount) by hemodialysis, and supplemental doses may need to be given after a dialysis session. Phenobarbital is significantly removed by hemoperfusion with a sieving coefficient equal to 0.8.[20,21] Supplemental dosing during hemoperfusion should be guided by serum concentration monitoring. Phenobarbital enters the breast milk so nursing infants should be monitored for possible adverse drug reactions.[22]

The primidone clearance rate (Cl/F) for older patients (≥12 years old) taking primidone alone is 35 mL/h/kg.[23] However, the primidone clearance rate increases to 50 mL/h/kg for older patients if they are receiving concurrent therapy with phenytoin or carbamazepine.[23] For children primidone clearance averages 125 mL/h/kg.[24] Primidone volume of distribution (V/F) equals 0.7 L/kg, and its half-life averages 8 hours in adults taking concurrent phenytoin or carbamazepine or children (<12 years old), and 15 hours in adults taking primidone alone.[11,23,24] Although no studies in patients with hepatic or renal disease are available, because almost equal amounts of primidone are eliminated by the liver and kidney, patients with renal or hepatic dysfunction receiving primidone should be closely monitored. A Child-Pugh score greater than 8 or creatinine clearance <30 mL/min are grounds for a decrease of 25%-50% in the initial daily drug dose for primidone. As in any patient with or without liver dysfunction, initial doses are meant as starting points for dosage titration based on patient response and avoidance of adverse effects. Primidone and phenobarbital serum concentrations as well as the presence of adverse drug effects should be monitored frequently in patients with liver or kidney disease taking primidone. Primidone is significantly removed (~30% of total body amount) by hemodialysis, and supplemental doses may need to be given after a dialysis session.

DRUG INTERACTIONS

Phenobarbital is a potent inducer of hepatic drug metabolism for the CYP1A2, CYP2C9, CYP2C19, and CYP3A4 enzyme systems.[13,25] Because phenobarbital is also a metabolite produced during primidone therapy, primidone has similar drug interaction potential.[13,25] Because phenobarbital is such a broad-based hepatic enzyme inducer, patients should be monitored closely for drug interactions whenever either of these agents are added to their therapeutic regimen. A brief list of the compounds whose metabolism and clearance are increased by concurrent phenobarbital treatment includes carbamazepine, lamotrigine, valproic acid, cyclosporin, nifedipine, diltiazem, verapamil, oral contraceptives, tricyclic antidepressants, quinidine, theophylline, and warfarin. Other anticonvulsants that decrease the metabolism and clearance of phenobarbital are felbamate and valproic acid. Phenytoin may also exhibit a co-interaction with phenobarbital where both agents change the metabolism and clearance of each other. The net result of this drug interaction is quite variable and can result in an increase, decrease, or no change in the steady-state concentration of both drugs. Primidone metabolism and clearance are increased by carbamazepine and phenytoin treatment while valproic acid therapy decreases primidone metabolism and clearance.

INITIAL DOSAGE DETERMINATION METHODS

Several methods to initiate phenobarbital or primidone therapy are available. The *Pharmacokinetic Dosing method* is the most flexible of the techniques. It allows individualized target serum concentrations to be chosen for a patient, and each pharmacokinetic parameter can be customized to reflect specific disease states and conditions present in the patient. *Literature-based Recommended Dosing* is a very commonly used method to prescribe initial doses of phenobarbital or primidone. Doses are based on those that commonly produce steady-state concentrations in the lower end of the therapeutic range, although there is a wide variation in the actual concentrations for a specific patient.

Pharmacokinetic Dosing Method

The goal of initial dosing of phenobarbital or primidone is to compute the best dose possible for the patient given their set of disease states and conditions that influence pharmacokinetics of the drugs and the epileptic disorder being treated. In order to do this, pharmacokinetic parameters for the patient will be estimated using average parameters measured in other patients with similar disease state and condition profiles.

Clearance Estimate

Phenobarbital is predominately metabolized by liver while primidone is about 50% hepatically eliminated. Unfortunately, there is no good way to estimate the elimination characteristics of liver-metabolized drugs using an endogenous marker of liver function in the same manner that serum creatinine and estimated creatinine clearance are used to estimate the elimination of agents that are renally eliminated. Because of this, a patient is categorized according to the disease states and conditions that are known to change drug clearance, and the clearance previously measured in these studies is used as an estimate of the current patient's clearance. For example, for a 70-kg adult patient, phenobarbital clearance would be assumed to equal 4 mL/h/kg: 70 kg • 4 mL/h/kg = 280 mL/h or 0.28 L/h. To produce the most conservative phenobarbital or primidone doses in patients with multiple concurrent disease states or conditions that affect their respective pharmacokinetics, the disease state or condition with the smallest clearance should be used to compute doses. This approach will avoid accidental overdosage has much as currently possible.

Volume of Distribution Estimate

The volume of distribution of both drugs is assumed to equal 0.7 L/kg for adults and children. Thus, for a 70-kg adult patient, the estimated volume of distribution would be 49 L: V = 0.7 L/kg • 70 kg = 49 L.

Half-Life and Elimination Rate Constant Estimate

Once the correct clearance and volume of distribution estimates are identified for the patient, they can be converted into the half-life ($t_{1/2}$) and elimination rate constant (k) estimates using the following equations: $t_{1/2} = (0.693 \cdot V)/Cl$, $k = 0.693/t_{1/2} = Cl/V$.

Selection of Appropriate Pharmacokinetic Model and Equations

Primidone and phenobarbital follow a one-compartment pharmacokinetic model. When oral therapy for either drug or intramuscular treatment with phenobarbital is required, both anticonvulsants have good bioavailability (assume F = 1), and once daily dosing for phenobarbital or multiple daily dosing for primidone provides a relatively smooth serum concentration-time curve that emulates an intravenous infusion. Because of this, a very simple pharmacokinetic equation that computes the average phenobarbital or primidone steady-state serum concentration (Css in μg/mL = mg/L) is widely used and allows maintenance dosage calculation: Css = [F(D/τ)]/Cl or D = (Css • Cl • τ)/F, where F is the bioavailability fraction for the oral dosage form (F = 1 for both drugs), D is the dose of the anticonvulsant in mg, Cl is anticonvulsant clearance in L/h, and τ is the dosage interval in hours.

When intravenous therapy with phenobarbital is required, a similar pharmacokinetic equation is widely used: Css = (D/τ)/Cl or D = Css • Cl • τ, where D is the dose of phenobarbital in mg, and τ is the dosage interval in hours. Cl is phenobarbital clearance in L/h. The equation used to calculate an intravenous loading dose for phenobarbital (LD in mg) is based on a simple one-compartment model: LD = Css • V, where Css is the desired phenobarbital steady-state concentration in μg/mL, which is equivalent to mg/L, and V is the phenobarbital volume of distribution. Intravenous phenobarbital doses should be administered no faster than 100 mg/minute.

EXAMPLE 1 ▶▶▶

GO is a 50-year-old, 75-kg (height = 5 ft 10 in) male with tonic-clonic seizures who requires therapy with oral phenobarbital. He has normal liver and renal function. Suggest an initial phenobarbital dosage regimen designed to achieve a steady-state concentration equal to 20 μg/mL.

1. *Estimate clearance and volume of distribution according to disease states and conditions present in the patient.*
   The clearance rate for an older patient is 4 mL/h/kg. Using this value, the estimated clearance would equal 0.3 L/h: Cl = 75 kg • 4 mL/h/kg = 300 mL/h or 0.3 L/h. The estimated volume of distribution would be 53 L: 75 kg • 0.7 L/kg = 53 L.

2. *Estimate half-life and elimination rate constant.*
   Once the correct clearance and volume of distribution estimates are identified for the patient, they can be converted into the phenobarbital half-life ($t_{1/2}$) and elimination rate constant (k) estimates using the following equations: $t_{1/2} = (0.693 \cdot V)/Cl = (0.693 \cdot 53 \text{ L})/0.3 \text{ L/h} = 122 \text{ h}$, $k = Cl/V = 0.3 \text{ L/h} / 53 \text{ L} = 0.0057 \text{ h}^{-1}$.

3. *Compute dosage regimen.*
   Oral phenobarbital tablets will be prescribed to this patient (F = 1). (Note: μg/mL = mg/L and this concentration unit was substituted for Css in the calculations so that unnecessary unit conversion was not required.) The dosage equation for oral phenobarbital is: D = (Css • Cl • τ)/F = (20 mg/L • 0.3 L/h • 24 h)/1 = 144 mg, rounded to 120 every 24 hours.

   A steady-state trough phenobarbital serum concentration should be measured after steady-state is attained in 3-5 half-lives. Since the patient is expected to have a half-life equal to 122 hours, the phenobarbital steady-state concentration could be obtained any time after 4 weeks of dosing (5 half-lives = 5 • 122 h = 610 h or 25 d). Phenobarbital serum concentrations should also be measured if the patient experiences an exacerbation of their epilepsy, or if the patient develops potential signs or symptoms of phenobarbital toxicity.

EXAMPLE 2 ▶ ▶ ▶

GO is a 50-year-old, 75-kg (height = 5 ft 10 in) male with tonic-clonic seizures who requires therapy with intravenous phenobarbital. He has normal liver and renal function. Suggest an initial phenobarbital dosage regimen designed to achieve a steady-state concentration equal to 20 μg/mL.

1. *Estimate clearance and volume of distribution according to disease states and conditions present in the patient.*
   The clearance rate for an older patient is 4 mL/h/kg. Using this value, the estimated clearance would equal 0.3 L/h: Cl = 75 kg • 4 mL/h/kg = 300 mL/h or 0.3 L/h. The estimated volume of distribution would be 53 L: 75 kg • 0.7 L/kg = 53 L.

2. *Estimate half-life and elimination rate constant.*
   Once the correct clearance and volume of distribution estimates are identified for the patient, they can be converted into the phenobarbital half-life ($t_{1/2}$) and elimination rate constant (k) estimates using the following equations: $t_{1/2} = (0.693 • V)/Cl = (0.693 • 53 L)/0.3 L/h = 122 h$, $k = Cl/V = 0.3 L/h / 53 L = 0.0057 h^{-1}$.

3. *Compute dosage regimen.*
   Intravenous phenobarbital will be prescribed to this patient. (Note: μg/mL = mg/L and this concentration unit was substituted for Css in the calculations so that unnecessary unit conversion was not required.) The dosage equation for intravenous phenobarbital is: $D = Css • Cl • \tau = 20 mg/L • 0.3 L/h • 24 h = 144 mg$, rounded to 120 every 24 hours. If needed, an intravenous loading dose could also be computed for the patient: LD = Css • V = 20 mg/L • 53 L = 1060 mg, rounded to 1000 mg. Intravenous loading doses should be administered no faster than 100 mg/min.

   A steady-state trough phenobarbital serum concentration should be measured after steady-state is attained in 3-5 half-lives. Since the patient is expected to have a half-life equal to 122 hours, the phenobarbital steady-state concentration could be obtained any time after 4 weeks of dosing (5 half-lives = 5 • 122 h = 610 h or 25 d). Phenobarbital serum concentrations should also be measured if the patient experiences an exacerbation of their epilepsy, or if the patient develops potential signs or symptoms of phenobarbital toxicity.

EXAMPLE 3 ▶ ▶ ▶

BI is a 23-year-old, 65-kg male with complex partial seizures who requires therapy with oral primidone. He has normal liver and renal function and takes carbamazepine. Suggest an initial primidone dosage regimen designed to achieve a steady-state primidone concentration equal to 6 μg/mL.

1. *Estimate clearance and volume of distribution according to disease states and conditions present in the patient.*
   The clearance rate for an adult patient taking carbamazepine is 50 mL/h/kg. Using this value, the estimated clearance would equal 3.25 L/h: Cl = 65 kg • 50 mL/h/kg = 3250 mL/h or 3.25 L/h. The estimated volume of distribution would be 46 L: 65 kg • 0.7 L/kg = 46 L.

2. *Estimate half-life and elimination rate constant.*
   Once the correct clearance and volume of distribution estimates are identified for the patient, they can be converted into the primidone half-life ($t_{1/2}$) and elimination rate constant (k) estimates using the following equations: $t_{1/2} = (0.693 • V)/Cl = (0.693 • 46 L)/3.25 L/h = 10 h$, $k = Cl/V = 3.25 L/h / 46 L = 0.071 h^{-1}$.

3. *Compute dosage regimen.*
   Oral primidone tablets will be prescribed to this patient (F = 1). (Note: μg/mL = mg/L and this concentration unit was substituted for Css in the calculations so that unnecessary unit conversion was not required.)

The dosage equation for oral primidone is: D = (Css • Cl • τ)/F = (6 mg/L • 3.25 L/h • 12 h)/1 = 234 mg, rounded to 250 mg every 12 hours. To avoid side effects, the starting dose would be 50% of this anticipated maintenance dose (125 mg every 12 hours) and would be titrated to the full dose over 1-2 weeks.

Steady-state trough primidone and phenobarbital serum concentrations should be measured after steady-state for both agents is attained in 3-5 half-lives. Since the patient is expected to have a phenobarbital half-life equal to 100 hours or more, the steady-state concentrations could be obtained any time after 3-4 weeks of dosing at the full primidone maintenance dose (5 phenobarbital half-lives = 5 • 100 h = 500 h or 21 d). Primidone and phenobarbital serum concentrations should also be measured if the patient experiences an exacerbation of their epilepsy, or if the patient develops potential signs or symptoms of primidone toxicity.

Literature-Based Recommended Dosing

Because of the large amount of variability in phenobarbital and primidone pharmacokinetics, even when concurrent disease states and conditions are identified, most clinicians believe that the use of standard drug doses for various situations are warranted. The original computation of these doses were based on the Pharmacokinetic Dosing methods, and subsequently modified based on clinical experience. In general, the expected steady-state serum concentrations used to compute these doses was in the lower end of the therapeutic range for each drug (Table 13-3). Phenobarbital is usually administered once or twice daily while primidone is given 2-4 times daily. To avoid side effects, primidone doses are started at 25%-50% of the ultimate desired maintenance dose with dosage increases made every 1-2 weeks depending on response and adverse effects. If the patient has significant hepatic dysfunction (Child-Pugh score ≥8) or renal disease (creatinine clearance <30 mL/min), maintenance doses prescribed using this method should be decreased by 25%-50% depending on how aggressive therapy is required to be for the individual.

To illustrate the similarities and differences between this method of dosage calculation and the Pharmacokinetic Dosing method, the same examples used in the previous section will be used.

EXAMPLE 4 ▶▶▶

GO is a 50-year-old, 75-kg (height = 5 ft 10 in) male with tonic-clonic seizures who requires therapy with oral phenobarbital. He has normal liver and renal function. Suggest an initial phenobarbital dosage regimen designed to achieve a steady-state concentration equal to 20 µg/mL.

1. *Estimate phenobarbital dose according to disease states and conditions present in the patient.*
   Oral phenobarbital tablets will be prescribed to this patient. The suggested initial maintenance dosage rate for phenobarbital in an adult patient is 1.5-2 mg/kg/d. Using 1.5 mg/kg/d, the dose would be: 75 kg • 1.5 mg/kg/d = 113 mg/d, rounded to 120 mg/d.

   Trough phenobarbital serum concentrations should be measured after steady-state is attained in 3-5 half-lives. Since the patient is expected to have a phenobarbital half-life equal to 100 hours or more, the steady-state concentrations could be obtained any time after a 3-4 weeks of dosing (5 phenobarbital half-lives = 5 • 100 h = 500 h or 21 d). Phenobarbital serum concentrations should also be measured if the patient experiences an exacerbation of their epilepsy, or if the patient develops potential signs or symptoms of phenobarbital toxicity.

TABLE 13-3   Literature-Based Initial Doses for Phenobarbital and Primidone

Patient Profile	Phenobarbital Dose (mg/kg/d)	Primidone Dose (mg/kg/d)
Neonate	2.5-5	12-20
Children	3-4.5	12-23
Adult	1.5-2	10-25

Note: intravenous loading doses for phenobarbital are 15-20 mg/kg for status epilepticus.

EXAMPLE 5 ▶ ▶ ▶

GO is a 50-year-old, 75-kg (height = 5 ft 10 in) male with tonic-clonic seizures who requires therapy with intravenous phenobarbital. He has normal liver and renal function. Suggest an initial phenobarbital dosage regimen designed to achieve a steady-state concentration equal to 20 µg/mL.

1. *Estimate phenobarbital dose according to disease states and conditions present in the patient.*

   Intravenous phenobarbital will be prescribed to this patient. The suggested initial maintenance dosage rate for phenobarbital in an adult patient is 1.5-2 mg/kg/d. Using 1.5 mg/kg/d, the maintenance dose would be: 75 kg • 1.5 mg/kg/d = 113 mg/d, rounded to 120 mg/d. If needed, the loading dose range is 15-20 mg/kg. Using 15 mg/kg, the loading dose would be: 75 kg • 15 mg/kg = 1125 mg, rounded to 1000 mg.

   A steady-state trough phenobarbital serum concentration should be measured after steady-state is attained in 3-4 weeks. Phenobarbital serum concentrations should also be measured if the patient experiences an exacerbation of their epilepsy, or if the patient develops potential signs or symptoms of phenobarbital toxicity.

EXAMPLE 6 ▶ ▶ ▶

BI is a 23-year-old, 65 kg male with complex partial seizures who requires therapy with oral primidone. He has normal liver and renal function and takes carbamazepine. Suggest an initial primidone dosage regimen designed to achieve a steady-state primidone concentration equal to 6 µg/mL.

1. *Estimate primidone dose according to disease states and conditions present in the patient.*

   Oral primidone tablets will be prescribed to this patient. The suggested initial maintenance dosage rate for primidone in an adult patient is 10-25 mg/kg/d. Because the patient is taking carbamazepine, which is known to induce primidone metabolism, a dose of 15 mg/kg/d will be used to compute the initial dose: 65 kg • 15 mg/kg/d = 975 mg/d, rounded to 1000 mg/d and given as 250 mg every 6 hours. To avoid side effects, the starting dose would be 50% of this anticipated maintenance dose (125 mg every 6 hours) and would be titrated to the full dose over 1-2 weeks according to response and adverse effects.

   Steady-state trough primidone and phenobarbital serum concentrations should be measured after steady-state for both agents is attained in 3-5 half-lives. Since the patient is expected to have a phenobarbital half-life equal to 100 hours or more, the steady-state concentrations could be obtained any time after a 3-4 weeks of dosing at the full primidone maintenance dose (5 phenobarbital half-lives = 5 • 100 h = 500 h or 21 d). Primidone and phenobarbital serum concentrations should also be measured if the patient experiences an exacerbation of their epilepsy, or if the patient develops potential signs or symptoms of primidone toxicity.

USE OF PHENOBARBITAL AND PRIMIDONE SERUM CONCENTRATIONS TO ALTER DOSES

Because of the large amount of pharmacokinetic variability among patients, it is likely that doses computed using patient population characteristics will not always produce phenobarbital or primidone serum concentrations that are expected or desirable. Because of pharmacokinetic variability, the narrow therapeutic index of phenobarbital and primidone, and the desire to avoid adverse side effects, measurement of serum concentrations for these anticonvulsants is conducted for most patients to insure that therapeutic, nontoxic levels are present. In addition to phenobarbital or primidone serum concentrations, important patient parameters (seizure frequency, potential side effects, etc) should be followed to confirm that the patient is responding to treatment and not developing adverse drug reactions.

When phenobarbital or primidone serum concentrations are measured in patients and a dosage change is necessary, clinicians should seek to use the simplest, most straightforward method available to determine a dose that will provide safe and effective treatment. In most cases, a simple dosage ratio can be used to change doses since phenobarbital and primidone follows *linear pharmacokinetics*. Sometimes, it is not possible to simply change the dose because of the limited number of oral dosage strengths, and the dosage interval must also be changed. In some situations, it may be necessary or desirable to compute the phenobarbital or primidone *pharmacokinetic parameters* for the patient and utilize these to calculate the best drug dose. Computerized methods that incorporate expected population pharmacokinetic characteristics (*Bayesian pharmacokinetic computer programs*) can be used in difficult cases where renal function is changing, serum concentrations are obtained at suboptimal times, or the patient was not at steady-state when serum concentrations were measured. An additional benefit of this dosing method is that a complete pharmacokinetic workup (determination of clearance, volume of distribution, and half-life) can be done with one or more measured concentrations that do not have to be at steady-state.

Linear Pharmacokinetics Method

Because phenobarbital and primidone follow linear, dose-proportional pharmacokinetics, steady-state serum concentrations change in proportion to dose according to the following equation: $D_{new}/C_{ss,new} = D_{old}/C_{ss,old}$ or $D_{new} = (C_{ss,new}/C_{ss,old})D_{old}$, where D is the dose, Css is the steady-state concentration, old indicates the dose that produced the steady-state concentration that the patient is currently receiving, and new denotes the dose necessary to produce the desired steady-state concentration. The advantages of this method are that it is quick and simple. The disadvantages are steady-state concentrations are required, and primidone may undergo some induction of its hepatic clearance at higher doses as phenobarbital concentrations increase. This method works for phenobarbital regardless of the route of administration. When primidone is administered to the patient, phenobarbital is produced as an active metabolite, and the new phenobarbital concentration resulting from a primidone dosage changes in a linear fashion. The phenobarbital concentration resulting from a primidone dosage change can be estimated using a rearrangement of the above equation: $C_{ss,new} = (D_{new}/D_{old})C_{ss,old}$, where D is the primidone dose, Css is the steady-state phenobarbital concentration, old indicates the primidone dose that produced the steady-state phenobarbital concentration that the patient is currently receiving, and new denotes the primidone dose necessary to produce the desired steady-state phenobarbital concentration.

EXAMPLE 7 ▶▶▶

LK is a 13-year-old, 47-kg (height = 5 ft 1 in) female with complex partial seizures who requires therapy with oral primidone. After dosage titration, the patient was prescribed 250 mg every 8 hours of primidone tablets (750 mg/d) for 1 month, and the steady-state primidone and phenobarbital steady-state concentrations equal

3 µg/mL and 15 µg/mL, respectively. The patient is assessed to be compliant with her dosage regimen. Suggest a primidone dosage regimen designed to achieve a steady-state primidone concentration of 6 µg/mL.

1. *Compute new dose to achieve desired serum concentration.*

   Using linear pharmacokinetics, the primidone dose necessary to cause the change in steady-state concentration would equal: $D_{new} = (Css_{new}/Css_{old})D_{old} = (6\,µg/mL\,/\,3\,µg/mL)\,750\,mg/d = 1500\,mg/d$, or 500 mg every 8 hours. The dosage regimen would be titrated to this value over a period of 1-2 weeks to avoid adverse effects. Using linear pharmacokinetics, the resulting steady-state phenobarbital serum concentration would equal: $C_{ss,new} = (D_{new}/D_{old})C_{ss,old} = (1500\,mg/d\,/\,750\,mg/d)\,15\,µg/mL = 30\,µg/mL$.

   A steady-state trough primidone and phenobarbital serum concentration should be measured after steady-state is attained in 3-4 weeks. Primidone and phenobarbital serum concentrations should also be measured if the patient experiences an exacerbation of their epilepsy, or if the patient develops potential signs or symptoms of primidone toxicity.

EXAMPLE 8 ▶▶▶

HI is a 42-year-old, 75-kg (height = 5 ft 10 in) male with tonic-clonic seizures who requires therapy with oral phenobarbital. After dosage titration, the patient was prescribed 120 mg daily of phenobarbital tablets for 1 month, and the steady-state phenobarbital concentration equals 20 µg/mL. The patient is assessed to be compliant with his dosage regimen. Suggest a phenobarbital dosage regimen designed to achieve a steady-state phenobarbital concentration of 30 µg/mL.

1. *Compute new dose to achieve desired serum concentration.*

   Using linear pharmacokinetics, the resulting steady-state phenobarbital serum concentration would equal: $D_{new} = (Css_{new}/Css_{old})\,D_{old} = (30\,µg/mL\,/\,20\,µg/mL)\,120\,mg/d = 180\,mg/d$.

   A steady-state trough phenobarbital serum concentration should be measured after steady-state is attained in 3-4 weeks. Phenobarbital serum concentrations should also be measured if the patient experiences an exacerbation of their epilepsy, or if the patient develops potential signs or symptoms of phenobarbital toxicity.

Pharmacokinetic Parameter Method

The Pharmacokinetic Parameter method of adjusting drug doses was among the first techniques available to change doses using serum concentrations. It allows the computation of an individual's own, unique pharmacokinetic constants and uses those to calculate a dose that achieves desired phenobarbital or primidone concentrations. For patients receiving oral phenobarbital, the Pharmacokinetic Parameter method requires that steady-state has been achieved and uses only a steady-state phenobarbital concentration (Css). Phenobarbital clearance (Cl) can be calculated using the following formula: $Cl = [F(D/\tau)]/Css$, where F is the bioavailability fraction for the oral dosage form (F = 1 for oral phenobarbital products), D is the dose of phenobarbital in mg, Css is the steady-state phenobarbital concentration in mg/L, and τ is the dosage interval in hours. Similarly, phenobarbital clearance during intravenous therapy can be computed using the equivalent formula: $Cl = (D/\tau)/Css$, where D is the dose of phenobarbital in mg, Css is the steady-state phenobarbital concentration in mg/L, and τ is the dosage interval in hours.

If the patient is receiving oral primidone, primidone clearance (Cl) is computed using the same equation: $Cl = [F(D/\tau)]/Css$, where F is the bioavailability fraction for the oral dosage form (F = 1 for oral primidone products), D is the dose of primidone in mg, Css is the steady-state primidone concentration in mg/L, and τ

is the dosage interval in hours. As with the Linear Pharmacokinetics method discussed previously, phenobarbital concentrations that occur during primidone treatment can be easily calculated. The phenobarbital concentration resulting from a primidone dosage change can be estimated using the following equation: $C_{ss,new} = (D_{new}/D_{old}) C_{ss,old}$, where D is the primidone dose, Css is the steady-state phenobarbital concentration, old indicates the primidone dose that produced the steady-state phenobarbital concentration that the patient is currently receiving, and new denotes the primidone dose necessary to produce the desired steady-state phenobarbital concentration.

To illustrate the similarities and differences between this method of dosage calculation and the Pharmacokinetic Parameter method, the same examples used in the previous section will be used.

EXAMPLE 9 ▶▶▶

LK is a 13-year-old, 47-kg (height = 5 ft 1 in) female with complex partial seizures who requires therapy with oral primidone. After dosage titration, the patient was prescribed 250 mg every 8 hours of primidone tablets (750 mg/d) for 1 month, and the steady-state primidone and phenobarbital steady-state concentrations equal 3 µg/mL and 15 µg/mL, respectively. The patient is assessed to be compliant with her dosage regimen. Suggest a primidone dosage regimen designed to achieve a steady-state primidone concentration of 6 µg/mL.

1. *Compute pharmacokinetic parameters.*

   The patient would be expected to achieve steady-state conditions for both primidone and phenobarbital after 3-4 weeks of therapy.

   Primidone clearance can be computed using a steady-state primidone concentration: Cl = [F(D/τ)]/Css = [1(250 mg/8 h)]/(3 mg/L) = 10 L/h. (Note: µg/mL = mg/L and this concentration unit was substituted for Css in the calculations so that unnecessary unit conversion was not required.)

2. *Compute primidone dose and resulting phenobarbital concentration.*

   Primidone clearance is used to compute the new dose: D = (Css • Cl • τ)/F = (6 mg/L • 10 L/h • 8 h)/1 = 480 mg, rounded to 500 mg every 8 hours. Using linear pharmacokinetics, the resulting steady-state phenobarbital serum concentration would equal: $C_{ss,new}$ = $(D_{new}/D_{old})C_{ss,old}$ = (1500 mg/d / 750 mg/d) 15 µg/mL = 30 µg/mL.

   Steady-state trough primidone and phenobarbital serum concentrations should be measured after steady-state is attained in 3-4 weeks. Primidone and phenobarbital serum concentrations should also be measured if the patient experiences an exacerbation of their epilepsy, or if the patient develops potential signs or symptoms of primidone toxicity.

EXAMPLE 10 ▶▶▶

HI is a 42-year-old, 75-kg (height = 5 ft 10 in) male with tonic-clonic seizures who requires therapy with oral phenobarbital. After dosage titration, the patient was prescribed 120 mg daily of phenobarbital tablets for 1 month, and the steady-state phenobarbital concentration equals 20 µg/mL. The patient is assessed to be compliant with his dosage regimen. Suggest a phenobarbital dosage regimen designed to achieve a steady-state phenobarbital concentration of 30 µg/mL.

1. *Compute pharmacokinetic parameters.*

   The patient would be expected to achieve steady-state conditions after 3-4 weeks of therapy.

   Phenobarbital clearance can be computed using a steady-state phenobarbital concentration: Cl = [F(D/τ)]/Css = [1(120 mg/24 h)]/(20 mg/L) = 0.25 L/h. (Note: µg/mL = mg/L and this concentration unit was substituted for Css in the calculations so that unnecessary unit conversion was not required.)

2. *Compute phenobarbital dose.*

Phenobarbital clearance is used to compute the new dose: D = (Css • Cl • τ)/F = (30 mg/L • 0.25 L/h • 24 h)/1 = 180 mg every 24 hours.

    A steady-state trough phenobarbital serum concentration should be measured after steady-state is attained in 3-4 weeks. Phenobarbital serum concentrations should also be measured if the patient experiences an exacerbation of their epilepsy, or if the patient develops potential signs or symptoms of phenobarbital toxicity.

BAYESIAN PHARMACOKINETIC COMPUTER PROGRAMS

Computer programs are available that can assist in the computation of pharmacokinetic parameters for patients. The most reliable computer programs use a nonlinear regression algorithm that incorporates components of Bayes theorem. Nonlinear regression is a statistical technique that uses an iterative process to compute the best pharmacokinetic parameters for a concentration/time data set. Briefly, the patient's drug dosage schedule and serum concentrations are input into the computer. The computer program has a pharmacokinetic equation preprogrammed for the drug and administration method (oral, intravenous bolus, intravenous infusion, etc). Typically, a one-compartment model is used, although some programs allow the user to choose among several different equations. Using population estimates based on demographic information for the patient (age, weight, gender, liver function, cardiac status, etc) supplied by the user, the computer program then computes estimated serum concentrations at each time there are actual serum concentrations. Kinetic parameters are then changed by the computer program, and a new set of estimated serum concentrations are computed. The pharmacokinetic parameters that generated the estimated serum concentrations closest to the actual values are remembered by the computer program, and the process is repeated until the set of pharmacokinetic parameters that result in estimated serum concentrations that are statistically closest to the actual serum concentrations are generated. These pharmacokinetic parameters can then be used to compute improved dosing schedules for patients. Bayes theorem is used in the computer algorithm to balance the results of the computations between values based solely on the patient's serum drug concentrations and those based only on patient population parameters. Results from studies that compare various methods of dosage adjustment have consistently found that these types of computer dosing programs perform at least as well as experienced clinical pharmacokineticists and clinicians and better than inexperienced clinicians.

    Some clinicians use Bayesian pharmacokinetic computer programs exclusively to alter drug doses based on serum concentrations. An advantage of this approach is that consistent dosage recommendations are made when several different practitioners are involved in therapeutic drug monitoring programs. However, since simpler dosing methods work just as well for patients with stable pharmacokinetic parameters and steady-state drug concentrations, many clinicians reserve the use of computer programs for more difficult situations. Those situations include serum concentrations that are not at steady-state, serum concentrations not obtained at the specific times needed to employ simpler methods, and unstable pharmacokinetic parameters. Many Bayesian pharmacokinetic computer programs are available to users, and most should provide answers similar to the one used in the following examples. The program used to solve problems in this book is DrugCalc written by Dr Dennis Mungall.[26] Currently, this program is available only for phenobarbital.

EXAMPLE 11 ▶▶▶

HI is a 42-year-old, 75-kg (height = 5 ft 10 in) male with tonic-clonic seizures who requires therapy with oral phenobarbital. After dosage titration, the patient was prescribed 120 mg daily of phenobarbital tablets for 1 month, and the steady-state phenobarbital concentration equals 20 μg/mL. The patient is assessed to be compliant with his dosage regimen. Suggest a phenobarbital dosage regimen designed to achieve a steady-state phenobarbital concentration of 30 μg/mL.

1. *Enter the patient's demographic, drug-dosing, and serum concentration/time data into the computer program.*

2. *Compute pharmacokinetic parameters for the patient using Bayesian pharmacokinetic computer program.*
   The pharmacokinetic parameters computed by the program are a volume of distribution of 51 L, a half-life equal to 185 h, and a clearance equal to 0.19 L/h.

3. *Compute dose required to achieve desired phenobarbital serum concentrations.*
   The one-compartment model first-order absorption equations used by the program to compute doses indicates that a dose of 180 mg every 24 hours will produce a steady-state phenobarbital concentration of 36 μg/mL.

EXAMPLE 12 ▶▶▶

JB is an 8-year-old, 35-kg male (height = 4 ft 2 in) with complex partial seizures who was started on phenobarbital syrup 100 mg every 24 hours. The phenobarbital concentration was 12 μg/mL before the 10th maintenance dose. What phenobarbital dose is needed to achieve Css = 25 μg/mL?

1. *Enter the patient's demographic, drug-dosing, and serum concentration/time data into the computer program.*
   In this patient case, it is unlikely that the patient is at steady-state so the Linear Pharmacokinetics method cannot be used.

2. *Compute pharmacokinetic parameters for the patient using Bayesian pharmacokinetic computer program.*
   The pharmacokinetic parameters computed by the program are a volume of distribution of 26 L, a half-life equal to 82 h, and clearance equal to 0.22 L/h.

3. *Compute dose required to achieve desired phenobarbital serum concentrations.*
   The one-compartment model oral equations used by the program to compute doses indicates that a dose of phenobarbital 175 mg every 24 hours will produce a steady-state concentration of 26 μg/mL.

DOSING STRATEGIES

Initial dose and dosage adjustment techniques using serum concentrations can be used in any combination as long as the limitations of each method are observed. Some dosing schemes link together logically when considered according to their basic approaches or philosophies. Dosage strategies that follow similar pathways are given in Table 13-4.

TABLE 13-4   Dosing Strategies

Dosing Approach/Philosophy	Initial Dosing	Use of Serum Concentrations to Alter Doses
Pharmacokinetic parameter/equations	Pharmacokinetic Dosing method	Pharmacokinetic Parameter method
Literature-based concept	Literature-based Recommended dosing method	Linear Pharmacokinetics method
Computerized	Bayesian computer program	Bayesian computer program

PROBLEMS

The following problems are intended to emphasize the computation of initial and individualized doses using clinical pharmacokinetic techniques. Clinicians should always consult the patient's chart to confirm that current anticonvulsant therapy is appropriate. Additionally, all other medications that the patient is taking, including prescription and nonprescription drugs, should be noted and checked to ascertain if a potential drug interaction with phenobarbital or primidone exists.

1. FH is a 37-year-old, 85-kg (height = 6 ft 1 in) male with tonic-clonic seizures who requires therapy with oral phenobarbital. He has normal liver and renal function. Suggest an initial phenobarbital dosage regimen designed to achieve a steady-state phenobarbital concentration equal to 15 μg/mL.

2. Patient FH (see problem 1) was prescribed 90 mg every 24 hours of phenobarbital tablets for 1 month, and the steady-state phenobarbital concentration equals 12 μg/mL. The patient is assessed to be compliant with his dosage regimen. Suggest a phenobarbital dosage regimen designed to achieve a steady-state phenobarbital concentration of 20 μg/mL.

3. AS is a 9-year-old, 35-kg female (height = 4 ft 6 in) with complex partial seizures who requires therapy with oral phenobarbital. She has normal liver and renal function. Suggest an initial phenobarbital dosage regimen designed to achieve a steady-state phenobarbital concentration equal to 20 μg/mL.

4. Patient AS (see problem 3) was prescribed 30 mg twice daily (60 mg/d) of phenobarbital elixir for 3 weeks, and the steady-state phenobarbital concentration equals 8.3 μg/mL. The patient is assessed to be compliant with her dosage regimen. Suggest a phenobarbital dosage regimen designed to achieve a steady-state phenobarbital concentration equal to 15 μg/mL.

5. FL is a 29-year-old, 75-kg (height = 5 ft 11 in) male with tonic-clonic seizures who requires therapy with oral primidone. He has normal liver function and is also receiving phenytoin therapy. Suggest an initial primidone dosage regimen designed to achieve a steady-state primidone concentration equal to 5 μg/mL.

6. Patient FL (see problem 5) was prescribed 500 mg every 12 hours of primidone tablets for 4 weeks, and the steady-state primidone and phenobarbital total concentrations equal 4.3 μg/mL and 11.6 μg/mL, respectively. The patient is assessed to be compliant with his dosage regimen. Suggest a primidone dosage regimen designed to achieve a steady-state primidone concentration of 6 μg/mL and estimate the resulting phenobarbital concentration.

7. PH is a 4-year-old, 22-kg male (height = 40 in) with tonic-clonic seizures who requires therapy with oral primidone. He has normal liver and renal function and is also treated with carbamazepine. Suggest an initial primidone dosage regimen designed to achieve a steady-state primidone concentration equal to 5 μg/mL.

8. Patient PH (see problem 7) was prescribed 75 mg three times daily (225 mg/d) of primidone tablets for 3 weeks, and the steady-state primidone and phenobarbital concentrations equal 5.5 μg/mL and 18 μg/mL, respectively. The patient is assessed to be compliant with his dosage regimen. Suggest a primidone dosage

regimen designed to achieve a steady-state primidone concentration of 8 µg/mL and estimate the resulting phenobarbital concentration.

9. PU is a 55-year-old, 68-kg (height = 5 ft 8 in) male with complex partial seizures who is receiving 90 mg daily of phenobarbital. He has normal liver and renal (bilirubin = 0.7 mg/dL, albumin = 4.0 gm/dL, serum creatinine = 1.1 mg/dL) function, and also takes 800 mg/d of carbamazepine. The phenobarbital concentration equals 14 µg/mL before the eighth dose. Compute a phenobarbital dose that will provide a steady-state concentration of 25 µg/mL.

10. LH is a 25-year-old, 60-kg (height = 5 ft 3 in) female with tonic-clonic seizures who was given a new prescription of 120 mg daily of phenobarbital tablets. She has normal liver and renal function and is also being treated with phenytoin. The trough phenobarbital concentration before the 10th dose equals 10 µg/mL. Compute a phenobarbital dose that will provide a steady-state concentration of 30 µg/mL.

ANSWERS TO PROBLEMS

1. *Answer to problem 1.*

Pharmacokinetic Dosing Method

1. *Estimate clearance and volume of distribution according to disease states and conditions present in the patient.*

    The clearance rate for an older patient is 4 mL/h/kg. Using this value, the estimated clearance would equal 0.34 L/h: Cl = 85 kg • 4 mL/h/kg = 340 mL/h or 0.34 L/h. The estimated volume of distribution would be 60 L: 85 kg • 0.7 L/kg = 60 L.

2. *Estimate half-life and elimination rate constant.*

    Once the correct clearance and volume of distribution estimates are identified for the patient, they can be converted into the phenobarbital half-life ($t_{1/2}$) and elimination rate constant (k) estimates using the following equations: $t_{1/2} = (0.693 • V)/Cl = (0.693 • 60 L)/0.34 L/h = 122 h$, $k = Cl/V = 0.34 L/h / 60 L = 0.0057 h^{-1}$.

3. *Compute dosage regimen.*

    Oral phenobarbital tablets will be prescribed to this patient (F = 1). (Note: µg/mL = mg/L and this concentration unit was substituted for Css in the calculations so that unnecessary unit conversion was not required). The dosage equation for oral phenobarbital is: $D = (Css • Cl • τ)/F = (15 mg/L • 0.34 L/h • 24 h)/1 = 122 mg$, rounded to 120 every 24 hours.

    A steady-state trough phenobarbital serum concentration should be measured after steady-state is attained in 3-5 half-lives. Since the patient is expected to have a half-life equal to 122 hours, the phenobarbital steady-state concentration could be obtained any time after 4 weeks of dosing (5 half-lives = 5 • 122 h = 610 h or 25 d). Phenobarbital serum concentrations should also be measured if the patient experiences an exacerbation of their epilepsy, or if the patient develops potential signs or symptoms of phenobarbital toxicity.

Literature-Based Recommended Dosing

1. *Estimate phenobarbital dose according to disease states and conditions present in the patient.*

    Oral phenobarbital tablets will be prescribed to this patient. The suggested initial maintenance dosage rate for phenobarbital in an adult patient is 1.5-2 mg/kg/d. Using 1.5 mg/kg/d, the dose would be: 85 kg • 1.5 mg/kg/d = 128 mg/d, rounded to 120 mg/d.

Trough phenobarbital serum concentrations should be measured after steady-state is attained in 3-5 half-lives. Since the patient is expected to have a phenobarbital half-life equal to 100 hours or more, the steady-state concentrations could be obtained any time after a 3-4 weeks of dosing (5 phenobarbital half-lives = 5 • 100 h = 500 h or 21 d). Phenobarbital serum concentrations should also be measured if the patient experiences an exacerbation of their epilepsy, or if the patient develops potential signs or symptoms of phenobarbital toxicity.

2. *Answer to problem 2.*

Linear Pharmacokinetics Method

1. *Compute new dose to achieve desired serum concentration.*

Using linear pharmacokinetics, the resulting steady-state phenobarbital serum concentration would equal: $D_{new} = (Css_{new}/Css_{old})D_{old} = (20 \mu g/mL / 12 \mu g/mL)$ 90 mg/d = 150 mg/d.

A steady-state trough phenobarbital serum concentration should be measured after steady-state is attained in 3-4 weeks. Phenobarbital serum concentrations should also be measured if the patient experiences an exacerbation of their epilepsy, or if the patient develops potential signs or symptoms of phenobarbital toxicity.

Pharmacokinetic Parameter Method

1. *Compute pharmacokinetic parameters.*

The patient would be expected to achieve steady-state conditions after 3-4 weeks of therapy.

Phenobarbital clearance can be computed using a steady-state phenobarbital concentration: $Cl = [F(D/\tau)]/Css = [1(90 \text{ mg}/24 \text{ h})]/(12 \text{ mg/L}) = 0.31$ L/h. (Note: $\mu g/mL = mg/L$ and this concentration unit was substituted for Css in the calculations so that unnecessary unit conversion was not required).

2. *Compute phenobarbital dose.*

Phenobarbital clearance is used to compute the new dose: $D = (Css • Cl • \tau)/F = (20 \text{ mg/L} • 0.31 \text{ L/h} • 24 \text{ h})/1 = 149$ mg, rounded to 150 mg every 24 hours.

A steady-state trough phenobarbital serum concentration should be measured after steady-state is attained in 3-4 weeks. Phenobarbital serum concentrations should also be measured if the patient experiences an exacerbation of their epilepsy, or if the patient develops potential signs or symptoms of phenobarbital toxicity.

3. *Answer to problem 3.*

Pharmacokinetic Dosing Method

1. *Estimate clearance and volume of distribution according to disease states and conditions present in the patient.*

The clearance rate for a pediatric patient is 8 mL/h/kg. Using this value, the estimated clearance would equal 0.28 L/h: Cl = 35 kg • 8 mL/h/kg = 280 mL/h or 0.28 L/h. The estimated volume of distribution would be 25 L: 35 kg • 0.7 L/kg = 25 L.

2. *Estimate half-life and elimination rate constant.*

Once the correct clearance and volume of distribution estimates are identified for the patient, they can be converted into the phenobarbital half-life ($t_{1/2}$) and elimination rate constant (k) estimates using the following equations: $t_{1/2} = (0.693 • V)/Cl = (0.693 • 25 \text{ L})/0.28 \text{ L/h} = 62$ h, $k = Cl/V = 0.28 \text{ L/h}/25 \text{ L} = 0.011$ h^{-1}.

3. *Compute dosage regimen.*

Oral phenobarbital elixir will be prescribed to this patient (F = 1). (Note: µg/mL = mg/L and this concentration unit was substituted for Css in the calculations so that unnecessary unit conversion was not required). The dosage equation for oral phenobarbital is: D = (Css • Cl • τ)/F = (20 mg/L • 0.28 L/h • 24 h)/1 = 134 mg, rounded to 120 every 24 hours.

A steady-state trough phenobarbital serum concentration should be measured after steady-state is attained in 3-5 half-lives. Since the patient is expected to have a half-life equal to 62 hours, the phenobarbital steady-state concentration could be obtained any time after 2 weeks of dosing (5 half-lives = 5 • 62 h = 310 h or 13 d). Phenobarbital serum concentrations should also be measured if the patient experiences an exacerbation of their epilepsy, or if the patient develops potential signs or symptoms of phenobarbital toxicity.

Literature-Based Recommended Dosing

1. *Estimate phenobarbital dose according to disease states and conditions present in the patient.*

Oral phenobarbital elixir will be prescribed to this patient. The suggested initial maintenance dosage rate for phenobarbital in a pediatric patient is 3-4.5 mg/kg/d. Using 3 mg/kg/d, the dose would be: 35 kg • 3 mg/kg/d = 105 mg/d, rounded to 100 mg/d.

Trough phenobarbital serum concentrations should be measured after steady-state is attained in 3-5 half-lives. Since the patient is expected to have a phenobarbital half-life equal to 60 hours, the steady-state concentrations could be obtained any time after 2 weeks of dosing (5 phenobarbital half-lives = 5 • 60 h = 300 h or 13 d). Phenobarbital serum concentrations should also be measured if the patient experiences an exacerbation of their epilepsy, or if the patient develops potential signs or symptoms of phenobarbital toxicity.

4. *Answer to problem 4.*

Linear Pharmacokinetics Method

1. *Compute new dose to achieve desired serum concentration.*

Using linear pharmacokinetics, the resulting steady-state phenobarbital serum concentration would equal: $D_{new} = (Css_{new}/Css_{old}) D_{old}$ = (15 µg/mL / 8.3 µg/mL) 60 mg/d = 108 mg/d, rounded to 100 mg every 24 hours.

A steady-state trough phenobarbital serum concentration should be measured after steady-state is attained in 2 weeks. Phenobarbital serum concentrations should also be measured if the patient experiences an exacerbation of their epilepsy, or if the patient develops potential signs or symptoms of phenobarbital toxicity.

Pharmacokinetic Parameter Method

1. *Compute pharmacokinetic parameters.*

The patient would be expected to achieve steady-state conditions after 2 weeks of therapy.

Phenobarbital clearance can be computed using a steady-state phenobarbital concentration: Cl = [F(D/τ)]/Css = [1(30 mg/12 h)]/(8.3 mg/L) = 0.30 L/h. (Note: µg/mL = mg/L and this concentration unit was substituted for Css in the calculations so that unnecessary unit conversion was not required.)

2. *Compute phenobarbital dose.*

Phenobarbital clearance is used to compute the new dose: D = (Css • Cl • τ)/F = (15 mg/L • 0.30 L/h • 12 h)/1 = 54 mg, rounded to 60 mg every 12 hours.

A steady-state trough phenobarbital serum concentration should be measured after steady-state is attained in 2 weeks. Phenobarbital serum concentrations should also be measured if the patient experiences an exacerbation of their epilepsy, or if the patient develops potential signs or symptoms of phenobarbital toxicity.

5. *Answer to problem 5.*

Pharmacokinetic Dosing Method

1. *Estimate clearance and volume of distribution according to disease states and conditions present in the patient.*

    The primidone clearance rate for an adult patient taking phenytoin is 50 mL/h/kg. Using this value, the estimated clearance would equal 3.75 L/h: Cl = 75 kg • 50 mL/h/kg = 3750 mL/h or 3.75 L/h. The estimated volume of distribution would be 53 L: 75 kg • 0.7 L/kg = 53 L.

2. *Estimate half-life and elimination rate constant.*

    Once the correct clearance and volume of distribution estimates are identified for the patient, they can be converted into the primidone half-life ($t_{1/2}$) and elimination rate constant (k) estimates using the following equations: $t_{1/2}$ = (0.693 • V)/Cl = (0.693 • 53 L)/3.75 L/h = 10 h, k = Cl/V = 3.75 L/h / 53 L = 0.071 h^{-1}.

3. *Compute dosage regimen.*

    Oral primidone tablets will be prescribed to this patient (F = 1). (Note: μg/mL = mg/L and this concentration unit was substituted for Css in the calculations so that unnecessary unit conversion was not required.) The dosage equation for oral primidone is: D = (Css • Cl • τ)/F = (5 mg/L • 3.75 L/h • 12 h)/1 = 225 mg, rounded to 250 mg every 12 hours. To avoid side effects, the starting dose would be 50% of this anticipated maintenance dose (125 mg every 12 hours) and would be titrated to the full dose over 1-2 weeks.

    Steady-state trough primidone and phenobarbital serum concentrations should be measured after steady-state for both agents is attained in 3-5 half-lives. Since the patient is expected to have a phenobarbital half-life equal to 100 hours or more, the steady-state concentrations could be obtained any time after 3-4 weeks of dosing at the full primidone maintenance dose (5 phenobarbital half-lives = 5 • 100 h = 500 h or 21 d). Primidone and phenobarbital serum concentrations should also be measured if the patient experiences an exacerbation of their epilepsy, or if the patient develops potential signs or symptoms of primidone toxicity.

Literature-Based Recommended Dosing

1. *Estimate primidone dose according to disease states and conditions present in the patient.*

    Oral primidone tablets will be prescribed to this patient. The suggested initial maintenance dosage rate for primidone in an adult patient is 10-25 mg/kg/d. Because the patient is taking phenytoin, which is known to induce primidone metabolism, a dose of 15 mg/kg/d will be used to compute the initial dose: 75 kg • 15 mg/kg/d = 1125 mg/d, rounded to 1000 mg/d and given as 250 mg every 6 hours. To avoid side effects, the starting dose would be 50% of this anticipated maintenance dose (125 mg every 6 hours) and would be titrated to the full dose over 1-2 weeks according to response and adverse effects.

    Steady-state trough primidone and phenobarbital serum concentrations should be measured after steady-state for both agents is attained in 3-5 half-lives. Since the patient is expected to have a phenobarbital half-life equal to 100 hours or more, the steady-state concentrations could be obtained any time after a 3-4 weeks of dosing at the full primidone maintenance dose (5 phenobarbital half-lives = 5 • 100 h = 500 h or 21 d). Primidone and phenobarbital serum concentrations should also be measured if the patient experiences an exacerbation of their epilepsy, or if the patient develops potential signs or symptoms of primidone toxicity.

6. *Answer to problem 6.*

Linear Pharmacokinetics Method

1. *Compute new dose to achieve desired serum concentration.*

Using linear pharmacokinetics, the primidone dose necessary to cause the change in steady-state concentration would equal: $D_{new} = (Css_{new}/Css_{old}) D_{old} = (6\ \mu g/mL\ /\ 4.3\ \mu g/mL)\ 1000\ mg/d = 1395\ mg/d$, rounded to 1500 mg/d or 500 mg every 8 hours. The dosage regimen would be titrated to this value over a period of 1-2 weeks to avoid adverse effects. Using linear pharmacokinetics, the resulting steady-state phenobarbital serum concentration would equal: $C_{ss,new} = (D_{new}/D_{old})\ C_{ss,old} = (1500\ mg/d\ /\ 1000\ mg/d)\ 11.6\ \mu g/mL = 17.4\ \mu g/mL$.

A steady-state trough primidone and phenobarbital serum concentration should be measured after steady-state is attained in 3-4 weeks. Primidone and phenobarbital serum concentrations should also be measured if the patient experiences an exacerbation of their epilepsy, or if the patient develops potential signs or symptoms of primidone toxicity.

Pharmacokinetic Parameter Method

1. *Compute pharmacokinetic parameters.*

The patient would be expected to achieve steady-state conditions for both primidone and phenobarbital after 3-4 weeks of therapy.

Primidone clearance can be computed using a steady-state primidone concentration: $Cl = [F(D/\tau)]/Css = [1(500\ mg/12\ h)]/(4.3\ mg/L) = 9.7\ L/h$. (Note: $\mu g/mL = mg/L$ and this concentration unit was substituted for Css in the calculations so that unnecessary unit conversion was not required.)

2. *Compute primidone dose and resulting phenobarbital concentration.*

Primidone clearance is used to compute the new dose: $D = (Css \bullet Cl \bullet \tau)/F = (6\ mg/L \bullet 9.7\ L/h \bullet 8\ h)/1 = 466\ mg$, rounded to 500 mg every 8 hours. Using linear pharmacokinetics, the resulting steady-state phenobarbital serum concentration would equal: $C_{ss,new} = (D_{new}/D_{old})\ C_{ss,old} = (1500\ mg/d\ /\ 1000\ mg/d)\ 11.6\ \mu g/mL = 17.4\ \mu g/mL$.

Steady-state trough primidone and phenobarbital serum concentrations should be measured after steady-state is attained in 3-4 weeks. Primidone and phenobarbital serum concentrations should also be measured if the patient experiences an exacerbation of their epilepsy, or if the patient develops potential signs or symptoms of primidone toxicity.

7. *Answer to problem 7.*

Pharmacokinetic Dosing Method

1. *Estimate clearance and volume of distribution according to disease states and conditions present in the patient.*

The clearance rate for a pediatric patient is 125 mL/h/kg. Using this value, the estimated clearance would equal 2.75 L/h: $Cl = 22\ kg \bullet 125\ mL/h/kg = 2750\ mL/h$ or 2.75 L/h. The estimated volume of distribution would be 15 L: $22\ kg \bullet 0.7\ L/kg = 15\ L$.

2. *Estimate half-life and elimination rate constant.*

Once the correct clearance and volume of distribution estimates are identified for the patient, they can be converted into the primidone half-life ($t_{1/2}$) and elimination rate constant (k) estimates using the following equations: $t_{1/2} = (0.693 \bullet V)/Cl = (0.693 \bullet 15\ L)/2.75\ L/h = 4\ h$, $k = Cl/V = 2.75\ L/h\ /\ 15\ L = 0.183\ h^{-1}$.

3. *Compute dosage regimen.*

Primidone tablets will be prescribed to this patient (F = 1). (Note: μg/mL = mg/L and this concentration unit was substituted for Css in the calculations so that unnecessary unit conversion was not required.) The dosage equation for oral primidone is: D = (Css • Cl • τ)/F = (5 mg/L • 2.75 L/h • 6 h)/1 = 82.5 mg, rounded to 100 mg every 6 hours. To avoid side effects, the starting dose would be 50% of this anticipated maintenance dose (50 mg every 6 hours) and would be titrated to the full dose over 1-2 weeks.

Steady-state trough primidone and phenobarbital serum concentrations should be measured after steady-state for both agents is attained in 3-5 half-lives. Since the patient is expected to have a phenobarbital half-life equal to 60 hours or more, the steady-state concentrations could be obtained any time after 2 weeks of dosing at the full primidone maintenance dose (5 phenobarbital half-lives = 5 • 60 h = 300 h or 13 d). Primidone and phenobarbital serum concentrations should also be measured if the patient experiences an exacerbation of their epilepsy, or if the patient develops potential signs or symptoms of primidone toxicity.

Literature-Based Recommended Dosing

1. *Estimate primidone dose according to disease states and conditions present in the patient.*

Primidone tablets will be prescribed to this patient. The suggested initial maintenance dosage rate for primidone in a pediatric patient is 12-23 mg/kg/d. Because the patient is taking phenytoin, which is known to induce primidone metabolism, a dose of 15 mg/kg/d will be used to compute the initial dose: 22 kg • 15 mg/kg/d = 330 mg/d, rounded to 300 mg/d and given as 100 mg every 8 hours. To avoid side effects, the starting dose would be 50% of this anticipated maintenance dose (50 mg every 8 hours) and would be titrated to the full dose over 1-2 weeks according to response and adverse effects.

Steady-state trough primidone and phenobarbital serum concentrations should be measured after steady-state for both agents is attained in 3-5 half-lives. Since the patient is expected to have a phenobarbital half-life equal to 60 hours or more, the steady-state concentrations could be obtained any time after 2 weeks of dosing at the full primidone maintenance dose (5 phenobarbital half-lives = 5 • 60 h = 300 h or 13 d). Primidone and phenobarbital serum concentrations should also be measured if the patient experiences an exacerbation of their epilepsy, or if the patient develops potential signs or symptoms of primidone toxicity.

8. *Answer to problem 8.*

Linear Pharmacokinetics Method

1. *Compute new dose to achieve desired serum concentration.*

Using linear pharmacokinetics, the primidone dose necessary to cause the change in steady-state concentration would equal: $D_{new} = (Css_{new}/Css_{old}) D_{old}$ = (8 μg/mL / 5.5 μg/mL) 225 mg/d = 327 mg/d, rounded to 300 mg/d or 100 mg every 8 hours. The dosage regimen would be titrated to this value over a period of 1-2 weeks to avoid adverse effects. Using linear pharmacokinetics, the resulting steady-state phenobarbital serum concentration would equal: $C_{ss,new} = (D_{new}/D_{old}) C_{ss,old}$ = (300 mg/d / 225 mg/d) 18 μg/mL = 24 μg/mL.

A steady-state trough primidone and phenobarbital serum concentration should be measured after steady-state is attained in 2 weeks. Primidone and phenobarbital serum concentrations should also be measured if the patient experiences an exacerbation of their epilepsy, or if the patient develops potential signs or symptoms of primidone toxicity.

Pharmacokinetic Parameter Method

1. *Compute pharmacokinetic parameters.*

   The patient would be expected to achieve steady-state conditions for both primidone and phenobarbital after 2 weeks of therapy.

   Primidone clearance can be computed using a steady-state primidone concentration: Cl = [F(D/τ)]/Css = [1(75 mg/8 h)]/(5.5 mg/L) = 1.7 L/h. (Note: μg/mL = mg/L and this concentration unit was substituted for Css in the calculations so that unnecessary unit conversion was not required.)

2. *Compute primidone dose and resulting phenobarbital concentration.*

   Primidone clearance is used to compute the new dose: D = (Css • Cl • τ)/F = (8 mg/L • 1.7 L/h • 8 h)/1 = 109 mg, rounded to 100 mg every 8 hours. Using linear pharmacokinetics, the resulting steady-state phenobarbital serum concentration would equal: $C_{ss,new} = (D_{new}/D_{old}) C_{ss,old}$ = (300 mg/d / 225 mg/d) 18 μg/mL = 24 μg/mL.

   Steady-state trough primidone and phenobarbital serum concentrations should be measured after steady-state is attained in 2 weeks. Primidone and phenobarbital serum concentrations should also be measured if the patient experiences an exacerbation of their epilepsy, or if the patient develops potential signs or symptoms of primidone toxicity.

9. *Answer to problem 9.*

   1. *Enter the patient's demographic, drug-dosing, and serum concentration/time data into the computer program.*

      After receiving phenobarbital for less than 4 weeks, it is unlikely the patient is at steady-state.

   2. *Compute pharmacokinetic parameters for the patient using Bayesian pharmacokinetic computer program.*

      The pharmacokinetic parameters computed by the program are a volume of distribution of 36 L, a half-life equal to 217 h, and a clearance equal to 0.11 L/h.

   3. *Compute dose required to achieve desired phenobarbital serum concentrations.*

      The one-compartment model first-order absorption equations used by the program to compute doses indicates that a dose of 60 mg every 24 hours will produce a steady-state phenobarbital concentration of 21 μg/mL.

10. *Answer to problem 10.*

    1. *Enter the patient's demographic, drug-dosing, and serum concentration/time data into the computer program.*

       After receiving phenobarbital for less than 4 weeks, it is unlikely that the patient is at steady-state.

    2. *Compute pharmacokinetic parameters for the patient using Bayesian pharmacokinetic computer program.*

       The pharmacokinetic parameters computed by the program are a volume of distribution of 44 L, a half-life equal to 97 h, and a clearance equal to 0.31 L/h.

    3. *Compute dose required to achieve desired phenobarbital serum concentrations.*

       The one-compartment model first-order absorption equations used by the program to compute doses indicates that a dose of 240 mg every 24 hours will produce a steady-state phenobarbital concentration of 29 μg/mL.

REFERENCES

1. Abramowicz M, Zuccotti G, Pflomm JM, eds. Drugs for epilepsy. *Treatment Guidelines From The Medical Letter.* 2013;11(126):9-18.
2. Anon. The epilepsies: the diagnosis and management of the epilepsies in adults and children in primary and secondary care. *UK National Institute for Health and Care Excellence.* http://www.nice.org.uk/nicemedia/live/13635/57779/57779.pdf. Accessed May 1, 2014.
3. French JA, Kanner AM, Bautista J, et al. Efficacy and tolerability of the new antiepileptic drugs I: treatment of new onset epilepsy: report of the Therapeutics and Technology Assessment Subcommittee and Quality Standards Subcommittee of the American Academy of Neurology and the American Epilepsy Society. *Neurology.* Apr 27 2004;62(8):1252-1260.
4. Glauser T, Ben-Menachem E, Bourgeois B, et al. Updated ILAE evidence review of antiepileptic drug efficacy and effectiveness as initial monotherapy for epileptic seizures and syndromes. *Epilepsia.* Mar 2013;54(3):551-563.
5. McNamara JO. Pharmacotherapy of the epilepsies. In: Brunton L, Chabner B, Knollman B, eds. *The Pharmacological Basis of Therapeutics.* 12th ed. New York, NY: McGraw-Hill; 2011:583-608.
6. Rogers SJ, Cavazos JE. Epilepsy. In: DiPiro JT, Talbert RL, Yee GC, Matzke GR, Wells BG, Posey LM, eds. *Pharmacotherapy.* 8th ed. New York, NY: McGraw-Hill; 2011:979-1005.
7. Porter RJ, Meldrum BS. Antiseizure drugs. In: Katzung BG, Masters SB, Trevor AJ, eds. *Basic & Clinical Pharmacology.* 12th ed. New York, NY: McGraw-Hill; 2012:403-428.
8. Glauser TA, Cnaan A, Shinnar S, et al. Ethosuximide, valproic acid, and lamotrigine in childhood absence epilepsy. *N Engl J Med.* Mar 4 2010;362(9):790-799.
9. Glauser TA, Cnaan A, Shinnar S, et al. Ethosuximide, valproic acid, and lamotrigine in childhood absence epilepsy: initial monotherapy outcomes at 12 months. *Epilepsia.* Jan 2013;54(1):141-155.
10. Smith DB. Primidone: clinical use. In: Levy R, Mattson R, Meldrum B, eds. *Antiepileptic Drugs.* 3rd ed. New York, NY: Raven Press; 1989:423-438.
11. Garnett WR. Antiepileptics. In: Schumacher GE, ed. *Therapeutic Drug Monitoring.* Stamford, CT: Appleton & Lange; 1995:345-395.
12. Browne TR, Evans JE, Szabo GK, Evans BA, Greenblatt DJ. Studies with stable isotopes II: phenobarbital pharmacokinetics during monotherapy. *J Clin Pharmacol.* 1985;25(1):51-58.
13. Hansten PD, Horn JR. *The Top 100 Drug Interactions.* Freeland, WA: H&H Publications; 2014.
14. Nelson E, Powell JR, Conrad K, et al. Phenobarbital pharmacokinetics and bioavailability in adults. *J Clin Pharmacol.* 1982;22(2-3):141-148.
15. Streete JM, Berry DJ, Pettit LI, Newbery JE. Phenylethylmalonamide serum levels in patients treated with primidone and the effects of other antiepileptic drugs. *Ther Drug Monit.* 1986;8(2):161-165.
16. Baumel IP, Gallagher BB, Mattson RH. Phenylethylmalonamide (PEMA): an important metabolite of primidone. *Arch Neurol.* 1972;27(1):34-41.
17. Heimann G, Gladtke E. Pharmacokinetics of phenobarbital in childhood. *Eur J Clin Pharmacol.* 1977;12(4):305-310.
18. Alvin J, McHorse T, Hoyumpa A, Bush MT, Schenker S. The effect of liver disease in man on the disposition of phenobarbital. *J Pharmacol Exp Ther.* 1975;192(1):224-235.
19. Pugh RN, Murray-Lyon IM, Dawson JL, Pietroni MC, Williams R. Transection of the oesophagus for bleeding oesophageal varices. *Br J Surg.* 1973;60(8):646-649.
20. Golper TA, Marx MA. Drug dosing adjustments during continuous renal replacement therapies. *Kidney Int Suppl.* May 1998;66:165S-168S.
21. Golper TA. Update on drug sieving coefficients and dosing adjustments during continuous renal replacement therapies. *Contrib Nephrol.* 2001;(132):349-353.
22. Rust RS, Dodson WE. Phenobarbital: absorption, distribution, and excretion. In: Levy RH, Mattson R, Meldrum B, eds. *Antiepileptic Drugs.* 3rd ed. New York, NY: Raven Press; 1989:293-304.
23. Cloyd JC, Miller KW, Leppik IE. Primidone kinetics: effects of concurrent drugs and duration of therapy. *Clin Pharmacol Ther.* 1981;29(3):402-407.
24. Kauffman RE, Habersang R, Lansky L. Kinetics of primidone metabolism and excretion in children. *Clin Pharmacol Ther.* 1977;22(2):200-205.
25. Hansten PD, Horn JR. *Drug Interactions Analysis and Management.* St. Louis, MO: Wolters Kluwer; 2014.
26. Wandell M, Mungall D. Computer assisted drug interpretation and drug regimen optimization. *Amer Assoc Clin Chem.* 1984;6:1-11.

14 Ethosuximide

INTRODUCTION

Ethosuximide is succinimide compound that is effective in the treatment of absence (petit mal) seizures (Table 14-1).[1-4] It is the product of an intense structure-activity research effort to find a specific agent to suppress absence seizures with a relatively low side effect profile. The antiepileptic effect of ethosuximide is thought to be due to its ability to decrease low-threshold calcium currents (T currents) in thalamic neurons.[5] The thalamus has a key role in the production of 3 Hz spike-wave rhythms that are a hallmark of absence seizures. Based on recent studies, ethosuximide is considered to be the best choice for initial monotherapy of absence seizures in children because of a high rate of efficacy combined with a low incidence of adverse effects.[6-8]

TABLE 14-1   International Classification of Epileptic Seizures With Recommended Therapies

Major Class	Subset of Class	Drug Treatment for Selected Seizure Type			
		2004 AAN/AES	**2013 Medical Letter**	**2012 NICE**	**2013 ILAE**[a]
Partial seizures (beginning locally)	1. Simple partial seizures (without impaired consciousness) a. with motor symptoms b. with somatosensory or special sensory symptoms c. with autonomic symptoms d. with psychological symptoms	Carbamazepine Phenytoin Valproate Phenobarbital Lamotrigine Gabapentin Oxcarbazepine Topiramate	Lamotrigine Carbamazepine Levetiracetam Oxcarbazepine *Alternatives:* Topiramate Valproate Gabapentin Zonisamide Phenytoin Pregabalin Lacosamide Ezogabine	Carbamazepine Lamotrigine Levetiracetam Oxcarbazepine Valproate *Adjunctive:* Carbamazepine Clobazam Gabapentin Lamotrigine Levetiracetam Oxcarbazepine Valproate Topiramate	*Adults:* Carbamazepine Levetiracetam Phenytoin Zonisamide Valproate *Children:* Oxcarbazepine Carbamazepine Phenobarbital Phenytoin Topiramate Valproate Vigabatrin *Elderly:* Gabapentin Lamotrigine Carbamazepine

(Continued)

TABLE 14-1 International Classification of Epileptic Seizures With Recommended Therapies (*Continued*)

Major Class	Subset of Class	Drug Treatment for Selected Seizure Type			
		2004 AAN/AES	**2013 Medical Letter**	**2012 NICE**	**2013 ILAE**[a]
	2. Complex partial seizures (with impaired consciousness) a. simple partial onset followed by impaired consciousness b. impaired consciousness at onset	Carbamazepine Phenytoin Valproate Phenobarbital Lamotrigine Gabapentin Oxcarbazepine Topiramate	Lamotrigine Carbamazepine Levetiracetam Oxcarbazepine *Alternatives:* Topiramate Valproate Gabapentin Zonisamide Phenytoin Pregabalin Lacosamide Ezogabine	Carbamazepine Lamotrigine Levetiracetam Oxcarbazepine Valproate *Adjunctive:* Carbamazepine Clobazam Gabapentin Lamotrigine Levetiracetam Oxcarbazepine Valproate Topiramate	*Adults:* Carbamazepine Levetiracetam Phenytoin Zonisamide Valproate *Children:* Oxcarbazepine Carbamazepine Phenobarbital Phenytoin Topiramate Valproate Vigabatrin *Elderly:* Gabapentin Lamotrigine Carbamazepine
	3. Partial seizures evolving into secondary generalized seizures	Carbamazepine Phenytoin Valproate Phenobarbital Lamotrigine Gabapentin Oxcarbazepine Topiramate	Lamotrigine Carbamazepine Levetiracetam Oxcarbazepine *Alternatives:* Topiramate Valproate Gabapentin Zonisamide Phenytoin Pregabalin Lacosamide Ezogabine	Carbamazepine Lamotrigine Levetiracetam Oxcarbazepine Valproate *Adjunctive:* Carbamazepine Clobazam Gabapentin Lamotrigine Levetiracetam Oxcarbazepine Valproate Topiramate	*Adults:* Carbamazepine Levetiracetam Phenytoin Zonisamide Valproate *Children:* Oxcarbazepine Carbamazepine Phenobarbital Phenytoin Topiramate Valproate Vigabatrin *Elderly:* Gabapentin Lamotrigine Carbamazepine
Generalized seizures (convulsive or nonconvulsive)	1. Absence seizures[b] (typical or atypical; also known as petit mal seizures)	*Children:*[c] Ethosuximide Valproate Lamotrigine	Ethosuximide Valproate *Alternatives:* Lamotrigine Clonazepam Zonisamide Levetiracetam	Ethosuximide Lamotrigine Valproate *Adjunctive:* Ethosuximide Lamotrigine Valproate	*Children:* Ethosuximide Valproate Lamotrigine

(*Continued*)

TABLE 14-1   International Classification of Epileptic Seizures With Recommended Therapies (Continued)

Major Class	Subset of Class	Drug Treatment for Selected Seizure Type			
		2004 AAN/AES	2013 Medical Letter	2012 NICE	2013 ILAE[a]
	2. Tonic-clonic seizures (also known as grand mal seizures)	Carbamazepine Phenytoin Valproate Phenobarbital Lamotrigine Oxcarbazepine Topiramate	Valproate Lamotrigine Levetiracetam *Alternatives:* Topiramate Zonisamide Phenytoin	Carbamazepine Lamotrigine Oxcarbazepine Valproate *Adjunctive:* Clobazam Lamotrigine Levetiracetam Valproate Topiramate	*Adults:* Carbamazepine Lamotrigine Oxcarbazepine Phenobarbital Phenytoin Topiramate Valproate Gabapentin Levetiracetam Vigabatrin
					Children: Carbamazepine Phenobarbital Phenytoin Topiramate Valproate Oxcarbazepine

[a]Only two highest available levels of evidence listed.
[b]Recent literature suggests either ethosuximide or valproic acid is a superior initial therapy compared to lamotrigine for absence seizures.[6,7]
[c]Lamotrigine added to previous recommendation per expert panel.
Abbreviations: ANN, American Academy of Neurology; AES, American Epilepsy Society; NICE, UK National Institute for Clinical Excellence; ILAE, International League Against Epilepsy.

THERAPEUTIC AND TOXIC CONCENTRATIONS

The therapeutic range for ethosuximide is defined by most laboratories as 40-100 μg/mL, although some clinicians suggest drug concentrations as high as 150 μg/mL with appropriate monitoring of serum concentrations and possible side effects.[9] The most common adverse effects of ethosuximide are gastric distress, nausea, vomiting, and anorexia, but these gastrointestinal problems appear to be due to local irritation of gastric mucosa. Generally, administration of smaller doses and more frequent dosing of the drug produce relief from these side effects. In the upper end of the therapeutic range (>70 μg/mL) some patients will begin to experience the concentration-dependent adverse effects of ethosuximide treatment: drowsiness, fatigue, lethargy, dizziness, ataxia, hiccups, euphoria, and headaches. Idiosyncratic side effects that are independent of concentration include rash, systemic lupus-like syndromes, and blood dyscrasias (leukopenia, pancytopenia).

CLINICAL MONITORING PARAMETERS

The goal of therapy with anticonvulsants is to reduce seizure frequency and maximize quality of life with a minimum of adverse drug effects. While it is desirable to entirely abolish all seizure episodes, it may not be possible to accomplish this in many patients. Patients should be monitored for concentration-related side effects (drowsiness, fatigue, lethargy, dizziness, ataxia, hiccups, euphoria, headaches) as well as gastrointestinal upset associated with local irritation of gastric mucosa (gastric distress, nausea, vomiting, anorexia). Serious, but rare, idiosyncratic side effects include systemic lupus-like syndromes, leukopenia, and pancytopenia.

Ethosuximide serum concentrations should be measured in most patients. Because epilepsy is an episodic disease state, patients do not experience seizures on a continuous basis. Thus, during dosage titration it is difficult to tell if the patient is responding to drug therapy or simply is not experiencing any abnormal central nervous system discharges at that time. Ethosuximide serum concentrations are also valuable tools to avoid adverse drug effects. Patients are more likely to accept drug therapy if adverse reactions are held to the absolute minimum.

BASIC CLINICAL PHARMACOKINETIC PARAMETERS

Ethosuximide is eliminated primarily by hepatic metabolism (70%-80%) via hydroxylation by CYP3A4 and then conjugated to inactive metabolites.[10,11] About 20%-30% of a ethosuximide dose is recovered as unchanged drug in the urine.[12] Ethosuximide is not significantly bound to plasma proteins. At concentrations exceeding 100 µg/mL, the drug may follow nonlinear pharmacokinetics, presumably due to Michaelis-Menten (concentration-dependent or saturable) metabolism.[13] Because an intravenous form of the drug is not commercially available, the absolute bioavailability in humans is not known. However, based on animal studies, ethosuximide oral bioavailability of capsules (250 mg) and syrup (250 mg/5 mL) is assumed to be 100%.[9] The typical maintenance dose for ethosuximide is 20 mg/kg/d for pediatric patients (<12 years old) and 15 mg/kg/d for older patients.[9]

EFFECTS OF DISEASE STATES AND CONDITIONS ON PHARMACOKINETICS AND DOSING

Ethosuximide oral clearance rate (Cl/F) for older children (≥12 years old) and adults is 12 mL/h/kg and for children is 16 mL/h/kg.[9] Ethosuximide volume of distribution (V/F) equals 0.7 L/kg, and its half-life averages 30 hours in children and 60 hours in adults.[9] Although studies in patients with hepatic disease are not available, 70%-80% of the drug is eliminated by hepatic metabolism. Because of this, patients with liver cirrhosis or acute hepatitis may have reduced ethosuximide clearance because of destruction of liver parenchyma. This loss of functional hepatic cells reduces the amount of enzymes available to metabolize the drug and decreases clearance. An index of liver dysfunction can be gained by applying the Child-Pugh clinical classification system to the patient (Table 14-2).[14] Child-Pugh scores are completely discussed in Chapter 3 (Drug Dosing in Special Populations: Renal and Hepatic Disease, Dialysis, Heart Failure, Obesity, and Drug Interactions), but will be

TABLE 14-2   Child-Pugh Scores for Patients With Liver Disease

Test/Symptom	Score 1 Point	Score 2 Points	Score 3 Points
Total bilirubin (mg/dL)	<2.0	2.0-3.0	>3.0
Serum albumin (g/dL)	>3.5	2.8-3.5	<2.8
Prothrombin time (seconds prolonged over control)	<4	4-6	>6
Ascites	Absent	Slight	Moderate
Hepatic encephalopathy	None	Moderate	Severe

Mild liver disease, 5-6 points; moderate liver disease, 7-9 points; severe liver disease, 10-15 points.

briefly discussed here. The Child-Pugh score consists of five laboratory tests or clinical symptoms: serum albumin, total bilirubin, prothrombin time, ascites, and hepatic encephalopathy. Each of these areas is given a score of 1 (normal) to 3 (severely abnormal; see Table 14-2), and the scores for the five areas are summed. The Child-Pugh score for a patient with normal liver function is 5 while the score for a patient with grossly abnormal serum albumin, total bilirubin, and prothrombin time values in addition to severe ascites and hepatic encephalopathy is 15. A Child-Pugh score greater than 8 is grounds for a decrease of 25%-50% in the initial daily drug dose for ethosuximide. As in any patient with or without liver dysfunction, initial doses are meant as starting points for dosage titration based on patient response and avoidance of adverse effects. Ethosuximide serum concentrations and the presence of adverse drug effects should be monitored frequently in patients with liver cirrhosis.

Similarly, a small amount (20%-30%) of ethosuximide is usually eliminated unchanged by the kidneys so patients with renal dysfunction (creatinine clearance <30 mL/min) receiving ethosuximide should be closely monitored.[12] Ethosuximide is significantly removed by hemodialysis, and supplemental doses may need to be given after a dialysis session.[15] The drug crosses into the placenta and enters breast milk, achieving concentrations at both sites similar to concurrent maternal serum concentrations.[16-18]

DRUG INTERACTIONS

Unlike other antiepileptic drugs, ethosuximide is not a hepatic enzyme inducer or inhibitor, and appears to cause no clinically important drug interactions.[19] Valproic acid can inhibit ethosuximide metabolism and increase steady-state concentrations, especially when ethosuximide serum concentrations are in the upper end of the therapeutic range.[13]

INITIAL DOSAGE DETERMINATION METHODS

Several methods to initiate ethosuximide therapy are available. The *Pharmacokinetic Dosing method* is the most flexible of the techniques. It allows individualized target serum concentrations to be chosen for a patient, and each pharmacokinetic parameter can be customized to reflect specific disease states and conditions present in the patient. *Literature-based Recommended dosing* is a very commonly used method to prescribe initial doses of ethosuximide. Doses are based on those that commonly produce steady-state concentrations in the lower end of the therapeutic range, although there is a wide variation in the actual concentrations for a specific patient.

Pharmacokinetic Dosing Method

The goal of initial dosing of ethosuximide is to compute the best dose possible for the patient, given their set of disease states and conditions that influence ethosuximide pharmacokinetics and the epileptic disorder being treated. In order to do this, pharmacokinetic parameters for the patient will be estimated using average parameters measured in other patients with similar disease state and condition profiles.

Clearance Estimate

Ethosuximide is predominately metabolized by liver. Unfortunately, there is no good way to estimate the elimination characteristics of liver-metabolized drugs using an endogenous marker of liver function in the same manner that serum creatinine and estimated creatinine clearance are used to estimate the elimination of agents that are renally eliminated. Because of this, a patient is categorized according to the disease states and conditions that are known to change ethosuximide clearance, and the clearance previously measured in these studies is used as an estimate of the current patient's clearance. For example, for a 20-kg pediatric patient, ethosuximide clearance would be assumed to equal 16 mL/h/kg: 20 kg • 16 mL/h/kg = 320 mL/h or 0.32 L/h. To produce the most conservative ethosuximide doses in patients with multiple concurrent disease states or conditions that affect ethosuximide pharmacokinetics, the disease state or condition with the smallest clearance should be used to compute doses. This approach will avoid accidental overdosage has much as currently possible.

Volume of Distribution Estimate

Ethosuximide volume of distribution is assumed to equal 0.7 L/kg for adults and children. Thus, for a 20-kg pediatric patient, the estimated ethosuximide volume of distribution would be 14 L: V = 0.7 L/kg • 20 kg = 14 L.

Half-Life and Elimination Rate Constant Estimate

Once the correct clearance and volume of distribution estimates are identified for the patient, they can be converted into the ethosuximide half-life ($t_{1/2}$) and elimination rate constant (k) estimates using the following equations: $t_{1/2} = (0.693 • V)/Cl$, $k = 0.693/t_{1/2} = Cl/V$.

Selection of Appropriate Pharmacokinetic Model and Equations

Ethosuximide follows a one-compartment pharmacokinetic model. When oral therapy is required, ethosuximide has good bioavailability (F = 1), and once or twice dosing provides a relatively smooth serum concentration-time curve that emulates an intravenous infusion. Because of this, a very simple pharmacokinetic equation that computes the average ethosuximide steady-state serum concentration (Css in µg/mL = mg/L) is widely used. This allows maintenance dosage calculation: $Css = [F(D/\tau)]/Cl$ or $D = (Css • Cl • \tau)/F$, where F is the bioavailability fraction for the oral dosage form (F = 1 for oral ethosuximide products), D is the dose of ethosuximide in mg, Cl is ethosuximide clearance in L/h, and τ is the dosage interval in hours.

EXAMPLE 1 ▶▶▶

LK is a 13-year-old, 47-kg (height = 5 ft 1 in) female with absence seizures who requires therapy with oral ethosuximide. She has normal liver and renal function. Suggest an initial ethosuximide dosage regimen designed to achieve a steady-state ethosuximide concentration equal to 50 µg/mL.

1. *Estimate the clearance and volume of distribution according to the disease states and conditions present in the patient.*
   The clearance rate for an older patient is 12 mL/h/kg. Using this value, the estimated clearance would equal 0.564 L/h: Cl = 47 kg • 12 mL/h/kg = 564 mL/h or 0.564 L/h. The estimated volume of distribution would be 33 L: 47 kg • 0.7 L/kg = 33 L.

2. *Estimate half-life and elimination rate constant.*
   Once the correct clearance and volume of distribution estimates are identified for the patient, they can be converted into the ethosuximide half-life ($t_{1/2}$) and elimination rate constant (k) estimates using the following equations: $t_{1/2} = (0.693 • V)/Cl = (0.693 • 33 L)/0.564 L/h = 41 h$, $k = Cl/V = 0.564 L/h / 33 L = 0.017 h^{-1}$.

3. *Compute dosage regimen.*
   Oral ethosuximide capsules will be prescribed to this patient (F = 1). (Note: µg/mL = mg/L and this concentration unit was substituted for Css in the calculations so that unnecessary unit conversion was not required.) The dosage equation for oral ethosuximide is: $D = (Css • Cl • \tau)/F = (50 mg/L • 0.564 L/h • 12 h)/1 = 338 mg$, rounded to 250 every 12 hours.

   A steady-state trough ethosuximide serum concentration should be measured after steady-state is attained in 3-5 half-lives. Since the patient is expected to have a half-life equal to 41 hours, the ethosuximide steady-state concentration could be obtained any time after the ninth day of dosing (5 half-lives = 5 • 41 h = 205 h or 9 d). Ethosuximide serum concentrations should also be measured if the patient experiences an exacerbation of their epilepsy, or if the patient develops potential signs or symptoms of ethosuximide toxicity.

EXAMPLE 2 ▶▶▶

CT is a 10 year old, 40 kg male with absence seizures who requires therapy with oral ethosuximide. He has normal liver and renal function. Suggest an initial ethosuximide dosage regimen designed to achieve a steady-state ethosuximide concentration equal to 50 µg/mL.

1. *Estimate clearance and volume of distribution according to disease states and conditions present in the patient.*

The clearance rate for a child is 16 mL/h/kg. Using this value, the estimated clearance would equal 0.640 L/h: Cl = 40 kg • 16 mL/h/kg = 640 mL/h or 0.640 L/h. Using 0.7 L/kg, the estimated volume of distribution would be 28 L: 40 kg • 0.7 L/kg = 28 L.

2. *Estimate half-life and elimination rate constant.*

Once the correct clearance and volume of distribution estimates are identified for the patient, they can be converted into the ethosuximide half-life ($t_{1/2}$) and elimination rate constant (k) estimates using the following equations: $t_{1/2}$ = (0.693 • V)/Cl = (0.693 • 28 L)/0.640 L/h = 30 h, k = Cl/V = 0.640 L/h / 28 L = 0.023 h^{-1}.

3. *Compute dosage regimen.*

Oral ethosuximide syrup will be prescribed to this patient (F = 1). (Note: µg/mL = mg/L and this concentration unit was substituted for Css in the calculations so that unnecessary unit conversion was not required.) The dosage equation for oral ethosuximide is: D = (Css • Cl • τ)/F = (50 mg/L • 0.640 L/h • 12 h)/1 = 384 mg, rounded to 400 mg every 12 h.

A steady-state trough ethosuximide serum concentration should be measured after steady-state is attained in 3-5 half-lives. Since the patient is expected to have a half-life equal to 30 hours, the ethosuximide steady-state concentration could be obtained any time after the sixth day of dosing (5 half-lives = 5 • 30 h = 150 h or 6 d). Ethosuximide serum concentrations should also be measured if the patient experiences an exacerbation of their epilepsy, or if the patient develops potential signs or symptoms of ethosuximide toxicity.

Literature-Based Recommended Dosing

Because of the large amount of variability in ethosuximide pharmacokinetics, even when concurrent disease states and conditions are identified, most clinicians believe that the use of standard ethosuximide doses for various situations is warranted. The original computation of these doses was based on the Pharmacokinetic Dosing methods, and was subsequently modified based on clinical experience. In general, the expected ethosuximide steady-state serum concentrations used to compute these doses was 40-50 µg/mL. The usual initial maintenance dose for pediatric patients (<12 years old) is 20 mg/kg/d. For older patients, the initial maintenance dose is 15 mg/kg/d. One or two divided daily doses are initially used for these total doses. To avoid gastrointestinal side effects, doses over 1500 mg given at one time should be avoided. Dosage increases of 3-7 mg/kg/d are made every 1-2 weeks depending on response and adverse effects. While maximal doses are 40 mg/kg/d for children less than 12 years old and 30 mg/kg/d for older patients, ethosuximide serum concentrations and adverse effects should be used to judge optimal response to the drug. If the patient has significant hepatic dysfunction (Child-Pugh score ≥8), maintenance doses prescribed using this method should be decreased by 25%-50% depending on how aggressive therapy is required to be for the individual.

To illustrate the similarities and differences between this method of dosage calculation and the Pharmacokinetic Dosing method, the same examples used in the previous section will be used.

EXAMPLE 3 ▶▶▶

LK is a 13-year-old, 47-kg (height = 5 ft 1 in) female with absence seizures who requires therapy with oral etho-suximide. She has normal liver and renal function. Suggest an initial ethosuximide dosage regimen designed to achieve a steady-state ethosuximide concentration equal to 50 μg/mL.

1. *Estimate ethosuximide dose according to disease states and conditions present in the patient.*

   Oral ethosuximide capsules will be prescribed to this patient. The suggested initial maintenance dosage rate for ethosuximide in an older patient is 15 mg/kg/d: 47 kg • 15 mg/kg/d = 705 mg/d, rounded to 750 mg/d. This dose could be given as 250 mg in the morning and 500 mg in the evening. This dose would be titrated upward in 3-7 mg/kg/d increments every 1-2 weeks while monitoring for adverse and therapeutic effects. The goals of therapy include maximal suppression of seizures and avoidance of side effects.

   A steady-state trough total ethosuximide serum concentration should be measured after steady-state is attained in 1-2 weeks. Ethosuximide serum concentrations should also be measured if the patient experiences an exacerbation of their epilepsy, or if the patient develops potential signs or symptoms of ethosuximide toxicity.

EXAMPLE 4 ▶▶▶

CT is a 10-year-old, 40-kg male with absence seizures who requires therapy with oral ethosuximide. He has nor-mal liver and renal function. Suggest an initial ethosuximide dosage regimen designed to achieve a steady-state ethosuximide concentration equal to 50 μg/mL.

1. *Estimate ethosuximide dose according to disease states and conditions present in the patient.*

   Oral ethosuximide syrup will be prescribed to this patient. The suggested initial maintenance dosage rate for ethosuximide for a child is 20 mg/kg/d: 40 kg • 20 mg/kg/d = 800 mg/d or 400 mg every 12 hours. This dose would be titrated upward in 3-7 mg/kg/d increments every 1-2 weeks while monitoring for adverse and ther-apeutic effects. The goals of therapy include maximal suppression of seizures and avoidance of side effects.

   A steady-state trough total ethosuximide serum concentration should be measured after steady-state is attained in 1-2 weeks. Ethosuximide serum concentrations should also be measured if the patient experiences an exacerbation of their epilepsy, or if the patient develops potential signs or symptoms of ethosuximide toxicity.

USE OF ETHOSUXIMIDE SERUM CONCENTRATIONS TO ALTER DOSES

Because of the large amount of pharmacokinetic variability among patients, it is likely that doses computed using patient population characteristics will not always produce ethosuximide serum concentrations that are expected or desirable. Because of pharmacokinetic variability, the possible nonlinear pharmacokinetics followed by the drug at high concentrations, the narrow therapeutic index of ethosuximide, and the desire to avoid adverse side effects of ethosuximide, measurement of ethosuximide serum concentrations is conducted for most patients to ensure that therapeutic, nontoxic levels are present. In addition to ethosuximide serum concentrations, important patient parameters (seizure frequency, potential ethosuximide side effects, etc) should be followed to confirm that the patient is responding to treatment and not developing adverse drug reactions.

When ethosuximide serum concentrations are measured in patients and a dosage change is necessary, clinicians should seek to use the simplest, most straightforward method available to determine a dose that will provide safe and effective treatment. In most cases, a simple dosage ratio can be used to change doses since ethosuximide follows *Linear Pharmacokinetics*. Sometimes, it is not possible to simply change the dose because of the limited number of oral dosage strengths, and the dosage interval must also be changed. In some situations, it may be necessary or desirable to compute the ethosuximide *pharmacokinetic parameters* for the patient and utilize these to calculate the best drug dose. Computerized methods that incorporate expected population pharmacokinetic characteristics (*Bayesian pharmacokinetic computer programs*) can be used in difficult cases where renal function is changing, serum concentrations are obtained at suboptimal times, or the patient was not at steady-state when serum concentrations were measured. An additional benefit of this method is that a complete pharmacokinetic workup (determination of clearance, volume of distribution, and half-life) can be done with one or more measured concentrations that do not have to be at steady-state.

Linear Pharmacokinetics Method

Because ethosuximide follows linear, dose-proportional pharmacokinetics in most patients with concentrations within and below the therapeutic range, steady-state serum concentrations change in proportion to dose according to the following equation: $D_{new}/C_{ss,new} = D_{old}/C_{ss,old}$ or $D_{new} = (C_{ss,new}/C_{ss,old})D_{old}$, where D is the dose, Css is the steady-state concentration, old indicates the dose that produced the steady-state concentration that the patient is currently receiving, and new denotes the dose necessary to produce the desired steady-state concentration. The advantages of this method are that it is quick and simple. The disadvantages are that steady-state concentrations are required and the assumption of linear pharmacokinetics may not be valid in all patients. When steady-state serum concentrations increase more than expected after a dosage increase or decrease less than expected after a dosage decrease, nonlinear ethosuximide pharmacokinetics is a possible explanation for the observation. Because of this, suggested dosage increases greater than 75% while using this method should be scrutinized by the prescribing clinician, and the risk versus benefit for the patient should be assessed before initiating large dosage increases (>75% over current dose).

EXAMPLE 5 ▶▶▶

LK is a 13-year-old, 47-kg (height = 5 ft 1 in) female with absence seizures who requires therapy with oral ethosuximide. After dosage titration, the patient was prescribed 500 mg every 12 hours of ethosuximide capsules (1000 mg/d) for 1 month, and the steady-state ethosuximide total concentration equals 38 μg/mL. The patient is assessed to be compliant with her dosage regimen. Suggest an ethosuximide dosage regimen designed to achieve a steady-state ethosuximide concentration of 80 μg/mL.

1. *Compute new dose to achieve desired serum concentration.*

   Using linear pharmacokinetics, the resulting total steady-state ethosuximide serum concentration would equal: $D_{new} = (Css_{new}/Css_{old})\,D_{old}$ = (80 μg/mL /38 μg/mL) 1000 mg/d = 2105 mg/d, rounded to 2000 mg/d or 1000 mg every 12 hours.

   A steady-state trough total ethosuximide serum concentration should be measured after steady-state is attained in 1-2 weeks. Ethosuximide serum concentrations should also be measured if the patient experiences an exacerbation of their epilepsy, or if the patient develops potential signs or symptoms of ethosuximide toxicity.

EXAMPLE 6 ▶▶▶

CT is a 10-year-old, 40-kg male with absence seizures who requires therapy with oral ethosuximide. After dosage titration, the patient was prescribed 500 mg twice daily (1000 mg/d) of ethosuximide syrup for 1 month, and the steady-state ethosuximide total concentration equals 130 μg/mL. The patient is assessed to be compliant with his dosage regimen. Suggest an ethosuximide dosage regimen designed to achieve a steady-state ethosuximide concentration of 75 μg/mL.

1. *Compute new dose to achieve desired serum concentration.*

   Using linear pharmacokinetics, the resulting total steady-state ethosuximide serum concentration would equal: $D_{new} = (Css_{new}/Css_{old}) D_{old} = (75\ \mu g/mL\ /\ 130\ \mu g/mL)\ 1000\ mg/d = 577\ mg/d$, rounded to 500 mg/d or 250 mg every 12 hours.

   A steady-state trough total ethosuximide serum concentration should be measured after steady-state is attained in 1-2 weeks. Ethosuximide serum concentrations should also be measured if the patient experiences an exacerbation of their epilepsy, or if the patient develops potential signs or symptoms of ethosuximide toxicity.

Pharmacokinetic Parameter Method

The Pharmacokinetic Parameter method of adjusting drug doses was among the first techniques available to change doses using serum concentrations. It allows the computation of an individual's own, unique pharmacokinetic constants and uses those to calculate a dose that achieves desired ethosuximide concentrations. The Pharmacokinetic Parameter method requires that steady-state has been achieved and uses only a steady-state ethosuximide concentration (Css). Ethosuximide clearance (Cl) can be calculated using the following formula: $Cl = [F(D/\tau)]/Css$, where F is the bioavailability fraction for the oral dosage form (F = 1 for oral ethosuximide products), D is the dose of ethosuximide in mg, Css is the steady-state ethosuximide concentration in mg/L, and τ is the dosage interval in hours.

To illustrate the similarities and differences between this method of dosage calculation and the Pharmacokinetic Parameter method, the same examples used in the previous section will be used.

EXAMPLE 7 ▶▶▶

LK is a 13-year-old, 47-kg (height = 5 ft 1 in) female with absence seizures who requires therapy with oral ethosuximide. After dosage titration, the patient was prescribed 500 mg every 12 hours of ethosuximide capsules (1000 mg/d) for 1 month, and the steady-state ethosuximide total concentration equals 38 μg/mL. The patient is assessed to be compliant with her dosage regimen. Suggest an ethosuximide dosage regimen designed to achieve a steady-state ethosuximide concentration of 80 μg/mL.

1. *Compute pharmacokinetic parameters.*

   The patient would be expected to achieve steady-state conditions after 1-2 weeks of therapy.

   Ethosuximide clearance can be computed using a steady-state ethosuximide concentration: $Cl = [F(D/\tau)]/Css = [1(500\ mg/12\ h)]/(38\ mg/L) = 1.1\ L/h$. (Note: μg/mL = mg/L and this concentration unit was substituted for Css in the calculations so that unnecessary unit conversion was not required.)

2. *Compute ethosuximide dose.*

   Ethosuximide clearance is used to compute the new dose: $D = (Css \bullet Cl \bullet \tau)/F = (80\ mg/L \bullet 1.1\ L/h \bullet 12\ h)/1 = 1056\ mg$, rounded to 1000 mg every 12 hours.

   A steady-state trough total ethosuximide serum concentration should be measured after steady-state is attained in 1-2 weeks. Ethosuximide serum concentrations should also be measured if the patient experiences an exacerbation of their epilepsy, or if the patient develops potential signs or symptoms of ethosuximide toxicity.

EXAMPLE 8 ▶▶▶

CT is a 10-year-old, 40-kg male with absence seizures who requires therapy with oral ethosuximide. After dosage titration, the patient was prescribed 500 mg twice daily (1000 mg/d) of ethosuximide syrup for 1 month, and the steady-state ethosuximide total concentration equals 130 µg/mL. The patient is assessed to be compliant with his dosage regimen. Suggest an ethosuximide dosage regimen designed to achieve a steady-state ethosuximide concentration of 75 µg/mL.

1. *Compute pharmacokinetic parameters.*

   The patient would be expected to achieve steady-state conditions after 1-2 weeks of therapy.

   Ethosuximide clearance can be computed using a steady-state ethosuximide concentration: Cl = [F(D/τ)]/Css = [1(500 mg/12 h)]/(130 mg/L) = 0.32 L/h. (Note: µg/mL = mg/L and this concentration unit was substituted for Css in the calculations so that unnecessary unit conversion was not required.)

2. *Compute ethosuximide dose.*

   Ethosuximide clearance is used to compute the new dose: D = (Css • Cl • τ)/F = (75 mg/L • 0.32 L/h • 12 h)/1 = 288 mg, rounded to 250 mg every 12 hours.

   A steady-state trough total ethosuximide serum concentration should be measured after steady-state is attained in 1-2 weeks. Ethosuximide serum concentrations should also be measured if the patient experiences an exacerbation of their epilepsy, or if the patient develops potential signs or symptoms of ethosuximide toxicity.

BAYESIAN PHARMACOKINETIC COMPUTER PROGRAMS

Computer programs are available that can assist in the computation of pharmacokinetic parameters for patients. The most reliable computer programs use a nonlinear regression algorithm that incorporates components of Bayes theorem.[20] Nonlinear regression is a statistical technique that uses an iterative process to compute the best pharmacokinetic parameters for a concentration/time data set. Briefly, the patient's drug dosage schedule and serum concentrations are input into the computer. The computer program has a pharmacokinetic equation preprogrammed for the drug and administration method (oral, intravenous bolus, intravenous infusion, etc). Typically, a one-compartment model is used, although some programs allow the user to choose among several different equations. Using population estimates based on demographic information for the patient (age, weight, gender, liver function, cardiac status, etc) supplied by the user, the computer program then computes estimated serum concentrations at each time there are actual serum concentrations. Kinetic parameters are then changed by the computer program, and a new set of estimated serum concentrations are computed. The pharmacokinetic parameters that generated the estimated serum concentrations closest to the actual values are remembered by the computer program, and the process is repeated until the set of pharmacokinetic parameters that result in estimated serum concentrations that are statistically closest to the actual serum concentrations are generated. These pharmacokinetic parameters can then be used to compute improved dosing schedules for patients. Bayes theorem is used in the computer algorithm to balance the results of the computations between values based solely on the patient's serum drug concentrations and those based only on patient population parameters. Results from studies that compare various methods of dosage adjustment have consistently found that these types of computer dosing programs perform at least as well as experienced clinical pharmacokineticists and clinicians and better than inexperienced clinicians.

Some clinicians use Bayesian pharmacokinetic computer programs exclusively to alter drug doses based on serum concentrations. An advantage of this approach is that consistent dosage recommendations are made when several different practitioners are involved in therapeutic drug-monitoring programs. However, since simpler dosing methods work just as well for patients with stable pharmacokinetic parameters and steady-state drug concentrations, many clinicians reserve the use of computer programs for more difficult situations. Those situations include serum concentrations that are not at steady-state, serum concentrations not obtained at the specific times needed to employ simpler methods, and unstable pharmacokinetic parameters. Many Bayesian pharmacokinetic computer programs are available to users, and most should provide answers similar to the one used in the following examples. The program used to solve problems in this book is DrugCalc written by Dr. Dennis Mungall.[20]

EXAMPLE 9 ▶▶▶

LK is a 13-year-old, 47-kg (height = 5 ft 1 in) female with absence seizures who requires therapy with oral ethosuximide. The patient has normal liver and renal function (bilirubin = 0.5 mg/dL, albumin 4.6 mg/dL, serum creatinine = 0.5 mg/dL). After dosage titration, the patient was prescribed 500 mg every 12 hours of ethosuximide capsules (1000 mg/d) for 2 weeks, and the steady-state ethosuximide total concentration equals 38 μg/mL. The patient is assessed to be compliant with her dosage regimen. Suggest an ethosuximide dosage regimen designed to achieve a steady-state ethosuximide concentration of 80 μg/mL.

1. *Enter the patient's demographic, drug-dosing, and serum concentration/time data into the computer program.*
2. *Compute pharmacokinetic parameters for the patient using Bayesian pharmacokinetic computer program.*
   The pharmacokinetic parameters computed by the program are a volume of distribution of 46 L, a half-life equal to 26 h, and a clearance equal to 1.24 L/h.
3. *Compute the dose required to achieve the desired ethosuximide serum concentrations.*
   The one-compartment model first-order absorption equations used by the program to compute doses indicates that a dose of 1000 mg every 12 hours will produce a steady-state ethosuximide concentration of 68 μg/mL.

EXAMPLE 10 ▶▶▶

JB is an 8-year-old, 35-kg male (height = 4 ft 2 in) with absence seizures who was started on ethosuximide syrup 350 mg every 12 hours. The ethosuximide concentration was 25 μg/mL before the fifth maintenance dose. What ethosuximide dose is needed to achieve Css = 75 μg/mL?

1. *Enter the patient's demographic, drug-dosing, and serum concentration/time data into the computer program.*
   In this patient case, it is unlikely that the patient is at steady-state so the Linear Pharmacokinetics method cannot be used.
2. *Compute the pharmacokinetic parameters for the patient using Bayesian pharmacokinetic computer program.*
   The pharmacokinetic parameters computed by the program are a volume of distribution of 30 L, a half-life equal to 18 h, and clearance equal to 1.12 L/h.
3. *Compute dose required to achieve desired ethosuximide serum concentrations.*
   The one-compartment model oral equations used by the program to compute doses indicates that a dose of ethosuximide 1000 mg every 12 hours will produce a steady-state concentration of 69 μg/mL.

TABLE 14-3 Dosing Strategies

Dosing Approach/Philosophy	Initial Dosing	Use of Serum Concentrations to Alter Doses
Pharmacokinetic parameter/equations	Pharmacokinetic Dosing method	Pharmacokinetic Parameter method
Literature-based concept	Literature-based Recommended dosing method	Linear Pharmacokinetics method
Computerized	Bayesian computer program	Bayesian computer program

DOSING STRATEGIES

Initial dose and dosage adjustment techniques using serum concentrations can be used in any combination as long as the limitations of each method are observed. Some dosing schemes link together logically when considered according to their basic approaches or philosophies. Dosage strategies that follow similar pathways are given in Table 14-3.

PROBLEMS

The following problems are intended to emphasize the computation of initial and individualized doses using clinical pharmacokinetic techniques. Clinicians should always consult the patient's chart to confirm that current anticonvulsant therapy is appropriate. Additionally, all other medications that the patient is taking, including prescription and nonprescription drugs, should be noted and checked to ascertain if a potential drug interaction with ethosuximide exists.

1. YH is a 4-year-old, 16-kg (height = 40 in) male with absence seizures who requires therapy with oral ethosuximide. He has normal liver function. Suggest an initial ethosuximide dosage regimen designed to achieve a steady-state ethosuximide concentration equal to 50 μg/mL.

2. Patient YH (see problem 1) was prescribed 300 mg every day of ethosuximide syrup for 1 month, and the steady-state ethosuximide total concentration equals 40 μg/mL. The patient is assessed to be compliant with his dosage regimen. Suggest an ethosuximide dosage regimen designed to achieve a steady-state ethosuximide concentration of 75 μg/mL.

3. FD is a 9-year-old, 35-kg female (height = 4 ft 6 in) with absence seizures who requires therapy with oral ethosuximide. She has normal liver function. Suggest an initial ethosuximide dosage regimen designed to achieve a steady-state ethosuximide concentration equal to 75 μg/mL.

4. Patient FD (see problem 3) was prescribed 350 mg every 12 hours (700 mg/d) of ethosuximide syrup for 2 weeks, and the steady-state ethosuximide total concentration equals 55 μg/mL. The patient is assessed to be compliant with her dosage regimen. Suggest an ethosuximide dosage regimen designed to achieve a steady-state ethosuximide concentration equal to 90 μg/mL.

5. LK is a 14-year-old, 60 kg male (height = 5 ft 6 in) with absence seizures who requires therapy with ethosuximide capsules. He has normal liver and renal function. Suggest an initial ethosuximide dosage regimen designed to achieve a steady-state ethosuximide concentration equal to 50 μg/mL.

6. Patient LK (see problem 5) was prescribed 500 mg every 12 hours (1000 mg/d) of ethosuximide capsules for 2 weeks, and the steady-state ethosuximide total concentration equals 40 μg/mL. The patient is assessed to be compliant with his dosage regimen. Suggest an ethosuximide dosage regimen designed to achieve a steady-state ethosuximide concentration of 60 μg/mL.

7. DG is a 15-year-old, 68-kg (height = 5 ft 8 in) male with absence seizures who is receiving 1000 mg daily of ethosuximide capsules. He has normal liver and renal function. The total ethosuximide concentration equals 22 μg/mL before the fourth dose. Compute an ethosuximide dose that will provide a steady-state concentration of 50 μg/mL.

8. YF is a 5-year-old, 20-kg (height = 42 in) female with absence seizures who was given a new prescription of 250 mg every 12 hours of oral ethosuximide syrup. She has normal liver and renal function. The trough ethosuximide concentration before the fifth dose equals 42 μg/mL. Compute an ethosuximide dose that will provide a total steady-state concentration of 75 μg/mL.

ANSWERS TO PROBLEMS

1. *Answer to problem 1.*

Pharmacokinetic Dosing Method

1. *Estimate the clearance and volume of distribution according to disease states and conditions present in the patient.*

The clearance rate for a pediatric patient is 16 mL/h/kg. Using this value, the estimated clearance would equal 0.256 L/h: Cl = 16 kg • 16 mL/h/kg = 256 mL/h or 0.256 L/h. Using 0.7 L/kg, the estimated volume of distribution would be 11 L: 16 kg • 0.7 L/kg = 11 L.

2. *Estimate the half-life and elimination rate constant.*

Once the correct clearance and volume of distribution estimates are identified for the patient, they can be converted into the ethosuximide half-life ($t_{1/2}$) and elimination rate constant (k) estimates using the following equations: $t_{1/2} = (0.693 • V)/Cl = (0.693 • 11 \text{ L})/0.256 \text{ L/h} = 30 \text{ h}$, $k = Cl/V = 0.256 \text{ L/h} /11 \text{ L} = 0.023 \text{ h}^{-1}$.

3. *Compute dosage regimen.*

Oral ethosuximide syrup will be prescribed to this patient (F = 1). (Note: μg/mL = mg/L and this concentration unit was substituted for Css in the calculations so that unnecessary unit conversion was not required.) The dosage equation for oral ethosuximide is: $D = (Css • Cl • τ)/F = (50 \text{ mg/L} • 0.256 \text{ L/h} • 12 \text{ h})/1 = 154 \text{ mg}$, rounded to 150 every 12 hours.

A steady-state trough ethosuximide serum concentration should be measured after steady-state is attained in 3-5 half-lives. Since the patient is expected to have a half-life equal to 30 hours, the ethosuximide steady-state concentration could be obtained any time after the sixth day of dosing (5 half-lives = 5 • 30 h = 150 h or 6 d). Ethosuximide serum concentrations should also be measured if the patient experiences an exacerbation of their epilepsy, or if the patient develops potential signs or symptoms of ethosuximide toxicity.

Literature-Based Recommended Dosing

1. *Estimate ethosuximide dose according to disease states and conditions present in the patient.*

Oral ethosuximide syrup will be prescribed to this patient. The suggested initial maintenance dosage rate for ethosuximide in a pediatric patient is 20 mg/kg/d: 16 kg • 20 mg/kg/d = 320 mg/d, rounded to 300 mg/d or 150 mg every 12 hours. This dose would be titrated upward in 3-7 mg/kg/d increments every 1-2 weeks while monitoring for adverse and therapeutic effects. The goals of therapy include maximal suppression of seizures and avoidance of side effects.

A steady-state trough total ethosuximide serum concentration should be measured after steady-state is attained in 1-2 weeks. Ethosuximide serum concentrations should also be measured if the patient experiences an exacerbation of their epilepsy, or if the patient develops potential signs or symptoms of ethosuximide toxicity.

2. *Answer to problem 2.*

Linear Pharmacokinetics Method

1. *Compute new dose to achieve desired serum concentration.*

Using linear pharmacokinetics, the resulting total steady-state ethosuximide serum concentration would equal: $D_{new} = (Css_{new}/Css_{old})\, D_{old} = $ (75 µg/mL /40 µg/mL) 300 mg/d = 563 mg/d, rounded to 600 mg/d.

A steady-state trough total ethosuximide serum concentration should be measured after steady-state is attained in 1-2 weeks. Ethosuximide serum concentrations should also be measured if the patient experiences an exacerbation of their epilepsy, or if the patient develops potential signs or symptoms of ethosuximide toxicity.

Pharmacokinetic Parameter Method

1. *Compute pharmacokinetic parameters.*

The patient would be expected to achieve steady-state conditions after 1-2 weeks of therapy.

Ethosuximide clearance can be computed using a steady-state ethosuximide concentration: $Cl = [F(D/\tau)]/ Css = $ [1(300 mg/24 h)]/(40 mg/L) = 0.31 L/h. (Note: µg/mL = mg/L and this concentration unit was substituted for Css in the calculations so that unnecessary unit conversion was not required.)

2. *Compute ethosuximide dose.*

Ethosuximide clearance is used to compute the new dose: $D = (Css \bullet Cl \bullet \tau)/F = $ (75 mg/L • 0.31 L/h • 24 h)/1 = 558 mg, rounded to 600 mg every 24 hours.

A steady-state trough total ethosuximide serum concentration should be measured after steady-state is attained in 1-2 weeks. Ethosuximide serum concentrations should also be measured if the patient experiences an exacerbation of their epilepsy, or if the patient develops potential signs or symptoms of ethosuximide toxicity.

Bayesian Pharmacokinetic Computer Programs

1. *Enter the patient's demographic, drug-dosing, and serum concentration/time data into the computer program.*

2. *Compute pharmacokinetic parameters for the patient using Bayesian pharmacokinetic computer program.*

The pharmacokinetic parameters computed by the program are a volume of distribution of 11.3 L, a half-life equal to 32 h, and a clearance equal to 0.24 L/h.

3. *Compute dose required to achieve desired ethosuximide serum concentrations.*

The one-compartment model first-order absorption equations used by the program to compute doses indicates that a dose of 500 mg every day will produce a steady-state ethosuximide concentration of 68 µg/mL.

3. *Answer to problem 3.*

Pharmacokinetic Dosing Method

1. *Estimate clearance and volume of distribution according to disease states and conditions present in the patient.*

The clearance rate for a pediatric patient is 16 mL/h/kg. Using this value, the estimated clearance would equal 0.560 L/h: Cl = 35 kg • 16 mL/h/kg = 560 mL/h or 0.560 L/h. Using 0.7 L/kg, the estimated volume of distribution would be 25 L: 35 kg • 0.7 L/kg = 25 L.

2. *Estimate half-life and elimination rate constant.*

Once the correct clearance and volume of distribution estimates are identified for the patient, they can be converted into the ethosuximide half-life ($t_{1/2}$) and elimination rate constant (k) estimates using the following equations: $t_{1/2} = (0.693 \bullet V)/Cl = (0.693 \bullet 25\ L)/0.560\ L/h = 31\ h$, $k = Cl/V = 0.560\ L/h/25\ L = 0.022\ h^{-1}$.

3. *Compute dosage regimen.*

Oral ethosuximide syrup will be prescribed to this patient (F = 1). (Note: µg/mL = mg/L and this concentration unit was substituted for Css in the calculations so that unnecessary unit conversion was not required.) The dosage equation for oral ethosuximide is: $D = (Css \bullet Cl \bullet \tau)/F = (75\ mg/L \bullet 0.560\ L/h \bullet 12\ h)/1 = 504\ mg$, rounded to 500 every 12 hours.

A steady-state trough ethosuximide serum concentration should be measured after steady-state is attained in 3-5 half-lives. Since the patient is expected to have a half-life equal to 31 hours, the ethosuximide steady-state concentration could be obtained any time after the sixth day of dosing (5 half-lives = 5 $\bullet$ 31 h = 155 h or 6 d). Ethosuximide serum concentrations should also be measured if the patient experiences an exacerbation of their epilepsy, or if the patient develops potential signs or symptoms of ethosuximide toxicity.

Literature-Based Recommended Dosing

1. *Estimate ethosuximide dose according to disease states and conditions present in the patient.*

Oral ethosuximide syrup will be prescribed to this patient. The suggested initial maintenance dosage rate for ethosuximide in a pediatric patient is 20 mg/kg/d: 35 kg $\bullet$ 20 mg/kg/d = 700 mg/d, 350 mg every 12 hours. This dose would be titrated upward in 3-7 mg/kg/d increments every 1-2 weeks while monitoring for adverse and therapeutic effects. The goals of therapy include maximal suppression of seizures and avoidance of side effects.

A steady-state trough total ethosuximide serum concentration should be measured after steady-state is attained in 1-2 weeks. Ethosuximide serum concentrations should also be measured if the patient experiences an exacerbation of their epilepsy, or if the patient develops potential signs or symptoms of ethosuximide toxicity.

4. *Answer to problem 4.*

Linear Pharmacokinetics Method

1. *Compute new dose to achieve the desired serum concentration.*

Using linear pharmacokinetics, the resulting total steady-state ethosuximide serum concentration would equal: $D_{new} = (Css_{new}/Css_{old})\ D_{old} = (90\ µg/mL\ /55\ µg/mL)\ 700\ mg/d = 1145\ mg/d$, rounded to 1100 mg/d or 550 mg every 12 hours.

A steady-state trough total ethosuximide serum concentration should be measured after steady-state is attained in 1-2 weeks. Ethosuximide serum concentrations should also be measured if the patient experiences an exacerbation of their epilepsy, or if the patient develops potential signs or symptoms of ethosuximide toxicity.

Pharmacokinetic Parameter Method

1. *Compute pharmacokinetic parameters.*

The patient would be expected to achieve steady-state conditions after 1-2 weeks of therapy.

Ethosuximide clearance can be computed using a steady-state ethosuximide concentration: $Cl = [F(D/\tau)]/Css = [1(350\ mg/12\ h)]/(55\ mg/L) = 0.53\ L/h$. (Note: µg/mL = mg/L and this concentration unit was substituted for Css in the calculations so that unnecessary unit conversion was not required.)

2. *Compute ethosuximide dose.*

Ethosuximide clearance is used to compute the new dose: D = (Css • Cl • τ)/F = (90 mg/L • 0.53 L/h • 12 h)/1 = 572 mg, rounded to 600 mg every 12 hours.

A steady-state trough total ethosuximide serum concentration should be measured after steady-state is attained in 1-2 weeks. Ethosuximide serum concentrations should also be measured if the patient experiences an exacerbation of their epilepsy, or if the patient develops potential signs or symptoms of ethosuximide toxicity.

Bayesian Pharmacokinetic Computer Programs

1. *Enter the patient's demographic, drug-dosing, and serum concentration/time data into the computer program.*

2. *Compute the pharmacokinetic parameters for the patient using Bayesian pharmacokinetic computer program.*

The pharmacokinetic parameters computed by the program are a volume of distribution of 25 L, a half-life equal to 36 h, and a clearance equal to 0.48 L/h.

3. *Compute the dose required to achieve the desired ethosuximide serum concentrations.*

The one-compartment model first-order absorption equations used by the program to compute doses indicates that a dose of 600 mg every 12 hours will produce a steady-state ethosuximide concentration of 95 µg/mL.

5. *Answer to problem 5.*

Pharmacokinetic Dosing Method

1. *Estimate clearance and volume of distribution according to the disease states and conditions present in the patient.*

The clearance rate for an older patient is 12 mL/h/kg. Using this value, the estimated clearance would equal 0.720 L/h: Cl = 60 kg • 12 mL/h/kg = 720 mL/h or 0.720 L/h. Using 0.7 L/kg, the estimated volume of distribution would be 42 L: 60 kg • 0.7 L/kg = 42 L.

2. *Estimate the half-life and elimination rate constant.*

Once the correct clearance and volume of distribution estimates are identified for the patient, they can be converted into the ethosuximide half-life ($t_{1/2}$) and elimination rate constant (k) estimates using the following equations: $t_{1/2}$ = (0.693 • V)/Cl = (0.693 • 42 L)/0.720 L/h = 40 h, k = Cl/V = 0.720 L/h /42 L = 0.017 h^{-1}.

3. *Compute dosage regimen.*

Oral ethosuximide capsules will be prescribed to this patient (F = 1). (Note: µg/mL = mg/L and this concentration unit was substituted for Css in the calculations so that unnecessary unit conversion was not required.) The dosage equation for oral ethosuximide is: D = (Css • Cl • τ)/F = (50 mg/L • 0.720 L/h • 24 h)/1 = 864 mg, rounded to 750 every day.

A steady-state trough ethosuximide serum concentration should be measured after steady-state is attained in 3-5 half-lives. Since the patient is expected to have a half-life equal to 40 hours, the ethosuximide steady-state concentration could be obtained any time after the sixth day of dosing (5 half-lives = 5 • 40 h = 200 h or 8 d). Ethosuximide serum concentrations should also be measured if the patient experiences an exacerbation of their epilepsy, or if the patient develops potential signs or symptoms of ethosuximide toxicity.

Literature-Based Recommended Dosing

1. *Estimate ethosuximide dose according to disease states and conditions present in the patient.*

   Oral ethosuximide capsules will be prescribed to this patient. The suggested initial maintenance dosage rate for ethosuximide in an older patient is 15 mg/kg/d: 60 kg • 15 mg/kg/d = 900 mg/d, rounded to 1000 mg daily. This dose would be titrated upward in 3-7 mg/kg/d increments every 1-2 weeks while monitoring for adverse and therapeutic effects. The goals of therapy include maximal suppression of seizures and avoidance of side effects.

   A steady-state trough total ethosuximide serum concentration should be measured after steady-state is attained in 1-2 weeks. Ethosuximide serum concentrations should also be measured if the patient experiences an exacerbation of their epilepsy, or if the patient develops potential signs or symptoms of ethosuximide toxicity.

6. *Answer to problem 6.*

Linear Pharmacokinetics Method

1. *Compute new dose to achieve desired serum concentration.*

   Using linear pharmacokinetics, the resulting total steady-state ethosuximide serum concentration would equal: $D_{new} = (Css_{new}/Css_{old}) D_{old} = (60 \ \mu g/mL \ /40 \ \mu g/mL) \ 1000 \ mg/d = 1500 \ mg/d$, or 750 mg every 12 hours.

   A steady-state trough total ethosuximide serum concentration should be measured after steady-state is attained in 1-2 weeks. Ethosuximide serum concentrations should also be measured if the patient experiences an exacerbation of their epilepsy, or if the patient develops potential signs or symptoms of ethosuximide toxicity.

Pharmacokinetic Parameter Method

1. *Compute pharmacokinetic parameters.*

   The patient would be expected to achieve steady-state conditions after 1-2 weeks of therapy.

   Ethosuximide clearance can be computed using a steady-state ethosuximide concentration: $Cl = [F(D/\tau)]/Css = [1(500 \ mg/12 \ h)]/(40 \ mg/L) = 1.0 \ L/h$. (Note: $\mu g/mL = mg/L$ and this concentration unit was substituted for Css in the calculations so that unnecessary unit conversion was not required.)

2. *Compute ethosuximide dose.*

   Ethosuximide clearance is used to compute the new dose: $D = (Css • Cl • \tau)/F = (60 \ mg/L • 1.0 \ L/h • 12 \ h)/1 = 720 \ mg$, rounded to 750 mg every 12 hours.

   A steady-state trough total ethosuximide serum concentration should be measured after steady-state is attained in 1-2 weeks. Ethosuximide serum concentrations should also be measured if the patient experiences an exacerbation of their epilepsy, or if the patient develops potential signs or symptoms of ethosuximide toxicity.

Bayesian Pharmacokinetic Computer Programs

1. *Enter the patient's demographic, drug-dosing, and serum concentration/time data into the computer program.*

2. *Compute the pharmacokinetic parameters for the patient using Bayesian pharmacokinetic computer program.*

   The pharmacokinetic parameters computed by the program are a volume of distribution of 42 L, a half-life equal to 32 h, and a clearance equal to 0.93 L/h.

3. *Compute the dose required to achieve the desired ethosuximide serum concentrations.*

The one-compartment model first-order absorption equations used by the program to compute doses indicates that a dose of 750 mg every 12 hours will produce a steady-state ethosuximide concentration of 61 µg/mL.

7. *Answer to problem 7.*

Bayesian Pharmacokinetic Computer Programs

1. *Enter the patient's demographic, drug-dosing, and serum concentration/time data into the computer program.*

This patient is not at steady-state, so linear pharmacokinetics cannot be used.

2. *Compute pharmacokinetic parameters for the patient using Bayesian pharmacokinetic computer program.*

The pharmacokinetic parameters computed by the program are a volume of distribution of 48 L, a half-life equal to 29 h, and a clearance equal to 1.2 L/h.

3. *Compute dose required to achieve the desired ethosuximide serum concentrations.*

The one-compartment model first-order absorption equations used by the program to compute doses indicates that a dose of 1750 mg every 24 hours will produce a steady-state ethosuximide concentration of 48 µg/mL. To avoid possible gastrointestinal side effects, this daily dose should be given as a divided dose of 750 mg in the morning and 1000 mg in the evening.

8. *Answer to problem 8.*

Bayesian Pharmacokinetic Computer Programs

1. *Enter the patient's demographic, drug-dosing, and serum concentration/time data into the computer program.*

2. *Compute the pharmacokinetic parameters for the patient using Bayesian pharmacokinetic computer program.*

The pharmacokinetic parameters computed by the program are a volume of distribution of 13 L, a half-life equal to 31 h, and a clearance equal to 0.30 L/h.

3. *Compute the dose required to achieve the desired ethosuximide serum concentrations.*

The one-compartment model first-order absorption equations used by the program to compute doses indicates that a dose of 300 mg every 12 hours will produce a steady-state ethosuximide concentration of 76 µg/mL.

REFERENCES

1. Abramowicz M, Zuccotti G, Pflomm JM, eds. Drugs for epilepsy. *Treatment Guidelines From The Medical Letter.* 2013;11(126):9-18.
2. Anon. The epilepsies: the diagnosis and management of the epilepsies in adults and children in primary and secondary care. *UK National Institute for Health and Care Excellence.* http://www.nice.org.uk/nicemedia/live/13635/57779/57779.pdf. Accessed May 1, 2014.
3. French JA, Kanner AM, Bautista J, et al. Efficacy and tolerability of the new antiepileptic drugs I: treatment of new onset epilepsy: report of the Therapeutics and Technology Assessment Subcommittee and Quality Standards Subcommittee of the American Academy of Neurology and the American Epilepsy Society. *Neurology.* Apr 27 2004;62(8):1252-1260.
4. Glauser T, Ben-Menachem E, Bourgeois B, et al. Updated ILAE evidence review of antiepileptic drug efficacy and effectiveness as initial monotherapy for epileptic seizures and syndromes. *Epilepsia.* Mar 2013;54(3):551-563.
5. McNamara JO. Pharmacotherapy of the epilepsies. In: Brunton L, Chabner B, Knollman B, eds. *The Pharmacological Basis of Therapeutics.* 12th ed. New York, NY: McGraw-Hill; 2011:583-608.

6. Glauser TA, Cnaan A, Shinnar S, et al. Ethosuximide, valproic acid, and lamotrigine in childhood absence epilepsy: initial monotherapy outcomes at 12 months. *Epilepsia.* Jan 2013;54(1):141-155.

7. Glauser TA, Cnaan A, Shinnar S, et al. Ethosuximide, valproic acid, and lamotrigine in childhood absence epilepsy. *N Engl J Med.* Mar 4, 2010;362(9):790-799.

8. Rogers SJ, Cavazos JE. Epilepsy. In: DiPiro JT, Talbert RL, Yee GC, Matzke GR, Wells BG, Posey LM, eds. *Pharmacotherapy.* 8th ed. New York, NY: McGraw-Hill; 2011:979-1005.

9. Garnett WR. Antiepileptics. In: Schumacher GE, ed. *Therapeutic Drug Monitoring.* Stamford, CT: Appleton & Lange; 1995:345-395.

10. Garnett WR, Anderson GD, Collins RJ. Antiepileptic drugs. In: Burton ME, Shaw LM, Schentag JJ, Evans WE, eds. *Applied Pharmacokinetics & Pharmacodynamics.* 4th ed. Philadelphia, PA: Lippincott Williams & Wilkins; 2006:491-511.

11. Chang T. Ethosuximide—biotransformation. In: Levy RH, Mattson R, Meldrum B, eds. *Antiepileptic Drugs.* 3rd ed. New York, NY: Raven Press; 1989:679-683.

12. Glazko AJ. Antiepileptic drugs: biotransformation, metabolism, and serum half-life. *Epilepsia.* 1975;16(2):367-391.

13. Bauer LA, Harris C, Wilensky AJ, Raisys VA, Levy RH. Ethosuximide kinetics: possible interaction with valproic acid. *Clin Pharmacol Ther.* 1982;31(6):741-745.

14. Pugh RN, Murray-Lyon IM, Dawson JL, Pietroni MC, Williams R. Transection of the oesophagus for bleeding oesophageal varices. *Br J Surg.* 1973;60(8):646-649.

15. Marbury TC, Lee CS, Perchalski RJ, Wilder BJ. Hemodialysis clearance of ethosuximide in patients with chronic renal disease. *Am J Hosp Pharm.* 1981;38(11):1757-1760.

16. Chang T. Ethosuximide—absorption, distribution, and excretion. In: Levy RH, Mattson R, Meldrum B, eds. *Antiepileptic Drugs.* 3rd ed. New York, NY: Raven Press; 1989:679-683.

17. Rane A, Tunell R. Ethosuximide in human milk and in plasma of a mother and her nursed infant. *Br J Clin Pharmacol.* 1981;12(6):855-858.

18. Koup JR, Rose JQ, Cohen ME. Ethosuximide pharmacokinetics in a pregnant patient and her newborn. *Epilepsia.* 1978;19(6):535-539.

19. Hansten PD, Horn JR. *Drug interactions analysis and management.* St. Louis, MO: Wolters Kluwer; 2014.

20. Wandell M, Mungall D. Computer assisted drug interpretation and drug regimen optimization. *Amer Assoc Clin Chem.* 1984;6:1-11.

15 Lamotrigine

INTRODUCTION

Lamotrigine is a phenyltriazine-based compound effective in the treatment of partial and generalized seizures (Table 15-1).[1-4] Although lamotrigine is listed as a recommended therapy for absence seizures by expert panels, recent literature suggests that ethosuximide or valproic acid may be more effective initial therapy for this epilepsy type.[5,6] It is also useful for the treatment of bipolar disorders, neurogenic pain, and Lennox-Gastaut syndrome.[7-9] While lamotrigine was originally developed as a antifolate agent, its therapeutic effects are not related to this property. The proposed mechanism of action in humans is the inhibition of voltage-sensitive sodium channels, which stabilizes neuronal membranes and modulates the presynaptic transmitter release of glutamate and aspartate.[9-12]

TABLE 15-1 International Classification of Epileptic Seizures With Recommended Therapies

| Major Class | Subset of Class | Drug Treatment for Selected Seizure Type | | | |
		2004 AAN/AES	2013 Medical Letter	2012 NICE	2013 ILAE[a]
Partial seizures (beginning locally)	1. Simple partial seizures (without impaired consciousness) a. with motor symptoms b. with somatosensory or special sensory symptoms c. with autonomic symptoms d. with psychological symptoms	Carbamazepine Phenytoin Valproate Phenobarbital Lamotrigine Gabapentin Oxcarbazepine Topiramate	Lamotrigine Carbamazepine Levetiracetam Oxcarbazepine *Alternatives:* Topiramate Valproate Gabapentin Zonisamide Phenytoin Pregabalin Lacosamide Ezogabine	Carbamazepine Lamotrigine Levetiracetam Oxcarbazepine Valproate *Adjunctive:* Carbamazepine Clobazam Gabapentin Lamotrigine Levetiracetam Oxcarbazepine Valproate Topiramate	*Adults:* Carbamazepine Levetiracetam Phenytoin Zonisamide Valproate *Children:* Oxcarbazepine Carbamazepine Phenobarbital Phenytoin Topiramate Valproate Vigabatrin *Elderly:* Gabapentin Lamotrigine Carbamazepine

(Continued)

TABLE 15-1 International Classification of Epileptic Seizures With Recommended Therapies *(Continued)*

Major Class	Subset of Class	Drug Treatment for Selected Seizure Type			
		2004 AAN/AES	**2013 Medical Letter**	**2012 NICE**	**2013 ILAE[a]**
	2. Complex partial seizures (with impaired consciousness) a. simple partial onset followed by impaired consciousness b. impaired consciousness at onset	Carbamazepine Phenytoin Valproate Phenobarbital Lamotrigine Gabapentin Oxcarbazepine Topiramate	Lamotrigine Carbamazepine Levetiracetam Oxcarbazepine *Alternatives:* Topiramate Valproate Gabapentin Zonisamide Phenytoin Pregabalin Lacosamide Ezogabine	Carbamazepine Lamotrigine Levetiracetam Oxcarbazepine Valproate *Adjunctive:* Carbamazepine Clobazam Gabapentin Lamotrigine Levetiracetam Oxcarbazepine Valproate Topiramate	*Adults:* Carbamazepine Levetiracetam Phenytoin Zonisamide Valproate *Children:* Oxcarbazepine Carbamazepine Phenobarbital Phenytoin Topiramate Valproate Vigabatrin *Elderly:* Gabapentin Lamotrigine Carbamazepine
	3. Partial seizures evolving into secondary generalized seizures	Carbamazepine Phenytoin Valproate Phenobarbital Lamotrigine Gabapentin Oxcarbazepine Topiramate	Lamotrigine Carbamazepine Levetiracetam Oxcarbazepine *Alternatives:* Topiramate Valproate Gabapentin Zonisamide Phenytoin Pregabalin Lacosamide Ezogabine	Carbamazepine Lamotrigine Levetiracetam Oxcarbazepine Valproate *Adjunctive:* Carbamazepine Clobazam Gabapentin Lamotrigine Levetiracetam Oxcarbazepine Valproate Topiramate	*Adults:* Carbamazepine Levetiracetam Phenytoin Zonisamide Valproate *Children:* Oxcarbazepine Carbamazepine Phenobarbital Phenytoin Topiramate Valproate Vigabatrin *Elderly:* Gabapentin Lamotrigine Carbamazepine
Generalized seizures (convulsive or nonconvulsive)	1. Absence seizures[b] (typical or atypical; also known as petit mal seizures)	*Children:[c]* Ethosuximide Valproate Lamotrigine	Ethosuximide Valproate *Alternatives:* Lamotrigine Clonazepam Zonisamide Levetiracetam	Ethosuximide Lamotrigine Valproate *Adjunctive:* Ethosuximide Lamotrigine Valproate	*Children:* Ethosuximide Valproate Lamotrigine

(Continued)

TABLE 15-1   International Classification of Epileptic Seizures With Recommended Therapies (*Continued*)

Major Class	Subset of Class	Drug Treatment for Selected Seizure Type			
		2004 AAN/AES	2013 Medical Letter	2012 NICE	2013 ILAE[a]
	2. Tonic-clonic seizures (also known as grand mal seizures)	Carbamazepine Phenytoin Valproate Phenobarbital Lamotrigine Oxcarbazepine Topiramate	Valproate Lamotrigine Levetiracetam *Alternatives:* Topiramate Zonisamide Phenytoin	Carbamazepine Lamotrigine Oxcarbazepine Valproate *Adjunctive:* Clobazam Lamotrigine Levetiracetam Valproate Topiramate	*Adults:* Carbamazepine Lamotrigine Oxcarbazepine Phenobarbital Phenytoin Topiramate Valproate Gabapentin Levetiracetam Vigabatrin *Children:* Carbamazepine Phenobarbital Phenytoin Topiramate Valproate Oxcarbazepine

[a]Only two highest available levels of evidence listed.
[b]Recent literature suggests either ethosuximide or valproic acid is a superior initial therapy compared to lamotrigine for absence seizures.[5,6]
[c]Lamotrigine added to previous recommendation per expert panel.
Abbreviations: ANN, American Academy of Neurology; AES, American Epilepsy Society; NICE, UK National Institute for Clinical Excellence; ILAE, International League Against Epilepsy.

THERAPEUTIC AND TOXIC CONCENTRATIONS

Unlike most of the older antiepileptic drugs, the therapeutic range of lamotrigine is not well defined.[13-16] However, lamotrigine serum concentration measurement can be a useful adjunct in addition to monitoring treatment for therapeutic response and adverse effects. The therapeutic range for epilepsy used by many laboratories for lamotrigine is 2-20 µg/mL. Some patients will experience a higher incidence of adverse effects at concentrations above 10-15 µg/mL, so the efficacy of lower serum concentrations should be assessed before moving to higher concentrations.[13-15] The most common concentration-dependent side effects of lamotrigine are diplopia, dizziness, ataxia, blurred vision, unsteadiness, and headache.[12]

CLINICAL MONITORING PARAMETERS

The goal of therapy with anticonvulsants is to reduce seizure frequency and maximize quality of life with a minimum of adverse drug effects.[12] While it is desirable to entirely abolish all seizure episodes, it may not be possible to accomplish this in many patients. The goal of therapy with lamotrigine for patients with bipolar disorder is to decrease the frequency and severity of mood episodes with a minimum of side effects. Patients should be monitored for concentration-related side effects (diplopia, dizziness, ataxia, blurred vision, unsteadiness, headache) as well as gastrointestinal upset (nausea, vomiting).[12,17,18] Somnolence, tremor, and rash are also common adverse events.[12,17,18] Typically, the rash caused by lamotrigine is classified as erythematous, generalized, and morbilliform.[9]

Serious, life-threatening rashes have been associated with lamotrigine treatment, and the prescribing information for the drug carries a black box warning for Stevens-Johnson syndrome, toxic epidermal necrolysis, and rash-related death.[17,18] These types of rashes usually occur early in therapy, typically in the first few months of use.[2,12] The manufacture recommends immediate discontinuation of lamotrigine upon development of a rash, unless the rash is proven to be not related to lamotrigine treatment. Some factors that may increase the risk of developing a rash include concurrent administration of valproate, administration of an initial dose of lamotrigine that exceeds the recommended starting dose, and titration to higher doses that exceed the recommended rate for lamotrigine.[17,18]

Because epilepsy is an episodic disease state, patients do not experience seizures continuously. Thus, during dosage titration it is difficult to tell if the patient is responding to drug therapy or simply is not experiencing any abnormal central nervous system discharges at that time. Similarly, bipolar disorder also occurs at irregular time intervals. Lamotrigine doses should be carefully titrated to individual patient response and tolerability. Serum concentrations of lamotrigine can be measured in patients as an adjunct to therapy.[13-16] Concentration monitoring is particularly useful if a therapeutic concentration has been established for a patient and a new clinical event (drug interaction, new disease state or condition, etc) changes the pharmacokinetics of the drug. Lamotrigine concentrations can also be measured to document patient adherence to drug treatment or when a patient is switched between the immediate-release and extended-release dosage forms to assure therapeutic levels are maintained.

BASIC CLINICAL PHARMACOKINETIC PARAMETERS

Lamotrigine is eliminated primarily via glucuronidation by the uridine 5'-diphospho-glucuronosyltransferase (UDP-glucuronosyltransferase or UGT) system. UGT1A4 appears to be the principle isoenzyme involved in the reaction.[19] After single doses of lamotrigine to normal subjects, 86% of the administered dose was recovered as glucuronidated metabolites (76% 2-N-glucuronide, 10% 5-N-glucuronide) and 10% was recovered as unchanged lamotrigine.[20-23] Lamotrigine follows linear pharmacokinetics within the typical dosage range.[11,24-26]

For oral use, lamotrigine is available in a variety of immediate-release tablets (tablets: 25 mg, 50 mg, 100 mg, 150 mg, 200 mg; chewable tablets: 2 mg, 5 mg, 25 mg; orally disintegrating tablets: 25 mg, 50 mg, 100 mg) and as extended-release tablets (25 mg, 50 mg, 100 mg, 200 mg, 250 mg, 300 mg). Chewable tablets can be swallowed whole, chewed, crushed, or dispersed in water or fruit juice for administration. Disintegrating tablets are placed on the tongue and then they are swished around in the mouth. If desired, water can be used to help swallow the medication after disintegration.

During multiple dosing, peak concentrations occur at about the same time (T_{max}) for all of immediate-release dosage forms (1.5-2.0 hours) when given twice daily.[25,27,28] For multiple doses of the extended-release dosage form administered once daily, T_{max} depends on the other medications that patients take.[17,29,30] During concurrent therapy with hepatic enzyme inducers (carbamazepine, phenytoin, phenobarbital, and/or primidone), the T_{max} for extended-release lamotrigine tablets is 4-6 hours. When given concomitantly with valproic acid, T_{max} for lamotrigine extended-release tablets equals 9-11 hours. When administered with other antiepileptic drugs, lamotrigine extended-release tablets have a T_{max} of 6-10 hours. If patients take other antiepileptic drugs that induce hepatic enzymes (such as carbamazepine, phenytoin, phenobarbital, or primidone) and switch from immediate-release lamotrigine to the identical daily dose of extended-release lamotrigine, area under the serum concentration curve may be reduced by clinically significant amounts (as much as 70%). When patients are switched between dosage forms, they should be closely monitored for changes in efficacy or toxicity, and measurement of lamotrigine serum concentrations should be considered before and after the change has been made.

Absorption of orally administered lamotrigine is nearly 100% and is not affected by concomitant administration with food.[16,31,32] Specific initial dosage titration is recommended to avoid adverse effects, so the manufacturers of lamotrigine provide special packaging of the medication in the form of starter packs or titration kits as an adherence aid for patients.

The plasma protein binding of lamotrigine is 55%, and the average volume of distribution ranges from 0.9 to 1.3 L/kg.[16,25,27,28,32,33] Lamotrigine crosses the placental barrier, and at birth the umbilical cord blood to maternal serum concentration ratio is approximately 1.0.[34-36] Lamotrigine also crosses into the breast milk of lactating mothers with a breast milk to maternal serum ratio of 0.59 (range: 0.35-0.86).[34,36] After breastfeeding from mothers taking lamotrigine (median maternal lamotrigine serum concentration = 9.0 μg/mL), the resulting median lamotrigine serum concentration in four newborns was 2.2 μg/mL.[36] In individual neonates and young infants, serum lamotrigine concentrations have been measured as high as 50% of the concurrent maternal amount in the serum.[17] The lamotrigine saliva-to-serum ratio after single doses is 0.46.[27]

EFFECTS OF DISEASES AND CONDITIONS ON PHARMACOKINETICS AND DOSING

Adults with normal liver and kidney function that take no hepatic enzyme inducers or inhibitors have an average half-life of 33 hours and an average clearance of 0.44 mL/min/kg for lamotrigine (Table 15-2).[27,37-40] The volume of distribution of lamotrigine is 0.9-1.3 L/kg. Because plasma protein binding is moderate (~55%), it is not altered to a large degree by the disease states or conditions that alter lamotrigine pharmacokinetics, and volume of distribution is similar for most patients.[16,25,27,28,32,33]

TABLE 15-2   Disease States and Conditions That Alter Lamotrigine Pharmacokinetics

Disease State/Condition	Half-Life	Clearance	Comment
Adult, normal liver and kidney function	33 h (range: 14-103 h)	0.44 mL/min/kg	Lamotrigine is eliminated by glucuronidation via the UGT system. UGT1A4 is the principle isoenzyme involved in lamotrigine elimination. About 10% of lamotrigine is eliminated unchanged in the urine.
Adults, chronic renal failure (average CrCl = 13 mL/min, range: 6-23 mL/min)	43-57 h	N/A	During 4 h hemodialysis period, ~20% (range: 6%-35%) of lamotrigine was removed. Half-life during hemodialysis averaged 13 h.
Adults, hepatic disease	*Mild hepatic disease:* 46 h	0.30 mL/min/kg	Severity of hepatic disease stratified using Child-Pugh scores (mild = 5-6 points, moderate = 7-9 points, severe = 10-15 points). Pharmacokinetic parameters highly variable in liver disease patients.
	Moderate hepatic disease: 72 h	0.24 mL/min/kg	
	Severe hepatic disease w/o ascites: 67 h	0.21 mL/min/kg	
	Severe hepatic disease with ascites: 100 h	0.15 mL/min/kg	

(Continued)

TABLE 15-2   Disease States and Conditions That Alter Lamotrigine Pharmacokinetics (*Continued*)

Disease State/Condition	Half-Life	Clearance	Comment
Adult, pregnant women (ages 23-37 y)	*Prepregnancy:* N/A	39 L/d	Pregnancy increases the clearance of lamotrigine compared to preconception values. The increase continues through the 2nd trimester and then stabilizes. After delivery, lamotrigine clearance declines quickly over a 2-wk period to prepregnancy levels.
	1st trimester N/A	77 L/d	
	2nd trimester N/A	92 L/d	
	3rd trimester N/A	97 L/d	
	Delivery N/A	103 L/d	
	1st wk postpartum N/A	85 L/d	
	2nd wk postpartum N/A	35 L/d	
Adult, elderly (ages 65-76 y)	31 h (range: 25-43 h)	0.40 mL/min/kg (range: 0.26-0.48 mL/min/kg)	Mean CrCl = 61 mL/min (range: 33-108)
Pediatric patients *Age: 10 mo-5.3 y*	*Taking phenytoin, carbamazepine, phenobarbital, or primidone:* 8 h	3.6 mL/min/kg	For the pediatric population, lamotrigine population pharmacokinetics has been determined while the patients took a variety of other antiepileptic drugs (AEDs). Many AEDs are inducers (phenytoin, carbamazepine, phenobarbital, or primidone) or inhibitors (valproate) of lamotrigine clearance.
	Taking other AEDs with no known influence on pharmacokinetics of lamotrigine: 19 h	1.2 mL/min/kg	
	Taking valproate: 45 h	0.47 mL/min/kg	
Age: 5-11 y	*Taking phenytoin, carbamazepine, phenobarbital, or primidone:* 7 h	2.5 mL/min/kg	
	Taking phenytoin, carbamazepine, phenobarbital, or primidone **in addition to** *valproate:* 19 h	0.89 mL/min/kg	
	Taking valproate: 66 h	0.24 mL/min/kg	
Age: 13-18 y	*Taking phenytoin, carbamazepine, phenobarbital, or primidone:* N/A	1.3 mL/min/kg	
	Taking phenytoin, carbamazepine, phenobarbital, or primidone **in addition to** *valproate:* N/A	0.5 mL/min/kg	
	Taking valproate: N/A	0.3 mL/min/kg	

TABLE 15-3   Child-Pugh Scores for Patients With Liver Disease

Test/Symptom	Score 1 Point	Score 2 Points	Score 3 Points
Total bilirubin (mg/dL)	<2.0	2.0-3.0	>3.0
Serum albumin (g/dL)	>3.5	2.8-3.5	<2.8
Prothrombin time (seconds prolonged over control)	<4	4-6	>6
Ascites	Absent	Slight	Moderate
Hepatic encephalopathy	None	Moderate	Severe

Mild liver disease, 5-6 points; moderate liver disease, 7-9 points; severe liver disease, 10-15 points.

Since a small amount of lamotrigine is eliminated unchanged in the urine (~10%), there is only a modest increase in average half-life for subjects with renal failure, and the range for these individuals falls within the range of adults with normal kidney function.[22,23,26,41] During a 4-hour hemodialysis session, about 20% of the total body amount of lamotrigine is removed, and the lamotrigine half-life during the procedure decreases to a mean value of 13 hours.[42,43] For hemodialysis patients receiving lamotrigine treatment, serum concentration measurement before and after the dialysis procedure can be helpful to ascertain the need for a posthemodialysis replacement dose.

The majority of a lamotrigine dose (~90%) is eliminated by glucuronidation via UGT, and UGT1A4 appears to be the principal isozyme involved.[19-23] Because of this, hepatic disease prolongs lamotrigine half-life and decreases lamotrigine clearance in a graded manner according to the degree of liver damage observed in the patient.[44] An index of liver dysfunction can be gained by applying the Child-Pugh clinical classification system to the patient (Table 15-3).[45] Child-Pugh scores are completely discussed in Chapter 3 (Drug Dosing in Special Populations: Renal and Hepatic Disease, Dialysis, Heart Failure, Obesity, and Drug Interactions), but will be briefly discussed here. The Child-Pugh score consists of five laboratory tests or clinical symptoms: serum albumin, total bilirubin, prothrombin time, ascites, and hepatic encephalopathy. Each of these areas is given a score of 1 (normal) to 3 (severely abnormal; see Table 15-2), and the scores for the five areas are summed. The Child-Pugh score for a patient with normal liver function is 5 while the score for a patient with grossly abnormal serum albumin, total bilirubin, and prothrombin time values in addition to severe ascites and hepatic encephalopathy is 15. The pharmacokinetic changes for lamotrigine range from modest ones (half-life = 46 hours, clearance = 0.30 mL/min/kg) for patients with mild liver disease (Child-Pugh score = 5-6 points) to large ones (half-life = 100 hours, clearance = 0.15 mL/min/kg) for patients with severe liver disease that includes ascites (Child-Pugh score = 10-15 points, that includes ascites as one of the scored characteristics).[17,18,44] Generally, no change in dose is needed for patients with mild liver disease. But, for patients with moderate or severe liver disease, decreases are needed for initial, escalation, and maintenance doses (~25% for moderate or severe liver disease without ascites, ~50% for severe liver disease with ascites). Escalation and maintenance doses should be titrated to clinical response, and measurement of lamotrigine serum concentrations can be a helpful adjunct. Because there is a large amount of variability in pharmacokinetics, patients with liver disease should be closely monitored for adverse effects due to lamotrigine therapy.

Pediatric patients taking lamotrigine for the treatment of seizures have been studied while taking other antiepileptics medications, so it is important to take concurrent medications into account when interpreting the findings of pharmacokinetic studies (see Table 15-2).[46-58] For children between the ages of 10 months and 5.3 years taking other antiepileptic drugs that are not thought to cause drug interactions with lamotrigine, the mean lamotrigine half-life was 19 hours and the mean lamotrigine clearance was 1.2 mL/min/kg. This pattern of higher clearance and shorter half-life compared to adults is observed with most other medications. The expected pattern of pharmacokinetic changes is also found in pediatric patients taking other antiepileptic drugs that are hepatic enzyme inducers (phenytoin, carbamazepine, phenobarbital, primidone: lamotrigine clearance = 3.6 mL/min/kg, lamotrigine half-life = 8 hours) or hepatic enzyme inhibitors (valproate: lamotrigine clearance = 0.47 mL/min/kg, lamotrigine half-life = 45 hours). Similar situations are observed with lamotrigine pharmacokinetics for older children aged 5-11 years and 13-18 years. When these age groups are administered lamotrigine concurrently with antiepileptics that are hepatic enzyme inducers, lamotrigine clearance is higher and lamotrigine half-life is shorter compared to adults, but there is a gradual change toward adult values as age increases, especially in teenaged patients. For the two older pediatric patient groups, it is also possible to see the effects of mixed coadministration of antiepileptic drugs that are hepatic enzyme inducers and inhibitors. In these cases, concomitant administration of valproate modulates the induction effect of phenytoin, carbamazepine, phenobarbital, or primidone therapy on lamotrigine pharmacokinetics.

Lamotrigine disposition has also been investigated in older adults (age range: 65-76 years, mean CrCl: 61 mL/min).[38] In this investigation, the pharmacokinetic parameters for lamotrigine was very similar to those measured in younger adults (see Table 15-2). Note that the subjects in this study had relatively good renal function for their age. Many elderly patients will have poorer renal function, and these individuals may have some moderate changes in the pharmacokinetics of lamotrigine.[59]

Using the FDA pregnancy classification system, lamotrigine is a Category C medication. So, lamotrigine is used to treat pregnant women when the potential benefits of drug therapy outweigh the potential risks. The clearance of lamotrigine is altered as the pregnancy progresses (see Table 15-2).[36] Compared to prepregnancy values, clearance increases through the first trimester and finally stabilizes during the second semester. Clearance remains increased until delivery, then starts to decline. By the second postpartum week, lamotrigine clearance returns to baseline values.

DRUG INTERACTIONS

Lamotrigine is eliminated via glucuronidation by the UGT system.[20-23] UGT1A4 is thought to be the principal isozyme involved in this reaction.[19] Lamotrigine pharmacokinetics are affected by enzyme inducers and inhibitors of this enzymatic pathway.[60,61] The principal enzyme inducers of lamotrigine clearance are the other antiepileptic drugs phenytoin, carbamazepine, phenobarbital, or primidone, and lamotrigine is commonly used in combination with these agents.[25,28,51,52,56,62] Valproate is the principal enzyme inhibitor of lamotrigine clearance.[28,40,51,52,56,62] Specific initial, escalation, and maintenance doses are recommended for patients taking combinations of one or more of these inducers and/or this inhibitor of lamotrigine clearance (Tables 15-4 to 15-6).[17,18] Obviously, these drug interactions may take place whether the patient is being treated for seizures or bipolar disorders.

Studies conducted in patients or subjects taking single or multiple doses of lamotrigine indicate that lamotrigine clearance is increased by 109%-150% when taken with phenytoin, carbamazepine, phenobarbital, or primidone (adults: mean Cl = 1.1-1.2 mL/min/kg, mean $t_{1/2}$ = 12-14 hours; children: see Table 15-2). However, when one of these other antiepileptic drugs is taken with valproate, lamotrigine clearance is decreased 20% from baseline (adults: mean Cl = 0.53 mL/min/kg, mean $t_{1/2}$ = 27 hours; children: see Table 15-2). When lamotrigine is taken only with valproate, lamotrigine clearance decreases by 32%-69% (adults: mean Cl = 0.28 mL/min/kg, mean $t_{1/2}$ = 59 hours; children: see Table 15-2). Clearly, valproate is such a potent inhibitor of lamotrigine elimination that it is able to negate the induction of metabolism due to several other antiepileptic drugs.

Other hepatic enzyme inducers of lamotrigine include efavirenz, nevirapine, oxcarbazepine, rifabutin, rifampin, rifapentine, and St. John's wort.[60] Oral contraceptives that contain an estrogen component (most commonly ethinyl estradiol) also induce lamotrigine clearance.[60,61] When taken concurrently with an ethinyl estradiol–containing oral contraceptive, lamotrigine clearance nearly doubled. However, during the placebo or drug-free week of oral contraceptive therapy in women taking the medication cyclically in order to induce

TABLE 15-4 Initial, Escalation, and Maintenance Doses of Lamotrigine for Initial Adjunctive Therapy of Epilepsy for Patients 13 Years or Older[a]

Time Frame	Immediate-Release Tablets			Extended-Release Tablets (*administered once daily*)		
	Taking Valproate Concurrently	Not Taking Enzyme Inducers[b] or Valproate	Taking Enzyme Inducers[b] and Not Taking Valproate	Taking Valproate Concurrently	Not Taking Enzyme Inducers[b] or Valproate	Taking Enzyme Inducers[b] and Not Taking Valproate
Weeks 1 and 2	25 mg every other day	25 mg/d	50 mg/d	25 mg every other day	25 mg/d	50 mg/d
Weeks 3 and 4	25 mg/d	50 mg/d	100 mg/d (give as 2 divided doses)	25 mg/d	50 mg/d	100 mg/d
Week 5	Increase by 25-50 mg/d every 1-2 wks until maintenance dose achieved (-week 8)	Increase by 50 mg/d every 1-2 wks until maintenance dose achieved (-week 8; give doses of 100 mg/d and above as 2 divided doses)	Increase by 100 mg/d every 1-2 wks until maintenance dose achieved (-week 8, give as 2 divided doses)	50 mg/d	100 mg/d	200 mg/d
Week 6	N/A	N/A	N/A	100 mg/d	150 mg/d	300 mg/d
Week 7	N/A	N/A	N/A	150 mg/d	200 mg/d	400 mg/d
Typical maintenance doses from week 8 and continuing	100-200 mg/d when taking with valproate alone or 100-400 mg/d when taking with valproate plus other inducers of glucuronidation. Give either regimen as 1-2 divided doses.	225-375 mg/d (give as 2 divided doses)	300-500 mg/d (give as 2 divided doses)	200-250 mg/d[c]	300-400 mg/d[c]	400-600 mg/d[c]

[a]Reduce initial, escalation, and maintenance doses by 25% for moderate (Child-Pugh score = 7-9 points) or severe (Child-Pugh score = 10-15 points) liver disease *without* ascites or by 50% for severe (Child-Pugh score = 10-15 points) liver disease *with* ascites.

[b]Enzyme inducers include phenytoin, carbamazepine, phenobarbital, or primidone.

[c]Additional dosage increases should not exceed 100 mg/d on a weekly basis.

TABLE 15-5   Escalation Doses of Lamotrigine for Initial Adjunctive Therapy of Epilepsy for Patients 2-12 Years[a]

Time Frame	Taking Valproate Concurrently[b]	Not Taking Enzyme Inducers[c] or Valproate[b] Concurrently	Taking Enzyme Inducers[c] and Not Taking Valproate[b] Concurrently
Weeks 1 and 2	0.15 mg/kg/d, given as 1-2 divided doses.	0.3 mg/kg/d, given as 1-2 divided doses.	0.6 mg/kg/d, given as 2 divided doses.
Weeks 3 and 4	0.3 mg/kg/d, given as 1-2 divided doses.	0.6 mg/kg/d, given in 2 divided doses.	1.2 mg/kg/d, given in 2 divided doses.
Week 5 to the time maintenance dose is established	Every 1-2 wks increase by 0.3 mg/kg/d, round increase to whole tablet amount, then add to previous dose. Give as 1-2 divided doses.	Every 1-2 wks increase by 0.6 mg/kg/d, round increase to whole tablet amount, then add to previous dose. Give as 2 divided doses.	Every 1-2 wks increase by 1.2 mg/kg/d, round increase to whole tablet amount, then add to previous dose. Give as 2 divided doses.
Typical maintenance dose	1-5 mg/kg/d (maximum dose 200 mg/d), given as 1-2 divided doses or 1-3 mg/kg/d with valproate alone, given as 1-2 divided doses.	4.5-7.5 mg/kg/d (maximum dose 300 mg/d), given as 2 divided doses.	5-15 mg/kg/d (maximum dose 400 mg/d), given as 2 divided doses.
Typical maintenance dose for patients with weight <30 kg	Dose might need to be increased by as much as 50% (in mg/kg/d), based on the clinical response of the patient.	Dose might need to be increased by as much as 50% (in mg/kg/d), based on the clinical response of the patient.	Dose might need to be increased by as much as 50% (in mg/kg/d), based on the clinical response of the patient.

[a]For patients weighing <30 kg, maintenance doses may need to be up to 50% higher for all ages and concurrent drug therapy categories.
[b]Only whole tablets should be used for dosing to avoid errors due to inaccurate splitting of tablets, and the smallest appropriate tablet for pediatric patients is 2 mg. Calculated doses should be rounded down to the nearest whole tablet amount.
[c]Enzyme inducers include phenytoin, carbamazepine, phenobarbital, or primidone.

withdrawal bleeding, lamotrigine concentrations increased twofold in 7 days. One recommended solution to this situation is to use an oral contraceptive with a different hormone composition.[60] Specific recommendations for maintenance doses of lamotrigine are available for patients starting, stopping, or taking estrogen-containing oral contraceptives (see *Initial Dosage Determination Methods* section).

TABLE 15-6   Escalation Doses of Immediate-Release Lamotrigine for Patients With Bipolar Disorder for Patients 18 Years and Older

Time Frame	Taking Valproate Concurrently	Not Taking Enzyme Inducers[a] or Valproate	Taking Enzyme Inducers[a] and Not Taking Valproate
Weeks 1 and 2	25 mg every other day	25 mg/d	50 mg/d
Weeks 3 and 4	25 mg/d	50 mg/d	100 mg/d, given twice daily
Week 5	50 mg/d	100 mg/d	200 mg/d, given twice daily
Week 6	100 mg/d	200 mg/d	300 mg/d, given twice daily
Week 7 (target dose)	100 mg/d	200 mg/d	Up to 400 mg/d, given twice daily

[a]Enzyme inducers include phenytoin, carbamazepine, phenobarbital, or primidone.

Lamotrigine therapy may increase the carbamazepine-10,11-epoxide to carbamazepine ratio in some patients.[63,64] Because the epoxide is an active metabolite with pharmacology similar to carbamazepine, patients taking lamotrigine and carbamazepine together may experience enhanced therapeutic effects or toxicities of carbamazepine with a decrease or no change in carbamazepine serum concentrations.[61]

INITIAL DOSAGE DETERMINATION METHODS

Although the risk factors for developing life-threatening rashes due to lamotrigine are not completely understood, there are suggestions in the literature that the incidence may be increased by concomitant administration of valproate, administration of initial lamotrigine doses that exceed the maximum recommended amount, or escalation of lamotrigine doses during the titration phase that exceeds the maximum recommended rate. Because of this, initial doses of lamotrigine are low, and the rate of dosage increase to target therapeutic amounts is slow. Additionally, initial dose and rate of dosage increase are adjusted to reflect changes in lamotrigine pharmacokinetics due to other drug therapy and disease states or conditions that the patient may have. While some clinicians prefer to use custom algorithms for initial doses and dosage titration of lamotrigine, many use the literature-based recommendations given in the prescribing information for lamotrigine because of the potential risk and ramifications of developing a rash during therapy (Tables 15-4 to 15-7).[17,18]

When used as adjunctive therapy for epilepsy, initial, escalation, and target doses for lamotrigine are stratified by age, dosage form, and concurrent drug therapy (see Tables 15-4 and 15-5). For pediatric patients weighing <30 kg, maintenance doses may need to be up to 50% higher for all ages and concurrent drug therapy categories (see Table 15-5). For initiation and escalation of lamotrigine as monotherapy, the recommendations for "not taking enzyme inducers or valproate" can be used.

Each category contains escalation dosage titrations that take several weeks to attain the target dosage. Because the titration process is complicated, some manufacturers have made available titration blister packs for the various dosage scenarios that may aid patient adherence to the regimen. Similarly, initial, escalation, and target doses of lamotrigine for bipolar disorders are stratified by concurrent drug therapy (see Table 15-6).

TABLE 15-7 Conversion to Monotherapy With Immediate-Release or Extended-Release Lamotrigine From Adjunctive Treatment With Concurrent Valproate for the Treatment of Epilepsy

Interval	Immediate-Release Lamotrigine (≥16 years old)	Extended-Release Lamotrigine (≥13 years old)	Concurrent Valproate
Step 1	Attain (if not already; use dosage escalation algorithm) or maintain dose of 200 mg/d	Attain (if not already; use dosage escalation algorithm) or maintain dose of 150 mg/d	Continue current maintenance dose.
Step 2	Continue 200 mg/d	Continue 150 mg/d	Decrease maintenance dose to 500 mg/d at a rate no >500 mg/d per week. Then, administer maintenance dose of 500 mg/d for 1 week.
Step 3	Increase dose to 300 mg/d and continue for 1 week	Increase dose to 200 mg/d and continue for 1 week	At same time as lamotrigine dosage increase, decrease valproate dose to 250 mg/d and continue for 1 week.
Step 4	Increase dose by 100 mg/d every week, until target maintenance dose of 500 mg/d is achieved	Increase dose to 250-300 mg/d	Discontinue valproate

Specific recommendations are available to convert epileptic patient drug therapy from concurrent therapy with lamotrigine and valproate to monotherapy with lamotrigine (see Table 15-7). Conversion of concurrent drug therapy with other antiepileptic drugs that are hepatic enzyme inducers (phenytoin, carbamazepine, phenobarbital, primidone) and lamotrigine to monotherapy with lamotrigine is conducted in two steps. First, using the recommendations in Table 15-4 for patients taking enzyme inducers with lamotrigine, establish a lamotrigine dose of 500 mg/d. Second, withdraw the other antiepileptic drug by reducing the dose by 20%, then continuing the same weekly decrease for 4 weeks until it is discontinued. For the extended-release tablets only, the target dose for lamotrigine monotherapy is 250-300 mg/d (compared to 500 mg/d for immediate-release lamotrigine tablets) so additional lamotrigine dosage titration is needed for this dosage form. After an additional 2 weeks have passed to allow hepatic enzyme induction to diminish, the lamotrigine extended-release dose may be decreased by 50-100 mg/d on a weekly basis, as needed, until the target dose is attained.

Although estrogen-containing oral contraceptives (principally those containing ethinyl estradiol, not progestin-only pills) are known to increase the clearance of lamotrigine, the recommended initial, escalation, and titration schedules for initiation of lamotrigine treatment should be followed in women taking these types of birth control pills (see Table 15-4). Eventually, maintenance doses for these individuals may need to be increased by as much as twofold according to clinical response. For women already receiving a stable maintenance dose of lamotrigine, starting estrogen-containing oral contraceptive therapy will probably require an increased maintenance dose of lamotrigine. When this is the case, lamotrigine dosage increases can be started at the same time as the estrogen-containing oral contraceptive, and the rate of dosage increase should be no greater than 50-100 mg/d on a weekly basis. Additionally, dose increases should not be greater than recommended by the disease state–specific escalation recommendations (see Tables 15-4 and 15-6) unless needed to maintain clinical response or effective lamotrigine serum concentrations. If the patient is taking cyclic estrogen-containing oral contraceptives with placebo or no tablets for a week, lamotrigine serum concentrations can increase during this time period, causing adverse effects. In this case, doses of lamotrigine may need to be decreased for the entire 28-day cycle. For patients already taking other inducers of glucuronidation (phenytoin, carbamazepine, phenobarbital, primidone, rifampin, etc), it may not be necessary to change maintenance doses of lamotrigine when oral contraceptive therapy is started.

When women stop taking estrogen-containing oral contraceptives, lamotrigine maintenance doses may need to be decreased by as much as 50%.[17,18] Doses should be decreased slowly in a stepwise fashion, no faster than 25% decrements per week over a 2-week time frame unless clinical response or lamotrigine serum concentrations support a different approach. For women taking other inducers of glucuronidation (phenytoin, carbamazepine, phenobarbital, primidone, rifampin, etc), it may not be necessary to alter maintenance doses of lamotrigine.

Generally, no change in dose is needed for patients with mild liver disease (Child-Pugh score = 5-6 points). But, for patients with moderate (Child-Pugh score = 7-9 points) or severe liver disease (Child-Pugh score = 10-15 points), decreases are needed for initial, escalation, and maintenance doses (~25% for moderate or severe liver disease without ascites, ~50% for severe liver disease with ascites). Escalation and maintenance doses should be titrated to clinical response, and measurement of lamotrigine serum concentrations can be a helpful adjunct. Of course, patients with liver disease should be closely monitored for adverse effects due to lamotrigine therapy.

Since only a small amount of lamotrigine is eliminated unchanged in the urine (~10%), dosing changes for patients with renal failure are usually not necessary. However, hemodialysis does clear lamotrigine from the body, and during a 4-hour hemodialysis session, about 20% of the total body amount of lamotrigine is removed. For hemodialysis patients receiving lamotrigine treatment, serum concentration measurement before and after the dialysis procedure can be helpful to ascertain the need for a posthemodialysis replacement dose.

If discontinuation of lamotrigine is necessary due to lack of therapeutic response or to development of adverse effects, the dosage should be tapered for patients taking the medication for either epilepsy or bipolar disorder. Unless the clinical situation dictates otherwise, lamotrigine doses should be decreased by about 50% per week over at least 2 weeks.

Literature-Based Recommended Dosing

The following examples illustrate the use of literature-based recommended dosing for different patient situations.

EXAMPLE 1 ▶▶▶

KL is a 51-year-old, 75-kg (height = 5 ft 10 in) male with complex partial seizures who requires adjunctive therapy with lamotrigine. He has normal liver and renal function and is currently taking carbamazepine (steady-state concentration = 9.2 µg/mL). Additional dosage increases have been tried with carbamazepine, but they have been unsuccessful due to development of adverse effects. Suggest an initial lamotrigine dosage regimen using immediate-release tablets for this patient.

1. *Estimate lamotrigine dose according to age, disease states and conditions, dosage form, and concurrent drug therapy.*
   For an adult patient taking carbamazepine who will be treated with immediate-release lamotrigine tablets, the initial doses given in Table 15-4 can be used.

   For the first 2 weeks, the initial dose should be 50 mg/d. For the next 2 weeks of therapy, the dose can be escalated to 100 mg/d, given as 50 mg twice daily. During week 5, the dose can be escalated by 100 mg/d to a total dose 200 mg/d, given as 100 mg twice daily. Subsequently, every 1-2 weeks the dose can be increased by 100 mg/d (eg, 300 mg/d as 150 mg twice daily, 400 mg/d as 200 mg twice daily, and 500 mg/d as 250 mg twice daily), until an effective target dose of 300-500 mg/d without adverse effects is attained.

   KL was titrated to a dose of lamotrigine 250 mg twice daily without any additional side effects and a decreased seizure frequency.

EXAMPLE 2 ▶▶▶

KL is a 51-year-old, 75-kg (height = 5 ft 10 in) male with complex partial seizures who requires monotherapy with lamotrigine. He has normal liver and renal function. Suggest an initial lamotrigine dosage regimen using immediate-release tablets for this patient. (*Note: This is a similar patient profile as example 1, except for no concurrent antiepileptic drug therapy, so that the differences can be contrasted.*)

1. *Estimate lamotrigine dose according to age, disease states and conditions, dosage form, and concurrent drug therapy.*
   For an adult patient taking no other antiepileptic drugs who will be treated with immediate-release lamotrigine tablets, the initial doses given in Table 15-4 can be used. (*Note: Lamotrigine is not FDA approved as initial monotherapy treatment for complex partial seizures, although it is considered to be one of the drugs of choice by several expert panels [see Table 15-1]*).

   For the first 2 weeks, the initial dose should be 25 mg/d. For the next 2 weeks of therapy, the dose can be escalated to 50 mg/d. During week 5, the dose can be escalated by 50 mg/d to a total dose 100 mg/d, given as 50 mg twice daily. Subsequently, every 1-2 weeks the dose can be increased by 50 mg/d (eg, 150 mg/d as 75 mg twice daily, 200 mg/d as 100 mg twice daily, etc), until an effective target dose of 225-375 mg/d without adverse effects is attained.

   KL was titrated to a dose of lamotrigine 125 mg twice daily (250 mg/d) without any side effects and a decreased seizure frequency.

EXAMPLE 3 ▶▶▶

KL is a 51-year-old, 75-kg (height = 5 ft 10 in) male with complex partial seizures who requires monotherapy with lamotrigine. He has normal liver and renal function. Suggest an initial lamotrigine dosage regimen using extended-release tablets for this patient. (*Note: This is a similar patient profile as example 2, except for use of extended-release tablets, so that the differences can be contrasted.*)

1. *Estimate lamotrigine dose according to age, disease states and conditions, dosage form, and concurrent drug therapy.*
For an adult patient taking no other antiepileptic drugs who will be treated with extended-release lamotrigine tablets, the initial doses given in Table 15-4 can be used. (*Note: Lamotrigine is not FDA approved as initial monotherapy treatment for complex partial seizures, although it is considered to be one of the drugs of choice by several expert panels [see Table 15-1]*).

For the first 2 weeks, the initial dose should be 25 mg/d (extended-release tablets administered once daily). For the next 2 weeks of therapy, the dose can be escalated to 50 mg/d. During week 5, the dose can be escalated by 50 mg/d to a total dose of 100 mg/d. During week 6 the dose can be advanced to 150 mg/d, and during week 7 the dose is increased to 200 mg/d. For week 8, the dose can be incremented again so that the lower target dose of 300 mg/d is attained, and, if needed, this can be increased to 400 mg/d the next week.

KL was titrated to a dose of lamotrigine extended-release tablets 400 mg/d without any side effects and a decreased seizure frequency.

EXAMPLE 4 ▶▶▶

AZ is a 9-year-old, 35-kg (height = 4 ft 6 in) female with simple partial seizures who requires adjunctive therapy with lamotrigine. She has normal liver and renal function and is currently taking carbamazepine (steady-state concentration = 10.4 µg/mL). Additional dosage increases have been tried with carbamazepine, but they have been unsuccessful due to development of adverse effects. Suggest an initial lamotrigine dosage regimen using immediate-release tablets for this patient.

1. *Estimate lamotrigine dose according to age, disease states and conditions, dosage form, and concurrent drug therapy.*
For a pediatric patient taking carbamazepine who will be treated with immediate-release lamotrigine tablets, the initial doses given in Table 15-5 can be used.

For the first 2 weeks, the initial dose should be 0.6 mg/kg/d or 10 mg twice daily (0.6 mg/kg/d • 35 kg = 21 mg/d, rounded down to 20 mg/d chewable tablets). For the next 2 weeks of therapy, the dose can be escalated to 1.2 mg/kg/d (1.2 mg/kg/d • 35 kg = 42 mg/d, rounded down to 40 mg/d chewable tablets), given as 20 mg twice daily. During week 5, the dose can be escalated by 1.2 mg/kg/d (additional 1.2 mg/kg/d • 35 kg = 42 mg/d, added to current dose and rounded down to 80 mg/d chewable tablets), given as 40 mg twice daily. Subsequently, every 1-2 weeks the dose can be increased by 1.2 mg/kg/d, until an effective target dose of 5-15 mg/kg/d (maximum dose 400 mg/d) without adverse effects is attained.

Over the next several weeks, AZ was titrated to a dose of lamotrigine chewable tablets 150 mg twice daily without any additional side effects and a decreased seizure frequency. Within 6 months, she was switched to lamotrigine tablets 150 mg twice daily when she could swallow whole tablets without any distress. Therapeutic response remained constant after the dosage form switch, with no change in seizure frequency or adverse effects.

EXAMPLE 5 ▶▶▶

MM is a 23-year-old, 55-kg (height = 5 ft 3 in) female with bipolar disorder that requires monotherapy with lamotrigine. She has normal liver and renal function, and she does not take oral contraceptives. Suggest an initial lamotrigine dosage regimen using immediate-release tablets for this patient.

1. *Estimate lamotrigine dose according to age, disease states and conditions, dosage form, and concurrent drug therapy.*
For a bipolar disorder patient taking lamotrigine immediate-release tablet monotherapy, the initial doses given in Table 15-6 can be used.

For the first 2 weeks, the lamotrigine dose should be 25 mg/d. For the next 2 weeks, the dose can be increased to 50 mg/d. During weeks 5 and 6, the dose is increased to 100 mg/d and 200 mg/d, respectively (maximum target dose: 200 mg/d).

MM was titrated to a dose of 200 mg/d of lamotrigine immediate-release tablets with a decrease in the frequency and severity of bipolar episodes and no adverse effects.

USE OF LAMOTRIGINE SERUM CONCENTRATIONS TO ALTER DOSES

A definitive therapeutic range for steady-state lamotrigine serum concentrations has not been established.[13-16] Because of this, serum concentration monitoring for lamotrigine plays only a supportive role in the dosing of the drug. Important patient parameters (seizure frequency or frequency/severity of mood episodes, potential lamotrigine side effects, etc) should be followed to confirm that the patient is responding to treatment and not developing adverse drug reactions.[8,12] However, there are clinical situations where lamotrigine serum concentration can be very helpful.

Once dosage titration has been conducted, and an effective dose of lamotrigine has been established by assessing therapeutic response and absence of adverse effects, many clinicians obtain a steady-state lamotrigine concentration to establish an individualized effective target value for the patient. When this is done, if seizure frequency changes or an adverse effect occurs, another lamotrigine serum concentration can be measured to ascertain potential solutions to the problem. For instance, if a patient suddenly has more seizures than usual, comparing the current lamotrigine serum concentration with the established effective target lamotrigine concentration can be helpful to decide a course of action. If the current lamotrigine concentration is lower than usual, reasons for the change can be explored (lack of adherence to therapy, drug interaction, etc), and, if appropriate, a lamotrigine dosage increase can be considered to reestablish effective concentrations. If the current lamotrigine concentration is about the same, changes to therapy may be warranted (increase lamotrigine dose, addition of other drug therapy, etc). Alternatively, if a patient suddenly develops adverse effects that could be due to lamotrigine therapy, and the current lamotrigine serum concentration is high, it may be appropriate to decrease the lamotrigine dose. Also, when an effective lamotrigine concentration has been established for a patient, the effects of new drug therapy that may cause drug interactions or of new disease states or conditions that can alter lamotrigine pharmacokinetics can be assessed prospectively by measuring current lamotrigine concentration before any clinical events occur.

Because a definitive therapeutic range for lamotrigine has not be firmly established, and the proposed causal relationship between the rate of lamotrigine dosage changes and the development of a rash, dosage increases are usually capped at 100 mg/d every week. When needed, dosage decreases are usually made using one of the smaller changes possible from available tablet strengths. Even if initial target doses have been successfully attained (see Tables 15-4 and 15-6), further dosage titration is usually limited to no more than 100 mg/d increases every 1-2 weeks. Thus, pharmacokinetic calculations are usually made to compute the expected steady-state concentration after a specific lamotrigine dosage change has been determined rather than computing a new dose based on a desired target concentration. Lamotrigine follows linear pharmacokinetics, the pharmacokinetic calculations involved during dosage titration are straightforward.

When a lamotrigine dosage change is made, sufficient time to attain steady-state conditions (~3-5 half-lives) should be allowed before assessing therapeutic outcome (see Table 15-2). Of course, any time adverse effects occur during dosage titration, measures should be taken to assess the likelihood that they are due to lamotrigine treatment and appropriate action should be taken when needed.

If lamotrigine serum concentrations are measured for patients in support of a dosage change, clinicians should seek to use the simplest, most straightforward method available to determine the steady-state concentration for the new regimen. In most cases, a simple dosage ratio can be used to change doses since lamotrigine follows *linear pharmacokinetics*. In some situations, it may be necessary or desirable to compute lamotrigine *pharmacokinetic parameters* for the patient and utilize these to calculate the steady-state concentration for a new dose.

SELECTION OF APPROPRIATE PHARMACOKINETIC MODEL AND EQUATIONS

Lamotrigine follows a one-compartment pharmacokinetic model. When oral therapy is required, lamotrigine has good bioavailability ($F = 1$) for all dosage forms, and once or twice dosing per day provides a relatively smooth serum concentration-time curve that approximates an intravenous infusion. Because of this, a very simple pharmacokinetic equation that computes the average lamotrigine steady-state serum concentration (Css in $\mu g/mL = mg/L$) is widely used and allows maintenance dosage calculation: $Css = [F(D/\tau)]/Cl$ or $D = (Css \bullet Cl \bullet \tau)/F$, where F is the bioavailability fraction for the oral dosage form ($F = 1$ for oral lamotrigine products), D is the dose of lamotrigine in mg, Cl is lamotrigine clearance in L/h, and τ is the dosage interval in hours.

Linear Pharmacokinetics Method

Because lamotrigine follows linear, dose-proportional pharmacokinetics, steady-state serum concentrations change in proportion to the dose according to the following equation: $D_{new}/C_{ss,new} = D_{old}/C_{ss,old}$ or $C_{ss,new} = (D_{new}/D_{old})C_{ss,old}$, where D is the dose, Css is the steady-state concentration, old indicates the dose that produced the steady-state concentration that the patient is currently receiving, and new denotes the steady-state concentration produced by the newly prescribed dose. The advantages of this method are that it is quick and simple. The disadvantage is steady-state concentrations are required.

EXAMPLE 6 ▶ ▶ ▶

KL is a 51-year-old, 75-kg (height = 5 ft 10 in) male with complex partial seizures who receives monotherapy with lamotrigine. He has normal liver and renal function. KL was titrated to a dose of lamotrigine 125 mg twice daily (250 mg/d) without any side effects and a decreased seizure frequency. At that time, a steady-state lamotrigine concentration was obtained before a dose and equaled 10.2 μg/mL. Several months ago, the patient was started on carbamazepine, and he has been on a stable dose for 4 weeks. Today, the steady-state lamotrigine concentration obtained before the next dose was 7.5 μg/mL. Suggest a new maintenance dosage regimen using immediate-release lamotrigine tablets to reestablish the original lamotrigine steady-state concentration for this patient.

1. *Use linear pharmacokinetics to compute the new concentration for a reasonable dosage increase.*

   Dosage increases for lamotrigine are usually made in increments of no more than 100 mg/d on a weekly basis. This patient is currently receiving 250 mg/d, so the maximum increase for the first week would be 350 mg/d: $C_{ss,new} = (D_{new}/D_{old})C_{ss,old} = (350 \text{ mg/d} / 250 \text{ mg/d})\ 7.5\ \mu g/mL = 10.5\ \mu g/mL$.

   To reestablish the original lamotrigine concentration for the patient, a dosage increase of 350 mg/d or 175 mg twice daily was prescribed. The patient should be carefully monitored for seizure frequency and adverse effects. If desired, steady-state lamotrigine serum concentrations can be measured 3-5 half-lives after the dosage change has been made ($\sim t_{1/2} = 14$ hours, $\sim$3-5 $t_{1/2}$ in 2-3 days).

2. *If the desired steady-state lamotrigine concentrations have not been attained with the first dosage increase, compute the new concentration for the next reasonable dosage increase. Continue titration until the desired steady-state concentration or optimal therapeutic response has been achieved.*

   The desired steady-state lamotrigine concentration has been reached, so this step is not necessary for this patient.

Pharmacokinetic Parameter Method

The Pharmacokinetic Parameter method of adjusting drug doses was among the first techniques available to change doses using serum concentrations. It allows the computation of an individual's own, unique pharmacokinetic constants and uses those to calculate the steady-state concentration that is achieved from a desired lamotrigine dosage regimen. For patients receiving oral lamotrigine, the Pharmacokinetic Parameter method requires that steady-state has been achieved and uses only a single steady-state lamotrigine concentration (Css). Lamotrigine clearance (Cl) can be calculated using the following formula: $Cl = [F(D/\tau)]/Css$, where F is the bioavailability fraction for the oral dosage form (F = 1 for oral lamotrigine products), D is the dose of lamotrigine in mg, Css is the steady-state lamotrigine concentration in mg/L, and τ is the dosage interval in hours.

To illustrate the similarities and differences between this method of dosage calculation and the Pharmacokinetic Parameter method, the same example used in the previous section will be used.

EXAMPLE 7 ▶▶▶

KL is a 51-year-old, 75-kg (height = 5 ft 10 in) male with complex partial seizures who receives monotherapy with lamotrigine. He has normal liver and renal function. KL was titrated to a dose of lamotrigine 125 mg twice daily (250 mg/d) without any side effects and a decreased seizure frequency. At that time, a steady-state lamotrigine concentration was obtained before a dose and equaled 10.2 µg/mL. Several months ago, the patient was started on carbamazepine, and he has been on a stable dose for 4 weeks. Today, the steady-state lamotrigine concentration obtained before the next dose was 7.5 µg/mL. Suggest a new maintenance dosage regimen using immediate-release lamotrigine tablets to reestablish the original lamotrigine steady-state concentration for this patient.

1. *Compute pharmacokinetic parameters.*

    Lamotrigine clearance can be computed using a steady-state lamotrigine concentration: $Cl = [F(D/\tau)]/Css = [1(250\ mg/d)]/(7.5\ mg/L) = 33.3$ L/d. (Note: µg/mL = mg/L and this concentration unit was substituted for Css in the calculations so that unnecessary unit conversion was not required.)

2. *Compute the new concentration for a reasonable lamotrigine dosage increase.*

    Dosage increases for lamotrigine are usually made in increments of no more than 100 mg/d on a weekly basis. This patient is currently receiving 250 mg/d, so the maximum increase for the first week would be 350 mg/d. Lamotrigine clearance is used to compute the steady-state concentration for the new dose: $Css = [F(D/\tau)]/Cl = [1(350\ mg/d)]/(33.3\ L/d) = 10.5$ mg/L.

    To reestablish the original lamotrigine concentration for the patient, a dosage increase of 350 mg/d or 175 mg twice daily was prescribed. The patient should be carefully monitored for seizure frequency and adverse effects. If desired, steady-state lamotrigine serum concentrations can be measured 3-5 half-lives after the dosage change has been made ($\sim t_{1/2} = 14$ hours, $\sim$3-5 $t_{1/2}$ in 2-3 days).

3. *If the desired steady-state lamotrigine concentrations have not been attained with the first dosage increase, compute the new concentration for the next reasonable dosage increase. Continue titration until the desired steady-state concentration or the optimal therapeutic response has been achieved.*

    The desired steady-state lamotrigine concentration has been reached, so this step is not necessary for this patient.

BAYESIAN PHARMACOKINETICS COMPUTER PROGRAMS

Computer programs are available that can assist in the computation of pharmacokinetic parameters for patients. The most reliable computer programs use a nonlinear regression algorithm that incorporates components of Bayes theorem. Nonlinear regression is a statistical technique that uses an iterative process to compute the best pharmacokinetic parameters for a concentration/time data set. Unfortunately, these types of computer programs are not as useful with lamotrigine compared to other antiepileptics due to complex initial dosage administration algorithms and the slow titration of maintenance doses. This dosage adjustment approach cannot be recommended for routine clinical use at this time because of these issues.

SPECIAL DOSING CONSIDERATIONS

Conversion of Patient Doses Between Dosage Forms

For patients stabilized on a maintenance dose of immediate-release lamotrigine tablets (usually administered twice daily), an initial dose of extended-release tablets can be determined by giving the same total daily amount of lamotrigine as a single daily dose. A patient taking a established maintenance dose of extended-release lamotrigine tablets may be converted to immediate-release tablets in a similar fashion. After conversion, patients should be monitored for therapeutic and adverse effects until steady-state is attained. Measurement of lamotrigine steady-state concentrations before and after the change is made may aid in the conversion process. Depending on the clinical response, maintenance doses may need to be readjusted into the target range (see Table 15-4). Patients taking other antiepileptic drugs that are hepatic enzyme inducers (phenytoin, carbamazepine, phenobarbital, primidone) may have lower lamotrigine serum concentrations after the conversion from immediate-release to extended-release lamotrigine, so this patient group should be closely monitored for loss of seizure control after the change is made.

PROBLEMS

The following problems are intended to emphasize the computation of initial and individualized doses using clinical pharmacokinetic techniques. Clinicians should always consult the patient's chart to confirm that current anticonvulsant therapy is appropriate. Additionally, all other medications that the patient is taking, including prescription and nonprescription drugs, should be noted and checked to ascertain if a potential drug interaction with lamotrigine exists.

1. YG is a 45-year-old, 67-kg (height = 5 ft 8 in) female with complex partial seizures who requires adjunctive therapy with lamotrigine. She has normal liver and renal function and is currently taking phenytoin (steady-state concentration = 18.2 μg/mL). Additional dosage increases have been tried with phenytoin, but they have been unsuccessful due to development of adverse effects. She does not take oral contraceptives. Suggest an initial lamotrigine dosage regimen using immediate-release tablets for this patient.

2. WR is a 22-year-old, 80-kg (height = 6 ft 0 in) male with simple partial seizures who requires monotherapy with lamotrigine. He has normal liver and renal function. Suggest an initial lamotrigine dosage regimen using immediate-release tablets for this patient.

3. PO is a 26-year-old, 55-kg (height = 5 ft 2 in) female with tonic-clonic seizures who requires monotherapy with lamotrigine. She has normal liver and renal function, and she does not take oral contraceptives. Suggest an initial lamotrigine dosage regimen using extended-release tablets for this patient.

4. Patient PO (see problem 3) has a new prescription for an estrogen-containing oral contraceptive. She has been taking lamotrigine extended-release tablets 400 mg/d for 6 months (steady-state concentration equals 15 μg/mL) and has an optimal clinical response. Suggest a new lamotrigine dosage regimen using extended-release tablets for this patient.

5. RW is a 56-year-old, 69-kg (height = 6 ft 0 in) male with simple partial seizures who requires monotherapy with lamotrigine. He has normal renal function, but he has severe liver disease (Child-Pugh score = 12, due to bilirubin = 3.2 mg/dL, serum albumin = 2.5 g/dL, prothrombin time = 8 seconds over control,

moderate ascites, and no hepatic encephalopathy). Suggest an initial lamotrigine dosage regimen using immediate-release tablets for this patient.

6. TF is a 33-year-old, 75-kg (height = 6 ft 1 in) male with bipolar disorder that requires monotherapy with lamotrigine. He has normal liver and renal function. Suggest an initial lamotrigine dosage regimen using immediate-release tablets for this patient.

7. FD is a 10-year-old, 35-kg (height = 4 ft 4 in) male with complex partial seizures who requires adjunctive therapy with lamotrigine. He has normal liver and renal function and is currently taking carbamazepine (steady-state concentration = 11.1 µg/mL). Additional dosage increases have been tried with carbamazepine, but they have been unsuccessful due to development of adverse effects. Suggest an initial lamotrigine dosage regimen using immediate-release tablets for this patient.

8. MK is a 41-year-old, 77-kg (height = 5 ft 9 in) male with tonic-clonic seizures who was started on monotherapy with lamotrigine a year ago. He has normal liver and renal function. MK was titrated to a dose of lamotrigine 125 mg twice daily (250 mg/d) without any side effects and a decreased seizure frequency. At that time, a steady-state lamotrigine concentration was obtained before a dose and equaled 10.2 µg/mL. A couple of months ago, the patient was started on carbamazepine, and he has been on a stable dose for 4 weeks (steady-state carbamazepine concentration = 8.9 µg/mL). Today, the steady-state lamotrigine concentration obtained before the next dose was 7.5 µg/mL. Suggest a new maintenance dosage regimen using immediate-release lamotrigine tablets to reestablish the original lamotrigine steady-state concentration for this patient.

9. OZ is a 29-year-old, 85-kg (height = 6 ft 2 in) male with complex partial seizures who was started on monotherapy with carbamazepine 9 months ago. He has normal liver and renal function. OZ has been on a stable carbamazepine dose for the last 8 weeks, and his steady-state carbamazepine concentration currently is 9.9 µg/mL. Two months ago, the patient was started on lamotrigine, and he has been on a stable dose of lamotrigine extended-release tablets 400 mg/d for 1 week. Today, the steady-state lamotrigine concentration obtained before the next dose was 5.2 µg/mL. Compute the expected lamotrigine steady-state concentration for a new dose of 500 mg/d.

ANSWERS TO PROBLEMS

1. *Answer to problem 1.*

Literature-Based Recommended Dosing

1. *Estimate lamotrigine dose according to age, disease states and conditions, dosage form, and concurrent drug therapy.*

For an adult patient taking phenytoin who will be treated with immediate-release lamotrigine tablets, the initial doses given in Table 15-4 can be used.

For the first 2 weeks, the initial dose should be 50 mg/d. For the next 2 weeks of therapy, the dose can be escalated to 100 mg/d, given as 50 mg twice daily. During week 5, the dose can be escalated by 100 mg/d to a total dose 200 mg/d, given as 100 mg twice daily. Subsequently, every 1-2 weeks the dose can be increased by 100 mg/d (eg, 300 mg/d as 150 mg twice daily, 400 mg/d as 200 mg twice daily, and 500 mg/d as 250 mg twice daily), until an effective target dose of 300-500 mg/d without adverse effects is attained.

YG was titrated to a dose of lamotrigine 250 mg twice daily without any additional side effects and a decreased seizure frequency.

2. *Answer to problem 2.*

Literature-Based Recommended Dosing

1. *Estimate lamotrigine dose according to age, disease states and conditions, dosage form, and concurrent drug therapy.*

For an adult patient taking no other antiepileptic drugs who will be treated with immediate-release lamotrigine tablets, the initial doses given in Table 15-4 can be used. (*Note: Lamotrigine is not FDA approved as initial monotherapy treatment for complex partial seizures, although it is considered to be one of the drugs of choice by several expert panels [see Table 15-1]*).

For the first 2 weeks, the initial dose should be 25 mg/d. For the next 2 weeks of therapy, the dose can be escalated to 50 mg/d. During week 5, the dose can be escalated by 50 mg/d to a total dose 100 mg/d, given as 50 mg twice daily. Subsequently, every 1-2 weeks the dose can be increased by 50 mg/d (eg, 150 mg/d as 75 mg twice daily, 200 mg/d as 100 mg twice daily, etc), until an effective target dose of 225-375 mg/d without adverse effects is attained.

WR was titrated to a dose of lamotrigine 125 mg twice daily (250 mg/d) without any side effects and a decreased seizure frequency.

3. *Answer to problem 3.*

Literature-Based Recommended Dosing

1. *Estimate lamotrigine dose according to age, disease states and conditions, dosage form, and concurrent drug therapy.*

For an adult patient taking carbamazepine who will be treated with extended-release lamotrigine tablets, the initial doses given in Table 15-4 can be used. (*Note: Lamotrigine is not FDA approved as initial monotherapy treatment for complex partial seizures, although it is considered to be one of the drugs of choice by several expert panels [see Table 15-1]*).

For the first 2 weeks, the initial dose should be 25 mg/d (extended-release tablets administered once daily). For the next 2 weeks of therapy, the dose can be escalated to 50 mg/d. During week 5, the dose can be escalated by 50 mg/d to a total dose of 100 mg/d. During week 6 the dose can be advanced to 150 mg/d, and during week 7 the dose is increased to 200 mg/d. For week 8, the dose can be incremented again so that the lower target dose of 300 mg/d is attained, and, if needed, this can be increased to 400 mg/d the next week.

PO was titrated to a dose of lamotrigine extended-release tablets 400 mg/d without any side effects and a decreased seizure frequency.

4. *Answer to problem 4.*

Literature-Based Recommended Dosing

1. *Estimate lamotrigine dose according to age, disease states and conditions, dosage form, and concurrent drug therapy.*

PO is currently taking lamotrigine extended-release tablets 400 mg/d without any side effects and a decreased seizure frequency. Before she begins taking the estrogen-containing oral contraceptive, a steady-state lamotrigine concentration is obtained, and it equals 15 µg/mL. This can be used as the new target-effective lamotrigine level for future dosing purposes.

PO plans to take the first dose of oral contraceptive tablets the next morning. At this time, she can increase her lamotrigine dose by 100 mg/d to a total dose of 500 mg/d (acceptable range: 50-100 mg/d increase on a weekly basis, maximum dose increase: twice the current, stable effective therapeutic dose). PO is monitored for changes in seizure frequency or new adverse effects.

This pattern is repeated until the end of the third week of oral conceptive therapy, at which time an additional lamotrigine serum concentration is obtained and compared with the initial concentration. If the new concentration is near the original concentration, and the therapeutic effect is acceptable, dosage titration may be completed. However, if the new concentration is much lower than the original concentration, and the therapeutic effect is not optimal, further dosage titration may be needed. Additional dosage increases should be suspended until the placebo week of the oral contraceptive cycle is completed.

5. *Answer to problem 5.*

Literature-Based Recommended Dosing

1. *Estimate lamotrigine dose according to age, disease states and conditions, dosage form, and concurrent drug therapy.*

For an adult patient taking no other antiepileptic drugs who will be treated with immediate-release lamotrigine tablets, the recommendations given in Table 15-4 can be used, but initial, escalation, and maintenance doses should be decreased by 50% for a severe liver disease patient with ascites. (*Note: Lamotrigine is not FDA approved as initial monotherapy treatment for complex partial seizures, although it is considered to be one of the drugs of choice by several expert panels [see Table 15-1]*).

For the first 2 weeks, the initial dose should be 12.5 mg/d. For the next 2 weeks of therapy, the dose can be escalated to 25 mg/d. During week 5, the dose can be escalated by 25 mg/d to a total dose of 50 mg/d given once daily. Subsequently, every 1-2 weeks the dose can be increased by 25 mg/d (eg, 75 mg/d once daily, 100 mg/d as 50 mg twice daily, etc), until an effective target dose of 100-175 mg/d without adverse effects is attained. (*Note: During the dosage titration phase, maintenance doses of 100 mg/d and above can be given twice daily so that a dose can be withheld if adverse effects arise. Once a stable dose has been achieved, consideration can be given to consolidating doses to once-daily administration to simplify dosage regimens.*)

RW was titrated to a dose of lamotrigine 75 mg twice daily (later converted to 150 mg daily) without any side effects and a decreased seizure frequency. Because of variability in lamotrigine pharmacokinetics for patients with liver disease, a steady-state concentration was measured (~$t_{1/2}$ = 100 hours, ~3-5 $t_{1/2}$ in 13-21 days) during once-daily dosing and equaled 12.9 µg/mL. This concentration can be used as a reference for future lamotrigine dosing if liver disease worsens, drug interactions occur, etc.

6. *Answer to problem 6.*

Literature-Based Recommended Dosing

1. *Estimate lamotrigine dose according to age, disease states and conditions, dosage form, and concurrent drug therapy.*

For a bipolar disorder patient taking lamotrigine immediate-release tablet monotherapy, the initial doses given in Table 15-6 can be used.

For the first 2 weeks, the lamotrigine dose should be 25 mg/d. For the next 2 weeks, the dose can be increased to 50 mg/d. During weeks 5 and 6, the dose is increased to 100 mg/d and 200 mg/d, respectively (maximum target dose: 200 mg/d).

TF was titrated to a dose of 200 mg/d of lamotrigine immediate-release tablets with a decrease in the frequency and severity of bipolar episodes and no adverse effects.

7. *Answer to problem 7.*

Literature-Based Recommended Dosing

1. *Estimate lamotrigine dose according to age, disease states and conditions, dosage form, and concurrent drug therapy.*

   For a pediatric patient taking carbamazepine who will be treated with immediate-release lamotrigine tablets, the initial doses given in Table 15-5 can be used.

   For the first 2 weeks, the initial dose should be 0.6 mg/kg/d or 10 mg twice daily (0.6 mg/kg/d • 35 kg = 21 mg/d, rounded down to 20 mg/d chewable tablets). For the next 2 weeks of therapy, the dose can be escalated to 1.2 mg/kg/d (1.2 mg/kg/d • 35 kg = 42 mg/d, rounded down to 40 mg/d chewable tablets), given as 20 mg twice daily. During week 5, the dose can be escalated by 1.2 mg/kg/d (additional 1.2 mg/kg/d • 35 kg = 42 mg/d, added to current dose and rounded down to 80 mg/d chewable tablets), given as 40 mg twice daily. Subsequently, every 1-2 weeks the dose can be increased by 1.2 mg/kg/d, until an effective target dose of 5-15 mg/kg/d (given twice daily, maximum dose 400 mg/d) without adverse effects is attained.

   Over the next several weeks, FD was titrated to a dose of lamotrigine chewable tablets 150 mg twice daily without any additional side effects and a decreased seizure frequency. Within 6 months, he was switched to lamotrigine tablets 150 mg twice daily when he could swallow whole tablets without any distress. Therapeutic response remained constant after the dosage form switch, with no change in seizure frequency or adverse effects.

8. *Answer to problem 8.*

Linear Pharmacokinetics Method

1. *Use linear pharmacokinetics to compute the new concentration for a reasonable dosage increase.*

   Dosage increases for lamotrigine are usually made in increments of no more than 100 mg/d on a weekly basis. This patient is currently receiving 250 mg/d, so the maximum increase for the first week would be 350 mg/d: $C_{ss,new} = (D_{new}/D_{old})C_{ss,old} = (350 \text{ mg/d}/250 \text{ mg/d})7.5 \text{ µg/mL} = 10.5 \text{ µg/mL}$.

   To reestablish the original lamotrigine concentration for the patient, a new dosage of 350 mg/d or 175 mg twice daily was prescribed. The patient should be carefully monitored for seizure frequency and adverse effects. If desired, steady-state lamotrigine serum concentrations can be measured 3-5 half-lives after the dosage change has been made ($\sim t_{1/2} = 14$ hours, $\sim$3-5 $t_{1/2}$ in 2-3 days).

2. *If the desired steady-state lamotrigine concentrations have not been attained with the first dosage increase, compute the new concentration for the next reasonable dosage increase. Continue titration until the desired steady-state concentration or optimal therapeutic response has been achieved.*

   The desired steady-state lamotrigine concentration has been reached, so this step is not necessary for this patient.

Pharmacokinetic Parameter Method

1. *Compute pharmacokinetic parameters.*

   Lamotrigine clearance can be computed using a steady-state lamotrigine concentration: $Cl = [F(D/\tau)]/Css = [1(250 \text{ mg/d})]/(7.5 \text{ mg/L}) = 33.3$ L/d. (Note: µg/mL = mg/L and this concentration unit was substituted for Css in the calculations so that unnecessary unit conversion was not required.)

2. *Compute the new concentration for a reasonable lamotrigine dosage increase.*

   Dosage increases for lamotrigine are usually made in increments of no more than 100 mg/d on a weekly basis. This patient is currently receiving 250 mg/d, so the maximum increase for the first week would be 350 mg/d. Lamotrigine clearance is used to compute the steady-state concentration for the new dose: Css = [F(D/τ)]/Cl = [1(350 mg/d)]/(33.3 L/d) = 10.5 mg/L.

To reestablish the original lamotrigine concentration for the patient, a dosage increase of 350 mg/d or 175 mg twice daily was prescribed. The patient should be carefully monitored for seizure frequency and adverse effects. If desired, steady-state lamotrigine serum concentrations can be measured 3-5 half-lives after the dosage change has been made ($\sim t_{1/2}$ = 14 hours, ~3-5 $t_{1/2}$ in 2-3 days).

3. *If the desired steady-state lamotrigine concentrations have not been attained with the first dosage increase, compute the new concentration for the next reasonable dosage increase. Continue titration until the desired steady-state concentration or optimal therapeutic response has been achieved.*

The desired steady-state lamotrigine concentration has been reached, so this step is not necessary for this patient.

9. *Answer to problem 9.*

Linear Pharmacokinetics Method

1. *Use linear pharmacokinetics to compute the new concentration for the dosage increase.*

Dosage increases for lamotrigine are usually made in increments of no more than 100 mg/d on a weekly basis. This patient is currently receiving 400 mg/d, so the maximum increased dose for the first week would be 500 mg/d: $C_{ss,new} = (D_{new}/D_{old})C_{ss,old}$ = (500 mg/d / 400 mg/d)5.2 µg/mL = 6.5 µg/mL.

The patient should be carefully monitored for seizure frequency and adverse effects. If desired, steady-state lamotrigine serum concentrations can be measured 3-5 half-lives after the dosage change has been made ($\sim t_{1/2}$ = 14 hours, ~3-5 $t_{1/2}$ in 2-3 days).

Pharmacokinetic Parameter Method

1. *Compute pharmacokinetic parameters.*

Lamotrigine clearance can be computed using a steady-state lamotrigine concentration: Cl = [F(D/τ)]/Css = [1(400 mg/d)]/(5.2 mg/L) = 76.9 L/d. (Note: µg/mL = mg/L and this concentration unit was substituted for Css in the calculations so that unnecessary unit conversion was not required.)

2. *Compute the new concentration for the dosage increase.*

Dosage increases for lamotrigine are usually made in increments of no more than 100 mg/d on a weekly basis. This patient is currently receiving 400 mg/d, so the maximum increased dose for the first week would be 500 mg/d. Lamotrigine clearance is used to compute the steady-state concentration for the new dose: Css = [F(D/τ)]/Cl = [1(500 mg/d)]/(76.9 L/d) = 6.5 mg/L.

The patient should be carefully monitored for seizure frequency and adverse effects. If desired, steady-state lamotrigine serum concentrations can be measured 3-5 half-lives after the dosage change has been made ($\sim t_{1/2}$ = 14 hours, ~3-5 $t_{1/2}$ in 2-3 days).

REFERENCES

1. French JA, Kanner AM, Bautista J, et al. Efficacy and tolerability of the new antiepileptic drugs I: treatment of new onset epilepsy: report of the Therapeutics and Technology Assessment Subcommittee and Quality Standards Subcommittee of the American Academy of Neurology and the American Epilepsy Society. *Neurology.* Apr 27, 2004;62(8):1252-1260.
2. Abramowicz M, Zuccotti G, Pflomm JM, eds. Drugs for epilepsy. *Treatment Guidelines From The Medical Letter.* 2013;11(126): 9-18.

3. Anon. The epilepsies: the diagnosis and management of the epilepsies in adults and children in primary and secondary care. *UK National Institute for Health and Care Excellence*. http://www.nice.org.uk/nicemedia/live/13635/57779/57779.pdf. Accessed May 5, 2014.

4. Glauser T, Ben-Menachem E, Bourgeois B, et al. Updated ILAE evidence review of antiepileptic drug efficacy and effectiveness as initial monotherapy for epileptic seizures and syndromes. *Epilepsia*. Mar 2013;54(3):551-563.

5. Glauser TA, Cnaan A, Shinnar S, et al. Ethosuximide, valproic acid, and lamotrigine in childhood absence epilepsy. *N Engl J Med*. Mar 4, 2010;362(9):790-799.

6. Glauser TA, Cnaan A, Shinnar S, et al. Ethosuximide, valproic acid, and lamotrigine in childhood absence epilepsy: initial monotherapy outcomes at 12 months. *Epilepsia*. Jan 2013;54(1):141-155.

7. Abramowicz M, Zuccotti G, Pflomm JM, eds. Drugs for depression and bipolar disorder. *Treatment Guidelines From The Medical Letter*. 2010;8(93):35-42.

8. Drayton SJ. Bipolar disorders. In: DiPiro JT, Talbert RL, Yee GC, Matzke GR, Wells BG, Posey LM, eds. *Pharmacotherapy*. 8th ed. New York, NY: McGraw-Hill; 2011:1191-1208.

9. McNamara JO. Pharmacotherapy of the epilepsies. In: Brunton L, Chabner B, Knollman B, eds. *The Pharmacological Basis of Therapeutics*. 12th ed. New York, NY: McGraw-Hill; 2011:583-608.

10. Leach MJ, Marden CM, Miller AA. Pharmacological studies on lamotrigine, a novel potential antiepileptic drug: II. Neurochemical studies on the mechanism of action. *Epilepsia*. Sep-Oct 1986;27(5):490-497.

11. Cheung H, Kamp D, Harris E. An in vitro investigation of the action of lamotrigine on neuronal voltage-activated sodium channels. *Epilepsy Res*. Nov 1992;13(2):107-112.

12. Rogers SJ, Cavazos JE. Epilepsy. In: DiPiro JT, Talbert RL, Yee GC, Matzke GR, Wells BG, Posey LM, eds. *Pharmacotherapy*. 8th ed. New York, NY: McGraw-Hill; 2011:979-1005.

13. Johannessen SI, Tomson T. Pharmacokinetic variability of newer antiepileptic drugs: when is monitoring needed? *Clin Pharmacokinet*. 2006;45(11):1061-1075.

14. Hirsch LJ, Weintraub D, Du Y, et al. Correlating lamotrigine serum concentrations with tolerability in patients with epilepsy. *Neurology*. Sep 28 2004;63(6):1022-1026.

15. Perucca E. Is there a role for therapeutic drug monitoring of new anticonvulsants? *Clin Pharmacokinet*. Mar 2000;38(3):191-204.

16. Rambeck B, Wolf P. Lamotrigine clinical pharmacokinetics. *Clin Pharmacokinet*. Dec 1993;25(6):433-443.

17. GlaxoSmithKline LLC [package insert]. Lamictal-XL prescribing information; 2012.

18. GlaxoSmithKline LLC [package insert]. Lamictal prescribing information; 2011.

19. Gulcebi MI, Ozkaynakci A, Goren MZ, Aker RG, Ozkara C, Onat FY. The relationship between UGT1A4 polymorphism and serum concentration of lamotrigine in patients with epilepsy. *Epilepsy Res*. Jun 2011;95(1-2):1-8.

20. Magdalou J, Herber R, Bidault R, Siest G. In vitro *N*-glucuronidation of a novel antiepileptic drug, lamotrigine, by human liver microsomes. *J Pharmacol Exp Ther*. Mar 1992;260(3):1166-1173.

21. Londero D, Lo Greco P. New micromethod for the determination of lamotrigine in human plasma by high-performance liquid chromatography. *J Chromatogr B Biomed Sci Appl*. Mar 28, 1997;691(1):139-144.

22. Doig MV, Clare RA. Use of thermospray liquid chromatography-mass spectrometry to aid in the identification of urinary metabolites of a novel antiepileptic drug, Lamotrigine. *J Chromatogr*. Aug 21, 1991;554(1-2):181-189.

23. Sinz MW, Remmel RP. Isolation and characterization of a novel quaternary ammonium-linked glucuronide of lamotrigine. *Drug Metab Dispos*. Jan-Feb 1991;19(1):149-153.

24. Peck AW. Clinical pharmacology of lamotrigine. *Epilepsia*. 1991;32(suppl 2):9S-12S.

25. Ramsay RE, Pellock JM, Garnett WR, et al. Pharmacokinetics and safety of lamotrigine (Lamictal) in patients with epilepsy. *Epilepsy Res*. Nov-Dec 1991;10(2-3):191-200.

26. Mikati MA, Schachter SC, Schomer DL, et al. Long-term tolerability, pharmacokinetic and preliminary efficacy study of lamotrigine in patients with resistant partial seizures. *Clin Neuropharmacol*. Aug 1989;12(4):312-321.

27. Cohen AF, Land GS, Breimer DD, Yuen WC, Winton C, Peck AW. Lamotrigine, a new anticonvulsant: pharmacokinetics in normal humans. *Clin Pharmacol Ther*. Nov 1987;42(5):535-541.

28. Jawad S, Yuen WC, Peck AW, Hamilton MJ, Oxley JR, Richens A. Lamotrigine: single-dose pharmacokinetics and initial 1 week experience in refractory epilepsy. *Epilepsy Res*. May 1987;1(3):194-201.

29. Naritoku DK, Warnock CR, Messenheimer JA, et al. Lamotrigine extended-release as adjunctive therapy for partial seizures. *Neurology*. Oct 16, 2007;69(16):1610-1618.

30. Tompson DJ, Ali I, Oliver-Willwong R, et al. Steady-state pharmacokinetics of lamotrigine when converting from a twice-daily immediate-release to a once-daily extended-release formulation in subjects with epilepsy (The COMPASS Study). *Epilepsia*. Mar 2008;49(3):410-417.

31. Yuen WC, Peck AW. Lamotrigine pharmacokinetics: oral and IV infusion in man. *Br J Clin Pharmacol*. 1988;26(suppl):242.

32. Dickins M, Chen C. Lamotrigine chemistry, biotransformation, and pharmacokinetics. In: Levy RH, Mattson RH, Meldrum BS, Perucca E, eds. *Antiepileptic Drugs*. 5th ed. Philadelphia, PA: Lippincott Williams & Wilkins; 2002:370-379.

33. Miller AA, Wheatley P, Sawyer DA, Baxter MG, Roth B. Pharmacological studies on lamotrigine, a novel potential antiepileptic drug: I. anticonvulsant profile in mice and rats. *Epilepsia.* Sep-Oct 1986;27(5):483-489.

34. Rambeck B, Kurlemann G, Stodieck SR, May TW, Jurgens U. Concentrations of lamotrigine in a mother on lamotrigine treatment and her newborn child. *Eur J Clin Pharmacol.* 1997;51(6):481-484.

35. Kacirova I, Grundmann M, Brozmanova H. Serum levels of lamotrigine during delivery in mothers and their infants. *Epilepsy Res.* Oct 2010;91(2-3):161-165.

36. Fotopoulou C, Kretz R, Bauer S, et al. Prospectively assessed changes in lamotrigine-concentration in women with epilepsy during pregnancy, lactation and the neonatal period. *Epilepsy Res.* Jul 2009;85(1):60-64.

37. Depot M, Powell JR, Messenheimer JA, Jr, Cloutier G, Dalton MJ. Kinetic effects of multiple oral doses of acetaminophen on a single oral dose of lamotrigine. *Clin Pharmacol Ther.* Oct 1990;48(4):346-355.

38. Posner J, Holdich T, Chrome P. Comparison of lamotrigine pharmacokinetics in young and elderly health volunteers. *J Pharmaceut Med.* 1991;1:121-128.

39. Posner J, Cohen AF, Land G, Winton C, Peck AW. The pharmacokinetics of lamotrigine (BW430C) in healthy subjects with unconjugated hyperbilirubinaemia (Gilbert's syndrome). *Br J Clin Pharmacol.* Jul 1989;28(1):117-120.

40. Yuen AW, Land G, Weatherley BC, Peck AW. Sodium valproate acutely inhibits lamotrigine metabolism. *Br J Clin Pharmacol.* May 1992;33(5):511-513.

41. Wootton R, Soul-Lawton J, Rolan PE, Sheung CT, Cooper JD, Posner J. Comparison of the pharmacokinetics of lamotrigine in patients with chronic renal failure and healthy volunteers. *Br J Clin Pharmacol.* Jan 1997;43(1):23-27.

42. Kaufman KR. Lamotrigine and hemodialysis in bipolar disorder: case analysis of dosing strategy with literature review. *Bipolar Disord.* Jun 2010;12(4):446-449.

43. Fillastre JP, Taburet AM, Fialaire A, Etienne I, Bidault R, Singlas E. Pharmacokinetics of lamotrigine in patients with renal impairment: influence of haemodialysis. *Drugs Exp Clin Res.* 1993;19(1):25-32.

44. Marcellin P, de Bony F, Garret C, et al. Influence of cirrhosis on lamotrigine pharmacokinetics. *Br J Clin Pharmacol.* May 2001; 51(5):410-414.

45. Pugh RN, Murray-Lyon IM, Dawson JL, Pietroni MC, Williams R. Transection of the oesophagus for bleeding oesophageal varices. *Br J Surg.* 1973;60(8):646-649.

46. He DK, Wang L, Qin J, et al. Population pharmacokinetics of lamotrigine in Chinese children with epilepsy. *Acta Pharmacol Sin.* Nov 2012;33(11):1417-1423.

47. Milovanovic JR, Jankovic SM. Population pharmacokinetics of lamotrigine in patients with epilepsy. *Int J Clin Pharmacol Ther.* Dec 2009;47(12):752-760.

48. Reimers A, Skogvoll E, Sund JK, Spigset O. Lamotrigine in children and adolescents: the impact of age on its serum concentrations and on the extent of drug interactions. *Eur J Clin Pharmacol.* Jul 2007;63(7):687-692.

49. Steinborn B. Pharmacokinetic interactions of carbamazepine with some antiepileptic drugs during epilepsy treatment in children and adolescents. *Rocz Akad Med Bialymst.* 2005;50 (suppl 1):9-15.

50. Battino D, Croci D, Granata T, Mamoli D, Messina S, Perucca E. Single-dose pharmacokinetics of lamotrigine in children: influence of age and antiepileptic comedication. *Ther Drug Monit.* Jun 2001;23(3):217-222.

51. Chen C. Validation of a population pharmacokinetic model for adjunctive lamotrigine therapy in children. *Br J Clin Pharmacol.* Aug 2000;50(2):135-145.

52. Armijo JA, Bravo J, Cuadrado A, Herranz JL. Lamotrigine serum concentration-to-dose ratio: influence of age and concomitant antiepileptic drugs and dosage implications. *Ther Drug Monit.* Apr 1999;21(2):182-190.

53. Furlan V, Demirdjian S, Bourdon O, Magdalou J, Taburet AM. Glucuronidation of drugs by hepatic microsomes derived from healthy and cirrhotic human livers. *J Pharmacol Exp Ther.* May 1999;289(2):1169-1175.

54. Chen C, Casale EJ, Duncan B, Culverhouse EH, Gilman J. Pharmacokinetics of lamotrigine in children in the absence of other antiepileptic drugs. *Pharmacotherapy.* Apr 1999;19(4):437-441.

55. Battino D, Croci D, Granata T, Estienne M, Pisani F, Avanzini G. Lamotrigine plasma concentrations in children and adults: influence of age and associated therapy. *Ther Drug Monit.* Dec 1997;19(6):620-627.

56. Bartoli A, Guerrini R, Belmonte A, Alessandri MG, Gatti G, Perucca E. The influence of dosage, age, and comedication on steady state plasma lamotrigine concentrations in epileptic children: a prospective study with preliminary assessment of correlations with clinical response. *Ther Drug Monit.* Jun 1997;19(3):252-260.

57. Vauzelle-Kervroedan F, Rey E, Cieuta C, et al. Influence of concurrent antiepileptic medication on the pharmacokinetics of lamotrigine as add-on therapy in epileptic children. *Br J Clin Pharmacol.* Apr 1996;41(4):325-330.

58. Battino D, Estienne M, Avanzini G. Clinical pharmacokinetics of antiepileptic drugs in paediatric patients. Part II. Phenytoin, carbamazepine, sulthiame, lamotrigine, vigabatrin, oxcarbazepine and felbamate. *Clin Pharmacokinet.* Nov 1995;29(5):341-369.

59. Punyawudho B, Ramsay RE, Macias FM, et al. Population pharmacokinetics of lamotrigine in elderly patients. *J Clin Pharmacol.* Apr 2008;48(4):455-463.

60. Hansten PD, Horn JR. *The Top 100 Drug Interactions.* Freeland, WA: H&H Publications; 2014.

61. Hansten PD, Horn JR. *Drug Interactions Analysis and Management.* St. Louis, MO: Wolters Kluwer; 2014.

62. Binnie CD, van Emde Boas W, Kasteleijn-Nolste-Trenite DG, et al. Acute effects of lamotrigine (BW430C) in persons with epilepsy. *Epilepsia.* May-Jun 1986;27(3):248-254.

63. Wolf P. Lamotrigine: preliminary clinical observations on pharmacokinetics and interactions with traditional antiepileptic drugs. *J Epilepsy.* 1992;5(2):73-79.

64. Warner T, Patsalos PN, Prevett M, Elyas AA, Duncan JS. Lamotrigine-induced carbamazepine toxicity: an interaction with carbamazepine-10,11-epoxide. *Epilepsy Res.* Apr 1992;11(2):147-150.

INTRODUCTION

Levetiracetam is a pyrrolidine-based compound effective in the management of partial and tonic-clonic seizures, and it is administered as the S-enantiomer of a stereoisomer pair (Table 16-1).[1-4] It is also useful for the treatment of myoclonic seizures in patients with juvenile myoclonic epilepsy. Levetiracetam does not exhibit antiseizure properties in all models used to screen antiepileptic drugs, and its exact mechanism of action is largely unknown. It does bind to a synaptic vesicle protein, SV2A, present in brain tissue, and this action is thought to be important to its therapeutic actions.[5,6]

TABLE 16-1 International Classification of Epileptic Seizures With Recommended Therapies

		Drug Treatment for Selected Seizure Type			
Major Class	**Subset of Class**	**2004 AAN/AES**	**2013 Medical Letter**	**2012 NICE**	**2013 ILAE[a]**
Partial seizures (beginning locally)	1. Simple partial seizures (without impaired consciousness) a. with motor symptoms b. with somatosensory or special sensory symptoms c. with autonomic symptoms d. with psychological symptoms	Carbamazepine Phenytoin Valproate Phenobarbital Lamotrigine Gabapentin Oxcarbazepine Topiramate	Lamotrigine Carbamazepine Levetiracetam Oxcarbazepine *Alternatives:* Topiramate Valproate Gabapentin Zonisamide Phenytoin Pregabalin Lacosamide Ezogabine	Carbamazepine Lamotrigine Levetiracetam Oxcarbazepine Valproate *Adjunctive:* Carbamazepine Clobazam Gabapentin Lamotrigine Levetiracetam Oxcarbazepine Valproate Topiramate	*Adults:* Carbamazepine Levetiracetam Phenytoin Zonisamide Valproate *Children:* Oxcarbazepine Carbamazepine Phenobarbital Phenytoin Topiramate Valproate Vigabatrin *Elderly:* Gabapentin Lamotrigine Carbamazepine

(Continued)

TABLE 16-1   International Classification of Epileptic Seizures With Recommended Therapies (*Continued*)

Major Class	Subset of Class	Drug Treatment for Selected Seizure Type			
		2004 AAN/AES	2013 Medical Letter	2012 NICE	2013 ILAE[a]
	2. Complex partial seizures (with impaired consciousness) a. simple partial onset followed by impaired consciousness b. impaired consciousness at onset	Carbamazepine Phenytoin Valproate Phenobarbital Lamotrigine Gabapentin Oxcarbazepine Topiramate	Lamotrigine Carbamazepine Levetiracetam Oxcarbazepine *Alternatives:* Topiramate Valproate Gabapentin Zonisamide Phenytoin Pregabalin Lacosamide Ezogabine	Carbamazepine Lamotrigine Levetiracetam Oxcarbazepine Valproate *Adjunctive:* Carbamazepine Clobazam Gabapentin Lamotrigine Levetiracetam Oxcarbazepine Valproate Topiramate	*Adults:* Carbamazepine Levetiracetam Phenytoin Zonisamide Valproate *Children:* Oxcarbazepine Carbamazepine Phenobarbital Phenytoin Topiramate Valproate Vigabatrin *Elderly:* Gabapentin Lamotrigine Carbamazepine
	3. Partial seizures evolving into secondary generalized seizures	Carbamazepine Phenytoin Valproate Phenobarbital Lamotrigine Gabapentin Oxcarbazepine Topiramate	Lamotrigine Carbamazepine Levetiracetam Oxcarbazepine *Alternatives:* Topiramate Valproate Gabapentin Zonisamide Phenytoin Pregabalin Lacosamide Ezogabine	Carbamazepine Lamotrigine Levetiracetam Oxcarbazepine Valproate *Adjunctive:* Carbamazepine Clobazam Gabapentin Lamotrigine Levetiracetam Oxcarbazepine Valproate Topiramate	*Adults:* Carbamazepine Levetiracetam Phenytoin Zonisamide Valproate *Children:* Oxcarbazepine Carbamazepine Phenobarbital Phenytoin Topiramate Valproate Vigabatrin *Elderly:* Gabapentin Lamotrigine Carbamazepine
Generalized seizures (convulsive or nonconvulsive)	1. Absence seizures[b] (typical or atypical; also known as petit mal seizures)	*Children:*[c] Ethosuximide Valproate Lamotrigine	Ethosuximide Valproate *Alternatives:* Lamotrigine Clonazepam Zonisamide Levetiracetam	Ethosuximide Lamotrigine Valproate *Adjunctive:* Ethosuximide Lamotrigine Valproate	*Children:* Ethosuximide Valproate Lamotrigine

(*Continued*)

TABLE 16-1   International Classification of Epileptic Seizures With Recommended Therapies (*Continued*)

Major Class	Subset of Class	Drug Treatment for Selected Seizure Type			
		2004 AAN/AES	**2013 Medical Letter**	**2012 NICE**	**2013 ILAE**[a]
	2. Tonic-clonic seizures (also known as grand mal seizures)	Carbamazepine Phenytoin Valproate Phenobarbital Lamotrigine Oxcarbazepine Topiramate	Valproate Lamotrigine Levetiracetam *Alternatives:* Topiramate Zonisamide Phenytoin	Carbamazepine Lamotrigine Oxcarbazepine Valproate *Adjunctive:* Clobazam Lamotrigine Levetiracetam Valproate Topiramate	*Adults:* Carbamazepine Lamotrigine Oxcarbazepine Phenobarbital Phenytoin Topiramate Valproate Gabapentin Levetiracetam Vigabatrin *Children:* Carbamazepine Phenobarbital Phenytoin Topiramate Valproate Oxcarbazepine

[a]Only two highest available levels of evidence listed.

[b]Recent literature suggests either ethosuximide or valproic acid is a superior initial therapy compared to lamotrigine for absence seizures.[7,8]

[c]Lamotrigine added to previous recommendation per expert panel.

Abbreviations: ANN, American Academy of Neurology; AES, American Epilepsy Society; NICE, UK National Institute for Clinical Excellence; ILAE, International League Against Epilepsy.

THERAPEUTIC AND TOXIC CONCENTRATIONS

Like many of the newer antiepileptic drugs, the therapeutic range of levetiracetam is not well defined.[9-11] However, levetiracetam serum concentration measurement can be a useful adjunct in addition to monitoring treatment for therapeutic response and adverse effects. The therapeutic range for epilepsy used by many laboratories for levetiracetam is 12-46 µg/mL, and predose steady-state trough concentrations are usually obtained for levetiracetam measurement. Some patients will experience a higher incidence of adverse effects in the upper end of these levels, so the efficacy of lower serum concentrations should be assessed before moving to higher concentrations. The most common concentration-dependent side effects of levetiracetam are sedation and behavioral disturbances.[6]

CLINICAL MONITORING PARAMETERS

The goals of therapy with anticonvulsants are to reduce seizure frequency and to maximize quality of life with a minimum of adverse drug effects.[6] While it is desirable to entirely abolish all seizure episodes, it may not be possible to accomplish this in many patients. Patients should be monitored for concentration-related side effects (sedation, behavioral disturbances). Somnolence, asthenia, and dizziness in adults and fatigue, aggression anorexia, and irritability in children are also common adverse events. Serious side effects include psychotic episodes (hallucinations, unusual behavior), mood changes (anxiety, depression, aggression, hostility), suicidal behavior, and muscle incoordination. Stevens-Johnson syndrome and toxic epidermal necrolysis have both been reported during levetiracetam therapy. Generally, these adverse effects occurred within 14-17 days of starting treatment, although some cases have happened as late as 4 months after beginning treatment. Should either of these dermatologic reactions develop, levetiracetam should be immediately discontinued and not restarted.[6,12]

Because epilepsy is an episodic disease state, patients do not experience seizures continuously. Thus, during dosage titration it is difficult to tell if the patient is responding to drug therapy or simply is not experiencing any abnormal central nervous system discharges at that time. Levetiracetam doses should be carefully titrated to individual patient response and tolerability. Steady-state serum concentrations of levetiracetam can be measured in patients as an adjunct to therapy.[10,11,13-15] Concentration monitoring is particularly useful if a therapeutic level has been established for a patient and a new clinical event (drug interaction, new disease state or condition, etc) changes the pharmacokinetics of the drug. Levetiracetam concentrations can also be measured to document patient adherence to drug treatment or when a patient is switched among the various dosage forms (immediate-release tablets, extended-release tablets, oral solution, or intravenous injection) to assure therapeutic levels are maintained.

BASIC CLINICAL PHARMACOKINETIC PARAMETERS

With normal renal function, levetiracetam is eliminated primarily as unchanged drug in the urine (~65% of administered dose, Table 16-2). The remainder of the drug is largely converted to a pharmacologically inactive metabolite and then eliminated into the urine (UBC L057, ~20% of dose). There are several other minor metabolites without antiseizure activity that account for the remainder of the dose. Metabolism of levetiracetam does not seem to be conducted principally by the cytochrome P-450 enzymes or the uridine 5'-diphosphoglucuronosyltransferase (UGT) systems. Enzymatic hydrolysis via type B esterases is a likely pathway for metabolite formation. The clearance, volume of distribution, and half-life for intravenous levetiracetam average about 0.95 mL/min/kg, 0.6 L/kg, and 7.3 hours, respectively. Levetiracetam follows linear pharmacokinetics within the usual dosage range.[3,9,16-19]

Levetiracetam is available in a variety of immediate-release tablets (tablets: 250 mg, 500 mg, 750 mg, 1000 mg) and as extended-release tablets (500 mg, 750 mg). An oral solution (100 mg/mL) and intravenous injection (500 mg/5 mL) are also available for administration. Bioavailability is ~92% for the various oral dosage forms, and if the intravenous injection is given intramuscularly, the bioavailability is 100%. Food intake does not appear to alter bioavailability for the oral dosage forms.[20,21]

For single doses, peak concentrations occur sooner (T_{max}) for the oral solution (~0.8 hours) compared to the immediate-release tablets (~1.5 hours).[17,22-25] For multiple doses of the extended-release dosage form administered twice daily, T_{max} occurs at about 4.5 hours. The steady-state maximum-to-minimum concentration ratio is 1.27 for immediate-release tablets given every 12 hours compared to 1.19 for extended-release tablets given once daily.[26] When patients are switched between dosage forms, they should be closely monitored for changes in efficacy or toxicity, and measurement of levetiracetam serum concentrations should be considered before and after the change has been made.

The plasma protein binding of levetiracetam is <10%.[17-19] Levetiracetam crosses the placental barrier, and at birth the umbilical cord blood to maternal serum concentration ratio is approximately 1.09. Levetiracetam also crosses into the breast milk of lactating mothers with a breast milk-to-maternal serum ratio of 1.05. After breast-feeding from mothers taking levetiracetam, the resulting range of levetiracetam serum concentration in newborns was 0.7-3.4 µg/mL.[13] The range of mean levetiracetam saliva to serum ratios in patients measured during multiple dosing is 0.36-0.41, and the correlation coefficient for concentrations in the two fluids is 0.86-0.87.[27]

TABLE 16-2   Disease States and Conditions That Alter Levetiracetam Pharmacokinetics

Disease State/Condition	Cl/F		V/F	$t_{1/2}$	Comment
Adult, normal kidney and liver function, immediate-release oral dosage forms	0.9 mL/min/kg 0.89 mL/min/kg 0.92 mL/min/kg 0.93 mL/min/kg 0.85 mL/min/kg 0.85 mL/min/kg		0.6 L/kg 0.57 L/kg N/A 0.57 L/kg 0.54 L/kg 0.52 L/kg	7.6 h 7.3 h 6.7 h 7.3 h 7.4 h 7.2 h	Levetiracetam is primarily eliminated by the kidneys as unchanged drug (~65% of dose). UCB L057, the primary metabolite, is also eliminated in the urine (~20% of dose). T_{max} averages 0.8 h for the oral solution and 1.5 h for the immediate release tablets. Oral bioavailability is 92% compared to intravenous drug. The steady-state peak-trough ratio is 0.94 for immediate-release tablets. The overall mean pharmacokinetic values are: Cl/F = 0.90 mL/min/kg, V/F = 0.56 L/kg, $t_{1/2}$ = 7.3 h
Adult, normal kidney and liver function, extended-release tablet	0.90 mL/min/kg		0.56 L/kg	7.3 h	T_{max} at steady-state equal to 4.5 h. Steady-state peak-trough ratio for extended-release tablet (1.19) given once daily similar to immediate-release (1.27) given twice daily. Bioavailability of extended-release tablet similar to immediate-release tablet.
Adult, variable renal function, normal liver function	**CrCl (mL/min)** 50-80 30-50 <30	**%Cl/F** 60% 50% 40%	N/A	N/A	To determine Cl/F for patient with decreased renal function, multiply the Cl/F value by percentage.
Adult, end-stage renal disease, normal liver function	18.2 mL/min/1.73 m²		0.5 L/kg	24.6 h	Hemodialysis clearances for levetiracetam and UCB L057 metabolite are 127 mL/min/1.73 m² and 99 mL/min/1.73 m², respectively. About ½ of levetiracetam is removed by 4 h hemodialysis with low-flux filter.

Adult, variable renal function, liver disease	*Healthy control*:
	  64.3 mL/min/1.73 m²
	
	Mild liver disease:
	  62.5 mL/min/1.73 m²
	
	Moderate liver disease:
	  55.4 mL/min/1.73 m²
	
	Severe liver disease:
	  29.2 mL/min/1.73 m²
			47.3 L
			
			49.1 L
			
			48.6 L
			
			44.6 L
				7.6 h
				
				7.6 h
				
				8.7 h
				
				18.4 h
					Severe liver disease group had lower renal function (63 mL/min/1.73 m² vs 100-121 mL/min/1.73 m² for other groups) and lower nonrenal Cl/F (12.4 mL/min/1.73 m² vs 19-21 mL/min/1.73 m² for the other groups). Decreased Cl/F and prolonged $t_{1/2}$ for severe liver function group is due to both decreased renal and liver elimination.

(Continued)

TABLE 16-2   Disease States and Conditions That Alter Levetiracetam Pharmacokinetics (*Continued*)

Disease State/Condition	Cl/F	V/F	$t_{1/2}$	Comment
Adult, normal kidney and liver function, variable concurrent AED therapy	**Concurrent AED** *Inducers (PHT, CBZ, OXC, PB, PRIM):* 1.03 mL/min/kg 1.17 mL/min/kg *VPA:* 0.70 mL/min/kg *Inducers + VPA:* 0.98 mL/min/kg	 N/A 0.6 L/kg N/A N/A	 7.4 h 6.1 h 11.5 h 9.4 h	Inducer AED increase the Cl/F and decrease the $t_{1/2}$ of levetiracetam. VPA decreases the Cl/F and increases the $t_{1/2}$ of levetiracetam. Administration of VPA with one or more inducer AED attenuates the changes.
Adult, elderly, variable concurrent other AED therapy	**Young (25 y) Elderly (64 y)** **(mL/min/kg)** *LEV only:* 1.39 0.56 *Inducers (PHT, CBZ, OXC, PB, PRIM):* 1.53 0.87 *Noninducer AED:* 1.21 0.74	 N/A N/A N/A	 N/A N/A N/A	Elderly patients have lower Cl/F compared to younger patients. Inducer AED increase Cl/F in both patient groups.
Adult, very elderly, variable concurrent other AED therapy	**Young Elderly Very Elderly** **(47 y) (73 y) (85 y)** **(mL/min/kg)** *LEV only:* 1.05 0.79 0.57 *Inducers (PHT, CBZ, OXC, PB, PRIM):* 1.43 0.93 1.09	 N/A N/A	 N/A N/A	Very elderly and elderly patients both have lower Cl/F values than younger adults for levetiracetam monotherapy. The oldest patients have the lowest overall Cl/F. Inducer AED increase Cl/F across the board and bring parity to Cl/F to the elderly groups.
Adult, normal kidney and liver function, intravenous drug	0.92 mL/min/kg 0.97 mL/min/kg	0.56 L/kg 0.66 L/kg	7.2 h 8.3 h	By definition, F = 1 for intravenous levetiracetam. Therefore, shown values are for Cl and V, not the hybrid constants. The overall mean pharmacokinetic values for intravenous drug are: Cl = 0.95 mL/min/kg, V = 0.6 L/kg, $t_{1/2}$ = 7.8 h
Adult, normal kidney and liver function, neurologic critical care, intravenous drug	1.09 mL/min/kg	0.43 L/kg	5.2 h	Clearance was higher in neurologic critical care patients with head trauma. By definition, F = 1 for intravenous levetiracetam. Therefore, shown values are for Cl and V, not the hybrid constants. V was calculated as Vss, which computationally is smaller than V calculated using the area method.
Adult, normal kidney and liver function, intramuscular administration	0.91 mL/min/kg	0.72 L/kg	9.4 h	Bioavailability for intramuscular injection was 100% compared to intravenous drug. T_{max} = 3.1 h.

(Continued)

TABLE 16-2   Disease States and Conditions That Alter Levetiracetam Pharmacokinetics (*Continued*)

Disease State/Condition	Cl/F	V/F	t$_{1/2}$	Comment
Adult females, normal kidney and liver function, pregnant	*Baseline (before pregnancy or > 1 mo after delivery):* 125 L/d	N/A	N/A	Levetiracetam steady-state levels decline during the first and second trimesters, but decrease precipitously in the third trimester. Umbilical cord/mother serum concentration ratio = 1.09. Breast milk/mother serum concentration ratio = 1.05.
	Third trimester: 427 L/d	N/A	N/A	
Neonates, 37-41 wks gestational age, 2.55-3.70 kg weight, single dose of intravenous PB 20 mg/kg given before levetiracetam	*Single dose, postnatal age 2 d:* 1.21 mL/min/kg	0.89 L/kg	8.9 h	Cl/F rapidly changes after birth. V/F is larger for neonates, which is similar to many other drugs. t$_{1/2}$ is longer for neonates than children and adults.
	Multiple dose for 7 d after birth: Day 1, 0.71 mL/min/kg	N/A	18.5 h	
	Day 7, 1.31 mL/min/kg	N/A	9.1 h	
Pediatric patients, normal kidney and liver function, variable concurrent other AED therapy	*Age 2.3-46.2 mo, mixed AED usage:* 1.46 mL/min/kg	0.63 L/kg	5.3 h	Generally, children taking inducer AED have higher Cl/F and V/F compared to adults. t$_{1/2}$ values are shorter.
	Age 6-12 y, mixed AED usage: 1.43 mL/min/kg	0.72 L/kg	6.0 h	
	Age 4-12 y old: w/CBZ, 1.23 mL/min/kg	N/A	4.4 h	
	w/VPA, 1.08 mL/min/kg	N/A	5.2 h	

Abbreviations: AED, antiepileptic drug; PHT, phenytoin; CBZ, carbamazepine; OXC, oxcarbazepine; PB, phenobarbital; PRIM, primidone; VPA, valproic acid.

EFFECTS OF DISEASES AND CONDITIONS ON PHARMACOKINETICS AND DOSING

Most investigations with levetiracetam have been conducted with oral dosage forms, so pharmacokinetic results are usually expressed as hybrid constants that include bioavailability (F) for clearance (Cl/F) and volume of distribution (V/F) as single values (see Table 16-2). Adults with normal liver and kidney function that take no hepatic enzyme inducers or inhibitors have an average half-life of 7.3 hours, a mean Cl/F equal to 0.90 mL/min/kg, and an average V/F of 0.56 L/kg for levetiracetam (see Table 16-2).[19,22-25] The clearance, volume of distribution, and half-life for intravenous levetiracetam average about 0.95 mL/min/kg, 0.6 L/kg, and 7.3 hours, respectively.[20,21] Because plasma protein binding is very low (<10%), it is not altered by any disease states or conditions that alter levetiracetam pharmacokinetics, and volume of distribution is similar for most patient categories.

The majority of a levetiracetam dose (~65%) is eliminated unchanged in the urine. Because of this, renal disease prolongs levetiracetam half-life and decreases levetiracetam clearance in a graded manner according to the degree of renal damage observed in the patient. Compared to adults with normal renal function, patients with a creatinine clearance (CrCl) of 50-80 mL/min have 60% of the normal Cl/F. Similarly, patients with CrCl equal to 30-50 mL/min have 50% of the normal Cl/F and patients with CrCl <30 mL/min have 40% of the normal Cl/F. Patients with end-stage renal disease have a levetiracetam clearance of 18.2 mL/min/1.73 m^2, a volume of distribution equal to 0.5 L/kg, and a half-life of 24.6 hours. The hemodialysis clearances for levetiracetam and UCB L057 (the major metabolite) are 127 mL/min/1.73 m^2 and 99 mL/min/1.73 m^2, respectively. During a 4-hour hemodialysis session with a low-flux filter, about one-half of levetiracetam is removed from the body.[28,29] For patients with renal dysfunction, levetiracetam doses should be titrated to clinical

TABLE 16-3 Child-Pugh Scores for Patients With Liver Disease

Test/Symptom	Score 1 Point	Score 2 Points	Score 3 Points
Total bilirubin (mg/dL)	<2.0	2.0-3.0	>3.0
Serum albumin (g/dL)	>3.5	2.8-3.5	<2.8
Prothrombin time (seconds prolonged over control)	<4	4-6	>6
Ascites	Absent	Slight	Moderate
Hepatic encephalopathy	None	Moderate	Severe

Child-Pugh Class A, mild liver disease: 5-6 points; Child-Pugh Class B, moderate liver disease: 7-9 points; Child-Pugh Class C, severe liver disease: 10-15 points.

response, and measurement of levetiracetam serum concentrations can be a helpful adjunct. Due to the variability in the pharmacokinetics for levetiracetam, patients with renal disease should be closely monitored for adverse effects due to levetiracetam therapy.

Since only a moderate amount of levetiracetam is eliminated by metabolic conversion (~35%) and the liver is not the principal site of metabolism, there is only a modest change in levetiracetam pharmacokinetics for subjects with hepatic disease. An index of liver dysfunction can be gained by applying the Child-Pugh clinical classification system to the patient (Table 16-3).[30] Child-Pugh scores are completely discussed in Chapter 3 (Drug Dosing in Special Populations: Renal and Hepatic Disease, Dialysis, Heart Failure, Obesity, and Drug Interactions), but will be briefly discussed here. The Child-Pugh score consists of five laboratory tests or clinical symptoms: serum albumin, total bilirubin, prothrombin time, ascites, and hepatic encephalopathy. Each of these areas is given a score of 1 (normal) to 3 (severely abnormal; see Table 16-3), and the scores for the five areas are summed. The Child-Pugh score for a patient with normal liver function is 5 while the score for a patient with grossly abnormal serum albumin, total bilirubin, and prothrombin time values in addition to severe ascites and hepatic encephalopathy is 15. The pharmacokinetic changes for levetiracetam range from modest ones (mild liver disease: none; moderate liver disease: half-life = 8.7 hours, Cl/F = 55.4 mL/min/1.73 m^2, V/F = 48.6 L) for patients with moderate liver disease (Child-Pugh score = 7-9 points) to larger ones (half-life = 18.4 hours, Cl/F = 29.2 mL/min/1.73 m^2) for patients with severe liver disease (Child-Pugh score = 10-15 points). Unfortunately, the patients with severe liver disease included in the research study also had decreased renal function compared to the other liver disease groups, so it is difficult to assign the entire change in levetiracetam pharmacokinetics to hepatic dysfunction. Generally, no change in dose is needed for patients with mild-moderate liver disease. But, for patients with severe liver disease (especially with a concurrent decline in renal function), an initial dosage decrease of 50% is recommended as a prudent change.[31] Doses of levetiracetam for liver disease patients should be titrated to clinical response, and measurement of serum concentrations can be a helpful adjunct. Because there is variability in the pharmacokinetics for the agent, patients with liver disease should be closely monitored for adverse effects due to levetiracetam therapy.

Adult and pediatric patients taking levetiracetam for the treatment of seizures have been studied while taking other antiepileptic drugs, and it is important to take concurrent medications into account when interpreting the findings of pharmacokinetic studies (see Table 16-2). Because the metabolism of levetiracetam does not include the cytochrome P-450 system or the UGT enzymes, the induction (phenytoin, carbamazepine, oxcarbazepine, phenobarbital, primidone) or inhibition (valproic acid and its derivatives) effects of other antiepileptics is moderated to a large extent compared to other antiseizure medications. For adults, taking other antiepileptic drugs that are inducers simultaneously with levetiracetam will increase Cl/F by about 15%-30% and decrease half-life by about 16% for levetiracetam. By comparison, taking valproic acid or one of its derivatives that are inhibitors concurrently with levetiracetam will decrease Cl/F by ~22% and increase half-life by ~58% for levetiracetam. When either inducers or inhibitors are coadministered alone with levetiracetam, V/F for levetiracetam will remain unchanged with concomitant antiepileptic therapy. If antiepileptic drugs from both the inducer and the inhibitor categories are given at the same time with levetiracetam, the effect on levetiracetam pharmacokinetics are largely neutral (~9% decrease in Cl/F, ~29% increase in half-life).[22,32] For the elderly and very elderly, the basic drug interaction pattern for levetiracetam with other antiepileptic drugs is the same, but adult patients over the age of 64 years have lower baseline levetiracetam Cl/F values for the effects to build upon.[33,34]

Pediatric patients taking other antiepileptic drugs that are inducers or inhibitors simultaneously with levetiracetam produces similar results for levetiracetam pharmacokinetic parameters. The inducer-class antiseizure medications (phenytoin, carbamazepine, oxcarbazepine, phenobarbital, primidone) increase Cl/F and decrease half-life for levetiracetam compared to patients taking levetiracetam monotherapy. The inhibitor-class antiseizure medications (valproic acid and its derivatives) decrease Cl/F and increase half-life for levetiracetam compared to patients taking levetiracetam monotherapy.[35-37]

Neonates (gestational age = 37-41 weeks, birth weight = 2550-3700 g) have been treated with intravenous levetiracetam to control seizures after delivery. Levetiracetam clearance on the first day of treatment was 0.71 mL/min/kg but rapidly increased over 7 days of therapy by 85%. During the same period, half-life decreased by 51% (see Table 16-2).

Intravenous levetiracetam has been investigated in normal individuals and patients with head trauma who were admitted to a neurologic critical care unit (see Table 16-2). Trauma patients are often hypermetabolic due to the physiologic demands placed on the body during the healing process. For this case, levetiracetam clearance is about 15% higher and half-life is about 33% shorter than normal adults.[20,21,38] If the intravenous dosage form is administered intramuscularly to normal adults, T_{max} averages 3.1 hours, and the bioavailability compared to intravenous drug is 100%.[21]

Using the FDA pregnancy classification system, levetiracetam is a Category C medication. Therefore, levetiracetam is used to treat pregnant women when the potential benefits of drug therapy outweigh the potential risks. Pregnancy alters the Cl/F of levetiracetam (see Table 16-2). Compared to baseline values, Cl/F continuously increases as the pregnancy progresses from the first to the second trimester, but a precipitous rise is noted during the third trimester. Clearance remains elevated until delivery, then starts to decline. By 1 month postpartum, levetiracetam clearance returns to baseline values. Levetiracetam crosses the placental barrier and is found in the breast milk of lactating mothers. At birth, the umbilical cord blood-to-maternal serum concentration ratio is approximately 1.09. The breast milk-to-maternal serum ratio is 1.05. After breastfeeding from mothers taking levetiracetam, the resulting range of levetiracetam serum concentration in newborns was 0.7-3.4 µg/mL.[13]

DRUG INTERACTIONS

Because the metabolism of levetiracetam does not involve the cytochrome P-450 system or the UGT enzymes, the induction (phenytoin, carbamazepine, oxcarbazepine, phenobarbital, primidone) or inhibition (valproic acid and its derivatives) effects of other antiepileptics on levetiracetam pharmacokinetics is moderate. Adult and pediatric patients taking levetiracetam for the treatment of seizures have been studied while taking other antiepileptic drugs, and it is important to take the effect of newly prescribed medications on levetiracetam pharmacokinetics into account when assessing a patient's therapy (see Table 16-2).[22,32-34] When other antiepileptic drugs are added to the treatment regimen of patients taking levetiracetam, patients should be monitored to ensure therapeutic effects are achieved and new adverse effects do not occur. Also, the effects of adding other common hepatic enzyme inducers or inhibitors to the therapeutic regimen of patients taking levetiracetam have not been thoroughly assessed. Measurement of levetiracetam steady-state concentrations can be a helpful adjunct when considering the effect of new therapies added to the medication regimen of epileptic patients.

INITIAL DOSAGE DETERMINATION METHODS

Several methods to initiate levetiracetam therapy are available. The *Pharmacokinetic Dosing method* is the most flexible of the techniques. It allows individualized target serum concentrations to be chosen for a patient, and each pharmacokinetic parameter can be customized to reflect specific disease states and conditions present in the patient. *Literature-based recommended dosing* is a very commonly used method to prescribe initial doses of levetiracetam. Doses are based on those that commonly produce steady-state concentrations in the lower end of the therapeutic range, although there is a wide variation in the actual concentrations for a specific patient (see Table 16-2).

Pharmacokinetic Dosing Method

The goal of initial dosing of levetiracetam is to compute the best dose possible for the patient given their set of disease states and conditions that influence levetiracetam pharmacokinetics and the epileptic disorder being treated. In order to do this, pharmacokinetic parameters for the patient will be estimated using average parameters measured in other patients with similar disease state and condition profiles.

Clearance, Volume of Distribution, and Half-Life Estimates

Levetiracetam is predominately eliminated unchanged by the kidney. Serum creatinine (S_{Cr}) and estimated creatinine clearance ($CrCl_{est}$) are used to estimate the elimination of agents that are renally eliminated, and there is a good correlation between creatinine clearance and levetiracetam clearance.[29,39-41] Unfortunately, the exact equation that best describes the relationship between $CrCl_{est}$ and levetiracetam clearance (Cl/F for orally administered drug, Cl for intravenously or intramuscularly administered drug) remains unpublished. Instead, clearance adjustments are used to account for decreased elimination for various $CrCl_{est}$ brackets (see Table 16-2). Because of this, a patient is categorized according to the disease states and conditions that are known to change levetiracetam clearance, and the clearance previously measured in these studies is used as an estimate of the current patient's levetiracetam clearance rate (see Table 16-2). Then, if the patient has a CrCl ≤80 mL/min, the clearance is adjusted for decreased renal function. For example, an adult epileptic patient with normal liver function that is to be initially treated with oral levetiracetam monotherapy (no other antiepileptic drug administration) would be assigned a levetiracetam Cl/F value equal to 0.90 mL/min/kg, a V/F value of 0.56 L/kg, and a $t_{1/2} = 7.3$ h.

If the patient has an estimated CrCl >80 mL/min, these estimates are used to compute levetiracetam dosages. If the patient has an estimated CrCl ≤80 mL/min, the clearance is adjusted for their renal function. To extend the current example, if the patient had a CrCl = 40 mL/min, the Cl/F value would be adjusted to 0.45 mL/min/kg (Cl/F = 0.50 • 0.90 mL/min/kg = 0.45 mL/min/kg), and the $t_{1/2}$ value would be adjusted to 14.4 hours ($t_{1/2} = [0.693(V/F)]/(Cl/F) = [0.693(0.56 \text{ L/kg})(1000 \text{ mL/L})]/[(0.45 \text{ mL/min/kg})(60 \text{ min/h})] = 14.4$ h, where 1000 mL/L and 60 min/h are unit conversion factors). If the patient is receiving intravenous or intramuscular levetiracetam (F = 1), the same type of adjustment for renal function is made using Cl instead of Cl/F.

Selection of Appropriate Pharmacokinetic Model and Equations

When oral therapy is required, levetiracetam is usually given once daily for extended-release tablets or twice daily for the other oral dosage forms. These dosage intervals provide a relatively smooth serum concentration-time curve that approximates an intravenous infusion. Because of this concentration-time profile, a very simple pharmacokinetic equation that calculates the average levetiracetam steady-state concentration (Css in μg/mL = mg/L) is widely used and allows maintenance dose computation: Css = (D/τ)/(Cl/F) or D = Css(Cl/F)τ, where D is the dose of levetiracetam in mg, Cl/F is the levetiracetam hybrid clearance/bioavailability parameter in L/h, and τ is the dosage interval in hours.

If intravenous dosing is needed, levetiracetam is usually given twice daily as a 15-minute infusion. For this route of administration, a predose steady-state trough concentration (Css_{min}) is usually maintained in the desired concentration range: $Css_{min} = (De^{-k\tau})/[V(1 - e^{-k\tau})]$ or $D = [Css_{min} V(1 - e^{-k\tau})]/(e^{-k\tau})$, where D is the dose of levetiracetam in mg, V is the volume of distribution in L, k is the elimination rate constant in h^{-1} [k = (0.693)/($t_{1/2}$)], and τ is the dosage interval in hours.

EXAMPLE 1 ▶▶▶

KL is a 50-year-old, 70-kg (height = 5 ft 10 in) male with complex partial seizures who requires therapy with levetiracetam. His serum creatinine equals 0.9 mg/dL. He has a normal liver function and is currently taking carbamazepine (steady-state concentration = 9.2 µg/mL). Additional dosage increases have been tried with carbamazepine, but they have been unsuccessful due to development of adverse effects. Suggest an initial levetiracetam dosage regimen using immediate-release tablets designed to achieve a steady-state levetiracetam concentration equal to 15 µg/mL.

1. *Estimate creatinine clearance.*

   This patient has a stable serum creatinine and is not obese. The Cockcroft-Gault equation can be used to estimate creatinine clearance:

   $$CrCl_{est} = [(140 - age)BW]/(72 \bullet S_{Cr}) = [(140 - 50 \, y)70 \, kg]/(72 \bullet 0.9 \, mg/dL) = 97 \, mL/min$$

   This patient has a $CrCl_{est}$ >80 mL/min, so levetiracetam clearance will not need to be adjusted for renal function (see Table 16-2).

2. *Estimate clearance, volume of distribution, and half-life according to disease states and conditions present in the patient.*
   The Cl/F rate for a patient taking carbamazepine is 1.17 mL/min/kg: Cl/F = (1.17 mL/min/kg)70 kg = 81.9 mL/min. The estimated V/F would be 0.6 L/kg, and the estimated half-life equals 6.1 h.

3. *Compute dosage regimen.*
   Levetiracetam immediate-release tablets will be prescribed to this patient. (Note: µg/mL = mg/L and this concentration unit was substituted for Css in the calculations so that unnecessary unit conversion was not required.) The dosage equation for oral levetiracetam is: D = Css(Cl/F)τ = (15 mg/L ● 81.9 mL/min ● 12 h ● 60 min/h)/(1000 mL/L) = 885 mg, rounded to 1000 mg every 12 hours.

   A steady-state trough levetiracetam serum concentration can be measured after steady-state is attained in 3-5 half-lives. Since the patient is expected to have a half-life equal to 6.1 hours, the levetiracetam steady-state concentration could be obtained any time after the second day of dosing (5 half-lives = 5 ● 6.1 h = 31 h or 1.3 d). Levetiracetam serum concentrations should also be measured if the patient experiences an exacerbation of their epilepsy or if the patient develops potential signs or symptoms of levetiracetam toxicity.

EXAMPLE 2 ▶▶▶

Same patient profile as in example 1, but serum creatinine is 1.8 mg/dL indicating renal impairment.

1. *Estimate creatinine clearance.*

   This patient has a stable serum creatinine and is not obese. The Cockcroft-Gault equation can be used to estimate creatinine clearance:

   $$CrCl_{est} = [(140 - age)BW]/(72 \bullet S_{Cr}) = [(140 - 50 \, y)70 \, kg]/(72 \bullet 1.8 \, mg/dL) = 49 \, mL/min$$

   This patient has a $CrCl_{est}$ = 30-50 mL/min, so levetiracetam clearance will be adjusted for renal function by multiplying Cl/F by 0.50 (see Table 16-2).

2. *Estimate clearance, volume of distribution, and half-life according to disease states and conditions present in the patient.*
   The Cl/F rate for a patient taking carbamazepine is 1.17 mL/min/kg, and the adjustment for renal dysfunction is 0.50: Cl/F = (0.50)1.17 mL/min/kg = 0.59 mL/min/kg: Cl/F = (0.59 mL/min/kg)70 kg = 41.3 mL/min. The estimated V/F would be 0.6 L/kg, and the estimated half-life equals: $t_{1/2}$ = [0.693(V/F)]/(Cl/F) = [0.693(0.6 L/kg)(1000 mL/L)]/[(0.59 mL/min/kg)(60 min/h)] = 11.7 h

3. *Compute dosage regimen.*

Levetiracetam immediate-release tablets will be prescribed to this patient. (Note: μg/mL = mg/L and this concentration unit was substituted for Css in the calculations so that unnecessary unit conversion was not required.) The dosage equation for oral levetiracetam is: D = Css(Cl/F)τ = (15 mg/L • 41.3 mL/min • 12 h • 60 min/h)/(1000 mL/L) = 446 mg, rounded to 500 mg every 12 hours.

A steady-state trough levetiracetam serum concentration can be measured after steady-state is attained in 3-5 half-lives. Since the patient is expected to have a half-life equal to 11.7 hours, the levetiracetam steady-state concentration could be obtained any time after the third day of dosing (5 half-lives = 5 • 11.7 h = 59 h or 2.5 d). Levetiracetam serum concentrations should also be measured if the patient experiences an exacerbation of their epilepsy or if the patient develops potential signs or symptoms of levetiracetam toxicity.

EXAMPLE 3 ▶▶▶

Same patient profile as in example 1, but patient not taking carbamazepine, and he will receive an intravenous levetiracetam dosage regimen designed to achieve a steady-state trough concentration equal to 15 μg/mL.

1. *Estimate creatinine clearance.*

This patient has a stable serum creatinine and is not obese. The Cockcroft-Gault equation can be used to estimate creatinine clearance:

$$CrCl_{est} = [(140 - age)BW]/(72 • S_{Cr}) = [(140 - 50 \text{ y})70 \text{ kg}]/(72 • 0.9 \text{ mg/dL}) = 97 \text{ mL/min}$$

This patient has a $CrCl_{est}$ > 80 mL/min, so levetiracetam clearance will not need to be adjusted for renal function (see Table 16-2).

2. *Estimate clearance, volume of distribution, and half-life according to disease states and conditions present in the patient.*

The Cl for a patient taking intravenous levetiracetam as monotherapy is 0.95 mL/min/kg: Cl = (0.95 mL/min/kg) 70 kg = 66.5 mL/min. The estimated V would be 0.6 L/kg: V = (0.6 L/kg)70 kg = 42 L. The estimated half-life equals 7.8 h, so k = (0.693)/(t$_{1/2}$) = (0.693)/(7.8 h) = 0.089 h^{-1}.

3. *Compute dosage regimen.*

Levetiracetam intravenous injection will be prescribed to this patient. (Note: μg/mL = mg/L and this concentration unit was substituted for Css in the calculations so that unnecessary unit conversion was not required.) The dosage equation for intravenous levetiracetam is: D = [Css$_{min}$ V(1 − e$^{-kτ}$)]/(e$^{-kτ}$) = [15 mg/L • 42 L (1 − e$^{-(0.089h^{-1})(12\,h)}$)]/(e$^{-(0.089h^{-1})(12\,h)}$) = 1203 mg, rounded to 1250 mg every 12 hours.

A steady-state trough levetiracetam serum concentration can be measured after steady-state is attained in 3-5 half-lives. Since the patient is expected to have a half-life equal to 7.8 hours, the levetiracetam steady-state concentration could be obtained any time after the second day of dosing (5 half-lives = 5 • 7.8 h = 39 h or 1.6 d). Levetiracetam serum concentrations should also be measured if the patient experiences an exacerbation of their epilepsy or if the patient develops potential signs or symptoms of levetiracetam toxicity.

Literature-Based Recommended Dosing

Because of the large amount of variability in levetiracetam pharmacokinetics, even when concurrent disease states and conditions are identified, most clinicians believe that the use of standard drug doses for various situations is warranted. The original computation of these doses were based on the Pharmacokinetic Dosing method, and subsequently modified based on clinical experience. In general, the expected steady-state serum concentrations used to compute these doses was in the lower end of the therapeutic range (12-15 μg/mL). For adults, the initial dose of levetiracetam is 1000 mg/d, administered once daily for the extended-release tablet and as divided

TABLE 16-4   Literature-Based Doses for Levetiracetam in Adult Patients With Renal Dysfunction

CrCl$_{est}$ (mL/min/1.73 m^2)	Dose
>80	500-1500 mg every 12 h
50-80	500-1000 mg every 12 h
30-50	250-750 mg every 12 h
<30	250-500 mg every 12 h

End-stage renal disease patients receiving hemodialysis: 500-1000 mg every 24 h maintenance dose, with a replacement supplemental dose of 250-500 mg after a dialysis session.

To normalize CrCl$_{est}$ (in mL/min) to a standard body surface area of 1.73 m^2 (mL/min/1.73 m^2), first compute the patient's own body surface area (BSA in m^2): BSA = 0.007184 • W$^{0.425}$ • H$^{0.725}$, where W is weight in kg and H is height in cm.[46] Then, apply the normalization equation: CrCl$_{est}$ (in mL/min/1.73 m^2) = (CrCl$_{est}$/BSA)1.73 m^2. Example: For a patient with a height = 173 cm, weight = 67 kg, CrCl$_{est}$ = 65 mL/min: BSA = 0.007184 • W$^{0.425}$ • H$^{0.725}$ = 0.007184 • (67 kg)$^{0.425}$ • (173 cm)$^{0.725}$ = 1.80 m^2, CrCl$_{est}$ (in mL/min/1.73 m^2) = [(CrCl$_{est}$)/(BSA)]1.73 m^2 = [(65 mL/min)/(1.80 m^2)]1.73 m^2 = 62.5 mL/min/1.73 m^2.

doses every 12 hours for the other oral dosage forms. The dose is titrated up 1000 mg/d every 2 weeks as needed, and the patient is monitored for seizure frequency and adverse drug effects. The maximum dose is usually 3000-4000 mg/d. Because the majority of levetiracetam is eliminated unchanged in the urine, doses are adjusted for renal dysfunction (Table 16-4). If the patient has severe hepatic dysfunction (Child-Pugh score ≥10), the prescribed maintenance dose can be decreased by 50%. For children, the dose varies according to age, and Table 16-5 lists initial doses, dosage increases during the titration period, and the maximum recommended dose.[42]

To illustrate the similarities and differences between this method of dosage calculation and the Pharmacokinetic Dosing method, the same examples used in the previous section will be used.

EXAMPLE 4 ▶▶▶

KL is a 50-year-old, 70-kg (height = 5 ft 10 in) male with complex partial seizures who requires therapy with levetiracetam. His serum creatinine equals 0.9 mg/dL. He has normal liver function and is currently taking carbamazepine (steady-state concentration = 9.2 µg/mL). Additional dosage increases have been tried with carbamazepine, but they have been unsuccessful due to development of adverse effects. Suggest an initial levetiracetam dosage regimen using immediate-release tablets designed to achieve a steady-state levetiracetam concentration equal to 15 µg/mL.

1. *Estimate creatinine clearance.*

   This patient has a stable serum creatinine and is not obese. The Cockcroft-Gault equation can be used to estimate creatinine clearance:

   $$CrCl_{est} = [(140 - age)BW]/(72 • S_{Cr}) = [(140 - 50 \text{ y})70 \text{ kg}]/(72 • 0.9 \text{ mg/dL}) = 97 \text{ mL/min}$$

   This patient has a CrCl$_{est}$ > 80 mL/min, so levetiracetam clearance will not need to be adjusted for renal function (see Table 16-4).

2. *Estimate levetiracetam dose according to disease states and conditions present in the patient.*

   For adults, the initial dose of levetiracetam is 1000 mg/d, administered as divided doses every 12 hours for immediate-release tablets. The dose is titrated up 1000 mg/d every 2 weeks as needed, and the patient is monitored for seizure frequency and adverse drug effects. The maximum dose is usually 3000-4000 mg/d.

   A steady-state trough levetiracetam serum concentration can be measured after steady-state is attained in 3-5 half-lives. Since the patient is expected to have a half-life equal to 6.1 hours, the levetiracetam steady-state concentration could be obtained any time after the second day of dosing (5 half-lives = 5 • 6.1 h = 31 h or 1.3 d). Levetiracetam serum concentrations should also be measured if the patient experiences an exacerbation of their epilepsy or if the patient develops potential signs or symptoms of levetiracetam toxicity.

TABLE 16-5   Literature-Based Initial Dose, Titration Rate, and Maximum Dose for Levetiracetam Immediate-Release Dosage Forms in Children

Age Group	Initial Dose (mg/kg/d, Given Every 12 hours)	Additional Titration Dose (mg/kg/d, Given Every 12 hours. This Dose is Added to Current Maintenance Dose Every 2 weeks, Based on Response and Adverse Effects)	Maximum Dose (mg/kg/d, Given Every 12 hours, Based on Response and Adverse Effects)
1-6 mo	14	14	42
6 mo to 4 y	20	20	50
4-16 y	20	20	60

EXAMPLE 5 ▶▶▶

Same patient profile as in example 1, but serum creatinine is 1.8 mg/dL indicating renal impairment.

1. *Estimate creatinine clearance.*

    This patient has a stable serum creatinine and is not obese. The Cockcroft-Gault equation can be used to estimate creatinine clearance:

$$CrCl_{est} = [(140 - age)BW]/(72 \bullet S_{Cr}) = [(140 - 50 \text{ y})70 \text{ kg}]/(72 \bullet 1.8 \text{ mg/dL}) = 49 \text{ mL/min}$$

    This patient has a $CrCl_{est}$ between 30 and 50 mL/min, so levetiracetam clearance will be adjusted for renal function according to the recommendations in Table 16-4.

2. *Estimate levetiracetam dose according to disease states and conditions present in the patient.*

    According to the guidelines given in Table 16-4, the initial dose for this patient should be 250 to 750 mg every 12 hours. Because the patient's renal function is in the upper area of the $CrCl_{est}$ adjustment range, the dose of 500 mg every 12 hours was prescribed.

    A steady-state trough levetiracetam serum concentration can be measured after steady-state is attained in 3-5 half-lives. Since the patient is expected to have a half-life equal to 11.7 hours, the levetiracetam steady-state concentration could be obtained any time after the third day of dosing (5 half-lives = 5 • 11.7 h = 59 h or 2.5 d). Levetiracetam serum concentrations should also be measured if the patient experiences an exacerbation of their epilepsy or if the patient develops potential signs or symptoms of levetiracetam toxicity.

EXAMPLE 6 ▶▶▶

Same patient profile as in example 1, but patient not taking carbamazepine, and he will receive an intravenous levetiracetam dosage regimen designed to achieve a steady-state trough concentration equal to 15 μg/mL.

1. *Estimate creatinine clearance.*

    This patient has a stable serum creatinine and is not obese. The Cockcroft-Gault equation can be used to estimate creatinine clearance:

$$CrCl_{est} = [(140 - age)BW]/(72 \bullet S_{Cr}) = [(140 - 50 \text{ y})70 \text{ kg}]/(72 \bullet 0.9 \text{ mg/dL}) = 97 \text{ mL/min}$$

    This patient has a $CrCl_{est}$ >80 mL/min, so levetiracetam clearance will not need to be adjusted for renal function (see Table 16-2).

2. *Estimate levetiracetam dose according to disease states and conditions present in the patient.*

For adults, the initial dose of levetiracetam is 1000 mg/d, administered intravenously as divided doses every 12 hours. The drug is infused over 15 minutes. The dose is titrated up 1000 mg/d every 2 weeks as needed, and the patient is monitored for seizure frequency and adverse drug effects. The maximum dose is usually 3000-4000 mg/d.

A steady-state trough levetiracetam serum concentration can be measured after steady-state is attained in 3-5 half-lives. Since the patient is expected to have a half-life equal to 7.8 hours, the levetiracetam steady-state concentration could be obtained any time after the second day of dosing (5 half-lives = 5 • 7.8 h = 39 h or 1.6 d). Levetiracetam serum concentrations should also be measured if the patient experiences an exacerbation of their epilepsy or if the patient develops potential signs or symptoms of levetiracetam toxicity.

USE OF LEVETIRACETAM SERUM CONCENTRATIONS TO ALTER DOSES

A definitive therapeutic range for steady-state levetiracetam serum concentrations has not been established.[9-11] Because of this, serum concentration monitoring for levetiracetam plays only a supportive role in the dosing of the drug. Important patient parameters (seizure frequency, potential levetiracetam side effects, etc) should be followed to confirm that the patient is responding to treatment and not developing adverse drug reactions.[6] However, there are clinical situations where levetiracetam serum concentrations can be very helpful.

Once dosage titration has been conducted, and an effective dose of levetiracetam has been established by assessing therapeutic response and absence of adverse effects, many clinicians obtain a steady-state trough levetiracetam concentration to establish an individualized effective target value for the patient. When this is done, if seizure frequency changes or an adverse effect occurs, another steady-state trough levetiracetam serum concentration can be measured to ascertain potential solutions to the problem. For instance, if a patient suddenly has more seizures than usual, comparing the current levetiracetam serum concentration with the established effective target levetiracetam concentration can be helpful to decide a course of action. If the current levetiracetam concentration is lower than usual, reasons for the change can be explored (lack of adherence to therapy, drug interaction, etc), and, if appropriate, a levetiracetam dosage increase can be considered to reestablish effective concentrations. If the current levetiracetam concentration is about the same, changes to therapy may be warranted (increase levetiracetam dose, addition of other drug therapy, etc). Alternatively, if a patient suddenly develops adverse effects that could be due to levetiracetam therapy, and the current levetiracetam serum concentration is high, it may be appropriate to decrease the levetiracetam dose. Also, when an effective levetiracetam concentration has been established for a patient, the effects of new drug therapy that may cause drug interactions or of new disease states or conditions that can alter levetiracetam pharmacokinetics can be assessed prospectively by measuring current levetiracetam concentration before any clinical events occur.

When a levetiracetam dosage change is made, sufficient time to attain steady-state conditions (~3-5 half-lives) should be allowed before assessing therapeutic outcome (see Table 16-2). Of course, any time adverse effects occur during dosage titration, measures should be taken to assess the likelihood that they are due to levetiracetam treatment and appropriate action should be taken when needed.

If levetiracetam serum concentrations are measured in patients and a dosage change is necessary, clinicians should seek to use the simplest, most straightforward method available to determine the steady-state concentration for the new regimen. In most cases, a simple dosage ratio can be used to change doses since levetiracetam follows *linear pharmacokinetics*. In some situations, it may be necessary or desirable to compute levetiracetam *pharmacokinetic parameters* for the patient and utilize these to calculate the steady-state concentration for a new dose. With two steady-state concentrations obtained before and after intravenous dose administration, it is possible to compute the levetiracetam pharmacokinetic parameters for a patient using the *One-Compartment Model*

Parameter method and utilize these to calculate the best drug dose. Finally, computerized methods that incorporate expected population pharmacokinetic characteristics (*Bayesian pharmacokinetic computer programs*) can be used in difficult cases where renal function is changing, serum concentrations are obtained at suboptimal times, or the patient was not at steady-state when serum concentrations were measured. An additional benefit of this method is that a complete pharmacokinetic workup (determination of clearance, volume of distribution, and half-life) can be done with one or more measured concentrations that do not have to be at steady-state.

Selection of Appropriate Pharmacokinetic Model and Equations

When oral therapy is required, levetiracetam is usually given once daily for extended-release tablets or twice daily for the other oral dosage forms. These dosage intervals provide a relatively smooth serum concentration-time curve that approximates an intravenous infusion. Because of this concentration-time profile, a very simple pharmacokinetic equation that computes the average levetiracetam steady-state serum concentration (Css in μg/mL = mg/L) is widely used and allows maintenance dosage calculation: Css = $(D/\tau)/(Cl/F)$ or D = Css(Cl/F)τ, where D is the dose of levetiracetam in mg, Cl/F is levetiracetam hybrid clearance/bioavailability parameter in L/h, and τ is the dosage interval in hours.

If intravenous dosing is needed, levetiracetam is usually given twice daily as a 15-minute infusion. For this route of administration, a predose steady-state trough concentration (Css$_{min}$) is usually maintained in the desired concentration range: Css$_{min}$ = $(De^{-k\tau})/[V(1 - e^{-k\tau})]$ or D = $[Css_{min} V(1 - e^{-k\tau})]/(e^{-k\tau})$, where D is the dose of levetiracetam in mg, V is the volume of distribution in L, k is the elimination rate constant in h^{-1} [k = $(0.693)/(t_{1/2})$], and τ is the dosage interval in hours.

Linear Pharmacokinetics Method

Because levetiracetam follows linear, dose-proportional pharmacokinetics, steady-state serum concentrations change in proportion to dose according to the following equation: $D_{new}/C_{ss,new} = D_{old}/C_{ss,old}$ or $D_{new} = (C_{ss,new}/C_{ss,old}) D_{old}$, where D is the dose, Css is the steady-state concentration, old indicates the dose that produced the steady-state concentration that the patient is currently receiving, and new denotes the steady-state concentration produced by the newly prescribed dose. The advantages of this method are that it is quick and simple. The disadvantage is steady-state concentrations are required. Additionally, this method can be used with any route of administration to adjust doses of levetiracetam if only a single steady-state concentration is available.

EXAMPLE 7 ▶▶▶

KL is a 51-year-old, 75-kg (height = 5 ft 10 in) male with complex partial seizures who receives monotherapy with levetiracetam. He has normal liver and renal function. KL was titrated to a dose of levetiracetam 1500 mg daily of extended-release tablets without any side effects and a decreased seizure frequency. At that time, a steady-state levetiracetam trough concentration was obtained before a dose and equaled 30.2 μg/mL. Several months ago, the patient was started on carbamazepine, and he has been on a stable dose for 4 weeks. Today, the steady-state levetiracetam trough concentration obtained before the next dose was 24.5 μg/mL. Suggest a new maintenance dosage regimen using extended-release levetiracetam tablets to reestablish the original levetiracetam steady-state concentration for this patient.

1. *Compute new dose to achieve the desired serum concentration.*

Using linear pharmacokinetics, the new levetiracetam dose would equal: D_{new} = (Css$_{new}$ /Css$_{old}$) D$_{old}$ = (30.2 μg/mL / 24.5 μg/mL) 1500 mg/d = 1849 mg/d, rounded to 1750 mg/d.

The patient should be carefully monitored for seizure frequency and adverse effects. If desired, steady-state levetiracetam trough serum concentrations can be measured 3-5 half-lives after the dosage change has been made (see Table 16-2: ~$t_{1/2}$ = 6.1 hours, ~3-5 $t_{1/2}$ in 1-2 days).

Pharmacokinetic Parameter Method

The Pharmacokinetic Parameter method of adjusting drug doses was among the first techniques available to change doses using serum concentrations. It allows the computation of an individual's own, unique pharmacokinetic constants and uses those to calculate the steady-state concentration that is achieved from a desired levetiracetam dosage regimen. For patients receiving oral levetiracetam, the Pharmacokinetic Parameter method requires that steady-state has been achieved and uses only a single steady-state levetiracetam concentration (Css). Levetiracetam Cl/F can be calculated using the following formula: $Cl/F = (D/\tau)/Css$, where D is the dose of levetiracetam in mg, Cl/F is levetiracetam hybrid clearance/bioavailability parameter in L/h, and τ is the dosage interval in hours. The corresponding equation used for intravenously administered drug is: $Cl = (D/\tau)/Css$.

To illustrate the similarities and differences between this method of dosage calculation and the Pharmacokinetic Parameter method, the same example used in the previous section will be used.

EXAMPLE 8 ▶▶▶

KL is a 51-year-old, 75-kg (height = 5 ft 10 in) male with complex partial seizures who receives monotherapy with levetiracetam. He has normal liver and renal function. KL was titrated to a dose of levetiracetam 1500 mg daily of extended-release tablets without any side effects and a decreased seizure frequency. At that time, a steady-state levetiracetam trough concentration was obtained before a dose and equaled 30.2 μg/mL. Several months ago, the patient was started on carbamazepine, and he has been on a stable dose for 4 weeks. Today, the steady-state levetiracetam trough concentration obtained before the next dose was 24.5 μg/mL. Suggest a new maintenance dosage regimen using extended-release levetiracetam tablets to reestablish the original levetiracetam steady-state concentration for this patient.

1. *Compute pharmacokinetic parameters.*

Levetiracetam Cl/F can be computed using a steady-state levetiracetam trough concentration: $Cl/F = (D/\tau)/Css = [(1500\ mg)/(24\ h)]/(24.5\ L) = 2.55\ L/h$. (Note: μg/mL = mg/L and this concentration unit was substituted for Css in the calculations so that unnecessary unit conversion was not required.)

2. *Compute the new levetiracetam dosage.*

Levetiracetam Cl/F is used to compute the new dose: $D = Css(Cl/F)\tau = 30.2\ mg/L(2.55\ L/h)\ 24\ h = 1848\ mg$, rounded to 1750 mg every 24 hours.

The patient should be carefully monitored for seizure frequency and adverse effects. If desired, steady-state levetiracetam trough serum concentrations can be measured 3-5 half-lives after the dosage change has been made (see Table 16-2: $\sim t_{1/2} = 6.1$ hours, $\sim$3-5 $t_{1/2}$ in 1-2 days).

One-Compartment Model Parameter Method

The One-Compartment Model Parameter method of adjusting drug doses was among the first techniques available to change doses using serum concentrations.[43] It allows the computation of an individual's own, unique pharmacokinetic constants and uses those to calculate a dose that achieves the desired levetiracetam concentrations. The standard One-Compartment Model Parameter method conducts a small pharmacokinetic experiment using three to four levetiracetam serum concentrations obtained during a dosage interval and does not require steady-state conditions. The Steady-State One-Compartment Model Parameter method assumes that steady-state has been achieved and requires only a steady-state peak and trough concentration pair obtained before and after a dose. One-compartment model intravenous bolus equations are used successfully to dose drugs that are given by infusion when the infusion time is less than the drug half-life.[44]

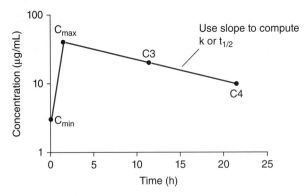

FIGURE 16-1   The One Compartment Model Parameter method for individualization of levetiracetam doses uses a trough (C_{min}), peak (C_{max}), and one to two additional postdose concentrations (C_3, C_4) to compute a patient's own, unique pharmacokinetic parameters. This version of the One Compartment Model Parameter method does not require steady-state conditions. The peak and trough concentrations are used to calculate the volume of distribution, and the postdose concentrations (C_{max}, C_3, C_4) are used to compute half-life. Once the volume of distribution and half-life have been measured, they can be used to compute the exact dose needed to achieve desired levetiracetam concentrations.

Standard One-Compartment Model Parameter Method

The standard version of the One-Compartment Model Parameter method does not require steady-state concentrations. A trough levetiracetam concentration is obtained before a dose, a peak levetiracetam concentration is obtained after the dose is infused (½ hour after a 15 minute infusion), and one to two additional postdose serum levetiracetam concentrations are obtained (Figure 16-1). Ideally, the one to two postdose concentrations should be obtained at least 1 estimated half-life from each other to minimize the influence of assay error. The postdose serum concentrations are used to calculate the levetiracetam elimination rate constant and half-life (see Figure 16-1). The half-life can be computed by graphing the postdose concentrations on semilogarithmic paper, drawing the best straight line through the data points, and determining the time needed for serum concentrations to decline by one-half. Once the half-life is known, the elimination rate constant (k) can be computed: $k = 0.693/(t_{1/2})$. Alternatively, the elimination rate constant can be directly calculated using the postdose serum concentrations [$k = (\ln C_1 - \ln C_2)/\Delta t$], where C_1 and C_2 are postdose serum concentrations and Δt is the time that expired between the times that C_1 and C_2 were obtained, and the half-life can be computed using the elimination rate constant ($t_{1/2} = 0.693/k$). The volume of distribution (V) is calculated using the following equation: $V = D/(C_{max} - C_{min})$ where D is the levetiracetam dose, C_{max} is the peak concentration and C_{min} is the trough concentration. The elimination rate constant and volume of distribution measured in this fashion are the patient's own, unique levetiracetam pharmacokinetic constants and can be used in one-compartment model intravenous bolus equations to compute the required dose to achieve any desired serum concentration.

Steady-State One-Compartment Model Parameter Method

If a steady-state peak and trough levetiracetam concentration pair is available for a patient, the One-Compartment Model Parameter method can be used to compute patient pharmacokinetic parameters and levetiracetam doses (Figure 16-2). Since the patient is at steady-state, the measured trough concentration obtained before the dose was given can be extrapolated to the next dosage time and used to compute the levetiracetam elimination rate constant [$k = (\ln Css_{max} - \ln Css_{min})/(\tau - t')$, where Css_{max} and Css_{min} are the

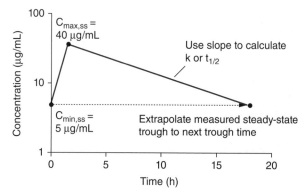

FIGURE 16-2 The steady-state version of the One Compartment Model Parameter method uses a steady-state peak (Css_{max}) and trough (Css_{min}) concentration pair to individualize levetiracetam therapy. Because the patient is at steady-state, consecutive trough concentrations will be identical, so the trough concentration can be extrapolated to the next predose time. The steady-state peak and trough concentrations are used to calculate the volume of distribution and half-life. Once the volume of distribution and half-life have been measured, they can be used to compute the exact dose needed to achieve the desired levetiracetam concentrations.

steady-state peak and trough serum concentrations and t' and τ are the combined infusion time plus waiting time and dosage interval, respectively], and the half-life can be computed using the elimination rate constant ($t_{1/2} = 0.693/k$). The volume of distribution (V) is calculated using the following equation: $V = D/(Css_{max} - Css_{min})$ where D is the levetiracetam dose, Css_{max} is the steady-state peak concentration, and Css_{min} is the steady-state trough concentration. The elimination rate constant and volume of distribution measured in this way are the patient's own, unique levetiracetam pharmacokinetic constants and can be used in one-compartment model intravenous bolus equations to compute the required dose to achieve any desired serum concentration. The dosage calculations are similar to those done in the initial dosage section of this chapter, except that the patient's real pharmacokinetic parameters are used in the equations instead of population pharmacokinetic estimates.

EXAMPLE 9 ▶▶▶

KL is a 50-year-old, 70-kg (height = 5 ft 10 in) male with complex partial seizures who requires therapy with levetiracetam. His serum creatinine equals 0.9 mg/dL. He has normal liver function and is currently taking carbamazepine (steady-state concentration = 9.2 μg/mL). Additional dosage increases have been tried with carbamazepine, but they have been unsuccessful due to development of adverse effects. The patient was started on an initial levetiracetam dosage regimen using intravenous drug of 1000 mg every 12 hours designed to achieve a steady-state trough levetiracetam concentration equal to 15 μg/mL 4 days ago, but seizure frequency did not markedly change. To assist in dosage adjustment, steady-state levetiracetam concentrations were drawn just before a dose (Css_{min} = 7.9 μg/mL) and 30 minutes after a 15-minute infusion (Css_{max} = 29.6 μg/mL). Compute a new intravenous levetiracetam dosage regimen designed to achieve a steady-state trough concentration equal to 12 μg/mL.

1. *Estimate creatinine clearance.*

This patient has a stable serum creatinine and is not obese. The Cockcroft-Gault equation can be used to estimate creatinine clearance:

$$CrCl_{est} = [(140 - age)BW]/(72 \cdot S_{Cr}) = [(140 - 50 \text{ y})70 \text{ kg}]/(72 \cdot 0.9 \text{ mg/dL}) = 97 \text{ mL/min}$$

This patient has a $CrCl_{est}$ >80 mL/min, so levetiracetam $t_{1/2}$ is expected to be 6.1 h (see Table 16-2). After 4 days of treatment with levetiracetam, the patient is at steady-state.

2. *Use Steady-State One-Compartment Model Parameter method to compute a new dose.*

A. *Compute the patient's elimination rate constant and half-life (note: t' = infusion time + waiting time of 15 minutes and ½ hour, respectively).*

$$k = (\ln Css_{max} - \ln Css_{min})/(\tau - t') = (\ln 29.6\ \mu g/mL - \ln 7.9\ \mu g/mL)/(12\ h - 0.75\ h) = 0.117\ h^{-1}$$
$$t_{1/2} = 0.693/k = 0.693/0.117\ h^{-1} = 5.9\ h$$

B. *Compute the patient's volume of distribution.*

$$V = D/(Css_{max} - Css_{min}) = 1000\ mg/(29.6\ mg/L - 7.9\ mg/L) = 46.1\ L$$

C. *Choose a new steady-state trough concentration.*

For the purposes of this example, the desired steady-state trough concentration will be 12 µg/mL.

D. *Determine the new dosage interval for the desired concentrations.*

For levetiracetam, a dosage interval of 12 hours is used for most patients (see Table 16-4).

E. *Determine the new dose for the desired concentrations.*

The dose is computed using the one-compartment model intravenous bolus equation utilized in the initial dosing section of this chapter:

$$D = [Css_{min}\ V(1 - e^{-k\tau})]/(e^{-k\tau}) = [12\ mg/L \bullet 46.1\ L\ (1 - e^{-(0.117\ h^{-1})(12\ h)})]/(e^{-(0.117\ h^{-1})(12\ h)}) = 1699\ mg,\ \text{rounded to } 1750$$

A dose of levetiracetam 1750 mg every 12 hours would be prescribed.

BAYESIAN PHARMACOKINETIC COMPUTER PROGRAMS

Computer programs are available that can assist in the computation of pharmacokinetic parameters for patients. The most reliable computer programs use a nonlinear regression algorithm that incorporates components of Bayes theorem.[45] Nonlinear regression is a statistical technique that uses an iterative process to compute the best pharmacokinetic parameters for a concentration-time data set. Briefly, the patient's drug dosage schedule and serum concentrations are input into the computer. The computer program has a pharmacokinetic equation preprogrammed for the drug and administration method (oral, intravenous bolus, intravenous infusion, etc). Typically, a one-compartment model is used, although some programs allow the user to choose among several different equations. Using population estimates based on demographic information for the patient (age, weight, gender, liver function, cardiac status, etc) supplied by the user, the computer program then computes estimated serum concentrations at each time there are actual serum concentrations. The computer program then changes kinetic parameters, and a new set of estimated serum concentrations are computed. The pharmacokinetic parameters that generated the estimated serum concentrations closest to the actual values are remembered by the computer program, and the process is repeated until the set of pharmacokinetic parameters that result in estimated serum concentrations that are statistically closest to the actual serum concentrations are generated. These pharmacokinetic parameters can then be used to compute improved dosing schedules for patients. Bayes theorem is used in the computer algorithm to balance the results of the computations between values based solely on the patient's serum drug concentrations and those based only on patient population parameters. Results from studies that compare various methods of dosage adjustment have consistently found that these types of computer-dosing programs perform at least as well as experienced clinical pharmacokineticists and clinicians and better than inexperienced clinicians.

Some clinicians use Bayesian pharmacokinetic computer programs exclusively to alter drug doses based on serum concentrations. An advantage of this approach is that consistent dosage recommendations are made when several different practitioners are involved in therapeutic drug monitoring programs. However, since simpler dosing methods work just as well for patients with stable pharmacokinetic parameters and steady-state drug concentrations, many clinicians reserve the use of computer programs for more difficult situations. Those situations include serum concentrations that are not at steady-state, serum concentrations not obtained at the specific times needed to employ simpler methods, and unstable pharmacokinetic parameters. Many Bayesian pharmacokinetic computer programs are available to users, and most should provide answers similar to the one used in the following examples. The program used to solve problems in this book is DrugCalc written by Dr Dennis Mungall.[45]

EXAMPLE 10 ▶▶▶

LK is a 13-year-old, 47-kg (height = 5 ft 1 in) female with partial seizures who requires therapy with oral leveti-racetam. The patient has normal liver and renal function (bilirubin = 0.5 mg/dL, albumin 4.6 mg/dL, serum creatinine = 0.5 mg/dL), and she is taking carbamazepine. After dosage titration, the patient was pre-scribed 750 mg every 12 hours of levetiracetam immediate-release tablets for 2 weeks, and the steady-state levetiracetam trough concentration equals 9.1 μg/mL. The patient is assessed to be adherent with her dosage regimen. Suggest a levetiracetam dosage regimen designed to achieve a steady-state levetiracetam trough con-centration of 15 μg/mL.

1. *Enter the patient's demographic, drug-dosing, and serum concentration/time data into the computer program.*
2. *Compute pharmacokinetic parameters for the patient using Bayesian pharmacokinetic computer program.*
   The pharmacokinetic parameters computed by the program are a volume of distribution of 33 L, a half-life equal to 4.7 h, and a clearance equal to 58 mL/min.
3. *Compute dose required to achieve the desired levetiracetam serum concentrations.*
   The one-compartment model first-order absorption equations used by the program to compute doses indi-cates that a dose of 1250 mg every 12 hours will produce a steady-state levetiracetam trough concentration of 15.8 μg/mL.

DOSING STRATEGIES

Initial dose and dosage adjustment techniques using serum concentrations can be used in any combination as long as the limitations of each method are observed. Some dosing schemes link together logically when con-sidered according to their basic approaches or philosophies. Dosage strategies that follow similar pathways are given in Table 16-6.

TABLE 16-6   Dosing Strategies

Dosing Approach/Philosophy	Initial Dosing	Use of Serum Concentrations to Alter Doses
Pharmacokinetic parameter/equations	Pharmacokinetic Dosing method	Pharmacokinetic Parameter method (any route) or One Compartment Model Parameter method (intravenous)
Literature-based/concept	Literature-based Recommended Dosing method	Linear Pharmacokinetics method
Computerized	Bayesian computer program	Bayesian computer program

SPECIAL DOSING CONSIDERATIONS

Conversion of Patient Doses Between Dosage Forms

The bioavailability of levetiracetam for oral solution, immediate-release tablets, and sustained-release tablets are all similar (F = 0.92). Because of this, patients can be switched between oral dosage forms using the same dose for each. However, since the absorption characteristics are different (T_{max} = 0.8 hour for oral solution, T_{max} = 1.5 hours for immediate release tablets, and T_{max} = 4.5 hours for extended-release tablets), there will be some small differences in steady-state trough levetiracetam concentrations. Because there is such a small difference between oral bioavailability and the bioavailability for the intravenous drug (F = 1), patients can be switched between any of the oral dosage forms and the intravenous form without dosage alteration. Should a patient experience increased seizure frequency or adverse effects attributable to levetiracetam after a dosage form change, a steady-state levetiracetam concentration can be measured to see if it has been altered by the conversion.

PROBLEMS

The following problems are intended to emphasize the computation of initial and individualized doses using clinical pharmacokinetic techniques. Clinicians should always consult the patient's chart to confirm that current anticonvulsant therapy is appropriate. Additionally, all other medications that the patient is taking, including prescription and nonprescription drugs, should be noted and checked to ascertain if a potential drug interaction with levetiracetam exists.

1. FH is a 37-year-old, 85-kg (height = 6 ft 1 in) male with tonic-clonic seizures who requires therapy with oral levetiracetam monotherapy. He has normal liver and renal function (S_{cr} = 1.1 mg/dL). Suggest an initial levetiracetam dosage regimen using extended-release tablets designed to achieve a steady-state levetiracetam concentration equal to 15 µg/mL.

2. Patient FH (see problem 1) was prescribed 1000 mg every 24 hours of levetiracetam extended-release tablets for 2 weeks, and the steady-state levetiracetam trough concentration equals 12.9 µg/mL. The patient is assessed to be adherent with his dosage regimen. Suggest a levetiracetam dosage regimen designed to achieve a steady-state levetiracetam trough concentration of 20 µg/mL.

3. AS is a 9-year-old, 35-kg female (height = 54 in) with complex partial seizures who requires therapy with oral levetiracetam immediate-release tablets. She has normal liver and renal function (S_{cr} = 0.6 mg/dL). AS also takes carbamazepine to treat her epilepsy. Suggest an initial levetiracetam dosage regimen designed to achieve a steady-state levetiracetam concentration equal to 20 µg/mL.

4. Patient AS (see problem 3) was prescribed 500 mg every 12 hours of levetiracetam immediate-release tablets for 3 weeks, and the steady-state levetiracetam trough concentration equals 8.3 µg/mL. The patient is assessed to be adherent with her dosage regimen. Suggest a levetiracetam dosage regimen designed to achieve a steady-state levetiracetam trough concentration equal to 15 µg/mL.

5. FL is a 29-year-old, 75-kg (height = 5 ft 11 in) male with simple partial seizures who requires therapy with oral levetiracetam immediate-release tablets. He has normal liver function, has impaired renal function (S_{cr} = 3.6 mg/dL), and is also receiving phenytoin therapy. Suggest an initial levetiracetam dosage regimen designed to achieve a steady-state levetiracetam concentration equal to 15 µg/mL.

6. Patient FL (see problem 5) was prescribed 500 mg every 12 hours of levetiracetam immediate-release tablets for 4 weeks, and the steady-state levetiracetam trough concentration equaled 15.7 µg/mL. The patient is assessed to be adherent with his dosage regimen. Suggest a levetiracetam dosage regimen designed to achieve a steady-state levetiracetam trough concentration of 24 µg/mL.

7. PH is a 4-year-old, 22-kg male (height = 40 in) with tonic-clonic seizures who requires therapy with levetiracetam oral solution. He has normal liver and renal function (Scr = 0.5 mg/dL) and is also treated with valproate sodium. Suggest an initial levetiracetam dosage regimen designed to achieve a steady-state levetiracetam concentration equal to 15 µg/mL.

8. Patient PH (see problem 7) was prescribed 300 mg every 12 hours of levetiracetam oral solution for 2 weeks, and the steady-state levetiracetam trough concentration equals 25.5 µg/mL. The patient is assessed to be adherent with his dosage regimen. Suggest a levetiracetam dosage regimen designed to achieve a steady-state levetiracetam trough concentration of 17 µg/mL.

9. HF is a 37-year-old, 85-kg (height = 6 ft 1 in) male with tonic-clonic seizures who requires therapy with oral levetiracetam monotherapy. He has severe liver disease (Child-Pugh score of 12) and a S_{cr} = 1.5 mg/dL. Suggest an initial levetiracetam dosage regimen using extended-release tablets designed to achieve a steady-state levetiracetam concentration equal to 15 µg/mL.

10. LK is a 50-year-old, 70-kg (height = 5 ft 10 in) male with complex partial seizures who requires therapy with levetiracetam. His serum creatinine equals 0.9 mg/dL. He has normal liver function and is currently taking phenytoin sodium capsules (steady-state concentration = 17.8 µg/mL). Additional dosage increases have been tried with phenytoin, but they have been unsuccessful due to development of adverse effects. The patient was started on an initial levetiracetam dosage regimen using intravenous drug of 1000 mg every 12 hours designed to achieve a steady-state trough levetiracetam concentration equal to 15 µg/mL 4 days ago, but seizure frequency did not markedly change. To assist in dosage adjustment, steady-state levetiracetam concentrations were drawn just before a dose (Css_{min} = 7.9 µg/mL) and 30 minutes after a 15 minute infusion (Css_{max} = 29.6 µg/mL). Compute a new intravenous levetiracetam dosage regimen designed to achieve a steady-state trough concentration equal to 15 µg/mL.

11. UP is a 55-year-old, 68-kg (height = 5 ft 8 in) male with complex partial seizures who was given a new prescription for 1000 mg daily of levetiracetam extended-release tablets. He has normal liver and renal (bilirubin = 0.7 mg/dL, albumin = 4.0 g/dL, serum creatinine = 1.1 mg/dL) function, and also takes 400 mg/d of phenytoin. The levetiracetam concentration at 6 hours after the third dose equals 8 µg/mL. Compute a levetiracetam dose that will provide a steady-state trough concentration of 20 µg/mL.

ANSWERS TO PROBLEMS

1. *Answer to problem 1.*

Pharmacokinetic Dosing Method

1. *Estimate creatinine clearance.*

    This patient has a stable serum creatinine and is not obese. The Cockcroft-Gault equation can be used to estimate creatinine clearance:

    $$CrCl_{est} = [(140 - age)BW]/(72 \bullet S_{Cr}) = [(140 - 37 \text{ y})85 \text{ kg}]/(72 \bullet 1.1 \text{ mg/dL}) = 111 \text{ mL/min}$$

    This patient has a $CrCl_{est}$ >80 mL/min, so levetiracetam clearance will not need to be adjusted for renal function (see Table 16-2).

2. *Estimate clearance, volume of distribution, and half-life according to disease states and conditions present in the patient.*

    The Cl/F rate for a patient taking levetiracetam monotherapy is 0.90 mL/min/kg: Cl/F = (0.90 mL/min/kg)85 kg = 76.5 mL/min. The estimated V/F would be 0.56 L/kg, and the estimated half-life equals 7.3 h.

3. *Compute dosage regimen.*

Levetiracetam extended-release tablets will be prescribed to this patient. (Note: μg/mL = mg/L and this concentration unit was substituted for Css in the calculations so that unnecessary unit conversion was not required.) The dosage equation for oral levetiracetam is: $D = Css(Cl/F)\tau = (15 \text{ mg/L} \bullet 76.5 \text{ mL/min} \bullet 24 \text{ h} \bullet 60 \text{ min/h})/(1000 \text{ mL/L}) = 1652$ mg, rounded to 1500 mg every 24 hours (dose rounded down to accommodate extended-release dosage form).

A steady-state trough levetiracetam serum concentration can be measured after steady-state is attained in 3-5 half-lives. Since the patient is expected to have a half-life equal to 7.3 hours, the levetiracetam steady-state concentration could be obtained any time after the second day of dosing (5 half-lives = 5 • 7.3 h = 36.5 h or 1.5 d). Levetiracetam serum concentrations should also be measured if the patient experiences an exacerbation of their epilepsy or if the patient develops potential signs or symptoms of levetiracetam toxicity.

Literature-Based Recommended Dosing

1. *Estimate creatinine clearance.*

This patient has a stable serum creatinine and is not obese. The Cockcroft-Gault equation can be used to estimate creatinine clearance:

$$CrCl_{est} = [(140 - age)BW]/(72 \bullet S_{Cr}) = [(140 - 37 \text{ y})85 \text{ kg}]/(72 \bullet 1.1 \text{ mg/dL}) = 111 \text{ mL/min}$$

This patient has a $CrCl_{est}$ >80 mL/min, so levetiracetam clearance will not need to be adjusted for renal function (see Table 16-4).

2. *Estimate levetiracetam dose according to disease states and conditions present in the patient.*

For adults, the initial dose of levetiracetam is 1000 mg/d, administered every 24 hours for extended-release tablets. The dose is titrated up 1000 mg/d every 2 weeks as needed, and the patient is monitored for seizure frequency and adverse drug effects. The maximum dose is usually 3000-4000 mg/d.

A steady-state trough levetiracetam serum concentration can be measured after steady-state is attained in 3-5 half-lives. Since the patient is expected to have a half-life equal to 7.3 hours, the levetiracetam steady-state concentration could be obtained any time after the second day of dosing (5 half-lives = 5 • 7.3 h = 36.5 h or 1.5 d). Levetiracetam serum concentrations should also be measured if the patient experiences an exacerbation of their epilepsy or if the patient develops potential signs or symptoms of levetiracetam toxicity.

2. *Answer to problem 2.*

Linear Pharmacokinetics Method

1. *Compute new dose to achieve the desired serum concentration.*

Using linear pharmacokinetics, the new levetiracetam dose would equal: $D_{new} = (Css_{new}/Css_{old}) D_{old} = (20.0 \text{ μg/mL} / 12.9 \text{ μg/mL}) 1000 \text{ mg/d} = 1550$ mg/d, rounded to 1500 mg/d. The new dose is 1500 mg every 24 hours.

The patient should be carefully monitored for seizure frequency and adverse effects. If desired, steady-state levetiracetam trough serum concentrations can be measured 3-5 half-lives after the dosage change has been made (see Table 16-2: ~$t_{1/2}$ = 7.3 hours, ~3-5 $t_{1/2}$ in 1-2 days).

Pharmacokinetic Parameter Method

1. *Compute pharmacokinetic parameters.*

Levetiracetam Cl/F can be computed using a steady-state levetiracetam trough concentration: $Cl/F = (D/\tau)/Css = [(1000 \text{ mg})/(24 \text{ h})]/(12.9 \text{ mg/L}) = 3.23$ L/h. (Note: μg/mL = mg/L and this concentration unit was substituted for Css in the calculations so that unnecessary unit conversion was not required.)

2. *Compute the new levetiracetam dosage.*

Levetiracetam Cl/F is used to compute the new dose: $D = Css(Cl/F)\tau = 20$ mg/L(3.23 L/h) 24 h = 1550 mg, rounded to 1500 mg every 24 hours.

The patient should be carefully monitored for seizure frequency and adverse effects. If desired, steady-state levetiracetam trough serum concentrations can be measured 3-5 half-lives after the dosage change has been made (see Table 16-2: $\sim t_{1/2} = 7.3$ hours, $\sim 3\text{-}5\ t_{1/2}$ in 1-2 days).

3. *Answer to problem 3.*

Pharmacokinetic Dosing Method

1. *Estimate creatinine clearance.*

This patient has a stable serum creatinine and is not obese. The equation for pediatric patients age 1-20 years is: $CrCl_{est}$ (in mL/min/1.73 m^2) = (0.55 • Ht)/S_{Cr}, where Ht is in cm and S_{Cr} is in mg/dL (Chapter 3):

$$Height = 54\ in\ (2.54\ cm/in) = 137\ cm$$

$$CrCl_{est}\ (in\ mL/min/1.73\ m^2) = (0.55 \bullet Ht)/S_{Cr} = (0.55 \bullet 137\ cm)/(0.6\ mg/dL) = 126\ mL/min/1.73\ m^2$$

This patient has a $CrCl_{est} > 80$ mL/min/1.73 m^2, so levetiracetam clearance will not need to be adjusted for renal function (see Table 16-2).

2. *Estimate clearance, volume of distribution, and half-life according to disease states and conditions present in the patient.*

The Cl/F rate for a pediatric patient taking levetiracetam concurrently with carbamazepine is 1.23 mL/min/kg: Cl/F = (1.23 mL/min/kg)35 kg = 43.1 mL/min. The estimated half-life equals 4.4 h.

3. *Compute dosage regimen.*

Levetiracetam immediate-release tablets will be prescribed to this patient. (Note: μg/mL = mg/L and this concentration unit was substituted for Css in the calculations so that unnecessary unit conversion was not required). The dosage equation for oral levetiracetam is: $D = Css(Cl/F)\tau = (20$ mg/L • 43.1 mL/min • 12 h • 60 min/h)/(1000 mL/L) = 621 mg, rounded to 500 mg every 12 hours.

A steady-state trough levetiracetam serum concentration can be measured after steady-state is attained in 3-5 half-lives. Since the patient is expected to have a half-life equal to 4.4 hours, the levetiracetam steady-state concentration could be obtained any time after the first day of dosing (5 half-lives = 5 • 4.4 h = 22 h or ~1 d). Levetiracetam serum concentrations should also be measured if the patient experiences an exacerbation of their epilepsy or if the patient develops potential signs or symptoms of levetiracetam toxicity.

Literature-Based Recommended Dosing

1. *Estimate creatinine clearance.*

This patient has a stable serum creatinine and is not obese. The equation for pediatric patients age 1-20 years is: $CrCl_{est}$ (in mL/min/1.73 m^2) = (0.55 • Ht)/S_{Cr}, where Ht is in cm and S_{Cr} is in mg/dL (Chapter 3):

$$Height = 54\ in\ (2.54\ cm/in) = 137\ cm$$

$$CrCl_{est}\ (in\ mL/min/1.73\ m^2) = (0.55 \bullet Ht)/S_{Cr} = (0.55 \bullet 137\ cm)/(0.6\ mg/dL) = 126\ mL/min/1.73\ m^2$$

This patient has a $CrCl_{est} > 80$ mL/min/1.73 m^2, so levetiracetam clearance will not need to be adjusted for renal function (see Table 16-2).

2. *Estimate levetiracetam dose according to disease states and conditions present in the patient.*

For children, the initial dose of levetiracetam is 20 mg/kg/d, administered as divided doses every 12 hours for immediate-release tablets (20 mg/kg/d • 35 kg = 700 mg/d, rounded to 250 mg every 12 hours). The dose is titrated up 20 mg/kg/d every 2 weeks as needed, and the patient is monitored for seizure frequency and adverse drug effects. The maximum dose is usually 60 mg/kg/d.

A steady-state trough levetiracetam serum concentration can be measured after steady-state is attained in 3-5 half-lives. Since the patient is expected to have a half-life equal to 4.4 hours, the levetiracetam steady-state concentration could be obtained any time after the first day of dosing (5 half-lives = 5 • 4.4 h = 22 h or ~1 d). Levetiracetam serum concentrations should also be measured if the patient experiences an exacerbation of their epilepsy or if the patient develops potential signs or symptoms of levetiracetam toxicity.

4. *Answer to problem 4.*

Linear Pharmacokinetics Method

1. *Compute new dose to achieve desired serum concentration.*

Using linear pharmacokinetics, the new levetiracetam dose would equal: $D_{new} = (Css_{new}/Css_{old})$ $D_{old} = (15.0\ \mu g/mL\ /\ 8.3\ \mu g/mL)\ 1000\ mg/d = 1807\ mg/d$, rounded to 2000 mg/d. The new dose is 1000 mg every 12 hours.

The patient should be carefully monitored for seizure frequency and adverse effects. If desired, steady-state levetiracetam trough serum concentrations can be measured 3-5 half-lives after the dosage change has been made (see Table 16-2: $\sim t_{1/2} = 4.4$ hours, ~3-5 $t_{1/2}$ in ~1 day).

Pharmacokinetic Parameter Method

1. *Compute pharmacokinetic parameters.*

Levetiracetam Cl/F can be computed using a steady-state levetiracetam trough concentration: $Cl/F = (D/\tau)/Css = [(500\ mg)/(12\ h)]/(8.3\ mg/L) = 5.02\ L/h$. (Note: $\mu g/mL = mg/L$ and this concentration unit was substituted for Css in the calculations so that unnecessary unit conversion was not required.)

2. *Compute the new levetiracetam dosage.*

Levetiracetam Cl/F is used to compute the new dose: $D = Css(Cl/F)\tau = 15\ mg/L(5.02\ L/h)12\ h = 904\ mg$, rounded to 1000 mg every 12 hours.

The patient should be carefully monitored for seizure frequency and adverse effects. If desired, steady-state levetiracetam trough serum concentrations can be measured 3-5 half-lives after the dosage change has been made (see Table 16-2: $\sim t_{1/2} = 4.4$ hours, ~3-5 $t_{1/2}$ in ~1 day).

5. *Answer to problem 5.*

Pharmacokinetic Dosing Method

1. *Estimate creatinine clearance.*

This patient has a stable serum creatinine and is not obese. The Cockcroft-Gault equation can be used to estimate creatinine clearance:

$$CrCl_{est} = [(140 - age)BW]/(72 \bullet S_{Cr}) = [(140 - 29\ y)75\ kg]/(72 \bullet 3.6\ mg/dL) = 32\ mL/min$$

This patient has a $CrCl_{est}$ <80 mL/min, so levetiracetam clearance will need to be adjusted for renal function (see Table 16-2). The clearance for this patient will be 50% of the normal value.

2. *Estimate clearance, volume of distribution, and half-life according to disease states and conditions present in the patient.*

The Cl/F rate for a patient taking levetiracetam with phenytoin is 1.17 mL/min/kg, and the Cl/F is adjusted for reduced renal function: Cl/F = 0.5(1.17 mL/min/kg)75 kg = 43.9 mL/min. The estimated V/F would be 0.6 L/kg, and the estimated half-life equals 11.8 h: $t_{1/2} = [0.693(V/F)]/(Cl/F) = [0.693(0.6 \text{ L/kg})(1000 \text{ mL/L})]/[0.5(1.17 \text{ mL/min/kg})(60 \text{ min/h})] = 11.8 \text{ h}$.

3. *Compute dosage regimen.*

Levetiracetam immediate-release tablets will be prescribed to this patient. (Note: μg/mL = mg/L and this concentration unit was substituted for Css in the calculations so that unnecessary unit conversion was not required.) The dosage equation for oral levetiracetam is: D = Css(Cl/F)τ = (15 mg/L • 43.9 mL/min • 12 h • 60 min/h)/(1000 mL/L) = 474 mg, rounded to 500 mg every 12 hours.

A steady-state trough levetiracetam serum concentration can be measured after steady-state is attained in 3-5 half-lives. Since the patient is expected to have a half-life equal to 11.8 hours, the levetiracetam steady-state concentration could be obtained any time after the third day of dosing (5 half-lives = 5 • 11.8 h = 59 h or 2.5 d). Levetiracetam serum concentrations should also be measured if the patient experiences an exacerbation of their epilepsy or if the patient develops potential signs or symptoms of levetiracetam toxicity.

Literature-Based Recommended Dosing

1. *Estimate creatinine clearance*

This patient has a stable serum creatinine and is not obese. The Cockcroft-Gault equation can be used to estimate creatinine clearance:

$$CrCl_{est} = [(140 - age)BW]/(72 • S_{Cr}) = [(140 - 29 \text{ y})75 \text{ kg}]/(72 • 3.6 \text{ mg/dL}) = 32 \text{ mL/min}$$

This patient has a $CrCl_{est}$ <80 mL/min, so levetiracetam clearance will need to be adjusted for renal function (see Table 16-4).

To normalize $CrCl_{est}$ (in mL/min) to a standard body surface area of 1.73 m^2 (mL/min/1.73 m^2), first compute the patient's own body surface area (BSA in m^2): BSA = 0.007184 • W$^{0.425}$ • H$^{0.725}$ = 0.007184 • (75 kg)$^{0.425}$ • [(71 in)(2.54 cm/in)]$^{0.725}$ = 1.95 m^2, $CrCl_{est}$ (in mL/min/1.73 m^2) = [(CrCl$_{est}$)/(BSA)]1.73 m^2 = [(32 mL/min)/(1.95 m^2)]1.73 m^2 = 28.4 mL/min/1.73 m^2).

2. *Estimate levetiracetam dose according to disease states and conditions present in the patient.*

For adults with $CrCl_{est}$ <30 mL/min/1.73 m^2, the initial dose of levetiracetam is reduced (see Table 16-4). For this patient, the dose of 500 mg every 12 hours for immediate-release tablets was selected because his renal function was in the upper end of the range. The dose is titrated up 500-1000 mg/d every 2-3 weeks as needed, and the patient is monitored for seizure frequency and adverse drug effects. The maximum dose is usually 3000-4000 mg/d, but may need to be adjusted due to renal dysfunction.

A steady-state trough levetiracetam serum concentration can be measured after steady-state is attained in 3-5 half-lives. Since the patient is expected to have a prolonged half-life, the levetiracetam steady-state concentration could be obtained any time after ~5-7 days of dosing. Levetiracetam serum concentrations should also be measured if the patient experiences an exacerbation of their epilepsy or if the patient develops potential signs or symptoms of levetiracetam toxicity.

6. *Answer to problem 6.*

Linear Pharmacokinetics Method

1. *Compute new dose to achieve the desired serum concentration.*

Using linear pharmacokinetics, the new levetiracetam dose would equal: $D_{new} = (Css_{new}/Css_{old})$ $D_{old} = (24.0 \ \mu g/mL/15.7 \ \mu g/mL) \ 1000 \ mg/d = 1529 \ mg/d$, rounded to 1500 mg/d. The new dose is 750 mg every 12 hours.

A steady-state trough levetiracetam serum concentration can be measured after steady-state is attained in 3-5 half-lives. Since the patient is expected to have a prolonged half-life, the levetiracetam steady-state concentration could be obtained any time after ~5-7 days of dosing. Levetiracetam serum concentrations should also be measured if the patient experiences an exacerbation of their epilepsy or if the patient develops potential signs or symptoms of levetiracetam toxicity.

Pharmacokinetic Parameter Method

1. *Compute pharmacokinetic parameters.*

Levetiracetam Cl/F can be computed using a steady-state levetiracetam trough concentration: $Cl/F = (D/\tau)/Css = [(500 \ mg)/(12 \ h)]/(15.7 \ mg/L) = 2.65 \ L/h$. (Note: $\mu g/mL = mg/L$ and this concentration unit was substituted for Css in the calculations so that unnecessary unit conversion was not required.)

2. *Compute the new levetiracetam dosage.*

Levetiracetam Cl/F is used to compute the new dose: $D = Css(Cl/F)\tau = 24 \ mg/L(2.65 \ L/h) \ 12 \ h = 763 \ mg$, rounded to 750 mg every 12 hours.

A steady-state trough levetiracetam serum concentration can be measured after steady-state is attained in 3-5 half-lives. Since the patient is expected to have a half-life equal to 11.8 hours, the levetiracetam steady-state concentration could be obtained any time after the third day of dosing (5 half-lives = $5 \bullet 11.8 \ h = 59 \ h$ or 2.5 d). Levetiracetam serum concentrations should also be measured if the patient experiences an exacerbation of their epilepsy or if the patient develops potential signs or symptoms of levetiracetam toxicity.

7. *Answer to problem 7.*

Pharmacokinetic Dosing Method

1. *Estimate creatinine clearance.*

This patient has a stable serum creatinine and is not obese. The equation for pediatric patients age 1-20 years: $CrCl_{est}$ (in mL/min/1.73 m^2) = $(0.55 \bullet Ht)/S_{Cr}$, where Ht is in cm and S_{Cr} is in mg/dL (Chapter 3):

$$Height = 40 \ in \ (2.54 \ cm/in) = 102 \ cm$$

$$CrCl_{est} \ (in \ mL/min/1.73 \ m^2) = (0.55 \bullet Ht)/S_{Cr} = (0.55 \bullet 102 \ cm)/(0.5 \ mg/dL) = 112 \ mL/min/1.73 \ m^2$$

This patient has a $CrCl_{est} > 80 \ mL/min/1.73 \ m^2$, so levetiracetam clearance will not need to be adjusted for renal function (see Table 16-2).

2. *Estimate clearance, volume of distribution, and half-life according to disease states and conditions present in the patient.*

The Cl/F rate for a pediatric patient taking levetiracetam concurrently with valproate sodium is 1.08 mL/min/kg: Cl/F = (1.08 mL/min/kg)22 kg = 23.8 mL/min. The estimated half-life equals 5.2 h.

3. *Compute dosage regimen.*

Levetiracetam oral solution will be prescribed to this patient. (Note: $\mu g/mL = mg/L$ and this concentration unit was substituted for Css in the calculations so that unnecessary unit conversion was not required.) The dosage equation for oral levetiracetam is: $D = Css(Cl/F)\tau = (15 \ mg/L \bullet 23.8 \ mL/min \bullet 12 \ h \bullet 60 \ min/h)/(1000 \ mL/L) = 257 \ mg$, rounded to 250 mg every 12 hours.

A steady-state trough levetiracetam serum concentration can be measured after steady-state is attained in 3-5 half-lives. Since the patient is expected to have a half-life equal to 5.2 hours, the levetiracetam steady-state concentration could be obtained any time after the second day of dosing (5 half-lives = 5 • 5.2 h = 26 h or ~1.1 d). Levetiracetam serum concentrations should also be measured if the patient experiences an exacerbation of their epilepsy or if the patient develops potential signs or symptoms of levetiracetam toxicity.

Literature-Based Recommended Dosing

1. *Estimate creatinine clearance.*

This patient has a stable serum creatinine and is not obese. The equation for pediatric patients age 1-20 years, $CrCl_{est}$ (in mL/min/1.73 m^2) = (0.55 • Ht)/S_{Cr}, where Ht is in cm and S_{Cr} is in mg/dL (Chapter 3):

$$Height = 40 \text{ in } (2.54 \text{ cm/in}) = 102 \text{ cm}$$

$$CrCl_{est} \text{ (in mL/min/1.73 m}^2) = (0.55 • Ht)/S_{Cr} = (0.55 • 102 \text{ cm})/(0.5 \text{ mg/dL}) = 112 \text{ mL/min/1.73 m}^2$$

This patient has a $CrCl_{est}$ greater than 80 mL/min/1.73 m^2, so levetiracetam clearance will not need to be adjusted for renal function (see Table 16-2).

2. *Estimate levetiracetam dose according to disease states and conditions present in the patient.*

For children, the initial dose of levetiracetam is 20 mg/kg/d, administered as divided doses every 12 hours for oral solution (20 mg/kg/d • 22 kg = 440 mg/d, rounded to 200 mg every 12 hours). The dose is titrated up 20 mg/kg/d every 2 weeks as needed, and the patient is monitored for seizure frequency and adverse drug effects. The maximum dose is usually 60 mg/kg/d.

A steady-state trough levetiracetam serum concentration can be measured after steady-state is attained in 3-5 half-lives. Since the patient is expected to have a half-life equal to 5.2 hours, the levetiracetam steady-state concentration could be obtained any time after the second day of dosing (5 half-lives = 5 • 5.2 h = 26 h or ~1.1 d). Levetiracetam serum concentrations should also be measured if the patient experiences an exacerbation of their epilepsy or if the patient develops potential signs or symptoms of levetiracetam toxicity.

8. *Answer to problem 8.*

Linear Pharmacokinetics Method

1. *Compute new dose to achieve desired serum concentration.*

Using linear pharmacokinetics, the new levetiracetam dose would equal: D_{new} = (Css_{new}/Css_{old}) D_{old} = (17 μg/mL / 25.5 μg/mL) 600 mg/d = 400 mg/d. The new dose is 200 mg every 12 hours.

The patient should be carefully monitored for seizure frequency and adverse effects. If desired, steady-state levetiracetam trough serum concentrations can be measured 3-5 half-lives after the dosage change has been made (see Table 16-2: ~$t_{1/2}$ = 5.2 hours, ~3-5 $t_{1/2}$ in ~1-2 days).

Pharmacokinetic Parameter Method

1. *Compute pharmacokinetic parameters.*

Levetiracetam Cl/F can be computed using a steady-state levetiracetam trough concentration: Cl/F = (D/τ)/Css = [(300 mg)/(12 h)]/(25.5 mg/L) = 0.98 L/h. (Note: μg/mL = mg/L and this concentration unit was substituted for Css in the calculations so that unnecessary unit conversion was not required.)

2. *Compute the new levetiracetam dosage.*

   Levetiracetam Cl/F is used to compute the new dose: D = Css(Cl/F)τ = 17 mg/L(0.98 L/h)12 h = 200 mg, dose is 200 mg every 12 hours.

   The patient should be carefully monitored for seizure frequency and adverse effects. If desired, steady-state levetiracetam trough serum concentrations can be measured 3–5 half-lives after the dosage change has been made (see Table 16-2: ~$t_{1/2}$ = 5.2 hours, ~3-5 $t_{1/2}$ in ~1-2 days).

9. *Answer to problem 9.*

Pharmacokinetic Dosing Method

1. *Estimate creatinine clearance.*

   This patient has a stable serum creatinine and is not obese. The Cockcroft-Gault equation can be used to estimate creatinine clearance:

$$CrCl_{est} = [(140 - age)BW]/(72 \bullet S_{Cr}) = [(140 - 37\ y)85\ kg]/(72 \bullet 1.5\ mg/dL) = 81.1\ mL/min$$

   This patient has a $CrCl_{est}$ >80 mL/min, so levetiracetam clearance will not need to be adjusted for renal function (see Table 16-2).

2. *Estimate clearance, volume of distribution, and half-life according to disease states and conditions present in the patient.*

   To compute the patient's own body surface area (BSA in m^2): BSA = 0.007184 $\bullet$ W$^{0.425}$ $\bullet$ H$^{0.725}$ = 0.007184 $\bullet$ (85 kg)$^{0.425}$ $\bullet$ [(73 in)(2.54 cm/in)]$^{0.725}$ = 2.09 m^2.

   The Cl/F rate for a patient taking levetiracetam monotherapy and severe liver disease is 29.2 mL/min/1.73 m^2: Cl/F = [(29.2 mL/min)/(1.73 m^2)] 2.09 m^2 = 35.3 mL/min. The estimated V/F would be ~45 L, and the estimated half-life equals 18.4 h.

3. *Compute dosage regimen.*

   Levetiracetam extended-release tablets will be prescribed to this patient. (Note: μg/mL = mg/L and this concentration unit was substituted for Css in the calculations so that unnecessary unit conversion was not required.) The dosage equation for oral levetiracetam is: D = Css(Cl/F)τ = (15 mg/L $\bullet$ 35.3 mL/min $\bullet$ 24 h $\bullet$ 60 min/h)/(1000 mL/L) = 762 mg, rounded to 750 mg every 24 hours.

   A steady-state trough levetiracetam serum concentration can be measured after steady-state is attained in 3-5 half-lives. Since the patient is expected to have a half-life equal to 18.4 hours, the levetiracetam steady-state concentration could be obtained any time after the fourth day of dosing (5 half-lives = 5 $\bullet$ 18.4 h = 92 h or 3.8 d). Levetiracetam serum concentrations should also be measured if the patient experiences an exacerbation of their epilepsy or if the patient develops potential signs or symptoms of levetiracetam toxicity.

Literature-Based Recommended Dosing

1. *Estimate creatinine clearance.*

   This patient has a stable serum creatinine and is not obese. The Cockcroft-Gault equation can be used to estimate creatinine clearance:

$$CrCl_{est} = [(140 - age)BW]/(72 \bullet S_{Cr}) = [(140 - 37\ y)85\ kg]/(72 \bullet 1.5\ mg/dL) = 81.1\ mL/min$$

   This patient has a $CrCl_{est}$ >80 mL/min, so levetiracetam clearance will not need to be adjusted for renal function (see Table 16-4).

2. *Estimate levetiracetam dose according to disease states and conditions present in the patient.*

For adults, the initial dose of levetiracetam is 1000 mg/d, administered every 24 hours for extended-release tablets. For patients with severe liver disease, this dose is reduced by half to 500 mg every 24 hours. The dose is titrated up 500-1000 mg/d every 2-3 weeks as needed, and the patient is monitored for seizure frequency and adverse drug effects. The maximum dose is usually 3000-4000 mg/d for patients with normal liver function, but these doses should be used with caution if severe liver disease is present.

A steady-state trough levetiracetam serum concentration can be measured after steady-state is attained in 3-5 half-lives. Since the patient is expected to have a half-life equal to 18.4 hours, the levetiracetam steady-state concentration could be obtained any time after the fourth day of dosing (5 half-lives = 5 • 18.4 h = 92 h or 3.8 d). Levetiracetam serum concentrations should also be measured if the patient experiences an exacerbation of their epilepsy or if the patient develops potential signs or symptoms of levetiracetam toxicity.

10. *Answer to problem 10.*

Linear Pharmacokinetics Method

1. *Compute new dose to achieve desired serum concentration.*

Using linear pharmacokinetics, the new levetiracetam dose would equal: $D_{new} = (Css_{new}/Css_{old})$ $D_{old} = (15\ \mu g/mL\ /\ 7.9\ \mu g/mL)\ 2000\ mg/d = 3797\ mg/d$, rounded to 4000 mg/d. The new dose is 2000 mg every 12 hours.

The patient should be carefully monitored for seizure frequency and adverse effects. If desired, steady-state levetiracetam trough serum concentrations can be measured 3-5 half-lives after the dosage change has been made (see Table 16-2: $\sim t_{1/2} = 6.1$ hours, ~ 3-5 $t_{1/2}$ in ~ 1-2 days).

Steady-State One-Compartment Model Parameter Method

1. *Estimate creatinine clearance.*

This patient has a stable serum creatinine and is not obese. The Cockcroft-Gault equation can be used to estimate creatinine clearance:

$$CrCl_{est} = [(140 - age)BW]/(72 \bullet S_{Cr}) = [(140 - 50\ y)70\ kg]/(72 \bullet 0.9\ mg/dL) = 97\ mL/min$$

This patient has a $CrCl_{est}$ >80 mL/min, so levetiracetam $t_{1/2}$ is expected to be 6.1 h (see Table 16-2). After 4 days of treatment with levetiracetam, the patient is at steady-state.

2. *Use Steady-State One-Compartment Model Parameter Method to Compute a New Dose.*

A. *Compute the patient's elimination rate constant and half-life (note: t′ = infusion time + waiting time of 15 minutes and ½ hour, respectively).*

$$k = (\ln Css_{max} - \ln Css_{min})/(\tau - t') = (\ln 29.6\ \mu g/mL - \ln 7.9\ \mu g/mL)/(12\ h - 0.75\ h) = 0.117\ h^{-1}$$
$$t_{1/2} = 0.693/k = 0.693/0.117\ h^{-1} = 5.9\ h$$

B. *Compute the patient's volume of distribution.*

$$V = D/(Css_{max} - Css_{min}) = 1000\ mg/(29.6\ mg/L - 7.9\ mg/L) = 46.1\ L$$

C. *Choose new steady-state trough concentration.*

The desired steady-state trough concentration will be 15 µg/mL.

D. *Determine the new dosage interval for the desired concentrations.*

For levetiracetam, a dosage interval of 12 hours is used for most patients (see Table 16-4).

E. *Determine the new dose for the desired concentrations.*

The dose is computed using the one-compartment model intravenous bolus equation:

$$D = [Css_{min} V(1 - e^{-k\tau})]/(e^{-k\tau}) = [15 \text{ mg/L} \bullet 46.1 \text{ L } (1 - e^{-(0.117 \text{ h}^{-1})(12 \text{ h})})]/(e^{-(0.117 \text{ h}^{-1})(12 \text{ h})}) = 2124 \text{ mg, rounded to } 2000$$

A dose of levetiracetam 2000 mg every 12 hours would be prescribed.

11. *Answer to problem 11.*

Bayesian Pharmacokinetic Computer Program

Patient is not at steady-state yet, and the levetiracetam concentration was obtained at mid-dosage interval. These factors make it difficult to use other methods to compute the best dose to achieve a target steady-state levetiracetam trough concentration.

1. *Enter the patient's demographic, drug-dosing, and serum concentration/time data into the computer program.*
2. *Compute pharmacokinetic parameters for the patient using Bayesian pharmacokinetic computer program.*

    The pharmacokinetic parameters computed by the program are a volume of distribution of 48 L, a half-life equal to 5.6 h, and a clearance equal to 88 mL/min.
3. *Compute dose required to achieve desired levetiracetam serum concentrations.*

    The one-compartment model first-order absorption equations used by the program to compute doses indicates that a dose of 2000 mg every 24 hours will produce a steady-state levetiracetam trough concentration of 20 μg/mL.

REFERENCES

1. Abramowicz M, Zuccotti G, Pflomm JM, eds. Drugs for epilepsy. *Treatment Guidelines From The Medical Letter.* 2013;11(126):9-18.
2. Anon. The epilepsies: the diagnosis and management of the epilepsies in adults and children in primary and secondary care. *UK National Institute for Health and Care Excellence.* http://www.nice.org.uk/nicemedia/live/13635/57779/57779.pdf. Accessed May 5, 2014.
3. French JA, Kanner AM, Bautista J, et al. Efficacy and tolerability of the new antiepileptic drugs I: treatment of new onset epilepsy: report of the Therapeutics and Technology Assessment Subcommittee and Quality Standards Subcommittee of the American Academy of Neurology and the American Epilepsy Society. *Neurology.* Apr 27 2004;62(8):1252-1260.
4. Glauser T, Ben-Menachem E, Bourgeois B, et al. Updated ILAE evidence review of antiepileptic drug efficacy and effectiveness as initial monotherapy for epileptic seizures and syndromes. *Epilepsia.* Mar 2013;54(3):551-563.
5. McNamara JO. Pharmacotherapy of the epilepsies. In: Brunton L, Chabner B, Knollman B, eds. *The Pharmacological Basis of Therapeutics.* 12th ed. New York, NY: McGraw-Hill; 2011:583-608.
6. Rogers SJ, Cavazos JE. Epilepsy. In: DiPiro JT, Talbert RL, Yee GC, Matzke GR, Wells BG, Posey LM, eds. *Pharmacotherapy.* 8th ed. New York, NY: McGraw-Hill; 2011:979-1005.
7. Glauser TA, Cnaan A, Shinnar S, et al. Ethosuximide, valproic acid, and lamotrigine in childhood absence epilepsy. *N Engl J Med.* Mar 4, 2010;362(9):790-799.
8. Glauser TA, Cnaan A, Shinnar S, et al. Ethosuximide, valproic acid, and lamotrigine in childhood absence epilepsy: initial monotherapy outcomes at 12 months. *Epilepsia.* Jan 2013;54(1):141-155.
9. Patsalos PN. Clinical pharmacokinetics of levetiracetam. *Clin Pharmacokinet.* 2004;43(11):707-724.

10. Perucca E. Is there a role for therapeutic drug monitoring of new anticonvulsants? *Clin Pharmacokinet.* Mar 2000;38(3):191-204.
11. Johannessen SI, Tomson T. Pharmacokinetic variability of newer antiepileptic drugs: when is monitoring needed? *Clin Pharmacokinet.* 2006;45(11):1061-1075.
12. UBC, Inc. [package insert]. Keppra prescribing information; 2011.
13. Tomson T, Palm R, Kallen K, et al. Pharmacokinetics of levetiracetam during pregnancy, delivery, in the neonatal period, and lactation. *Epilepsia.* Jun 2007;48(6):1111-1116.
14. Tomson T, Battino D. Pharmacokinetics and therapeutic drug monitoring of newer antiepileptic drugs during pregnancy and the puerperium. *Clin Pharmacokinet.* 2007;46(3):209-219.
15. Italiano D, Perucca E. Clinical pharmacokinetics of new-generation antiepileptic drugs at the extremes of age: an update. *Clin Pharmacokinet.* May 3, 2013.
16. Slatter JG, Su P, Sams JP, Schaaf LJ, Wienkers LC. Bioactivation of the anticancer agent CPT-11 to SN-38 by human hepatic microsomal carboxylesterases and the in vitro assessment of potential drug interactions. *Drug Metab Dispos.* Oct 1997;25(10):1157-1164.
17. Strolin Benedetti M, Whomsley R, Nicolas JM, Young C, Baltes E. Pharmacokinetics and metabolism of 14C-levetiracetam, a new antiepileptic agent, in healthy volunteers. *Eur J Clin Pharmacol.* Nov 2003;59(8-9):621-630.
18. Radtke RA. Pharmacokinetics of levetiracetam. *Epilepsia.* 2001;42(suppl 4):24-27.
19. Patsalos PN. Pharmacokinetic profile of levetiracetam: toward ideal characteristics. *Pharmacol Ther.* Feb 2000;85(2):77-85.
20. Ramael S, De Smedt F, Toublanc N, et al. Single-dose bioavailability of levetiracetam intravenous infusion relative to oral tablets and multiple-dose pharmacokinetics and tolerability of levetiracetam intravenous infusion compared with placebo in healthy subjects. *Clin Ther.* May 2006;28(5):734-744.
21. Leppik IE, Goel V, Rarick J, Nixdorf DR, Cloyd JC. Intramuscular and intravenous levetiracetam in humans: safety and pharmacokinetics. *Epilepsy Res.* Oct 2010;91(2-3):289-292.
22. Freitas-Lima P, Alexandre V, Jr, Pereira LR, Feletti F, Perucca E, Sakamoto AC. Influence of enzyme inducing antiepileptic drugs on the pharmacokinetics of levetiracetam in patients with epilepsy. *Epilepsy Res.* Mar 2011;94(1-2):117-120.
23. Coupez R, Nicolas JM, Browne TR. Levetiracetam, a new antiepileptic agent: lack of in vitro and in vivo pharmacokinetic interaction with valproic acid. *Epilepsia.* Feb 2003;44(2):171-178.
24. Coupez R, Straetemans R, Sehgal G, Stockis A, Lu ZS. Levetiracetam: relative bioavailability and bioequivalence of a 10% oral solution (750 mg) and 750-mg tablets. *J Clin Pharmacol.* Dec 2003;43(12):1370-1376.
25. Ragueneau-Majlessi I, Levy RH, Meyerhoff C. Lack of effect of repeated administration of levetiracetam on the pharmacodynamic and pharmacokinetic profiles of warfarin. *Epilepsy Res.* Nov 2001;47(1-2):55-63.
26. Rouits E, Burton I, Guenole E, Troenaru MM, Stockis A, Sargentini-Maier ML. Pharmacokinetics of levetiracetam XR 500 mg tablets. *Epilepsy Res.* Apr 2009;84(2-3):224-231.
27. Grim SA, Ryan M, Miles MV, et al. Correlation of levetiracetam concentrations between serum and saliva. *Ther Drug Monit.* Feb 2003;25(1):61-66.
28. Baltez E, Coupez R. Levetiracetam dose adjustment for patients on hemodialysis (Abstract). *Epilepsia.* 2000;41(suppl 7):254.
29. French J. Use of levetiracetam in special populations. *Epilepsia.* 2001;42(suppl 4):40-43.
30. Pugh RN, Murray-Lyon IM, Dawson JL, Pietroni MC, Williams R. Transection of the oesophagus for bleeding oesophageal varices. *Br J Surg.* 1973;60(8):646-649.
31. Brockmoller J, Thomsen T, Wittstock M, Coupez R, Lochs H, Roots I. Pharmacokinetics of levetiracetam in patients with moderate to severe liver cirrhosis (Child-Pugh Classes A, B, and C): characterization by dynamic liver function tests. *Clin Pharmacol Ther.* Jun 2005;77(6):529-541.
32. Perucca E, Gidal BE, Baltes E. Effects of antiepileptic comedication on levetiracetam pharmacokinetics: a pooled analysis of data from randomized adjunctive therapy trials. *Epilepsy Res.* Feb 2003;53(1-2):47-56.
33. Contin M, Mohamed S, Albani F, Riva R, Baruzzi A. Levetiracetam clinical pharmacokinetics in elderly and very elderly patients with epilepsy. *Epilepsy Res.* Feb 2012;98(2-3):130-134.
34. Hirsch LJ, Arif H, Buchsbaum R, et al. Effect of age and comedication on levetiracetam pharmacokinetics and tolerability. *Epilepsia.* Jul 2007;48(7):1351-1359.
35. Pellock JM, Glauser TA, Bebin EM, et al. Pharmacokinetic study of levetiracetam in children. *Epilepsia.* Dec 2001;42(12):1574-1579.
36. Glauser TA, Mitchell WG, Weinstock A, et al. Pharmacokinetics of levetiracetam in infants and young children with epilepsy. *Epilepsia.* Jun 2007;48(6):1117-1122.
37. Fountain NB, Conry JA, Rodriguez-Leyva I, et al. Prospective assessment of levetiracetam pharmacokinetics during dose escalation in 4- to 12-year-old children with partial-onset seizures on concomitant carbamazepine or valproate. *Epilepsy Res.* Apr 2007;74(1):60-69.
38. Spencer DD, Jacobi J, Juenke JM, Fleck JD, Kays MB. Steady-state pharmacokinetics of intravenous levetiracetam in neurocritical care patients. *Pharmacotherapy.* Oct 2011;31(10):934-941.
39. Cockcroft DW, Gault MH. Prediction of creatinine clearance from serum creatinine. *Nephron.* 1976;16:31-41.

40. Salazar DE, Corcoran GB. Predicting creatinine clearance and renal drug clearance in obese patients from estimated fat-free body mass. *Am J Med.* 1988;84:1053-1060.

41. Traub SL, Johnson CE. Comparison of methods of estimating creatinine clearance in children. *Am J Hosp Pharm.* 1980;37:195-201.

42. Tschudy MM, Arcara KM. *The Harriet Lane Handbook: A Manual for Pediatric House Officers.* 19th ed. Philadelphia, PA: Mosby Elsevier; 2012.

43. Shargel L, Wu-Pong S, Yu A. *Applied Biopharmaceutics and Pharmacokinetics.* 6th ed. New York, NY: McGraw-Hill; 2012.

44. Murphy JE, Winter ME. Clinical pharmacokinetic pearls: bolus versus infusion equations. *Pharmacotherapy.* 1996;16(4):698-700.

45. Wandell M, Mungall D. Computer assisted drug interpretation and drug regimen optimization. *Amer Assoc Clin Chem.* 1984;6:1-11.

46. Du Bois D, Du Bois EF. A formula to estimate the approximate surface area if height and weight be known. *Arch Intern Med.* Jun 1916;17(6):863-871.

17 Oxcarbazepine/Eslicarbazepine

INTRODUCTION

Oxcarbazepine is an iminostilbene derivative related to the tricyclic antidepressants that is used in the treatment of tonic-clonic (grand mal), partial, or secondarily generalized seizures (Table 17-1).[1-4] Lack of an intravenous dosage form has limited its use in the treatment of acute seizures. Thus, the drug is used primarily as a prophylactic agent in the chronic therapy of epilepsy. Oxcarbazepine is also a useful agent to treat bipolar affective disorders and neurogenic pain (trigeminal neuralgia, diabetic neuropathy, etc) after carbamazepine has been considered.[5-8]

Oxcarbazepine (10,11-dihydro-10-oxo-carbazepine) is chemically related to carbamazepine, differing from carbamazepine by only a double-bonded oxygen on the central ring. Therefore, it is the 10-keto analog of carbamazepine. Upon oral administration, oxcarbazepizne is rapidly metabolized via a reduction reaction to a 10-hydroxy metabolite (10,11-dihydro-10-hydroxy-carbazepine, known as the monohydroxy derivative or MHD). MHD is present in the blood as a stereoisomer: (S)-(+)-MHD and (R)-(−)-MHD. The antiseizure activity of oxcarbazepine is due to MHD and is related to the ability of MHD to decrease transmission

TABLE 17-1 International Classification of Epileptic Seizures With Recommended Therapies

Major Class	Subset of Class	Drug Treatment for Selected Seizure Type			
		2004 AAN/AES	**2013 Medical Letter**	**2012 NICE**	**2013 ILAE**[a]
Partial seizures (beginning locally)	1. Simple partial seizures (without impaired consciousness) a. with motor symptoms b. with somato-sensory or special sensory symptoms c. with autonomic symptoms d. with psy-chological symptoms	Carbamazepine Phenytoin Valproate Phenobarbital Lamotrigine Gabapentin Oxcarbazepine Topiramate	Lamotrigine Carbamazepine Levetiracetam Oxcarbazepine *Alternatives:* Topiramate Valproate Gabapentin Zonisamide Phenytoin Pregabalin Lacosamide Ezogabine	Carbamazepine Lamotrigine Levetiracetam Oxcarbazepine Valproate *Adjunctive:* Carbamazepine Clobazam Gabapentin Lamotrigine Levetiracetam Oxcarbazepine Valproate Topiramate	*Adults:* Carbamazepine Levetiracetam Phenytoin Zonisamide Valproate *Children:* Oxcarbazepine Carbamazepine Phenobarbital Phenytoin Topiramate Valproate Vigabatrin *Elderly:* Gabapentin Lamotrigine Carbamazepine

(Continued)

TABLE 17-1 International Classification of Epileptic Seizures With Recommended Therapies (Continued)

Major Class	Subset of Class	Drug Treatment for Selected Seizure Type			
		2004 AAN/AES	**2013 Medical Letter**	**2012 NICE**	**2013 ILAE[a]**
	2. Complex partial seizures (with impaired consciousness) a. simple partial onset followed by impaired consciousness b. impaired consciousness at onset	Carbamazepine Phenytoin Valproate Phenobarbital Lamotrigine Gabapentin Oxcarbazepine Topiramate	Lamotrigine Carbamazepine Levetiracetam Oxcarbazepine *Alternatives:* Topiramate Valproate Gabapentin Zonisamide Phenytoin Pregabalin Lacosamide Ezogabine	Carbamazepine Lamotrigine Levetiracetam Oxcarbazepine Valproate *Adjunctive:* Carbamazepine Clobazam Gabapentin Lamotrigine Levetiracetam Oxcarbazepine Valproate Topiramate	*Adults:* Carbamazepine Levetiracetam Phenytoin Zonisamide Valproate *Children:* Oxcarbazepine Carbamazepine Phenobarbital Phenytoin Topiramate Valproate Vigabatrin *Elderly:* Gabapentin Lamotrigine Carbamazepine
	3. Partial seizures evolving into secondary gener-alized seizures	Carbamazepine Phenytoin Valproate Phenobarbital Lamotrigine Gabapentin Oxcarbazepine Topiramate	Lamotrigine Carbamazepine Levetiracetam Oxcarbazepine *Alternatives:* Topiramate Valproate Gabapentin Zonisamide Phenytoin Pregabalin Lacosamide Ezogabine	Carbamazepine Lamotrigine Levetiracetam Oxcarbazepine Valproate *Adjunctive:* Carbamazepine Clobazam Gabapentin Lamotrigine Levetiracetam Oxcarbazepine Valproate Topiramate	*Adults:* Carbamazepine Levetiracetam Phenytoin Zonisamide Valproate *Children:* Oxcarbazepine Carbamazepine Phenobarbital Phenytoin Topiramate Valproate Vigabatrin *Elderly:* Gabapentin Lamotrigine Carbamazepine
Generalized seizures (convulsive or nonconvulsive)	1. Absence seizures[b] (typical or atypi-cal; also known as petit mal seizures)	*Children:[c]* Ethosuximide Valproate Lamotrigine	Ethosuximide Valproate *Alternatives:* Lamotrigine Clonazepam Zonisamide Levetiracetam	Ethosuximide Lamotrigine Valproate *Adjunctive:* Ethosuximide Lamotrigine Valproate	*Children:* Ethosuximide Valproate Lamotrigine

(Continued)

TABLE 17-1   International Classification of Epileptic Seizures With Recommended Therapies (Continued)

Major Class	Subset of Class	Drug Treatment for Selected Seizure Type			
		2004 AAN/AES	2013 Medical Letter	2012 NICE	2013 ILAE[a]
	2. Tonic-clonic seizures (also known as grand mal seizures)	Carbamazepine Phenytoin Valproate Phenobarbital Lamotrigine Oxcarbazepine Topiramate	Valproate Lamotrigine Levetiracetam Alternatives: Topiramate Zonisamide Phenytoin	Carbamazepine Lamotrigine Oxcarbazepine Valproate Adjunctive: Clobazam Lamotrigine Levetiracetam Valproate Topiramate	Adults: Carbamazepine Lamotrigine Oxcarbazepine Phenobarbital Phenytoin Topiramate Valproate Gabapentin Levetiracetam Vigabatrin Children: Carbamazepine Phenobarbital Phenytoin Topiramate Valproate Oxcarbazepine

[a]Only two highest available levels of evidence listed.

[b]Recent literature suggests ethosuximide or valproic acid is superior initial therapy compared to lamotrigine for absence seizures.[9,10]

[c]Lamotrigine added to previous recommendation per expert panel.

Abbreviations: ANN, American Academy of Neurology; AES, American Epilepsy Society; NICE, UK National Institute for Clinical Excellence; ILAE, International League Against Epilepsy.

in the nucleus ventralis anterior section of the thalamus, an area of the brain thought to be involved with the generalization and propagation of epileptic discharges.[5,11] Although the exact cellular mechanism of action is unclear, inhibition of voltage-gated sodium channels appears to be involved. Additionally, MHD depresses posttetanic potentiation and may prevent increases in cyclic AMP. In this regard, MHD has pharmacologic properties that are almost identical to carbamazepine.

As the drug development cycle moved into a new generation of anticonvulsants, it was suggested that MHD be developed in its own right as a new drug. This effort came to fruition in 2009 when the European Medicines Agency approved eslicarbazepine acetate (eslicarbazepine is (S)-(+)-MHD, also known as S-licarbazepine) for use as a prescription drug in the European Union. In 2013, a revised New Drug Application was submitted in the United States to the Food and Drug Administration, and it was approved in November of that year as a prescription-only agent for the treatment of partial seizures. The S-enantiomer was chosen as the sole component because it is the predominate isomer in the blood after oral administration of oxcarbazepine. Eslicarbazepine acetate is rapidly converted to eslicarbazepine, which, of course, has the same pharmacokinetic properties and pharmacodynamic effects as (S)-(+)-MHD produced after the administration of oxcarbazepine.

Because oxcarbazepine and eslicarbazepine acetate share an active moiety (known as either (S)-(+)-MHD, S-licarbazepine, or eslicarbazepine in various research studies), they are considered together in this chapter. Oxcarbazepine is covered in the first major section of the chapter, and eslicarbazepine is discussed in the second major section of the chapter. Because oxcarbazepine has been available for much longer period of time, it is to be expected that more is known about MHD after its administration compared to eslicarbazepine. But, in general, most of what is written about (S)-(+)-MHD in the oxcarbazepine section directly applies to eslicarbazepine.

OXCARBAZEPINE

THERAPEUTIC AND TOXIC CONCENTRATIONS

Unlike most of the older antiepileptic drugs, the therapeutic range of oxcarbazepine is not well defined.[12-14] However, serum concentration monitoring during oxcarbazepine treatment can be a useful adjunct in addition to monitoring treatment for therapeutic response and adverse effects. Although oxcarbazepine is measurable in the serum after oral administration of the drug, MHD (monohydroxy derivative), which is the active metabolite of oxcarbazepine, is the moiety that is actually monitored in clinical practice. After oral administration of oxcarbazepine, stereoisomers of MHD are produced by presystemic metabolism and additional hepatic clearance of oxcarbazepine in the ratio of about 4:1 [(S)-(+)-MHD:(R)-(−)-MHD].[15-18] The therapeutic range for epilepsy used by many laboratories for MHD (MHD = (S)-(+)-MHD + (R)-(−)-MHD) is 3-35 μg/mL. Some patients will experience a higher incidence of adverse effects at concentrations in the upper end of the therapeutic range, so the efficacy of lower MHD serum concentrations should be assessed before moving to higher concentrations.[12-14] The most common dose- or concentration-dependent side effects of oxcarbazepine are sedation, somnolence, fatigue, dizziness, ataxia, nausea, and headache.[11,19]

CLINICAL MONITORING PARAMETERS

The goal of therapy with anticonvulsants is to reduce seizure frequency and maximize quality of life with a minimum of adverse drug effects. While it is desirable to entirely abolish all seizure episodes, it may not be possible to accomplish this in many patients. Patients should be monitored for concentration-related side effects of oxcarbazepine therapy (sedation, somnolence, fatigue, dizziness, ataxia, nausea, headache). Other potential adverse reactions include diplopia, abnormal vision, abdominal pain, vomiting, dyspepsia, tremor, abnormal gait, and suicidal ideation or behavior. Some patients may develop hyponatremia during chronic therapy with oxcarbazepine, and serum sodium concentrations can be periodically measured to detect this problem.[11,19-23]

Severe allergic reactions, including anaphylaxis and angioedema, have been reported both after the first dose and after multiple doses of oxcarbazepine. Skin rashes can occur during oxcarbazepine therapy, and about 25%-30% of patients who developed a rash with carbamazepine will also develop a rash during oxcarbazepine treatment. Stevens-Johnson syndrome and toxic epidermal necrolysis have both been reported during oxcarbazepine therapy. Generally, these severe dermatologic adverse effects occur within 19 days of starting treatment. The incidence of these serious skin rashes is 0.5-6 cases per million-patient years. Should either of these dermatologic reactions develop, oxcarbazepine should be immediately discontinued and not restarted.[11,19,23]

Because epilepsy is an episodic disease state, patients do not experience seizures continuously. Thus, during dosage titration it is difficult to tell if the patient is responding to drug therapy or simply is not experiencing any abnormal central nervous system discharges at that time. Similarly, bipolar disorder also occurs at irregular time intervals. Oxcarbazepine doses should be carefully titrated to individual patient response and tolerability. Serum concentrations of MHD can be measured in patients as an adjunct to therapy.[12-14] Concentration monitoring is particularly useful if a therapeutic concentration has been established for a patient and a new clinical event (drug interaction, new disease state or condition, etc) changes the pharmacokinetics of the drug. MHD concentrations can also be measured to document patient adherence to drug treatment or when a patient is switched between the oral dosage forms of oxcarbazepine to assure therapeutic levels are maintained.

BASIC CLINICAL PHARMACOKINETIC PARAMETERS

After oral administration, oxcarbazepine is extensively converted by presystemic metabolism and subsequent hepatic clearance via cytosol arylketone reductase to a monohydroxy derivative (MHD) in a stereospecific manner [(S)-(+)-MHD and (R)-(−)-MHD]. When oxcarbazepine is given orally, the ratio of (S)-(+)-MHD:(R)-(−)-MHD in the serum is about 4:1. MHD is further metabolized to glucuronide conjugates, which are principally eliminated by the kidney and to an inactive metabolite via oxidation that is a dihydroxy derivative known as DHD. Glucuronidation is undertaken by the UDP-glucuronosyltransferase (UGT) family of enzymes. After a single oral dose of oxcarbazepine, the urine contained the following compounds (expressed as percent of administered dose of oxcarbazepine): (S)-(+)-MHD = 22%, (S)-(+)-MHD-glucuronide = 39%, (R)-(−)-MHD = 5%, (R)-(−)-MHD-glucuronide = 6%, DHD = 3%, oxcarbazepine = undetectable.[15-18] The range of typical half-life ($t_{1/2}$) values for orally administered oxcarbazepine in adult subjects or patients with normal renal function and not taking enzyme inducers is 2.2-3.7 hours. For the same conditions, the range of typical half-lives is 13.0-17.0 hours for racemic MHD. For (S)-(+)-MHD and (R)-(−)-MHD, half-lives are 11.2 hours and 15.8 hours, respectively, after oral oxcarbazepine administration.[15,17,24-26] Oxcarbazepine and (R)-(−)-MHD, but not (S)-(+)-MHD, appear to be substrates for P-glycoprotein transport using a mouse small intestine model.[27]

After intravenous administration of oxcarbazepine, presystemic metabolism obviously does not occur, and the drug is only eliminated by hepatic clearance. Since there is no hepatic first-pass effect for oxcarbazepine when given intravenously, the ratio of (S)-(+)-MHD:(R)-(−)-MHD in the serum is different and equals about 1.4:1. The distribution of compounds in the urine is also different after intravenous administration (expressed as percent of administered dose of oxcarbazepine): (S)-(+)-MHD = 16%, (S)-(+)-MHD-glucuronide = 32%, (R)-(−)-MHD = 12%, (R)-(−)-MHD-glucuronide = 13%, DHD = 4%, oxcarbazepine = undetectable. For (S)-(+)-MHD and (R)-(−)-MHD, half-lives are 10.6 hours and 9.0 hours, respectively, after intravenous administration of MHD.[17]

An injectable form of oxcarbazepine is not available for clinical use. For oral use, the drug is available as immediate-release tablets (150 mg, 300 mg, 600 mg), extended-release tablets (150 mg, 300 mg, 600 mg), and suspension (300 mg/5 mL). Oral bioavailability of oxcarbazepine is 100% using MHD concentrations as a comparator.[17] The immediate-release dosage forms are rapidly absorbed from the gastrointestinal tract resulting in oxcarbazepine peak concentrations between 1.5 and 2 hours, MHD peak concentrations between 4 and 6 hours, and DHD peak concentrations 12-24 hours after a single dose of oxcarbazepine tablets.[28-30] During multiple dose studies with oxcarbazepine tablets given every 12 hours, peak concentrations occur in about 1 hour for oxcarbazepine, in about 3 hours for MHD, and in about 4-6 hours for DHD.[31,32] Peak concentrations of MHD after multiple doses of the extended-release tablet given once daily are observed about 7 hours after administration. During administration of multiple doses of 600 mg/d, the area under the concentration-time curve (AUC) and C_{max} are approximately equivalent for immediate-release tablets given every 12 hours and extended-release tablets given once daily. But at a dosage rate of 1200 mg/d administered as multiple doses, the AUC and C_{max} were about 19% lower for the extended-release tablets compared to the immediate-release tablets. Giving the extended-release tablet with meals, especially meals with a high fat content, can result in higher C_{max} concentrations than a comparable dose of immediate-release tablets. Because of this, extended-release tablets should only be taken on an empty stomach (at least 1 hour before or at least 2 hours after meals).[33,34] Rectal administration of an extemporaneously compounded oxcarbazepine fatty suppository or of oxcarbazepine oral suspension results in subtherapeutic MHD concentrations, so this route of administration with these dosage forms is not recommended.[35,36]

The AUC for MHD is proportional to the dose of oxcarbazepine that is administered, so doubling the dose of oxcarbazepine will double the AUC of MHD for a patient. In this sense, oxcarbazepine follows linear pharmacokinetics.[25,26,37-39] The plasma protein binding of MHD is 35%-40%, and the average volume of distribution of MHD after intravenous administration in normal-weight adults is 47.9 L and 54.7 L for (S)-(+)-MHD and (R)-(−)-MHD, respectively.[17,26,39-42] Oxcarbazepine is listed as a Category C medication using the FDA rating system for the use of drugs during pregnancy.

Oxcarbazepine, MHD, and DHD cross the placental barrier, and at birth the umbilical cord blood-to-maternal serum concentration ratio for each compound is approximately 1.0.[43] Oxcarbazepine and MHD are transferred across the human placenta within about 15 minutes of maternal exposure, and placental tissue can convert oxcarbazepine into MHD.[44] At birth, maternal and neonatal blood concentrations of both oxcarbazepine and MHD are equal. But after birth, serum concentrations of both compounds fell in a newborn who breastfed, so that 12% of the original concentration for oxcarbazepine ($t_{1/2}$ = ~22 hours) and 7% of the original concentration for MHD ($t_{1/2}$ = ~17 hours) were present by 5 days postpartum. The decline occurred despite continued consumption of oxcarbazepine by the mother. Oxcarbazepine and MHD cross into the breast milk of lactating mothers with a breast milk-to-maternal serum ratio of 0.50 for both agents.[45]

The blood/plasma, CSF/plasma, and saliva/plasma ratios for MHD during oxcarbazepine therapy are 1.3, 0.61, and 1.0, respectively.[26,40,46,47] The concentration of MHD is about 14% lower in the human neocortex of the brain when compared to the concurrent serum concentration.[19] Single-volume plasmapheresis conducted over a 3-hour time period removes 3%-4% of the daily oxcarbazepine dose and 5%-6% of the total body stores of MHD, so replacement doses of oxcarbazepine are not warranted.[48] Oral activated charcoal (50 g, mixed with water) administered within 30 minutes of an oral oxcarbazepine dose decreased oxcarbazepine and MHD AUC values to 4% and 8%, respectively, of control values. Four repeated doses of oral activated charcoal (20 g, mixed with water) administered 12, 24, 36, and 48 hours after oxcarbazepine was given decreases MHD AUC and $t_{1/2}$ values to 46% and 45%, respectively, of control values. Either of these modes of administration may be of use in acute overdose situations, depending upon the clinical scenario.[49]

EFFECTS OF DISEASE STATES AND CONDITIONS ON PHARMACOKINETICS AND DOSING

Assessing the effects of disease states and conditions on oxcarbazepine dosing and MHD pharmacokinetics is fraught with challenges. First and foremost is the obvious obstacle of the administration of a prodrug while tracking active metabolite concentrations and attempting to associate those concentrations to the ultimate therapeutic effect. Fortunately, the AUC for MHD is proportional to the dose of oxcarbazepine that is administered, so doubling the dose of oxcarbazepine will double the AUC of MHD for a patient. Using this framework, oxcarbazepine functionally follows linear pharmacokinetics with regard to MHD concentrations.[25,26,37-39] However, the pharmacokinetic parameters for MHD are difficult to calculate because for most of the dosage interval MHD is being continually produced by metabolic conversion of oxcarbazepine. So, in most multiple dose cases, there is never a time during the dosage interval where there is a clear elimination phase for MHD. Especially for single dose studies done when oxcarbazepine was a new entity, serum concentrations for both oxcarbazepine and MHD were at or near the ability of the assay limits to detect the compounds, so accurate determination of pharmacokinetic parameters was difficult. Thus, it is unusual to have clearance, volume of distribution, or half-life values for MHD during oxcarbazepine administration. In most studies involving oxcarbazepine, only AUC, C_{max}, C_{min}, and T_{max} are reported during multiple dose investigations. Finally, MHD is actually present in the body as the distinct stereoisomers, (S)-(+)-MHD and (R)-(−)-MHD, but most research articles simply report total MHD serum concentrations (total MHD = (S)-(+)-MHD + (R)-(−)-MHD. Due to these limitations, it is only possible to report semiquantitative findings in this section of the book.

The majority of a oxcarbazepine dose (60%-70%) is eliminated as MHD (30%-40%) or MHD-glucuronide (20%-40%) in the urine. Because of this, renal disease prolongs MHD half-life and decreases MHD clearance in a graded manner according to the degree of renal damage observed in the patient. Compared to adults with normal renal function (CrCl >90 mL/min), patients with a creatinine clearance (CrCl) of 30-80 mL/min have a 66% higher MHD AUC, patients with CrCl equal to 10-30 mL/min have a 147% higher MHD AUC, and patients with CrCl <10 mL/min have a 134% higher MHD AUC. The $t_{1/2}$ of MHD progressively rises through the CrCl classifications (CrCl >90 mL/min, $t_{1/2}$ = 10 hours; CrCl of 30-80 mL/min, $t_{1/2}$ = 12 hours; CrCl of 10-30 mL/min, $t_{1/2}$ = 16 hours; CrCl <10 mL/min, $t_{1/2}$ = 19 hours). For MHD-glucuronide, the AUC values are 259%, 1392%, and 3512% higher than control for each of the respective CrCl categories. The AUC for oxcarbazepine also increases with decreasing renal function. While the prescribing information for oxcarbazepine recommends a 50% dosage decrease for patients with CrCl <30 mL/min and a slower titration rate, the results of this research study suggest that a 40% decrease in dose for patients with a CrCl = 30-80 (especially in the CrCl = 30-50 mL/min range) and a 60% decrease in dose for patients with a CrCl = 10-30 mL/min may be appropriate. The large store of MHD-glucuronide in patients with renal dysfunction is worth noting because similar metabolites for other drugs have been known to regenerate the active drug via de-glucuronidation. Because of this, caution is advised for patients taking oxcarbazepine with CrCl <10 mL/min. For patients with renal dysfunction, oxcarbazepine doses should be titrated to clinical response, and measurement of MHD serum concentrations can be a helpful adjunct. Due to the variability in the pharmacokinetics for MHD, patients with renal disease should be closely monitored for adverse effects due to oxcarbazepine therapy.[23,50]

After oral administration, oxcarbazepine is extensively converted by presystemic metabolism and subsequent hepatic clearance via cytosol arylketone reductase in a stereospecific manner ((S)-(+)-MHD:(R)-(−)-MHD serum ratio about 4:1). After an intravenous administration of oxcarbazepine, presystemic metabolism obviously does not occur, and the drug is only metabolized by hepatic clearance. Since there is no first-pass effect when oxcarbazepine is given intravenously, the ratio of (S)-(+)-MHD:(R)-(−)-MHD in the serum is different and equals about 1.4:1. Glucuronidation of MHD is undertaken by the UDP-glucuronosyl transferase family of enzymes.[15,17,24-26] Oxcarbazepine and (R)-(−)-MHD, but not (S)-(+)-MHD, appear to be substrates for P-glycoprotein transport using a mouse small intestine model.[27]

Based on this pattern of metabolism, one would expect liver dysfunction to alter oxcarbazepine and MHD pharmacokinetics. However, the only unpublished research article to evaluate oxcarbazepine therapy in patients with hepatic disease recommends no change in oxcarbazepine dosing in patients with mild or moderate hepatic dysfunction but did not include patients with severe liver disease.[23,51] Because of this uncertainty for patients with hepatic dysfunction, oxcarbazepine doses should be titrated to clinical response, and measurement of MHD serum concentrations can be a helpful adjunct. Due to the variability in the pharmacokinetics for MHD, patients with hepatic disease should be closely monitored for adverse effects due to oxcarbazepine therapy. An index of liver dysfunction can be gained by applying the Child-Pugh clinical classification system to the patient (Table 17-2).[52] Child-Pugh scores are completely discussed in Chapter 3 (Drug Dosing in Special Populations: Renal and Hepatic Disease, Dialysis, Heart Failure, Obesity, and Drug Interactions), but will be briefly discussed here. The Child-Pugh score consists of five laboratory tests or clinical symptoms: serum albumin, total bilirubin, prothrombin time, ascites, and hepatic encephalopathy. Each of these areas is given a score of 1 (normal) to 3 (severely abnormal; see Table 17-2), and the scores for the five areas are summed. The Child-Pugh score for a patient with normal liver function is 5 while the score for a patient with grossly abnormal serum albumin, total bilirubin, and prothrombin time values in addition to severe ascites and hepatic encephalopathy is 15.

Adult and pediatric patients taking oxcarbazepine for the treatment of seizures have been studied while taking other antiepileptic drugs, and it is important to take concurrent medications into account when interpreting the

TABLE 17-2 Child-Pugh Scores for Patients With Liver Disease

Test/Symptom	Score 1 Point	Score 2 Points	Score 3 Points
Total bilirubin (mg/dL)	<2.0	2.0-3.0	>3.0
Serum albumin (g/dL)	>3.5	2.8-3.5	<2.8
Prothrombin time (seconds prolonged over control)	<4	4-6	>6
Ascites	Absent	Slight	Moderate
Hepatic encephalopathy	None	Moderate	Severe

Child-Pugh Class A, mild liver disease: 5-6 points; Child-Pugh Class B, moderate liver disease: 7-9 points; Child-Pugh Class C, severe liver disease: 10-15 points.

findings of pharmacokinetic studies. Because the metabolism of oxcarbazepine does not include the cytochrome P-450 system, the induction (phenytoin, carbamazepine, phenobarbital, primidone) or inhibition (valproic acid and its derivatives) effects of other antiepileptics is moderated to some extent compared to other antiseizure medications. For adults, taking other antiepileptic drugs that are inducers simultaneously with oxcarbazepine decreases MHD AUC by about 30%-35% and decreases half-life by about 13%-18% for MHD. By comparison, taking valproic acid or one of its derivatives that are inhibitors concurrently with oxcarbazepine had little effect on oxcarbazepine or MHD concentrations.[24,37] When lamotrigine was coadministered with oxcarbazepine, there were only slight decreases in oxcarbazepine and MHD AUC values (6-9%).[32] For patients taking oxcarbazepine concurrently with valproic acid, there may be a small increase in the free fraction of MHD (64% for cotherapy, 57% for oxcarbazepine monotherapy), and there may be a slight impact of the volume of distribution for MHD in this situation.[41] When other inducers or inhibitors are coadministered alone with oxcarbazepine, volume of distribution for MHD will likely remain unchanged due to the relatively low plasma protein binding for MHD.

For children taking oxcarbazepine, MHD clearance is about 50%-60% higher than in adults for the age range of 1 month to 3 years and is about 30%-160% higher than adults for older children. Pediatric patients taking other antiepileptic drugs that are inducers or inhibitors simultaneously with oxcarbazepine produces similar results for MHD pharmacokinetic parameters as in adults. The inducer-class antiseizure medications (phenytoin, carbamazepine, phenobarbital, primidone) increase clearance and decrease half-life for MHD compared to patients taking oxcarbazepine monotherapy. Less is known for the inhibitor-class antiseizure medications (valproic acid and its derivatives) in the pediatric population.[53-56]

For elderly men and women taking oxcarbazepine, the basic pattern compared with younger adults is similar to other antiepileptic drugs. For older women (age: 60-79 years), the AUC for MHD was 33% higher and $t_{1/2}$ for MHD was 16% longer compared to younger women. Similarly, the AUC for MHD was 53% higher and $t_{1/2}$ for MHD was 87% longer for older men (age: 61-82 years) compared to younger men. These results are consistent with the age-associated decreases measured in CrCl for the older population.[23,57] These results suggest that initial doses for oxcarbazepine should be decreased by 33%-50% for elderly adults.

Using the FDA pregnancy classification system, oxcarbazepine is a Category C medication. Thus, oxcarbazepine is used to treat pregnant women when the potential benefits of drug therapy outweigh the potential risks. Pregnancy alters the steady-state concentrations of MHD in women taking oxcarbazepine. Compared to baseline values, MHD steady-state concentrations decrease during pregnancy by the following amounts: 72% during first trimester, 74% during second trimester, and 64% during third trimester. Postpartum, MHD steady-state concentrations return to baseline values (mean time 109 days postdelivery). Oxcarbazepine, MHD, and DHD cross the placental barrier, and at birth the umbilical cord blood-to-maternal serum concentration ratio for each compound is approximately 1.0.[43] Oxcarbazepine and MHD are transferred across the human placenta within about 15 minutes of maternal exposure, and placental tissue can convert oxcarbazepine into MHD.[44] At birth, maternal and neonatal blood concentrations of both oxcarbazepine and MHD are equal. But after birth, serum concentrations of both compounds fell in a newborn who were breastfed, so that 12% of the original concentration for oxcarbazepine ($t_{1/2}$ = ~22 hours) and 7% of the original concentration for MHD ($t_{1/2}$ = ~17 hours) were present by 5 days postpartum. The decline occurred despite continued consumption of oxcarbazepine by the mother.[45] Oxcarbazepine and MHD cross into the breast milk of lactating mothers with a breast milk-to-maternal serum ratio of 0.50 for both agents.[45]

DRUG INTERACTIONS

After oral administration, oxcarbazepine is extensively converted by presystemic metabolism and subsequent hepatic clearance via cytosol arylketone reductase in a stereospecific manner (S)-(+)-MHD:(R)-(−)-MHD serum ratio about 4:1. After intravenous administration of oxcarbazepine, presystemic metabolism obviously does not occur, and the drug is metabolized solely by hepatic clearance. Since there is no first-pass effect when oxcarbazepine is given intravenously, the ratio of (S)-(+)-MHD:(R)-(−)-MHD in the serum is different than for orally administered oxcarbazepine and equals about 1.4:1. Glucuronidation of MHD is conducted by the UDP-glucuronosyl transferase family of enzymes.[15,17,24-26] Additionally, oxcarbazepine and (R)-(−)-MHD, but not (S)-(+)-MHD, are substrates for P-glycoprotein transport using a mouse small intestine model.[27] Because of this complex elimination pattern, there are ample opportunities for drug interactions.

Adult and pediatric patients taking oxcarbazepine for the treatment of seizures have been studied while taking other antiepileptic drugs. Because the metabolism of oxcarbazepine does not include the cytochrome P-450 system, the induction (phenytoin, carbamazepine, phenobarbital, primidone) or inhibition (valproic acid and its derivatives) effects of other antiepileptics is modulated to some extent compared to other anticonvulsants. For adults, taking other antiepileptic drugs that are inducers simultaneously with oxcarbazepine will decrease MHD AUC by about 30%-35% and decrease half-life by about 13%-18% for MHD. By comparison, taking valproic acid or one of its derivatives that are inhibitors concurrently with oxcarbazepine has little effect on oxcarbazepine or MHD concentrations.[24,37,58] When lamotrigine was coadministered with oxcarbazepine, there were only slight decreases in oxcarbazepine and MHD AUC values (6%-9%).[32] For patients taking oxcarbazepine concurrently with valproic acid, there may be a small increase in the free fraction of MHD (64% for cotherapy, 57% for oxcarbazepine monotherapy), and there may be a slight impact on the volume of distribution for MHD in this situation.[41] When other inducers or inhibitors are coadministered alone with oxcarbazepine, volume of distribution for MHD will likely remain unchanged due to the relatively low plasma protein binding for MHD.

Pediatric patients taking other antiepileptic drugs that are inducers or inhibitors simultaneously with oxcarbazepine produces similar results for MHD pharmacokinetic parameters as in adults. The inducer-class antiseizure medications (phenytoin, carbamazepine, phenobarbital, primidone) increase clearance and decrease half-life for MHD compared to patients taking oxcarbazepine monotherapy. Less is known for the inhibitor-class antiseizure medications (valproic acid and its derivatives) in the pediatric population.[53-56]

Oxcarbazepine has the potential to alter the concentrations and pharmacokinetics of other drugs due to its ability to induce or inhibit the cytochrome P-450 system. Early in the development of oxcarbazepine, it was noted that oxcarbazepine 300 mg administered orally twice daily could increase the elimination of two marker agents, antipyrine and 6β-OH-cortosol, which are used as broad-based indicators of liver enzyme induction.[59] At about the same time, a similar study that administered oxcarbazepine orally at a rate of 1500-2400 mg/d altered antipyrine clearance and half-life even more than lower doses of oxcarbazepine.[60] Subsequent to these investigations, oxcarbazepine was found to be an inducer for CYP3A4.[61] Oxcarbazepine therapy decreases the steady-state concentrations of many drugs, including ethinyl estradiol, levonorgestrel, rufinamide, lamotrigine, levetiracetam, pregabalin, and topiramate.[32,62,67] In contrast to the effect on CYP3A4, oxcarbazepine and MHD arc inhibitors of thc CYP2C19 systcm and decrease the elimination of phenytoin.[68]

INITIAL DOSAGE DETERMINATION METHODS

Oxcarbazepine dosing is usually initiated using a "start low, go slow" type of titration process.[11,19,23,34,69] This is a rational and preferred way to instigate dosing with the agent because the complex metabolic and elimination pattern yields widely different MHD concentrations depending on a variety of factors (patient age, concurrent antiepileptic therapy, etc), and it avoids the development of adverse effects early in treatment. Achieving a therapeutic effect without the development of side effects will improve patient adherence with oxcarbazepine therapy. There are several ways to start oxcarbazepine treatment, and one of the many recommended methods will be discussed in this section of the book as *Literature-Based Recommended Dosing*.[11,19,23,34,69,70]

For adults, oxcarbazepine treatment is usually started at a rate of 300-600 mg/d (immediate-release oral dosage forms given as equal, divided doses every 12 hours; extended-release tablets given once daily on an empty stomach). Every 1-2 weeks the dosage rate may be advanced by giving an additional 300-600 mg/d, and patients should be simultaneously monitored for seizure frequency and adverse drug effects. This dosage titration scheme can be used for adjunctive therapy with oxcarbazepine, oxcarbazepine monotherapy, or conversion from other antiepileptics to oxcarbazepine monotherapy. For patients that are undergoing conversion to oxcarbazepine monotherapy, the other anticonvulsants can be tapered off over a 3-6-week time frame, while the expected dose of oxcarbazepine is being ramped up during the first 2-4 weeks of this time period. The aim of this procedure is to ensure that effective amounts of oxcarbazepine will be prescribed early in the conversion process, before the other antiepileptic drugs are discontinued. Maximum tolerated doses of oxcarbazepine are usually in the 2400-3000 mg/d range.

For children, aged 4-16 years the initial dose of oxcarbazepine is 8-10 mg/kg/d for adjunctive therapy, conversion to oxcarbazepine monotherapy, or oxcarbazepine monotherapy. For adjunctive therapy with oxcarbazepine, the dose is slowly titrated to the recommended maximum over a 2-3-week time period (patient weight with maximum oxcarbazepine dosage: 20-29 kg, 900 mg/d; 29-39 kg, 1200 mg/d; ≥40 kg, 1800 mg/d). For conversion to oxcarbazepine monotherapy, oxcarbazepine doses are advanced at a rate of 10 mg/kg/d weekly, while the concomitantly administered antiepileptic therapy is tapered off over 3-6 weeks. For oxcarbazepine monotherapy, the dose is also slowly titrated, but at a rate of 5 mg/kg/d every 3-7 days. The maximum dose of oxcarbazepine monotherapy (either converted from other antiepileptic drugs or as initial therapy) is determined by patient weight: 900 mg/d for 20 kg, 1200 mg/d for 25-30 kg, 1500 mg/d for 35-45 kg, 1800 mg/d for 50-55 kg, 2100 mg/d for 60-70 kg. For younger children aged 2-3 years, the initial dose of oxcarbazepine for the adjunctive treatment is also 8-10 mg/kg/d, but if the patient weighs under 20 kg a dose of 16-20 mg/kg/d can be used. For younger patients, the dose of oxcarbazepine can be titrated over 2-4 weeks, and the dose should not exceed 60 mg/kg/d given in two divided doses.

For adult patients with severe renal dysfunction (CrCl <30 mL/min) the initial dose of oxcarbazepine should be reduced by ½ to 300 mg/d. Adults suffering from liver disease with mild to moderate hepatic impairment (see Table 17-2) can be started on the typical dose, but the dosage of oxcarbazepine for patients with severe liver dysfunction is unknown. Dosage adjustments for elderly patients should be made on the basis of their renal function (CrCl).

Literature-Based Recommended Dosing

EXAMPLE 1 ▶▶▶

SO is a 51-year-old, 75-kg (height = 5 ft 10 in) male with complex partial seizures who requires adjunctive therapy with oxcarbazepine. He has a normal liver and renal function and is currently taking phenytoin (steady-state concentration = 18.2 μg/mL). Additional dosage increases have been tried with phenytoin, but they have been unsuccessful due to development of adverse effects. Suggest an initial oxcarbazepine dosage regimen using immediate-release tablets for this patient.

1. *Estimate oxcarbazepine dose according to age, disease states and conditions, dosage form, and concurrent drug therapy.*

   For an adult patient taking phenytoin and treated with immediate-release oxcarbazepine tablets, the initial dose is 300-600 mg/d given as a divided dose every 12 hours.

   For the first 2 weeks, the initial dose of 150 mg every 12 hours was chosen. Every 1-2 weeks of therapy, the dose can be escalated by an additional 300-600 mg/d to a maximum of 2400-3000 mg/d. The patient should be closely monitored for seizure frequency and adverse drug effects.

   SO was titrated to a dose of oxcarbazepine 1200 mg every 12 hours without any additional side effects and a decreased seizure frequency.

EXAMPLE 2 ▶▶▶

SO is a 51-year-old, 75-kg (height = 5 ft 10 in) male with complex partial seizures who requires monotherapy with oxcarbazepine. He has normal liver and renal function. Suggest an initial oxcarbazepine dosage regimen using immediate-release tablets for this patient. (*Note: This is a similar patient profile as Example 1, except for no concurrent antiepileptic drug therapy, so that the differences can be contrasted.*)

1. *Estimate oxcarbazepine dose according to age, disease states and conditions, dosage form, and concurrent drug therapy.*

For an adult patient taking oxcarbazepine as monotherapy using immediate-release tablets, the initial dose is 300-600 mg/d given as a divided dose every 12 hours.

For the first 2 weeks, the initial dose of 300 mg every 12 hours was chosen. Every 1-2 weeks of therapy, the dose can be escalated by an additional 300-600 mg/d to a maximum of 2400-3000 mg/d. The patient should be closely monitored for seizure frequency and adverse drug effects.

SO was titrated to a dose of oxcarbazepine 1500 mg every 12 hours without any side effects and a decreased seizure frequency.

EXAMPLE 3 ▶▶▶

SO is a 51-year-old, 75-kg (height = 5 ft 10 in) male with complex partial seizures who requires monotherapy with oxcarbazepine. He has normal liver and renal function. Suggest an initial oxcarbazepine dosage regimen using extended-release tablets for this patient. (*Note: This is a similar patient profile as Example 2, except for use of extended-release tablets, so that the differences can be contrasted.*)

1. *Estimate oxcarbazepine dose according to age, disease states and conditions, dosage form, and concurrent drug therapy.*

For an adult patient taking oxcarbazepine as monotherapy using extended-release tablets, the initial dose is 300-600 mg/d given once daily on an empty stomach.

For the first 2 weeks, the initial dose of 600 mg daily was chosen. Every 1-2 weeks of therapy, the dose can be escalated by an additional 300-600 mg/d to a maximum of 2400-3000 mg/d. The patient should be closely monitored for seizure frequency and adverse drug effects.

SO was titrated to a dose of oxcarbazepine 1800 mg daily without any side effects and a decreased seizure frequency.

EXAMPLE 4 ▶▶▶

JX is a 9-year-old 35-kg (height = 4 ft 6 in) female with simple partial seizures who requires adjunctive therapy with oxcarbazepine. She has normal liver and renal function and is currently taking valproate (steady-state concentration = 81.7 µg/mL). Additional dosage increases have been tried with valproate, but they have been unsuccessful due to development of adverse effects. Suggest an initial oxcarbazepine dosage regimen using oral suspension for this patient.

1. *Estimate oxcarbazepine dose according to age, disease states and conditions, dosage form, and concurrent drug therapy.*

For a pediatric patient taking valproate and treated with oxcarbazepine oral suspension, the initial dose is 8-10 mg/kg/d given as two divided doses every 12 hours.

For the first 1-2 weeks, the initial dose of 150 mg every 12 hours was chosen (35 kg • 9 mg/kg/d = 315 mg, rounded to 300 mg/d). Every 1-2 weeks of therapy, the dose can be escalated by an additional 150-300 mg/d to a target dose of 1200 mg/d. The patient should be closely monitored for seizure frequency and adverse drug effects.

SO was titrated to a dose of oxcarbazepine 600 mg every 12 hours without any side effects and a decreased seizure frequency. Within 6 months, she was switched to oxcarbazepine tablets 600 mg every 12 hours when she could swallow whole tablets without any distress. Therapeutic response remained constant after the dosage form switch, with no change in seizure frequency or adverse effects.

USE OF MHD SERUM CONCENTRATIONS TO ALTER DOSES OF OXCARBAZEPINE

A definitive therapeutic range for steady-state MHD serum concentrations during oxcarbazepine treatment has not been established.[12-14] Because of this, serum concentration monitoring for oxcarbazepine plays only a supportive role in the dosing of the drug. Important patient parameters (seizure frequency or frequency/severity of mood episodes, potential oxcarbazepine side effects, etc) should be followed to confirm that the patient is responding to treatment and not developing adverse drug reactions.[8,11] However, there are clinical situations where MHD steady-state serum concentration monitoring of trough levels can be very helpful.

Once dosage titration has been conducted, and an effective dose of oxcarbazepine has been established by assessing therapeutic response and absence of adverse effects, many clinicians obtain a steady-state MHD concentration to establish an individualized effective target value for the patient. When this is done, if seizure frequency changes or an adverse effect occurs, another MHD serum concentration can be measured to ascertain potential solutions to the problem. For instance, if a patient suddenly has more seizures than usual, comparing the current MHD serum concentration with the established effective target MHD concentration can be helpful to decide a course of action. If the current MHD concentration is lower than usual, reasons for the change can be explored (lack of adherence to therapy, drug interaction, etc), and, if appropriate, an oxcarbazepine dosage increase can be considered to reestablish effective concentrations. If the current MHD concentration is about the same, changes to therapy may be warranted (increase oxcarbazepine dose, addition of other drug therapy, etc). Alternatively, if a patient suddenly develops adverse effects that could be due to oxcarbazepine therapy, and the current MHD serum concentration is high, it may be appropriate to decrease the oxcarbazepine dose. Also, when an effective MHD concentration has been established for a patient, the effects of new drug therapy that may cause drug interactions or of new disease states or conditions that can alter oxcarbazepine or MHD pharmacokinetics can be assessed prospectively by measuring the current MHD concentration before any clinical events occur.

Because a definitive therapeutic range for MHD has not been firmly established, and a "start low, go slow" dosage titration strategy has been established for the drug, oxcarbazepine dose increases are usually capped at the rate noted in the initial dosing section. When needed, dosage decreases are usually made using one of the smaller changes possible from available tablet strengths. Thus, pharmacokinetic calculations are usually made to compute the expected steady-state concentration after a specific oxcarbazepine dosage change has been determined rather than computing a new dose based on a desired target concentration. Because MHD follows linear pharmacokinetics during oxcarbazepine treatment, the pharmacokinetic calculations involved during dosage titration are straightforward.

When an oxcarbazepine dosage change is made, sufficient time to attain steady-state conditions (~3-5 half-lives) should be allowed before assessing therapeutic outcome. Of course, any time adverse effects occur during dosage titration, measures should be taken to assess the likelihood that they are due to oxcarbazepine treatment and appropriate action should be taken when needed.

If MHD serum concentrations are measured for patients in support of a dosage change, clinicians should seek to use the simplest, most straightforward method available to determine the steady-state concentration for the new regimen. In this case, a simple dosage ratio can be used to change doses since MHD follows *linear pharmacokinetics* during oxcarbazepine therapy.

Linear Pharmacokinetics Method

Because oxcarbazepine follows linear, dose-proportional pharmacokinetics, steady-state serum concentrations change in proportion to dose according to the following equation: $D_{new}/C_{ss,new} = D_{old}/C_{ss,old}$ or $C_{ss,new} = (D_{new}/D_{old}) C_{ss,old}$, where D is the dose, C_{ss} is the steady-state concentration, old indicates the dose that produced the steady-state concentration that the patient is currently receiving, and new denotes the steady-state concentration produced by the newly prescribed dose. The advantages of this method are that it is quick and simple. The disadvantage is steady-state concentrations are required.

EXAMPLE 5 ▶▶▶

EY is a 51-year-old, 75-kg (height = 5 ft 10 in) male with complex partial seizures who receives monotherapy with oxcarbazepine. He has normal liver and renal function. EY was titrated to a dose of oxcarbazepine 900 mg every 12 hours (1800 mg/d) without any side effects and a decreased seizure frequency. At that time, a steady-state MHD concentration was obtained before a dose and equaled 10.2 μg/mL. Several months ago, the patient was started on phenytoin, and he has been on a stable dose for 4 weeks. Today, the steady-state MHD concentration obtained before the next dose was 7.5 μg/mL. Suggest a new maintenance dosage regimen using immediate-release oxcarbazepine tablets to reestablish the original MHD steady-state concentration for this patient.

1. *Use linear pharmacokinetics to compute the new concentration for a reasonable dosage increase.*
   Dosage increases for oxcarbazepine are usually made in increments of no more than 300-600 mg/d every 1-2 weeks. This patient is currently receiving 1800 mg/d, so the maximum increase for the first week would be 600 mg/d: $C_{ss,new} = (D_{new}/D_{old})C_{ss,old} = (2400 \text{ mg/d} / 1800 \text{ mg/d})7.5 \text{ μg/mL} = 10.0 \text{ μg/mL}$.
   To reestablish the original MHD concentration for the patient, a dosage increase of 2400 mg/d or 1200 mg every 12 hours was prescribed. The patient should be carefully monitored for seizure frequency and adverse effects. If desired, steady-state MHD serum concentrations can be measured 3-5 half-lives after the dosage change has been made ($\sim t_{1/2} = 15$ hours, $\sim$3-5 $t_{1/2}$ in 2-3 days).

2. *If desired steady-state MHD concentrations have not been attained with the first dosage increase, compute the new concentration for the next reasonable dosage increase. Continue titration until the desired steady-state concentration or optimal therapeutic response has been achieved.*
   The desired steady-state MHD concentration has been reached, so this step is not necessary for this patient.

BAYESIAN PHARMACOKINETICS COMPUTER PROGRAMS

Computer programs are available that can assist in the computation of pharmacokinetic parameters for patients. The most reliable computer programs use a nonlinear regression algorithm that incorporates components of Bayes theorem. Nonlinear regression is a statistical technique that uses an iterative process to compute the best pharmacokinetic parameters for a concentration-time data set. Unfortunately, these types of computer programs are not as useful with oxcarbazepine compared to other antiepileptics due to complex initial dosage administration algorithms, the slow titration of maintenance doses, and the use of a prodrug as the administered agent. This dosage adjustment approach cannot be recommended for routine clinical use at this time because of these issues.

ESLICARBAZEPINE

INTRODUCTION

As the drug development cycle moved into a new generation of anticonvulsants, it was suggested that the active metabolite of oxcarbazepine, MHD for monohydroxy derivative of oxcarbazepine, be developed in its own right as a new drug. This effort came to fruition in 2009 when the European Medicines Agency approved eslicarbazepine acetate [eslicarbazepine is (S)-(+)-MHD, also known as S-licarbazepine] for use as a prescription drug in the European Union. In 2013, a revised New Drug Application was submitted in the United States to the Food and Drug Administration, and shortly thereafter eslicarbazepine was approved as a prescription-only agent. The S-enantiomer was chosen as the sole component because it is the predominate isomer in the blood after oral administration of oxcarbazepine. Eslicarbazepine acetate is rapidly converted to eslicarbazepine, which, of course, has the same pharmacokinetic properties and pharmacodynamic effects as (S)-(+)-MHD produced after the administration of oxcarbazepine.

Because oxcarbazepine and eslicarbazepine acetate share an active moiety (known as either (S)-(+)-MHD, S-licarbazepine, or eslicarbazepine in various research studies), they are considered together in this chapter. Oxcarbazepine is covered in the first major section of the chapter, and eslicarbazepine is discussed in the second major section of the chapter. Because oxcarbazepine has been available for much longer period of time, it is to be expected that more is known about MHD after its administration compared to eslicarbazepine. But, in general, most of what is written about (S)-(+)-MHD in the oxcarbazepine section directly applies to eslicarbazepine.

THERAPEUTIC AND TOXIC CONCENTRATIONS

Unlike most of the older antiepileptic drugs, the therapeutic range of eslicarbazepine is not well defined. However, serum concentration monitoring during eslicarbazepine acetate treatment can be a useful adjunct in addition to monitoring treatment for therapeutic response and adverse effects. Although eslicarbazepine acetate is measurable in the serum after oral administration of the drug, in normal subjects and patients with normal kidney and hepatic function this prodrug is often near the assay limits for detecting its serum concentration. Eslicarbazepine (also known as (S)-(+)-MHD or S-licarbazepine), which is the active metabolite of eslicarbazepine acetate, is the moiety that is predominate in the serum of humans. After oral administration of eslicarbazepine acetate, eslicarbazepine is produced by presystemic metabolism via hydrolase cleavage of the acetate group so that about 95% of the total exposure of the administered drug is eslicarbazepine. The remainder of the prodrug is present in the serum as (R)-licarbazepine (also known as (R)-(−)-MHD, ~4%) and oxcarbazepine (~1%). (R)-licarbazepine is most likely produced via metabolic conversion of oxcarbazepine.[71-77]

The therapeutic range for epilepsy used by many laboratories for MHD [MHD = (S)-(+)-MHD + (R)-(−)-MHD which is the same as eslicarbazepine + (R)-licarbazepine] during oxcarbazepine treatment is 3-35 µg/mL, but for orally administered oxcarbazepine the ratio of the S- to R-enantiomer is 4:1. In other words, 80% of metabolite in the serum is the S-enantiomer. The typical assay for MHD is not stereospecific for the individual enantiomers. Also, from the results of population pharmacokinetic analysis of oral eslicarbazepine acetate for the treatment of partial seizures, it is known that there is a 33% chance of response at an eslicarbazepine steady-state concentration of 4.6 µg/mL, a 38% chance of response at an eslicarbazepine steady-state concentration equal to 10.7 µg/mL, and a 40% chance of response with an eslicarbazepine steady-state concentration of 17.0 µg/mL.[78]

Keeping this information in mind, the preliminary therapeutic range for eslicarbazepine acetate oral dosage forms will also be 3-35 µg/mL, but it is likely this will be refined in the future with more clinical experience, and, possibly, the routine use of a stereospecific assay. Some patients will experience a higher incidence of adverse effects at concentrations in the upper end of the therapeutic range, so the efficacy of lower eslicarbazepine serum concentrations should be assessed before moving to higher concentrations. The most common dose- or concentration-dependent side effects of eslicarbazepine are sedation, somnolence, fatigue, dizziness, ataxia, nausea, and headache.[79]

CLINICAL MONITORING PARAMETERS

The goal of therapy with anticonvulsants is to reduce seizure frequency and maximize quality of life with a minimum of adverse drug effects. While it is desirable to entirely abolish all seizure episodes, it may not be possible to accomplish this in many patients. Patients should be monitored for concentration-related side effects of eslicarbazepine treatment (sedation, somnolence, fatigue, dizziness, ataxia, nausea, headache). Other potential adverse reactions include diplopia, blurred vision, diarrhea, vomiting, lack of attention, tremor, abnormal gait, prolongation of the PR interval, and skin rash. A few patients (<1% incidence) may develop hyponatremia during chronic therapy with eslicarbazepine, and serum sodium concentrations can be periodically measured to detect this problem.[79]

Because epilepsy is an episodic disease state, patients do not experience seizures continuously. Thus, during dosage titration it is difficult to tell if the patient is responding to drug therapy or simply is not experiencing any abnormal central nervous system discharges at that time. Eslicarbazepine acetate doses should be carefully titrated to individual patient response and tolerability. Serum concentrations of eslicarbazepine can be measured in patients as an adjunct to therapy. Concentration monitoring is particularly useful if a therapeutic concentration has been established for a patient and a new clinical event (drug interaction, new disease state or condition, etc) changes the pharmacokinetics of the drug. Eslicarbazepine concentrations can also be measured to document patient adherence to drug treatment or when a patient is switched between the oral dosage forms of eslicarbazepine to assure therapeutic levels are maintained.

BASIC CLINICAL PHARMACOKINETIC PARAMETERS

After oral administration of eslicarbazepine acetate, eslicarbazepine is produced by extensive presystemic metabolism via hydrolase cleavage of the acetate group so that about 95% of the total systemic exposure of the administered drug is eslicarbazepine. The remainder of the prodrug is present in the serum as (R)-licarbazepine (also known as (R)-(−)-MHD, ~4%) and oxcarbazepine (~1%). (R)-licarbazepine is most likely produced via metabolic conversion of oxcarbazepine. After absorption of the prodrug, these three metabolites undergo some interconversion, with oxcarbazepine being the intermediary between eslicarbazepine and (R)-licarbazepine by chiral metabolism via arylketone reductase. Ultimately, all three of these species are glucuronidated by the UDP-glucuronosyl transferase (UGT) system and eliminated in the urine. The final percentages of metabolites recovered in the urine are: ~62% unchanged eslicarbazepine, ~30% eslicarbazepine glucuronide, ~4% oxcarbazepine glucuronide, ~3% (R)-licarbazepine, ~2% oxcarbazepine, <1% both oxcarbazepine glucuronide and (R)-licarbazepine glucuronide.[71-77] For eslicarbazepine and (R)-licarbazepine, half-lives are 10.6 hours and 9.0 hours, respectively, after intravenous administration of racemic licarbazepine.[17]

In vitro studies have shown that eslicarbazepine is glucuronidated by the following UGT family of enzymes: UGT1A4, UGT1A9, UGT2B4, UGT2B7, and UGT2B17. Of these, UGT2B4 has the highest affinity for eslicarbazepine, and there is a good correlation between eslicarbazepine glucuronidatation and other substrates of UGT1A4.[80] The range of typical half-life ($t_{1/2}$) values for eslicarbazepine at steady-state during orally administered eslicarbazepine acetate treatment in adult subjects or patients with normal renal function and not taking enzyme inducers is 13-20 hours using a stereospecific assay method.[81,82] Oxcarbazepine and (R)-licarbazepine, but not eslicarbazepine, appear to be substrates for P-glycoprotein transport using a mouse small intestine model.[27]

An injectable form of eslicarbazepine is not available for clinical use. For oral use, eslicarbazepine acetate is available as immediate-release tablets (200 mg, 400 mg, 600 mg, 800 mg) and a suspension is under development.[83] Oral bioavailability of eslicarbazepine acetate is >90% using the mass balance of administered dose recovered as metabolites in the urine as a comparator.[71-77] The immediate-release dosage forms of eslicarbazepine acetate are rapidly absorbed from the gastrointestinal tract resulting in eslicarbazepine peak concentrations at steady-state between 1.5 and 3 hours. Eslicarbazepine acetate can be given on an empty stomach or with food without altering bioavailability.[77]

The AUC for eslicarbazepine is proportional to the dose of eslicarbazepine acetate that is administered, so doubling the dose of eslicarbazepine acetate will double the AUC of eslicarbazepine for a patient. In this sense, eslicarbazepine follows linear pharmacokinetics.[72,83,84] The plasma protein binding in humans of both eslicarbazepine and (R)-licarbazepine is identical at 30%, with more binding occurring to albumin (19%-20%) and less binding occurring to α_1-acid glycoprotein (2%-4%).[85,86] The average volume of distribution of these metabolites after intravenous administration of an experimental racemic mixture in normal weight adults is 47.9 L and 54.7 L for eslicarbazepine and (R)-licarbazepine, respectively.[17] The CSF-plasma ratio using AUC measurements in both fluids during eslicarbazepine acetate oral therapy at steady-state is 32% for eslicarbazepine, 61% for (R)-licarbazepine, and 38% for oxcarbazepine.[87]

EFFECTS OF DISEASE STATES AND CONDITIONS ON PHARMACOKINETICS AND DOSING

Assessing the effects of disease states and conditions on eslicarbazepine acetate dosing and eslicarbazepine pharmacokinetics is fraught with challenges. First and foremost is the obvious obstacle of the administration of a prodrug while tracking active metabolite concentrations and attempting to associate those concentrations to the ultimate therapeutic effect. Fortunately, the AUC for eslicarbazepine is proportional to the dose of eslicarbazepine acetate that is administered, so doubling the dose of eslicarbazepine acetate will double the AUC of eslicarbazepine for a patient. Using this framework, eslicarbazepine acetate functionally follows linear pharmacokinetics with regard to eslicarbazepine concentrations.[72,83,84] However, the pharmacokinetic parameters for eslicarbazepine are difficult to calculate because for most of the dosage interval eslicarbazepine is being continually produced by metabolic conversion of eslicarbazepine acetate, and the interconversion of eslicarbazepine, oxcarbazepine, and (R)-licarbazepine that occurs simultaneously. So, in most multiple dose cases, there is never a time during the dosage interval where there is a clear elimination phase for eslicarbazepine. Especially for single-dose studies done when eslicarbazepine was a new entity, serum concentrations for both oxcarbazepine and (R)-licarbazepine were at or near the ability of the assay limits to detect the compounds, so accurate determination of pharmacokinetic parameters was difficult. Thus, it is unusual to have accurate clearance, volume of distribution, or half-life values for eslicarbazepine during eslicarbazepine acetate administration. In most studies involving eslicarbazepine, only AUC, C_{max}, C_{min}, and T_{max} are reported during multiple-dose investigations. Finally, eslicarbazepine and (R)-licarbazepine are actually present in the body as distinct stereoisomers, but some research articles simply report total MHD serum concentrations (total MHD = (S)-(+)-MHD + (R)-(−)-MHD or eslicarbazepine + (R)-licarbazepine). Due to these limitations, it is only possible to report semiquantitative findings in this section of the book.

The majority of a eslicarbazepine acetate dose (~92%) is eliminated as unchanged eslicarbazepine (~62%) or eslicarbazepine-glucuronide (~30%) in the urine. Because of this, renal disease prolongs eslicarbazepine half-life and decreases eslicarbazepine renal clearance in a graded manner according to the degree of renal damage observed in the patient. Compared to adults with normal renal function (CrCl >80 mL/min) acting as the control in a single-dose study, patients with a creatinine clearance (CrCl) of 50-80 mL/min have 59% of the control renal clearance for eslicarbazepine, patients with CrCl equal to 30-50 mL/min have 21% of the control renal clearance, and patients with CrCl <30 mL/min have 9% of the control renal clearance. The $t_{1/2}$ of eslicarbazepine progressively rose through the CrCl classifications (CrCl >80 mL/min = 10.7 hours, CrCl of 50-80 mL/min = 10.6 hours, CrCl of 30-50 mL/min = 17.9 hours, CrCl <30 mL/min = 28.3 hours). The renal clearance for oxcarbazepine, (R)-licarbazepine, and their respective glucuronides also decrease with declining renal function. Because of these findings, the prescribing information for eslicarbazepine acetate recommends a 50% initial dosage decrease to 200 mg/d for patients with CrCl values of 30-60 mL/min followed by a slow titration to 400 mg/d after 2 weeks of therapy, if appropriate. The large stores of the three glucuronide metabolites in patients with severe renal dysfunction are worth noting because similar metabolites for other drugs have been known to regenerate the active drug via deglucuronidation. Because of this, caution is advised for patients taking eslicarbazepine with CrCl <30 mL/min. For patients with renal dysfunction, eslicarbazepine acetate doses should be titrated to clinical response, and measurement of eslicarbazepine serum concentrations can be a helpful adjunct. Due to the variability in the pharmacokinetics for eslicarbazepine, patients with renal disease should be closely monitored for adverse effects due to eslicarbazepine therapy. For patients with end-stage renal disease, hemodialysis of 4 hours duration every other day with a low-flux filter decreased concentrations of the metabolites, but it wasn't until after the second dialysis session that concentrations approached the lower limits of the assay.[88]

After oral administration of eslicarbazepine acetate, eslicarbazepine is produced by extensive presystemic metabolism via hydrolase cleavage of the acetate group so that about 95% of the total systemic exposure of the administered drug is eslicarbazepine. The remainder of the prodrug is present in the serum as (R)-licarbazepine (~4%) and oxcarbazepine (~1%). (R)-licarbazepine is most likely produced via metabolic conversion of oxcarbazepine. After absorption of the prodrug, these three metabolites undergo some interconversion, with oxcarbazepine being the intermediary between eslicarbazepine and (R)-licarbazepine by chiral metabolism via arylketone reductase. Ultimately, all three of these species are glucuronidated by the UDP-glucuronosyl transferase (UGT) system and eliminated in the urine.[71-77] Oxcarbazepine and (R)-licarbazepine, but not eslicarbazepine, appear to be substrates for P-glycoprotein transport using a mouse small intestine model.[27]

Based on this pattern of metabolism, one would expect liver dysfunction to alter the pharmacokinetics of eslicarbazepine acetate and its metabolites. However, the only research article to evaluate eslicarbazepine therapy in patients with moderate hepatic disease recommends no change in eslicarbazepine acetate dosing in patients with either mild or moderate hepatic dysfunction but did not include patients with severe liver disease.[89] While it is true that mean AUC, C_{maxss}, and C_{minss} for eslicarbazepine in moderate liver disease patients were not significantly different than those computed for the normal control group, the variability for those parameters in the liver disease patients was about double that found for the normal subjects. Additionally, there was a 19% increase in half-life for the patients with moderate liver damage. Because of this uncertainty for patients with hepatic dysfunction, eslicarbazepine acetate doses should be titrated to clinical response, and measurement of eslicarbazepine serum concentrations can be a helpful adjunct. Due to the variability in the pharmacokinetics for eslicarbazepine, patients with hepatic disease should be closely monitored for adverse effects due to eslicarbazepine acetate therapy. An index of liver dysfunction can be gained by applying the Child-Pugh clinical classification system to the patient (see Table 17-2).[52] Child-Pugh scores are completely discussed in Chapter 3 (Drug Dosing in Special Populations: Renal and Hepatic Disease, Dialysis, Heart Failure, Obesity, and Drug Interactions), but will be briefly discussed here. The Child-Pugh score consists of five laboratory tests or clinical symptoms: serum albumin, total bilirubin, prothrombin time, ascites, and hepatic encephalopathy. Each of these areas is given a score of 1 (normal) to 3 (severely abnormal; see Table 17-2), and the scores for the five areas are summed. The Child-Pugh score for a patient with normal liver function is 5 while the score for a patient with grossly abnormal serum albumin, total bilirubin, and prothrombin time values in addition to severe ascites and hepatic encephalopathy is 15.

Adult and pediatric patients taking eslicarbazepine acetate for the treatment of seizures have been studied while taking other antiepileptic drugs, and it is important to take concurrent medications into account when interpreting the findings of pharmacokinetic studies. Because the metabolism of eslicarbazepine doesn't include the cytochrome P-450 system, the induction (phenytoin, carbamazepine, phenobarbital) effects of other antiepileptics is moderated to some extent compared to other antiseizure medications. For adults, taking phenytoin or phenobarbital simultaneously with eslicarbazepine acetate decreases eslicarbazepine steady-state concentrations by about 33%-66%. Similarly, taking carbamazepine changes eslicarbazepine clearance in a dose-dependent manner. This produces an increase in eslicarbazepine clearance of 13% while taking 200 mg/d of carbamazepine and an increase in eslicarbazepine clearance of 150% a day when taking 2400 mg/d of carbamazepine.[78,84,90] By comparison, taking valproic acid or one of its derivatives, lamotrigine, or topiramate concurrently with eslicarbazepine acetate had little to no effect on eslicarbazepine steady-state concentrations.[78,84,90] When other antiepileptic agents are coadministered with eslicarbazepine acetate, the volume of distribution for eslicarbazepine will likely remain unchanged due to the relatively low plasma protein binding for eslicarbazepine.

For children taking eslicarbazepine acetate, the effects of other antiseizure medication on eslicarbazepine pharmacokinetics appear similar to that found in adults. Additionally, the pattern of higher clearance rates (~48% greater) and shorter half-lives (~38% less) for younger children (2-6 years) compared to older children (7-11 years) and adolescents (12-17 years) that is found for many other drugs holds true for eslicarbazepine. Eslicarbazepine AUC values change proportionally with eslicarbazepine acetate for children, as is the case for adults. Thus, the drug follows linear pharmacokinetics for the pediatric population.[83]

For elderly men and women taking eslicarbazepine acetate, there is no change in eslicarbazepine pharmacokinetics values compared to those calculated for younger adults. Initial doses for eslicarbazepine acetate do not need to be adjusted for age in older adults.[73] Eslicarbazepine acetate has not been studied during pregnancy, so it is not recommended for use in pregnant women. However, during treatment with oxcarbazepine, it is known that MHD [the active metabolite of oxcarbazepine, which is a racemic mixture of eslicarbazepine and (R)-licarbazepine] does cross the placenta into umbilical cord blood during pregnancy and does enter the breast milk of lactating mothers.[43-45]

DRUG INTERACTIONS

After oral administration, eslicarbazepine acetate is extensively converted by presystemic metabolism via hydrolase cleavage of the acetate group so that about 95% of the total systemic exposure of the administered drug is eslicarbazepine. The remainder of the prodrug is present in the serum as (R)-licarbazepine (~ 4%) and oxcarbazepine (~ 1%). (R)-licarbazepine is most likely produced via metabolic conversion of oxcarbazepine. After absorption of the prodrug, these three metabolites undergo some interconversion, with oxcarbazepine being the intermediary between eslicarbazepine and (R)-licarbazepine by chiral metabolism via arylketone reductase. Ultimately, all three of these species are glucuronidated by the UDP-glucuronosyl transferase (UGT) system and eliminated in the urine.[71-77] In vitro studies have shown that eslicarbazepine is glucuronidated by the following UGT family of enzymes: UGT1A4, UGT1A9, UGT2B4, UGT2B7, and UGT2B17. Oxcarbazepine and (R)-licarbazepine, but not eslicarbazepine, appear to be substrates for P-glycoprotein transport using a mouse small intestine model.[27] Because of this complex elimination pattern, there are ample opportunities for drug interactions.

Adult and pediatric patients taking eslicarbazepine acetate for the treatment of seizures have been studied while taking other antiepileptic drugs. Because the metabolism of eslicarbazepine does not include the cytochrome P-450 system, the induction (phenytoin, carbamazepine, phenobarbital) effects of other antiepileptics is moderated to some extent compared to other antiseizure medications.

For adults, taking phenytoin or phenobarbital simultaneously with eslicarbazepine acetate decreases eslicarbazepine steady-state concentrations by about 33%-66%. Similarly, taking carbamazepine changes eslicarbazepine clearance in a dose-dependent manner, producing an increase in eslicarbazepine clearance of 13% while taking 200 mg/d of carbamazepine and escalating to an increase in eslicarbazepine clearance of 150% a day when taking 2400 mg/d of carbamazepine.[78,84,90] By comparison, taking valproic acid or one of its derivatives, lamotrigine, or topiramate concurrently with eslicarbazepine acetate had little to no effect on eslicarbazepine steady-state concentrations.[78,84,90] When other antiepileptic agents are coadministered with eslicarbazepine acetate, the volume of distribution for eslicarbazepine will likely remain unchanged due to the relatively low plasma protein binding for eslicarbazepine. For children taking eslicarbazepine acetate, the effects of other antiseizure medication on eslicarbazepine pharmacokinetics appear similar to that found in adults.[83]

Eslicarbazepine has the potential to alter the concentrations and pharmacokinetics of other drugs due to its ability to induce or inhibit the cytochrome P-450 system. Eslicarbazepine is an inducer of CYP3A4. Eslicarbazepine therapy decreases the steady-state concentrations of many drugs, including ethinyl estradiol, levonorgestrel, (S)-warfarin, simvastatin, rosuvastatin, carbamazepine, lamotrigine, and topiramate.[78,79,81,82,86,91] In contrast to the effect on CYP3A4, eslicarbazepine inhibits the CYP2C19 system and decreases the elimination of phenytoin and phenobarbital.[78,90] (R)-warfarin, digoxin, levetiracetam, metformin, and valproic acid concentrations are not appreciably altered by coadministration of eslicarbazepine acetate.[86,90,92,93]

INITIAL DOSAGE DETERMINATION METHODS

Eslicarbazepine dosing is usually initiated using a "start low, go slow" type of titration process.[94,95] This is a rational and preferred way to instigate dosing with the agent because the complex metabolic and elimination pattern yields widely different eslicarbazepine concentrations depending on a variety of factors (patient age, concurrent antiepileptic therapy, etc), and it avoids the development of adverse effects early in treatment. *Literature-Based Recommended Dosing* will achieve a therapeutic effect without the development of side effects and, thus, will improve patient adherence with eslicarbazepine acetate therapy.[79,90,94,95]

For adults requiring adjunctive treatment for partial seizures, eslicarbazepine treatment is usually started at a rate of 400 mg/d, and patients should be simultaneously monitored for seizure frequency and adverse drug effects. In 1-2 weeks the dosage rate may be advanced to 800 mg/d while monitoring continues. Finally, in an additional 1-2 weeks, the dose can be increased to 1200 mg/d if the patient tolerates the lower doses and additional antiseizure effect is desired.

The majority of an eslicarbazepine acetate dose (~92%) is eliminated as unchanged eslicarbazepine (~62%) or eslicarbazepine-glucuronide (~30%) in the urine. Because of this, the prescribing information for eslicarbazepine acetate recommends a 50% initial dosage decrease to 200 mg/d for patients with CrCl values of 30-60 mL/min followed by a slow titration to 400 mg/d after 2 weeks of therapy, if appropriate. Since large stores of the three glucuronide metabolites accumulate in patients with severe renal dysfunction, caution is advised for patients taking eslicarbazepine acetate with CrCl <30 mL/min. For patients with renal dysfunction, eslicarbazepine acetate doses should be titrated to clinical response, and measurement of eslicarbazepine serum concentrations can be a helpful adjunct. Due to the variability in the pharmacokinetics for eslicarbazepine, patients with renal disease should be closely monitored for adverse effects due to eslicarbazepine therapy.[88]

Literature-Based Recommended Dosing

EXAMPLE 6 ▶▶▶

SO is a 51-year-old, 75-kg (height = 5 ft 10 in) male with complex partial seizures who requires adjunctive therapy with eslicarbazepine acetate. He has normal liver and renal function and is currently taking phenytoin (steady-state concentration = 18.2 μg/mL). Additional dosage increases have been tried with phenytoin, but they have been unsuccessful due to development of adverse effects. Suggest an initial eslicarbazepine acetate dosage regimen using immediate-release tablets for this patient.

1. *Estimate eslicarbazepine acetate dose according to age, disease states and conditions, dosage form, and concurrent drug therapy.*

    For an adult patient taking phenytoin and treated with immediate-release eslicarbazepine acetate tablets, the initial dose is 400 mg/d given as a single daily dose. The patient was closely monitored for seizure frequency and adverse drug effects. Serum concentrations of phenytoin were measured during the first week of therapy, and a phenytoin dosage adjustment was made due to rising levels.

    After the first 2 weeks of treatment, the eslicarbazepine acetate dose was increased to 800 mg daily with continued monitoring.

EXAMPLE 7 ▶▶▶

SO is a 51-year-old, 75-kg (height = 5 ft 10 in) male with complex partial seizures taking phenytoin (steady-state concentration = 18.2 μg/mL, free fraction = 11%) who requires adjunctive therapy with eslicarbazepine acetate. He has normal liver function, but his CrCl$_{est}$ = 42 mL/min. Suggest an initial eslicarbazepine acetate dosage regimen using immediate-release tablets for this patient. (*Note: This is a similar patient profile as Example 6, except for renal dysfunction, so that the differences can be contrasted.*)

1. *Estimate eslicarbazepine acetate dose according to age, disease states and conditions, dosage form, and concurrent drug therapy.*

    For an adult patient with renal dysfunction taking phenytoin and treated with immediate-release eslicarbazepine acetate tablets, the initial dose is 200 mg/d given as a single daily dose. The patient was closely monitored for seizure frequency and adverse drug effects. Serum concentrations of phenytoin were measured during the first week of therapy, and a phenytoin dosage adjustment was made due to rising levels.

    After the first 2 weeks of treatment, an eslicarbazepine steady-state trough concentration was 10.3 μg/mL, and the eslicarbazepine acetate dose was increased to 400 mg daily with continued monitoring.

USE OF SERUM CONCENTRATIONS TO ALTER DOSES OF ESLICARBAZEPINE

A definitive therapeutic range for steady-state eslicarbazepine serum concentrations during eslicarbazepine acetate treatment has not been established. Because of this, serum concentration monitoring for eslicarbazepine plays only a supportive role in the dosing of the drug. Important patient parameters (seizure frequency, potential eslicarbazepine side effects, etc) should be followed to confirm that the patient is responding to treatment and not developing adverse drug reactions.[94,95] However, there are clinical situations where measuring eslicarbazepine steady-state trough serum concentrations can be very helpful.

Once dosage titration has been conducted, and an effective dose of eslicarbazepine acetate has been established by assessing therapeutic response and absence of adverse effects, many clinicians obtain a steady-state eslicarbazepine concentration to establish an individualized effective target value for the patient. When this is done, if seizure frequency changes or an adverse effect occurs, another eslicarbazepine serum concentration can be measured to ascertain potential solutions to the problem. For instance, if a patient suddenly has more seizures than usual, comparing the current eslicarbazepine serum concentration with the established effective target eslicarbazepine concentration can be helpful to decide a course of action. If the current eslicarbazepine concentration is lower than usual, reasons for the change can be explored (lack of adherence to therapy, drug interaction, etc), and, if appropriate, an eslicarbazepine acetate dosage increase can be considered to reestablish effective concentrations. If the current eslicarbazepine concentration is about the same, changes to therapy may be warranted (increase eslicarbazepine acetate dose, addition of other drug therapy, etc). Alternatively, if a patient suddenly develops adverse effects that could be due to eslicarbazepine acetate therapy, and the current eslicarbazepine serum concentration is high, it may be appropriate to decrease the eslicarbazepine acetate dose. Also, when an effective eslicarbazepine concentration has been established for a patient, the effects of new drug therapy that may cause drug interactions or of new disease states or conditions that can alter eslicarbazepine pharmacokinetics can be assessed prospectively by measuring current eslicarbazepine concentrations before any clinical events occur.

Because a definitive therapeutic range for eslicarbazepine has not be firmly established, and a "start low, go slow" dosage titration strategy has been established for the drug, eslicarbazepine acetate dose increases are made at the rate noted in the initial dosing section. When needed, dosage decreases are usually made using one of the smaller changes possible from available tablet strengths. Thus, pharmacokinetic calculations are usually made to compute the expected steady-state concentration after a specific eslicarbazepine acetate dosage change has been determined rather than computing a new dose based on a desired target concentration. Because eslicarbazepine follows linear pharmacokinetics during eslicarbazepine acetate treatment, the pharmacokinetic calculations involved during dosage titration are straightforward.

When a dosage change in eslicarbazepine acetate is made, sufficient time to attain steady-state conditions (~3-5 half-lives) should be allowed before assessing therapeutic outcome. Of course, any time adverse effects occur during dosage titration, measures should be taken to assess the likelihood that they are due to eslicarbazepine treatment and appropriate action should be taken when needed.

If eslicarbazepine serum concentrations are measured for patients in support of a dosage change, clinicians should seek to use the simplest, most straightforward method available to determine the steady-state concentration for the new regimen. In this case, a simple dosage ratio can be used to change doses since eslicarbazepine follows *linear pharmacokinetics* during eslicarbazepine acetate therapy.

Linear Pharmacokinetics Method

Because eslicarbazepine follows linear, dose-proportional pharmacokinetics, steady-state serum concentrations change in proportion to dose according to the following equation: $D_{new}/C_{ss,new} = D_{old}/C_{ss,old}$ or $C_{ss,new} = (D_{new}/D_{old})C_{ss,old}$, where D is the dose, C_{ss} is the steady-state concentration, old indicates the dose that produced the steady-state concentration that the patient is currently receiving, and new denotes the steady-state concentration produced by the newly prescribed dose. The advantages of this method are that it is quick and simple. The disadvantage is steady-state concentrations are required.

EXAMPLE 8 ▶▶▶

EY is a 51-year-old, 75-kg (height = 5 ft 10 in) male with complex partial seizures who receives therapy with carbamazepine and eslicarbazepine acetate. He has normal liver and renal function. EY was titrated to a dose of eslicarbazepine acetate 800 mg daily without any side effects and a decreased seizure frequency. At that time, a steady-state eslicarbazepine trough concentration was obtained before a dose and equaled 10.2 μg/mL. Several months ago, the patient was started on phenytoin, and he has been on a stable dose for 4 weeks. Today, the steady-state eslicarbazepine trough concentration obtained before the next dose was 7.5 μg/mL. Suggest a new maintenance dosage regimen using immediate-release eslicarbazepine acetate tablets to reestablish the original eslicarbazepine steady-state concentration for this patient.

1. *Use linear pharmacokinetics to compute the new concentration for a reasonable dosage increase.*
   This patient is currently receiving 800 mg/d, so the maximum increase for the first week would be an additional 400 mg/d: $C_{ss,new} = (D_{new}/D_{old})C_{ss,old} = (1200 \text{ mg/d} / 800 \text{ mg/d})7.5 \text{ μg/mL} = 11.3 \text{ μg/mL}$.
   To reestablish the original eslicarbazepine concentration for the patient, a dosage increase of 1200 mg/d or 1200 mg once daily was prescribed. The patient should be carefully monitored for seizure frequency and adverse effects. If desired, steady-state eslicarbazepine serum concentrations can be measured 3-5 half-lives after the dosage change has been made ($\sim t_{1/2} = 15$ hours, $\sim$3-5 $t_{1/2}$ in 2-3 days).

2. *If the desired steady-state eslicarbazepine concentrations have not been attained with the first dosage increase, compute the new concentration for the next reasonable dosage increase. Continue titration until the desired steady-state concentration or optimal therapeutic response has been achieved.*
   The desired steady-state eslicarbazepine concentration has been reached, so this step is not necessary for this patient.

BAYESIAN PHARMACOKINETICS COMPUTER PROGRAMS

Computer programs are available that can assist in the computation of pharmacokinetic parameters for patients. The most reliable computer programs use a nonlinear regression algorithm that incorporates components of Bayes theorem. Nonlinear regression is a statistical technique that uses an iterative process to compute the best pharmacokinetic parameters for a concentration/time data set. Unfortunately, these types of computer programs aren't as useful with eslicarbazepine compared to other antiepileptics due to fixed initial dosage administration algorithms, the slow titration of maintenance doses, and the use of a prodrug as the administered agent. This dosage adjustment approach cannot be recommended for routine clinical use at this time because of these issues.

PROBLEMS

The following problems are intended to emphasize the computation of initial and individualized doses using clinical pharmacokinetic techniques. Clinicians should always consult the patient's chart to confirm that current anticonvulsant therapy is appropriate. Additionally, all other medications that the patient is taking, including prescription and nonprescription drugs, should be noted and checked to ascertain if a potential drug interaction with oxcarbazepine, MHD, or eslicarbazepine exists.

OXCARBAZEPINE

1. YG is a 45-year-old, 67-kg (height = 5 ft 8 in) female with complex partial seizures who requires adjunctive therapy with oxcarbazepine. She has normal liver and renal function and is currently taking phenytoin (steady-state concentration = 18.2 μg/mL). Additional dosage increases have been tried with phenytoin, but they have been unsuccessful due to development of adverse effects. She does not take oral contraceptives. Suggest an initial oxcarbazepine dosage regimen using immediate-release tablets for this patient.

2. RW is a 56-year-old, 69-kg (height = 6 ft) male with simple partial seizures who requires monotherapy with oxcarbazepine. He has renal dysfunction ($CrCl_{est}$ = 25 mL/min), but he has normal liver function. Suggest an initial oxcarbazepine dosage regimen using immediate-release tablets for this patient.

3. FD is a 10-year-old, 35-kg (height = 4 ft 4 in) male with complex partial seizures who requires adjunctive therapy with oxcarbazepine. He has normal liver and renal function and is currently taking phenobarbital (steady-state concentration = 31.1 µg/mL). Additional dosage increases have been tried with phenobarbital, but they have been unsuccessful due to development of adverse effects. Suggest an initial oxcarbazepine dosage regimen using immediate-release tablets for this patient.

4. AL is a 24-year-old, 82-kg (height = 6 ft 1 in) male with complex partial seizures who receives monotherapy with oxcarbazepine. He has normal liver and renal function. AL was titrated to a dose of oxcarbazepine 1800 mg every day without any side effects and a decreased seizure frequency. At that time, a steady-state MHD concentration was obtained before a dose and equaled 25.7 µg/mL. Several months ago, the patient was started on phenytoin, and he has been on a stable dose for 4 weeks. Today, the steady-state MHD concentration obtained before the next oxcarbazepine dose was 17.5 µg/mL. Suggest a new maintenance dosage regimen using extended-release oxcarbazepine tablets to reestablish the original MHD steady-state concentration for this patient.

ESLICARBAZEPINE

5. RX is a 39-year-old, 78-kg (height = 5 ft 8 in) male with complex partial seizures who requires adjunctive therapy with eslicarbazepine acetate. He has normal liver and renal function and is currently taking lamotrigine. Additional dosage increases have been tried with lamotrigine, but they have been unsuccessful due to development of adverse effects. Suggest an initial eslicarbazepine acetate dosage regimen using immediate-release tablets for this patient.

6. JS is a 22-year-old, 87-kg (height = 6 ft 3 in) male with complex partial seizures taking valproic acid (steady-state concentration = 80.2 µg/mL, free fraction = 8%) who requires adjunctive therapy with eslicarbazepine acetate. He has normal liver function, but his $CrCl_{est}$ = 42 mL/min. Suggest an initial eslicarbazepine acetate dosage regimen using immediate-release tablets for this patient.

7. WS is a 24-year-old, 68-kg (height = 5 ft 11 in) male with complex partial seizures who receives therapy with topiramate and eslicarbazepine acetate. He has normal liver and renal function. WS was titrated to a dose of eslicarbazepine acetate 800 mg daily without any side effects and a decreased seizure frequency. At that time, a steady-state eslicarbazepine trough concentration was obtained before a dose and equaled 20.4 µg/mL. Several months ago, the patient was started on carbamazepine, and he has been on a stable dose for 4 weeks. Today, the steady-state eslicarbazepine trough concentration obtained before the next dose was 15.2 µg/mL. Suggest a new maintenance dosage regimen using immediate-release eslicarbazepine acetate tablets to reestablish the original eslicarbazepine steady-state concentration for this patient.

ANSWERS TO PROBLEMS

OXCARBAZEPINE

1. *Answer to problem 1.*

Literature-Based Recommended Dosing

1. *Estimate oxcarbazepine dose according to age, disease states and conditions, dosage form, and concurrent drug therapy.*

For an adult patient taking phenytoin and treated with immediate-release oxcarbazepine tablets, the initial dose is 300-600 mg/d given as a divided dose every 12 hours.

For the first 2 weeks, the initial dose of 150 mg every 12 hours was chosen. Every 1-2 weeks of therapy, the dose can be escalated by an additional 300-600 mg/d to a maximum of 2400-3000 mg/d. The patient should be closely monitored for seizure frequency and adverse drug effects.

The patient was titrated to a dose of oxcarbazepine 1200 mg every 12 hours without any additional side effects and a decreased seizure frequency.

2. *Answer to problem 2.*

Literature-Based Recommended Dosing

1. *Estimate oxcarbazepine dose according to age, disease states and conditions, dosage form, and concurrent drug therapy.*

For an adult patient with normal renal function taking oxcarbazepine monotherapy and treated with immediate-release tablets, the initial dose is 300-600 mg/d given as a divided dose every 12 hours. However, for patients with CrCl <30 mL/min, the maximum starting dose should be reduced to 300 mg/d.

For the first 2 weeks, the initial dose of 150 mg every 12 hours was chosen. Every 1-2 weeks of therapy, the dose can be escalated by an additional 150-300 mg/d to a maximum of 1200-1500 mg/d. The patient should be closely monitored for seizure frequency and adverse drug effects.

The patient was titrated to a dose of oxcarbazepine 600 mg every 12 hours without any additional side effects and a decreased seizure frequency. The measured MHD steady-state trough concentration at that time was 17.3 µg/mL.

3. *Answer to problem 3.*

Literature-Based Recommended Dosing

1. *Estimate oxcarbazepine dose according to age, disease states and conditions, dosage form, and concurrent drug therapy.*

For a pediatric patient taking oxcarbazepine as adjunctive therapy using oral suspension, the initial dose is 8-10 mg/kg/d given as two divided doses every 12 hours.

For the first 2 weeks, the initial dose of 150 mg every 12 hours was chosen (35 kg • 9 mg/kg/d = 315 mg, rounded to 300 mg/d). Every 1-2 weeks of therapy, the dose can be escalated by an additional 150-300 mg/d to a target dose of 1200 mg/d. The patient should be closely monitored for seizure frequency and adverse drug effects.

The patient was titrated to a dose of oxcarbazepine 600 mg every 12 hours without any side effects and a decreased seizure frequency. Within 6 months, he was switched to oxcarbazepine tablets 600 mg every 12 hours when he could swallow whole tablets without any distress. Therapeutic response remained constant after the dosage form switch, with no change in seizure frequency or adverse effects.

4. *Answer to problem 4.*

Linear Pharmacokinetics Method

1. *Use linear pharmacokinetics to compute the new concentration for a reasonable dosage increase.*

Dosage increases for oxcarbazepine are usually made in increments of no more than 300-600 mg/d every 1-2 weeks. This patient is currently receiving 1800 mg/d, so the maximum increase for the first week would be 600 mg/d: $C_{ss,new} = (D_{new}/D_{old})C_{ss,old} = (2400 \text{ mg/d} / 1800 \text{ mg/d})17.5 \text{ µg/mL} = 23.3 \text{ µg/mL}$.

To reestablish the original MHD concentration for the patient, a dosage increase of 2400 mg daily was prescribed. The patient should be carefully monitored for seizure frequency and adverse effects. If desired, steady-state MHD serum concentrations can be measured 3-5 half-lives after the dosage change has been made ($\sim t_{1/2}$ = 15 hours, $\sim$3-5 $t_{1/2}$ in 2-3 days).

2. *If the desired steady-state MHD concentrations have not been attained with the first dosage increase, compute the new concentration for the next reasonable dosage increase. Continue titration until the desired steady-state concentration or optimal therapeutic response has been achieved.*

The desired steady-state MHD concentration has been reached, so this step is not necessary for this patient.

Eslicarbazepine

5. *Answer to problem 5.*

Literature-Based Recommended Dosing

1. *Estimate eslicarbazepine acetate dose according to age, disease states and conditions, dosage form, and concurrent drug therapy.*

For an adult patient taking lamotrigine and treated with immediate-release eslicarbazepine acetate tablets, the initial dose is 400 mg/d given as a single daily dose. The patient was closely monitored for seizure frequency and adverse drug effects. Serum concentrations of lamotrigine were measured during the first week of therapy, and no lamotrigine dosage adjustment was necessary.

After the first 2 weeks of treatment, the eslicarbazepine acetate dose was increased to 800 mg daily with continued monitoring.

6. *Answer to problem 6.*

Literature-Based Recommended Dosing

1. *Estimate eslicarbazepine acetate dose according to age, disease states and conditions, dosage form, and concurrent drug therapy.*

For an adult patient with renal dysfunction taking valproic acid and treated with immediate-release eslicarbazepine acetate tablets, the initial dose is 200 mg/d given as a single daily dose. The patient was closely monitored for seizure frequency and adverse drug effects. Serum concentrations of valproic acid were measured during the first week of therapy, and a valproic acid dosage adjustment was not needed.

After the first 2 weeks of treatment, an eslicarbazepine steady-state trough concentration was 7.7 µg/mL, and the eslicarbazepine acetate dose was increased to 400 mg daily with continued monitoring.

7. *Answer to problem 7.*

Linear Pharmacokinetics Method

1. *Use linear pharmacokinetics to compute the new concentration for a reasonable dosage increase.*

This patient is currently receiving 800 mg/d, so the maximum increase for the first week would be an additional 400 mg/d: $C_{ss,new} = (D_{new}/D_{old})C_{ss,old}$ = (1200 mg/d / 800 mg/d)15.2 µg/mL = 22.8 µg/mL.

To reestablish the original eslicarbazepine concentration for the patient, a dosage increase of 1200 mg/d or 1200 mg once daily was prescribed. The patient should be carefully monitored for seizure frequency and adverse effects. If desired, steady-state eslicarbazepine serum concentrations can be measured 3-5 half-lives after the dosage change has been made ($\sim t_{1/2} = 15$ hours, $\sim$3-5 $t_{1/2}$ in 2-3 days).

2. *If the desired steady-state eslicarbazepine concentrations have not been attained with the first dosage increase, compute the new concentration for the next reasonable dosage increase. Continue titration until desired steady-state concentration or optimal therapeutic response has been achieved.*

The desired steady-state eslicarbazepine concentration has been reached, so this step is not necessary for this patient.

REFERENCES

1. Abramowicz M, Zuccotti G, Pflomm JM, eds. Drugs for epilepsy. *Treatment Guidelines From The Medical Letter.* 2013;11(126):9-18.
2. Anon. The epilepsies: the diagnosis and management of the epilepsies in adults and children in primary and secondary care. *UK National Institute for Health and Care Excellence.* Available at: http://www.nice.org.uk/nicemedia/live/13635/57779/57779.pdf. Accessed May 5, 2014.
3. French JA, Kanner AM, Bautista J, et al. Efficacy and tolerability of the new antiepileptic drugs I: treatment of new onset epilepsy: report of the Therapeutics and Technology Assessment Subcommittee and Quality Standards Subcommittee of the American Academy of Neurology and the American Epilepsy Society. *Neurology.* Apr 27, 2004;62(8):1252-1260.
4. Glauser T, Ben-Menachem E, Bourgeois B, et al. Updated ILAE evidence review of antiepileptic drug efficacy and effectiveness as initial monotherapy for epileptic seizures and syndromes. *Epilepsia.* Mar 2013;54(3):551-563.
5. McNamara JO. Pharmacotherapy of the epilepsies. In: Brunton L, Chabner B, Knollman B, eds. *The Pharmacological Basis of Therapeutics.* 12th ed. New York, NY: McGraw-Hill; 2011:583-608.
6. Abramowicz M, Zuccotti G, Pflomm JM, eds. Drugs for depression and bipolar disorder. *Treatment Guidelines From The Medical Letter.* 2010;8(93):35-42.
7. Baumann TJ, Strickland JM, Herndon CM. Pain management. In: DiPiro JT, Talbert RL, Yee GC, Matzke GR, Wells BG, Posey LM, eds. *Pharmacotherapy.* 8th ed. New York, NY: McGraw-Hill; 2011:1045-1059.
8. Drayton SJ. Bipolar disorders. In: DiPiro JT, Talbert RL, Yee GC, Matzke GR, Wells BG, Posey LM, eds. *Pharmacotherapy.* 8th ed. New York, NY: McGraw-Hill; 2011:1191-1208.
9. Glauser TA, Cnaan A, Shinnar S, et al. Ethosuximide, valproic acid, and lamotrigine in childhood absence epilepsy: initial monotherapy outcomes at 12 months. *Epilepsia.* Jan 2013;54(1):141-155.
10. Glauser TA, Cnaan A, Shinnar S, et al. Ethosuximide, valproic acid, and lamotrigine in childhood absence epilepsy. *N Engl J Med.* Mar 4, 2010;362(9):790-799.
11. Rogers SJ, Cavazos JE. Epilepsy. In: DiPiro JT, Talbert RL, Yee GC, Matzke GR, Wells BG, Posey LM, eds. *Pharmacotherapy.* 8th ed. New York, NY: McGraw-Hill; 2011:979-1005.
12. Italiano D, Perucca E. Clinical pharmacokinetics of new-generation antiepileptic drugs at the extremes of age: an update. *Clin Pharmacokinet.* May 3, 2013.
13. Johannessen SI, Tomson T. Pharmacokinetic variability of newer antiepileptic drugs: when is monitoring needed? *Clin Pharmacokinet.* 2006;45(11):1061-1075.
14. Perucca E. Is there a role for therapeutic drug monitoring of new anticonvulsants? *Clin Pharmacokinet.* Mar 2000;38(3):191-204.
15. Volosov A, Xiaodong S, Perucca E, Yagen B, Sintov A, Bialer M. Enantioselective pharmacokinetics of 10-hydroxycarbazepine after oral administration of oxcarbazepine to healthy Chinese subjects. *Clin Pharmacol Ther.* Dec 1999;66(6):547-553.
16. Flesch G, Francotte E, Hell F, Degen PH. Determination of the R-(−) and S-(+) enantiomers of the monohydroxylated metabolite of oxcarbazepine in human plasma by enantioselective high-performance liquid chromatography. *J Chromatogr.* Oct 2, 1992;581(1):147-151.
17. Flesch G, Czendlik C, Renard D, Lloyd P. Pharmacokinetics of the monohydroxy derivative of oxcarbazepine and its enantiomers after a single intravenous dose given as racemate compared with a single oral dose of oxcarbazepine. *Drug Metab Dispos.* Jun 2011;39(6):1103-1110.
18. Schutz H, Feldmann KF, Faigle JW, Kriemler HP, Winkler T. The metabolism of 14C-oxcarbazepine in man. *Xenobiotica.* Aug 1986;16(8):769-778.
19. May TW, Korn-Merker E, Rambeck B. Clinical pharmacokinetics of oxcarbazepine. *Clin Pharmacokinet.* 2003;42(12):1023-1042.

20. Holtmann M, Krause M, Opp J, Tokarzewski M, Korn-Merker E, Boenigk HE. Oxcarbazepine-induced hyponatremia and the regulation of serum sodium after replacing carbamazepine with oxcarbazepine in children. *Neuropediatrics.* Dec 2002;33(6):298-300.

21. Isojarvi JI, Huuskonen UE, Pakarinen AJ, Vuolteenaho O, Myllyla VV. The regulation of serum sodium after replacing carbamazepine with oxcarbazepine. *Epilepsia.* Jun 2001;42(6):741-745.

22. Sachdeo RC, Wasserstein A, Mesenbrink PJ, D'Souza J. Effects of oxcarbazepine on sodium concentration and water handling. *Ann Neurol.* May 2002;51(5):613-620.

23. Novartis Pharmaceuticals Corporation [package insert]. Trileptal prescribing information; 2011.

24. McKee PJ, Blacklaw J, Forrest G, et al. A double-blind, placebo-controlled interaction study between oxcarbazepine and carbamazepine, sodium valproate and phenytoin in epileptic patients. *Br J Clin Pharmacol.* Jan 1994;37(1):27-32.

25. Dickinson RG, Hooper WD, Dunstan PR, Eadie MJ. First dose and steady-state pharmacokinetics of oxcarbazepine and its 10-hydroxy metabolite. *Eur J Clin Pharmacol.* 1989;37(1):69-74.

26. Jung H, Noguez A, Mayet L, Fuentes I, Gonzalez-Esquivel DF. The distribution of 10-hydroxy carbazepine in blood compartments. *Biopharm Drug Dispos.* Jan 1997;18(1):17-23.

27. Fortuna A, Alves G, Falcao A, Soares-da-Silva P. Evaluation of the permeability and P-glycoprotein efflux of carbamazepine and several derivatives across mouse small intestine by the Ussing chamber technique. *Epilepsia.* Mar 2012;53(3):529-538.

28. Tartara A, Galimberti CA, Manni R, et al. The pharmacokinetics of oxcarbazepine and its active metabolite 10-hydroxy-carbazepine in healthy subjects and in epileptic patients treated with phenobarbitone or valproic acid. *Br J Clin Pharmacol.* Oct 1993;36(4):366-368.

29. Keranen T, Jolkkonen J, Jensen PK, Menge GP, Andersson P. Absence of interaction between oxcarbazepine and erythromycin. *Acta Neurol Scand.* Aug 1992;86(2):120-123.

30. Keranen T, Jolkkonen J, Klosterskov-Jensen P, Menge GP. Oxcarbazepine does not interact with cimetidine in healthy volunteers. *Acta Neurol Scand.* Apr 1992;85(4):239-242.

31. Hulsman JA, Rentmeester TW, Banfield CR, et al. Effects of felbamate on the pharmacokinetics of the monohydroxy and dihydroxy metabolites of oxcarbazepine. *Clin Pharmacol Ther.* Oct 1995;58(4):383-389.

32. Theis JG, Sidhu J, Palmer J, Job S, Bullman J, Ascher J. Lack of pharmacokinetic interaction between oxcarbazepine and lamotrigine. *Neuropsychopharmacology.* Dec 2005;30(12):2269-2274.

33. Leppik IE, Hovinga CA. Extended-release antiepileptic drugs: a comparison of pharmacokinetic parameters relative to original immediate-release formulations. *Epilepsia.* Jan 2013;54(1):28-35.

34. Supernus Pharmaceuticals, Inc. [package insert]. Oxtellar XR prescribing information; 2013.

35. van der Kuy PH, Koppejan EH, Wirtz JJ. Rectal absorption of oxcarbazepine. *Pharm World Sci.* Aug 2000;22(4):165-166.

36. Clemens PL, Cloyd JC, Kriel RL, Remmel RP. Relative bioavailability, metabolism and tolerability of rectally administered oxcarbazepine suspension. *Clin Drug Investig.* 2007;27(4):243-250.

37. Van Parys JA, Hop W, Vulto A, Edelbroek P. Steady-state pharmacokinetics of oxcarbazepine in adults. *Epilepsia.* 1998;39(suppl 6):47.

38. Viola MS, Bercellini MA, Saidon P, Rubio MC. Pharmacokinetic variability of oxcarbazepine in epileptic patients. *Medicina (B Aires).* 2000;60(6):914-918.

39. Patsalos PN, Elyas AA, Zakrzewska JM. Protein binding of oxcarbazepine and its primary active metabolite, 10-hydroxycarbazepine, in patients with trigeminal neuralgia. *Eur J Clin Pharmacol.* 1990;39(4):413-415.

40. Klitgaard NA, Kristensen O. Use of saliva for monitoring oxcarbazepine therapy in epileptic patients. *Eur J Clin Pharmacol.* 1986;31(1):91-94.

41. May TW, Rambeck B, Salke-Kellermann A. Fluctuations of 10-hydroxy-carbazepine during the day in epileptic patients. *Acta Neurol Scand.* Jun 1996;93(6):393-397.

42. Gonzalez-Esquivel DF, Ortega-Gavilan M, Alcantara-Lopez G, Jung-Cook H. Plasma level monitoring of oxcarbazepine in epileptic patients. *Arch Med Res.* Mar-Apr 2000;31(2):202-205.

43. Myllynen P, Pienimaki P, Jouppila P, Vahakangas K. Transplacental passage of oxcarbazepine and its metabolites in vivo. *Epilepsia.* Nov 2001;42(11):1482-1485.

44. Pienimaki P, Lampela E, Hakkola J, Arvela P, Raunio H, Vahakangas K. Pharmacokinetics of oxcarbazepine and carbamazepine in human placenta. *Epilepsia.* Mar 1997;38(3):309-316.

45. Bulau P, Paar WD, von Unruh GE. Pharmacokinetics of oxcarbazepine and 10-hydroxy-carbazepine in the newborn child of an oxcarbazepine-treated mother. *Eur J Clin Pharmacol.* 1988;34(3):311-313.

46. Theisohn M, Heimann G. Disposition of the antiepileptic oxcarbazepine and its metabolites in healthy volunteers. *Eur J Clin Pharmacol.* 1982;22(6):545-551.

47. Christensen J, Hojskov CS, Dam M, Poulsen JH. Plasma concentration of topiramate correlates with cerebrospinal fluid concentration. *Ther Drug Monit.* Oct 2001;23(5):529-535.

48. Christensen J, Balslev T, Villadsen J, Heinsvig EM, Dam M, Poulsen JH. Removal of 10-hydroxycarbazepine by plasmapheresis. *Ther Drug Monit.* Aug 2001;23(4):374-379.

49. Keranen T, Sorri A, Moilanen E, Ylitalo P. Effects of charcoal on the absorption and elimination of the antiepileptic drugs lamotrigine and oxcarbazepine. *Arzneimittelforschung.* 2010;60(7):421-426.

50. Rouan MC, Lecaillon JB, Godbillon J, et al. The effect of renal impairment on the pharmacokinetics of oxcarbazepine and its metabolites. *Eur J Clin Pharmacol.* 1994;47(2):161-167.

51. Glauser TA. Oxcarbazepine in the treatment of epilepsy. *Pharmacotherapy.* Aug 2001;21(8):904-919.

52. Pugh RN, Murray-Lyon IM, Dawson JL, Pietroni MC, Williams R. Transection of the oesophagus for bleeding oesophageal varices. *Br J Surg.* 1973;60(8):646-649.

53. Pariente-Khayat A, Fran A, Vauzelle-Kervroedan F, et al. Pharmacokinetics of oxcarbazepine as add-on therapy in children. *Epilepsia.* 1994;35 (suppl 8):119.

54. Rey E, Bulteau C, Motte J, et al. Oxcarbazepine pharmacokinetics and tolerability in children with inadequately controlled epilepsy. *J Clin Pharmacol.* Nov 2004;44(11):1290-1300.

55. Sallas WM, Milosavljev S, D'Souza J, Hossain M. Pharmacokinetic drug interactions in children taking oxcarbazepine. *Clin Pharmacol Ther.* Aug 2003;74(2):138-149.

56. Northam RS, Hernandez AW, Litzinger MJ, et al. Oxcarbazepine in infants and young children with partial seizures. *Pediatr Neurol.* Nov 2005;33(5):337-344.

57. van Heiningen PN, Eve MD, Oosterhuis B, et al. The influence of age on the pharmacokinetics of the antiepileptic agent oxcarbazepine. *Clin Pharmacol Ther.* Oct 1991;50(4):410-419.

58. Johannessen Landmark C, Baftiu A, Tysse I, et al. Pharmacokinetic variability of four newer antiepileptic drugs, lamotrigine, levetiracetam, oxcarbazepine, and topiramate: a comparison of the impact of age and comedication. *Ther Drug Monit.* Aug 2012;34(4):440-445.

59. Larkin JG, McKee PJ, Forrest G, et al. Lack of enzyme induction with oxcarbazepine (600 mg daily) in healthy subjects. *Br J Clin Pharmacol.* Jan 1991;31(1):65-71.

60. Patsalos PN, Zakrzewska JM, Elyas AA. Dose dependent enzyme induction by oxcarbazepine? *Eur J Clin Pharmacol.* 1990;39(2):187-188.

61. Andreasen AH, Brosen K, Damkier P. A comparative pharmacokinetic study in healthy volunteers of the effect of carbamazepine and oxcarbazepine on cyp3a4. *Epilepsia.* Mar 2007;48(3):490-496.

62. May TW, Boor R, Rambeck B, Jurgens U, Korn-Merker E, Brandt C. Serum concentrations of rufinamide in children and adults with epilepsy: the influence of dose, age, and comedication. *Ther Drug Monit.* Apr 2011;33(2):214-221.

63. May TW, Rambeck B, Jurgens U. Serum concentrations of Levetiracetam in epileptic patients: the influence of dose and co-medication. *Ther Drug Monit.* Dec 2003;25(6):690-699.

64. May TW, Rambeck B, Neb R, Jurgens U. Serum concentrations of pregabalin in patients with epilepsy: the influence of dose, age, and comedication. *Ther Drug Monit.* Dec 2007;29(6):789-794.

65. May TW, Rambeck B, Jurgens U. Serum concentrations of topiramate in patients with epilepsy: influence of dose, age, and comedication. *Ther Drug Monit.* Jun 2002;24(3):366-374.

66. May TW, Rambeck B, Jurgens U. Influence of oxcarbazepine and methsuximide on lamotrigine concentrations in epileptic patients with and without valproic acid comedication: results of a retrospective study. *Ther Drug Monit.* Apr 1999;21(2):175-181.

67. Fattore C, Cipolla G, Gatti G, et al. Induction of ethinylestradiol and levonorgestrel metabolism by oxcarbazepine in healthy women. *Epilepsia.* Jun 1999;40(6):783-787.

68. Lakehal F, Wurden CJ, Kalhorn TF, Levy RH. Carbamazepine and oxcarbazepine decrease phenytoin metabolism through inhibition of CYP2C19. *Epilepsy Res.* Dec 2002;52(2):79-83.

69. Schmidt D, Arroyo S, Baulac M, et al. Recommendations on the clinical use of oxcarbazepine in the treatment of epilepsy: a consensus view. *Acta Neurol Scand.* Sep 2001;104(3):167-170.

70. Tschudy MM, Arcara KM. *The Harriet Lane Handbook: A Manual for Pediatric House Officers.* 19th ed. Philadelphia, PA: Mosby; 2012.

71. Almeida L, Soares-da-Silva P. Safety, tolerability and pharmacokinetic profile of BIA 2-093, a novel putative antiepileptic agent, during first administration to humans. *Drugs R D.* 2003;4(5):269-284.

72. Almeida L, Soares-da-Silva P. Safety, tolerability, and pharmacokinetic profile of BIA 2-093, a novel putative antiepileptic, in a rising multiple-dose study in young healthy humans. *J Clin Pharmacol.* Aug 2004;44(8):906-918.

73. Almeida L, Falcao A, Maia J, Mazur D, Gellert M, Soares-da-Silva P. Single-dose and steady-state pharmacokinetics of eslicarbazepine acetate (BIA 2-093) in healthy elderly and young subjects. *J Clin Pharmacol.* Sep 2005;45(9):1062-1066.

74. Falcao A, Maia J, Almeida L, Mazur D, Gellert M, Soares-da-Silva P. Effect of gender on the pharmacokinetics of eslicarbazepine acetate (BIA 2-093), a new voltage-gated sodium channel blocker. *Biopharm Drug Dispos.* Jul 2007;28(5):249-256.

75. Fontes-Ribeiro C, Nunes T, Falcao A, et al. Eslicarbazepine acetate (BIA 2-093): relative bioavailability and bioequivalence of 50 mg/mL oral suspension and 200 mg and 800 mg tablet formulations. *Drugs R D.* 2005;6(5):253-260.

76. Hainzl D, Parada A, Soares-da-Silva P. Metabolism of two new antiepileptic drugs and their principal metabolites S(+)- and R(−)-10,11-dihydro-10-hydroxy carbamazepine. *Epilepsy Res.* May 2001;44(2-3):197-206.

77. Maia J, Vaz-da-Silva M, Almeida L, et al. Effect of food on the pharmacokinetic profile of eslicarbazepine acetate (BIA 2-093). *Drugs R D*. 2005;6(4):201-206.
78. Falcao A, Fuseau E, Nunes T, Almeida L, Soares-da-Silva P. Pharmacokinetics, drug interactions and exposure-response relationship of eslicarbazepine acetate in adult patients with partial-onset seizures: population pharmacokinetic and pharmacokinetic/pharmacodynamic analyses. *CNS Drugs*. Jan 1, 2012;26(1):79-91.
79. BIAL-Portela & Ca, S.A. [package insert]. Zebinix prescribing information; 2009.
80. Loureiro AI, Fernandes-Lopes C, Bonifacio MJ, Wright LC, Soares-da-Silva P. Hepatic UDP-glucuronosyltransferase is responsible for eslicarbazepine glucuronidation. *Drug Metab Dispos*. Sep 2011;39(9):1486-1494.
81. Nunes T, Sicard E, Almeida L, et al. Pharmacokinetic interaction study between eslicarbazepine acetate and topiramate in healthy subjects. *Curr Med Res Opin*. Jun 2010;26(6):1355-1362.
82. Almeida L, Nunes T, Sicard E, et al. Pharmacokinetic interaction study between eslicarbazepine acetate and lamotrigine in healthy subjects. *Acta Neurol Scand*. Apr 2010;121(4):257-264.
83. Almeida L, Minciu I, Nunes T, et al. Pharmacokinetics, efficacy, and tolerability of eslicarbazepine acetate in children and adolescents with epilepsy. *J Clin Pharmacol*. Aug 2008;48(8):966-977.
84. Perucca E, Elger C, Halasz P, Falcao A, Almeida L, Soares-da-Silva P. Pharmacokinetics of eslicarbazepine acetate at steady-state in adults with partial-onset seizures. *Epilepsy Res*. Sep 2011;96(1-2):132-139.
85. Fortuna A, Alves G, Falcao A, Soares-da-Silva P. Binding of licarbazepine enantiomers to mouse and human plasma proteins. *Biopharm Drug Dispos*. Jul 2010;31(5-6):362-366.
86. Vaz-da-Silva M, Almeida L, Falcao A, et al. Effect of eslicarbazepine acetate on the steady-state pharmacokinetics and pharmacodynamics of warfarin in healthy subjects during a three-stage, open-label, multiple-dose, single-period study. *Clin Ther*. Jan 2010;32(1):179-192.
87. Nunes T, Rocha JF, Falcao A, Almeida L, Soares-da-Silva P. Steady-state plasma and cerebrospinal fluid pharmacokinetics and tolerability of eslicarbazepine acetate and oxcarbazepine in healthy volunteers. *Epilepsia*. Jan 2013;54(1):108-116.
88. Maia J, Almeida L, Falcao A, et al. Effect of renal impairment on the pharmacokinetics of eslicarbazepine acetate. *Int J Clin Pharmacol Ther*. Mar 2008;46(3):119-130.
89. Almeida L, Potgieter JH, Maia J, Potgieter MA, Mota F, Soares-da-Silva P. Pharmacokinetics of eslicarbazepine acetate in patients with moderate hepatic impairment. *Eur J Clin Pharmacol*. Mar 2008;64(3):267-273.
90. Anon. *CHMP Assessment Report for Zebinix*. London: European Medicines Agency; 2009.
91. Falcao A, Vaz-da-Silva M, Gama H, Nunes T, Almeida L, Soares-da-Silva P. Effect of eslicarbazepine acetate on the pharmacokinetics of a combined ethinylestradiol/levonorgestrel oral contraceptive in healthy women. *Epilepsy Res*. 2013 Aug;105(3):368-76 [Epub Apr 6, 2013].
92. Vaz da Silva M, Costa R, Soares E, et al. Effect of eslicarbazepine acetate on the pharmacokinetics of digoxin in healthy subjects. *Fundam Clin Pharmacol*. Aug 2009;23(4):509-514.
93. Rocha JF, Vaz-da-Silva M, Almeida L, et al. Effect of eslicarbazepine acetate on the pharmacokinetics of metformin in healthy subjects. *Int J Clin Pharmacol Ther*. Apr 2009;47(4):255-261.
94. Rauchenzauner M, Luef G. Eslicarbazepine acetate for partial-onset seizures. *Expert Rev Neurother*. Dec 2011;11(12):1673-1681.
95. Patsalos PN, Berry DJ. Pharmacotherapy of the third-generation AEDs: lacosamide, retigabine and eslicarbazepine acetate. *Expert Opin Pharmacother*. Apr 2012;13(5):699-715.

V IMMUNOSUPPRESSANTS

18 Cyclosporine

INTRODUCTION

Cyclosporine is a cyclic polypeptide calcineurin inhibitor with immunosuppressant properties that is used for the prevention of graft-versus-host disease in hematopoietic stem cell transplantation patients, for the prevention of graft rejection in solid organ transplant patients, and for the treatment of psoriasis, rheumatoid arthritis, and a variety of other autoimmune diseases.[1-3] The immunomodulating properties of cyclosporine are due to its ability to block the production of interleukin-2 and other cytokines secreted by T lymphocytes.[1-3] Cyclosporine binds to cyclophilin, an intracellular cytoplasmic protein found in T cells. The cyclosporine-cyclophilin complex interacts with calcineurin, inhibits the catalytic activity of calcineurin, and prevents the production of intermediaries involved with the expression of genes regulating the production of cytokines.

THERAPEUTIC AND TOXIC CONCENTRATIONS

The therapeutic range of cyclosporine used by clinicians varies greatly according to the type of assay used to measure cyclosporine and whether blood or serum concentrations are determined by the clinical laboratory (Table 18-1).[1,3-5] Because cyclosporine is bound to red blood cells, blood concentrations are higher that simultaneously measured serum or plasma concentrations. High-pressure liquid chromatography (HPLC) assay techniques are specific for cyclosporine measurement in blood, serum, or plasma. However, older polyclonal immunoassays are nonspecific and measure both cyclosporine and its metabolites. Newer monoclonal immunoassays (various) are now available that are relatively specific for cyclosporine and produce results similar to the HPLC assay. As a result, cyclosporine concentrations measured simultaneously in a patient using the specific high pressure liquid chromatography technique or one of the specific immunoassays will be lower than that determined using a nonspecific immunoassay. Since cyclosporine metabolites are excreted in the bile,

TABLE 18-1 Cyclosporine Therapeutic Concentrations for Different Assay Techniques and Biologic Fluids

Assay	Biologic Fluid	Therapeutic Concentrations (ng/mL)
High-pressure liquid chromatography (HPLC), monoclonal immunoassay	Blood	100-400
High-pressure liquid chromatography (HPLC), monoclonal immunoassay	Plasma	50-150
Polyclonal immunoassay	Blood	200-800
Polyclonal immunoassay	Plasma	100-400

liver transplant patients who are immediately posttransplant surgery can have very high cyclosporine metabolite concentrations in the blood, serum, and plasma because bile production has not begun yet in the newly transplanted organ. If nonspecific immunoassays are used to measure cyclosporine concentrations in liver transplant patients immediately after surgery before the graft has begun to produce bile, the predominate species measured with this assay methodology may be cyclosporine metabolites and not cyclosporine. One reason some laboratories favor the use of immunoassays for the measurement of cyclosporine concentrations, even though they are less specific for the parent compound, is that it takes less time to conduct the technique so that cyclosporine concentrations can be returned to clinicians more rapidly. For the purposes of the pharmacokinetic calculations and problems presented in this book, cyclosporine concentrations in the blood using the cyclosporine-specific high-pressure liquid chromatograph assay results will be used.

Desired cyclosporine concentrations differ between the various types of transplants, change with time during the posttransplantation phase, and are often determined by protocols specific to the transplantation service and institution.[1,3,4,6-10] Thus, it is especially important for clinicians to be aware of these various factors, as acceptable cyclosporine concentrations under these different circumstances may be different than those listed by their clinical laboratory or those given in this text.

For patients receiving cyclosporine after a hematopoietic stem cell transplantation, the goal of therapy is to prevent graft-versus-host disease while avoiding adverse effects of immunosuppressant therapy.[3,10] Graft-versus-host disease is a result of donor T-lymphocytes detecting antigens on host tissues and producing an immunologic response against these antigens and host tissues. Acute graft-versus-host disease usually occurs within the first 100 days after transplantation of donor cells, and causes epithelial tissue damage in organs. The most common tissues attacked are skin, gastrointestinal tract, and liver. To prevent acute graft-versus-host disease from occurring in allogenic hematopoietic stem cell transplantation patients with HLA-matched donors, cyclosporine therapy is usually instituted a few days before or on the day of stem cell transplant (day 0), and doses are adjusted to provide therapeutic trough concentrations. Methotrexate or glucocorticoids are usually also given in conjunction with cyclosporine treatment to hematopoietic stem cell transplantation patients. If prophylaxis of acute graft-versus-host disease is successful, cyclosporine doses start to be tapered between posttransplant day 50 and 100, with the goal of drug discontinuation by about posttransplant day 180. For allogeneic hematopoietic stem cell transplantation patients with HLA-mismatched or HLA-matched unrelated donors, the risk of acute graft-versus-host disease is higher, so cyclosporine therapy may be more prolonged for these patients. After posttransplantation day 100, chronic graft-versus-host disease may occur, and severe cases or patients with systemic signs and symptoms of the disease are usually treated with prednisone.

For patients receiving solid organ transplants such as kidney, liver, heart, lung, or heart-lung transplantation, the goal of cyclosporine therapy is to prevent acute or chronic rejection of the transplanted organ while minimizing drug side effects.[1,6-9] In this case, the recipient's immune system detects foreign antigens on the donor organ which produces an immunologic response against the graft. This leads to inflammatory and cytotoxic effects directed against the transplanted tissue, and produces the risk of organ tissue damage and failure. In the case of a rejected kidney transplant, it is possible to remove the graft and place the patient on a form of dialysis to sustain their life. However, for other solid organ transplantation patients, graft rejection can result in death. Because cyclosporine can cause nephrotoxicity, some centers delay cyclosporine therapy in renal transplant patients for a few days or until the kidney begins functioning to avoid untoward effects on the newly transplanted organ. Also, desired cyclosporine concentrations in renal transplant patients are generally lower to avoid toxicity in the new renal graft than for other transplant patients (typically 100-200 ng/mL versus 150-300 ng/mL using whole blood with a specific, high-pressure liquid chromatograph assay). For other solid organ transplant patients, cyclosporine therapy may be started several hours before surgery or, for patients with poor kidney function, held until after transplantation to avoid nephrotoxicity. During the immediate postoperative phase, intravenous cyclosporine may be given to these patients. For long-term management of immunosuppression in solid organ tissue transplant patients, cyclosporine doses are gradually tapered to the lowest concentration and dose possible over a 6- to 12-month time period as long as rejection episodes do not occur. In some cases, it may be possible to completely discontinue cyclosporine therapy.

Hypertension, nephrotoxicity, hyperlipidemia, tremor, hirsutism, and gingival hyperplasia are all typical adverse effects of cyclosporine treatment.[1-4] Hypertension is the most common side effect associated with cyclosporine therapy, and is treated with traditional antihypertensive drug therapy. Nephrotoxicity is separated into acute and chronic varieties. Acute nephrotoxicity is concentration- or dose-dependent and reverses with a dosage decrease. Renal damage in this situation is thought to be due to renal vasoconstriction, which results in increased renal vascular resistance, decreased renal blood flow, and reduced glomerular filtration rate. Chronic nephrotoxicity is accompanied by kidney tissue damage, including interstitial fibrosis, nonspecific tubular vacuolization, and structural changes in arteries, arterioles, and proximal tubular epithelium. Increased serum creatinine and blood urea nitrogen (BUN) values, hyperkalemia, hyperuricemia, proteinuria, and increased renal sodium excretion occur with cyclosporine-induced nephrotoxicity. The clinical features of cyclosporine nephrotoxicity and acute graft rejection in renal transplant patients are similar, so renal biopsies may be conducted to differentiate between these possibilities.[1] Because biopsy findings are similar between cyclosporine-induced nephrotoxicity and chronic rejection of kidney transplants, this technique is of less help in this situation. Hyperlipidemia is treated using dietary counseling and antilipid drug therapy. Cyclosporine dosage decreases may be necessary to decrease tremor associated with drug therapy while hirsutism is usually addressed using patient counseling. Gingival hyperplasia can be minimized through the use of appropriate and regular dental hygiene and care.

CLINICAL MONITORING PARAMETERS

Hematopoietic stem cell transplantation patients should be monitored for the signs and symptoms associated with graft-versus-host disease.[3] These include a generalized maculopapular skin rash, diarrhea, abdominal pain, ileus, hyperbilirubinemia, and increased liver function tests (alkaline phosphatase and serum transaminases). Patients with severe chronic graft-versus-host disease may have involvement of the skin, liver, eyes, mouth, esophagus, or other organs similar to what might be seen with systemic autoimmune diseases.

Solid organ transplant patients should be monitored for graft rejection consistent with the transplanted organ. For renal transplant patients, increased serum creatinine, azotemia, hypertension, edema, weight gain secondary to fluid retention, graft tenderness, fever, and malaise may be due to an acute rejection episode. Hypertension, proteinuria, a continuous decline in renal function (increases in serum creatinine and blood urea nitrogen levels), and uremia are indicative of chronic rejection in renal transplant patients.[1,6] For hepatic transplant patients, acute rejection signs and symptoms include fever, lethargy, graft tenderness, increased white blood cell count, change in bile color or amount, hyperbilirubinemia, and increased liver function tests. Chronic rejection in a liver transplant patient may be accompanied only by increased liver function tests and jaundice.[1,7] For heart transplant patients, acute rejection is accompanied by low-grade fever, malaise, heart failure (presence of S_3 heart sound), or atrial arrhythmia. Chronic rejection in heart transplant patients, also known as cardiac allograft vasculopathy, is characterized by accelerated coronary artery atherosclerosis and may include the following symptoms: arrhythmias, decreased left ventricular function, heart failure, myocardial infarction, and sudden cardiac death.[1,9] For lung transplant patients, acute rejection may result in no or nonspecific symptoms (cough, dyspnea, hypoxemia, low-grade fever, inspiratory crackles, interstitial infiltrates, declining lung function). Chronic rejection in lung transplant patients, also called bronchiolitis obliterans syndrome, is characterized by decreased airflow and can resemble acute bronchitis.[8] For all solid organ transplant patients, tissue biopsies may be taken from the transplanted tissue to confirm the diagnosis of organ rejection.[1,6-9]

Typical adverse effects of cyclosporine treatment include hypertension, nephrotoxicity, hyperlipidemia, tremor, hirsutism, and gingival hyperplasia.[1-4] The management of these more common drug side effects are discussed in the previous section. Other cyclosporine adverse drug reactions that occur less frequently include gastrointestinal side effects (nausea, vomiting, diarrhea), headache, hepatotoxicity, hyperglycemia, acne, leukopenia, hyperkalemia, and hypomagnesemia.

Because of the pivotal role that cyclosporine plays as an immunosuppressant in transplant patients, as well as the severity of its concentration- and dose-dependent side effects, cyclosporine concentrations should be measured in every patient receiving the drug. If a patient experiences signs or symptoms of graft-versus-host disease or organ rejection, a cyclosporine concentration should be checked to ensure that levels have not fallen below the therapeutic range. If a patient encounters a possible clinical problem that could be an adverse drug effect of cyclosporine therapy, a cyclosporine concentration should be measured to determine if levels are in the toxic range. During the immediate posttransplantation phase, cyclosporine concentrations are measured daily in most patients even though steady-state may not yet have been achieved in order to prevent acute rejection in solid organ transplant patients or acute graft-versus-host disease in hematopoietic stem cell transplantation patients.

After discharge from the hospital, cyclosporine concentrations continue to be obtained at most clinic visits. In patients receiving allogeneic hematopoietic stem cell transplantations from HLA-matched donors, it is usually possible to decrease cyclosporine doses and concentrations about 2 months after the transplant and stop cyclosporine therapy altogether after about 6 months posttransplant if no or mild acute rejection episodes have taken place. However, in allogeneic hematopoietic stem cell transplantation patients with HLA-mismatched related or HLA-identical unrelated donors and most solid organ transplant patients, chronic cyclosporine therapy is usually required. In these cases, cyclosporine doses and concentrations are decreased to the minimum required level to prevent graft-versus-host reactions or rejection episodes in order to decrease drug adverse effects. Methods to adjust cyclosporine doses using cyclosporine concentrations are discussed later in this chapter. Although newer data is available that suggests determination of cyclosporine area under the concentration-time curve using multiple concentrations[11-15] or 2-hour postdose cyclosporine concentrations[16-19] may provide better outcomes for some transplant types, many transplant centers continue to use predose trough cyclosporine concentration determinations to adjust drug doses.

BASIC CLINICAL PHARMACOKINETIC PARAMETERS

Cyclosporine is almost completely eliminated by hepatic metabolism (>99%).[20] Hepatic metabolism is mainly via the CYP3A4 enzyme system, and the drug is a substrate for p-glycoprotein. There are more than 25 identified cyclosporine metabolites.[5,21] None of these metabolites appear to have significant immunosuppressive effects in humans. Most of the metabolites are eliminated in the bile. Less than 1% of a cyclosporine dose is recovered as unchanged drug in the urine. Within the therapeutic range, cyclosporine follows linear pharmacokinetics.[22]

There is a large amount of intrasubject variability in cyclosporine concentrations obtained on a day-to-day basis, even when the patient should be at steady-state. There are many reasons for this variability. Cyclosporine has low water solubility, and its gastrointestinal absorption can be influenced by many variables.[5,21,23,24] To improve the consistency of absorption rate and bioavailability for original dosage form (Sandimmune, Novartis), a microemulsion version of the drug (Neoral, Novartis) was marketed to help reduce absorption variability. While use of microemulsion cyclosporine does decrease steady-state concentration variability (10%-30% for Neoral versus 16%-38% for Sandimmune for trough concentrations), there are still substantial day-to-day changes in cyclosporine concentrations regardless of the dosage form used.[25] The fat content of meals has an influence on the absorption of oral cyclosporine.[26] Food containing a large amount of fat enhances the absorption of cyclosporine. Oral cyclosporine solution is prepared with olive oil and alcohol to enhance the solubility of the drug. The solution is mixed in milk, chocolate milk, or orange juice using a glass container immediately before swallowing. When the entire dose has been given, the glass container should be rinsed with the diluting liquid and immediately consumed. If microemulsion cyclosporine solution is administered, it should be mixed in a similar fashion using apple or orange juice. In either case, grapefruit juice should not be used since this vehicle inhibits CYP3A4 and/or p-glycoprotein contained in the gastrointestinal tract and markedly increases bioavailability. Variation in cyclosporine solution absorption is dependent on how accurately the administration technique for each dose is reproduced. After liver transplantation, bile production and flow may not begin immediately, or bile flow may be diverted from the gastrointestinal tract using a T tube.[27,28] In the absence of bile salts, the absorption of cyclosporine can be greatly decreased. Bile appears to assist in the dissolution of cyclosporine which increases the absorption of the drug. Diarrhea also impairs cyclosporine absorption,[29,30] and hematopoietic stem cell transplantation patients may experience diarrhea as a part of graph-versus-host disease.[3] Other drug therapy can also increase or decrease the intestinal first-pass clearance of cyclosporine.[31]

Cyclosporine is a low-to-moderate hepatic extraction ratio drug with an average liver extraction ratio of ~30%.[32] Because of this, its hepatic clearance is influenced by unbound fraction in the blood (f_B), intrinsic clearance (Cl'_{int}), and liver blood flow (LBF). Cyclosporine binds primarily to erythrocytes and lipoproteins, yielding unbound fractions in the blood that are highly variable (1.4%-12%).[33-38] Erythrocyte concentrations vary in transplant patients, especially those who have received hematopoietic stem cell transplantation or kidney transplants. Lipoprotein concentrations also vary among patients, and hyperlipidemia is an adverse effect of cyclosporine. Hepatic intrinsic clearance is different among individuals, and there is a large amount of variability in this value within individual liver transplant patients that changes according to the viability of the graft and time after transplantation surgery. Other drug therapy can also increase or decrease the hepatic intrinsic clearance of cyclosporine.[31] Liver blood flow exhibits a great deal of day-to-day intrasubject variability which will also change the hepatic clearance of cyclosporine. Of course, changing the unbound fraction in the blood, hepatic intrinsic clearance, or liver blood flow will also change the hepatic first-pass metabolism of cyclosporine. Taking all of these possible factors into consideration that alter absorption and clearance allows one to gain a better appreciation of why cyclosporine concentrations change on a day-to-day basis.

Cyclosporine capsules and solution are available in regular (25-mg and 100-mg capsules; 100-mg/mL solution) and microemulsion (25-mg, 50-mg, and 100-mg capsules; 100-mg/mL solution) form. Although the oral absorption characteristics are more consistent and bioavailability higher for microemulsion forms of cyclosporine, it is recommended that patients who switched from cyclosporine to microemulsion cyclosporine have doses converted on a 1:1 basis. Subsequent microemulsion cyclosporine dosage adjustments are based on concentration monitoring. Cyclosporine injection for intravenous administration is available at a concentration of 50 mg/mL. Before administration, each milliliter of the concentrate should be diluted in 20-100 mL of normal saline or 5% dextrose, and the total dose infused over 2-6 hours. For patients stabilized on oral cyclosporine, the initial intravenous dose should be about 33% of the oral dose. Anaphylactic reactions have occurred with this dosage form, possibly due to the castor oil diluent used to enhance dissolution of the drug. The initial dose of cyclosporine varies greatly among various transplant centers. Cyclosporine therapy is commonly started 4-12 hours before the transplantation procedure. According to a survey of transplant centers in the United States, the average initial oral dose (± standard deviation) for renal, liver, and heart transplant patients were 9 ± 3 mg/kg/d, 8 ± 4 mg/kg/d, and 7 ± 3 mg/kg/d.[25] For both rheumatoid arthritis and psoriasis, the recommended initial dose is 2.5 mg/kg/d administered twice daily as divided doses with maximal recommended doses of 4 mg/kg/d.

EFFECTS OF DISEASE STATES AND CONDITIONS ON CYCLOSPORINE PHARMACOKINETICS AND DOSING

Transplantation type does not appear to have a substantial effect on cyclosporine pharmacokinetics. The overall mean for all transplant groups is a clearance of 6 mL/min/kg, a volume of distribution equal to 5 L/kg, and a half-life of 10 hours for adults.[5,21,23,24] Average clearance is higher (10 mL/min/kg) and mean half-life is shorter (6 hours) in children (≤16 years old).[5,21,23,24] The determination of cyclosporine half-life is difficult for patients receiving the drug on a twice daily dosage schedule because only a few concentrations can be measured in the postabsorption, postdistribution phase. Because of this, half-life measurements were taken from studies that allowed at least 24 hours between doses. These results, as with the other pharmacokinetic parameters discussed in this chapter, are based on a specific high-pressure liquid chromatography assay method conducted using whole blood samples. As discussed in a previous section, nonspecific cyclosporine assays measure metabolite concentrations in addition to parent drug, and concurrently measured plasma or serum concentrations are lower than whole blood concentrations.

Because the drug is primarily eliminated by hepatic metabolism, clearance is lower (3 mL/min/kg) and half-life prolonged (20 hours) in patients with liver failure.[5,21,39] Immediately after liver transplantation, cyclosporine metabolism is depressed until the graft begins functioning in a stable manner. Additionally, patients with transient liver dysfunction, regardless of transplantation type, will have decreased cyclosporine clearance and increased half-life values. Immediately after transplantation surgery, oral absorption of cyclosporine, especially in liver transplant patients with T tubes, is highly variable.[27,28] Obesity does not influence cyclosporine pharmacokinetics, so doses should be based on ideal body weight for these individuals.[40-44] Renal failure does not change cyclosporine pharmacokinetics, and the drug is not significantly removed by hemodialysis or peritoneal dialysis.[45-47] The hemofiltration sieving coefficient for cyclosporine is 0.58, which indicates significant removal.[48,49] Replacement doses during hemoperfusion should be determined using cyclosporine concentrations.

DRUG INTERACTIONS

Drug interactions with cyclosporine fall into two basic categories. The first are agents known to cause nephrotoxicity when administered by themselves.[31] The fear is that administration of a known nephrotoxin with cyclosporine will increase the incidence of renal damage over that observed when cyclosporine or the other agent are given separately. Drugs in this category of drug interactions include aminoglycoside antibiotics, vancomycin, cotrimoxazole (trimethoprim-sulfamethoxazole), amphotericin B, and anti-inflammatory drugs (azapropazone, diclofenac, naproxen, other nonsteroidal anti-inflammatory drugs). Other agents are melphalan, ketoconazole, cimetidine, ranitidine, and tacrolimus.

The second category of drug interactions involves inhibition or induction of cyclosporine metabolism. Cyclosporine is metabolized by CYP3A4 and is a substrate for p-glycoprotein, so the potential for many pharmacokinetic drug interactions exists with agents that inhibit these pathways or are also cleared by these mechanisms.[31] Because both of these drug elimination systems also exist in the gastrointestinal tract, inhibition drug interactions may also enhance cyclosporine oral bioavailability by diminishing the intestinal and hepatic first-pass effects. Drugs that inhibit cyclosporine clearance include the calcium channel blockers (verapamil, diltiazem, nicardipine), azole antifungals (fluconazole, itraconazole, ketoconazole), macrolide antibiotics (erythromycin, clarithromycin), antivirals (indinavir, nelfinavir, ritonavir, saquinavir), steroids (methylprednisolone, oral contraceptives, androgens), psychotropic agents (fluvoxamine, nefazodone), and as well as other agents (amiodarone, chloroquine, allopurinol, bromocriptine, metoclopramide, cimetidine, grapefruit juice). Inducing agents include other antibiotics (nafcillin, rifampin, rifabutin), anticonvulsants (phenytoin, carbamazepine, phenobarbital, primidone), barbiturates, aminoglutethimide, troglitazone, octreotide, and ticlopidine. Because of the large number of interacting agents, and the critical nature of the drugs involved in the treatment of transplant patients, complete avoidance of drug interactions with cyclosporine is not possible. Thus, most drug interactions with cyclosporine are managed using appropriate cyclosporine dosage modification with cyclosporine concentration monitoring as a guide.

Cyclosporine can also change the clearance of other drugs via competitive inhibition of CYP3A4 and/or p-glycoprotein.[31] Drugs that may experience decreased clearance and increased serum concentrations when given with cyclosporine include prednisolone, digoxin, calcium channel blockers (verapamil, diltiazem, bepridil, nifedipine and most other dihydropyridine analogues, sildenafil), statins (atorvastatin, simvastatin, lovastatin, and rosuvastatin), ergot alkaloids, and vinca alkaloids.

INITIAL DOSAGE DETERMINATION METHODS

Several methods to initiate cyclosporine therapy are available. The *Pharmacokinetic Dosing method* is the most flexible of the techniques. It allows individualized target serum concentrations to be chosen for a patient, and each pharmacokinetic parameter can be customized to reflect specific disease states and conditions present in the patient. *Literature-based recommended dosing* is a very commonly used method to prescribe initial doses of cyclosporine. Doses are based on those that commonly produce steady-state concentrations in the lower end of the therapeutic range, although there is a wide variation in the actual concentrations for a specific patient.

Pharmacokinetic Dosing Method

The goal of initial dosing of cyclosporine is to compute the best dose possible for the patient in order to prevent graft rejection or graft-versus-host disease given their set of disease states and conditions that influence cyclosporine pharmacokinetics, while avoiding adverse drug reactions. In order to do this, pharmacokinetic parameters for the patient will be estimated using average parameters measured in other patients with similar disease state and condition profiles.

Clearance Estimate

Cyclosporine is almost completely metabolized by the liver. Unfortunately, there is no good way to estimate the elimination characteristics of liver-metabolized drugs using an endogenous marker of liver function in the same fashion that serum creatinine and estimated creatinine clearance are used to estimate the elimination of agents that are renally eliminated. Because of this, a patient is categorized according to the disease states and conditions that are known to change cyclosporine clearance, and the clearance previously measured in these studies is used as an estimate of the current patient's clearance rate. For example, an adult transplant patient with normal liver function would be assigned a cyclosporine clearance rate equal to 6 mL/min/kg, while a pediatric transplant patient with the same profile would be assumed to have a cyclosporine clearance of 10 mL/min/kg.

Selection of Appropriate Pharmacokinetic Model and Equations

When given by intravenous infusion or orally, cyclosporine follows a two-compartment model.[47] When oral therapy is chosen, the drug is often erratically absorbed with variable absorption rates, and some patients may have a "double-peak" phenomenon occur where a maximum concentration is achieved 2-3 hours after dosage administration with a second maximum concentration 2-4 hours after that.[26,50] Because of the complex absorption profile and the fact that the drug is usually administered twice daily, a very simple pharmacokinetic equation that calculates the average cyclosporine steady-state serum concentration (Css in ng/mL = μg/L) is widely used and allows maintenance dose computation: $Css = [F(D/\tau)]/Cl$ or $D = (Css \bullet Cl \bullet \tau)/F$, where F is the bioavailability fraction for the oral dosage form (F averages 0.3 or 30% for most patient populations and oral dosage forms), D is the dose of cyclosporine in mg, Cl is cyclosporine clearance in L/h, and τ is the dosage interval in hours. If the drug is to be given intravenously as intermittent infusions, the equivalent equation for that route of administration is $Css = (D/\tau)/Cl$ or $D = Css \bullet Cl \bullet \tau$. If the drug is to be given as a continuous intravenous infusion, the equation for that method of administration is $Css = k_o/Cl$, or $k_o = Css \bullet Cl$, where k_o is the infusion rate.

Steady-State Concentration Selection

The generally accepted therapeutic ranges for cyclosporine in blood, serum, or plasma using various specific and nonspecific (parent drug + metabolite) assays are given in Table 18-1. More important than these general guidelines are the specific requirements for each graft type as defined by the transplant center where the surgery was conducted. Clinicians should become familiar with the cyclosporine protocols used at the various institutions at which they practice. Although it is unlikely that steady-state has been achieved, cyclosporine concentrations are usually obtained on a daily basis, even when dosage changes were made the previous day, due to the critical nature of the therapeutic effect provided by the drug.

EXAMPLE 1 ▶▶▶

HO is a 50-year-old, 75-kg (height = 5 ft 10 in) male renal transplant patient 2 days posttransplant surgery. The patient's liver function tests are normal. Suggest an initial oral cyclosporine dose designed to achieve a steady-state cyclosporine trough blood concentration equal to 250 ng/mL.

1. *Estimate clearance according to disease states and conditions present in the patient.*
   The mean cyclosporine clearance for adult patients is 6 mL/min/kg. The cyclosporine blood clearance for this patient is expected to be 27 L/h: Cl = 6 mL/min/kg • 75 kg • (60 min/h / 1000 mL/L) = 27 L/h.
2. *Compute dosage regimen.*
   A 12-hour dosage interval will be used for this patient. (Note: ng/mL = μg/L and this concentration was substituted for Css in the calculations so that unnecessary unit conversion was not required. Also, a conversion constant of 1000 μg/mg is used to change the dose amount to mg.) The dosage equation for oral cyclosporine is: D = (Css • Cl • τ)/F = (250 μg/L • 27 L/h • 12 h)/(0.3 • 1000 μg/mg) = 270 mg, rounded to 300 mg every 12 hours.

   Cyclosporine serum concentrations would be obtained on a daily basis with steady-state expected to occur in about 2 days (5 half-lives = 5 • 10 h = 50 h, or ~2 days).

EXAMPLE 2 ▶▶▶

Same patient as in example 1, except compute an initial dose using intravenous cyclosporine.

1. *Estimate clearance according to disease states and conditions present in the patient.*
   The mean cyclosporine clearance for adult patients is 6 mL/min/kg. The cyclosporine blood clearance for this patient is expected to be 27 L/h: Cl = 6 mL/min/kg • 75 kg • (60 min/h / 1000 mL/L) = 27 L/h.
2. *Compute dosage regimen.*
   A 12-hour dosage interval will be used for this patient. (Note: ng/mL = μg/L and this concentration was substituted for Css in the calculations so that unnecessary unit conversion was not required. Also, a conversion constant of 1000 μg/mg is used to change the dose amount to mg.) The dosage equation for intravenous cyclosporine is: D = Css • Cl • τ = (250 μg/L • 27 L/h • 12 h)/(1000 μg/mg) = 81 mg, rounded to 75 mg every 12 hours.

If the cyclosporine dose is given as a continuous infusion instead of intermittent infusions, the dosage equation is $k_o = Css \bullet Cl = (250\ \mu g/L \bullet 27\ L/h)/(1000\ \mu g/mg) = 6.8\ mg/h$, rounded to 7 mg/h.

Cyclosporine serum concentrations would be obtained on a daily basis with steady-state expected to occur in about 2 days (5 half-lives = $5 \bullet 10\ h = 50\ h$, or ~2 days).

Literature-Based Recommended Dosing

Because of the large amount of variability in cyclosporine pharmacokinetics, even when concurrent disease states and conditions are identified, many clinicians believe that the use of standard cyclosporine doses for various situations is warranted. Indeed, most transplant centers use doses that are determined using a cyclosporine dosage protocol. The original computation of these doses were based on the Pharmacokinetic Dosing method described in the previous section, and subsequently modified based on clinical experience. In general, the expected cyclosporine steady-state concentration used to compute these doses is dependent upon the type of transplanted tissue and the posttransplantation time line. Generally speaking, initial oral doses of 8-18 mg/kg/d or intravenous doses of 3-6 mg/kg/d (1/3 the oral dose to account for ~ 30% oral bioavailability) are used and vary greatly from institution to institution.[1-4] For obese individuals (> 30% over ideal body weight), ideal body weight should be used to compute initial doses.[40-44] Initial doses for children are 15 mg/kg/d orally or 5-6 mg/kg/d intravenously infused over 2-6 hours.[51] If the drug is started intravenously, pediatric patients are converted to an oral dose as soon as feasible. Then, the oral dose is tapered by 5% per week until it equals 3-10 mg/kg/d administered once or twice daily. To illustrate how this technique is used, the same patient examples utilized in the previous section will be repeated for this dosage approach for comparison purposes.

EXAMPLE 3 ▶▶▶

HO is a 50-year-old, 75-kg (height = 5 ft 10 in) male renal transplant patient 2 days posttransplant surgery. The patient's liver function tests are normal. Suggest an initial oral cyclosporine dose designed to achieve a steady-state cyclosporine trough blood concentration within the therapeutic range.

1. *Choose cyclosporine dose based on disease states and conditions present in the patient and transplant type.*
   The cyclosporine oral dosage range for adult patients is 8-18 mg/kg/d. Because this is a renal transplant patient, a dose in the lower end of the range (8 mg/kg/d) will be used in order to avoid nephrotoxicity. The initial cyclosporine dose for this patient is 600 mg/d given as 300 mg every 12 hours: Dose = 8 mg/kg/d • 75 kg = 600 mg/d or 300 mg every 12 hours.

   Cyclosporine serum concentrations would be obtained on a daily basis with steady-state expected to occur after 2 days (5 half-lives = $5 \bullet 10\ h = 50\ h$, or ~2 days) of treatment.

EXAMPLE 4 ▶▶▶

Same patient as in example 3, except compute an initial dose using intravenous cyclosporine.

1. *Choose cyclosporine dose based on disease states and conditions present in the patient and transplant type.*
   The cyclosporine intravenous dosage range for adult patients is 3-6 mg/kg/d. Because this is a renal transplant patient, a dose in the lower end of the range (3 mg/kg/d) will be used in order to avoid nephrotoxicity. The initial cyclosporine dose for this patient is 200 mg/d given as 100 mg every 12 hours: Dose = 3 mg/kg/d • 75 kg = 225 mg/d, rounded to 200 mg/d or 100 mg every 12 hours.

If the cyclosporine dose is given as a continuous infusion instead of intermittent infusions, the infusion rate is k_o = (3 mg/kg/d • 75 kg)/(24 h/d) = 9.4 mg/h, rounded to 9 mg/h.

Cyclosporine serum concentrations would be obtained on a daily basis with steady-state expected to occur after 2 days (5 half-lives = 5 • 10 h = 50 h, or ~2 days) of treatment.

USE OF CYCLOSPORINE CONCENTRATIONS TO ALTER DOSES

Because of the large amount of pharmacokinetic variability among patients, it is likely that doses computed using patient population characteristics will not always produce cyclosporine concentrations that are expected or desirable. Because of pharmacokinetic variability, the narrow therapeutic index of cyclosporine, and the severity of cyclosporine adverse side effects, measurement of cyclosporine concentrations is mandatory for patients to ensure that therapeutic, nontoxic levels are present. In addition to cyclosporine concentrations, important patient parameters (transplanted organ function tests or biopsies, clinical signs and symptoms of graft rejection or graft-versus-host disease, potential cyclosporine side effects, etc) should be followed to confirm that the patient is responding to treatment and not developing adverse drug reactions.

For hematopoietic stem cell transplantation patients, steady-state trough concentrations are typically measured for cyclosporine. For solid organ transplant patients, the optimal times and strategies for measurement of steady-state concentrations are somewhat controversial.[4,52] At first, it was assumed that the predose trough concentration would be best as it represents the lowest concentration during the dosage interval. However, recent studies have found that the steady-state cyclosporine concentration 2 hours after a dose (C2) reflects cyclosporine area under the curve better than a trough concentration. Finally, some clinicians believe that since cyclosporine is such a critical component of transplant therapy, that multiple postdose cyclosporine concentrations should be measured to obtain the best estimate of area under the curve that is possible. Currently, most transplant centers measure a single steady-state cyclosporine concentration as either a predose trough or 2 hours postdose, while some conduct multiple measurements to determine cyclosporine area under the curve estimates.

When cyclosporine concentrations are measured in patients and a dosage change is necessary, clinicians should seek to use the simplest, most straightforward method available to determine a dose that will provide safe and effective treatment. In most cases, a simple dosage ratio can be used to change cyclosporine doses assuming the drug follows *linear pharmacokinetics*. Sometimes, it is useful to compute cyclosporine pharmacokinetic constants for a patient and base dosage adjustments on these. In this case, it may be possible to calculate and use *pharmacokinetic parameters* to alter the cyclosporine dose. Another approach involves measuring several postdose steady-state cyclosporine concentrations to estimate the *area under the concentration-time curve (AUC)* and adjusting the cyclosporine dose to attain a target AUC. Finally, computerized methods that incorporate expected population pharmacokinetic characteristics (*Bayesian pharmacokinetic computer programs*) can be used in difficult cases where concentrations are obtained at suboptimal times or the patient was not at steady-state when concentrations were measured.

Linear Pharmacokinetics Method

Because cyclosporine follows linear, dose-proportional pharmacokinetics,[22] steady-state concentrations change in proportion to dose according to the following equation: $D_{new}/C_{ss,new} = D_{old}/C_{ss,old}$ or $D_{new} = (C_{ss,new}/C_{ss,old}) D_{old}$, where D is the dose, Css is the steady-state concentration, old indicates the dose that produced the steady-state concentration that the patient is currently receiving, and new denotes the dose necessary to produce the

TABLE 18-2   Recommended 2-h (+/− 15 min) Postdose Steady-State Cyclosporine Concentrations (C2) for Various Solid Organ Transplant Types and Posttransplant Times[53-55]

Renal Transplant	
Posttransplant Time (months)	**C2 Level (ng/mL)**
1	1500-2000
2	1500
3	1300
4-6	1100
7-12	900
>12	800
Liver Transplant	
Posttransplant Time (months)	**C2 Level (ng/mL)**
0-3	1000
4-6	800
>6	600

desired steady-state concentration. The C_{ss} can be either a steady-state trough concentration or a steady-state concentration measured 2 hours (+/−15 minutes) after a dose (C2). When C2 levels are used, recommended concentrations vary according to transplant type and posttransplant time (Table 18-2). The advantages of this method are that it is quick and simple. The disadvantage is steady-state concentrations are required.

EXAMPLE 5A ▶▶▶

LK is a 50-year-old, 75-kg (height = 5 ft 10 in) male renal transplant recipient who is receiving 400 mg every 12 hours of oral cyclosporine capsules. He has normal liver function. The current steady-state cyclosporine blood concentration equals 375 ng/mL. Compute a cyclosporine dose that will provide a steady-state concentration of 200 ng/mL.

1. *Compute new dose to achieve the desired concentration.*

The patient would be expected to achieve steady-state conditions after the second day (5 $t_{1/2}$ = 5 • 10 h = 50 h) of therapy.

Using linear pharmacokinetics, the new dose to attain the desired concentration should be proportional to the old dose that produced the measured concentration (total daily dose = 400 mg/dose • 2 doses/d = 800 mg/d):

$$D_{new} = (C_{ss,new}/C_{ss,old})D_{old} = (200 \text{ ng/mL} / 375 \text{ ng/mL}) \, 800 \text{ mg/d} = 427 \text{ mg/d, rounded to } 400 \text{ mg/d}$$

The new suggested dose would be 400 mg/d or 200 mg every 12 hours of cyclosporine capsules to be started at the next scheduled dosing time.

A steady-state trough cyclosporine serum concentration should be measured after steady-state is attained in 3-5 half-lives. Since the patient is expected to have a half-life equal to 10 hours, the cyclosporine steady-state concentration could be obtained any time after the second day of dosing (5 half-lives = 5 • 10 h = 50 h). Cyclosporine concentrations should also be measured if the patient experiences signs or symptoms of graft rejection, or if the patient develops potential signs or symptoms of cyclosporine toxicity.

EXAMPLE 5B ▶▶▶

LK is a 50-year-old, 75-kg (height = 5 ft 10 in) male renal transplant recipient who is 5 months posttransplant and receiving 400 mg every 12 hours of oral cyclosporine capsules. He has normal liver function. The current C2 steady-state cyclosporine blood concentration equals 1500 ng/mL. Compute a cyclosporine dose that will provide a C2 steady-state concentration of 800 ng/mL. (*Note: this is the same case as in example 5A in order to illustrate differences between trough and C2 level monitoring.*)

1. *Compute new dose to achieve the desired concentration.*

The patient would be expected to achieve steady-state conditions after the second day (5 $t_{1/2}$ = 5 • 10 h = 50 h) of therapy.

Using linear pharmacokinetics, the new dose to attain the desired concentration should be proportional to the old dose that produced the measured concentration (total daily dose = 400 mg/dose • 2 doses/d = 800 mg/d):

$$D_{new} = (C_{ss,new}/C_{ss,old})D_{old} = (800 \text{ ng/mL} / 1500 \text{ ng/mL}) \, 800 \text{ mg/d} = 427 \text{ mg/d, rounded to } 400 \text{ mg/d}$$

The new suggested dose would be 400 mg/d or 200 mg every 12 hours of cyclosporine capsules to be started at the next scheduled dosing time.

A steady-state trough cyclosporine serum concentration should be measured after steady-state is attained in 3-5 half-lives. Since the patient is expected to have a half-life equal to 10 hours, the cyclosporine steady-state concentration could be obtained any time after the second day of dosing (5 half-lives = 5 • 10 h = 50 h). Cyclosporine concentrations should also be measured if the patient experiences signs or symptoms of graft rejection, or if the patient develops potential signs or symptoms of cyclosporine toxicity.

EXAMPLE 6 ▶▶▶

FD is a 60-year-old, 85-kg (height = 6 ft 1 in) male liver transplant patient who is receiving 75 mg every 12 hours of intravenous cyclosporine. The current steady-state cyclosporine concentration equals 215 ng/mL. Compute a cyclosporine dose that will provide a steady-state concentration of 350 ng/mL.

1. *Compute new dose to achieve the desired concentration.*

The patient recently received a liver transplantation and would be expected to have a longer cyclosporine half-life if the organ is not yet functioning at an optimal level ($t_{1/2}$ = 20 h). Because of this, it could take up to 4 days of consistent cyclosporine therapy to achieve steady-state conditions (5 $t_{1/2}$ = 5 • 20 h = 100 h or ~4 d).

Using linear pharmacokinetics, the new dose to attain the desired concentration should be proportional to the old dose that produced the measured concentration (total daily dose = 75 mg/dose • 2 doses/d = 150 mg/d):

$$D_{new} = (C_{ss,new}/C_{ss,old})D_{old} = (350 \text{ ng/mL} / 215 \text{ ng/mL}) \, 150 \text{ mg/d} = 244 \text{ mg/d, rounded to } 250 \text{ mg/d}$$
$$\text{or } 125 \text{ mg every 12 hours.}$$

A steady-state trough cyclosporine serum concentration should be measured after steady-state is attained in 3-5 half-lives. Since the patient is expected to have a half-life up to 20 hours, the cyclosporine steady-state concentration could be obtained any time after the fourth day of dosing (5 half-lives = 5 • 20 h = 100 h or 4 days). Cyclosporine concentrations should also be measured if the patient experiences signs or symptoms of graft rejection, or if the patient develops potential signs or symptoms of cyclosporine toxicity.

If the patient in example 6 received cyclosporine as a continuous infusion at a rate of 6 mg/h, the equivalent dosage adjustment computation would be:

$$D_{new} = (C_{ss,new}/C_{ss,old})D_{old} = (350 \text{ ng/mL} / 215 \text{ ng/mL}) \, 6 \text{ mg/h} = 9.8 \text{ mg/h, rounded to } 10 \text{ mg/h}$$

Pharmacokinetic Parameter Method

The Pharmacokinetic Parameter method of adjusting drug doses was among the first techniques available to change doses using drug concentrations. It allows the computation of an individual's own, unique pharmacokinetic constants and uses those to calculate a dose that achieves desired cyclosporine concentrations. The Pharmacokinetic Parameter method requires that steady-state has been achieved and uses only a steady-state cyclosporine concentration. Cyclosporine clearance can be measured using a single steady-state cyclosporine concentration and the following formula for orally administered drug: $Cl = [F(D/\tau)]/Css$, where Cl is cyclosporine clearance in L/h, F is the bioavailability factor for cyclosporine (F = 0.3), τ is the dosage interval in hours, and Css is the cyclosporine steady-state concentration in ng/mL which also equals µg/L. If cyclosporine is administered intravenously, it is not necessary to take bioavailability into account: $Cl = (D/\tau)/Css$, where Cl is cyclosporine clearance in L/h, τ is the dosage interval in hours, and Css is the cyclosporine steady-state concentration in ng/mL which also equals µg/L. Although this method does allow computation of cyclosporine clearance, it yields exactly the same cyclosporine dose as that supplied using linear pharmacokinetics. As a result, most clinicians prefer to directly calculate the new dose using the Simpler Linear Pharmacokinetics method. To demonstrate this point, the patient cases used to illustrate the linear pharmacokinetics method will be used as examples for the Pharmacokinetic Parameter method.

EXAMPLE 7 ▶▶▶

LK is a 50-year-old, 75-kg (height = 5 ft 10 in) male renal transplant recipient who is receiving 400 mg every 12 hours of oral cyclosporine capsules. He has normal liver function. The current steady-state cyclosporine blood concentration equals 375 ng/mL. Compute a cyclosporine dose that will provide a steady-state concentration of 200 ng/mL.

1. *Compute pharmacokinetic parameters.*

The patient would be expected to achieve steady-state conditions after the second day (5 $t_{1/2}$ = 5 • 10 h = 50 h or 2 days) of therapy.

Cyclosporine clearance can be computed using a steady-state cyclosporine concentration: $Cl = [F(D/\tau)]/Css = [0.3 • (400 \text{ mg}/12 \text{ h}) • 1000 \text{ µg/mg}]/(375 \text{ µg/L}) = 26.7 \text{ L/h}$. (Note: µg/L = ng/mL and this concentration unit was substituted for Css in the calculations so that unnecessary unit conversion was not required.)

2. *Compute cyclosporine dose.*

Cyclosporine clearance is used to compute the new dose: $D = (Css • Cl • \tau)/F = (200 \text{ µg/L} • 26.7 \text{ L/h} • 12 \text{ h})/(0.3 • 1000 \text{ µg/mg}) = 214 \text{ mg}$, rounded to 200 mg every 12 hours.

A steady-state trough cyclosporine serum concentration should be measured after steady-state is attained in 3-5 half-lives. Since the patient is expected to have a half-life equal to 10 hours, the cyclosporine steady-state concentration could be obtained any time after the second day of dosing (5 half-lives = 5 • 10 h = 50 h). Cyclosporine concentrations should also be measured if the patient experiences signs or symptoms of graft rejection, or if the patient develops potential signs or symptoms of cyclosporine toxicity.

EXAMPLE 8 ▶▶▶

FD is a 60-year-old, 85-kg (height = 6 ft 1 in) male liver transplant patient who is receiving 75 mg every 12 hours of intravenous cyclosporine. The current steady-state cyclosporine concentration equals 215 ng/mL. Compute a cyclosporine dose that will provide a steady-state concentration of 350 ng/mL.

1. *Compute pharmacokinetic parameters.*

   The patient recently received a liver transplantation and would be expected to have a longer cyclosporine half-life if the organ is not yet functioning at an optimal level ($t_{1/2} = 20$ h). Because of this, it could take up to 4 days of consistent cyclosporine therapy to achieve steady-state conditions ($5\ t_{1/2} = 5 \bullet 20$ h $= 100$ h or ~4 d).

   Cyclosporine clearance can be computed using a steady-state cyclosporine concentration: $Cl = (D/\tau)/Css = [(75$ mg/12 h$) \bullet 1000\ \mu g/mg]/(215\ \mu g/L) = 29.1$ L/h. (Note: $\mu g/L = $ ng/mL and this concentration unit was substituted for Css in the calculations so that unnecessary unit conversion was not required.)

2. *Compute cyclosporine dose.*

   Cyclosporine clearance is used to compute the new dose: $D = Css \bullet Cl \bullet \tau = (350\ \mu g/L \bullet 29.1$ L/h $\bullet$ 12h$)/1000\ \mu g/mg = 122$ mg, rounded to 125 mg every 12 hours.

   A steady-state trough cyclosporine serum concentration should be measured after steady-state is attained in 3-5 half-lives. Since the patient is expected to have a half-life up to 20 hours, the cyclosporine steady-state concentration could be obtained any time after the fourth day of dosing (5 half-lives $= 5 \bullet 20$ h $= 100$ h or 4 days). Cyclosporine concentrations should also be measured if the patient experiences signs or symptoms of graft rejection, or if the patient develops potential signs or symptoms of cyclosporine toxicity.

   If the patient in example 8 received cyclosporine as a continuous infusion at a rate of 6 mg/h, the equivalent clearance and dosage adjustment computations would be:

   $$Cl = k_o/Css = (6\text{ mg/h} \bullet 1000\ \mu g/mg)/(215\ \mu g/L) = 27.9\text{ L/h}$$

   $$k_o = Css \bullet Cl = (350\ \mu g/L \bullet 27.9\text{ L/h})/(1000\ \mu g/mg) = 9.8\text{ mg/h, rounded to 10 mg/h}$$

Area Under the Concentration-Time Curve (AUC) Method

Some solid organ transplant centers believe that measurement or estimation of cyclosporine area under the concentration-time curve (AUC) is the best way to optimize cyclosporine therapy. While AUC can be measured using hourly postdose cyclosporine levels, studies have shown that there is a strong correlation between 3 and 4 cyclosporine concentrations and the total AUC. Based on this finding, most centers utilizing this method measure several steady-state cyclosporine concentrations and use a published regression equation determined in other patients receiving the same transplanted organ and similar drug therapy (to account for possible drug interactions) in order to convert the concentrations to an estimated AUC. Then, if necessary, adjust the cyclosporine dose using linear pharmacokinetics to achieve the target AUC: $D_{new}/AUC_{new} = D_{old}/AUC_{old}$ or $D_{new} = (AUC_{new}/AUC_{old})D_{old}$, where D is the dose, AUC is the steady-state area under the concentration-time curve, old indicates the dose that produced the steady-state area under the concentration-time curve that the patient is currently receiving, and new denotes the dose necessary to produce the desired steady-state area under the concentration-time curve.

There are many regression equations from which to choose based on the target transplant population and other concurrent therapy that may cause drug interactions with cyclosporine. The one used for the examples and problems in this book is for renal transplant patients in the immediate 3 month posttransplant period that received a variety of other immunosuppressants (prednisone plus mycophenolate mofetil or rapamycin).[56] In this investigation, the steady-state AUC from time 0 hours (predose) to 4 hours after the dose (AUC_{0-4h}) strongly correlated with the total steady-state AUC during the dosage interval and was used to adjust cyclosporine doses: AUC_{0-4h} [in ($\mu g \bullet$ h)/L] $= 256 + C_{1h} + (0.9 \bullet C_{2h}) + (1.4 \bullet C_{3h})$, where C_{1h}, C_{2h}, and C_{3h} are steady-state cyclosporine concentrations in $\mu g/L$ obtained 1, 2, and 3 hours, respectively, after a dose. The dose is then adjusted to produce a new steady-state AUC equal to 4400-5500 ($\mu g \bullet$ h)/L using linear pharmacokinetics.[13]

EXAMPLE 9 ▶▶▶

GQ is a 47-year-old, 78-kg (height = 6 ft 1 in) male who has undergone renal transplantation. He is receiving 400 mg every 12 hours of oral cyclosporine. The following cyclosporine steady-state concentrations have been measured to determine an estimated AUC_{0-4h}: C_{1h} = 412 ng/ml, C_{2h} = 1251 ng/mL, C_{3h} = 1009 ng/mL. Compute a cyclosporine dose that will provide a steady-state AUC_{0-4h} of 5000 (μg • h)/L.

1. *Compute pharmacokinetic parameters.*

   Cyclosporine AUC_{0-4h} can be estimated using the steady-state cyclosporine concentrations: AUC_{0-4h} = 256 + C_{1h} + (0.9 • C_{2h}) + (1.4 • C_{3h}) = 256 + (412 μg/L) + (0.9 • 1251 μg/L) + (1.4 • 1009 μg/L) = 3206 (μg • h)/L. (Note: μg/L = ng/mL and this concentration unit was substituted for Css in the calculations.)

2. *Compute cyclosporine dose.*

   Linear pharmacokinetics is used to compute the new dose (total daily dose = 400 mg/dose • 2 doses/d = 800 mg/d): D_{new} = (AUC_{new}/AUC_{old})D_{old} = {[5000 (μg • h)/L]/[3206 (μg • h)/L)]}(800 mg/d) = 1258 mg/d, rounded to 600 mg every 12 hours.

   Steady-state cyclosporine serum concentrations should be measured after steady-state is attained in 3-5 half-lives. Cyclosporine concentrations should also be measured if the patient experiences signs or symptoms of graft rejection, or if the patient develops potential signs or symptoms of cyclosporine toxicity.

BAYESIAN PHARMACOKINETIC COMPUTER PROGRAMS

Computer programs are available that can assist in the computation of pharmacokinetic parameters for patients.[57-59] The most reliable computer programs use a nonlinear regression algorithm that incorporates components of Bayes theorem. Nonlinear regression is a statistical technique that uses an iterative process to compute the best pharmacokinetic parameters for a concentration/time data set. Briefly, the patient's drug dosage schedule and serum concentrations are input into the computer. The computer program has a pharmacokinetic equation preprogrammed for the drug and administration method (oral, intravenous bolus, intravenous infusion, etc). Typically, a one-compartment model is used, although some programs allow the user to choose among several different equations. Using population estimates based on demographic information for the patient (age, weight, gender, liver function, cardiac status, etc) supplied by the user, the computer program then computes estimated serum concentrations at each time there are actual serum concentrations. Kinetic parameters are then changed by the computer program, and a new set of estimated serum concentrations are computed. The pharmacokinetic parameters that generated the estimated serum concentrations closest to the actual values are remembered by the computer program, and the process is repeated until the set of pharmacokinetic parameters that result in estimated serum concentrations that are statistically closest to the actual serum concentrations are generated. These pharmacokinetic parameters can then be used to compute improved dosing schedules for patients. Bayes theorem is used in the computer algorithm to balance the results of the computations between values based solely on the patient's serum drug concentrations and those based only on patient population parameters. Results from studies that compare various methods of dosage adjustment have consistently found that these types of computer-dosing programs perform at least as well as experienced clinical pharmacokineticists and clinicians and better than inexperienced clinicians.

Some clinicians use Bayesian pharmacokinetic computer programs exclusively to alter drug doses based on serum concentrations. An advantage of this approach is that consistent dosage recommendations are made when several different practitioners are involved in therapeutic drug-monitoring programs. However, since simpler dosing methods work just as well for patients with stable pharmacokinetic parameters and steady-state drug concentrations, many clinicians reserve the use of computer programs for more difficult situations.

Those situations include serum concentrations that are not at steady-state, serum concentrations not obtained at the specific times needed to employ simpler methods, and unstable pharmacokinetic parameters. When only a limited number of cyclosporine steady-state concentrations are available, Bayesian pharmacokinetic computer programs can be used to compute a complete patient pharmacokinetic profile that includes clearance, volume of distribution, and half-life.

Many Bayesian pharmacokinetic computer programs are available to users, and most should provide answers similar to the one used in the following examples. The program used to solve problems in this book is DrugCalc written by Dr Dennis Mungall.[60]

EXAMPLE 10 ▶▶▶

LK is a 50-year-old, 75-kg (height = 5 ft 10 in) male renal transplant recipient who is receiving 400 mg every 12 hours of oral cyclosporine capsules. He has normal liver (bilirubin = 0.7 mg/dL, albumin = 4.0 g/dL). The current steady-state cyclosporine blood concentration equals 375 ng/mL. Compute a cyclosporine dose that will provide a steady-state concentration of 200 ng/mL.

1. *Enter the patient's demographic, drug-dosing, and serum concentration/time data into the computer program.*
2. *Compute pharmacokinetic parameters for the patient using Bayesian pharmacokinetic computer program.*
   The pharmacokinetic parameters computed by the program are a volume of distribution of 403 L, a half-life equal to 17.6 h, and a clearance equal to 15.9 L/h.
3. *Compute dose required to achieve the desired cyclosporine serum concentrations.*
   The one-compartment model first-order absorption equations used by the program to compute doses indicates that a dose of 200 mg every 12 hours will produce a steady-state cyclosporine concentration of 210 ng/mL. Using the Linear Pharmacokinetics and Pharmacokinetic Parameter methods previously described in the chapter produced the same answer for this patient.

EXAMPLE 11 ▶▶▶

FD is a 60-year-old, 85-kg (height = 6 ft 1 in) male liver transplant patient who is receiving 75 mg every 12 hours of intravenous cyclosporine. He has elevated liver function tests (bilirubin = 3.2 mg/dL, albumin = 2.5 g/dL). The current steady-state cyclosporine concentration equals 215 ng/mL. Compute a cyclosporine dose that will provide a steady-state concentration of 350 ng/mL.

1. *Enter the patient's demographic, drug-dosing, and serum concentration/time data into the computer program.*
2. *Compute pharmacokinetic parameters for the patient using Bayesian pharmacokinetic computer program.*
   The pharmacokinetic parameters computed by the program are a volume of distribution of 403 L, a half-life equal to 13.8 h, and a clearance equal to 20.3 L/h.
3. *Compute dose required to achieve the desired cyclosporine serum concentrations.*
   The one-compartment model first-order absorption equations used by the program to compute doses indicates that a dose of 125 mg every 12 hours will produce a steady-state cyclosporine concentration of 380 ng/mL. Using the Linear Pharmacokinetics and Pharmacokinetic Parameter methods previously described in the chapter produced the same answer for this patient.

TABLE 18-3   Dosing Strategies

Dosing Approach/Philosophy	Initial Dosing	Use of Serum Concentrations to Alter Doses
Pharmacokinetic parameter/equations	Pharmacokinetic Dosing method	Pharmacokinetic Parameter method
Literature-based concept	Literature-based Recommended Dosing method	Linear Pharmacokinetics or AUC method
Computerized	Bayesian computer program	Bayesian computer program

EXAMPLE 12 ▶▶▶

YT is a 25-year-old, 55-kg (height = 5 ft 2 in) female hematopoietic stem cell transplantation recipient who received 300 mg every 12 hours of oral cyclosporine capsules for two doses after transplant, but because her renal function decreased, her dose was empirically changed to 200 mg every 12 hours. She has normal liver function (bilirubin = 0.9 mg/dL, albumin = 3.9 g/dL). The cyclosporine blood concentration obtained 12 hours after her first dose of the lower dosage regimen equaled 280 ng/mL. Compute a cyclosporine dose that will provide a steady-state concentration of 250 ng/mL.

1. *Enter the patient's demographic, drug-dosing, and serum concentration/time data into the computer program.*
2. *Compute pharmacokinetic parameters for the patient using Bayesian pharmacokinetic computer program.*
   The pharmacokinetic parameters computed by the program are a volume of distribution of 401 L, a half-life equal to 35 h, and a clearance equal to 8 L/h.
3. *Compute dose required to achieve the desired cyclosporine serum concentrations.*
   The one-compartment model first-order absorption equations used by the program to compute doses indicates that a dose of 100 mg every 12 hours will produce a steady-state cyclosporine concentration of 250 ng/mL.

DOSING STRATEGIES

Initial dose and dosage adjustment techniques using serum concentrations can be used in any combination as long as the limitations of each method are observed. Some dosing schemes link together logically when considered according to their basic approaches or philosophies. Dosage strategies that follow similar pathways are given in Table 18-3.

PROBLEMS

The following problems are intended to emphasize the computation of initial and individualized doses using clinical pharmacokinetic techniques. Clinicians should always consult the patient's chart to confirm that current immunosuppressive therapy is appropriate. Additionally, all other medications that the patient is taking, including prescription and nonprescription drugs, should be noted and checked to ascertain if a potential drug interaction with cyclosporine exists.

1. VI is a 37-year-old, 85-kg (height = 6 ft 1 in) male heart transplant patient who requires therapy with oral cyclosporine. He has normal liver function. Suggest an initial dosage regimen designed to achieve a steady-state cyclosporine concentration equal to 300 ng/mL.

2. Patient VI (see problem 1) was prescribed 400 mg every 12 hours of cyclosporine capsules for 4 days, and the steady-state cyclosporine concentration equals 426 ng/mL. The patient is assessed to be compliant with his dosage regimen. Suggest a cyclosporine dosage regimen designed to achieve a steady-state cyclosporine concentration of 300 ng/mL.

3. AS is a 9-year-old, 35-kg female (height = 4 ft 6 in) hematopoietic stem cell transplantation patient who requires therapy with oral cyclosporine. She has normal liver function. Suggest an initial cyclosporine dosage regimen designed to achieve a steady-state cyclosporine concentration equal to 250 ng/mL.

4. Patient AS (see problem 3) was prescribed 150 mg every 12 hours of cyclosporine solution for 3 days, and the steady-state cyclosporine concentration equals 173 ng/mL. The patient is assessed to be compliant with her dosage regimen. Suggest an oral cyclosporine dosage regimen designed to achieve a steady-state cyclosporine concentration equal to 250 ng/mL.

5. FL is a 29-year-old, 78-kg (height = 5 ft 11 in) male liver transplant patient who requires therapy with oral cyclosporine. He has poor liver function because of his liver disease. Suggest an initial cyclosporine dosage regimen to be started 24 hours before transplant surgery designed to achieve a steady-state cyclosporine concentration equal to 300 ng/mL.

6. Patient FL (see problem 5) is 10 days postsurgery for a liver transplantation. He was prescribed 400 mg every 12 hours of cyclosporine capsules since transplantation, and the steady-state cyclosporine concentration equals 531 ng/mL. The patient is assessed to be compliant with his dosage regimen. Suggest a cyclosporine dosage regimen designed to achieve a steady-state cyclosporine concentration of 250 ng/mL.

7. PH is a 22-year-old, 67-kg female (height = 5 ft 5 in) renal transplant patient who requires therapy with oral cyclosporine. She is 36 hours posttransplantation procedure, and the transplanted kidney is beginning to function normally. Her liver function is normal. Suggest an initial cyclosporine dosage regimen designed to achieve a steady-state cyclosporine concentration equal to 200 ng/mL.

8. Patient PH (see problem 7) was prescribed 200 mg every 12 hours of cyclosporine capsules for 3 days, and the steady-state cyclosporine concentration equals 125 ng/mL. The patient is assessed to be compliant with her dosage regimen. Suggest a cyclosporine dosage regimen designed to achieve a steady-state cyclosporine concentration of 200 ng/mL.

9. PU is a 55-year-old, 68-kg (height = 5 ft 8 in) male heart transplant patient who received two intravenous cyclosporine doses (125 mg every 12 hours) and was switched to oral cyclosporine capsules 300 mg every 12 hours. He has normal liver (bilirubin = 0.7 mg/dL, albumin = 4.0 g/dL) function. The cyclosporine concentration equals 190 ng/mL 12 hours after the first oral dose of the drug. Compute a cyclosporine dose that will provide a steady-state concentration of 250 ng/mL.

10. LH is a 25-year-old, 60-kg (height = 5 ft 3 in) female renal transplant patient who was given a new prescription for cyclosporine capsules 200 mg every 12 hours 2 days after transplantation surgery. She has normal liver function (bilirubin = 0.4 mg/dL, albumin = 3.7 g/dL) and is also being treated with phenytoin. The trough cyclosporine concentration before the third dose equals 90 ng/mL. Compute a cyclosporine dose that will provide a steady-state concentration of 200 ng/mL.

11. UT is a 28-year-old, 75-kg (height = 5 ft 11 in) male liver transplant patient who is 20 days postsurgery. He was prescribed 400 mg every 12 hours of cyclosporine capsules, and the steady-state C2 cyclosporine concentration equals 2124 ng/mL. The patient is assessed to be compliant with his dosage regimen. Suggest a cyclosporine dosage regimen designed to achieve a steady-state C2 cyclosporine concentration of 1000 ng/mL.

12. KL is a 21-year-old, 67-kg female (height = 5 ft 6 in) renal transplant patient who is 4 months postsurgery. She was prescribed 200 mg every 12 hours of cyclosporine capsules, and the steady-state C2 cyclosporine concentration equals 688 ng/mL. The patient is assessed to be compliant with her dosage regimen. Suggest a cyclosporine dosage regimen designed to achieve a steady-state C2 cyclosporine concentration of 1100 ng/mL.

13. QG is a 51-year-old, 78-kg (height = 6 ft 1 in) male who has undergone renal transplantation. He is receiving 400 mg every 12 hours of oral cyclosporine. The following cyclosporine steady-state concentrations have been measured to determine an estimated AUC_{0-4h}: C_{1h} = 525 ng/mL, C_{2h} = 1399 ng/mL, C_{3h} = 1250 ng/mL. Compute a cyclosporine dose that will provide a steady-state AUC_{0-4h} of 5000 ($\mu g \bullet h$)/L.

ANSWERS TO PROBLEMS

1. *Answer to problem 1.*

Pharmacokinetic Dosing Method

1. *Estimate clearance according to disease states and conditions present in the patient.*
    The mean cyclosporine clearance for adult patients is 6 mL/min/kg. The cyclosporine blood clearance for this patient is expected to be 30.6 L/h: Cl = 6 mL/min/kg $\bullet$ 85 kg $\bullet$ (60 min/h / 1000 mL/L) = 30.6 L/h.

2. *Compute dosage regimen.*
    A 12-hour dosage interval will be used for this patient. (Note: ng/mL = μg/L and this concentration was substituted for Css in the calculations so that unnecessary unit conversion was not required. Also, a conversion constant of 1000 μg/mg is used to change the dose amount to mg.) The dosage equation for oral cyclosporine is: D = (Css $\bullet$ Cl $\bullet$ τ)/F = (300 μg/L $\bullet$ 30.6 L/h $\bullet$ 12 h)/ (0.3 $\bullet$ 1000 μg/mg) = 367 mg, rounded to 400 mg every 12 hours.
    Cyclosporine serum concentrations would be obtained on a daily basis with steady-state expected to occur in about 2 days (5 half-lives = 5 $\bullet$ 10 h = 50 h, or ~2 days).

Literature-Based Recommended Dosing

1. *Choose cyclosporine dose based on disease states and conditions present in the patient and transplant type.*
    The cyclosporine oral dosage range for adult patients is 8-18 mg/kg/d. Because this is a heart transplant patient, a dose in the middle of the range (10 mg/kg/d) will be used in order to avoid graft rejection. The initial cyclosporine dose for this patient is 800 mg/d given as 400 mg every 12 hours: Dose = 10 mg/kg/d $\bullet$ 85 kg = 850 mg/d, rounded to 800 mg/d or 400 mg every 12 hours.
    Cyclosporine serum concentrations would be obtained on a daily basis with steady-state expected to occur after 2 days (5 half-lives = 5 $\bullet$ 10 h = 50 h, or ~2 days) of treatment.

2. *Answer to problem 2.*

Linear Pharmacokinetics Method

1. *Compute new dose to achieve the desired concentration.*
    The patient would be expected to achieve steady-state conditions after the second day (5 $t_{1/2}$ = 5 $\bullet$ 10 h = 50 h) of therapy.
    Using linear pharmacokinetics, the new dose to attain the desired concentration should be proportional to the old dose that produced the measured concentration (total daily dose = 400 mg/dose $\bullet$ 2 doses/d = 800 mg/d):

$$D_{new} = (C_{ss,new}/C_{ss,old})D_{old} = (300 \text{ ng/mL} / 426 \text{ ng/mL}) \text{ } 800 \text{ mg/d} = 563 \text{ mg/d, rounded to } 600 \text{ mg/d}$$

The new suggested dose would be 600 mg/d or 300 mg every 12 hours of cyclosporine capsules to be started at the next scheduled dosing time.

A steady-state trough cyclosporine serum concentration should be measured after steady-state is attained in 3-5 half-lives. Since the patient is expected to have a half-life equal to 10 hours, the cyclosporine steady-state concentration could be obtained any time after the second day of dosing (5 half-lives = 5 • 10 h = 50 h). Cyclosporine concentrations should also be measured if the patient experiences signs or symptoms of graft rejection, or if the patient develops potential signs or symptoms of cyclosporine toxicity.

Pharmacokinetic Parameter Method

1. *Compute pharmacokinetic parameters.*

The patient would be expected to achieve steady-state conditions after the second day (5 $t_{1/2}$ = 5 • 10 h = 50 h or 2 days) of therapy.

Cyclosporine clearance can be computed using a steady-state cyclosporine concentration: Cl = [F(D/τ)]/Css = [0.3 • (400 mg/12 h) •1000 μg/mg]/(426 μg/L) = 23.5 L/h. (Note: μg/L = ng/ml and this concentration unit was substituted for Css in the calculations so that unnecessary unit conversion was not required.)

2. *Compute cyclosporine dose.*

Cyclosporine clearance is used to compute the new dose: D = (Css • Cl • τ)/F = (300 μg/L • 23.5 L/h • 12 h)/(0.3 • 1000 μg/mg) = 282 mg, rounded to 300 mg every 12 hours.

A steady-state trough cyclosporine serum concentration should be measured after steady-state is attained in 3-5 half-lives. Since the patient is expected to have a half-life equal to 10 hours, the cyclosporine steady-state concentration could be obtained any time after the second day of dosing (5 half-lives = 5 • 10 h = 50 h). Cyclosporine concentrations should also be measured if the patient experiences signs or symptoms of graft rejection, or if the patient develops potential signs or symptoms of cyclosporine toxicity.

3. *Answer to problem 3.*

Pharmacokinetic Dosing Method

1. *Estimate clearance according to disease states and conditions present in the patient.*

The mean cyclosporine clearance for pediatric patients is 10 mL/min/kg. The cyclosporine blood clearance for this patient is expected to be 21 L/h: Cl = 10 mL/min/kg • 35 kg • (60 min/h / 1000 mL/L) = 21 L/h.

2. *Compute dosage regimen.*

A 12-hour dosage interval will be used for this patient. (Note: ng/mL = μg/L and this concentration was substituted for Css in the calculations so that unnecessary unit conversion was not required. Also, a conversion constant of 1000 μg/mg is used to change the dose amount to mg.) The dosage equation for oral cyclosporine is: D = (Css • Cl • τ)/F = (250 μg/L • 21 L/h • 12 h)/(0.3 • 1000 μg/mg) = 210 mg, rounded to 200 mg every 12 hours of cyclosporine solution.

Cyclosporine serum concentrations would be obtained on a daily basis with steady-state expected to occur in about 1-2 days (5 half-lives = 5 • 6 h = 30 h).

Literature-Based Recommended Dosing

1. *Choose cyclosporine dose based on disease states and conditions present in the patient and transplant type.*

The cyclosporine oral dosage range is 8-18 mg/kg/d. Because this is a pediatric patient, a dose in the middle of the range (12 mg/kg/d) will be used in order to avoid graft-versus-host disease. The initial cyclosporine dose for this patient is 400 mg/d given as 200 mg every 12 hours: Dose = 12 mg/kg/d • 35 kg = 420 mg/d, rounded to 400 mg/d or 200 mg every 12 hours of cyclosporine solution.

Cyclosporine serum concentrations would be obtained on a daily basis with steady-state expected to occur in about 1-2 days (5 half-lives = 5 • 6 h = 30 h) of treatment.

4. *Answer to problem 4.*

Linear Pharmacokinetics Method

1. *Compute new dose to achieve the desired concentration.*

The patient would be expected to achieve steady-state conditions by the second day (5 $t_{1/2}$ = 5 • 6 h = 30 h) of therapy.

Using linear pharmacokinetics, the new dose to attain the desired concentration should be proportional to the old dose that produced the measured concentration (total daily dose = 150 mg/dose • 2 doses/d = 300 mg/d):

$$D_{new} = (C_{ss,new}/C_{ss,old})D_{old} = (250 \text{ ng/mL} / 173 \text{ ng/mL}) \, 300 \text{ mg/d} = 434 \text{ mg/d, rounded to } 400 \text{ mg/d}$$

The new suggested dose would be 400 mg/d or 200 mg every 12 hours of cyclosporine solution to be started at the next scheduled dosing time.

A steady-state trough cyclosporine serum concentration should be measured after steady-state is attained in 3-5 half-lives. Since the patient is expected to have a half-life equal to 6 hours, the cyclosporine steady-state concentration could be obtained any time after the first day of dosing (5 half-lives = 5 • 6 h = 30 h). Cyclosporine concentrations should also be measured if the patient experiences signs or symptoms of graft rejection, or if the patient develops potential signs or symptoms of cyclosporine toxicity.

Pharmacokinetic Parameter Method

1. *Compute pharmacokinetic parameters.*

The patient would be expected to achieve steady-state conditions after the second day (5 $t_{1/2}$ = 5 • 6 h = 30 h) of therapy.

Cyclosporine clearance can be computed using a steady-state cyclosporine concentration: Cl = [F(D/τ)]/Css = [0.3 • (150 mg/12 h) • 1000 μg/mg]/(173 μg/L) = 21.7 L/h. (Note: μg/L = ng/mL and this concentration unit was substituted for Css in the calculations so that unnecessary unit conversion was not required.)

2. *Compute cyclosporine dose.*

Cyclosporine clearance is used to compute the new dose: D = (Css • Cl • τ)/F = (250 μg/L • 21.7 L/h • 12 h)/(0.3 • 1000 μg/mg) = 217 mg, rounded to 200 mg every 12 hours of cyclosporine solution.

A steady-state trough cyclosporine serum concentration should be measured after steady-state is attained in 3-5 half-lives. Since the patient is expected to have a half-life equal to 6 hours, the cyclosporine steady-state concentration could be obtained any time after the first day of dosing (5 half-lives = 5 • 6 h = 30 h). Cyclosporine concentrations should also be measured if the patient experiences signs or symptoms of graft rejection, or if the patient develops potential signs or symptoms of cyclosporine toxicity.

5. *Answer to problem 5.*

Pharmacokinetic Dosing Method

1. *Estimate clearance according to disease states and conditions present in the patient.*

The mean cyclosporine clearance for adult patients is 6 mL/min/kg. The cyclosporine blood clearance for this patient is expected to be 28.1 L/h: Cl = 6 mL/min/kg • 78 kg • (60 min/h/ 1000 mL/L) = 28.1 L/h

2. *Compute dosage regimen.*

A 12-hour dosage interval will be used for this patient. (Note: ng/mL = μg/L and this concentration was substituted for Css in the calculations so that unnecessary unit conversion was not required. Also, a conversion constant of 1000 μg/mg is used to change the dose amount to mg.) The dosage equation for oral cyclosporine is: D = (Css • Cl • τ)/F = (300 μg/L • 28.1 L/h • 12 h)/ (0.3 • 1000 μg/mg) = 337 mg, rounded to 300 mg every 12 hours.

Cyclosporine serum concentrations would be obtained on a daily basis with steady-state expected to occur in about 2 days (5 half-lives = 5 • 10 h = 50 h, or ~2 days).

Literature-Based Recommended Dosing

1. *Choose cyclosporine dose based on disease states and conditions present in the patient and transplant type.*

The cyclosporine oral dosage range for adult patients is 8-18 mg/kg/d. Because this is a liver transplant patient, a dose in the middle of the range (10 mg/kg/d) will be used in order to avoid graft rejection. The initial cyclosporine dose for this patient is 800 mg/d given as 400 mg every 12 hours: Dose = 10 mg/kg/d • 78 kg = 780 mg/d, rounded to 800 mg/d or 400 mg every 12 hours.

Cyclosporine serum concentrations would be obtained on a daily basis with steady-state expected to occur after 2 days (5 half-lives = 5 • 10 h = 50 h, or ~2 days) of treatment.

6. *Answer to problem 6.*

Linear Pharmacokinetics Method

1. *Compute new dose to achieve the desired concentration.*

The patient would be expected to achieve steady-state conditions after the second day (5 $t_{1/2}$ = 5 • 10 h = 50 h) of therapy.

Using linear pharmacokinetics, the new dose to attain the desired concentration should be proportional to the old dose that produced the measured concentration (total daily dose = 400 mg/dose • 2 doses/d = 800 mg/d):

$$D_{new} = (C_{ss,new}/C_{ss,old})D_{old} = (250\ ng/mL\ /\ 531\ ng/mL)\ 800\ mg/d = 377\ mg/d, \text{rounded to } 400\ mg/d$$

The new suggested dose would be 400 mg/d or 200 mg every 12 hours of cyclosporine capsules to be started at the next scheduled dosing time.

A steady-state trough cyclosporine serum concentration should be measured after steady-state is attained in 3-5 half-lives. Since the patient is expected to have a half-life equal to 10 hours, the cyclosporine steady-state concentration could be obtained any time after the second day of dosing (5 half-lives = 5 • 10 h = 50 h). Cyclosporine concentrations should also be measured if the patient experiences signs or symptoms of graft rejection, or if the patient develops potential signs or symptoms of cyclosporine toxicity.

Pharmacokinetic Parameter Method

1. *Compute pharmacokinetic parameters.*

   The patient would be expected to achieve steady-state conditions after the second day ($5 \; t_{1/2} =$ 5 • 10 h = 50 h or 2 days) of therapy.

   Cyclosporine clearance can be computed using a steady-state cyclosporine concentration: Cl = [F(D/τ)]/ Css = [0.3 • (400 mg/12 h) •1000 μg/mg]/ (531 μg/L) = 18.8 L/h. (Note: μg/L = ng/mL and this concentration unit was substituted for Css in the calculations so that unnecessary unit conversion was not required.)

2. *Compute cyclosporine dose.*

   Cyclosporine clearance is used to compute the new dose: D = (Css • Cl • τ)/F = (250 μg/L • 18.8 L/h • 12 h)/(0.3 • 1000 μg/mg) = 188 mg, rounded to 200 mg every 12 hours.

   A steady-state trough cyclosporine serum concentration should be measured after steady-state is attained in 3-5 half-lives. Since the patient is expected to have a half-life equal to 10 hours, the cyclosporine steady-state concentration could be obtained any time after the second day of dosing (5 half-lives = 5 • 10 h = 50 h). Cyclosporine concentrations should also be measured if the patient experiences signs or symptoms of graft rejection, or if the patient develops potential signs or symptoms of cyclosporine toxicity.

7. *Answer to problem 7.*

Pharmacokinetic Dosing Method

1. *Estimate clearance according to disease states and conditions present in the patient.*

   The mean cyclosporine clearance for adult patients is 6 mL/min/kg. The cyclosporine blood clearance for this patient is expected to be 24.1 L/h: Cl = 6 mL/min/kg • 67 kg • (60 min/h/ 1000 mL/L) = 24.1 L/h.

2. *Compute dosage regimen.*

   A 12-hour dosage interval will be used for this patient. (Note: ng/mL = μg/L and this concentration was substituted for Css in the calculations so that unnecessary unit conversion was not required. Also, a conversion constant of 1000 μg/mg is used to change the dose amount to mg.) The dosage equation for oral cyclosporine is: D = (Css • Cl • τ)/F = (200 μg/L • 24.1 L/h • 12 h)/ (0.3 • 1000 μg/mg) = 193 mg, rounded to 200 mg every 12 hours.

   Cyclosporine serum concentrations would be obtained on a daily basis with steady-state expected to occur in about 2 days (5 half-lives = 5 • 10 h = 50 h, or ~2 days).

Literature-Based Recommended Dosing

1. *Choose cyclosporine dose based on disease states and conditions present in the patient and transplant type.*

   The cyclosporine oral dosage range for adult patients is 8-18 mg/kg/d. Because this is a kidney transplant patient, a dose in the lower end of the range (8 mg/kg/d) will be used in order to avoid nephrotoxicity. The initial cyclosporine dose for this patient is 500 mg/d: Dose = 8 mg/ kg/d • 67 kg = 536 mg/d, rounded to 500 mg/d or 200 mg every morning and 300 mg every evening.

   Cyclosporine serum concentrations would be obtained on a daily basis with steady-state expected to occur after 2 days (5 half-lives = 5 • 10 h = 50 h, or ~2 days) of treatment.

8. *Answer to problem 8.*

Linear Pharmacokinetics Method

1. *Compute new dose to achieve the desired concentration.*

   The patient would be expected to achieve steady-state conditions after the second day (5 $t_{1/2}$ = 5 • 10 h = 50 h) of therapy.

   Using linear pharmacokinetics, the new dose to attain the desired concentration should be proportional to the old dose that produced the measured concentration (total daily dose = 200 mg/dose • 2 doses/d = 400 mg/d):

   $$D_{new} = (C_{ss,new}/C_{ss,old})D_{old} = (200 \text{ ng/mL} / 125 \text{ ng/mL}) 400 \text{ mg/d} = 640 \text{ mg/d, rounded to } 600 \text{ mg/d}$$

   The new suggested dose would be 600 mg/d or 300 mg every 12 hours of cyclosporine capsules to be started at the next scheduled dosing time.

   A steady-state trough cyclosporine serum concentration should be measured after steady-state is attained in 3-5 half-lives. Since the patient is expected to have a half-life equal to 10 hours, the cyclosporine steady-state concentration could be obtained any time after the second day of dosing (5 half-lives = 5 • 10 h = 50 h). Cyclosporine concentrations should also be measured if the patient experiences signs or symptoms of graft rejection, or if the patient develops potential signs or symptoms of cyclosporine toxicity.

Pharmacokinetic Parameter Method

1. *Compute pharmacokinetic parameters.*

   The patient would be expected to achieve steady-state conditions after the second day (5 $t_{1/2}$ = 5 • 10 h = 50 h or 2 days) of therapy.

   Cyclosporine clearance can be computed using a steady-state cyclosporine concentration: Cl = [F(D/τ)]/Css = [0.3 • (200 mg/12 h) • 1000 μg/mg]/(125 μg/L) = 40 L/h. (Note: μg/L = ng/mL and this concentration unit was substituted for Css in the calculations so that unnecessary unit conversion was not required.)

2. *Compute cyclosporine dose.*

   Cyclosporine clearance is used to compute the new dose: D = (Css • Cl • τ)/F = (200 μg/L • 40 L/h • 12 h)/(0.3 • 1000 μg/mg) = 320 mg, rounded to 300 mg every 12 hours.

   A steady-state trough cyclosporine serum concentration should be measured after steady-state is attained in 3-5 half-lives. Since the patient is expected to have a half-life equal to 10 hours, the cyclosporine steady-state concentration could be obtained any time after the second day of dosing (5 half-lives = 5 • 10 h = 50 h). Cyclosporine concentrations should also be measured if the patient experiences signs or symptoms of graft rejection, or if the patient develops potential signs or symptoms of cyclosporine toxicity.

9. *Answer to problem 9.*

Bayesian Pharmacokinetic Computer Program

1. *Enter the patient's demographic, drug-dosing, and serum concentration/time data into the computer program.*

2. *Compute pharmacokinetic parameters for the patient using Bayesian pharmacokinetic computer program.*

The pharmacokinetic parameters computed by the program are a volume of distribution of 401 L, a half-life equal to 35 h, and a clearance equal to 8 L/h.

3. *Compute dose required to achieve the desired cyclosporine serum concentrations.*

The one-compartment model first-order absorption equations used by the program to compute doses indicates that a dose of 100 mg every 12 hours will produce a steady-state cyclosporine concentration of 250 ng/mL.

10. *Answer to problem 10.*

Bayesian Pharmacokinetic Computer Program

1. *Enter the patient's demographic, drug-dosing, and serum concentration/time data into the computer program.*

Because the patient is also being treated with phenytoin, an enzyme-induction drug interaction for cyclosporine should be entered into the program at the appropriate place.

2. *Compute pharmacokinetic parameters for the patient using Bayesian pharmacokinetic computer program.*

The pharmacokinetic parameters computed by the program are a volume of distribution of 240 L, a half-life equal to 7 h, and a clearance equal to 23.7 L/h.

3. *Compute dose required to achieve desired cyclosporine serum concentrations.*

The one-compartment model first-order absorption equations used by the program to compute doses indicates that a dose of 400 mg every 12 hours will produce a steady-state cyclosporine concentration of 200 ng/mL.

11. *Answer to problem 11.*

Linear Pharmacokinetics Method

1. *Compute new dose to achieve the desired concentration.*

Using linear pharmacokinetics, the new dose to attain the desired C2 concentration should be proportional to the old dose that produced the measured concentration (total daily dose = 400 mg/dose • 2 doses/d = 800 mg/d):

$$D_{new} = (C_{ss,new}/C_{ss,old})D_{old} = (1000 \text{ ng/mL} / 2124 \text{ ng/mL}) \, 800 \text{ mg/d} = 377 \text{ mg/d, rounded to 400 mg/d}$$

The new suggested dose would be 400 mg/d or 200 mg every 12 hours of cyclosporine capsules to be started at the next scheduled dosing time.

A steady-state trough cyclosporine serum concentration should be measured after steady-state is attained. Cyclosporine concentrations should also be measured if the patient experiences signs or symptoms of graft rejection, or if the patient develops potential signs or symptoms of cyclosporine toxicity.

12. *Answer to problem 12.*

Linear Pharmacokinetics Method

1. *Compute new dose to achieve the desired concentration.*

Using linear pharmacokinetics, the new dose to attain the desired C2 concentration should be proportional to the old dose that produced the measured concentration (total daily dose = 200 mg/dose • 2 doses/d = 400 mg/d):

$$D_{new} = (C_{ss,new}/C_{ss,old})D_{old} = (1100 \text{ ng/mL} / 688 \text{ ng/mL}) \, 400 \text{ mg/d} = 640 \text{ mg/d, rounded to 600 mg/d}$$

The new suggested dose would be 600 mg/d or 300 mg every 12 hours of cyclosporine capsules to be started at the next scheduled dosing time.

A steady-state trough cyclosporine serum concentration should be measured after steady-state is attained. Cyclosporine concentrations should also be measured if the patient experiences signs or symptoms of graft rejection, or if the patient develops potential signs or symptoms of cyclosporine toxicity.

13. *Answer to problem 13.*

Area Under the Concentration-Time Curve Method

1. *Compute pharmacokinetic parameters.*

Cyclosporine AUC_{0-4h} can be estimated using the steady-state cyclosporine concentrations: $AUC_{0-4h} = 256 + C_{1h} + (0.9 \bullet C_{2h}) + (1.4 \bullet C_{3h}) = 256 + (525 \ \mu g/L) + (0.9 \bullet 1399 \ \mu g/L) + (1.4 \bullet 1250 \ \mu g/L) = 3790 \ (\mu g \bullet h)/L$. (Note: $\mu g/L = ng/mL$ and this concentration unit was substituted for Css in the calculations.)

2. *Compute cyclosporine dose.*

Linear pharmacokinetics is used to compute the new dose (total daily dose $= 400$ mg/dose $\bullet$ 2 doses/d $= 800$ mg/d): $D_{new} = (AUC_{new}/AUC_{old})D_{old} = \{[5000 \ (\mu g \bullet h)/L]/[3790 \ (\mu g \bullet h)/L)]\}$ (800 mg/d) $= 1055$ mg/d, rounded to 500 mg every 12 hours.

Steady-state cyclosporine serum concentrations should be measured after steady-state is attained in 3-5 half-lives. Cyclosporine concentrations should also be measured if the patient experiences signs or symptoms of graft rejection, or if the patient develops potential signs or symptoms of cyclosporine toxicity.

REFERENCES

1. Johnson HJ, Schonder KS. Solid-organ transplantation. In: DiPiro JT, Talbert RL, Yee GC, Matzke GR, Wells BG, Posey LM, eds. *Pharmacotherapy*. 8th ed. New York, NY: McGraw-Hill; 2011:1547-1558.
2. Krensky AM, Bennett WM, Vincenti F. Immunosuppressants, tolerogens, and immunostimulants. In: Brunton LL, Lazo JS, Parker KL, eds. *The Pharmacological Basis of Therapeutics*. 12th ed. New York, NY: McGraw-Hill; 2011:1005-1030.
3. Perkins JB, Yee GC. Hematopoietic stem cell transplantation. In: DiPiro JT, Talbert RL, Yee GC, Matzke GR, Wells BG, Posey LM, eds. *Pharmacotherapy*. 8th ed. New York, NY: McGraw-Hill; 2011:2455-2472.
4. Johnston A, Holt DW. Cyclosporine. In: Burton ME, Shaw LM, Schentag JJ, Evans WE, eds. *Applied Pharmacokinetics and Pharmacodynamics*. 4th ed. Philadelphia, PA: Lippincott Williams & Wilkens; 2006:512-528.
5. Min DI. Cyclosporine. In: Schumacher GE, ed. *Therapeutic Drug Monitoring*. Stamford, CT: Appleton & Lange; 1995:449-468.
6. Chandraker A, Milford EL, Sayegh MH. Transplantation in the treatment of renal failure. In: Longo DL, Fauci AS, Kasper DL, Hauser SL, Jameson JL, Loscalzo J, eds. *Principles of Internal Medicine*. 18th ed. New York, NY: McGraw-Hill; 2012:2327-2333.
7. Dienstag JL, Chung RT. Liver transplantation. In: Longo DL, Fauci AS, Kasper DL, Hauser SL, Jameson JL, Loscalzo J, eds. *Principles of Internal Medicine*. 18th ed. New York, NY: McGraw-Hill; 2012:2606-2614.
8. Trulock EP. Lung transplantation. In: Longo DL, Fauci AS, Kasper DL, Hauser SL, Jameson JL, Loscalzo J, eds. *Principles of Internal Medicine*. 18th ed. New York, NY: McGraw-Hill; 2012:2189-2195.
9. Hunt SA, Mallidi HR. Cardiac transplantation and prolonged assisted circulation. In: Longo DL, Fauci AS, Kasper DL, Hauser SL, Jameson JL, Loscalzo J, eds. *Principles of Internal Medicine*. 18th ed. New York, NY: McGraw-Hill; 2012:1916-1919.
10. Appelbaum F. Hematopoietic cell transplantation. In: Longo DL, Fauci AS, Kasper DL, Hauser SL, Jameson JL, Loscalzo J, eds. *Principles of Internal Medicine*. 18th ed. New York, NY: McGraw-Hill; 2012:958-964.
11. Primmett DR, Levine M, Kovarik JM, Mueller EA, Keown PA. Cyclosporine monitoring in patients with renal transplants: two- or three-point methods that estimate area under the curve are superior to trough levels in predicting drug exposure. *Ther Drug Monit.* Jun 1998;20(3):276-283.
12. Morris RG, Russ GR, Cervelli MJ, Juneja R, McDonald SP, Mathew TH. Comparison of trough, 2-hour, and limited AUC blood sampling for monitoring cyclosporin (Neoral) at day 7 post-renal transplantation and incidence of rejection in the first month. *Ther Drug Monit.* Aug 2002;24(4):479-486.

13. Mahalati K, Belitsky P, West K, et al. Approaching the therapeutic window for cyclosporine in kidney transplantation: a prospective study. *J Am Soc Nephrol.* Apr 2001;12(4):828-833.

14. Wacke R, Rohde B, Engel G, et al. Comparison of several approaches of therapeutic drug monitoring of cyclosporin A based on individual pharmacokinetics. *Eur J Clin Pharmacol.* 2000;56:43-48.

15. Grevel J. Area-under-the-curve versus trough level monitoring of cyclosporine concentration: critical assessment of dosage adjustment practices and measurement of clinical outcome. *Ther Drug Monit.* 1993;15(6):488-491.

16. Stefoni S, Midtved K, Cole E, et al. Efficacy and safety outcomes among de novo renal transplant recipients managed by C2 monitoring of cyclosporine a microemulsion: results of a 12-month, randomized, multicenter study. *Transplantation.* Mar 15, 2005; 79(5):577-583.

17. Nashan B, Cole E, Levy G, Thervet E. Clinical validation studies of Neoral C(2) monitoring: a review. *Transplantation.* May 15, 2002;73(suppl 9): 3S-11S.

18. Levy G, Burra P, Cavallari A, et al. Improved clinical outcomes for liver transplant recipients using cyclosporine monitoring based on 2-hr post-dose levels (C2). *Transplantation.* Mar 27, 2002;73(6):953-959.

19. Grant D, Kneteman N, Tchervenkov J, et al. Peak cyclosporine levels (Cmax) correlate with freedom from liver graft rejection: results of a prospective, randomized comparison of neoral and sandimmune for liver transplantation (NOF-8). *Transplantation.* 1999;67(8):1133-1137.

20. Kronbach T, Fischer V, Meyer UA. Cyclosporine metabolism in human liver: identification of a cytochrome P-450III gene family as the major cyclosporine-metabolizing enzyme explains interactions of cyclosporine with other drugs. *Clin Pharmacol Ther.* 1988; 43(6):630-635.

21. Yee GC, Salomon DR. Cyclosporine. In: Evans WE, Schentag JJ, Jusko WJ, Relling MV, eds. *Applied Pharmacokinetics.* 3rd ed. Vancouver, WA: Applied Therapeutics; 1992:28-21-28-40.

22. Grevel J, Welsh MS, Kahan BD. Linear cyclosporine phamacokinetics. *Clin Pharmacol Ther.* 1988;43:175.

23. Lindholm A. Factors influencing the pharmacokinetics of cyclosporine in man. *Ther Drug Monit.* 1991;13(6):465-477.

24. Fahr A. Cyclosporin clinical pharmacokinetics. *Clin Pharmacokinet.* 1993;24(6):472-495.

25. Anon. *Neoral Package Insert.* East Hanover, NJ: Novartis Pharmaceuticals; 2005.

26. Gupta SK, Manfro RC, Tomlanovich SJ, Gambertoglio JG, Garovoy MR, Benet LZ. Effect of food on the pharmacokinetics of cyclosporine in healthy subjects following oral and intravenous administration. *J Clin Pharmacol.* 1990;30(7):643-653.

27. Naoumov NV, Tredger JM, Steward CM, et al. Cyclosporin A pharmacokinetics in liver transplant recipients in relation to biliary T-tube clamping and liver dysfunction. *Gut.* 1989;30(3):391-396.

28. Tredger JM, Naoumov NV, Steward CM, et al. Influence of biliary T tube clamping on cyclosporine pharmacokinetics in liver transplant recipients. *Transplant Proc.* 1988;20(2) suppl 2):512-515.

29. Burckart GJ, Starzl T, Williams L. Cyclosporine monitoring and pharmacokinetics in pediatric liver transplant patients. *Transplant Proc.* 1985;17:1172.

30. Atkinson K, Britton K, Paull P. Detrimental effect of intestinal disease on absorption of orally administered cyclosporine. *Transplant Proc.* 1983;15:2446.

31. Hansten PD, Horn JR. *Drug Interactions Analysis and Management.* St. Louis, MO: Wolters Kluwer; 2014.

32. Wu CY, Benet LZ, Hebert MF, et al. Differentiation of absorption and first-pass gut and hepatic metabolism in humans: studies with cyclosporine. *Clin Pharmacol Ther.* 1995;58(5):492-497.

33. Legg B, Rowland M. Cyclosporin: measurement of fraction unbound in plasma. *J Pharm Pharmacol.* 1987;39(8):599-603.

34. Legg B, Gupta SK, Rowland M, Johnson RW, Solomon LR. Cyclosporin: pharmacokinetics and detailed studies of plasma and erythrocyte binding during intravenous and oral administration. *Eur J Clin Pharmacol.* 1988;34(5):451-460.

35. Lemaire M, Tillement JP. Role of lipoproteins and erythrocytes in the in vitro binding and distribution of cyclosporin A in the blood. *J Pharm Pharmacol.* 1982;34(11):715-718.

36. Rosano TG. Effect of hematocrit on cyclosporine (cyclosporin A) in whole blood and plasma of renal-transplant patients. *Clin Chem.* 1985;31(3):410-412.

37. Sgoutas D, MacMahon W, Love A, Jerkunica I. Interaction of cyclosporin A with human lipoproteins. *J Pharm Pharmacol.* 1986;38(8):583-588.

38. Henricsson S. A new method for measuring the free fraction of cyclosporin in plasma by equilibrium dialysis. *J Pharm Pharmacol.* 1987;39(5):384-385.

39. Ptachcinski RJ, Venkataramanan R, Burckart GJ. Clinical pharmacokinetics of cyclosporin. *Clin Pharmacokinet.* 1986;11(2): 107-132.

40. Flechner SM, Kolbeinsson MC, Lum B, Tam J, Moran T. The effect of obesity on cyclosporine pharmacokinetics in uremic patients. *Transplant Proc.* 1989;21(1, pt 2):1446-1448.

41. Flechner SM, Kolbeinsson ME, Tam J, Lum B. The impact of body weight on cyclosporine pharmacokinetics in renal transplant recipients. *Transplantation.* 1989;47(5):806-810.

42. Flechner SM, Haug M, Fisher RK, Modlin CS. Cyclosporine disposition and long-term renal function in a 500-pound kidney transplant recipient. *Am J Kidney Dis.* 1998;32(4):E4.

43. Yee GC, McGuire TR, Gmur DJ, Lennon TP, Deeg HJ. Blood cyclosporine pharmacokinetics in patients undergoing marrow transplantation. Influence of age, obesity, and hematocrit. *Transplantation.* 1988;46(3):399-402.

44. Yee GC, Lennon TP, Gmur DJ, Cheney CL, Oeser D, Deeg HJ. Effect of obesity on cyclosporine disposition. *Transplantation.* 1988;45(3):649-651.

45. Swan SK, Bennett WM. Drug dosing guidelines in patients with renal failure. *West J Med.* 1992;156(6):633-638.

46. Bennett WM. Guide to drug dosage in renal failure. *Clin Pharmacokinet.* 1988;15(5):326-354.

47. Follath F, Wenk M, Vozeh S, et al. Intravenous cyclosporine kinetics in renal failure. *Clin Pharmacol Ther.* 1983;34(5):638-643.

48. Golper TA, Marx MA. Drug dosing adjustments during continuous renal replacement therapies. *Kidney Int Suppl.* May 1998;66:165S-168S.

49. Golper TA. Update on drug sieving coefficients and dosing adjustments during continuous renal replacement therapies. *Contrib Nephrol.* 2001;(132):349-353.

50. Lindholm A, Henricsson S, Lind M, Dahlqvist R. Intraindividual variability in the relative systemic availability of cyclosporin after oral dosing. *Eur J Clin Pharmacol.* 1988;34(5):461-464.

51. Tschudy MM, Arcara KM. *The Harriet Lane Handbook: A Manual for Pediatric House Officers.* 19th ed. Philadelphia, PA: Mosby; 2012.

52. Keown PA. New concepts in cyclosporine monitoring. *Curr Opin Nephrol Hypertens.* Nov 2002;11(6):619-626.

53. Cole E, Midtvedt K, Johnston A, Pattison J, O'Grady C. Recommendations for the implementation of Neoral C(2) monitoring in clinical practice. *Transplantation.* May 15, 2002;73(suppl 9):19S-22S.

54. Levy G, Thervet E, Lake J, Uchida K. Patient management by Neoral C(2) monitoring: an international consensus statement. *Transplantation.* May 15, 2002;73(suppl 9):12S-18S.

55. Levy GA. C2 monitoring strategy for optimising cyclosporin immunosuppression from the Neoral formulation. *BioDrugs.* 2001;15(5):279-290.

56. Mahalati K, Belitsky P, Sketris I, West K, Panek R. Neoral monitoring by simplified sparse sampling area under the concentration-time curve: its relationship to acute rejection and cyclosporine nephrotoxicity early after kidney transplantation. *Transplantation.* Jul 15, 1999;68(1):55-62.

57. Anderson JE, Munday AS, Kelman AW, et al. Evaluation of a Bayesian approach to the pharmacokinetic interpretation of cyclosporin concentrations in renal allograft recipients. *Ther Drug Monit.* 1994;16(2):160-165.

58. Kahan BD, Kramer WG, Williams C, Wideman CA. Application of Bayesian forecasting to predict appropriate cyclosporine dosing regimens for renal allograft recipients. *Transplant Proc.* 1986;18(6) (suppl 5):200-203.

59. Ruggeri A, Martinelli M. A program for the optimization of cyclosporine therapy using population kinetics modeling. *Comput Methods Programs Biomed.* 2000;61(1):61-69.

60. Wandell M, Mungall D. Computer assisted drug interpretation and drug regimen optimization. *Amer Assoc Clin Chem.* 1984;6:1-11.

19 Tacrolimus

INTRODUCTION

Tacrolimus (also known as FK506) is a macrolide-based calcineurin inhibitor, with immunosuppressant actions, that is used for the prevention of graft rejection in solid organ transplant patients.[1] Currently, it is approved for use in heart, liver, and renal transplant patients. It is also used in lung, heart-lung, and other solid organ transplant recipients, as well as the treatment of graft-versus-host disease in hematopoietic stem cell transplant patients.[1,2] The immunomodulating effects of tacrolimus are due to its ability to block the production of interleukin-2 and other cytokines produced by T lymphocytes.[1-3] Tacrolimus binds to FK-binding protein-12 (FKPB-12), an intracellular cytoplasmic protein found in T cells. The tacrolimus-FKPB complex interacts with calcineurin, inhibits the catalytic activity of calcineurin, and blocks the production of intermediaries involved with the expression of genes regulating the production of cytokines.

THERAPEUTIC AND TOXIC CONCENTRATIONS

The therapeutic range for tacrolimus used by most transplantation centers is 5-20 ng/mL in blood.[1,4,5] Although, plasma tacrolimus concentrations have been measured and an equivalent therapeutic range in this matrix suggested (0.5-2 ng/mL), the most widely used assays for the drug use blood samples.[4,5] Because tacrolimus is extensively bound to erythrocytes, blood concentrations average about 15 times greater than concurrently measured serum or plasma concentrations.[5] Using blood as the assay matrix, specific immuno-assay systems are in widespread use.[6-8] For the purposes of the pharmacokinetic computations and problems presented in this book, tacrolimus concentrations in the blood determined with these specific immunoassay systems or high-pressure liquid chromatography (HPLC) will be used. Because predose trough steady-state concentrations correlate well with steady-state area under the concentration/time curve (AUC) measurements, tacrolimus trough concentrations are used in patient-monitoring situations.[5,9,10]

Desired tacrolimus concentrations differ between the various types of transplants, change with time during the posttransplantation phase, and are determined by protocols specific to the transplantation service and institution.[1,2,11-15] Because of these factors, it is very important for clinicians to be aware of these situations since acceptable tacrolimus concentrations under these different circumstances may be different than those given by the clinical laboratory or those suggested in this textbook.

For patients receiving solid organ transplants such as kidney, liver, heart, lung, or heart-lung transplantation, the goal of tacrolimus therapy is to prevent acute or chronic rejection of the transplanted organ while minimizing drug side effects.[1,12-15] In this case, the recipient's immune system detects foreign antigens on the donor organ which produces an immunologic response against the graft. This leads to inflammatory and cyto-toxic effects directed against the transplanted tissue, and produces the risk of organ tissue damage and failure. In the case of a rejected kidney transplant, it is possible to remove the graft and place the patient on a form of dialysis to sustain their life. However, for other solid organ transplantation patients, graft rejection can result in death. Because tacrolimus can cause nephrotoxicity, some centers delay tacrolimus therapy in renal transplant patients for a few days or until the kidney begins functioning to avoid untoward effects on the newly transplanted organ. Also, desired tacrolimus concentrations in renal transplant patients are generally lower to avoid toxicity in the new renal graft than for other transplant patients (typically 5-15 ng/mL vs 5-20 ng/mL using whole blood). For other solid organ transplant patients, tacrolimus therapy may be started several hours before the surgery. During the immediate postoperative phase, intravenous tacrolimus may be given to these patients. For long-term management of immunosuppression in solid organ tissue transplant patients, tacrolimus doses are gradually tapered to the lowest concentration and dose possible over a 6- to 12-month time period as long as rejection episodes do not occur. In some cases, it may be possible to completely discontinue tacrolimus therapy.

For patients receiving tacrolimus after a hematopoietic stem cell transplant, the goal of therapy is to prevent graft-versus-host disease while avoiding adverse effects of immunosuppressant therapy.[2,11] Graft-versus-host disease is a result of donor T lymphocytes detecting antigens on host tissues and producing an immunologic response against these antigens and host tissues. Acute graft-versus-host disease usually occurs within the first 100 days after transplantation of donor stem cells, and causes epithelial tissue damage in organs. The most common tissues attacked are skin, gastrointestinal tract, and liver. To prevent acute graft-versus-host disease from occurring in allogenic hematopoietic stem cell transplant patients with HLA-matched donors, tacrolimus therapy is usually instituted a few days before or on the day of stem cell transplant (day 0), and doses are adjusted to provide therapeutic trough concentrations. Methotrexate or glucocorticoids are usually also given in conjunction with tacrolimus treatment to hematopoietic stem cell transplantation patients. If prophylaxis of acute graft-versus-host disease is successful, tacrolimus doses are tapered between posttransplant days 50 and 100, with the goal of drug discontinuation by about posttransplant day 180. For allogeneic hematopoietic stem cell transplant patients with HLA-mismatched or HLA-identical unrelated donors, the risk of acute graft-versus-host disease is higher, so tacrolimus therapy may be more prolonged for these patients. After posttransplantation day 100, chronic graft-versus-host disease may occur, and severe cases or patients with systemic signs and symptoms of the disease are usually treated with prednisone. Tacrolimus is used as an adjunctive agent to treat this type of immunologic response.

Neurotoxicity (coma, delirium, psychosis, encephalopathy, seizures, tremor, confusion, headaches, paresthesias, insomnia, nightmares, photophobia, anxiety), nephrotoxicity, hypertension, electrolyte imbalances (hyperkalemia, hypomagnesemia), glucose intolerance, gastrointestinal upset (diarrhea, nausea, vomiting, anorexia), hepatotoxicity, pruritus, alopecia, and leukocytosis are all typical adverse effects of tacrolimus treatment.[1-3] Neurologic side effects tend to be associated with high ($\geq$25 ng/mL) tacrolimus blood concentrations and usually respond to dosage decreases. Hypertension is a common side effect associated with tacrolimus therapy, and is treated with traditional antihypertensive drug therapy. Glucose intolerance can range from mild increases in glucose concentrations to insulin-dependent posttransplant diabetes mellitus in ~10%-20% of patients. Nephrotoxicity is similar to that seen with cyclosporine, and is separated into acute and chronic varieties. Acute nephrotoxicity is concentration- or dose-dependent and reverses with a dosage decrease. Chronic nephrotoxicity is accompanied by kidney tissue damage, including interstitial fibrosis, nonspecific tubular vacuolization, and structural changes in arteries, arterioles, and proximal tubular epithelium. Increased serum creatinine and blood urea nitrogen (BUN) values and hyperkalemia occur with tacrolimus-induced nephrotoxicity. The clinical features of tacrolimus nephrotoxicity and acute graft rejection in renal transplant patients are similar, so renal biopsies may be conducted to differentiate between these possibilities. Because biopsy findings are similar between tacrolimus-induced nephrotoxicity and chronic rejection of kidney transplants, this technique is less helpful in this situation.[1] Dosage decreases may be necessary to limit adverse drug effects associated with tacrolimus therapy.

CLINICAL MONITORING PARAMETERS

Solid organ transplant patients should be monitored for graft rejection consistent with the transplanted organ.[1] For renal transplant patients, increased serum creatinine, azotemia, hypertension, edema, weight gain secondary to fluid retention, graft tenderness, fever, and malaise may be due to an acute rejection episode. Hypertension, proteinuria, a continuous decline in renal function (increases in serum creatinine and blood urea nitrogen levels), and uremia are indicative of chronic rejection in renal transplant patients.[1,15] For hepatic transplant patients, acute rejection signs and symptoms include fever, lethargy, graft tenderness, increased white blood cell count, change in bile color or amount, hyperbilirubinemia, and increased liver function tests. Chronic rejection in a liver transplant patient may be accompanied only by increased liver function tests and jaundice.[1,14] For heart transplant patients, acute rejection is accompanied by low-grade fever, malaise, heart failure (presence of S_3 heart sound), or atrial arrhythmia. Chronic rejection in heart transplant patients, also known as cardiac allograft vasculopathy which is characterized by accelerated coronary artery atherosclerosis, may include the following symptoms: arrhythmias, decreased left ventricular function, heart failure, myocardial infarction, and sudden cardiac death.[1,12] For lung transplant patients, acute rejection may result in no or nonspecific symptoms (cough, dyspnea, hypoxemia, low-grade fever, inspiratory crackles, interstitial infiltrates, declining lung function). Chronic rejection in lung transplant patients, also called bronchiolitis obliterans syndrome, is characterized by decreased airflow and can resemble acute bronchitis.[13] For all solid organ transplant patients, tissue biopsies may be taken from the transplanted tissue to confirm the diagnosis of organ rejection.[1]

Hematopoietic stem cell transplant patients should be monitored for the signs and symptoms associated with graft-versus-host disease.[2,11] These include a generalized maculopapular skin rash, diarrhea, abdominal pain, ileus, hyperbilirubinemia, and increased liver function tests (alkaline phosphatase and serum transaminases). Patients with severe chronic graft-versus-host disease may have involvement of the skin, liver, eyes, mouth, esophagus, or other organs similar to what might be seen with systemic autoimmune diseases.

Typical adverse effects of tacrolimus treatment include neurotoxicity, nephrotoxicity, hypertension, hyperkalemia, hypomagnesemia, glucose intolerance, gastrointestinal upset, hepatotoxicity, pruritus, alopecia, and leukocytosis.[1-3] The management of these more common drug side effects are discussed in the previous section. Other tacrolimus adverse drug reactions that occur less frequently include hyperlipidemia and thrombocytopenia.

Because of the pivotal role that tacrolimus plays as an immunosuppressant in transplant patients, as well as the severity of its concentration- and dose-dependent side effects, tacrolimus concentrations should be measured in every patient receiving the drug. If a patient experiences signs or symptoms of organ rejection or graft-versus-host disease, a tacrolimus concentration should be checked to ensure that levels have not fallen below the therapeutic range. If a patient encounters a possible clinical problem that could be an adverse drug effect of tacrolimus therapy, a tacrolimus concentration should be measured to determine if levels are in the toxic range. During the immediate posttransplantation phase, tacrolimus concentrations are measured daily in most patients even though steady-state may not yet have been achieved in order to prevent acute rejection in solid organ transplant patients or acute graft-versus-host disease in hematopoietic stem cell transplant patients.

After discharge from the hospital, tacrolimus concentrations continue to be obtained at most clinic visits. In patients receiving allogeneic hematopoietic stem cell transplants from HLA-matched donors, it is usually possible to decrease tacrolimus doses and concentrations about 2 months after the transplant and stop tacrolimus therapy altogether after about 6 months posttransplant if no or mild acute rejection episodes have taken place. However, in allogeneic hematopoietic stem cell transplant patients with HLA-mismatched related or HLA-identical unrelated donors and most solid organ transplant patients, chronic tacrolimus therapy is usually required. In these cases, tacrolimus doses and concentrations are decreased to the minimum level required to prevent graft-versus-host reactions or rejection episodes in order to decrease drug adverse effects.

Methods to adjust tacrolimus doses using tacrolimus concentrations are discussed later in this chapter. Because of a good correlation with the tacrolimus steady-state area under the concentration/time curve, pre-dose steady-state trough tacrolimus concentration determinations are used by most transplant centers to adjust drug doses.[5,9,10] Because of the success found in using area under the concentration-time curve (AUC) measurements with cyclosporine, some investigators are beginning to suggest that determination of tacrolimus AUC using multiple concentrations may be a useful monitoring technique.[16-19]

BASIC CLINICAL PHARMACOKINETIC PARAMETERS

Tacrolimus is almost completely eliminated by hepatic metabolism (>99%). Hepatic metabolism is mainly via the CYP3A4 enzyme system, and the drug is a substrate for p-glycoprotein.[20-23] There are more than 15 identified tacrolimus metabolites.[5] None of these metabolites appear to have significant immunosuppressive effects in humans. Most of the metabolites are eliminated in the bile.[24] Less than 1% of a tacrolimus dose is recovered as unchanged drug in the urine.[25]

There is a large amount of intrasubject variability in tacrolimus concentrations obtained on a day-to-day basis, even when the patient should be at steady-state.[5] There are many reasons for this variability. Tacrolimus has low water solubility, and its gastrointestinal absorption can be influenced by many variables. While oral absorption rate is generally fast for most patients (times to maximum concentration between 0.5 and 1 h), some patients absorb tacrolimus very slowly which yields a flat concentration-time profile.[9,25-27] Additionally, absorption lag times of up to 2 hours have been reported in liver transplant patients.[9] While the average oral bioavailability is 25%, there is a large amount of variation in this parameter among patients (4%-89%).[5] Renal transplant patients may have reduced oral bioavailability for tacrolimus. When given with meals, especially with high fat content food, oral bioavailability of tacrolimus decreases.[5] To avoid the possible effect of food on tacrolimus bioavailability, the drug should be given at a constant time in relation to meals. Oral tacrolimus should not be taken with grapefruit juice since this vehicle inhibits CYP3A4 and/or p-glycoprotein contained in the gastrointestinal tract and markedly increases bioavailability.[28] After liver transplantation, bile production and flow may not begin immediately, or bile flow may be diverted from the gastrointestinal tract using a T tube. Unlike cyclosporine, tacrolimus gastrointestinal absorption does not seem to be influenced by the presence or absence of bile.[25,29] Other drug therapy can also increase or decrease the intestinal first-pass clearance of tacrolimus.[28]

Tacrolimus is a low hepatic extraction ratio drug.[5] Because of this, its hepatic clearance is influenced by unbound fraction in the blood (f_B) and intrinsic clearance (Cl'_{int}). Tacrolimus binds primarily to erythrocytes, α_1-acid glycoprotein, and albumin.[30-33] The exact value for protein binding (72%-99%) depends on the technique used and matrix tested, and these factors have resulted in a large range of reported values for unbound fractions in the blood.[5] Erythrocyte concentrations vary in transplant patients, especially those who have received hematopoietic stem cell or kidney transplants. α_1-Acid glycoprotein concentrations also vary greatly among patients. Hepatic intrinsic clearance is different among individuals, and there is a large amount of variability in this value that changes according to the viability of the graft and time after transplantation surgery among individual liver transplant patients. Other drug therapy can also increase or decrease the hepatic intrinsic clearance of tacrolimus.[28] Taking all of these possible factors into consideration that alter absorption and clearance allows one to gain a better appreciation of why tacrolimus concentrations change on a day-to-day basis.

Tacrolimus capsules are available in 0.5, 1, and 5 mg strengths. Tacrolimus injection for intravenous administration is available at a concentration of 5 mg/mL. Before administration, it should be diluted in normal saline or 5% dextrose to a concentration between 0.004 and 0.02 mg/L, and the drug should be given as a continuous infusion. Anaphylactic reactions have occurred with this dosage form, possibly due to the castor oil diluent used to enhance dissolution of the drug. The initial dose of tacrolimus varies greatly among various transplant centers with a range of 0.1-0.3 mg/kg/d given twice daily for orally administered drug and

0.05-0.1 mg/kg/d for intravenously administered drug.[1,5] For patients with liver dysfunction, these doses may be reduced by 25%-50%.[29,34,35] Tacrolimus therapy may be started before the transplantation procedure.[1,2] Recommended initial oral doses of tacrolimus are 0.2 mg/kg/d for adult kidney transplant patients, 0.10-0.15 mg/kg/d for adult liver transplant patients, 0.15-0.2 mg/kg/d for pediatric hepatic transplant recipients, and 0.075 mg/kg/d for adult heart transplant patients. Oral tacrolimus is usually given in two divided daily doses given every 12 hours.

EFFECTS OF DISEASE STATES AND CONDITIONS ON TACROLIMUS PHARMACOKINETICS AND DOSING

Transplantation type does not appear to have a substantial effect on tacrolimus pharmacokinetics.[5] The overall mean for all transplant groups is a clearance of 0.06 L/h/kg, a volume of distribution equal to 1 L/kg, and a half-life of 12 hours for adults.[5] In children (≤16 years old), average clearance and volume of distribution are higher (0.138 L/h/kg and 2.6 L/kg, respectively) but the mean half-life is about the same as adults (12 hours).[5] The determination of tacrolimus half-life is difficult for patients receiving the drug on a twice-daily dosage schedule because only a few concentrations can be measured in the postabsorption, postdistribution phase. These results, as with the other pharmacokinetic parameters discussed in this chapter, are based on specific immunoassay or HPLC results which were conducted using whole blood samples. As discussed in a previous section, concurrently measured plasma or serum concentrations are lower than whole blood concentrations.

Because the drug is primarily eliminated by hepatic metabolism, average clearance is lower (0.04 L/h/kg) in adult patients with liver dysfunction.[29,34,35] Also, mean volume of distribution is larger (3 L/kg) and half-life prolonged and variable (mean = 60 hours, range 28-141 h) in this patient population. Immediately after liver transplantation, tacrolimus metabolism is depressed until the graft begins functioning in a stable manner. Additionally, patients with transient liver dysfunction, regardless of transplantation type, will have decreased tacrolimus clearance and increased half-life values. Renal failure does not significantly change tacrolimus pharmacokinetics, and tacrolimus dosage adjustments are not necessary for patients receiving hemodialysis or peritoneal dialysis.[36,37]

DRUG INTERACTIONS

Compared with cyclosporine, tacrolimus drug interactions are not as well documented, and many drug interactions that are reported with cyclosporine are assumed to also occur with tacrolimus.[28] Drug interactions with tacrolimus fall into two basic categories. The first are agents known to cause nephrotoxicity when administered by themselves. The fear is that administration of a known nephrotoxin with tacrolimus will increase the incidence of renal damage over that observed when tacrolimus or the other agents are given separately. Compounds in this category of drug interactions include aminoglycoside antibiotics, vancomycin, cotrimoxazole (trimethoprim-sulfamethoxazole), amphotericin B, cisplatin, and nonsteroidal anti-inflammatory drugs. Coadministration of tacrolimus with cyclosporine has resulted in augmented nephrotoxic side effects.

The second category of drug interactions involves inhibition or induction of tacrolimus metabolism.[28] Tacrolimus is metabolized by CYP3A4 and is a substrate for p-glycoprotein, so the potential for many pharmacokinetic drug interactions exists with agents that inhibit these pathways or are also cleared by these mechanisms. Because both of these drug elimination systems also exist in the gastrointestinal tract, inhibition drug interactions may also enhance tacrolimus oral bioavailability by diminishing the intestinal and hepatic first-pass effects. Drugs that may inhibit tacrolimus clearance include the calcium channel blockers (verapamil, diltiazem, nicardipine), azole antifungals (fluconazole, itraconazole, ketoconazole), macrolide antibiotics (erythromycin, clarithromycin, troleandomycin), antivirals (indinavir, nelfinavir, ritonavir, saquinavir), steroids (methylprednisolone, oral contraceptives, androgens), and psychotropic agents (fluvoxamine, nefazodone) as well as other compounds (cimetidine, lansoprazole, grapefruit juice). Inducing agents include other antibiotics (nafcillin, caspofungin, rifampin, rifabutin), anticonvulsants (phenytoin, carbamazepine, phenobarbital, primidone), barbiturates, aminoglutethimide, St. John's Wort, sirolimus, and troglitazone. Because of the large number of potentially interacting agents, and the critical nature of the drugs involved in the treatment of transplant patients, complete avoidance of drug interactions with tacrolimus is not possible. Thus, most drug interactions with tacrolimus are managed using appropriate tacrolimus dosage modification with tacrolimus concentration monitoring as a guide.

If given with antacids, tacrolimus concentrations may decrease.[28] The mechanisms of action for this drug interaction appear to be pH-mediated destruction of tacrolimus for sodium bicarbonate or magnesium oxide and physical adsorption of tacrolimus to the antacid for aluminum hydroxide gel. Gastrointestinal prokinetic agents (cisapride, metoclopramide) may increase tacrolimus concentrations. Tacrolimus also has the potential to change the clearance of other drugs via competitive inhibition of CYP3A4 and/or p-glycoprotein.[28]

INITIAL DOSAGE DETERMINATION METHODS

Several methods to initiate tacrolimus therapy are available. The *Pharmacokinetic Dosing method* is the most flexible of the techniques. It allows individualized target serum concentrations to be chosen for a patient, and each pharmacokinetic parameter can be customized to reflect specific disease states and conditions present in the patient. *Literature-based recommended dosing* is a very commonly used method to prescribe initial doses of tacrolimus. Doses are based on those that commonly produce steady-state concentrations in the lower end of the therapeutic range, although there is a wide variation in the actual concentrations for a specific patient.

Pharmacokinetic Dosing Method

The goal of initial dosing of tacrolimus is to compute the best dose possible for the patient in order to prevent graft rejection or graft-versus-host disease given their set of disease states and conditions that influence tacrolimus pharmacokinetics, while avoiding adverse drug reactions. In order to do this, pharmacokinetic parameters for the patient will be estimated using average parameters measured in other patients with similar disease state and condition profiles.

Clearance Estimate

Tacrolimus is almost completely metabolized by the liver. Unfortunately, there is no good way to estimate the elimination characteristics of liver-metabolized drugs using an endogenous marker of liver function in the same fashion that serum creatinine and estimated creatinine clearance are used to estimate the elimination of agents that are renally eliminated. Because of this, a patient is categorized according to the disease states and conditions that are known to change tacrolimus clearance, and the clearance previously measured in these studies is used as an estimate of the current patient's clearance rate. For example, an adult transplant patient with normal liver function would be assigned a tacrolimus clearance rate equal to 0.06 L/h/kg, while a pediatric transplant patient with the same profile would be assumed to have a tacrolimus clearance of 0.138 L/h/kg.

Selection of Appropriate Pharmacokinetic Model and Equations

When given by intravenous infusion or orally, tacrolimus follows a two-compartment model. When oral therapy is chosen, the drug is often erratically absorbed with variable absorption rates. Because of the complex absorption profile and the fact that the drug is usually administered twice daily, a very simple pharmacokinetic equation that calculates the average tacrolimus steady-state concentration (Css in ng/mL = μg/L) is widely used and allows maintenance dose computation: $Css = [F(D/\tau)]/Cl$ or $D = (Css \bullet Cl \bullet \tau)/F$, where F is the bioavailability fraction for the oral dosage form (F averages 0.25 or 25% for most patient populations), D is the dose of tacrolimus in mg, Cl is tacrolimus clearance in L/h, and τ is the dosage interval in hours. If the drug is to be given as a continuous intravenous infusion, the equivalent equation for that route of administration is $Css = k_o/Cl$ or $k_o = Css \bullet Cl$, where k_o is the infusion rate in mg/h.

Steady-State Concentration Selection

The generally accepted therapeutic range for tacrolimus in the blood is 5-20 ng/mL. More important than these general guidelines are the specific requirements for each graft type as defined by the transplant center where the surgery was conducted. Clinicians should become familiar with the tacrolimus protocols used at the various institutions at which they practice. Although it is unlikely that steady-state has been achieved, tacrolimus concentrations are usually obtained on a daily basis, even when dosage changes were made the previous day, due to the critical nature of the therapeutic effect provided by the drug.

EXAMPLE 1 ▶▶▶

HO is a 50-year-old, 75-kg (height = 5 ft 10 in) male renal transplant patient 2 days posttransplant surgery. The patient's liver function tests are normal. Suggest an initial oral tacrolimus dose designed to achieve a steady-state tacrolimus trough blood concentration equal to 15 ng/mL.

1. *Estimate clearance according to disease states and conditions present in the patient.*
The mean tacrolimus clearance for adult patients is 0.06 L/h/kg. The tacrolimus blood clearance for this patient is expected to be 4.5 L/h: Cl = 0.06 L/h/kg $\bullet$ 75 kg = 4.5 L/h.

2. *Compute dosage regimen.*
A 12-hour dosage interval will be used for this patient. (Note: ng/mL = μg/L and this concentration was substituted for Css in the calculations so that unnecessary unit conversion was not required. Also, a conversion constant of 1000 μg/mg is used to change the dose amount to mg.) The dosage equation for oral tacrolimus is:
D = (Css $\bullet$ Cl $\bullet$ τ)/F = (15 μg/L $\bullet$ 4.5 L/h $\bullet$ 12 h)/(0.25 $\bullet$ 1000 μg/mg) = 3.2 mg, rounded to 3 mg every 12 hours.
Tacrolimus concentrations would be obtained on a daily basis with steady-state expected to occur in about 3 days (5 half-lives = 5 $\bullet$ 12 h = 60 h).

EXAMPLE 2 ▶▶▶

Same patient as in example 1, except compute an initial dose using intravenous tacrolimus.

1. *Estimate clearance according to disease states and conditions present in the patient.*
The mean tacrolimus clearance for adult patients is 0.06 L/h/kg. The tacrolimus blood clearance for this patient is expected to be 4.5 L/h: Cl = 0.06 L/h/kg $\bullet$ 75 kg = 4.5 L/h.

2. *Compute dosage regimen.*
A continuous infusion will be used for this patient. (Note: ng/mL = μg/L and this concentration was substituted for Css in the calculations so that unnecessary unit conversion was not required. Also, a conversion constant of 1000 μg/mg is used to change the dose amount to mg.) The dosage equation for intravenous tacrolimus is: k_o = Css $\bullet$ Cl = (15 μg/L $\bullet$ 4.5 L/h)/(1000 μg/mg) = 0.07 mg/h.
Tacrolimus concentrations would be obtained on a daily basis with steady-state expected to occur in about 3 days (5 half-lives = 5 $\bullet$ 12 h = 60 h).

Literature-Based Recommended Dosing

Because of the large amount of variability in tacrolimus pharmacokinetics, even when concurrent disease states and conditions are identified, many clinicians believe that the use of standard tacrolimus doses for various situations is warranted. Indeed, most transplant centers use doses that are determined using a tacrolimus dosage protocol. The original computation of these doses were based on the Pharmacokinetic Dosing method described in the previous section, and subsequently modified based on clinical experience. In general, the expected tacrolimus steady-state concentration used to compute these doses is dependent upon the type of transplanted tissue and the posttransplantation time line. Generally speaking, initial oral doses of 0.1-0.3 mg/kg/d given twice daily are needed to achieve therapeutic tacrolimus steady-state concentrations.[1,5] Usual initial continuous infusion intravenous doses are 0.05-0.1 mg/kg/d.[1,5] For patients with liver dysfunction, these doses may be reduced by 25%-50%.[29,34,35] Initial doses for children undergoing liver transplantation are 0.15-0.2 mg/kg/d orally administered twice daily or 0.03-0.15 mg/kg/d by continuous intravenous infusion. If the drug is started intravenously, pediatric patients are converted to an oral doses as soon as feasible.[38] To illustrate how this technique is used, the same patient examples utilized in the previous section will be repeated for this dosage approach for comparison purposes.

EXAMPLE 3 ▶▶▶

HO is a 50-year-old, 75-kg (height = 5 ft 10 in) male renal transplant patient 2 days posttransplant surgery. The patient's liver function tests are normal. Suggest an initial oral tacrolimus dose designed to achieve a steady-state tacrolimus trough blood concentration within the therapeutic range.

1. *Choose tacrolimus dose based on disease states and conditions present in the patient and transplant type.*
   The tacrolimus oral dosage range for adult patients is 0.1-0.3 mg/kg/d. Because this is a renal transplant patient, a dose in the lower end of the range (0.1 mg/kg/d) will be used in order to avoid nephrotoxicity. The initial tacrolimus dose for this patient is 8 mg/d given as 4 mg every 12 hours: Dose = 0.1 mg/kg/d • 75 kg = 7.5 mg/d, rounded to 8 mg/d or 4 mg every 12 hours

   Tacrolimus concentrations would be obtained on a daily basis with steady-state expected to occur after 3 days (5 half-lives = 5 • 12 h = 60 h) of treatment.

EXAMPLE 4 ▶▶▶

Same patient as in example 3, except compute an initial dose using intravenous tacrolimus.

1. *Choose tacrolimus dose based on disease states and conditions present in the patient and transplant type.*
   The tacrolimus intravenous dosage range for adult patients is 0.03-0.1 mg/kg/d. Because this is a renal transplant patient, a dose in the lower end of the range (0.03 mg/kg/d) will be used in order to avoid nephrotoxicity. The initial tacrolimus intravenous infusion dose for this patient is 0.09 mg/h: Dose = (0.03 mg/kg/d • 75 kg)/(24 h/d) = 0.09 mg/h.

   Tacrolimus concentrations would be obtained on a daily basis with steady-state expected to occur after 3 days (5 half-lives = 5 • 12 h = 60 h) of treatment.

USE OF TACROLIMUS CONCENTRATIONS TO ALTER DOSES

Because of the large amount of pharmacokinetic variability among patients, it is likely that doses computed using patient population characteristics will not always produce tacrolimus concentrations that are expected or desirable. Because of pharmacokinetic variability, the narrow therapeutic index of tacrolimus, and the severity of tacrolimus adverse side effects, measurement of tacrolimus concentrations is mandatory for patients to ensure that therapeutic, nontoxic levels are present. In addition to tacrolimus concentrations, important patient parameters (transplanted organ function tests or biopsies, clinical signs and symptoms of graft rejection or graft-versus-host disease, potential tacrolimus side effects, etc) should be followed to confirm that the patient is responding to treatment and not developing adverse drug reactions.

For most patients, predose steady-state trough tacrolimus concentrations are typically measured. Since alternate methods to monitor cyclosporine concentrations have met with some success, investigators have begun suggesting similar methods for tacrolimus. Of these methods, estimation of tacrolimus area under the concentration-time curve (AUC) using several measured steady-state concentrations is the one that is gaining use in some transplant centers.

When tacrolimus concentrations are measured in patients and a dosage change is necessary, clinicians should seek to use the simplest, most straightforward method available to determine a dose that will provide safe and effective treatment. In most cases, a simple dosage ratio can be used to change tacrolimus doses assuming the drug follows *linear pharmacokinetics*. Sometimes, it is useful to compute tacrolimus pharmacokinetic constants for a patient and base dosage adjustments on these. In this case, it may be possible to calculate and use *pharmacokinetic parameters* to alter the tacrolimus dose. Another approach involves measuring several postdose steady-state tacrolimus concentrations to estimate the *area under the concentration-time curve (AUC)* and adjusting the tacrolimus dose to attain a target AUC. Finally, computerized methods that incorporate expected population pharmacokinetic characteristics (*Bayesian pharmacokinetic computer programs*) can be used in difficult cases where concentrations are obtained at suboptimal times or the patient was not at steady-state when concentrations were measured.

Linear Pharmacokinetics Method

Assuming tacrolimus follows linear, dose-proportional pharmacokinetics,[39] steady-state concentrations change in proportion to dose according to the following equation: $D_{new}/C_{ss,new} = D_{old}/C_{ss,old}$ or $D_{new} = (C_{ss,new}/C_{ss,old})D_{old}$, where D is the dose, Css is the steady-state concentration, old indicates the dose that produced the steady-state concentration that the patient is currently receiving, and new denotes the dose necessary to produce the desired steady-state concentration. The advantages of this method are that it is quick and simple. The disadvantage is steady-state concentrations are required.

EXAMPLE 5 ▶▶▶

LK is a 50-year-old, 75-kg (height = 5 ft 10 in) male renal transplant recipient who is receiving 5 mg every 12 hours of oral tacrolimus capsules. He has normal liver function. The current steady-state tacrolimus blood concentration equals 24 ng/mL. Compute a tacrolimus dose that will provide a steady-state concentration of 15 ng/mL.

1. *Compute new dose to achieve desired concentration.*

The patient would be expected to achieve steady-state conditions after the third day ($5\,t_{1/2} = 5 \bullet 12\,h = 60\,h$) of therapy.

Using linear pharmacokinetics, the new dose to attain the desired concentration should be proportional to the old dose that produced the measured concentration (total daily dose = 5 mg/dose • 2 doses/d = 10 mg/d):

$$D_{new} = (C_{ss,new}/C_{ss,old})D_{old} = (15\ ng/mL\,/\,24\ ng/mL)\ 10\ mg/d = 6.3\ mg/d, \text{ rounded to } 6\ mg/d$$

The new suggested dose would be 6 mg/d or 3 mg every 12 hours of tacrolimus capsules to be started at the next scheduled dosing time.

A steady-state trough tacrolimus concentration should be measured after steady-state is attained in 3-5 half-lives. Since the patient is expected to have a half-life equal to 12 hours, the tacrolimus steady-state concentration could be obtained any time after the third day of dosing (5 half-lives = 5 • 12 h = 60 h). Tacrolimus concentrations should also be measured if the patient experiences signs or symptoms of graft rejection, or if the patient develops potential signs or symptoms of tacrolimus toxicity.

EXAMPLE 6 ▶▶▶

FD is a 60-year-old, 85-kg (height = 6 ft 1 in) male liver transplant patient who is receiving 0.15 mg/h of intravenous tacrolimus as a continuous infusion. The current steady-state tacrolimus concentration equals 9 ng/mL. Compute a tacrolimus dose that will provide a steady-state concentration of 15 ng/mL.

1. *Compute new dose to achieve the desired concentration.*

The patient would be expected to achieve steady-state conditions after the third day (5 $t_{1/2}$ = 5 • 12 h = 60 h) of therapy.

Using linear pharmacokinetics, the new dose to attain the desired concentration should be proportional to the old dose that produced the measured concentration:

$$D_{new} = (C_{ss,new}/C_{ss,old})D_{old} = (15 \text{ ng/mL} / 9 \text{ ng/mL}) \, 0.15 \text{ mg/h} = 0.25 \text{ mg/h}$$

A tacrolimus concentration should be measured after steady-state is attained in 3-5 half-lives. Since the patient is expected to have a half-life equal to 12 hours, the tacrolimus steady-state concentration could be obtained any time after the third day of dosing (5 half-lives = 5 • 12 h = 60 h). Tacrolimus concentrations should also be measured if the patient experiences signs or symptoms of graft rejection, or if the patient develops potential signs or symptoms of tacrolimus toxicity.

Pharmacokinetic Parameter Method

The Pharmacokinetic Parameter method of adjusting drug doses was among the first techniques available to change doses using drug concentrations. It allows the computation of an individual's own, unique pharmacokinetic constants and uses those to calculate a dose that achieves desired tacrolimus concentrations. The pharmacokinetic parameter method requires that steady-state has been achieved and uses only a steady-state tacrolimus concentration. Tacrolimus clearance can be measured using a single steady-state tacrolimus concentration and the following formula for orally administered drug: $Cl = [F(D/\tau)]/Css$, where Cl is tacrolimus clearance in L/h, F is the bioavailability factor for tacrolimus (F = 0.25), τ is the dosage interval in hours, and Css is the tacrolimus steady-state concentration in ng/mL, which also equals μg/L. If tacrolimus is administered intravenously, it is not necessary to take bioavailability into account: $Cl = k_o/Css$, where Cl is tacrolimus clearance in L/h, k_o is the tacrolimus infusion rate in mg/h, and Css is the tacrolimus steady-state concentration in ng/mL which also equals μg/L. Although this method does allow computation of tacrolimus clearance, it yields exactly the same tacrolimus dose as that supplied using linear pharmacokinetics. As a result, most clinicians prefer to directly calculate the new dose using the Simpler Linear Pharmacokinetics method. To demonstrate this point, the patient cases used to illustrate the Linear Pharmacokinetics method will be used as examples for the Pharmacokinetic Parameter method.

EXAMPLE 7 ▶▶▶

LK is a 50-year-old, 75-kg (height = 5 ft 10 in) male renal transplant recipient who is receiving 5 mg every 12 hours of oral tacrolimus capsules. He has normal liver function. The current steady-state tacrolimus blood concentration equals 24 ng/mL. Compute a tacrolimus dose that will provide a steady-state concentration of 15 ng/mL.

1. *Compute pharmacokinetic parameters.*

The patient would be expected to achieve steady-state conditions after the third day (5 $t_{1/2}$ = 5 • 12 h = 60 h) of therapy.

Tacrolimus clearance can be computed using a steady-state tacrolimus concentration:

$$Cl = [F(D/\tau)]/Css = [0.25 \bullet (5 \text{ mg}/12 \text{ h}) \bullet 1000 \text{ } \mu g/mg]/(24 \text{ } \mu g/L) = 4.3 \text{ L/h}.$$

(Note: $\mu g/L$ = ng/mL and this concentration unit was substituted for Css in the calculations so that unnecessary unit conversion was not required.)

2. *Compute tacrolimus dose.*

Tacrolimus clearance is used to compute the new dose: D = (Css • Cl • τ)/F = (15 $\mu g/L$ • 4.3 L/h • 12 h)/(0.25 • 1000 $\mu g/mg$) = 3.1 mg, rounded to 3 mg every 12 hours.

A steady-state trough tacrolimus concentration should be measured after steady-state is attained in 3-5 half-lives. Since the patient is expected to have a half-life equal to 12 hours, the tacrolimus steady-state concentration could be obtained any time after the third day of dosing (5 half-lives = 5 • 12 h = 60 h). Tacrolimus concentrations should also be measured if the patient experiences signs or symptoms of graft rejection, or if the patient develops potential signs or symptoms of tacrolimus toxicity.

EXAMPLE 8 ▶▶▶

FD is a 60-year-old, 85-kg (height = 6 ft 1 in) male liver transplant patient who is receiving 0.15 mg/h of intravenous tacrolimus as a continuous infusion. The current steady-state tacrolimus concentration equals 9 ng/mL. Compute a tacrolimus dose that will provide a steady-state concentration of 15 ng/mL.

1. *Compute pharmacokinetic parameters.*

The patient would be expected to achieve steady-state conditions after the third day (5 $t_{1/2}$ = 5 • 12 h = 60 h) of therapy.

Tacrolimus clearance can be computed using a steady-state tacrolimus concentration: Cl = k_0/Css = (0.15 mg/h • 1000 $\mu g/mg$)/(9 $\mu g/L$) = 16.7 L/h.

(Note: $\mu g/L$ = ng/mL and this concentration unit was substituted for Css in the calculations so that unnecessary unit conversion was not required.)

2. *Compute tacrolimus dose.*

Tacrolimus clearance is used to compute the new dose: k_0 = Css • Cl = (15 $\mu g/L$ • 16.7 L/h)/1000 $\mu g/mg$ = 0.25 mg/h.

A steady-state trough tacrolimus concentration should be measured after steady-state is attained in 3-5 half-lives. Since the patient is expected to have a half-life equal to 12 hours, the tacrolimus steady-state concentration could be obtained any time after the third day of dosing (5 half-lives = 5 • 12 h = 60 h). Tacrolimus concentrations should also be measured if the patient experiences signs or symptoms of graft rejection, or if the patient develops potential signs or symptoms of tacrolimus toxicity.

Area Under the Concentration-Time Curve Method

Some solid organ transplant centers believe that measurement or estimation of tacrolimus area under the concentration-time curve (AUC) is the best way to optimize tacrolimus therapy. While AUC can be measured using hourly postdose tacrolimus levels, studies have shown that there is a strong correlation between 3 and 4 tacrolimus concentrations and the total AUC. Based on this finding, most centers utilizing this method measure several steady-state tacrolimus concentrations and use a published regression equation determined in other patients receiving the same transplanted organ and similar drug therapy (to account for possible drug interactions) in order to convert the concentrations to an estimated AUC. Then, if necessary, adjust the tacrolimus dose using linear pharmacokinetics to achieve the target AUC: $D_{new}/AUC_{new} = D_{old}/AUC_{old}$ or $D_{new} = (AUC_{new}/AUC_{old})D_{old}$, where D is the dose, AUC is the steady-state area under the concentration-time curve, old indicates the dose that produced the steady-state area under the concentration-time curve that the patient is currently receiving, and new denotes the dose necessary to produce the desired steady-state area under the concentration-time curve.

There are many regression equations from which to choose based on the target transplant population and other concurrent therapy that may cause drug interactions with tacrolimus. The one used for the examples and problems in this book is for renal transplant patients treated with tacrolimus for at least 6 months that received other immunosuppressants (prednisone plus azathioprine).[19] In this investigation, the steady-state AUC over the dosage interval [from time 0 hours (predose) to 12 hours after the dose, AUC_{0-12h}] strongly correlated with four steady-state concentrations, and this relationship was used to adjust tacrolimus doses: AUC_{0-12h} (in [ng • h]/mL) = $10 + (1.4 • C_{0h}) + (0.8 • C_{1h}) + (1.6 • C_{2h}) + (5.5 • C_{4h})$, where C_{0h}, C_{1h}, C_{2h}, C_{4h} are steady-state tacrolimus concentrations in ng/mL obtained 0, 1, 2, and 4 hours, respectively, after a dose. The dose is then adjusted to produce a new steady-state AUC_{0-12h} equal to 104 ± 33 (ng • h)/mL using linear pharmacokinetics.[18]

EXAMPLE 9 ▶▶▶

DR is a 47-year-old, 78-kg (height = 6 ft 1 in) male who has undergone renal transplantation. He is receiving 5 mg every 12 hours of oral tacrolimus. The following tacrolimus steady-state concentrations have been measured to determine an estimated AUC_{0-12h}: C_{0h} = 4 ng/mL, C_{1h} = 8 ng/mL, C_{2h} = 10 ng/mL, C_{3h} = 8 ng/mL. Compute a tacrolimus dose that will provide a steady-state AUC_{0-12h} of 100 (ng • h)/mL.

1. *Compute pharmacokinetic parameters.*

Tacrolimus AUC_{0-12h} can be estimated using the steady-state tacrolimus concentrations: AUC_{0-12h} [in (ng • h)/mL] = $10 + (1.4 • C_{0h}) + (0.8 • C_{1h}) + (1.6 • C_{2h}) + (5.5 • C_{4h})$ = $10 + (1.4 • 4$ ng/mL$) + (0.8 • 8$ ng/mL$) + (1.6 • 10$ ng/mL$) + (5.5 • 8$ ng/mL$)$ = 82 (ng • h)/mL.

2. *Compute tacrolimus dose.*

Linear pharmacokinetics is used to compute the new dose (total daily dose = 5 mg/dose • 2 doses/d = 10 mg/d): $D_{new} = (AUC_{new}/AUC_{old})D_{old}$ = {[100 (ng • h)/mL]/[82 (ng • h)/mL)]}(10 mg/d) = 12 mg/d, or 6 mg every 12 hours.

Steady-state tacrolimus serum concentrations should be measured after steady-state is attained in 3-5 half-lives. Tacrolimus concentrations should also be measured if the patient experiences signs or symptoms of graft rejection, or if the patient develops potential signs or symptoms of tacrolimus toxicity.

BAYESIAN PHARMACOKINETIC COMPUTER PROGRAMS

Computer programs are available that can assist in the computation of pharmacokinetic parameters for patients. The most reliable computer programs use a nonlinear regression algorithm that incorporates components of Bayes theorem. Nonlinear regression is a statistical technique that uses an iterative process to compute the best pharmacokinetic parameters for a concentration/time data set. Briefly, the patient's drug dosage schedule and drug concentrations are input into the computer. The computer program has a pharmacokinetic equation pre-programmed for the drug and administration method (oral, intravenous bolus, intravenous infusion, etc). Typically, a one-compartment model is used; although some programs allow the user to choose among several different equations. Using population estimates based on demographic information for the patient (age, weight, gender, liver function, cardiac status, etc) supplied by the user, the computer program then computes estimated drug concentrations at each time there are actual drug concentrations. Kinetic parameters are then changed by the computer program, and a new set of estimated drug concentrations are computed. The pharmacokinetic parameters that generated the estimated drug concentrations closest to the actual values are remembered by the computer program, and the process is repeated until the set of pharmacokinetic parameters that result in esti-mated drug concentrations that are statistically closest to the actual drug concentrations are generated. These pharmacokinetic parameters can then be used to compute improved dosing schedules for patients. Bayes theorem is used in the computer algorithm to balance the results of the computations between values based solely on the patient's drug concentrations and those based only on patient population parameters. Results from studies that compare various methods of dosage adjustment have consistently found that these types of computer dosing programs perform at least as well as experienced clinical pharmacokineticists and clinicians and better than inexperienced clinicians.

Some clinicians use Bayesian pharmacokinetic computer programs exclusively to alter drug doses based on drug concentrations. An advantage of this approach is that consistent dosage recommendations are made when several different practitioners are involved in therapeutic drug-monitoring programs. However, since simpler dosing methods work just as well for patients with stable pharmacokinetic parameters and steady-state drug concentrations, many clinicians reserve the use of computer programs for more difficult situations. Those situations include drug concentrations that are not at steady-state, drug concentrations not obtained at the specific times needed to employ simpler methods, and unstable pharmacokinetic parameters. When only a limited number of tacrolimus steady-state concentrations are available, Bayesian pharmacokinetic com-puter programs can be used to compute a complete patient pharmacokinetic profile that includes clearance, volume of distribution, and half-life. Many Bayesian pharmacokinetic computer programs are available to users, and most should provide answers similar to the one used in the following examples.[40]

EXAMPLE 10 ▶▶▶

LK is a 50-year-old, 75-kg (height = 5 ft 10 in) male renal transplant recipient who is receiving 5 mg every 12 hours of oral tacrolimus capsules. He has normal liver (bilirubin = 0.7 mg/dL, albumin = 4.0 g/dL). The current steady-state tacrolimus blood concentration equals 24 ng/mL. Compute a tacrolimus dose that will provide a steady-state concentration of 15 ng/mL.

1. *Enter the patient's demographic, drug-dosing, and concentration/time data into the computer program.*

2. *Compute pharmacokinetic parameters for the patient using Bayesian pharmacokinetic computer program.*
   The pharmacokinetic parameters computed by the program are a volume of distribution of 76 L, a half-life equal to 15.8 h, and a clearance equal to 3.3 L/h.

3. *Compute dose required to achieve the desired tacrolimus concentrations.*
   The one-compartment model first-order absorption equations used by the program to compute doses indi-cates that a dose of 2 mg every 12 hours will produce a steady-state tacrolimus concentration of 15 ng/mL. Using the Linear Pharmacokinetics and Pharmacokinetic Parameter methods previously described in the chapter produced a similar answer for this patient.

EXAMPLE 11 ▶▶▶

FD is a 60-year-old, 85-kg (height = 6 ft 1 in) male liver transplant patient who is receiving 0.15 mg/h of intravenous tacrolimus as a continuous infusion. He has normal liver function tests (bilirubin = 1.1 mg/dL, albumin = 3.5 g/dL). The current steady-state tacrolimus concentration equals 9 ng/mL. Compute a tacrolimus dose that will provide a steady-state concentration of 15 ng/mL.

1. *Enter the patient's demographic, drug-dosing, and concentration/time data into the computer program.*
2. *Compute pharmacokinetic parameters for the patient using Bayesian pharmacokinetic computer program.*
   The pharmacokinetic parameters computed by the program are a volume of distribution of 85 L, a half-life equal to 3.6 h, and a clearance equal to 16.3 L/h.
3. *Compute dose required to achieve the desired tacrolimus concentrations.*
   The one-compartment model continuous infusion equations used by the program to compute doses indicates that a dose of 0.24 mg/h will produce a steady-state tacrolimus concentration of 15 ng/ml. Using the Linear Pharmacokinetics and Pharmacokinetic Parameter methods previously described in the chapter produced a similar answer for this patient.

EXAMPLE 12 ▶▶▶

YT is a 25-year-old, 55-kg (height = 5 ft 2 in) female renal transplant recipient who received 4 mg every 12 hours of oral tacrolimus capsules for two doses after transplant, but because her renal function decreased, her dose was empirically changed to 2 mg every 12 hours. She has normal liver function (bilirubin = 0.9 mg/dL, albumin = 3.9 g/dL). The tacrolimus blood concentration obtained 12 hours after her first dose of the lower dosage regimen equaled 22 ng/mL. Compute a tacrolimus dose that will provide a steady-state concentration of 15 ng/mL.

1. *Enter the patient's demographic, drug-dosing, and concentration/time data into the computer program.*
2. *Compute pharmacokinetic parameters for the patient using Bayesian pharmacokinetic computer program.*
   The pharmacokinetic parameters computed by the program are a volume of distribution of 54 L, a half-life equal to 1.8 h, and a clearance equal to 21 L/h.
3. *Compute dose required to achieve the desired tacrolimus concentrations.*
   The one-compartment model first-order absorption equations used by the program to compute doses indicates that a dose of 1 mg every 12 hours will produce a steady-state tacrolimus concentration of 15 ng/mL.

DOSING STRATEGIES

Initial dose and dosage adjustment techniques using serum concentrations can be used in any combination as long as the limitations of each method are observed. Some dosing schemes link together logically when considered according to their basic approaches or philosophies. Dosage strategies that follow similar pathways are given in Table 19-1.

TABLE 19-1   Dosing Strategies

Dosing Approach/Philosophy	Initial Dosing	Use of Serum Concentrations to Alter Doses
Pharmacokinetic parameter/equations	Pharmacokinetic Dosing method	Pharmacokinetic Parameter method
Literature-based concept	Literature-based Recommended Dosing method	Linear Pharmacokinetics or area under the concentration-time curve (AUC) method
Computerized	Bayesian computer program	Bayesian computer program

PROBLEMS

The following problems are intended to emphasize the computation of initial and individualized doses using clinical pharmacokinetic techniques. Clinicians should always consult the patient's chart to confirm that current immunosuppressive therapy is appropriate. Additionally, all other medications that the patient is taking, including prescription and nonprescription drugs, should be noted and checked to ascertain if a potential drug interaction with tacrolimus exists.

1. VI is a 37-year-old, 85-kg (height = 6 ft 1 in) male heart transplant patient who requires therapy with oral tacrolimus. He has normal liver function. Suggest an initial dosage regimen designed to achieve a steady-state tacrolimus concentration equal to 15 ng/mL.

2. Patient VI (see problem 1) was prescribed 5 mg every 12 hours of tacrolimus capsules for 4 days, and the steady-state tacrolimus concentration equals 28 ng/mL. The patient is assessed to be compliant with his dosage regimen. Suggest a tacrolimus dosage regimen designed to achieve a steady-state tacrolimus concentration of 15 ng/mL.

3. AS is a 9-year-old, 35-kg female (height = 4 ft 6 in) hematopoietic stem cell transplantation patient who requires therapy with oral tacrolimus. She has normal liver function. Suggest an initial tacrolimus dosage regimen designed to achieve a steady-state tacrolimus concentration equal to 12 ng/mL.

4. Patient AS (see problem 3) was prescribed 3 mg every 12 hours of tacrolimus capsules for 3 days, and the steady-state tacrolimus concentration equals 9 ng/mL. The patient is assessed to be compliant with her dosage regimen. Suggest an oral tacrolimus dosage regimen designed to achieve a steady-state tacrolimus concentration equal to 12 ng/mL.

5. FL is a 29-year-old, 78-kg (height = 5 ft 11 in) male liver transplant patient who requires therapy with oral tacrolimus. He has poor liver function because of his liver disease. Suggest an initial tacrolimus dosage regimen to be started 24 hours before transplant surgery designed to achieve a steady-state tacrolimus concentration equal to 15 ng/mL.

6. Patient FL (see problem 5) is 10 days postsurgery for a liver transplantation. He was prescribed 4 mg every 12 hours of tacrolimus capsules since transplantation, and the steady-state tacrolimus concentration equals 33 ng/mL. The patient is assessed to be compliant with his dosage regimen. Suggest a tacrolimus dosage regimen designed to achieve a steady-state tacrolimus concentration of 15 ng/mL.

7. PH is a 22-year-old, 67-kg female (height = 5 ft 5 in) renal transplant patient who requires therapy with oral tacrolimus. She is 36 hours posttransplantation procedure, and the transplanted kidney is beginning to function normally. Her liver function is normal. Suggest an initial tacrolimus dosage regimen designed to achieve a steady-state tacrolimus concentration equal to 15 ng/mL.

8. Patient PH (see problem 7) was prescribed 3 mg every 12 hours of tacrolimus capsules for 3 days, and the steady-state tacrolimus concentration equals 11 ng/mL. The patient is assessed to be compliant with her dosage regimen. Suggest a tacrolimus dosage regimen designed to achieve a steady-state tacrolimus concentration of 15 ng/mL.

9. PU is a 55-year-old, 68-kg (height = 5 ft 8 in) male heart transplant patient who received a continuous intravenous infusion of tacrolimus (0.25 mg/h for 24 hours) and was switched to oral tacrolimus capsules 3 mg every 12 hours. He has normal liver (bilirubin = 0.7 mg/dL, albumin = 4.0 g/dL) function. The tacrolimus concentration equals 25 ng/mL 12 hours after the first oral dose of the drug. Compute a tacrolimus dose that will provide a steady-state concentration of 20 ng/mL.

10. LH is a 25-year-old, 60-kg (height = 5 ft 3 in) female renal transplant patient who was given a new prescription for tacrolimus capsules 4 mg every 12 hours 2 days after transplantation surgery. She has normal liver function (bilirubin = 0.4 mg/dL, albumin = 3.7 g/dL) and is also being treated with phenytoin. The trough tacrolimus concentration before the fourth dose equals 10 ng/mL. Compute a tacrolimus dose that will provide a steady-state concentration of 20 ng/mL.

11. GY is a 36-year-old, 71-kg (height = 5 ft 11 in) male who has undergone renal transplantation. He is receiving 8 mg every 12 hours of oral tacrolimus. The following tacrolimus steady-state concentrations have been measured to determine an estimated AUC_{0-12h}: C_{0h} = 6 ng/mL, C_{1h} = 13 ng/mL, C_{2h} = 16 ng/mL, C_{3h} = 12 ng/mL. Compute a tacrolimus dose that will provide a steady-state AUC_{0-12h} of 100 (ng • h)/mL.

ANSWERS TO PROBLEMS

1. *Answer to problem 1.*

Pharmacokinetic Dosing Method

1. *Estimate clearance according to disease states and conditions present in the patient.*

   The mean tacrolimus clearance for adult patients is 0.06 L/h/kg. The tacrolimus blood clearance for this patient is expected to be: Cl = 0.06 L/h/kg • 85 kg = 5.1 L/h.

2. *Compute dosage regimen.*

   A 12-hour dosage interval will be used for this patient. (Note: ng/mL = µg/L and this concentration was substituted for Css in the calculations so that unnecessary unit conversion was not required. Also, a conversion constant of 1000 µg/mg is used to change the dose amount to mg.) The dosage equation for oral tacrolimus is: D = (Css • Cl • τ)/F = (15 µg/L • 5.1 L/h • 12 h)/(0.25 • 1000 µg/mg) = 3.7 mg, rounded to 4 mg every 12 hours.

   Tacrolimus concentrations would be obtained on a daily basis with steady-state expected to occur after about 3 days of therapy (5 half-lives = 5 • 12 h = 60 h).

Literature-Based Recommended Dosing

1. *Choose tacrolimus dose based on disease states and conditions present in the patient and transplant type.*

   The tacrolimus oral dosage range for adult patients is 0.1-0.3 mg/kg/d. Because this is a heart transplant patient, a dose in the middle of the range (0.15 mg/kg/d) will be used in order to avoid graft rejection. The initial tacrolimus dose for this patient is: Dose = 0.15 mg/kg/d • 85 kg = 12.8 mg/d, rounded to 12 mg/d or 6 mg every 12 hours.

   Tacrolimus concentrations would be obtained on a daily basis with steady-state expected to occur after 3 days (5 half-lives = 5 • 12 h = 60 h) of treatment.

2. *Answer to problem 2.*

Linear Pharmacokinetics Method

1. *Compute new dose to achieve desired concentration.*

   The patient would be expected to achieve steady-state conditions after the third day (5 $t_{1/2}$ = 5 • 12 h = 60 h) of therapy.

   Using linear pharmacokinetics, the new dose to attain the desired concentration should be proportional to the old dose that produced the measured concentration (total daily dose = 5 mg/dose • 2 doses/d = 10 mg/d):

   $$D_{new} = (C_{ss,new}/C_{ss,old})D_{old} = (15 \text{ ng/mL}/28 \text{ ng/mL}) \ 10 \text{ mg/d} = 5.4 \text{ mg/d, rounded to 6 mg/d}$$

   The new suggested dose would be 6 mg/d or 3 mg every 12 hours of tacrolimus capsules to be started at the next scheduled dosing time.

A steady-state trough tacrolimus concentration should be measured after steady-state is attained in 3-5 half-lives. Since the patient is expected to have a half-life equal to 12 hours, the tacrolimus steady-state concentration could be obtained any time after the third day of dosing (5 half-lives = 5 • 12 h = 60 h). Tacrolimus concentrations should also be measured if the patient experiences signs or symptoms of graft rejection, or if the patient develops potential signs or symptoms of tacrolimus toxicity.

Pharmacokinetic Parameter Method

1. *Compute pharmacokinetic parameters.*

The patient would be expected to achieve steady-state conditions after the third day (5 $t_{1/2}$ = 5 • 12 h = 60 h) of therapy.

Tacrolimus clearance can be computed using a steady-state tacrolimus concentration: Cl = [F(D/τ)]/Css = [0.25 • (5 mg/12 h) • 1000 μg/mg]/(28 μg/L) = 3.7 L/h. (Note: μg/L = ng/mL and this concentration unit was substituted for Css in the calculations so that unnecessary unit conversion was not required).

2. *Compute tacrolimus dose.*

Tacrolimus clearance is used to compute the new dose: D = (Css • Cl • τ)/F = (15 μg/L • 3.7 L/h • 12 h)/(0.25 • 1000 μg/mg) = 2.7 mg, rounded to 3 mg every 12 hours.

A steady-state trough tacrolimus concentration should be measured after steady-state is attained in 3-5 half-lives. Since the patient is expected to have a half-life equal to 12 hours, the tacrolimus steady-state concentration could be obtained any time after the third day of dosing (5 half-lives = 5 • 12 h = 60 h). Tacrolimus concentrations should also be measured if the patient experiences signs or symptoms of graft rejection, or if the patient develops potential signs or symptoms of tacrolimus toxicity.

3. *Answer to problem 3.*

Pharmacokinetic Dosing Method

1. *Estimate clearance according to disease states and conditions present in the patient.*

The mean tacrolimus clearance for pediatric patients is 0.138 L/h/kg. The tacrolimus blood clearance for this patient is expected to be: Cl = 0.138 L/h/kg • 35 kg = 4.8 L/h.

2. *Compute dosage regimen.*

A 12-hour dosage interval will be used for this patient. (Note: ng/mL = μg/L and this concentration was substituted for Css in the calculations so that unnecessary unit conversion was not required. Also, a conversion constant of 1000 μg/mg is used to change the dose amount to mg.) The dosage equation for oral tacrolimus is: D = (Css • Cl • τ)/F = (12 μg/L • 4.8 L/h • 12 h)/(0.25 • 1000 μg/mg) = 2.8 mg, rounded to 3 mg every 12 hours of tacrolimus capsules.

Tacrolimus concentrations would be obtained on a daily basis with steady-state expected to occur after about 3 days (5 half-lives = 5 • 12 h = 60 h).

Literature-Based Recommended Dosing

1. *Choose tacrolimus dose based on disease states and conditions present in the patient and transplant type.*

The tacrolimus oral dosage range is 0.1-0.3 mg/kg/d. Because this is a pediatric patient, a dose in the middle of the range (0.15 mg/kg/d) will be used in order to avoid graft-versus-host disease. The initial tacrolimus dose for this patient is: Dose = 0.15 mg/kg/d • 35 kg = 5.3 mg/d, rounded to 6 mg/d or 3 mg every 12 hours of tacrolimus capsules.

Tacrolimus concentrations would be obtained on a daily basis with steady-state expected to occur after about 3 days (5 half-lives = 5 • 12 h = 60 h) of treatment.

4. *Answer to problem 4.*

Linear Pharmacokinetics Method

1. *Compute new dose to achieve desired concentration.*

The patient would be expected to achieve steady-state conditions by the third day (5 $t_{1/2}$ = 5 • 12 h = 60 h) of therapy.

Using linear pharmacokinetics, the new dose to attain the desired concentration should be proportional to the old dose that produced the measured concentration (total daily dose = 3 mg/dose • 2 doses/d = 6 mg/d):

$$D_{new} = (C_{ss,new}/C_{ss,old})D_{old} = (12 \text{ ng/mL}/9 \text{ ng/mL}) \ 6 \text{ mg/d} = 8 \text{ mg/d}$$

The new suggested dose would be 8 mg/d or 4 mg every 12 hours of tacrolimus capsules to be started at the next scheduled dosing time.

A steady-state trough tacrolimus concentration should be measured after steady-state is attained in 3-5 half-lives. Since the patient is expected to have a half-life equal to 12 hours, the tacrolimus steady-state concentration could be obtained any time after the third day of dosing (5 half-lives = 5 • 12 h = 60 h). Tacrolimus concentrations should also be measured if the patient experiences signs or symptoms of graft rejection, or if the patient develops potential signs or symptoms of tacrolimus toxicity.

Pharmacokinetic Parameter Method

1. *Compute pharmacokinetic parameters.*

The patient would be expected to achieve steady-state conditions after the third day (5 $t_{1/2}$ = 5 • 12 h = 60 h) of therapy.

Tacrolimus clearance can be computed using a steady-state tacrolimus concentration: Cl = [F(D/τ)]/Css = [0.25 • (3 mg/12 h) •1000 μg/mg]/(9 μg/L) = 6.9 L/h. (Note: μg/L = ng/mL and this concentration unit was substituted for Css in the calculations so that unnecessary unit conversion was not required.)

2. *Compute tacrolimus dose.*

Tacrolimus clearance is used to compute the new dose: D = (Css • Cl • τ)/F = (12 μg/L • 6.9 L/h • 12 h)/(0.25 • 1000 μg/mg) = 4 mg, given as 4 mg every 12 hours of tacrolimus capsules.

A steady-state trough tacrolimus concentration should be measured after steady-state is attained in 3-5 half-lives. Since the patient is expected to have a half-life equal to 12 hours, the tacrolimus steady-state concentration could be obtained any time after the third day of dosing (5 half-lives = 5 • 12 h = 60 h). Tacrolimus concentrations should also be measured if the patient experiences signs or symptoms of graft rejection, or if the patient develops potential signs or symptoms of tacrolimus toxicity.

5. *Answer to problem 5.*

Pharmacokinetic Dosing Method

1. *Estimate clearance according to disease states and conditions present in the patient.*

The mean tacrolimus clearance for adult patients with liver dysfunction is 0.04 L/h/kg. The tacrolimus blood clearance for this patient is expected to be: Cl = 0.04 L/h/kg • 78 kg = 3.1 L/h.

2. *Compute dosage regimen.*

A 12-hour dosage interval will be used for this patient. (Note: ng/mL = μg/L and this concentration was substituted for Css in the calculations so that unnecessary unit conversion was not required. Also, a conversion constant of 1000 μg/mg is used to change the dose amount to mg.) The dosage equation for oral tacrolimus is: D = (Css • Cl • τ)/F = (15 μg/L • 3.1 L/h • 12 h)/ (0.25 • 1000 μg/mg) = 2.2 mg, rounded to 2 mg every 12 hours.

Tacrolimus concentrations would be obtained on a daily basis with steady-state expected to occur after about 12 days of therapy (5 half-lives = 5 • 60 h = 300 h or 12.5 d). However, this patient is scheduled to receive his transplant the next day.

Literature-Based Recommended Dosing

1. *Choose tacrolimus dose based on disease states and conditions present in the patient and transplant type.*

The tacrolimus oral dosage range for adult patients is 0.1-0.3 mg/kg/d. Because this patient has liver dysfunction, a dose in the lower end of the range (0.1 mg/kg/d) will be used in order to avoid graft rejection. The initial tacrolimus dose for this patient is: Dose = 0.1 mg/kg/d • 78 kg = 7.8 mg/d, rounded to 8 mg/d. Because this patient has liver dysfunction, this dose should be empirically reduced by 50%: 8 mg/d • 0.5 = 4 mg/d or 2 mg every 12 hours.

Tacrolimus concentrations would be obtained on a daily basis with steady-state expected to occur after about 12 days of therapy (5 half-lives = 5 • 60 h = 300 h or 12.5 d). However, this patient is scheduled to receive his transplant the next day.

6. *Answer to problem 6.*

Linear Pharmacokinetics Method

1. *Compute new dose to achieve the desired concentration.*

The patient would be expected to achieve steady-state conditions after the third day (5 $t_{1/2}$ = 5 • 12 h = 60 h) of therapy.

Using linear pharmacokinetics, the new dose to attain the desired concentration should be proportional to the old dose that produced the measured concentration (total daily dose = 4 mg/dose • 2 doses/d = 8 mg/d):

$$D_{new} = (C_{ss,new}/C_{ss,old})D_{old} = (15 \text{ ng/mL} / 33 \text{ ng/mL}) \, 8 \text{ mg/d} = 3.6 \text{ mg/d, rounded to 4 mg/d}$$

The new suggested dose would be 4 mg/d or 2 mg every 12 hours of tacrolimus capsules to be started at the next scheduled dosing time.

A steady-state trough tacrolimus concentration should be measured after steady-state is attained in 3-5 half-lives. Since the patient is expected to have a half-life equal to 12 hours, the tacrolimus steady-state concentration could be obtained any time after the third day of dosing (5 half-lives = 5 • 12 h = 60 h). Tacrolimus concentrations should also be measured if the patient experiences signs or symptoms of graft rejection, or if the patient develops potential signs or symptoms of tacrolimus toxicity.

Pharmacokinetic Parameter Method

1. *Compute pharmacokinetic parameters.*

The patient would be expected to achieve steady-state conditions after the third day (5 $t_{1/2}$ = 5 • 12 h = 60 h) of therapy.

Tacrolimus clearance can be computed using a steady-state tacrolimus concentration: $Cl = [F(D/\tau)]/Css = [0.25 \bullet (4 \text{ mg}/12 \text{ h}) \bullet 1000 \text{ μg/mg}]/(33 \text{ μg/L}) = 2.5 \text{ L/h}$. (Note: μg/L = ng/mL and this concentration unit was substituted for Css in the calculations so that unnecessary unit conversion was not required.)

2. *Compute tacrolimus dose.*

Tacrolimus clearance is used to compute the new dose: $D = (Css \bullet Cl \bullet \tau)/F = (15 \text{ μg/L} \bullet 2.5 \text{ L/h} \bullet 12 \text{ h})/(0.25 \bullet 1000 \text{ μg/mg}) = 1.8 \text{ mg}$, rounded to 2 mg every 12 hours.

A steady-state trough tacrolimus concentration should be measured after steady-state is attained in 3-5 half-lives. Since the patient is expected to have a half-life equal to 12 hours, the tacrolimus steady-state concentration could be obtained any time after the third day of dosing (5 half-lives = 5 $\bullet$ 12 h = 60 h). Tacrolimus concentrations should also be measured if the patient experiences signs or symptoms of graft rejection, or if the patient develops potential signs or symptoms of tacrolimus toxicity.

7. *Answer to problem 7.*

Pharmacokinetic Dosing Method

1. *Estimate clearance according to disease states and conditions present in the patient.*

The mean tacrolimus clearance for adult patients is 0.06 L/h/kg. The tacrolimus blood clearance for this patient is expected to be: $Cl = 0.06 \text{ L/h/kg} \bullet 67 \text{ kg} = 4.0 \text{ L/h}$

2. *Compute dosage regimen.*

A 12-hour dosage interval will be used for this patient. (Note: ng/mL = μg/L and this concentration was substituted for Css in the calculations so that unnecessary unit conversion was not required. Also, a conversion constant of 1000 μg/mg is used to change the dose amount to mg.) The dosage equation for oral tacrolimus is: $D = (Css \bullet Cl \bullet \tau)/F = (15 \text{ μg/L} \bullet 4.0 \text{ L/h} \bullet 12 \text{ h})/(0.25 \bullet 1000 \text{ μg/mg}) = 2.9 \text{ mg}$, rounded to 3 mg every 12 hours.

Tacrolimus concentrations would be obtained on a daily basis with steady-state expected to occur after about 3 days of therapy (5 half-lives = 5 $\bullet$ 12 h = 60 h).

Literature-Based Recommended Dosing

1. *Choose tacrolimus dose based on disease states and conditions present in the patient and transplant type.*

The tacrolimus oral dosage range for adult patients is 0.1-0.3 mg/kg/d. Because this is a kidney transplant patient, a dose in the lower end of the range (0.1 mg/kg/d) will be used in order to avoid nephrotoxicity. The initial tacrolimus dose for this patient is: Dose = 0.1 mg/kg/d $\bullet$ 67 kg = 6.7 mg/d, rounded to 6 mg/d or 3 mg every 12 hours.

Tacrolimus concentrations would be obtained on a daily basis with steady-state expected to occur after 3 days (5 half-lives = 5 $\bullet$ 12 h = 60 h) of treatment.

8. *Answer to problem 8.*

Linear Pharmacokinetics Method

1. *Compute new dose to achieve the desired concentration.*

The patient would be expected to achieve steady-state conditions after the third day (5 $t_{1/2}$ = 5 $\bullet$ 12 h = 60 h) of therapy.

Using linear pharmacokinetics, the new dose to attain the desired concentration should be proportional to the old dose that produced the measured concentration (total daily dose = 3 mg/dose • 2 doses/d = 6 mg/d):

$$D_{new} = (C_{ss,new}/C_{ss,old})D_{old} = (15 \text{ ng/mL} / 11 \text{ ng/mL}) \, 6 \text{ mg/d} = 8.2 \text{ mg/d, rounded to 8 mg/d}$$

The new suggested dose would be 8 mg/d or 4 mg every 12 hours of tacrolimus capsules to be started at the next scheduled dosing time.

A steady-state trough tacrolimus concentration should be measured after steady-state is attained in 3-5 half-lives. Since the patient is expected to have a half-life equal to 12 hours, the tacrolimus steady-state concentration could be obtained any time after the third day of dosing (5 half-lives = 5 • 12 h = 60 h). Tacrolimus concentrations should also be measured if the patient experiences signs or symptoms of graft rejection, or if the patient develops potential signs or symptoms of tacrolimus toxicity.

Pharmacokinetic Parameter Method

1. *Compute pharmacokinetic parameters.*

The patient would be expected to achieve steady-state conditions after the third day (5 $t_{1/2}$ = 5 • 12 h = 60 h) of therapy.

Tacrolimus clearance can be computed using a steady-state tacrolimus concentration: Cl = [F(D/τ)]/Css = [0.25 • (3 mg/12 h) • 1000 μg/mg]/(11 μg/L) = 5.7 L/h. (Note: μg/L = ng/mL and this concentration unit was substituted for Css in the calculations so that unnecessary unit conversion was not required.)

2. *Compute tacrolimus dose.*

Tacrolimus clearance is used to compute the new dose: D = (Css • Cl • τ)/F = (15 μg/L • 5.7 L/h • 12 h)/(0.25 • 1000 μg/mg) = 4.1 mg, rounded to 4 mg every 12 hours.

A steady-state trough tacrolimus concentration should be measured after steady-state is attained in 3-5 half-lives. Since the patient is expected to have a half-life equal to 12 hours, the tacrolimus steady-state concentration could be obtained any time after the third day of dosing (5 half-lives = 5 • 12 h = 60 h). Tacrolimus concentrations should also be measured if the patient experiences signs or symptoms of graft rejection, or if the patient develops potential signs or symptoms of tacrolimus toxicity.

9. *Answer to problem 9.*

Bayesian Pharmacokinetic Computer Program

1. *Enter the patient's demographic, drug-dosing, and concentration/time data into the computer program.*

2. *Compute pharmacokinetic parameters for the patient using Bayesian pharmacokinetic computer program.*

The pharmacokinetic parameters computed by the program are a volume of distribution of 69 L, a half-life equal to 14 h, and a clearance equal to 3.4 L/h.

3. *Compute dose required to achieve the desired tacrolimus concentrations.*

The one-compartment model infusion and first-order absorption equations used by the program to compute doses indicates that a dose of 4 mg every 12 hours will produce a steady-state tacrolimus concentration of 20 ng/mL.

10. *Answer to problem 10.*

Bayesian Pharmacokinetic Computer Program

1. *Enter the patient's demographic, drug-dosing, and concentration/time data into the computer program.*

Because the patient is also being treated with phenytoin, an enzyme-induction drug interaction for tacrolimus should be entered into the program at the appropriate place.

2. *Compute pharmacokinetic parameters for the patient using Bayesian pharmacokinetic computer program.*

The pharmacokinetic parameters computed by the program are a volume of distribution of 60 L, a half-life equal to 9 h, and a clearance equal to 4.5 L/h.

3. *Compute dose required to achieve the desired tacrolimus concentrations.*

The one-compartment first-order absorption equations used by the program to compute doses indicates that a dose of 6 mg every 12 hours will produce a steady-state tacrolimus concentration of 20 ng/mL.

11. *Answer to problem 11.*

Area Under the Concentration-Time Curve Method

1. *Compute pharmacokinetic parameters.*

Tacrolimus AUC_{0-12h} can be estimated using the steady-state tacrolimus concentrations: AUC_{0-12h} [in (ng • h)/mL] $= 10 + (1.4 • C_{0h}) + (0.8 • C_{1h}) + (1.6 • C_{2h}) + (5.5 • C_{4h}) = 10 + (1.4 • 6 \text{ ng/mL}) + (0.8 • 13 \text{ ng/mL}) + (1.6 • 16 \text{ ng/mL}) + (5.5 • 12 \text{ ng/mL}) = 120$ (ng • h)/mL.

2. *Compute tacrolimus dose*

Linear pharmacokinetics is used to compute the new dose (total daily dose $= 8$ mg/dose • 2 doses/d $= 16$ mg/d): $D_{new} = (AUC_{new}/AUC_{old})D_{old} = \{[100 \text{ (ng • h)/mL}]/[120 \text{ (ng • h)/mL}]\}$ (16 mg/d) $= 13.3$ mg/d, rounded to 14 mg/d or 7 mg every 12 hours.

Steady-state tacrolimus serum concentrations should be measured after steady-state is attained in 3-5 half-lives. Tacrolimus concentrations should also be measured if the patient experiences signs or symptoms of graft rejection, or if the patient develops potential signs or symptoms of tacrolimus toxicity.

REFERENCES

1. Johnson HJ, Schonder KS. Solid-organ transplantation. In: DiPiro JT, Talbert RL, Yee GC, Matzke GR, Wells BG, Posey LM, eds. *Pharmacotherapy*. 8th ed. New York, NY: McGraw-Hill; 2011:1547-1558.
2. Perkins JB, Yee GC. Hematopoietic stem cell transplantation. In: DiPiro JT, Talbert RL, Yee GC, Matzke GR, Wells BG, Posey LM, eds. *Pharmacotherapy*. 8th ed. New York, NY: McGraw-Hill; 2011:2455-2472.
3. Krensky AM, Bennett WM, Vincenti F. Immunosuppressants, tolerogens, and immunostimulants. In: Brunton LL, Lazo JS, Parker KL, eds. *The Pharmacological Basis of Therapeutics*. 12th ed. New York, NY: McGraw-Hill; 2011:1005-1030.
4. Jusko WJ, Thomson AW, Fung J, et al. Consensus document: therapeutic monitoring of tacrolimus (FK-506). *Ther Drug Monit*. 1995;17(6):606-614.
5. Venkataramanan R, Swaminathan A, Prasad T, et al. Clinical pharmacokinetics of tacrolimus. *Clin Pharmacokinet*. 1995;29(6):404-430.
6. D'Ambrosio R, Girzaitis N, Jusko WJ. Multicenter comparison of tacrolimus (FK 506) whole blood concentrations as measured by the Abbott IMX analyzer and enzyme immunoassay with methylene chloride extraction. *Ther Drug Monit*. 1994;16(3):287-292.
7. Matsunami H, Tada A, Makuuchi M, Lynch SV, Strong RW. New technique for measuring tacrolimus concentrations in blood [letter]. *Am J Hosp Pharm*. 1994;51(1):123.
8. Winkler M, Christians U, Stoll K, Baumann J, Pichlmayr R. Comparison of different assays for the quantitation of FK 506 levels in blood or plasma. *Ther Drug Monit*. 1994;16(3):281-286.

9. Jusko WJ, Piekoszewski W, Klintmalm GB, et al. Pharmacokinetics of tacrolimus in liver transplant patients. *Clin Pharmacol Ther.* 1995;57(3):281-290.

10. Regazzi MB, Rinaldi M, Molinaro M, et al. Clinical pharmacokinetics of tacrolimus in heart transplant recipients. *Ther Drug Monit.* 1999;21(1):2-7.

11. Appelbaum F. Hematopoietic cell transplantation. In: Longo DL, Fauci AS, Kasper DL, Hauser SL, Jameson JL, Loscalzo J, eds. *Principles of Internal Medicine.* 18th ed. New York, NY: McGraw-Hill; 2012:958-964.

12. Hunt SA, Mallidi HR. Cardiac transplantation and prolonged assisted circulation. In: Longo DL, Fauci AS, Kasper DL, Hauser SL, Jameson JL, Loscalzo J, eds. *Principles of Internal Medicine.* 18th ed. New York, NY: McGraw-Hill; 2012:1916-1919.

13. Trulock EP. Lung transplantation. In: Longo DL, Fauci AS, Kasper DL, Hauser SL, Jameson JL, Loscalzo J, eds. *Principles of Internal Medicine.* 18th ed. New York, NY: McGraw-Hill; 2012:2189-2195.

14. Dienstag JL, Chung RT. Liver transplantation. In: Longo DL, Fauci AS, Kasper DL, Hauser SL, Jameson JL, Loscalzo J, eds. *Principles of Internal Medicine.* 18th ed. New York, NY: McGraw-Hill; 2012:2606-2614.

15. Chandraker A, Milford EL, Sayegh MH. Transplantation in the treatment of renal failure. In: Longo DL, Fauci AS, Kasper DL, Hauser SL, Jameson JL, Loscalzo J, eds. *Principles of Internal Medicine.* 18th ed. New York, NY: McGraw-Hill; 2012:2327-2333.

16. Scholten EM, Cremers SC, Schoemaker RC, et al. AUC-guided dosing of tacrolimus prevents progressive systemic overexposure in renal transplant recipients. *Kidney Int.* Jun 2005;67(6):2440-2447.

17. Ragette R, Kamler M, Weinreich G, Teschler H, Jakob H. Tacrolimus pharmacokinetics in lung transplantation: new strategies for monitoring. *J Heart Lung Transplant.* Sep 2005;24(9):1315-1319.

18. Filler G, Grygas R, Mai I, et al. Pharmacokinetics of tacrolimus (FK 506) in children and adolescents with renal transplants. *Nephrol Dial Transplant.* Aug 1997;12(8):1668-1671.

19. Wong KM, Shek CC, Chau KF, Li CS. Abbreviated tacrolimus area-under-the-curve monitoring for renal transplant recipients. *Am J Kidney Dis.* Apr 2000;35(4):660-666.

20. Floren LC, Bekersky I, Benet LZ, et al. Tacrolimus oral bioavailability doubles with coadministration of ketoconazole. *Clin Pharmacol Ther.* 1997;62(1):41-49.

21. Hebert MF, Fisher RM, Marsh CL, Dressler D, Bekersky I. Effects of rifampin on tacrolimus pharmacokinetics in healthy volunteers. *J Clin Pharmacol.* 1999;39(1):91-96.

22. Sattler M, Guengerich FP, Yun CH, Christians U, Sewing KF. Cytochrome P-450 3A enzymes are responsible for biotransformation of FK506 and rapamycin in man and rat. *Drug Metab Dispos.* 1992;20(5):753-761.

23. Karanam BV, Vincent SH, Newton DJ, Wang RW, Chiu SH. FK 506 metabolism in human liver microsomes: investigation of the involvement of cytochrome P450 isozymes other than CYP3A4 [published erratum appears in *Drug Metab Dispos.* Nov-Dec 1994; 22(6):979]. *Drug Metab Dispos.* 1994;22(5):811-814.

24. Iwasaki K, Shiraga T, Nagase K, Hirano K, Nozaki K, Noda K. Pharmacokinetic study of FK 506 in the rat. *Transplant Proc.* 1991; 23(6):2757-2759.

25. Venkataramanan R, Jain A, Warty VS, et al. Pharmacokinetics of FK 506 in transplant patients. *Transplant Proc.* 1991;23(6):2736-2740.

26. Gruber SA, Hewitt JM, Sorenson AL, et al. Pharmacokinetics of FK506 after intravenous and oral administration in patients awaiting renal transplantation. *J Clin Pharmacol.* 1994;34(8):859-864.

27. Venkataramanan R, Jain A, Warty VW, et al. Pharmacokinetics of FK 506 following oral administration: a comparison of FK 506 and cyclosporine. *Transplant Proc.* 1991;23(1, pt 2):931-933.

28. Hansten PD, Horn JR. *Drug Interactions Analysis and Management.* St. Louis, MO: Wolters Kluwer; 2014.

29. Jain AB, Venkataramanan R, Cadoff E, et al. Effect of hepatic dysfunction and T tube clamping on FK 506 pharmacokinetics and trough concentrations. *Transplant Proc.* 1990;22(1):57-59.

30. Kobayashi M, Tamura K, Katayama N, et al. FK 506 assay past and present—characteristics of FK 506 ELISA. *Transplant Proc.* 1991;23(6):2725-2729.

31. Kay JE, Sampare-Kwateng E, Geraghty F, Morgan GY. Uptake of FK 506 by lymphocytes and erythrocytes. *Transplant Proc.* 1991;23(6):2760-2762.

32. Piekoszewski W, Jusko WJ. Plasma protein binding of tacrolimus in humans. *J Pharm Sci.* 1993;82(3):340-341.

33. Nagase K, Iwasaki K, Nozaki K, Noda K. Distribution and protein binding of FK506, a potent immunosuppressive macrolide lactone, in human blood and its uptake by erythrocytes. *J Pharm Pharmacol.* 1994;46(2):113-117.

34. Winkler M, Ringe B, Rodeck B, et al. The use of plasma levels for FK 506 dosing in liver-grafted patients. *Transpl Int.* 1994;7(5):329-333.

35. Jain AB, Abu-Elmagd K, Abdallah H, et al. Pharmacokinetics of FK506 in liver transplant recipients after continuous intravenous infusion [see comments]. *J Clin Pharmacol.* 1993;33(7):606-611.

36. Bennett WM. Guide to drug dosage in renal failure. *Clin Pharmacokinet.* 1988;15(5):326-354.

37. Swan SK, Bennett WM. Drug dosing guidelines in patients with renal failure. *West J Med.* 1992;156(6):633-638.

38. Tschudy MM, Arcara KM. *The Harriet Lane Handbook: A Manual for Pediatric House Officers.* 19th ed. Philadelphia, PA: Mosby; 2012.

39. Bekersky I, Dressler D, Mekki QA. Dose linearity after oral administration of tacrolimus 1-mg capsules at doses of 3, 7, and 10 mg. *Clin Ther.* 1999;21(12):2058-2064.

40. Wandell M, Mungall D. Computer assisted drug interpretation and drug regimen optimization. *Amer Assoc Clin Chem.* 1984;6:1-11.

20 Sirolimus

INTRODUCTION

Sirolimus (also known as rapamycin) is a macrocyclic lactone-based mTOR (mammalian target of rapamycin) inhibitor that is used for the prevention of graft rejection in solid organ transplant patients.[1] It is currently approved for use in renal transplant patients. It is also used to prevent rejection in other solid organ transplant recipients as well as the treatment of graft-versus-host disease in hematopoietic stem cell transplant patients.[1,2] The immunomodulating properties of sirolimus are due to its ability to block the effects of interleukin-2 on T-lymphocyte activation and proliferation.[1,3] Sirolimus binds to FK-binding protein-12 (FKPB-12), an intracellular cytoplasmic protein found in T cells. The sirolimus-FKPB complex then binds to mTOR, which inhibits the reaction of the T cell to interleukin-2 binding to its outer cell wall. This action prevents T-cell proliferation and progression of the cell cycle.

Because the calcineurin inhibitors (cyclosporine and tacrolimus) are nephrotoxic, sirolimus is used by many transplant centers as part of calcineurin inhibitor avoidance regimens or calcineurin inhibitor conversion protocols in order to avoid drug-induced renal damage.[1,2,4]

THERAPEUTIC AND TOXIC CONCENTRATIONS

The therapeutic range of sirolimus used by clinicians varies greatly according to the type of assay used to measure the drug.[5-8] For the purposes of the pharmacokinetic calculations and problems presented in this book, sirolimus concentrations in the blood using a sirolimus-specific chromatograph assay methodology will be used, and the therapeutic range for steady-state sirolimus concentrations of 5-15 ng/mL will be assumed to be appropriate. For renal transplant patients, sirolimus concentrations <5 ng/mL are associated with acute rejection episodes and sirolimus concentrations >15 ng/mL are related to the development of adverse effects.[9]

Desired sirolimus concentrations differ between the various types of transplants, change with time during the posttransplantation phase, and are determined by protocols specific to the transplantation service and institution where the patient is treated.[1,2,4,8] It is very important for clinicians to be aware of these factors since acceptable sirolimus concentrations under various circumstances may be different than those given by a specific clinical laboratory or those suggested in this textbook.

For patients receiving solid organ transplants, the goal of sirolimus therapy is to prevent acute or chronic rejection of the transplanted organ while minimizing drug side effects.[1,10-13] In this case, the recipient's immune system detects foreign antigens on the donor organ which produces an immunologic response against the graft. This leads to inflammatory and cytotoxic effects directed against the transplanted tissue, and produces the risk of organ tissue damage and failure. In the case of a rejected kidney transplant, it is possible to remove the graft and place the patient on a form of dialysis to sustain their life. However, for other solid organ transplantation patients, graft rejection can result in death.

Because tacrolimus and cyclosporine can cause nephrotoxicity, many transplant centers include sirolimus as part of calcineurin inhibitor avoidance regimens or calcineurin conversion protocols. Calcineurin inhibitor avoidance regimens involve a combination of immunosuppressant drugs, but cyclosporine or tacrolimus are not prescribed as part of the therapy. Calcineurin conversion protocols start as posttransplant therapy with tacrolimus or cyclosporine as part of the treatment regimen, but eventually replace them with sirolimus therapy.

The implementation of these strategies is best established for renal transplant patients. The usage pattern for sirolimus is stratified by patient immunologic risk. For patients with a low or moderate immunologic risk, sirolimus therapy (recommended: 6 mg loading dose, followed by 2 mg/d) is initiated with cyclosporine and corticosteroids for 2-4 months, and therapeutic steady-state sirolimus (typically 10-15 ng/mL) and cyclosporine concentrations should be maintained. If an adequate response has been attained during that time frame, the cyclosporine dose is tapered off over 4-8 weeks, and the sirolimus dose is adjusted to maintain therapeutic steady-state concentrations. Because cyclosporine inhibits sirolimus metabolism, the sirolimus dose usually needs to be increased while cyclosporine doses are decreased. For this clinical scenario, the recommended sirolimus steady-state concentrations after cyclosporine withdrawal are 16-24 ng/mL for the first year after transplantation and 12-20 ng/mL thereafter.[4,8] For patients with a high immunologic risk (defined as Black transplant recipients, past transplant recipients with a failed kidney graft due to an immunologic etiology, or patients with lab results indicating high panel-reactive antibodies), sirolimus therapy (recommended: up to 15-mg loading dose, followed by 5 mg/d) is initiated with cyclosporine and corticosteroids for 1 year following transplantation. Therapeutic steady-state sirolimus (typically 10-15 ng/mL) and cyclosporine concentrations should be maintained. If an adequate response has been attained during that time frame, adjustments to the dosage regimens for the individual medications are based on the clinical response of the patient and may include reduction of the cyclosporine dose.[4,8] If tacrolimus is prescribed as the calcineurin inhibitor, the same dosage approaches can be used.

For patients receiving sirolimus after a hematopoietic stem cell transplant, the goal of therapy is to prevent graft-versus-host disease while avoiding adverse effects of immunosuppressant therapy.[2,14] Graft-versus-host disease is a result of donor T lymphocytes detecting antigens on host tissues and producing an immunologic response against these antigens and host tissues. Acute graft-versus-host disease usually occurs within the first 100 days after transplantation of donor stem cells, and causes epithelial tissue damage in organs. The most common tissues attacked are skin, gastrointestinal tract, and liver. To prevent acute graft-versus-host disease from occurring in allogenic hematopoietic stem cell transplant patients with HLA-matched donors, tacrolimus or cyclosporine therapy is usually instituted a few days before or on the day of stem cell transplant (day 0), and doses are adjusted to provide therapeutic trough concentrations. Methotrexate or glucocorticoids are usually also given in conjunction with tacrolimus or cyclosporine treatment to hematopoietic stem cell transplantation patients. If prophylaxis of acute graft-versus-host disease is successful, calcineurin inhibitor (cyclosporine or tacrolimus) doses start to be tapered between posttransplant days 50-100, with the goal of drug discontinuation by about posttransplant day 180. For allogeneic hematopoietic stem cell transplant patients with HLA-mismatched or HLA-identical unrelated donors, the risk of acute graft-versus-host disease is higher, so calcineurin inhibitor therapy may be more prolonged for these patients. After posttransplantation day 100, chronic graft-versus-host disease may occur, and severe cases or patients with systemic signs and symptoms of the disease are usually treated with prednisone. Sirolimus is currently used as an adjunctive agent to treat both acute and chronic graft-versus-host disease at many transplant centers, and several investigations are under way to define its optimal use in hematopoietic stem cell transplant patients.[15]

Myelosuppression, hyperlipidemia, delayed wound healing, peripheral edema, mouth ulcers, increased liver function tests, hypertension, rash, acne, diarrhea, and arthralgia are all typical adverse effects of sirolimus therapy.[1,4,8] Dose-related myelosuppression consists of thrombocytopenia (usually within 2 weeks of initiation of therapy), leucopenia, and anemia, and it is associated with sirolimus concentrations above 15 ng/mL. Myelosuppression is usually transient and typically improves even though treatment with sirolimus is continued.[9,16,17] Hypercholesterolemia and hypertriglyceridemia are usually managed by reducing the dose of sirolimus or by treating the patient with antilipid therapy. Development of hypercholesterolemia is also related to sirolimus concentrations in excess of 15 ng/mL.[9]

The prescribing information for sirolimus contains a black box warning that identifies several important issues. Patients taking sirolimus are more susceptible to infections and to the development of malignancies, including lymphoma. Liver transplant patients may have a higher death rate, experience loss of the transplanted organ, or develop hepatic artery thrombosis while on sirolimus therapy. Lung patients may develop bronchial anastomotic dehiscence during sirolimus treatment.

CLINICAL MONITORING PARAMETERS

Solid organ transplant patients should be monitored for graft rejection consistent with the transplanted organ.[1] Sirolimus is most often used for the treatment of renal transplantation, but it is also used for other solid organ transplants. For renal transplant patients, increased serum creatinine, azotemia, hypertension, edema, weight gain secondary to fluid retention, graft tenderness, fever and malaise may be due to an acute rejection episode. Hypertension, proteinuria, a continuous decline in renal function (increases in serum creatinine and blood urea nitrogen levels), and uremia are indicative of chronic rejection in renal transplant patients.[1, 13] For hepatic transplant patients, acute rejection signs and symptoms include fever, lethargy, graft tenderness, increased white blood cell count, change in bile color or amount, hyperbilirubinemia, and increased liver function tests. Chronic rejection in a liver transplant patient may be accompanied only by increased liver function tests and jaundice.[1, 12] For heart transplant patients, acute rejection is accompanied by low-grade fever, malaise, heart failure (presence of S_3 heart sound), or atrial arrhythmia. Chronic rejection in heart transplant patients, also known as cardiac allograft vasculopathy which is characterized by accelerated coronary artery atherosclerosis, may include the following symptoms: arrhythmias, decreased left ventricular function, heart failure, myocardial infarction, and sudden cardiac death.[1, 10] For lung transplant patients, acute rejection may result in no or nonspecific symptoms (cough, dyspnea, hypoxemia, low-grade fever, inspiratory crackles, interstitial infiltrates, declining lung function). Chronic rejection in lung transplant patients, also called bronchiolitis obliterans syndrome, is characterized by decreased airflow and can resemble acute bronchitis.[11] For all solid organ transplant patients, tissue biopsies may be taken from the transplanted tissue to confirm the diagnosis of organ rejection.[1]

Hematopoietic stem cell transplant patients should be monitored for the signs and symptoms associated with graft-versus-host disease.[2, 14] These include a generalized maculopapular skin rash, diarrhea, abdominal pain, ileus, hyperbilirubinemia, and increased liver function tests (alkaline phosphatase and serum transaminases). Patients with severe chronic graft-versus-host disease may have involvement of the skin, liver, eyes, mouth, esophagus, or other organs similar to what might be seen with systemic autoimmune diseases.

Typical adverse effects of sirolimus treatment include myelosuppression, hyperlipidemia, delayed wound healing, peripheral edema, mouth ulcers, increased liver function tests, hypertension, rash, acne, diarrhea, and arthralgia.[1,4,8,16,17] The management of these common drug side effects is discussed in the previous section. The serious problems listed in the black box warning found in the prescribing information for sirolimus (development of infection or malignancy, specific issues regarding liver or lung transplantation) need to be carefully considered by prescribers to ensure the benefits of therapy outweigh the risks.

Because of the pivotal role that sirolimus plays as an immunosuppressant in transplant patients, as well as the severity of its concentration- and dose-dependent side effects, sirolimus concentrations should be measured in every patient receiving the drug. If a patient experiences signs or symptoms of organ rejection or graft-versus-host disease, a sirolimus concentration should be checked to ensure that levels have not fallen below the therapeutic range. If a patient encounters a possible clinical problem that could be an adverse drug effect of sirolimus therapy, a sirolimus concentration should be measured to determine if levels are in the toxic range. During the early posttransplantation phase, sirolimus concentrations are measured at least every

5-7 days in most patients during dosage initiation or after a dosage adjustment in solid organ transplant patients or graft-versus-host disease in hematopoietic stem cell transplant patients.

After discharge from the hospital, sirolimus concentrations continue to be obtained at most clinic visits. Sirolimus doses and concentrations are decreased to the minimum required to prevent graft-versus-host reactions or rejection episodes in order to decrease drug adverse effects. Methods to adjust sirolimus doses using sirolimus concentrations are discussed later in this chapter. When a dosage change is necessary, a steady-state sirolimus concentration should be measured 5-7 days later to confirm that levels are within the therapeutic range. Because of a good correlation with the sirolimus steady-state area under the concentration-time curve (AUC), predose steady-state trough sirolimus concentration determinations are used by most transplant centers to adjust drug doses.[1,9] Because of the success found in using area under the concentration-time curve (AUC) measurements with cyclosporine, some investigators are beginning to suggest that determination of sirolimus AUC using multiple concentrations may be a useful monitoring technique.[18,19]

BASIC CLINICAL PHARMACOKINETIC PARAMETERS

Sirolimus is extensively eliminated by hepatic metabolism. Hepatic metabolism is mainly via the CYP3A4 enzyme system, and the drug is a substrate for p-glycoprotein.[20-22] There are at least seven identified sirolimus metabolites.[8,23,24] None of these metabolites appear to have significant immunosuppressive effects in humans. Most of the metabolites are eliminated in the bile.[25] About 2% of a sirolimus dose is recovered in the urine.[25]

There is a large amount of intrasubject variability in sirolimus concentrations obtained on a day-to-day basis, even when the patient should be at steady-state.[9,26] There are many reasons for this variability. Sirolimus has low water solubility, and its gastrointestinal absorption can be influenced by many variables. The oral absorption rate is generally fast for most patients, with average times to maximum concentration (T_{max}) during multiple dosing equal to 2 hours for the oral solution and 3 hours for the tablet.[27,28] The ratio of maximum-to-minimum steady-state sirolimus concentrations ($C_{max_{ss}}/C_{min_{ss}}$) is approximately 2 with once daily dosing.[8,9] The average bioavailability is 14% for the oral solution and 17% for the tablets.[29,30] When administered with meals containing high fat content food, oral bioavailability of sirolimus oral solution increases by 34%.[31] To avoid the possible effect of food on sirolimus bioavailability, the drug should be given at a constant time in relation to meals. Sirolimus should not be taken with grapefruit juice since this vehicle inhibits CYP3A4 and/or p-glycoprotein contained in the gastrointestinal tract and markedly increases bioavailability.[20] Other drug therapy can also increase or decrease the intestinal first-pass clearance of sirolimus.[20,32]

Sirolimus is removed from the body almost exclusively by hepatic metabolism. Its hepatic clearance is influenced by unbound fraction in the blood (f_B), intrinsic clearance (Cl'_{int}), and liver blood flow. Sirolimus distributes extensively into erythrocytes (~95% of drug contained in blood), and only about 3% of drug in the blood is found in the plasma.[33] Within the plasma, the majority of sirolimus is bound to albumin (~97%) with the remainder bound to α_1-acid glycoprotein and lipoproteins.[8] Erythrocyte concentrations vary in transplant patients, especially those who have received hematopoietic stem cell or kidney transplants. Albumin and α_1-acid glycoprotein concentrations also vary greatly among transplant patients. Hepatic intrinsic clearance is different among all individuals, and there is a large amount of variability in this value among individual liver transplant patients. This value changes according to the viability of the graft and time after transplantation surgery. Other drug therapy can also increase or decrease the hepatic intrinsic clearance of sirolimus, and many transplant patients take cyclosporine concomitantly which inhibits the hepatic metabolism of sirolimus.[32] Liver blood flow is quite variable for patients and changes throughout the day. Taking all of these possible factors that alter absorption and clearance into consideration allows one to gain a better appreciation of why sirolimus concentrations change on a day-to-day basis.

Sirolimus tablets are available in 0.5, 1, and 2 mg strengths. Sirolimus oral solution is available at a concentration of 1 mg/mL. Before administration, the oral solution should be diluted in at least 60 mL of water or orange juice, stirred immediately for 1 minute, and drunk by the patient right away. The initial dose of sirolimus varies greatly among various transplant centers.[1,4] Recommended initial doses for renal transplant patients with a low-to-moderate immunologic risk are a loading dose of 6 mg followed by a maintenance dose of 2 mg daily. For renal transplant patients with a high immunologic risk (defined as Black transplant recipients, past transplant recipients with a failed kidney graft due to an immunologic etiology, or patients with lab results indicating high panel-reactive antibodies) the initial doses consist of a loading dose of up to 15 mg followed by a maintenance dose equal to 5 mg daily.[1,4,8] Because the steady-state-to-single dose accumulation ratio for sirolimus is ~3, recommended loading doses are usually three times the prescribed maintenance dose.[8] Many transplant centers omit loading doses and commence dosing only with the maintenance dose.[4] For patients with liver dysfunction, maintenance doses should be reduced by 33%-50%.[28,34] Because such a small amount of drug is excreted in the urine, it is assumed that renal failure does not substantially change sirolimus pharmacokinetics.[8,25] A limited number of studies in special populations with concurrent renal dysfunction have been conducted and compared to literature controls.[35,36] The results of these studies support the notion that sirolimus doses do not need adjustment for renal failure. Oral sirolimus is administered on a once-daily schedule.

EFFECTS OF DISEASE STATES AND CONDITIONS ON SIROLIMUS PHARMACOKINETICS AND DOSING

Because there is no intravenous dosage form generally available for comparison, bioavailability for the different transplant types is unknown, so hybrid pharmacokinetic parameters are usually reported in pharmacokinetic studies. Using this approach, a combined clearance (Cl) and bioavailability (F) parameter (Cl/F) is calculated as a surrogate for clearance and a similar hybrid parameter (V/F) is computed as a substitute for volume of distribution (V). When changes are calculated for Cl/F, either clearance changed, bioavailability changed, or both changed simultaneously. Likewise, if there is an alteration in V/F, volume of distribution may have changed, bioavailability may have changed, or both may have changed concurrently. For example, if Cl/F increased, it could be due to a rise in clearance, a decline in bioavailability, a simultaneous increase in clearance and decrease in bioavailability, or both parameters could change so that the quotient results in a net increase. Under multiple-dosing conditions, there often are not enough postabsorption, postdistribution sirolimus blood concentrations during a long enough period to accurately determine half-life. In these cases, the mean residence time (MRT) is calculated as a measure of drug persistence in the body.

When assessing individual research reports, it is important to ascertain concurrent drug therapy for potential drug interactions that might change pharmacokinetic parameters. In the case of sirolimus, the type of calcineurin inhibitor therapy is particularly important to note because cyclosporine inhibits the hepatic metabolism of sirolimus but tacrolimus has little, if any, effect on sirolimus pharmacokinetics.[20,32,37]

Of all of the solid organ transplantation types that sirolimus is used as an immunosuppressant, the most pharmacokinetic information is available for renal transplant patients (Table 20-1).[38-44] For adult renal transplant patients taking cyclosporine, the Cl/F is about 240 mL/h/kg, the V/F is about 10 L/kg, and the half-life is about 60 hours. Adult renal transplant patients receiving concurrent tacrolimus therapy have a Cl/F of 310 mL/h/kg, a V/F of about 8 L/kg, and an MRT of 27 hours. As is the case for many other drugs administered to children, pediatric renal transplant patients eliminate sirolimus faster than similar adult patients, but this effect diminishes as age approaches 18 years. The situation is similar for pediatric renal transplant patients taking sirolimus whether calcineurin inhibitor therapy is prescribed or not.

Adult liver transplant patients taking a calcineurin inhibitor (patients not stratified by type of calcineurin inhibitor) had a sirolimus Cl/F of 146 mL/h/kg after 1 month of therapy, while pediatric liver transplant patients being treated with tacrolimus had a sirolimus Cl/F equal to 401 mL/h/kg and a half-life equal to 21.2 hours.

TABLE 20-1   Select Transplant Patients With Pharmacokinetic Parameters

Patient Characteristics	Cl/F	V/F	$t_{1/2}$ or MRT	Comment
Adult, renal transplant, treated with cyclosporine	8.9 L/h 208 mL/h/kg 147 mL/h/kg 240 mL/h/kg 281 mL/h/kg 323 mL/h/kg	452 L 12 L/kg 8.3 L/kg 12 L/kg N/D N/D	$t_{1/2}$ = 63 h $t_{1/2}$ = 62.3 h $t_{1/2}$ = 57 h $t_{1/2}$ = 62 h N/D $t_{1/2}$ = 57 h	With no reference intravenous dosage form generally available, clearance (Cl) and bioavailability (F) parameters are combined to form Cl/F, and volume of distribution (V) and bioavailability parameters are combined to form V/F. Half-life is large, so steady-state concentrations are not attained until 7-12 d of consistent dosing, and sirolimus doses can be administered once daily. Patients taking cyclosporine concurrently have decreased sirolimus Cl/F and increased $t_{1/2}$. The overall averages for this series of patients are: Cl/F = 240 mL/h/kg, V/F = 10 L/kg, $t_{1/2}$ = 60 h.
Adult, renal transplant, treated with cyclosporine or tacrolimus	210 mL/h/kg with cyclosporine 310 mL/h/kg with tacrolimus	5 L/kg 7.7 L/kg	MRT = 24 h MRT = 27 h	Patients treated concurrently with cyclosporine have a decreased sirolimus Cl/F. Tacrolimus therapy has little to no effect on sirolimus pharmacokinetics for most patients.
Pediatric, renal transplant, treated with cyclosporine (compared with adults treated at same institution)	485 mL/h/kg, children 376 mL/h/kg, adolescents 208 mL/h/kg, adults	N/D N/D N/D	$t_{1/2}$ = 49.1 h $t_{1/2}$ = 70.3 h $t_{1/2}$ = 62.0 h	Children have higher Cl/F and lower $t_{1/2}$ compared to adults, and pediatric patients may require twice daily dosing. Adolescents have intermediate pharmacokinetic parameter values for sirolimus that approach adult values.
Pediatric, renal transplant, treated with cyclosporine, tacrolimus, or no calcineurin inhibitor	Treated with cyclosporine (L/h per mg/m²) ——————— 9.2 (0-5 y) 4.4 (6-11 y) 4.8 (12-18 y) Treated with tacrolimus (L/h per mg/m²) ——————— 26.0 (0-5 y) 10.6 (6-11 y) 15.4 (12-18 y) Not treated with calcineurin inhibitor (L/h per mg/m²) ——————— 49.2 (0-5 y) 27.1 (6-11 y) 27.4 (12-18 y)	 N/D N/D N/D N/D N/D N/D N/D N/D N/D	 MRT = 9.7 h MRT = 10.9 h MRT = 10.2 h MRT = 5.1 h MRT = 4.9 h MRT = 5.3 h N/D N/D N/D	The effects of age and type of calcineurin inhibitor therapy are that younger patients have higher Cl/F values, faster elimination, and cyclosporine therapy decreases sirolimus Cl/F. As pediatric patients approach puberty, the pharmacokinetic parameters for sirolimus attain adult values. Patients in the youngest age group may require twice daily dosing to maintain therapeutic $C_{min_{ss}}$ values.

(Continued)

TABLE 20-1   Select Transplant Patients With Pharmacokinetic Parameters (*Continued*)

Patient Characteristics	Cl/F	V/F	$t_{1/2}$ or MRT	Comment
Pediatric, chronic renal failure with dialysis, no calcineurin inhibitor treatment	273-726 mL/h/kg, children 316-631 mL/h/kg, adolescents	22.1-35.8 L/kg 20.0-34.4 L/kg	$t_{1/2}$ = 52.4-107 h $t_{1/2}$ = 47.8-65.5 h	Renal failure doesn't appear to substantially change sirolimus pharmacokinetics for pediatric patients.
Adult, liver transplant, treated with cyclosporine or tacrolimus (combined group)	146 mL/h/kg at 1 mo 128 mL/h/kg at 3 mo	N/D N/D	N/D N/D	Liver transplant patients may have lower Cl/F compared to renal transplant patients. Because patients were not stratified by type of calcineurin inhibitor treatment, the effects of concomitant therapy can't be determined.
Pediatric, liver transplant, treated with tacrolimus	401 mL/h/kg	N/D	$t_{1/2}$ = 21.2 h MRT = 25.3 h	As with other transplant types, pediatric liver transplant patients have higher Cl/F and lower $t_{1/2}$ compared to similar adults.
Pediatric, small bowel transplant, treated with tacrolimus	729 mL/h/kg	N/D	$t_{1/2}$ = 19.3 h MRT = 26.2 h	Pediatric small bowel transplant patients have higher Cl/F values than other pediatric transplant patients.
Pediatric, bone marrow transplant, treated with tacrolimus (some treated with fluconazole)	190 mL/h/kg without fluconazole 190 mL/h/kg with fluconazole	6.6 L/kg 4.3-5.8 L/kg	N/D N/D	Pediatric bone marrow transplant patients have lower Cl/F values than other pediatric patients.

Cl/F, hybrid clearance/bioavailability; MRT, mean residence time; N/D, not determined; $t_{1/2}$, half-life; V/F, hybrid volume of distribution/bioavailability.

The posttransplant time was 6-144 months for the adults, and the median posttransplant time equaled 8.3 months for the children. If administered immediately after liver transplantation, sirolimus metabolism may be depressed until the graft begins functioning in a stable manner.

Pediatric small bowel transplant patients receiving therapy with tacrolimus had a Cl/F of 729 mL/h/kg, a half-life of 19.3 hours, and an MRT of 26.2 hours. The median posttransplant time was 25.4 months for these patients when sirolimus pharmacokinetic parameters were determined, so the small bowel graft was likely stable with consistent sirolimus oral absorption. For small bowel transplant patients, if the graft is not functioning optimally, malabsorption of sirolimus can cause a decrease in bioavailability, which would make Cl/F increase.

Pediatric bone marrow transplant patients treated with tacrolimus had a Cl/F equal to 190 mL/min/kg and a V/F equal to 4.3-6.6 L/kg. Some of these patients were taking fluconazole concurrently, which can inhibit sirolimus hepatic metabolism.[20, 32]

Because the drug is primarily eliminated by hepatic metabolism, average clearance is lower in adult patients with liver dysfunction.[45,46] Using the Child-Pugh rating system (Table 20-2), patients with mild liver disease had a sirolimus Cl/F of 147 mL/h/kg, patients with moderate liver disease had a sirolimus Cl/F equal to 137 mL/h/kg, and patients with severe liver disease had a sirolimus Cl/F of 98.1 mL/h/kg (Table 20-3). Also, mean volume of distribution was larger, and mean residence time was prolonged and variable in this

TABLE 20-2   Child-Pugh Scores for Patients With Liver Disease[47]

Test/Symptom	Score 1 Point	Score 2 Points	Score 3 Points
Total bilirubin (mg/dL)	<2.0	2.0-3.0	>3.0
Serum albumin (g/dL)	>3.5	2.8-3.5	<2.8
Prothrombin time (seconds prolonged over control)	<4	4-6	>6
Ascites	Absent	Slight	Moderate
Hepatic encephalopathy	None	Moderate	Severe

Mild liver disease (Grade A), 5-6 points; moderate liver disease (Grade B), 7-9 points; severe liver disease (Grade C): 10-15 points.

TABLE 20-3   Sirolimus Pharmacokinetics in Patients With Hepatic Dysfunction

Pharmacokinetic Parameter	Controls With Normal Liver Function	Mild Hepatic Disease (Child-Pugh Grade A)	Moderate Hepatic Disease (Child-Pugh Grade B)	Severe Hepatic Disease (Child-Pugh Grade C)
Cl/F (mL/h/kg)	215	147	137	98.1
V_{ss}/F (L/kg)	17.4	16.1	21.2	29.1
MRT (h)	82.4	116	185	280

patient population. Immediately after liver transplantation, sirolimus metabolism may be depressed until the graft begins functioning in a stable manner. Additionally, patients with transient liver dysfunction, regardless of transplantation type, will have decreased sirolimus clearance and increased half-life values. Because only a small amount of sirolimus is eliminated in the urine, it is unlikely that renal failure substantially alters its clearance.[8] Since sirolimus is a relatively large molecule (molecular weight = 914.2 Da), very lipophilic, and highly bound in the blood, it is probable that it is not highly removed by various renal dialysis techniques. Sirolimus pharmacokinetics in renal failure patients and patients undergoing dialysis requires further investigation to provide a definitive answer for the best dosing of the drug in these groups.

DRUG INTERACTIONS

Compared with cyclosporine, sirolimus drug interactions are not as well documented, and many drug interactions that are reported with calcineurin inhibitors are assumed to also occur with sirolimus.[8,20,32] Drug interactions with sirolimus involve inhibition or induction of its metabolism by other drugs.[32] Sirolimus is metabolized by CYP3A4 and is a substrate for p-glycoprotein, so the potential for many pharmacokinetic drug interactions exists with agents that inhibit these pathways or are also cleared by these mechanisms. Because both of these drug elimination systems also exist in the gastrointestinal tract, inhibition drug interactions may also enhance sirolimus oral bioavailability by diminishing the intestinal and hepatic first-pass effects. Drugs that may inhibit sirolimus metabolism include the calcium channel blockers (verapamil, diltiazem, nicardipine), azole antifungals (clotrimazole, fluconazole, itraconazole, ketoconazole, posaconazole, voriconazole), macrolide antibiotics (erythromycin, clarithromycin, azithromycin, troleandomycin), antivirals (atazanavir, darunavir, indinavir, nelfinavir, ritonavir, saquinavir, telaprevir, delavirdine), antiarrhythmics (amiodarone, dronedarone), psycho-tropic agents (fluvoxamine, nefazodone) as well as other compounds (quinupristin, telithromycin, aprepitant, berberine, conivaptan, grapefruit juice). Inducing agents include other antibiotics (rifampin, rifabutin, rifapen-tine), other antivirals (efavirenz, nevirapine), anticonvulsants (phenytoin, carbamazepine, oxcarbazepine, phenobarbital, primidone), barbiturates, bosentan, and St. John's Wort. Because of the large number of poten-tially interacting agents, and the critical nature of the drugs involved in the treatment of transplant patients, complete avoidance of drug interactions with sirolimus is not possible. Thus, most drug interactions with sirolimus are managed using appropriate sirolimus dosage modification with sirolimus concentration monitor-ing as a guide.

   Sirolimus is frequently administered with calcineurin inhibitors, and tacrolimus coadministration does not appear to have a significant effect on sirolimus pharmacokinetics.[37,48] However, cyclosporine is a potent inhibitor of sirolimus metabolism.[8,20,32] This effect can be mitigated by administering sirolimus about 4 hours after the cyclosporine dose is given, but steady-state concentrations of both immunosuppressants should be monitored with doses adjusted appropriately.[38,49] For patients receiving concomitant cyclosporine and siroli-mus treatment, sirolimus steady-state concentrations may fall if cyclosporine therapy is discontinued. If cyclo-sporine treatment is halted, sirolimus concentrations should be measured, and the sirolimus dose increased if levels decline below therapeutic amounts.

INITIAL DOSAGE DETERMINATION METHODS

Several methods to initiate sirolimus therapy are available. The *Pharmacokinetic Dosing method* is the most flexible of the techniques. It allows individualized target serum concentrations to be chosen for a patient, and each pharmacokinetic parameter can be customized to reflect specific disease states and conditions present in the patient. *Literature-based recommended dosing* is the most common method used to prescribe initial doses of sirolimus. Doses are based on those that commonly produce steady-state concentrations in the therapeutic range, although there is a wide variation in the actual concentrations for a specific patient.

Pharmacokinetic Dosing Method

The goal of initial dosing of sirolimus is to compute the best dose possible for the patient in order to prevent graft rejection or graft-versus-host disease given their set of disease states and conditions that influence siro-limus pharmacokinetics, while avoiding adverse drug reactions. In order to do this, pharmacokinetic param-eters for the patient will be estimated using average parameters measured in other patients with similar disease state and condition profiles.

Clearance Estimate

Sirolimus is almost completely metabolized by the liver. Unfortunately, there is no good way to estimate the elimination characteristics of liver-metabolized drugs using an endogenous marker of liver function in the same fashion that serum creatinine and estimated creatinine clearance are used to estimate the elimination of agents that are renally eliminated. Because of this, a patient is categorized according to the disease states and conditions that are known to change sirolimus clearance, and the clearance previously measured in these stud-ies is used as an estimate of the current patient's clearance rate (see Table 20-1). For example, an adult trans-plant patient with normal liver function treated concomitantly with cyclosporine would be assigned a sirolimus Cl/F value equal to 240 mL/h/kg and a V/F value of 10 L/kg, while a pediatric transplant patient in the child age group with the same profile would be assumed to have a sirolimus Cl/F of 485 mL/h/kg (V/F value not determined).

Selection of Appropriate Pharmacokinetic Model and Equations

When oral therapy is chosen for agents with a large first-pass metabolism, the drug is often erratically absorbed with variable absorption rates. Because of the complex absorption profile and the fact that the drug is usually administered once daily for adults and twice daily for younger children, a very simple pharmacokinetic equation that calculates the average sirolimus steady-state concentration (Css in ng/mL = μg/L) is widely used and allows maintenance dose computation: Css = (D/τ)/(Cl/F) or D = Css(Cl/F)τ, where D is the dose of sirolimus in mg, Cl/F is sirolimus hybrid clearance/bioavailability parameter in L/h, and τ is the dosage interval in hours. If a loading dose (LD) of the drug is to be given, the equation that computes it is LD = Css(V/F), where V/F is the sirolimus hybrid volume of distribution/bioavailability parameter in L.

Steady-State Concentration Selection

The generally accepted therapeutic range for sirolimus in the blood is 5-15 ng/mL. For renal transplant patients with a low or moderate immunologic risk, recommended therapeutic steady-state sirolimus (typically 10-15 ng/mL) and cyclosporine concentrations should be maintained. If an adequate response has been attained during that time frame, the cyclosporine dose is tapered off over 4-8 weeks, and the sirolimus dose is adjusted to maintain therapeutic steady-state concentrations. Because cyclosporine inhibits sirolimus metabolism, the sirolimus dose usually needs to be increased while cyclosporine doses are decreased. For this clinical scenario, the recommended sirolimus steady-state concentrations after cyclosporine withdrawal are 16-24 ng/mL for the first year after transplantation and 12-20 ng/mL thereafter.[4,8] For renal transplant patients with a high immunologic risk (defined as Black transplant recipients, past transplant recipients with a failed kidney graft due to an immunologic etiology, or patients with lab results indicating high panel-reactive antibodies), sirolimus therapy is initiated with cyclosporine and corticosteroids for 1 year following transplantation. Therapeutic steady-state sirolimus (typically 10-15 ng/mL) and cyclosporine concentrations should be maintained. If an adequate response has been attained during that time frame, adjustments to the dosage regimens for the individual medications are based on the clinical response of the patient and may include reduction of the cyclosporine dose.[4,8] If tacrolimus is prescribed as the calcineurin inhibitor, the same dosage approaches can be used.

More important than these general guidelines are the specific requirements for each graft type as defined by the transplant center where the surgery was conducted. Clinicians should become familiar with the sirolimus protocols used at the various institutions at which they practice. During the early posttransplantation phase, sirolimus concentrations are measured at least every 5-7 days in most patients during dosage initiation or after a dosage adjustment in solid organ transplant patients or graft-versus-host disease in hematopoietic stem cell transplant patients. After discharge from the hospital, sirolimus concentrations continue to be obtained at most clinic visits.

EXAMPLE 1 ▶ ▶ ▶

HO is a 50-year-old, 70-kg (height = 5 ft 10 in) male renal transplant patient. The patient's liver function tests are normal, and the patient is taking cyclosporine. Suggest an oral loading dose and an initial oral maintenance dose for sirolimus designed to achieve a steady-state sirolimus trough blood concentration equal to 5 ng/mL.

1. *Estimate pharmacokinetic parameters according to disease states and conditions present in the patient.*
   The mean sirolimus Cl/F for adult renal transplant patients taking cyclosporine is 240 mL/h/kg and the mean V/F is 10 L/kg. The sirolimus Cl/F for this patient is: Cl/F = (240 mL/h/kg • 70 kg)/(1000 mL/L) = 16.8 L/h. The sirolimus V/F for this patient is: V/F = 10 L/kg • 70 kg = 700 L.

2. *Compute dosage regimen.*

Loading dose: (Note: ng/mL = μg/L and this concentration was substituted for Css in the calculations so that unnecessary unit conversion was not required. Also, a conversion constant of 1000 μg/mg is used to change the dose amount to mg.) The dosage equation for oral sirolimus is: LD = Css(V/F) = (5 μg/L • 700 L)/(1000 μg/mg) = 3.5 mg, rounded to 4 mg.

Maintenance dose: A 24-hour dosage interval will be used for this patient. (Note: ng/mL = μg/L and this concentration was substituted for Css in the calculations so that unnecessary unit conversion was not required. Also, a conversion constant of 1000 μg/mg is used to change the dose amount to mg.) The dosage equation for oral sirolimus is: D = Css(Cl/F)τ = (5 μg/L • 16.8 L/h • 24 h)/(1000 μg/mg) = 2 mg. Dosage regimen is 2 mg every 24 hours.

Sirolimus concentrations would be obtained in about 7 days with steady-state expected to occur in about 7-12 days (3 half-lives = 3 • 60 h = 180 h, 180 h/(24 h/d) = 7.5 d).

EXAMPLE 2 ▶ ▶ ▶

PP is a 3-year-old, 15-kg (height = 30 in) male renal transplant patient. The patient's liver function tests are normal, and the patient is taking cyclosporine. Suggest an initial oral maintenance dose for sirolimus designed to achieve a steady-state sirolimus trough blood concentration equal to 5 ng/mL.

1. *Estimate pharmacokinetic parameters according to disease states and conditions present in the patient.*

The mean sirolimus Cl/F for younger pediatric renal transplant patients taking cyclosporine is 485 mL/h/kg. The sirolimus CL/F for this patient is: Cl = (485 mL/h/kg • 15 kg)/(1000 mL/L) = 7.3 L/h.

2. *Compute dosage regimen.*

Maintenance dose: A 12-hour dosage interval will be used for this patient. (Note: ng/mL = μg/L and this concentration was substituted for Css in the calculations so that unnecessary unit conversion was not required. Also, a conversion constant of 1000 μg/mg is used to change the dose amount to mg.) The dosage equation for oral sirolimus is: D = Css(Cl/F)τ = (5 μg/L • 7.3 L/h • 12 h)/(1000 μg/mg) = 0.44 mg. Dosage regimen is 0.44 mg every 12 hours.

Sirolimus concentrations would be obtained in about 7 days with steady-state expected to occur in about 7-12 days (3 half-lives = 3 • 49.1 h = 147 h, 147 h/(24 h/d) = 6.1 d).

Literature-Based Recommended Dosing

Because of the large amount of variability in sirolimus pharmacokinetics, even when concurrent disease states and conditions are identified, many clinicians believe that the use of standard sirolimus doses for various situations is warranted. Indeed, most transplant centers use doses that are determined using a sirolimus dosage protocol. The original computations of these doses were based on the Pharmacokinetic Dosing method described in the previous section, and subsequently modified based on clinical experience. In general, the expected sirolimus steady-state concentration used to compute these doses is dependent upon the type of transplanted tissue and the posttransplantation time line. Because the steady-state-to-single dose accumulation ratio for sirolimus is ~3, recommended loading doses are usually three times the prescribed maintenance dose.[8] Many transplant centers omit loading doses and commence dosing only with the maintenance dose.[4]

The implementation of these strategies is best established for renal transplant patients 13 years old and above. The dosage for sirolimus is stratified by the patient's immunologic risk. For patients with a low or moderate immunologic risk, sirolimus therapy is initiated using a 6-mg loading dose, followed by 2 mg/d with concomitant cyclosporine and corticosteroids therapy for 2-4 months. Therapeutic steady-state siroli-mus (typically 10-15 ng/mL) and cyclosporine concentrations should be maintained. If an adequate response has been attained during that time frame, the cyclosporine dose is tapered off over 4-8 weeks, and the siro-limus dose is adjusted to maintain therapeutic steady-state concentrations. Because cyclosporine inhibits sirolimus metabolism, the sirolimus dose usually needs to be increased while cyclosporine doses are decreased. For this clinical scenario, the recommended sirolimus steady-state concentrations after cyclospo-rine withdrawal are 16-24 ng/mL for the first year after transplantation and 12-20 ng/mL thereafter.[4,8]

For patients with a high immunologic risk (defined as Black transplant recipients, past transplant recipients with a failed kidney graft due to an immunologic etiology, or patients with lab results indicating high panel-reactive antibodies), sirolimus therapy is initiated using a loading dose up to 15 mg, followed by 5 mg/d with concurrent cyclosporine and corticosteroids treatment for 1 year following transplantation. Therapeutic steady-state sirolimus (typically 10-15 ng/mL) and cyclosporine concentrations should be maintained. If an adequate response has been attained during that time frame, adjustments to the dosage regimens for the individual medi-cations are based on the clinical response of the patient and may include reduction of the cyclosporine dose.[4,8] If tacrolimus is prescribed as the calcineurin inhibitor, the same dosage approaches can be used.

Sirolimus doses for adolescents 13 years old or older with low body weight (<40 kg) undergoing renal transplantation should be computed using body surface area. The recommended amounts are a loading dose of 3 mg/m^2 and an initial maintenance equal to 1 mg/m^2/d. Body surface area (BSA in m^2) can be estimated using the following formula[50]: BSA = 0.007184 • W$^{0.425}$ • H$^{0.725}$, where W is weight in kg and H is height in cm.

EXAMPLE 3 ▶▶▶

HO is a 50-year-old, 70-kg (height = 5 ft 10 in) male renal transplant patient with a low immunologic risk of rejec-tion. The patient's liver function tests are normal, and the patient is taking cyclosporine. Suggest an oral loading dose and an initial oral maintenance dose for sirolimus designed to achieve a steady-state sirolimus trough blood concentration within the therapeutic range.

1. *Choose sirolimus dose based on disease states and conditions present in the patient and transplant type.*
   For adult patients with a low or moderate immunologic risk, sirolimus therapy is initiated using a 6-mg load-ing dose, followed by 2 mg/d with concomitant cyclosporine and corticosteroids therapy for 2-4 months.
   Sirolimus concentrations would be obtained in about 7 days with steady-state expected to occur in about 7-12 days [3 half-lives = 3 • 60 h = 180 h, 180 h/(24 h/d) = 7.5 d].

EXAMPLE 4 ▶▶▶

Same patient profile as in example 3, except there is a high immunologic risk of rejection due to a Black ethnic background and a past kidney graft that was lost due to acute rejection.

1. *Choose sirolimus dose based on disease states and conditions present in the patient and transplant type.*
   For patients with a high immunologic risk (defined as Black transplant recipients, past transplant recipients with a failed kidney graft due to an immunologic etiology, or patients with lab results indicating high panel-reactive antibodies), sirolimus therapy is initiated using a loading dose up to 15 mg, followed by a main-tenance dose of 5 mg/d. Because this patient has multiple immunologic risk factors, a loading dose in the higher range is selected. The patient was prescribed a loading dose of 15 mg and a maintenance dose of 5 mg every 24 hours.
   Sirolimus concentrations would be obtained in about 7 days with steady-state expected to occur in about 7-12 days (3 half-lives = 3 • 60 h = 180 h, 180 h/(24 h/d) = 7.5 d).

USE OF SIROLIMUS CONCENTRATIONS TO ALTER DOSES

Because of the large amount of pharmacokinetic variability among patients, it is likely that doses computed using patient population characteristics will not always produce sirolimus concentrations that are expected or desirable. Because of pharmacokinetic variability, the narrow therapeutic index of sirolimus, and the severity of sirolimus adverse side effects, measurement of sirolimus concentrations is mandatory for patients to ensure that therapeutic, nontoxic levels are present. In addition to sirolimus concentrations, important patient parameters (transplanted organ function tests or biopsies, clinical signs and symptoms of graft rejection or graft-versus-host disease, potential sirolimus side effects, etc) should be followed to confirm that the patient is responding to treatment and not developing adverse drug reactions.

For most patients, predose steady-state trough sirolimus concentrations are typically measured. Since alternate methods to monitor cyclosporine concentrations have met with some success, investigators have begun suggesting similar methods for sirolimus. Of these methods, estimation of sirolimus area under the concentration-time curve (AUC) using several measured steady-state concentrations is the one that is used in some transplant centers.

When sirolimus concentrations are measured in patients and a dosage change is necessary, clinicians should seek to use the simplest, most straightforward method available to determine a dose that will provide safe and effective treatment. In most cases, a simple dosage ratio can be used to change sirolimus doses assuming the drug follows *linear pharmacokinetics*. Sometimes, it is useful to compute sirolimus pharmacokinetic constants for a patient and base dosage adjustments on these. In this case, it may be possible to calculate and use *pharmacokinetic parameters* to alter the sirolimus dose. Another approach involves measuring several postdose steady-state sirolimus concentrations to estimate the *area under the concentration-time curve (AUC)* and adjusting the sirolimus dose to attain a target AUC. Finally, computerized methods that incorporate expected population pharmacokinetic characteristics (*Bayesian pharmacokinetic computer programs*) can be used in difficult cases where concentrations are obtained at suboptimal times or the patient was not at steady-state when concentrations were measured.

Linear Pharmacokinetics Method

Assuming sirolimus follows linear, dose-proportional pharmacokinetics, steady-state concentrations change in proportion to dose according to the following equation:[1,4,9] $D_{new}/C_{ss,new} = D_{old}/C_{ss,old}$ or $D_{new} = (C_{ss,new}/C_{ss,old}) D_{old}$, where D is the dose, Css is the steady-state concentration, old indicates the dose that produced the steady-state concentration that the patient is currently receiving, and new denotes the dose necessary to produce the desired steady-state concentration. The advantages of this method are that it is quick and simple. The disadvantage is steady-state concentrations are required.

EXAMPLE 5 ▶▶▶

LK is a 49-year-old, 75-kg (height = 5 ft 10 in) male renal transplant recipient who is receiving 5 mg every 24 hours of oral sirolimus tablets. He has normal liver function and is taking cyclosporine. The current steady-state sirolimus blood concentration equals 24 ng/mL. Compute a sirolimus dose that will provide a steady-state concentration of 15 ng/mL.

1. *Compute new dose to achieve desired concentration.*

The patient would be expected to achieve steady-state conditions after the seventh day (3 $t_{1/2}$ = 3 • 60 h = 180 h or 7.5 d) of therapy.

Using linear pharmacokinetics, the new dose to attain the desired concentration should be proportional to the old dose that produced the measured concentration:

$$D_{new} = (C_{ss,new}/C_{ss,old})D_{old} = (15 \text{ ng/mL} / 24 \text{ ng/mL})5 \text{ mg/d} = 3.1 \text{ mg/d, rounded to 3 mg/d}$$

The new dose would be 3 mg every 24 hours of sirolimus tablets to be started at the next scheduled dosing time.

A steady-state trough sirolimus concentration should be measured after steady-state is attained in 3-5 half-lives. Since the patient is expected to have a half-life equal to 60 hours, the sirolimus steady-state concentration could be obtained any time after the seventh day of dosing ($3 \text{ t}_{1/2} = 3 \bullet 60 \text{ h} = 180 \text{ h or 7.5 d}$). Sirolimus concentrations should also be measured if the patient experiences signs or symptoms of graft rejection, or if the patient develops potential signs or symptoms of sirolimus toxicity.

EXAMPLE 6 ▶ ▶ ▶

FD is a 15-year-old, 55-kg (height = 5 ft 3 in) male liver transplant patient who is receiving 2 mg every 24 hours of oral sirolimus tablets. The graft is functioning and stable. The current steady-state sirolimus concentration equals 3 ng/mL. Compute a sirolimus dose that will provide a steady-state concentration of 6 ng/mL.

1. *Compute new dose to achieve desired concentration.*

   The patient would be expected to achieve steady-state conditions after the seventh day ($3 \text{ t}_{1/2} = 3 \bullet 60 \text{ h} = 180 \text{ h or 7.5 d}$) of therapy.

   Using linear pharmacokinetics, the new dose to attain the desired concentration should be proportional to the old dose that produced the measured concentration:

$$D_{new} = (C_{ss,new}/C_{ss,old})D_{old} = (6 \text{ ng/mL} / 3 \text{ ng/mL})2 \text{ mg/d} = 4 \text{ mg/d}$$

The new dose would be 4 mg every 24 hours of sirolimus tablets to be started at the next scheduled dosing time.

A sirolimus concentration should be measured after steady-state is attained in 3-5 half-lives. Since the patient is expected to have a half-life equal to 60 hours, the sirolimus steady-state concentration could be obtained any time after the seventh day of dosing (3 half-lives = $3 \bullet 60 \text{ h} = 180 \text{ h or 7.5 d}$). Sirolimus concentrations should also be measured if the patient experiences signs or symptoms of graft rejection, or if the patient develops potential signs or symptoms of sirolimus toxicity.

Pharmacokinetic Parameter Method

The Pharmacokinetic Parameter method of adjusting drug doses was among the first techniques available to change doses using drug concentrations. It allows the computation of an individual's own, unique pharmacokinetic constants and uses those to calculate a dose that achieves desired sirolimus concentrations. The Pharmacokinetic Parameter method requires that steady-state has been achieved and uses only a steady-state sirolimus concentration. Sirolimus clearance can be measured using a single steady-state sirolimus concentration and the following formula for orally administered drug: Cl/F = (D/τ)/Css, where Cl/F is the sirolimus clearance/bioavailability hybrid constant in L/h, τ is the dosage interval in hours, and Css is the sirolimus steady-state concentration in ng/mL which also equals μg/L. Although this method does allow computation of sirolimus Cl/F, it yields exactly the same sirolimus dose as that supplied using linear pharmacokinetics. As a result, most clinicians prefer to directly calculate the new dose using the Simpler Linear Pharmacokinetics method. To demonstrate this point, the patient cases used to illustrate the linear pharmacokinetics method will be used as examples for the Pharmacokinetic Parameter method.

EXAMPLE 7 ▶▶▶

LK is a 49-year-old, 75-kg (height = 5 ft 10 in) male renal transplant recipient who is receiving 5 mg every 24 hours of oral sirolimus tablets. He has normal liver function. The current steady-state sirolimus blood concentration equals 24 ng/mL. Compute a sirolimus dose that will provide a steady-state concentration of 15 ng/mL.

1. *Compute pharmacokinetic parameters.*
   The patient would be expected to achieve steady-state conditions after the seventh day (3 $t_{1/2}$ = 3 • 60 h = 180 h or 7.5 d) of therapy.

   Sirolimus Cl/F can be computed using a steady-state sirolimus concentration: Cl/F = (D/τ)/Css = [(5 mg/24 h) • 1000 μg/mg]/ (24 μg/L) = 8.7 L/h. (Note: μg/L = ng/mL and this concentration unit was substituted for Css in the calculations so that unnecessary unit conversion was not required.)

2. *Compute sirolimus dose.*
   Sirolimus Cl/F is used to compute the new dose: D = Css(Cl/F)τ = (15 μg/L • 8.7 L/h • 24 h)/(1000 μg/mg) = 3.1 mg, rounded to 3 mg every 24 hours.

   A steady-state trough sirolimus concentration should be measured after steady-state is attained in 3-5 half-lives. Since the patient is expected to have a half-life equal to 60 hours, the sirolimus steady-state concentration could be obtained any time after the seventh day of dosing (3 half-lives = 3 • 60 h = 180 h or 7.5 d). Sirolimus concentrations should also be measured if the patient experiences signs or symptoms of graft rejection, or if the patient develops potential signs or symptoms of sirolimus toxicity.

EXAMPLE 8 ▶▶▶

FD is a 15-year-old, 55-kg (height = 5 ft 3 in) male liver transplant patient who is receiving 2 mg every 24 hours of oral sirolimus tablets. The graft is functioning and stable. The current steady-state sirolimus concentration equals 3 ng/mL. Compute a sirolimus dose that will provide a steady-state concentration of 6 ng/mL.

1. *Compute pharmacokinetic parameters.*
   The patient would be expected to achieve steady-state conditions after the seventh day (3 $t_{1/2}$ = 3 • 60 h = 180 h or 7.5 d) of therapy.

   Sirolimus Cl/F can be computed using a steady-state sirolimus concentration: Cl/F = (D/τ)/Css = [(2 mg / 24 h) • 1000 μg/mg]/(3 μg/L) = 27.8 L/h. (Note: μg/L = ng/mL and this concentration unit was substituted for Css in the calculations so that unnecessary unit conversion was not required.)

2. *Compute sirolimus dose.*
   Sirolimus Cl/F is used to compute the new dose: D = Css(Cl/F)τ = (6 μg/L • 27.8 L/h • 24 h)/(1000 μg/mg) = 4 mg. The new dose is sirolimus tablets 4 mg every 24 hours.

A steady-state trough sirolimus concentration should be measured after steady-state is attained in 3-5 half-lives. Since the patient is expected to have a half-life equal to 60 hours, the sirolimus steady-state concentration could be obtained any time after the seventh day of dosing (3 half-lives = 3 • 60 h = 180 h or 7.5 d). Sirolimus concentrations should also be measured if the patient experiences signs or symptoms of graft rejection, or if the patient develops potential signs or symptoms of sirolimus toxicity.

Area Under the Concentration-Time Curve (AUC) Method

Some solid organ transplant centers believe that measurement or estimation of sirolimus area under the concentration-time curve (AUC) is the best way to optimize sirolimus therapy. While AUC can be measured using hourly postdose sirolimus levels, studies have shown that there is a strong correlation between 2 and 4 sirolimus concentrations and the total AUC. Based on this finding, most centers utilizing this method measure several steady-state sirolimus concentrations and use a published regression equation determined in other patients receiving the same transplanted organ and similar drug therapy (to account for possible drug interactions) in order to convert the concentrations to an estimated AUC. Then, if necessary, adjust the sirolimus dose using linear pharmacokinetics to achieve the target AUC: $D_{new}/AUC_{new} = D_{old}/AUC_{old}$ or $D_{new} = (AUC_{new}/AUC_{old})D_{old}$, where D is the dose, AUC is the steady-state area under the concentration-time curve, old indicates the dose that produced the steady-state area under the concentration-time curve that the patient is currently receiving, and new denotes the dose necessary to produce the desired steady-state area under the concentration-time curve. Desired sirolimus AUC values differ between the various types of transplants, change with time during the posttransplantation phase, and are determined by protocols specific to the transplantation service and institution where the patient is treated. It is very important for clinicians to be aware of these factors since acceptable sirolimus AUC values under various circumstances may be different than those given by a specific clinical laboratory or those suggested in this textbook.

There are many regression equations from which to choose based on the target transplant population and other concurrent therapy that may cause drug interactions with sirolimus. The ones used for the examples and problems in this book are for renal transplant patients. For adults, the equation was derived using patients who were not treated with a calcineurin inhibitor.[18] In this investigation, the steady-state AUC over the dosage interval [from time 0 hours (predose) to 24 hours after the dose, AUC_{0-24h}] strongly correlated with two steady-state concentrations, and this relationship was used to adjust sirolimus doses: AUC_{0-24h} [in (ng • h)/mL] = $(19.35 • C_{0h}) + (4.55 • C_{2h}) + 45.87$, where C_{0h} and C_{2h} are steady-state sirolimus concentrations in ng/mL obtained 0 and 2 hours, respectively, after a dose. The dose is then adjusted to produce a new steady-state AUC_{0-24h} equal to 310 ± 90 (ng • h)/mL using linear pharmacokinetics.

For the pediatrics population, one equation is for younger patients that received sirolimus every 12 hours, and the other equation is for older patients that received sirolimus every 24 hours.[19] For pediatric patients dosed every 12 hours, the steady-state AUC over the dosage interval [from time 0 hours (predose) to 12 hours after the dose, AUC_{0-12h}] strongly correlated with four steady-state concentrations, and this relationship was used to adjust sirolimus doses: AUC_{0-12h} [in (ng • h)/mL] = $10^{[1.085 + (0.117 • logC_{0h}) + (0.164 • logC_{1h}) - (0.131 • logC_{2h}) + (0.823 • logC_{4h})]}$, where C_{0h}, C_{1h}, C_{2h}, and C_{4h} are steady-state sirolimus concentrations in ng/mL obtained 0, 1, 2, and 4 hours, respectively, after a dose. The dose is then adjusted to produce a new steady-state AUC_{0-12h} equal to ~146 (ng • h)/mL using linear pharmacokinetics. For the derivation of this equation, there was a mixture of patients included that received tacrolimus, cyclosporine, or no calcineurin inhibitor.

For pediatric patients dosed every 24 hours, the steady-state AUC over the dosage interval [from time 0 hours (predose) to 24 hours after the dose, AUC_{0-24h}] strongly correlated with two steady-state concentrations, and this relationship was used to adjust sirolimus doses: AUC_{0-24h} [in (ng • h)/mL] = $10^{[1.100 + (0.115 • logC_{0h}) + (0.803 • logC_{4h})]}$, where C_{0h} and C_{4h} are steady-state sirolimus concentrations in ng/mL obtained 0 and 4 hours, respectively, after a dose. The dose is then adjusted to produce a new steady-state AUC_{0-24h} equal to ~177 (ng • h)/mL using linear pharmacokinetics. For the derivation of this equation, the included patients did not take concurrent calcineurin inhibitors.

EXAMPLE 9 ▶ ▶ ▶

SD is a 37-year-old, 78-kg (height = 6 ft 1 in) male who has undergone renal transplantation. He is receiving 5 mg every 24 hours of oral sirolimus. The following sirolimus steady-state concentrations have been measured to determine an estimated AUC_{0-24h}: $C_{0h} = 17$ ng/mL, $C_{2h} = 34$ ng/mL. Compute a sirolimus dose that will provide a steady-state AUC_{0-24h} of 310 (ng • h)/mL.

1. *Compute pharmacokinetic parameters.*

   Sirolimus AUC_{0-24h} can be estimated using the steady-state sirolimus concentrations: AUC_{0-24h} [in (ng • h)/mL] = $(19.35 • C_{0h}) + (4.55 • C_{2h}) + 45.87 = (19.35 • 17$ ng/mL$) + (4.55 • 34$ ng/mL$) + 45.87 = 530$ (ng • h)/mL.

2. *Compute sirolimus dose.*

   Linear pharmacokinetics is used to compute the new dose: $D_{new} = (AUC_{new}/AUC_{old})D_{old} = \{[310$ (ng • h)/mL]/$[530$ (ng • h)/mL]$\}(5$ mg/d$) = 2.9$ mg/d, rounded to 3 mg every 24 hours.

   Steady-state sirolimus serum concentrations should be measured after steady-state is attained in 3-5 half-lives. Sirolimus concentrations should also be measured if the patient experiences signs or symptoms of graft rejection, or if the patient develops potential signs or symptoms of sirolimus toxicity.

BAYESIAN PHARMACOKINETIC COMPUTER PROGRAMS

Computer programs are available that can assist in the computation of pharmacokinetic parameters for patients. The most reliable computer programs use a nonlinear regression algorithm that incorporates components of Bayes theorem. Nonlinear regression is a statistical technique that uses an iterative process to compute the best pharmacokinetic parameters for a concentration/time data set. Briefly, the patient's drug dosage schedule and drug concentrations are input into the computer. The computer program has a pharmacokinetic equation preprogrammed for the drug and administration method (oral, intravenous bolus, intravenous infusion, etc). Typically, a one-compartment model is used, although some programs allow the user to choose among several different equations. Using population estimates based on demographic information for the patient (age, weight, gender, liver function, cardiac status, etc) supplied by the user, the computer program then computes estimated drug concentrations at each time there are actual drug concentrations. Kinetic parameters are then changed by the computer program, and a new set of estimated drug concentrations are computed. The pharmacokinetic parameters that generated the estimated drug concentrations closest to the actual values are remembered by the computer program, and the process is repeated until the set of pharmacokinetic parameters that result in estimated drug concentrations that are statistically closest to the actual drug concentrations are generated. These pharmacokinetic parameters can then be used to compute improved dosing schedules for patients. Bayes theorem is used in the computer algorithm to balance the results of the computations between values based solely on the patient's drug concentrations and those based only on patient population parameters. Results from studies that compare various methods of dosage adjustment have consistently found that these types of computer-dosing programs perform at least as well as experienced clinical pharmacokineticists and clinicians and better than inexperienced clinicians.

Some clinicians use Bayesian pharmacokinetic computer programs exclusively to alter drug doses based on drug concentrations. An advantage of this approach is that consistent dosage recommendations are made when several different practitioners are involved in therapeutic drug monitoring programs. However, since simpler dosing methods work just as well for patients with stable pharmacokinetic parameters and steady-state drug concentrations, many clinicians reserve the use of computer programs for more difficult situations. Those situations include drug concentrations that are not at steady-state, drug concentrations not obtained at the specific times needed to employ simpler methods, and unstable pharmacokinetic parameters. When only a limited number of cyclosporine steady-state concentrations are available, Bayesian pharmacokinetic computer programs can be used to compute a complete patient pharmacokinetic profile that includes clearance, volume of distribution, and half-life. Many Bayesian pharmacokinetic computer programs are available to users, and most should provide answers similar to the one used in the following examples.[51]

EXAMPLE 10 ▶ ▶ ▶

MB is a 52-year-old, 73-kg (height = 5 ft 9 in) male renal transplant recipient who is receiving 5 mg every 24 hours of oral sirolimus tablets. He has normal liver function (bilirubin = 0.7 mg/dL, albumin = 4.0 g/dL), and takes cyclosporine. The current steady-state predose sirolimus blood concentration equals 24 ng/mL. Compute a sirolimus dose that will provide a steady-state concentration of 15 ng/mL.

1. *Enter the patient's demographic, drug-dosing, and concentration/time data into the computer program.*
2. *Compute pharmacokinetic parameters for the patient using Bayesian pharmacokinetic computer program.*
   The pharmacokinetic parameters computed by the program are a V/F of 712 L, a half-life equal to 65 h, and a Cl/F equal to 8.6 L/h.
3. *Compute dose required to achieve the desired sirolimus concentrations.*
   The one-compartment model first-order absorption equations used by the program to compute doses indicates that a dose of 3 mg every 24 hours will produce a steady-state sirolimus concentration of 15 ng/mL.

DOSING STRATEGIES

Initial dose and dosage adjustment techniques using serum concentrations can be used in any combination as long as the limitations of each method are observed. Some dosing schemes link together logically when considered according to their basic approaches or philosophies. Dosage strategies that follow similar pathways are given in Table 20-4.

PROBLEMS

The following problems are intended to emphasize the computation of initial and individualized doses using clinical pharmacokinetic techniques. Clinicians should always consult the patient's chart to confirm that current immunosuppressive therapy is appropriate. Additionally, all other medications that the patient is

TABLE 20-4   Dosing Strategies

Dosing Approach/Philosophy	Initial Dosing	Use of Serum Concentrations to Alter Doses
Pharmacokinetic parameter/equations	Pharmacokinetic Dosing method	Pharmacokinetic Parameter method
Literature-based concept	Literature-based Recommended Dosing method	Linear Pharmacokinetics or area under the concentration-time curve (AUC) method
Computerized	Bayesian computer program	Bayesian computer program

taking, including prescription and nonprescription drugs, should be noted and checked to ascertain if a potential drug interaction with sirolimus exists.

1. IV is a 37-year-old, 85-kg (height = 6 ft 1 in) male renal transplant patient with a low immunologic risk of rejection who requires therapy with oral sirolimus. He has normal liver function, and he is taking tacrolimus. Suggest an initial maintenance dosage regimen designed to achieve a steady-state sirolimus concentration equal to 7 ng/mL.

2. Patient IV (see problem 1) was prescribed 5 mg every 24 hours of sirolimus tablets for 14 days, and the steady-state sirolimus concentration equals 21 ng/mL. The patient is assessed to be compliant with his dosage regimen. Suggest a sirolimus dosage regimen designed to achieve a steady-state sirolimus concentration of 10 ng/mL.

3. DF is a 29-year-old, 68-kg (height = 5 ft 8 in) male renal transplant patient with a high immunologic risk of rejection who requires therapy with oral sirolimus. He has normal liver function, and he is taking cyclosporine. Suggest an initial loading dose and maintenance dosage regimen designed to achieve a steady-state sirolimus concentration equal to 15 ng/mL.

4. Patient DF (see problem 3) was prescribed 6 mg every 24 hours of sirolimus tablets for 14 days, and the steady-state sirolimus concentration equals 9 ng/mL. The patient is assessed to be compliant with his dosage regimen. Suggest a sirolimus dosage regimen designed to achieve a steady-state sirolimus concentration of 15 ng/mL.

5. WQ is a 14-year-old, 35-kg female (height = 4 ft 9 in) renal transplantation patient with a low immunologic risk of rejection who requires therapy with oral sirolimus. She has normal liver function and is being treated with cyclosporine. Suggest an initial sirolimus maintenance dosage regimen designed to achieve a steady-state sirolimus concentration equal to 5 ng/mL.

6. Patient WQ (see problem 5) was prescribed 2 mg every 24 hours of sirolimus tablets for 14 days, and the steady-state sirolimus concentration equals 15 ng/mL. The patient is assessed to be compliant with her dosage regimen. Suggest an oral sirolimus dosage regimen designed to achieve a steady-state sirolimus concentration equal to 7 ng/mL.

7. NH is a 56-year-old, 71-kg (height = 6 ft 2 in) male liver transplant patient who requires therapy with oral sirolimus. His graft is functioning normally, and he is taking tacrolimus. Suggest an initial maintenance dosage regimen designed to achieve a steady-state sirolimus concentration equal to 10 ng/mL.

8. Patient NH (see problem 7) was prescribed 2 mg every 24 hours of sirolimus tablets for 14 days, and the steady-state sirolimus concentration equals 7 ng/mL. The patient is assessed to be compliant with his dosage regimen. Suggest a sirolimus dosage regimen designed to achieve a steady-state sirolimus concentration of 10 ng/mL.

9. UI is a 43-year-old, 64-kg (height = 5 ft 8 in) male who has undergone renal transplantation. He is receiving 3 mg every 24 hours of oral sirolimus. The following sirolimus steady-state concentrations have been measured to determine an estimated AUC_{0-24h}: $C_{0h} = 3$ ng/mL, $C_{2h} = 7$ ng/mL. Compute a sirolimus dose that will provide a steady-state AUC_{0-24h} of 310 (ng • h)/mL.

10. FH is a 12-year-old, 36-kg (height = 4 ft 6 in) male who has undergone renal transplantation. He is receiving 3 mg every 24 hours of oral sirolimus. The following sirolimus steady-state concentrations have been measured to determine an estimated AUC_{0-24h}: $C_{0h} = 15$ ng/mL, $C_{2h} = 30$ ng/mL. Compute a sirolimus dose that will provide a steady-state AUC_{0-24h} of 177 (ng • h)/mL.

11. LI is a 57-year-old, 67-kg (height = 5 ft 9 in) male renal transplant recipient who just received his first prescription for sirolimus: 5 mg every 24 hours of oral sirolimus tablets. He has normal liver function (bilirubin = 0.6 mg/dL, albumin = 4.2 g/dL), and takes cyclosporine. After the third dose, the predose sirolimus blood concentration equals 6 ng/mL. Compute a sirolimus dose that will provide a steady-state concentration of 15 ng/mL.

ANSWERS TO PROBLEMS

1. *Answer to problem 1.*

Pharmacokinetic Dosing Method

1. *Estimate pharmacokinetic parameters according to disease states and conditions present in the patient.*

   The mean sirolimus Cl/F for adult renal transplant patients taking tacrolimus is 310 mL/h/kg and the mean V/F is 7.7 L/kg. The sirolimus CL/F for this patient is: Cl/F = (310 mL/h/kg • 85 kg)/(1000 mL/L) = 26.4 L/h. The sirolimus V/F for this patient is: V/F = 7.7 L/kg • 85 kg = 655 L.

2. *Compute dosage regimen.*

   Maintenance dose: A 24-hour dosage interval will be used for this patient. (Note: ng/mL = µg/L and this concentration was substituted for Css in the calculations so that unnecessary unit conversion was not required. Also, a conversion constant of 1000 µg/mg is used to change the dose amount to mg.) The dosage equation for oral sirolimus is: D = Css(Cl/F)τ = (7 µg/L • 26.4 L/h • 24 h)/(1000 µg/mg) = 4.4 mg, rounded to 4.5 mg every 24 hours.

   Sirolimus concentrations would be obtained in about 7 days with steady-state expected to occur in about 7-12 days (half-life not known for this population; assuming 3 half-lives = 3 • 60 h = 180 h, 180 h/(24 h/d) = 7.5 d).

Literature-Based Recommended Dosing

1. *Choose sirolimus dose based on disease states and conditions present in the patient and transplant type.*

   For adult patients with a low or moderate immunologic risk, sirolimus therapy is initiated using a 6-mg loading dose, followed by 2 mg/d with concomitant cyclosporine and corticosteroids therapy for 2-4 months. A specific literature-based recommended dose for patients taking tacrolimus is not available, so the doses for patients taking cyclosporine are often used.

   Sirolimus concentrations would be obtained in about 7 days with steady-state expected to occur in about 7-12 days (half-life not known for this population; assuming 3 half-lives = 3 • 60 h = 180 h, 180 h/(24 h/d) = 7.5 d).

2. *Answer to problem 2.*

Linear Pharmacokinetics Method

1. *Compute new dose to achieve the desired concentration.*

   Assuming a $t_{1/2}$ = 60 h, the patient would be expected to achieve steady-state conditions after the seventh day (half-life not known for this population; assuming 3 $t_{1/2}$ = 3 • 60 h = 180 h or 7.5 d) of therapy.

   Using linear pharmacokinetics, the new dose to attain the desired concentration should be proportional to the old dose that produced the measured concentration:

   $$D_{new} = (C_{ss,new}/C_{ss,old})D_{old} = (10\ ng/mL\ /\ 21\ ng/mL)\ 5\ mg/d = 2.4\ mg/d, \text{ rounded to } 2.5\ mg/d$$

   The new dose would be 2.5 mg every 24 hours of sirolimus tablets to be started at the next scheduled dosing time.

A steady-state trough sirolimus concentration should be measured after steady-state is attained in 3-5 half-lives. Since the patient is assumed to have a half-life equal to 60 hours, the sirolimus steady-state concentration could be obtained any time after the seventh day of dosing (3 $t_{1/2}$ = 3 • 60 h = 180 h or 7.5 d). Sirolimus concentrations should also be measured if the patient experiences signs or symptoms of graft rejection, or if the patient develops potential signs or symptoms of sirolimus toxicity.

Pharmacokinetic Parameter Method

1. *Compute pharmacokinetic parameters.*

The patient would be expected to achieve steady-state conditions after the seventh day (half-life not known for this population; assuming 3 $t_{1/2}$ = 3 • 60 h = 180 h or 7.5 days) of therapy.

Sirolimus Cl/F can be computed using a steady-state sirolimus concentration: Cl/F = (D/τ)/Css = [(5 mg/24 h) •1000 μg/mg]/(21 μg/L) = 9.9 L/h. (Note: μg/L = ng/mL and this concentration unit was substituted for Css in the calculations so that unnecessary unit conversion was not required.)

2. *Compute sirolimus dose.*

Sirolimus Cl/F is used to compute the new dose: D = Css(Cl/F)τ = (10 μg/L• 9.9 L/h • 24 h)/ (1000 μg/mg) = 2.4 mg, rounded to 2.5 mg every 24 hours.

A steady-state trough sirolimus concentration should be measured after steady-state is attained in 3-5 half-lives. Since the patient is expected to have a half-life equal to 60 hours, the sirolimus steady-state concentration could be obtained any time after the seventh day of dosing (half-life not known for this population; assuming three half-lives = 3 • 60 h = 180 h or 7.5 d). Sirolimus concentrations should also be measured if the patient experiences signs or symptoms of graft rejection, or if the patient develops potential signs or symptoms of sirolimus toxicity.

3. *Answer to problem 3.*

Pharmacokinetic Dosing Method

1. *Estimate pharmacokinetic parameters according to disease states and conditions present in the patient.*

The mean sirolimus Cl/F for adult renal transplant patients taking cyclosporine is 240 mL/ h/kg and the mean V/F is 10 L/kg. The sirolimus CL/F for this patient is: Cl/F = (240 mL/h/kg • 68 kg)/(1000 mL/L) = 16.3 L/h. The sirolimus V/F for this patient is: V/F = 10 L/kg • 68 kg = 680 L.

2. *Compute dosage regimen.*

Loading dose: (Note: ng/mL = μg/L and this concentration was substituted for Css in the calculations so that unnecessary unit conversion was not required. Also, a conversion constant of 1000 μg/mg is used to change the dose amount to mg.) The dosage equation for oral sirolimus is: LD = Css(V/F) = (15 μg/L • 680 L)/(1000 μg/mg) = 10.2 mg, rounded to 10 mg.

Maintenance dose: A 24-hour dosage interval will be used for this patient. (Note: ng/mL = μg/L and this concentration was substituted for Css in the calculations so that unnecessary unit conversion was not required. Also, a conversion constant of 1000 μg/mg is used to change the dose amount to mg.) The dosage equation for oral sirolimus is: D = Css(Cl/F)τ = (15 μg/L • 16.3 L/h • 24 h)/(1000 μg/mg) = 5.9 mg, rounded to 6 mg every 24 hours.

Sirolimus concentrations would be obtained in about 7 days with steady-state expected to occur in about 7-12 days ($t_{1/2}$ = 60 h: 3 half-lives = 3 • 60 h = 180 h, 180 h/(24 h/d) = 7.5 d).

Literature-Based Recommended Dosing

1. *Choose sirolimus dose based on disease states and conditions present in the patient and transplant type.*

   For patients with a high immunologic risk (defined as Black transplant recipients, past transplant recipients with a failed kidney graft due to an immunologic etiology, or patients with lab results indicating high panel-reactive antibodies), sirolimus therapy is initiated using a loading dose up to 15 mg, followed by a maintenance dose of 5 mg/d. The patient was prescribed a loading dose of 15 mg and a maintenance dose of 5 mg every 24 hours.

   Sirolimus concentrations would be obtained in about 7 days with steady-state expected to occur in about 7-12 days (3 half-lives = 3 • 60 h = 180 h, 180 h/(24 h/d) = 7.5 d).

4. *Answer to problem 4.*

Linear Pharmacokinetics Method

1. *Compute new dose to achieve the desired concentration.*

   Assuming a $t_{1/2} = 60$ h, the patient would be expected to achieve steady-state conditions after the seventh day (3 $t_{1/2} = 3 \cdot 60$ h = 180 h or 7.5 d) of therapy.

   Using linear pharmacokinetics, the new dose to attain the desired concentration should be proportional to the old dose that produced the measured concentration:

$$D_{new} = (C_{ss,new}/C_{ss,old})D_{old} = (15 \text{ ng/mL}/9 \text{ ng/mL}) \, 6 \text{ mg/d} = 10 \text{ mg/d}$$

   The new dose would be 10 mg every 24 hours of sirolimus tablets to be started at the next scheduled dosing time.

   A steady-state trough sirolimus concentration should be measured after steady-state is attained in 3-5 half-lives. Since the patient is expected to have a half-life equal to 60 hours, the sirolimus steady-state concentration could be obtained any time after the seventh day of dosing ($3t_{1/2} = 3 \cdot 60$ h = 180 h or 7.5 d). Sirolimus concentrations should also be measured if the patient experiences signs or symptoms of graft rejection, or if the patient develops potential signs or symptoms of sirolimus toxicity.

Pharmacokinetic Parameter Method

1. *Compute pharmacokinetic parameters.*

   The patient would be expected to achieve steady-state conditions after the seventh day (3 $t_{1/2} =$ 3 • 60 h = 180 h or 7.5 days) of therapy.

   Sirolimus Cl/F can be computed using a steady-state sirolimus concentration: Cl/F = $(D/\tau)/Css = [(6 \text{ mg/24 h}) \cdot 1000 \, \mu\text{g/mg}]/(9 \, \mu\text{g/L}) = 27.8$ L/h. (Note: μg/L = ng/mL and this concentration unit was substituted for Css in the calculations so that unnecessary unit conversion was not required.)

2. *Compute sirolimus dose.*

   Sirolimus Cl/F is used to compute the new dose: D = Css(Cl/F)τ = (15 μg/L• 27.8 L/h • 24 h)/ (1000 μg/mg) = 10 mg, the new dose is 10 mg every 24 hours.

   A steady-state trough sirolimus concentration should be measured after steady-state is attained in 3-5 half-lives. Since the patient is expected to have a half-life equal to 60 hours, the sirolimus steady-state concentration could be obtained any time after the seventh day of dosing (3 half-lives = 3 • 60 h = 180 h or 7.5 d). Sirolimus concentrations should also be measured if the patient experiences signs or symptoms of graft rejection, or if the patient develops potential signs or symptoms of sirolimus toxicity.

5. *Answer to problem 5.*

Pharmacokinetic Dosing Method

1. *Estimate pharmacokinetic parameters according to disease states and conditions present in the patient.*

The mean sirolimus Cl/F for adolescent renal transplant patients taking cyclosporine is 376 mL/h/kg. The sirolimus CL/F for this patient is: Cl/F = (376 mL/h/kg • 35 kg)/(1000 mL/L) = 13.2 L/h.

2. *Compute dosage regimen.*

Maintenance dose: A 24-hour dosage interval will be used for this patient. (Note: ng/mL = µg/L and this concentration was substituted for Css in the calculations so that unnecessary unit conversion was not required. Also, a conversion constant of 1000 µg/mg is used to change the dose amount to mg.) The dosage equation for oral sirolimus is: D = Css(Cl/F)τ = (5 µg/L • 13.2 L/h • 24 h)/(1000 µg/mg) = 1.6 mg, rounded to 1.5 mg every 24 hours.

Sirolimus concentrations would be obtained in about 7 days with steady-state expected to occur in about 7-12 days (3 half-lives = 3 • 70.3 h = 211 h, 211 h/(24 h/d) = 8.8 d).

Literature-Based Recommended Dosing

1. *Choose sirolimus dose based on disease states and conditions present in the patient and transplant type.*

For adolescents with a low body weight (<40 kg), sirolimus therapy is initiated using a loading dose of 3 mg/m^2 and an initial maintenance equal to 1 mg/m^2/d. Body surface area (BSA in m^2) can be estimated using the following formula: BSA (in m^2) = 0.007184 • W$^{0.425}$ • H$^{0.725}$, where W is weight in kg and H is height in cm (height 4 ft 9 in = 57 in; 57 in • 2.54 cm/in = 145 cm). For this patient: BSA = 0.007184 • (35 kg)$^{0.425}$ • (145 cm)$^{0.725}$ = 1.2 m^2.

The loading dose is 3 mg/m^2: LD = (3 mg/m^2)(1.2 m^2) = 3.6 mg, rounded to 3.5 mg.

The initial maintenance equal to 1 mg/m^2/d: D = (1 mg/m^2/d)(1.2 m^2) = 1.2 mg/d, rounded to 1 mg every 24 h.

Sirolimus concentrations would be obtained in about 7 days with steady-state expected to occur in about 7-12 days (3 half-lives = 3 • 70.3 h = 211 h, 211 h/(24 h/d) = 8.8 d).

6. *Answer to problem 6.*

Linear Pharmacokinetics Method

1. *Compute new dose to achieve the desired concentration.*

Assuming a $t_{1/2}$ = 70.3 h, the patient would be expected to achieve steady-state conditions after the ninth day (3 $t_{1/2}$ = 3 • 70.3 h = 211 h or 8.8 d) of therapy.

Using linear pharmacokinetics, the new dose to attain the desired concentration should be proportional to the old dose that produced the measured concentration:

$$D_{new} = (C_{ss,new}/C_{ss,old})D_{old} = (7 \text{ ng/mL}/15 \text{ ng/mL}) \text{ } 2 \text{ mg/d} = 0.93 \text{ mg/d, rounded to 1 mg/d}$$

The new dose would be 1 mg every 24 hours of sirolimus tablets to be started at the next scheduled dosing time.

A steady-state trough sirolimus concentration should be measured after steady-state is attained in 3-5 half-lives. Since the patient is expected to have a half-life equal to 70.3 hours, the sirolimus steady-state concentration could be obtained any time after the ninth day of dosing (3 $t_{1/2}$ = 3 • 70.3 h = 211 h or 8.8 d). Sirolimus concentrations should also be measured if the patient experiences signs or symptoms of graft rejection, or if the patient develops potential signs or symptoms of sirolimus toxicity.

Pharmacokinetic Parameter Method

1. *Compute pharmacokinetic parameters.*

Assuming a $t_{1/2} = 70.3$ h, the patient would be expected to achieve steady-state conditions after the ninth day ($3\ t_{1/2} = 3 \bullet 70.3$ h $= 211$ h or 8.8 d) of therapy.

Sirolimus Cl/F can be computed using a steady-state sirolimus concentration: Cl/F = (D/τ)/Css = [(2 mg/24 h) $\bullet$ 1000 µg/mg]/(15 µg/L) = 5.6 L/h. (Note: µg/L = ng/mL and this concentration unit was substituted for Css in the calculations so that unnecessary unit conversion was not required).

2. *Compute sirolimus dose.*

Sirolimus Cl/F is used to compute the new dose: D = Css(Cl/F)τ = (7 µg/L $\bullet$ 5.6 L/h $\bullet$ 24 h)/(1000 µg/mg) = 0.94 mg, rounded to 1 mg every 24 hours.

A steady-state trough sirolimus concentration should be measured after steady-state is attained in 3-5 half-lives. Since the patient is expected to have a half-life equal to 70.3 hours, the sirolimus steady-state concentration could be obtained any time after the ninth day of dosing ($3\ t_{1/2} = 3 \bullet 70.3$ h $= 211$ h or 8.8 d). Sirolimus concentrations should also be measured if the patient experiences signs or symptoms of graft rejection, or if the patient develops potential signs or symptoms of sirolimus toxicity.

7. *Answer to problem 7.*

Pharmacokinetic Dosing Method

1. *Estimate pharmacokinetic parameters according to disease states and conditions present in the patient.*

The mean sirolimus Cl/F for adult liver transplant patients taking tacrolimus is 146 mL/h/kg. The sirolimus CL/F for this patient is: Cl/F = (146 mL/h/kg $\bullet$ 71 kg)/(1000 mL/L) = 10.4 L/h.

2. *Compute dosage regimen.*

Maintenance dose: A 24-hour dosage interval will be used for this patient. (Note: ng/mL = µg/L and this concentration was substituted for Css in the calculations so that unnecessary unit conversion was not required. Also, a conversion constant of 1000 µg/mg is used to change the dose amount to mg.) The dosage equation for oral sirolimus is: D = Css(Cl/F)τ = (10 µg/L $\bullet$ 10.4 L/h $\bullet$ 24 h)/(1000 µg/mg) = 2.5 mg, maintenance dose is 2.5 mg every 24 hours.

Sirolimus concentrations would be obtained in about 7 days with steady-state expected to occur in about 7-12 days [assuming $t_{1/2} = 60$ h for this population: 3 half-lives = 3 $\bullet$ 60 h = 180 h, 180 h/(24 h/d) = 7.5 d].

Literature-Based Recommended Dosing

1. *Choose sirolimus dose based on disease states and conditions present in the patient and transplant type.*

For adult renal failure patients with a low or moderate immunologic risk, sirolimus therapy is initiated using a 6-mg loading dose, followed by 2 mg/d. While a specific literature-based recommended dose for liver transplant patients taking tacrolimus is not available, this dose is oftentimes used for this population.

Sirolimus concentrations would be obtained in about 7 days with steady-state expected to occur in about 7-12 days [assuming $t_{1/2} = 60$ h for this population: 3 half-lives = 3 $\bullet$ 60 h = 180 h, 180 h/(24 h/d) = 7.5 d].

8. *Answer to problem 8.*

Linear Pharmacokinetics Method

1. *Compute new dose to achieve desired concentration.*

Assuming a $t_{1/2} = 60$ h, the patient would be expected to achieve steady-state conditions after the seventh day ($3\ t_{1/2} = 3 \bullet 60$ h $= 180$ h or 7.5 d) of therapy.

Using linear pharmacokinetics, the new dose to attain the desired concentration should be proportional to the old dose that produced the measured concentration:

$$D_{new} = (C_{ss,new}/C_{ss,old})D_{old} = (10\ \text{ng/mL}/7\ \text{ng/mL})\ 2\ \text{mg/d} = 2.9\ \text{mg/d, rounded to 3 mg/d}$$

The new dose would be 3 mg every 24 hours of sirolimus tablets to be started at the next scheduled dosing time.

A steady-state trough sirolimus concentration should be measured after steady-state is attained in 3-5 half-lives. Since the patient is assumed to have a half-life equal to 60 hours, the sirolimus steady-state concentration could be obtained any time after the seventh day of dosing ($3\ t_{1/2} = 3 \bullet 60$ h $= 180$ h or 7.5 d). Sirolimus concentrations should also be measured if the patient experiences signs or symptoms of graft rejection, or if the patient develops potential signs or symptoms of sirolimus toxicity.

Pharmacokinetic Parameter Method

1. *Compute pharmacokinetic parameters.*

Assuming a $t_{1/2} = 60$ h, the patient would be expected to achieve steady-state conditions after the seventh day ($3\ t_{1/2} = 3 \bullet 60$ h $= 180$ h or 7.5 d) of therapy.

Sirolimus Cl/F can be computed using a steady-state sirolimus concentration: $Cl/F = (D/\tau)/Css = [(2\ \text{mg}/24\ \text{h}) \bullet 1000\ \mu\text{g/mg}]/(7\ \mu\text{g/L}) = 11.9$ L/h. (Note: μg/L = ng/mL and this concentration unit was substituted for Css in the calculations so that unnecessary unit conversion was not required.)

2. *Compute sirolimus dose.*

Sirolimus Cl/F is used to compute the new dose: $D = Css(Cl/F)\tau = (10\ \mu\text{g/L} \bullet 11.9\ \text{L/h} \bullet 24\ \text{h})/(1000\ \mu\text{g/mg}) = 2.9$ mg, rounded to 3 mg every 24 hours.

A steady-state trough sirolimus concentration should be measured after steady-state is attained in 3-5 half-lives. Since the patient is assumed to have a half life equal to 60 hours, the sirolimus steady-state concentration could be obtained any time after the seventh day of dosing (3 half-lives = $3 \bullet 60$ h $= 180$ h or 7.5 d). Sirolimus concentrations should also be measured if the patient experiences signs or symptoms of graft rejection, or if the patient develops potential signs or symptoms of sirolimus toxicity.

9. *Answer to problem 9.*

Area Under the Concentration-Time Curve Method

1. *Compute pharmacokinetic parameters.*

Sirolimus AUC_{0-24h} can be estimated using the steady-state sirolimus concentrations: AUC_{0-24h} (in [ng $\bullet$ h]/mL) $= (19.35 \bullet C_{0h}) + (4.55 \bullet C_{2h}) + 45.87 = (19.35 \bullet 3\ \text{ng/mL}) + (4.55 \bullet 7\ \text{ng/mL}) + 45.87 = 136$ (ng $\bullet$ h)/mL.

2. *Compute sirolimus dose.*

Linear pharmacokinetics is used to compute the new dose: $D_{new} = (AUC_{new}/AUC_{old})D_{old} = $ {[310 (ng • h)/mL] / [136 (ng • h)/mL]}(3 mg/d) = 6.8 mg/d, rounded to 7 mg every 24 hours.

Steady-state sirolimus serum concentrations should be measured after steady-state is attained in 3-5 half-lives. Sirolimus concentrations should also be measured if the patient experiences signs or symptoms of graft rejection, or if the patient develops potential signs or symptoms of sirolimus toxicity.

10. *Answer to problem 10.*

Area Under the Concentration-Time Curve Method

1. *Compute pharmacokinetic parameters.*

Sirolimus AUC_{0-24h} can be estimated using the steady-state sirolimus concentrations: AUC_{0-24h} [in (ng • h)/mL] $= 10^{[1.100 + (0.115 \cdot \log C_{0h}) + (0.803 \cdot \log C_{4h})]} = 10^{\{1.100 + [0.115 \cdot \log(15\,ng/mL)] + [0.803 \cdot \log(30\,ng/mL)]\}} = $ 264 (ng • h)/mL.

2. *Compute sirolimus dose.*

Linear pharmacokinetics is used to compute the new dose: $D_{new} = (AUC_{new}/AUC_{old})D_{old} = $ {[177 (ng • h)/mL]/[264 (ng • h)/mL]}(3 mg/d) = 2 mg/d, new dose is 2 mg every 24 hours.

Steady-state sirolimus serum concentrations should be measured after steady-state is attained in 3-5 half-lives. Sirolimus concentrations should also be measured if the patient experiences signs or symptoms of graft rejection, or if the patient develops potential signs or symptoms of sirolimus toxicity.

11. *Answer to problem 11.*

Bayesian Pharmacokinetic Computer Program Method

This patient is not at steady-state yet, so methods that require a steady-state sirolimus concentration cannot be used. A method must be used that can compute a dose using the available information.

1. *Enter the patient's demographic, drug-dosing, and concentration/time data into the computer program.*

2. *Compute pharmacokinetic parameters for the patient using Bayesian pharmacokinetic computer program.*

The pharmacokinetic parameters computed by the program are a V/F of 712 L, a half-life equal to 65 h, and a Cl/F equal to 8.6 L/h.

3. *Compute dose required to achieve the desired sirolimus concentrations.*

The one-compartment model first-order absorption equations used by the program to compute doses indicates that a dose of 3 mg every 24 hours will produce a steady-state sirolimus concentration of 15 ng/mL.

REFERENCES

1. Johnson HJ, Schonder KS. Solid-organ transplantation. In: DiPiro JT, Talbert RL, Yee GC, Matzke GR, Wells BG, Posey LM, eds. *Pharmacotherapy.* 8th ed. New York, NY: McGraw-Hill; 2011:1547-1558.

2. Perkins JB, Yee GC. Hematopoietic stem cell transplantation. In: DiPiro JT, Talbert RL, Yee GC, Matzke GR, Wells BG, Posey LM, eds. *Pharmacotherapy.* 8th ed. New York, NY: McGraw-Hill; 2011:2455-2472.

3. Krensky AM, Bennett WM, Vincenti F. Immunosuppressants, tolerogens, and immunostimulants. In: Brunton LL, Lazo JS, Parker KL, eds. *The Pharmacological Basis of Therapeutics.* 12th ed. New York, NY: McGraw-Hill; 2011:1005-1030.

4. Lee RA, Gabardi S. Current trends in immunosuppressive therapies for renal transplant recipients. *Am J Health Syst Pharm.* Nov 15, 2012;69(22):1961-1975.

5. Johnson-Davis KL, De S, Jimenez E, McMillin GA, De BK. Evaluation of the Abbott ARCHITECT i2000 sirolimus assay and comparison with the Abbott IMx sirolimus assay and an established liquid chromatography-tandem mass spectrometry method. *Ther Drug Monit.* Aug 2011;33(4):453-459.

6. Davis DL, Murthy JN, Napoli KL, et al. Comparison of steady-state trough sirolimus samples by HPLC and a radioreceptor assay. *Clin Biochem.* Feb 2000;33(1):31-36.

7. Westley IS, Morris RG, Taylor PJ, Salm P, James MJ. CEDIA sirolimus assay compared with HPLC-MS/MS and HPLC-UV in transplant recipient specimens. *Ther Drug Monit.* Jun 2005;27(3):309-314.

8. Anon. *Rapamune Prescribing Information.* Philadelphia, PA: Wyeth Pharmaceuticals; 2012.

9. Kahan BD, Napoli KL, Kelly PA, et al. Therapeutic drug monitoring of sirolimus: correlations with efficacy and toxicity. *Clin Transplant.* Apr 2000;14(2):97-109.

10. Hunt SA, Mallidi HR. Cardiac transplantation and prolonged assisted circulation. In: Longo DL, Fauci AS, Kasper DL, Hauser SL, Jameson JL, Loscalzo J, eds. *Principles of Internal Medicine.* 18th ed. New York, NY: McGraw-Hill; 2012:1916-1919.

11. Trulock EP. Lung transplantation. In: Longo DL, Fauci AS, Kasper DL, Hauser SL, Jameson JL, Loscalzo J, eds. *Principles of Internal Medicine.* 18th ed. New York, NY: McGraw-Hill; 2012:2189-2195.

12. Dienstag JL, Chung RT. Liver transplantation. In: Longo DL, Fauci AS, Kasper DL, Hauser SL, Jameson JL, Loscalzo J, eds. *Principles of Internal Medicine.* 18th ed. New York, NY: McGraw-Hill; 2012:2606-2614.

13. Chandraker A, Milford EL, Sayegh MH. Transplantation in the treatment of renal failure. In: Longo DL, Fauci AS, Kasper DL, Hauser SL, Jameson JL, Loscalzo J, eds. *Principles of Internal Medicine.* 18th ed. New York, NY: McGraw-Hill; 2012:2327-2333.

14. Appelbaum F. Hematopoietic cell transplantation. In: Longo DL, Fauci AS, Kasper DL, Hauser SL, Jameson JL, Loscalzo J, eds. *Principles of Internal Medicine.* 18th ed. New York, NY: McGraw-Hill; 2012:958-964.

15. Abouelnasr A, Roy J, Cohen S, Kiss T, Lachance S. Defining the role of sirolimus in the management of graft-versus-host disease: from prophylaxis to treatment. *Biol Blood Marrow Transplant.* Jan 2013;19(1):12-21.

16. Augustine JJ, Bodziak KA, Hricik DE. Use of sirolimus in solid organ transplantation. *Drugs.* 2007;67(3):369-391.

17. Monchaud C, Marquet P. Pharmacokinetic optimization of immunosuppressive therapy in thoracic transplantation: part II. *Clin Pharmacokinet.* 2009;48(8):489-516.

18. Cattaneo D, Cortinovis M, Baldelli S, Gotti E, Remuzzi G, Perico N. Limited sampling strategies for the estimation of sirolimus daily exposure in kidney transplant recipients on a calcineurin inhibitor-free regimen. *J Clin Pharmacol.* Jul 2009;49(7):773-781.

19. Forbes N, Schachter AD, Yasin A, Sharma AP, Filler G. Limited sampling strategies for sirolimus after pediatric renal transplantation. *Pediatr Transplant.* Dec 2009;13(8):1020-1026.

20. Hansten PD, Horn JR. *The Top 100 Drug Interactions.* Freeland, WA: H&H Publications; 2014.

21. Sattler M, Guengerich FP, Yun CH, Christians U, Sewing KF. Cytochrome P-450 3A enzymes are responsible for biotransformation of FK506 and rapamycin in man and rat. *Drug Metab Dispos.* Sep-Oct 1992;20(5):753-761.

22. Wacher VJ, Silverman JA, Wong S, et al. Sirolimus oral absorption in rats is increased by ketoconazole but is not affected by D-alpha-tocopheryl poly(ethylene glycol 1000) succinate. *J Pharmacol Exp Ther.* Oct 2002;303(1):308-313.

23. Nickmilder MJ, Latinne D, Verbeeck RK, Janssens W, Svoboda D, Lhoest GJ. Isolation and identification of new rapamycin dihydrodiol metabolites from dexamethasone-induced rat liver microsomes. *Xenobiotica.* Sep 1997;27(9):869-883.

24. Streit F, Christians U, Schiebel HM, Meyer A, Sewing KF. Structural identification of three metabolites and a degradation product of the macrolide immunosuppressant sirolimus (rapamycin) by electrospray-MS/MS after incubation with human liver microsomes. *Drug Metab Dispos.* Nov 1996;24(11):1272-1278.

25. Kumi KA. Sirolimus (Rapamycin) oral solution clinical pharmacology/biopharmacuetics review application number 21083. *FDA Center for Drug Evaluation and Research.* http://www.accessdata.fda.gov/drugsatfda_docs/nda/99/21083A_Rapamune_clinphrmr.pdf. Accessed February 11, 2014.

26. Djebli N, Rousseau A, Hoizey G, et al. Sirolimus population pharmacokinetic/pharmacogenetic analysis and bayesian modelling in kidney transplant recipients. *Clin Pharmacokinet.* 2006;45(11):1135-1148.

27. Kelly PA, Napoli K, Kahan BD. Conversion from liquid to solid rapamycin formulations in stable renal allograft transplant recipients. *Biopharm Drug Dispos.* Jul 1999;20(5):249-253.

28. Zimmerman JJ, Kahan BD. Pharmacokinetics of sirolimus in stable renal transplant patients after multiple oral dose administration. *J Clin Pharmacol.* May 1997;37(5):405-415.

29. Zimmerman JJ. Exposure-response relationships and drug interactions of sirolimus. *AAPS J.* 2004;6(4):e28.

30. Yatscoff RW, Wang P, Chan K, Hicks D, Zimmerman J. Rapamycin: distribution, pharmacokinetics, and therapeutic range investigations. *Ther Drug Monit.* Dec 1995;17(6):666-671.

31. Zimmerman JJ, Ferron GM, Lim HK, Parker V. The effect of a high-fat meal on the oral bioavailability of the immunosuppressant sirolimus (rapamycin). *J Clin Pharmacol.* Nov 1999;39(11):1155-1161.

32. Hansten PD, Horn JR. *Drug Interactions Analysis and Management.* St. Louis, MO: Wolters Kluwer; 2014.

33. Yatscoff R, LeGatt D, Keenan R, Chackowsky P. Blood distribution of rapamycin. *Transplantation.* Nov 1993;56(5):1202-1206.

34. MacDonald A, Scarola J, Burke JT, Zimmerman JJ. Clinical pharmacokinetics and therapeutic drug monitoring of sirolimus. *Clin Ther.* 2000;22 (suppl B): 101B-121B.

35. Rogers CC, Alloway RR, Alexander JW, Cardi M, Trofe J, Vinks AA. Pharmacokinetics of mycophenolic acid, tacrolimus and sirolimus after gastric bypass surgery in end-stage renal disease and transplant patients: a pilot study. *Clin Transplant.* May-Jun 2008;22(3):281-291.

36. Tejani A, Alexander S, Ettenger R, et al. Safety and pharmacokinetics of ascending single doses of sirolimus (Rapamune, rapamycin) in pediatric patients with stable chronic renal failure undergoing dialysis. *Pediatr Transplant.* Apr 2004;8(2):151-160.

37. Tortorici MA, Parks V, Matschke K, Korth-Bradley J, Patat A. The evaluation of potential pharmacokinetic interaction between sirolimus and tacrolimus in healthy volunteers. *Eur J Clin Pharmacol.* Apr 2013;69(4):835-842.

38. Wu FL, Tsai MK, Chen RR, et al. Effects of calcineurin inhibitors on sirolimus pharmacokinetics during staggered administration in renal transplant recipients. *Pharmacotherapy.* May 2005;25(5):646-653.

39. Schachter AD, Benfield MR, Wyatt RJ, et al. Sirolimus pharmacokinetics in pediatric renal transplant recipients receiving calcineurin inhibitor co-therapy. *Pediatr Transplant.* Dec 2006;10(8):914-919.

40. Schubert M, Venkataramanan R, Holt DW, et al. Pharmacokinetics of sirolimus and tacrolimus in pediatric transplant patients. *Am J Transplant.* May 2004;4(5):767-773.

41. Ettenger RB, Grimm EM. Safety and efficacy of TOR inhibitors in pediatric renal transplant recipients. *Am J Kidney Dis.* Oct 2001;38(4) (suppl 2): 22S-28S.

42. Gallant-Haidner HL, Trepanier DJ, Freitag DG, Yatscoff RW. Pharmacokinetics and metabolism of sirolimus. *Ther Drug Monit.* Feb 2000;22(1):31-35.

43. Mahalati K, Kahan BD. Clinical pharmacokinetics of sirolimus. *Clin Pharmacokinet.* 2001;40(8):573-585.

44. Brattstrom C, Sawe J, Tyden G, et al. Kinetics and dynamics of single oral doses of sirolimus in sixteen renal transplant recipients. *Ther Drug Monit.* Aug 1997;19(4):397-406.

45. Zimmerman JJ, Lasseter KC, Lim HK, et al. Pharmacokinetics of sirolimus (rapamycin) in subjects with mild to moderate hepatic impairment. *J Clin Pharmacol.* Dec 2005;45(12):1368-1372.

46. Zimmerman JJ, Patat A, Parks V, Moirand R, Matschke K. Pharmacokinetics of sirolimus (rapamycin) in subjects with severe hepatic impairment. *J Clin Pharmacol.* Mar 2008;48(3):285-292.

47. Pugh RN, Murray-Lyon IM, Dawson JL, Pietroni MC, Williams R. Transection of the oesophagus for bleeding oesophageal varices. *Br J Surg.* 1973;60(8):646-649.

48. McAlister VC, Mahalati K, Peltekian KM, Fraser A, MacDonald AS. A clinical pharmacokinetic study of tacrolimus and sirolimus combination immunosuppression comparing simultaneous to separated administration. *Ther Drug Monit.* Jun 2002;24(3):346-350.

49. Kaplan B, Meier-Kriesche HU, Napoli KL, Kahan BD. The effects of relative timing of sirolimus and cyclosporine microemulsion formulation coadministration on the pharmacokinetics of each agent. *Clin Pharmacol Ther.* Jan 1998;63(1):48-53.

50. Du Bois D, Du Bois EF. A formula to estimate the approximate surface area if height and weight be known. *Arch Intern Med.* Jun 1916;17(6):863-871.

51. Wandell M, Mungall D. Computer assisted drug interpretation and drug regimen optimization. *Amer Assoc Clin Chem.* 1984;6:1-11.

VI   OTHER DRUGS

21

Lithium

INTRODUCTION

Lithium is an alkali metal that is administered as a monovalent cation (Li^+) for the treatment of bipolar disorder. In the United States, orally administered carbonate and citrate salts of lithium are available. While lithium is still used as a primary mood stabilizer for bipolar disorders, valproic acid, carbamazepine, or lamotrigine are also reasonable choices.[1,2] Although this drug has been used in psychiatric medicine since the 1940s, the mechanism of action of lithium is largely unknown. Among the current theories are competition with other cations at receptor and tissue sites, dopamine-receptor supersensitivity blockage, decreased stimulation of β-receptor–induced adenylate cyclase, and enhanced sensitivity to serotonin (5-HT), acetylcholine, and γ-aminobutyric acid (GABA).[1,2]

THERAPEUTIC AND TOXIC CONCENTRATIONS

The general therapeutic range for lithium is 0.6-1.5 mmol/L. Because lithium is a monovalent cation, the therapeutic range expressed in mEq/L is identical to these values (ie, 0.6-1.5 mEq/L). However, most clinicians apply different therapeutic concentration ranges depending on the clinical situation of the patient.[3,4] For individuals with acute mania, a minimum lithium concentration of 0.8 mmol/L is usually recommended. The usual desired range for these individuals is 0.8-1 mmol/L. If patients with acute mania do not respond to these levels, it is necessary to occasionally use lithium concentrations of 1-1.2 mmol/L and in some instances concentrations as high as 1.2-1.5 mmol/L are needed. For long-term maintenance use, the usual desired range is 0.6-0.8 mmol/L. If patients do not respond to these levels during maintenance treatment, occasional use of lithium concentrations equal to 0.9-1 mmol/L is required and in some cases concentrations as high as 1-1.2 mmol/L are necessary to gain an adequate outcome.

These therapeutic ranges are based on steady-state lithium serum concentrations obtained 12 hours after a dose. The adoption of a standardized 12-hour postdose lithium concentration to assess dose and response has been paramount in establishing the aforementioned therapeutic ranges for the agent.[5] After oral administration, lithium concentrations follow a complex concentration-time curve that is best described using multicompartment models (Figure 21-1).[5-9] There is a great deal of variability among patients in the time needed for distribution between serum and tissues to occur, and under these conditions using a uniform time for the determination of steady-state serum concentrations is important. When lithium serum concentration monitoring is anticipated for an individual, the patient needs to understand that it is important to take their medication as instructed for 2-3 days before the blood sample is obtained, to have the blood sample withdrawn 12 ± 0.5 h after the last dose, and to report any discrepancies in compliance and blood sampling time to their care provider.

Short-term side effects observed when starting lithium or after a dosage increase include muscle weakness, lethargy, polydipsia, polyuria, nocturia, headache, impairment of memory or concentration, confusion, impaired fine motor performance, and hand tremors.[1,2] Many of these adverse effects will diminish with

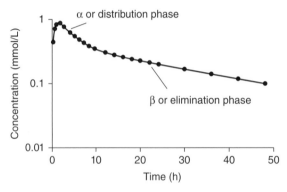

FIGURE 21-1   Lithium ion serum concentration-time curve after a single 900-mg oral dose of lithium carbonate (24.4 mmol or mEq of lithium ion) rapid-release capsules. Maximum serum concentrations occur 2-3 hours after the dose is given. After the peak concentration is achieved, the distribution phase lasts for 6-10 hours, followed by the elimination phase. In patients with good renal function (creatinine clearance >80 mL/min), the average elimination half-life for lithium is 24 hours. Because of the long distribution phase, lithium serum concentrations used for dosage adjustment purposes should be obtained no sooner than 12 hours after dosage administration.

continued dosing of lithium. However, some intervention may be needed for the tremor including a shorter dosage interval using the same total daily dose in order to decrease peak lithium concentrations, a decreased lithium dose, or concurrent treatment with a β-blocker. Long-term adverse effects include a drug-induced diabetes insipidus, renal toxicity (glomerulosclerosis, renal tubular atrophy, interstitial nephritis, urinary casts), hypothyroidism with or without goiter formation, electrocardiographic abnormalities, leukocytosis, weight gain, and dermatologic changes.[1,2]

At lithium serum concentrations within the upper end of the therapeutic range (1.2-1.5 mmol/L), the following adverse effects can be noted in patients: decreased memory and concentration, drowsiness, fine hand tremor, weakness, lack of coordination, nausea, diarrhea, vomiting, or fatigue.[1,2] At concentrations just above the therapeutic range (1.5-3 mmol/L), confusion, giddiness, agitation, slurred speech, lethargy, blackouts, ataxia, dysarthria, nystagmus, blurred vision, tinnitus, vertigo, hyperreflexia, hypertonia, dysarthria, coarse hand tremors, and muscle fasciculations may occur in patients. If concentrations exceed 3 mmol/L, severe toxicity occurs with choreoathetosis, seizures, irreversible brain damage, arrhythmias, hypotension, respiratory and cardiovascular complications, stupor, coma, and death. At toxic lithium concentrations, lithium can cause a nonspecific decrease in glomerular filtration which, in turn, decreases lithium clearance. The decrease in lithium clearance will cause a further increase in the lithium serum concentration. This phenomenon can cause a viscous circle of decreased clearance leading to increased lithium serum concentration, which leads to additional decreases in lithium clearance and so on. Because of this and the severe toxic side effects, lithium concentrations above 3.5-4 mmol/L may require hemodialysis to remove the drug as quickly as possible.[1,2,4]

CLINICAL MONITORING PARAMETERS

The signs and symptoms of bipolar disease include both those of depression (depressed affect, sad mood, decreased interest and pleasure in normal activities, decreased appetite and weight loss, insomnia or hypersomnia, psychomotor retardation or agitation, decreased energy or fatigue, feelings of worthlessness or guilt, impaired decision making and concentration, suicidal ideation or attempts) and mania (abnormal and persistently elevated mood, grandiosity, decreased need for sleep, pressure of speech, flight of ideas, distractible with poor attention span, increased activity or agitation, excessive involvement in high-risk activities).[1,2,4]

Generally, onset of action for lithium is 1-2 weeks, and a 4- to 6-week treatment period is required to assess complete therapeutic response to the drug.[1,2,4]

Before initiating lithium therapy, patients should undergo a complete physical examination, and a general serum chemistry panel (including serum electrolytes and serum creatinine), complete blood cell count with differential, thyroid function tests, urinalysis (including osmolality and specific gravity), and urine toxicology screen for substances of abuse should also be obtained. For patients with renal dysfunction (measured 24-hour creatinine clearance) or baseline cardiac disease (electrocardiogram) additional testing is recommended. Clinicians should consider ordering a pregnancy test for females of childbearing age. Follow-up testing in the following areas should be conducted every 6-12 months: serum electrolytes, serum creatinine (measured 24-hour creatinine clearance in patients with renal dysfunction), thyroid function tests, complete blood cell count with differential. If urine output exceeds 3 L/d, a urinalysis with osmolality and specific gravity should also be measured.

Lithium serum concentrations should be measured in every patient receiving the drug. As previously discussed, dosage schedules should be arranged so that serum samples for lithium measurement are obtained 12 ± 0.5 hours after a dose.[5] Usually this requires administration of the drug every 12 hours for twice daily dosing. For three times a day dosing, it is necessary to give the drug so that there is a 12-hour time period overnight. Examples of two common dosage schemes are 0900 H, 1500 H, and 2100 H or 0800 H, 1400 H, and 2000 H. Obviously, the choice should be individualized based upon the patient's lifestyle. Upon initiation of therapy, serum concentrations can be measured every 2-3 days for safety reasons in patients that are predisposed to lithium toxicity even though steady-state has not yet been achieved. Once the desired steady-state lithium concentration has been achieved, lithium concentrations should be rechecked every 1-2 weeks for approximately 2 months or until concentrations have stabilized. Because patients with acute mania can have increased lithium clearance, lithium concentrations should be remeasured in these patients once the manic episode is over and clearance returns to normal. Otherwise, lithium concentrations may accumulate to toxic levels due to the decrease in lithium clearance. During lithium maintenance therapy, steady-state lithium serum concentrations should be repeated every 3-6 months. This time period should be altered to every 6-12 months for patients whose mood is stable or every 1-2 months for patients with frequent mood alterations. If lithium dosage alterations are needed, or therapy with another drug known to interact with lithium is added, lithium serum concentrations should be measured within 1-2 weeks after the change.

After patients have been stabilized on a multiple dose per day regimen, it is possible to consider once daily administration of lithium for those receiving a total dose of 1800 mg/d or less.[4] However, the change in dosage interval will alter the 12 hour lithium concentration, and further dosage titration may be needed to re-establish desired levels.[4]

BASIC CLINICAL PHARMACOKINETIC PARAMETERS

Lithium is eliminated almost completely (>95%) unchanged in the urine.[9] The ion is filtered freely at the glomerulus, and subsequently 60%-80% of the amount filtered is reabsorbed by the proximal tubule of the nephron. Lithium eliminated in the saliva, sweat, and feces accounts for less than 5% of the administered dose.[10] On average, lithium clearance is approximately 20% of the patient's creatinine clearance.[10-12] Lithium is administered orally as carbonate or citrate salts. Lithium carbonate capsules (150, 300, 600 mg) and tablets (rapid release: 300 mg; sustained release: 300, 450 mg) are available. There are 8.12 mmol (or 8.12 mEq) of lithium in 300 mg of lithium carbonate. Lithium citrate syrup (8 mmol or mEq/5 mL) is another oral dosage form. Oral bioavailability is good for all lithium salts and dosage forms and equals 100%.[13,14] The peak lithium concentration occurs 15-30 minutes after a dose of lithium citrate syrup, 1-3 hours after a dose of rapid-release lithium carbonate tablets or capsules, and 4-8 hours after a dose of sustained-release lithium carbonate tablets. Lithium ion is not plasma protein bound. The typical dose of lithium carbonate is 900-2400 mg/d in adult patients with normal renal function.

EFFECTS OF DISEASE STATES AND CONDITIONS ON LITHIUM PHARMACOKINETICS

Adults with normal renal function (creatinine clearance >80 mL/min) have an average elimination half-life of 24 hours, volume of distribution equal to 0.9 L/kg, and clearance of 20 mL/min for lithium.[5-9] During an acute manic phase, lithium clearance can increase by as much as 50% which produces a half-life that is about ½ the normal value.[15] In children 9-12 years of age, average elimination half-life equals 18 hours, volume of distribution is 0.9 L/kg, and clearance equals 40 mL/min for the ion.[16] Because glomerular filtration and creatinine clearance decrease with age, lithium clearance can be decreased in elderly patients, producing half-lives up to 36 hours.[11,12] Because of the circadian rhythm of glomerular filtration, lithium clearance is about 30% higher during daytime hours.[17]

Because lithium is eliminated almost exclusively by the kidney, renal dysfunction is the most important disease state that effects lithium pharmacokinetics. Lithium clearance rate decreases in proportion to creatinine clearance. In adults, the lithium clearance-creatinine clearance ratio is 20%, but during a manic phase increases to about 30%.[11,12,15] This relationship between renal function and lithium clearance will form the basis for initial dosage computation later in the chapter. Because of the decrease in clearance, the average lithium half-life is 40-50 hours in renal failure patients.

The renal clearance of lithium for a patient is influenced by the state of sodium balance and fluid hydration in that individual. Lithium is reabsorbed in the proximal tubule of the nephron via the same mechanisms used to maintain sodium balance.[5] Thus, when a patient is in negative sodium balance, the kidney increases sodium reabsorption as a compensatory maneuver and lithium reabsorption increases as a result. The kidney also increases sodium reabsorption when a patient becomes dehydrated, and, again, lithium reabsorption increases. In both cases, increased lithium reabsorption leads to decreased lithium clearance. Some common things that cause sodium depletion and/or dehydration include sodium-restricted diets for the treatment of other conditions; vomiting, diarrhea, or fever that might be due to viral or other illnesses; heavy or intense exercise; excessive sweating; use of saunas or hot tubs; and hot weather. Overuse of coffee, tea, soft drinks, or other caffeine-containing liquids and ethanol should be avoided by patients taking lithium. Patients should be advised to maintain adequate fluid intake at all times (2.5-3 L/d) and to increase fluid intake as needed.[2]

During periods of acute mania, lithium clearance can be increased by as much as 50%.[15] Lithium is generally not used in the first trimester due to possible teratogenic effects on the fetus.[1,2,4] Due to increased glomerular filtration, lithium clearance may be increased in pregnant women, especially during the third trimester. Lithium crosses the placenta, and human milk concentrations are 30%-100% that of concurrent serum concentrations.[18]

Lithium is removed from the body by hemodialysis, peritoneal dialysis, and arteriovenous hemodiafiltration with clearance values of 30-50 mL/min, 13-15 mL/min, and 21 mL/min, respectively.[10,19,20] The sieving coefficient for lithium during hemofiltration is 0.90.[21,22] Replacement doses of lithium during dialysis or hemofiltration should be determined using serum concentration monitoring.

DRUG INTERACTIONS

Many diuretics have drug interactions with lithium.[23] Thiazide diuretics cause sodium and water depletion which leads to increased sodium reabsorption in the proximal tubule of the kidney as a compensatory mechanism. Since lithium is reabsorbed by the same mechanisms as sodium, lithium reabsorption increases and lithium clearance decreases by 40%-50% during treatment with thiazide diuretics. Other diuretics that work at the site of the distal tubule of the kidney may cause a similar interaction with lithium (chlorthalidone, metolazone). Although there are case reports of loop diuretics causing a similar interaction, there are also reports of no drug interaction between lithium and these agents. Because of this, many clinicians favor the use of a loop diuretic, with careful monitoring of adverse effects and lithium serum concentrations, in patients taking lithium. Amiloride has also been reported to have minimal effects on lithium clearance.

Nonsteroidal anti-inflammatory agents (NSAIDs) also decrease lithium clearance and increase lithium concentrations. The probable mechanism is an NSAID-induced decrease in renal blood flow via inhibition of prostaglandins. Of these agents, sulindac and aspirin appear to have little or no drug interaction with lithium.

Angiotensin-converting enzyme inhibitors (ACEIs) and angiotensin receptor blockers (ARBs) have been reported to inhibit the elimination of lithium by an undefined mechanism. Of the two classes of drugs, more documentation exists for the ACEIs where lithium serum concentrations have increased by as much as 200%-300% from pretreatment levels.

Some serotonin-specific reuptake inhibitors (SSRIs) have been reported to cause a serotonergic hyper-arousal syndrome when taken in conjunction with lithium. Case report of this problem are currently available for fluoxetine, sertraline, and fluvoxamine. In addition to elevated lithium concentrations, patients have developed stiffness of arms and legs, course tremors, dizziness, ataxia, dysarthric speech, and seizures when taking these SSRI agents with lithium. Although there are also literature reports of these combinations used safely, caution should be exercised when concurrent treatment with SSRIs and lithium is indicated.

Theophylline increases the lithium clearance-creatinine clearance ratio by as much as 58% resulting in an average decrease of 21% in steady-state lithium concentrations. A rare, but severe, drug interaction between lithium and antipsychotic drugs has been reported where patients are more susceptible to the development of extrapyramidal symptoms or irreversible brain damage. Again, although there are reports of using antipsychotic agents and lithium together successfully, patients requiring this combination therapy should be closely monitored for adverse drug reactions.

INITIAL DOSAGE DETERMINATION METHODS

Several methods to initiate lithium therapy are available. The *Pharmacokinetic Dosing method* is the most flexible of the techniques. It allows individualized target serum concentrations to be chosen for a patient, and each pharmacokinetic parameter can be customized to reflect specific disease states and conditions present in the patient. However, it is computationally intensive. *Literature-based recommended dosing* is a very commonly used method to prescribe initial doses of lithium. Doses are based on those that commonly produce steady-state concentrations in the lower end of the therapeutic range, although there is a wide variation in the actual concentrations for a specific patient. *Test dose methods* use concentrations measured after one or more lithium test doses to rapidly individualize lithium therapy.

Pharmacokinetic Dosing Method

The goal of initial dosing of lithium is to compute the best dose possible for the patient given their set of disease states and conditions that influence lithium pharmacokinetics and the type and severity of their bipolar disease. In order to do this, pharmacokinetic parameters for the patient will be estimated using average parameters measured in other patients with similar disease state and condition profiles.

Clearance Estimate

Lithium ion is almost totally eliminated unchanged in the urine, and there is a consistent relationship between lithium clearance and creatinine clearance with a ratio of 20% between the two (lithium clearance-creatinine clearance).[10-12] This relationship allows the estimation of lithium clearance for a patient which can be used to compute an initial dose of the drug. Mathematically, the equation for the straight line shown in Figure 21-2 is: $Cl = 0.2(CrCl)$, where Cl is lithium clearance in mL/min and CrCl is creatinine clearance in mL/min. For dosing purposes, it is more useful to have lithium clearance expressed in L/d. The equation converted to

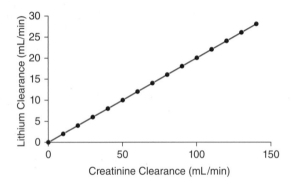

FIGURE 21-2   The ratio between lithium clearance and creatinine clearance is 0.2 for patients requiring maintenance therapy with lithium. This relationship is used to estimate lithium clearance for patients requiring initial dosing with the drug.

these units is: Cl = 0.288(CrCl), where Cl is lithium clearance in L/d and CrCl is creatinine clearance in mL/min. For patients with acute mania, lithium clearance is increased by about 50%, and the corresponding equation for these individuals is: Cl = 0.432(CrCl), where Cl is lithium clearance in L/d and CrCl is creatinine clearance in mL/min.[15]

Selection of Appropriate Pharmacokinetic Model and Equation

When given orally, lithium follows a two-compartment model (see Figure 21-1).[5-9] After the peak concentration is achieved, serum concentrations drop rapidly because of distribution of drug from blood to tissues (α or distribution phase). By 6-10 hours after administration of the drug, lithium concentrations decline more slowly, and the elimination rate constant for this segment of the concentration-time curve is the one that varies with renal function (β or elimination phase). While this model is the most correct from a strict pharmacokinetic viewpoint, it cannot easily be used clinically because of its mathematical complexity. During the elimination phase of the concentration-time curve, lithium serum concentrations drop very slowly due to the long elimination half-life (24 hours with normal renal function, up to 50 hours with end-stage renal disease). Because of this, a very simple pharmacokinetic equation that computes the average lithium steady-state serum concentration (Css in mmol/L = mEq/L) is widely used and allows maintenance dosage calculation: Css = [F(D/τ)]/Cl or D/τ = (Css • Cl)/F, where F is the bioavailability fraction for the oral dosage form (F = 1 for oral lithium), D is the lithium dose in mmoles, τ is the dosage interval in days, and Cl is lithium clearance in L/d. Because this equation computes lithium ion requirement and lithium carbonate doses are prescribed in mg, the ratio of lithium ion content to lithium carbonate salt (8.12 mmol Li$^+$/300 mg lithium carbonate) is used to convert the result from this equation into a lithium carbonate dose. Total daily amounts of lithium are usually given as near-equally divided doses twice or three times a day, and single doses above 1200 mg/d of lithium carbonate are usually not given in order to avoid gastrointestinal upset.

Steady-State Concentration Selection

Lithium serum concentrations are selected based on the presence or absence of acute mania and titrated to response.[3] For individuals with acute mania, a minimum lithium concentration of 0.8 mmol/L is usually recommended. The usual desired range for these individuals is 0.8-1 mmol/L. If patients with acute mania do not respond to these levels, it is necessary to occasionally use lithium concentrations of 1-1.2 mmol/L and in some instances concentrations as high as 1.2-1.5 mmol/L are needed. For long-term maintenance use, the usual desired range is 0.6-0.8 mmol/L. If patients do not respond to these levels during maintenance treatment, occasional use of lithium concentrations equal to 0.9-1 mmol/L is required and in some cases concentrations as high as 1-1.2 mmol/L are necessary to gain an adequate outcome.

EXAMPLE 1 ▶▶▶

MJ is a 50-year-old, 70-kg (height = 5 ft 10 in) male with bipolar disease. He is not currently experiencing an episode of acute mania. His serum creatinine is 0.9 mg/dL. Compute an oral lithium dose for this patient for maintenance therapy.

1. *Estimate creatinine clearance.*

This patient has a stable serum creatinine and is not obese. The Cockcroft-Gault equation can be used to estimate creatinine clearance:

$$CrCl_{est} = [(140 - age)BW]/(72 \bullet S_{Cr}) = [(140 - 50\ y)70\ kg]/(72 \bullet 0.9\ mg/dL)$$

$$CrCl_{est} = 97\ mL/min$$

2. *Estimate clearance.*

The drug clearance versus creatinine clearance relationship is used to estimate the lithium clearance for this patient:

$$Cl = 0.288(CrCl) = 0.288(97\ mL/min) = 27.9\ L/d$$

3. *Use average steady-state concentration equation to compute lithium maintenance dose.*

For a patient requiring maintenance therapy for bipolar disease, the desired lithium concentration would be 0.6-0.8 mmol/L. A serum concentration equal to 0.6 mmol/L will be chosen for this patient, and oral lithium carbonate will be used (F = 1, 8.12 mmol Li$^+$/300 mg of lithium carbonate).

$$D/\tau = (Css \bullet Cl)/F = (0.6\ mmol/L \bullet 27.9\ L/d)/1 = 16.7\ mmol/d$$

D/τ = (300 mg lithium carbonate/8.12 mmol Li$^+$) 16.7 mmol/d = 617 mg/d, rounded to 600 mg/d of lithium carbonate. This dose would be given as 300 mg of lithium carbonate every 12 hours.

Upon initiation of therapy, serum concentrations can be measured every 2-3 days for safety reasons in patients that are predisposed to lithium toxicity even though steady-state has not yet been achieved. Once the desired steady-state lithium concentration has been achieved, lithium concentrations should be rechecked every 1-2 weeks for approximately 2 months or until concentrations have stabilized.

EXAMPLE 2 ▶▶▶

Same patient profile as in example 1, but serum creatinine is 3.5 mg/dL indicating renal impairment.

1. *Estimate creatinine clearance.*

This patient has a stable serum creatinine and is not obese. The Cockcroft-Gault equation can be used to estimate creatinine clearance:

$$CrCl_{est} = [(140 - age)BW]/(72 \bullet S_{Cr}) = [(140 - 50\ y)70\ kg]/(72 \bullet 3.5\ mg/dL)$$

$$CrCl_{est} = 25\ mL/min$$

2. *Estimate clearance.*
The drug clearance versus creatinine clearance relationship is used to estimate the lithium clearance for this patient:

$$Cl = 0.288(CrCl) = 0.288(25 \text{ mL/min}) = 7.2 \text{ L/d}$$

3. *Use average steady-state concentration equation to compute lithium maintenance dose.*
For a patient requiring maintenance therapy for bipolar disease, the desired lithium concentration would be 0.6-0.8 mmol/L. A serum concentration equal to 0.6 mmol/L will be chosen for this patient, and oral lithium carbonate will be used (F = 1, 8.12 mmol Li^+/300 mg of lithium carbonate).

$$D/\tau = (Css \bullet Cl)/F = (0.6 \text{ mmol/L} \bullet 7.2 \text{ L/d})/1 = 4.3 \text{ mmol/d}$$

$D/\tau = (300 \text{ mg lithium carbonate}/8.12 \text{ mmol } Li^+)$ 4.3 mmol/d = 159 mg/d, rounded to 150 mg/d of lithium carbonate. This dose would be given as 150 mg of lithium carbonate daily.

Upon initiation of therapy, serum concentrations can be measured every 2-3 days for safety reasons in patients that are predisposed to lithium toxicity even though steady-state has not yet been achieved. Once the desired steady-state lithium concentration has been achieved, lithium concentrations should be rechecked every 1-2 weeks for approximately 2 months or until concentrations have stabilized.

EXAMPLE 3 ▶▶▶

Same patient profile as in example 1, but serum creatinine is 0.9 mg/dL, and the patient is being treated for acute mania. Compute an oral lithium carbonate dose for this patient.

1. *Estimate creatinine clearance.*
This patient has a stable serum creatinine and is not obese. The Cockcroft-Gault equation can be used to estimate creatinine clearance:

$$CrCl_{est} = [(140 - age)BW]/(72 \bullet S_{cr}) = [(140 - 50 \text{ y})70 \text{ kg}]/(72 \bullet 0.9 \text{ mg/dL})$$
$$CrCl_{est} = 97 \text{ mL/min}$$

2. *Estimate clearance.*
The drug clearance versus creatinine clearance relationship is used to estimate the lithium clearance for this patient:

$$Cl = 0.432 (CrCl) = 0.432 (97 \text{ mL/min}) = 41.9 \text{ L/d}$$

3. *Use average steady-state concentration equation to compute lithium maintenance dose.*
For a patient requiring therapy for the acute manic phase of bipolar disease, the desired lithium concentration would be 0.8 mmol/L. Oral lithium carbonate will be used (F = 1, 8.12 mmol Li^+/300 mg of lithium carbonate).

$$D/\tau = (Css \bullet Cl)/F = (0.8 \text{ mmol/L} \bullet 41.9 \text{ L/d})/1 = 33.5 \text{ mmol/d}$$

$D/\tau = (300 \text{ mg lithium carbonate}/8.12 \text{ mmol } Li^+)$ 33.5 mmol/d = 1238 mg/d, rounded to 1200 mg/d of lithium carbonate. This dose would be given as 600 mg of lithium carbonate every 12 hours.

Upon initiation of therapy, serum concentrations can be measured every 2-3 days for safety reasons in patients that are predisposed to lithium toxicity even though steady-state has not yet been achieved. Once the desired steady-state lithium concentration has been achieved, lithium concentrations should be rechecked every 1-2 weeks for approximately 2 months or until concentrations have stabilized. Because patients with acute mania can have increased lithium clearance, lithium concentrations should be remeasured in these patients once the manic episode is over and clearance returns to normal.

Literature-Based Recommended Dosing

Because of the large amount of variability in lithium pharmacokinetics, even when concurrent disease states and conditions are identified, many clinicians believe that the use of standard lithium doses for various situations are warranted. The original computation of these doses was based on the Pharmacokinetic Dosing method described in the previous section, and subsequently modified based on clinical experience. For the treatment of acute mania, initial doses are usually 900-1200 mg/d of lithium carbonate.[1,2,4] If the drug is being used for bipolar disease prophylaxis, an initial dose of 600 mg/d lithium carbonate is recommended.[1,2,4] In both cases, the total daily dose is given in 2-3 divided daily doses. To avoid adverse side effects, lithium doses are slowly increased by 300-600 mg/d every 2-3 days according to clinical response and lithium serum concentrations. Renal dysfunction is the major condition that alters lithium pharmacokinetics and dosage.[24-27] If creatinine clearance is 10-50 mL/min, the prescribed initial dose is 50%-75% of that recommended for patients with normal renal function. For creatinine clearance values below 10 mL/min, the prescribed dose should be 25%-50% of the usual dose in patients with good renal function. Recommended doses for children and adolescents with normal renal function are 15-60 mg/kg/d and 600-1800 mg/d, respectively, with doses administered 3-4 times daily.[28]

Zetin and associates have developed a multiple regression equation that computes lithium carbonate doses for patients based on hospitalization status, age, gender, and weight of the patient as well as the presence or absence of concurrent tricyclic use by the patient.[29,30] However, since renal function was not assessed as an independent parameter in their study population, this dosage method is not presented.

To illustrate the similarities and differences between this method of initial dosage calculation and the Pharmacokinetic Dosing method, the same examples used in the previous section will be used.

EXAMPLE 4 ▶▶▶

MJ is a 50-year-old, 70-kg (height = 5 ft 10 in) male with bipolar disease. He is not currently experiencing an episode of acute mania. His serum creatinine is 0.9 mg/dL. Recommend an oral lithium dose for this patient for maintenance therapy.

1. *Estimate creatinine clearance.*

This patient has a stable serum creatinine and is not obese. The Cockcroft-Gault equation can be used to estimate creatinine clearance:

$$CrCl_{est} = [(140 - age)BW]/(72 \bullet S_{Cr}) = [(140 - 50\ y)70\ kg]/(72 \bullet 0.9\ mg/dL)$$

$$CrCl_{est} = 97\ mL/min$$

2. *Chose lithium dose based on disease states and conditions present in the patient.*
The patient requires prophylactic lithium therapy for bipolar disease, and has good renal function. A lithium carbonate dose of 600 mg/d, given as 300 mg every 12 hours, is recommended as the initial amount. The dosage rate will be increased 300-600 mg/d every 2-3 days as needed to provide adequate therapeutic effect, avoid adverse effects, and produce therapeutic lithium steady-state concentrations.

EXAMPLE 5 ▶▶▶

Same patient profile as in example 4, but serum creatinine is 3.5 mg/dL indicating renal impairment.
1. *Estimate creatinine clearance*
This patient has a stable serum creatinine and is not obese. The Cockcroft-Gault equation can be used to estimate creatinine clearance:

$$CrCl_{est} = [(140 - age)BW]/(72 \bullet S_{Cr}) = [(140 - 50 \text{ y})70 \text{ kg}]/(72 \bullet 3.5 \text{ mg/dL})$$
$$CrCl_{est} = 25 \text{ mL/min}$$

2. *Chose lithium dose based on disease states and conditions present in the patient.*
The patient requires prophylactic lithium therapy for bipolar disease, and has moderate renal function. With an estimated creatinine clearance of 25 mL/min, lithium carbonate doses should be 50%-75% of the usual amount. A lithium carbonate dose of 300 mg/d, given as 150 mg every 12 hours, is recommended as the initial amount. The dosage rate will be increased 150-300 mg/d every 5-7 days as needed to provide adequate therapeutic effect, avoid adverse effects, and produce therapeutic lithium steady-state concentrations.

EXAMPLE 6 ▶▶▶

Same patient profile as in example 4, but serum creatinine is 0.9 mg/dL, and the patient is being treated for the acute mania phase of bipolar disease. Compute an oral lithium carbonate dose for this patient.
1. *Estimate creatinine clearance.*
This patient has a stable serum creatinine and is not obese. The Cockcroft-Gault equation can be used to estimate creatinine clearance:

$$CrCl_{est} = [(140 - age)BW]/(72 \bullet S_{Cr}) = [(140 - 50 \text{ y})70 \text{ kg}]/(72 \bullet 0.9 \text{ mg/dL})$$
$$CrCl_{est} = 97 \text{ mL/min}$$

2. *Chose lithium dose based on disease states and conditions present in the patient.*
The patient requires lithium therapy for acute mania, and has good renal function. A lithium carbonate dose of 900 mg/d, given as 300 mg at 0800 H, 1400 H, and 2000 H, is recommended as the initial amount. The dosage rate will be increased 300-600 mg/d every 2-3 days as needed to provide adequate therapeutic effect, avoid adverse effects, and produce therapeutic lithium steady-state concentrations.

TABLE 21-1   Cooper Nomogram for Lithium Dosing[31,32]
(Lithium Carbonate Dosage Required to Produce Steady-State Lithium Serum Concentrations Between 0.6 and 1.2 mmol/L)[a]

Lithium Serum Concentration 24 h After the Test Dose (mmol/L)	Lithium Carbonate Dosage Requirement[b]
<0.05	1200 mg three times daily (3600 mg/d)[c]
0.05-0.09	900 mg three times daily (2700 mg/d)
0.10-0.14	600 mg three times daily (1800 mg/d)
0.15-0.19	300 mg four times daily (1200 mg/d)
0.20-0.23	300 mg three times daily (900 mg/d)
0.24-0.30	300 mg twice daily (600 mg/d)
>0.30	300 mg twice daily[d] (600 mg/d)

[a]Lithium dosage requirements should be reassessed with changes in clinical status (mania versus maintenance treatment), renal function, or other factors that alter lithium pharmacokinetics.
[b]Dosage schedule determined to provide minimum fluctuation in lithium serum concentration and maximum patient compliance. A change in dosage interval can be made by the prescribing clinician, but the total daily dose should remain the same.
[c]Use extreme caution. Patient appears to have an increased clearance and short half-life for lithium which would require large lithium carbonate maintenance doses. However, such a large maintenance dose requires careful patient monitoring for response and adverse side effects.
[d]Use extreme caution. Patient appears to have a reduced clearance and long half-life for lithium, and may accumulate steady-state lithium concentrations above the therapeutic range.

Test Dose Methods to Assess Initial Lithium Dosage Requirements

Several methods to assess initial lithium dosage requirement using one or most lithium test doses and one or more lithium serum concentrations are available for clinical use.

Cooper Nomogram

The Cooper nomogram of lithium maintenance dosage assessment requires the administration of a single test dose of 600 mg lithium carbonate and a single lithium serum concentration measured 24 hours later.[31,32] The 24-hour lithium serum concentration is compared to a table that converts the observed concentration into the lithium carbonate dose required to produced a steady-state lithium concentration between 0.6 and 1.2 mmol/L (Table 21-1). The theoretical basis for this dosage approach lies in the relationship between the serum concentration of a drug obtained about 1 half-life after dosage and the elimination rate constant for the drug in a patient. This nomogram can also be expressed as an equation for the total daily lithium dosage requirement (D in mmol/d): $D = e^{(4.80 - 7.5C_{test})}$, where C_{test} is the 24-hour postdose lithium concentration for a 600-mg lithium carbonate dose.[10] Perry and associates have suggested a similar nomogram that employs a larger test dose of 1200 mg lithium carbonate.[4,33,34] An important requirement for these methods is an accurate lithium assay that can reproducibly measure the lithium concentrations that occur after a single dose of the drug. Additionally, at the time the lithium carbonate test dose is given, the lithium serum concentration in the patient must equal zero.

EXAMPLE 7 ▶▶▶

LK is a 47-year-old, 65-kg (height = 5 ft 5 in) female with bipolar disease. She is not currently experiencing an episode of acute mania. Her serum creatinine is 0.9 mg/dL. Compute an oral lithium dose for this patient during maintenance therapy using the Cooper nomogram.

1. *Administer 600-mg lithium carbonate test dose and measure 24-hour postdose lithium concentration. Use nomogram to recommend lithium carbonate maintenance dose.*

After the test dose was given, the 24-hour lithium concentration was 0.12 mmol/L. The recommended lithium carbonate maintenance dose is 600 mg three times daily. The doses would be given at 0900 H, 1500 H and 2100 H to allow a 12 hour window after the evening dose so that lithium serum concentration measurements can be made.

Upon initiation of therapy, serum concentrations can be measured every 2-3 days for safety reasons in patients that are predisposed to lithium toxicity even though steady-state has not yet been achieved. Once the desired steady-state lithium concentration has been achieved, lithium concentrations should be rechecked every 1-2 weeks for approximately 2 months or until concentrations have stabilized. Because patients with acute mania can have increased lithium clearance, lithium concentrations should be remeasured in these patients once the manic episode is over and clearance returns to normal.

Perry Method

This technique conducts a small pharmacokinetic experiment in a patient after the administration of a lithium carbonate test dose.[35] First, a test dose (600-1500 mg) of lithium carbonate is given to the patient. Then, lithium serum concentrations are measured 12 and 36 hours after the test dose was given. The two lithium concentrations are used to compute the elimination rate constant for the individual: $k_e = (\ln C_{12h} - \ln C_{36h})/\Delta t$, where k_e is the elimination rate constant in h^{-1} for lithium, C_{12h} and C_{36h} are the lithium concentrations in mmol/L (or mEq/L) at 12 and 36 hours, respectively, after the test dose was given, and Δt is the difference between times (24 hours) that the two serum concentrations were obtained. With knowledge of the elimination rate constant (k_e), the accumulation ratio (R) can be computed for any dosage interval: $R = 1/(1 - e^{-k_e\tau})$, where τ is the dosage interval in hours. The accumulation ratio (R) is also equal to the ratio of the concentration at any time, t, after a single dose ($C_{SD,t}$ in mmol/L) and the steady-state concentration at that same time after the dose during multiple dosing ($C_{ss,t}$ in mmol/L): $R = C_{ss,t}/C_{SD,t}$ or $C_{ss,t} = R \bullet C_{SD,t}$. Once a steady-state concentration can be computed for a dosage regimen, linear pharmacokinetic principles can be used to compute the dose required to achieve a target lithium steady-state serum concentration: $D_{new} = (C_{ss,new}/C_{ss,old})D_{old}$, where D is the dose, Css is the steady-state concentration, old indicates the dose that produced the steady-state concentration that the patient is currently receiving, and new denotes the dose necessary to produce the desired steady-state concentration. As with the Cooper nomogram, the lithium serum concentration must be zero before the test dose is administered.

EXAMPLE 8 ▶ ▶ ▶

HG is a 32-year-old, 58-kg (height = 5 ft 1 in) female with bipolar disease. She is not currently experiencing an episode of acute mania. Her serum creatinine is 0.9 mg/dL. A single test dose of lithium (1200 mg) was given to the patient, and lithium concentrations were measured as 0.6 mmol/L and 0.3 mmol/L at 12 hours and 36 hours, respectively, after the drug was given. Compute an oral lithium dose for this patient which will produce a steady-state serum concentration of 0.8 mmol/L using the Perry Method.

1. *Administer lithium carbonate test dose and measure 12 and 36 hour postdose lithium concentrations. Compute the lithium elimination rate constant and accumulation ratio for the patient.*

The lithium elimination rate constant is computed using the two serum concentrations: $k_e = (\ln C_{12h} - \ln C_{36h})/\Delta t = [\ln (0.6 \text{ mmol/L}) - \ln (0.3 \text{ mmol/L})]/24 \text{ h} = 0.0289 \text{ h}^{-1}$. The lithium accumulation ratio is computed using the elimination rate constant and desired lithium dosage interval of 12 hours: $R = 1/(1 - e^{-k_e\tau}) = 1/(1 - e^{-(0.0289 h^{-1})(12h)}) = 3.4$.

2. *Compute the estimated lithium concentration at steady-state for the test dose that was given. Use this relationship to compute the dosage regimen for the patient.*

   Using the lithium concentration at 12 hours, the steady-state lithium concentration for 1200 mg every 12 hours can be computed: $C_{ss,t} = R \cdot C_{SD,t} = 3.4 \cdot 0.6 \text{ mmol/L} = 2.0 \text{ mmol/L}$. Linear pharmacokinetic principles can be used to compute the dose required to achieve the target lithium steady-state serum concentration: $D_{new} = (0.8 \text{ mmol/L} /2 \text{ mmol/L})1200 \text{ mg} = 480 \text{ mg}$, rounded to 450 mg every 12 hours of lithium carbonate.

   Upon initiation of therapy, serum concentrations can be measured every 2-3 days for safety reasons in patients that are predisposed to lithium toxicity even though steady-state has not yet been achieved. Once the desired steady-state lithium concentration has been achieved, lithium concentrations should be rechecked every 1-2 weeks for approximately 2 months or until concentrations have stabilized. Because patients with acute mania can have increased lithium clearance, lithium concentrations should be remeasured in these patients once the manic episode is over and clearance returns to normal.

Repeated One-Point or Ritschel Method

The method to individualize lithium dose proposed by Ritschel and associates utilizes another way to compute the elimination rate constant for a patient.[36,37] In this case, two equal lithium doses are administered apart from each other by the desired dosage interval (usually 12 hours). A single serum concentration is obtained before the second test dose is given and another is gathered after the second dose is given at a time equaling the anticipated dosage interval. These are used to compute the elimination rate constant (k_e in h^{-1}) for the patient: $k_e = \{\ln [C_1/(C_2 - C_1)]\}/\tau$, where C_1 is the lithium concentration in mmol/L obtained after the first test dose, C_2 is the lithium concentration in mmol/L obtained after the second test dose, and τ is the expected dosage interval in hours for lithium dosing and is also the postdose time at which the lithium concentrations were obtained.

With knowledge of the elimination rate constant (k_e), the accumulation ratio (R) can be computed for the dosage interval: $R = 1/(1 - e^{-k_e\tau})$, where τ is the dosage interval in hours. The accumulation ratio (R) is also equal to the ratio of the concentration at any time, t, after a single dose ($C_{SD,t}$ in mmol/L) and the steady-state concentration at that same time after the dose is administered as multiple doses ($C_{ss,t}$ in mmol/L): $R = C_{ss,t}/C_{SD,t}$ or $C_{ss,t} = R \cdot C_{SD,t}$. Once a steady-state concentration can be computed for a dosage regimen, linear pharmacokinetic principles can be used to compute the dose required to achieve a target lithium steady-state serum concentration: $D_{new} = (C_{ss,new}/C_{ss,old})D_{old}$, where D is the dose, Css is the steady-state peak or trough concentration, old indicates the dose that produced the steady-state concentration that the patient is currently receiving, and new denotes the dose necessary to produce the desired steady-state concentration. As with the Cooper and Perry methods, the lithium serum concentration must be zero before the test dose is administered.

EXAMPLE 9 ▶▶▶

CB is a 27-year-old, 75-kg (height = 6 ft 2 in) male with bipolar disease. He is currently experiencing an episode of acute mania. His serum creatinine is 1.0 mg/dL. Two test doses of lithium (600 mg each, 12 hours apart) were given to the patient, and lithium concentrations were measured as 0.3 mmol/L and 0.5 mmol/L 12 hours after the first and second doses, respectively. Compute an oral lithium dose for this patient which will produce a steady-state serum concentration of 1.2 mmol/L using the Ritschel Repeated One-Point method.

1. *Administer lithium carbonate test doses and measure lithium concentrations. Compute the lithium elimination rate constant and accumulation ratio for the patient.*

   The lithium elimination rate constant is computed using the two serum concentrations: $k_e = \{\ln [C_1/(C_2 - C_1)]\}/\tau = \ln [(0.3 \text{ mmol/L})/(0.5 \text{ mmol/L} - 0.3 \text{ mmol/L})]/12 \text{ h} = 0.0338 \text{ h}^{-1}$. The lithium accumulation ratio is computed using the elimination rate constant and desired lithium dosage interval of 12 hours: $R = 1/(1 - e^{-k_e\tau}) = 1/(1 - e^{-(0.0338h^{-1})(12h)}) = 3.0$.

2. *Compute the estimated lithium concentration at steady-state for the test dose that was given. Use this relationship to compute the dosage regimen for the patient.*

   Using the lithium concentration at 12 hours, the steady-state lithium concentration for 600 mg every 12 hours can be computed: $C_{ss,t} = R \bullet C_{SD,t} = 3.0 \bullet 0.3 \text{ mmol/L} = 0.9 \text{ mmol/L}$. Linear pharmacokinetic principles can be used to compute the dose required to achieve the target lithium steady-state serum concentration: $D_{new} = (1.2 \text{ mmol/L} / 0.9 \text{ mmol/L})600 \text{ mg} = 800 \text{ mg}$, rounded to 900 mg every 12 hours of lithium carbonate.

   Upon initiation of therapy, serum concentrations can be measured every 2-3 days for safety reasons in patients that are predisposed to lithium toxicity even though steady-state has not yet been achieved. Once the desired steady-state lithium concentration has been achieved, lithium concentrations should be rechecked every 1-2 weeks for approximately 2 months or until concentrations have stabilized. Because patients with acute mania can have increased lithium clearance, lithium concentrations should be remeasured in these patients once the manic episode is over and clearance returns to normal.

USE OF LITHIUM SERUM CONCENTRATIONS TO ALTER DOSAGES

Because of pharmacokinetic variability among patients, it is likely that doses computed using patient population characteristics will not always produce lithium serum concentrations that are expected. Because of this, lithium serum concentrations are measured in all patients to ensure that therapeutic, nontoxic levels are present. Additionally, important patient parameters should be followed to confirm that the patient is responding to treatment and not developing adverse drug reactions.

When lithium serum concentrations are measured in patients and a dosage change is necessary, clinicians should seek to use the simplest, most straightforward method available to determine a dose that will provide safe and effective treatment. In most cases, a simple dosage ratio can be used to change lithium doses since this drug follows *linear pharmacokinetics*.

Also, computerized methods that incorporate expected population pharmacokinetic characteristics (*Bayesian pharmacokinetic computer programs*) can be used in difficult cases where renal function is changing, serum concentrations are obtained at suboptimal times, or the patient was not at steady-state when serum concentrations were measured. An additional benefit of this method is that a complete pharmacokinetic workup (determination of clearance, volume of distribution, and half-life) can be done with one or more measured concentrations that do not have to be at steady-state.

Linear Pharmacokinetics Method

Because lithium follows linear, dose-proportional pharmacokinetics, steady-state serum concentrations change in proportion to dose according to the following equation: $D_{new}/C_{ss,new} = D_{old}/C_{ss,old}$ or $D_{new} = (C_{ss,new}/C_{ss,old})D_{old}$, where D is the dose, Css is the steady-state peak or trough concentration, old indicates the dose that produced the steady-state concentration that the patient is currently receiving, and new denotes the dose necessary to produce the desired steady-state concentration. The advantages of this method are that it is quick and simple. The principle disadvantage is steady-state concentrations are required.

EXAMPLE 10 ▶▶▶

YC is a 37-year-old, 55-kg (height = 5 ft 1 in) female with bipolar disease. She is currently not experiencing an episode of acute mania and requires prophylactic treatment with lithium. Her serum creatinine is 0.6 mg/dL. The patient is receiving 900 mg of lithium carbonate at 0800 H, 1400 H, and 2000 H, and her 12-hour postdose steady-state lithium serum concentration equals 1.1 mmol/L. Compute a new lithium dose to achieve a steady-state concentration of 0.6 mmol/L

1. *Compute new dose to achieve the desired serum concentration.*

   Using linear pharmacokinetics, the new dose to attain the desired concentration should be proportional to the old dose (2700 mg/d) that produced the measured concentration:

   $$D_{new} = (C_{ss,new}/C_{ss,old})D_{old} = (0.6 \text{ mmol/L} / 1.1 \text{ mmol/L}) \, 2700 \text{ mg/d} = 1473 \text{ mg/d, round to } 1500 \text{ mg/d}$$

   The patient would be administered 600 mg of lithium carbonate at 0800 H and 2000 H, and 300 mg of lithium carbonate at 1400 H.

   When lithium dosage alterations are needed, lithium serum concentrations should be measured within 1-2 weeks after the change. During lithium maintenance therapy, steady-state lithium serum concentrations should be repeated every 3-6 months. This time period should be altered to every 6-12 months for patients whose mood is stable or every 1-2 months for patients with frequent mood alterations.

Bayesian Pharmacokinetic Computer Programs

Computer programs are available that can assist in the computation of pharmacokinetic parameters for patients.[15] The most reliable computer programs use a nonlinear regression algorithm that incorporates components of Bayes theorem. Nonlinear regression is a statistical technique that uses an iterative process to compute the best pharmacokinetic parameters for a concentration/time data set. Briefly, the patient's drug dosage schedule and serum concentrations are input into the computer. The computer program has a pharmacokinetic equation preprogrammed for the drug and administration method (oral, intravenous bolus, intravenous infusion, etc). Typically, a one-compartment model is used, although some programs allow the user to choose among several different equations. Using population estimates based on demographic information for the patient (age, weight, gender, renal function, etc) supplied by the user, the computer program then computes estimated serum concentrations at each time there are actual serum concentrations. Kinetic parameters are then changed by the computer program, and a new set of estimated serum concentrations are computed. The pharmacokinetic parameters that generated the estimated serum concentrations closest to the actual values are remembered by the computer program, and the process is repeated until the set of pharmacokinetic parameters that result in estimated serum concentrations that are statistically closest to the actual serum concentrations are generated. These pharmacokinetic parameters can then be used to compute improved dosing schedules for patients. Bayes theorem is used in the computer algorithm to balance the results of the computations between values based solely on the patient's serum drug concentrations and those based only on patient population parameters. Results from studies that compare various methods of dosage adjustment have consistently found that these types of computer dosing programs perform at least as well as experienced clinical pharmacokineticists and clinicians and better than inexperienced clinicians.

Some clinicians use Bayesian pharmacokinetic computer programs exclusively to alter drug doses based on serum concentrations. An advantage of this approach is that consistent dosage recommendations are made when several different practitioners are involved in therapeutic drug-monitoring programs. However, since simpler dosing methods work just as well for patients with stable pharmacokinetic parameters and steady-state drug concentrations, many clinicians reserve the use of computer programs for more difficult situations. Those situations include serum concentrations that are not at steady-state, serum concentrations not obtained at the specific times needed to employ simpler methods, and unstable pharmacokinetic parameters. Many Bayesian pharmacokinetic computer programs are available to users, and most should provide answers similar to the one used in the following examples. The program used to solve problems in this book is DrugCalc written by Dr Dennis Mungall.[38]

For comparison purposes, three cases presented previously using other dosage methods are managed using a Bayesian pharmacokinetic computer program.

EXAMPLE 11 ▶▶▶

YC is a 37-year-old, 55-kg (height = 5 ft 1 in) female with bipolar disease. She is currently not experiencing an episode of acute mania and requires prophylactic treatment with lithium. Her serum creatinine is 0.6 mg/dL. The patient is receiving 900 mg of lithium carbonate at 0800 H, 1400 H, and 2000 H, and her steady-state lithium serum concentration equals 1.1 mmol/L. Compute a new lithium dose to achieve a steady-state concentration of 0.6 mmol/L

1. *Enter the patient's demographic, drug-dosing, and serum concentration/time data into the computer program.*
   Lithium doses must be entered into DrugCalc as mmoles of lithium ion; 900 mg of lithium carbonate provides 24.4 mmol of lithium ion: 900 mg (8.12 mmol Li^+/300 mg lithium carbonate) = 24.4 mmol Li^+

2. *Compute pharmacokinetic parameters for the patient using Bayesian pharmacokinetic computer program.*
   The pharmacokinetic parameters computed by the program are a volume of distribution of 38 L, a half-life equal to 17.9 hours, and a clearance equal to 1.48 L/h.

3. *Compute dose required to achieve the desired lithium serum concentrations.*
   The one-compartment first-order absorption equations used by the program to compute doses indicates that a dose of 13 mmol Li^+ every 12 hours will produce a steady-state concentration of 0.6 mmol/L. This dose is equivalent to 480 mg of lithium carbonate [13 mmol (300 mg lithium carbonate/8.12 mmol Li^+) = 480 mg lithium carbonate]. Rounding this dose to an amount available as an oral dosage form, 450 mg of lithium carbonate would be given every 12 hours.

EXAMPLE 12 ▶▶▶

LK is a 47-year-old, 65-kg (height = 5 ft 5 in) female with bipolar disease. She is not currently experiencing an episode of acute mania. Her serum creatinine is 0.9 mg/dL. After the test dose of 600-mg lithium carbonate was given, the 24-hour lithium concentration was 0.12 mmol/L. Compute an oral lithium dose for this patient for maintenance therapy that would achieve a steady-state concentration equal to 0.6 mmol/L.

1. *Enter the patient's demographic, drug-dosing, and serum concentration/time data into the computer program.*
   Lithium doses must be entered into DrugCalc as mmoles of lithium ion; 600 mg of lithium carbonate provides 16.2 mmol of lithium ion: 600 mg (8.12 mmol Li^+/300 mg lithium carbonate) = 16.2 mmol Li^+

2. *Compute pharmacokinetic parameters for the patient using Bayesian pharmacokinetic computer program.*
   The pharmacokinetic parameters computed by the program are a volume of distribution of 77 L, a half-life equal to 38 hours, and a clearance equal to 1.42 L/h.

3. *Compute dose required to achieve desired lithium serum concentrations.*

The one-compartment first-order absorption equations used by the program to compute doses indicates that a dose of 10 mmol Li^+ every 8 hours will produce a steady-state concentration of 0.8 mmol/L. This dose is equivalent to 369 mg of lithium carbonate [10 mmol (300 mg lithium carbonate/8.12 mmol Li^+) = 369 mg lithium carbonate]. Rounding this dose to an amount available as an oral dosage form, 300 mg of lithium carbonate would be given three times daily at 0800 H, 1400 H, and 2000 H to provide a 12-hour window for serum concentration monitoring after the evening dose.

EXAMPLE 13 ▶▶▶

CB is a 27-year-old, 75-kg (height = 6 ft 2 in) male with bipolar disease. He is currently experiencing an episode of acute mania. His serum creatinine is 1.0 mg/dL. Two test doses of lithium (600 mg each) were given to the patient at 0800 H and 2000 H, and lithium concentrations were measured as 0.3 mmol/L and 0.5 mmol/L 12 hours after the first and second doses, respectively. Compute an oral lithium dose for this patient which will produce a steady-state serum concentration of 1.2 mmol/L.

1. *Enter the patient's demographic, drug-dosing, and serum concentration/time data into the computer program.*

Lithium doses must be entered into DrugCalc as mmoles of lithium ion; 600 mg of lithium carbonate provides 16.2 mmol of lithium ion: 600 mg (8.12 mmol Li^+/300 mg lithium carbonate) = 16.2 mmol Li^+

2. *Compute pharmacokinetic parameters for the patient using Bayesian pharmacokinetic computer program.*

The pharmacokinetic parameters computed by the program are a volume of distribution of 38 L, a half-life equal to 19.2 hours, and a clearance equal to 1.37 L/h.

3. *Compute dose required to achieve the desired lithium serum concentrations.*

The one-compartment first-order absorption equations used by the program to compute doses indicates that a dose of 22 mmol Li^+ every 12 hours will produce a steady-state concentration of 1.2 mmol/L. This dose is equivalent to 813 mg of lithium carbonate [22 mmol (300 mg lithium carbonate/8.12 mmol Li^+) = 813 mg lithium carbonate]. Rounding this dose to an amount available as an oral dosage form, 900 mg of lithium carbonate would be given every 12 hours.

When lithium dosage alterations are needed, lithium serum concentrations should be measured within 1-2 weeks after the change. During lithium maintenance therapy, steady-state lithium serum concentrations should be repeated every 3-6 months. This time period should be altered to every 6-12 months for patients whose mood is stable or every 1-2 months for patients with frequent mood alterations.

DOSING STRATEGIES

Initial dose and dosage adjustment techniques using serum concentrations can be used in any combination as long as the limitations of each method are observed. Some dosing schemes link together logically when considered according to their basic approaches or philosophies. Dosage strategies that follow similar pathways are given in Table 21-2.

TABLE 21-2   Dosing Strategies

Dosing Approach/Philosophy	Initial Dosing	Use of Serum Concentrations to Alter Doses
Pharmacokinetic parameter/equations	Pharmacokinetic Dosing method	Linear Pharmacokinetics method
Literature-based concept	Literature-based Recommended Dosing method	Linear Pharmacokinetics method
Test dose	Cooper nomogram or Perry method or Repeated one-point method	Linear Pharmacokinetics method
Computerized	Bayesian computer program	Bayesian computer program

PROBLEMS

The following problems are intended to emphasize the computation of initial and individualized doses using clinical pharmacokinetic techniques. Clinicians should always consult the patient's chart to confirm that current therapy is appropriate. Additionally, all other medications that the patient is taking, including prescription and nonprescription drugs, should be noted and checked to ascertain if a potential drug interaction with lithium exists.

1. PG is a 67-year-old, 72-kg (height = 6 ft 1 in, serum creatinine = 1.2 mg/dL) male with bipolar disease requiring maintenance therapy with oral lithium. Suggest an initial lithium carbonate dosage regimen designed to achieve a steady-state lithium concentration equal to 0.6 mmol/L.

2. Patient PG (see problem 1) was prescribed lithium carbonate 900 mg orally every 12 hours. The current 12-hour postdose steady-state lithium concentration equals 1.0 mmol/L. Compute a new lithium carbonate dose that will provide a steady-state concentration of 0.6 mmol/L.

3. DU is a 21-year-old, 70-kg (height = 5 ft 9 in, serum creatinine = 0.8 mg/dL) female with bipolar disease who requires therapy with lithium. She is currently experiencing an episode of acute mania. Suggest an initial lithium carbonate dosage regimen designed to achieve a steady-state lithium concentration equal to 0.8 mmol/L.

4. Patient DU (see problem 3) was prescribed lithium carbonate 600 mg orally at 0800 H, 1400 H, and 2000 H. The current 12-hour postdose steady-state lithium concentration equals 0.6 mmol/L. Compute a new oral lithium dose that will provide a steady-state concentration of 1 mmol/L.

5. JH is a 35-year-old, 60-kg (height = 5 ft 2 in, serum creatinine = 0.8 mg/dL) female with bipolar disease requiring maintenance treatment with lithium. She was administered a test dose of lithium carbonate 600 mg, and the 24-hour postdose lithium concentration is 0.07 mmol/L. Suggest an initial lithium dosage regimen designed to achieve a steady-state concentration equal to 0.8 mmol/L.

6. Patient JH (see problem 5) was prescribed lithium carbonate 600 mg orally every 12 hours starting 12 hours after the concentration for the test dose was measured. A lithium serum concentration was obtained just before the 10th dose of this regimen and equaled 0.4 mmol/L. Compute a new oral lithium carbonate dose that will provide a steady-state concentration of 0.6 mmol/L.

7. PZ is a 24-year-old, 80-kg (height = 5 ft 11 in, serum creatinine = 1.1 mg/dL) male in the acute manic phase of bipolar disease who requires therapy with oral lithium. He was administered a test dose of

lithium carbonate 600 mg at 0800 H, and the 24-hour postdose lithium concentration is 0.21 mmol/L. Suggest an initial lithium dosage regimen designed to achieve a steady-state concentration equal to 0.8 mmol/L.

8. Patient PZ (see problem 7) was prescribed lithium carbonate 600 mg orally at 0800, 1400 H, and 2000 H (first dose at 1400 H on the same day the lithium test dose concentration was obtained). A lithium serum concentration was obtained just before the 12th dose of this regimen and equaled 1.5 mmol/L. Compute a new lithium carbonate dose that will provide a steady-state concentration of 1 mmol/L.

9. WG is a 41-year-old, 130-kg (height = 5 ft 11 in, serum creatinine = 1.2 mg/dL) male in the acute phase of bipolar disease that requires treatment with lithium carbonate. He was given a test dose of lithium carbonate 1200 mg at 0800 H, and lithium concentrations were obtained 12 and 36 hours postdose. The lithium concentrations were 0.42 mmol/L and 0.28 mmol/L. Suggest an initial lithium carbonate dosage regimen designed to achieve a steady-state concentration equal to 1 mmol/L.

10. FY is a 32-year-old, 68-kg (height = 5 ft 4 in, serum creatinine = 0.9 mg/dL) female with bipolar disease that requires maintenance treatment with lithium carbonate. She was given a test dose of lithium carbonate 900 mg at 0800 H, and lithium concentrations were obtained 12 and 36 hours postdose. The lithium concentrations were 0.3 mmol/L and 0.11 mmol/L. Suggest an initial lithium carbonate dosage regimen designed to achieve a steady-state concentration equal to 1.0 mmol/L.

11. MW is a 22-year-old, 81-kg (height = 6 ft 2 in) male with bipolar disease. He is currently experiencing an episode of acute mania. His serum creatinine is 0.9 mg/dL. Two test doses of lithium (900 mg each, 12 hours apart) were given to the patient, and lithium concentrations were measured as 0.19 mmol/L and 0.31 mmol/L 12 hours after the first and second doses, respectively. Compute an oral lithium dose for this patient which will produce a steady-state serum concentration of 1 mmol/L.

12. YT is a 42-year-old, 66-kg (height = 5 ft 0 in) female with bipolar disease. She requires prophylactic treatment for bipolar disease. Her serum creatinine is 1.4 mg/dL. Two test doses of lithium (300 mg each, 12 hours apart) were given to the patient, and lithium concentrations were measured as 0.11 mmol/L and 0.2 mmol/L 12 hours after the first and second doses, respectively. Compute an oral lithium dose for this patient which will produce a steady-state serum concentration of 0.6 mmol/L.

ANSWERS TO PROBLEMS

1. *Answer to problem 1.*

Pharmacokinetic Dosing Method

1. *Estimate creatinine clearance.*

   This patient has a stable serum creatinine and is not obese. The Cockcroft-Gault equation can be used to estimate creatinine clearance:

   $$CrCl_{est} = [(140 - age)BW]/(72 \cdot S_{Cr}) = [(140 - 67\ y)72\ kg]/(72 \cdot 1.2\ mg/dL)$$
   $$CrCl_{est} = 61\ ml/min$$

2. *Estimate clearance.*

   The drug clearance versus creatinine clearance relationship is used to estimate the lithium clearance for this patient:

   $$Cl = 0.288(CrCl) = 0.288(61\ mL/min) = 17.6\ L/d$$

3. *Use average steady-state concentration equation to compute lithium maintenance dose.*

For a patient requiring maintenance therapy for bipolar disease the desired lithium concentration would be 0.6-0.8 mmol/L. A serum concentration equal to 0.6 mmol/L will be chosen for this patient, and oral lithium carbonate will be used (F = 1, 8.12 mmol Li^+/300 mg of lithium carbonate).

$$D/\tau = (Css \bullet Cl)/F = (0.6 \text{ mmol/L} \bullet 17.6 \text{ L/d})/1 = 10.6 \text{ mmol/d}$$

D/τ = (300 mg lithium carbonate/8.12 mmol Li^+) 10.6 mmol/d = 392 mg/d, rounded to 450 mg/d of lithium carbonate. This dose would be given as 150 mg of lithium carbonate in the morning and 300 mg of lithium carbonate in the evening.

Upon initiation of therapy, serum concentrations can be measured every 2-3 days for safety reasons in patients that are predisposed to lithium toxicity even though steady-state has not yet been achieved. Once the desired steady-state lithium concentration has been achieved, lithium concentrations should be rechecked every 1-2 weeks for approximately 2 months or until concentrations have stabilized.

Literature-Based Recommended Dosing

1. *Estimate creatinine clearance.*

This patient has a stable serum creatinine and is not obese. The Cockcroft-Gault equation can be used to estimate creatinine clearance:

$$CrCl_{est} = [(140 - age)BW]/(72 \bullet S_{Cr}) = [(140 - 67 \text{ y})72 \text{ kg}]/(72 \bullet 1.2 \text{ mg/dL})$$
$$CrCl_{est} = 61 \text{ mL/min}$$

2. *Choose lithium dose based on disease states and conditions present in the patient.*

The patient requires prophylactic lithium therapy for bipolar disease and has good renal function. A lithium carbonate dose of 600 mg/d, given as 300 mg every 12 hours, is recommended as the initial amount. The dosage rate will be increased 300-600 mg/d every 2-3 days as needed to provide adequate therapeutic effect, avoid adverse effects, and produce therapeutic lithium steady-state concentrations.

2. *Answer to problem 2.*

Linear Pharmacokinetics Method

1. *Compute new dose to achieve desired serum concentration.*

Using linear pharmacokinetics, the new dose to attain the desired concentration should be proportional to the old dose (1800 mg/d) that produced the measured concentration:

$$D_{new} = (C_{ss,new}/C_{ss,old})D_{old} = (0.6 \text{ mmol/L} / 1.0 \text{ mmol/L}) 1800 \text{ mg/d} = 1080 \text{ mg/d},$$
round to 900 mg/d

The patient would be administered 450 mg of lithium carbonate every 12 hours.

When lithium dosage alterations are needed, lithium serum concentrations should be measured within 1-2 weeks after the change. During lithium maintenance therapy, steady-state lithium serum concentrations should be repeated every 3-6 months. This time period should be altered to every 6-12 months for patients whose mood is stable or every 1-2 months for patients with frequent mood alterations.

3. *Answer to problem 3.*

Pharmacokinetic Dosing Method

1. *Estimate creatinine clearance.*

This patient has a stable serum creatinine and is not obese. The Cockcroft-Gault equation can be used to estimate creatinine clearance:

$$CrCl_{est} = \{[(140 - age)BW]/(72 \bullet S_{Cr})\} \bullet 0.85 = \{[(140 - 21 \; y)70 \; kg]/(72 \bullet 0.8 \; mg/dL)\} \bullet 0.85$$
$$CrCl_{est} = 123 \; mL/min$$

2. *Estimate clearance.*

The drug clearance versus creatinine clearance relationship for a patient with acute mania is used to estimate the lithium clearance for this patient:

$$Cl = 0.432(CrCl) = 0.432(123 \; mL/min) = 53.1 \; L/d$$

3. *Use average steady-state concentration equation to compute lithium maintenance dose.*

For a patient requiring therapy for the acute mania phase of bipolar disease the desired lithium concentration would be 0.8-1 mmol/L. A serum concentration equal to 0.8 mmol/L was chosen for this patient, and oral lithium carbonate will be used (F = 1, 8.12 mmol Li^+/300 mg of lithium carbonate).

$$D/\tau = (Css \bullet Cl)/F = (0.8 \; mmol/L \bullet 53.1 \; L/d)/1 = 42.5 \; mmol/d$$

D/τ = (300 mg lithium carbonate/8.12 mmol Li^+) 42.5 mmol/d = 1570 mg/d, rounded to 1500 mg/d of lithium carbonate. This dose would be given as 600 mg of lithium carbonate at 0800 H and 2000 H and 300 mg of lithium carbonate at 1400 H.

Upon initiation of therapy, serum concentrations can be measured every 2-3 days for safety reasons in patients that are predisposed to lithium toxicity even though steady-state has not yet been achieved. Once the desired steady-state lithium concentration has been achieved, lithium concentrations should be rechecked every 1-2 weeks for approximately 2 months or until concentrations have stabilized.

Literature-Based Recommended Dosing

1. *Estimate creatinine clearance.*

This patient has a stable serum creatinine and is not obese. The Cockcroft-Gault equation can be used to estimate creatinine clearance:

$$CrCl_{est} = \{[(140 - age)BW]/(72 \bullet S_{Cr})\} \bullet 0.85 = \{[(140 - 21 \; y)70 \; kg]/(72 \bullet 0.8 \; mg/dL)\} \bullet 0.85$$
$$CrCl_{est} = 123 \; mL/min$$

2. *Choose lithium dose based on disease states and conditions present in the patient.*

The patient requires acute lithium therapy for the treatment of the acute manic phase of bipolar disease, and has good renal function. A lithium carbonate dose of 1200 mg/d, given as 600 mg every 12 hours, is recommended as the initial amount. The dosage rate will be increased 300-600 mg/d every 2-3 days as needed to provide adequate therapeutic effect, avoid adverse effects, and produce therapeutic lithium steady-state concentrations.

4. *Answer to problem 4.*

Linear Pharmacokinetics Method

1. *Compute new dose to achieve desired serum concentration.*

Using linear pharmacokinetics, the new dose to attain the desired concentration should be proportional to the old dose (1800 mg/d) that produced the measured concentration:

$$D_{new} = (C_{ss,new}/C_{ss,old})D_{old} = (1 \text{ mmol/L} / 0.6 \text{ mmol/L})1800 \text{ mg/d} = 3000 \text{ mg/d},$$
round to 2700 mg/d

The patient would be administered 900 mg of lithium carbonate at 0800 H, 1400 H, and 2000 H.
When lithium dosage alterations are needed, lithium serum concentrations should be measured within 1-2 weeks after the change. During lithium maintenance therapy, steady-state lithium serum concentrations should be repeated every 3-6 months. This time period should be altered to every 6-12 months for patients whose mood is stable or every 1-2 months for patients with frequent mood alterations.

5. *Answer to problem 5.*

Cooper Nomogram

1. *Administer 600 mg lithium carbonate test dose and measure 24-hour postdose lithium concentration. Use Cooper nomogram to recommend lithium carbonate maintenance dose.*

After the test dose was given, the 24-hour postdose lithium concentration was 0.07 mmol/L. The recommended lithium carbonate maintenance dose is 900 mg three times daily. The doses would be given at 0900 H, 1500 H and 2100 H to allow a 12-hour window after the evening dose so that lithium serum concentration measurements can be made.

Upon initiation of therapy, serum concentrations can be measured every 2-3 days for safety reasons in patients that are predisposed to lithium toxicity even though steady-state has not yet been achieved. Once the desired steady-state lithium concentration has been achieved, lithium concentrations should be rechecked every 1-2 weeks for approximately 2 months or until concentrations have stabilized.

Bayesian Pharmacokinetic Computer Program

1. *Enter the patient's demographic, drug-dosing, and serum concentration/time data into the computer program.*

Lithium doses must be entered into DrugCalc as mmoles of lithium ion; 600 mg of lithium carbonate provides 16.2 mmol of lithium ion: 600 mg (8.12 mmol Li^+/300 mg lithium carbonate) = 16.2 mmol Li^+.

2. *Compute pharmacokinetic parameters for the patient using Bayesian pharmacokinetic computer program.*

The pharmacokinetic parameters computed by the program are a volume of distribution of 99 L, a half-life equal to 27 hours, and a clearance equal to 2.53 L/h.

3. *Compute dose required to achieve the desired lithium serum concentrations.*

The one-compartment first-order absorption equations used by the program to compute doses indicates that a dose of 34 mmol Li^+ every 12 hours will produce a steady-state concentration of 0.8 mmol/L. This dose is equivalent to 1256 mg of lithium carbonate [34 mmol (300 mg lithium carbonate/8.12 mmol Li^+) = 1256 mg lithium carbonate]. Rounding this dose to an amount available as an oral dosage form, 1200 mg of lithium carbonate would be given every 12 hours.

Upon initiation of therapy, serum concentrations can be measured every 2-3 days for safety reasons in patients that are predisposed to lithium toxicity even though steady-state has not yet been achieved. Once the desired steady-state lithium concentration has been achieved, lithium concentrations should be rechecked every 1-2 weeks for approximately 2 months or until concentrations have stabilized.

6. *Answer to problem 6.*

Linear Pharmacokinetics Method

1. *Compute new dose to achieve the desired serum concentration.*

Using linear pharmacokinetics, the new dose to attain the desired concentration should be proportional to the old dose (1200 mg/d) that produced the measured concentration:

$$D_{new} = (C_{ss,new}/C_{ss,old})D_{old} = (0.6\ mmol/L\ /\ 0.4\ mmol/L)1200\ mg/d = 1800\ mg/d$$

The patient would be administered 900 mg of lithium carbonate every 12 hours.

When lithium dosage alterations are needed, lithium serum concentrations should be measured within 1-2 weeks after the change. During lithium maintenance therapy, steady-state lithium serum concentrations should be repeated every 3-6 months. This time period should be altered to every 6-12 months for patients whose mood is stable or every 1-2 months for patients with frequent mood alterations.

Bayesian Pharmacokinetic Computer Program

1. *Enter the patient's demographic, drug-dosing, and serum concentration/time data into the computer program.*

Lithium doses must be entered into DrugCalc as mmoles of lithium ion; 600 mg of lithium carbonate provides 16.2 mmol of lithium ion: 600 mg ($8.12\ mmol\ Li^+/300\ mg$ lithium carbonate) = 16.2 mmol Li^+. In this case, the concentration after the test dose (problem 5) as well as the concentration just before the 10th dose can be used in the program.

2. *Compute pharmacokinetic parameters for the patient using Bayesian pharmacokinetic computer program.*

The pharmacokinetic parameters computed by the program are a volume of distribution of 112 L, a half-life equal to 35 hours, and a clearance equal to 2.22 L/h.

3. *Compute dose required to achieve the desired lithium serum concentrations.*

The one-compartment first-order absorption equations used by the program to compute doses indicates that a dose of 21 mmol Li^+ every 12 hours will produce a steady-state concentration of 0.8 mmol/L. This dose is equivalent to 776 mg of lithium carbonate [21 mmol (300 mg lithium carbonate/$8.12\ mmol\ Li^+$) = 776 mg lithium carbonate]. Rounding this dose to an amount available as an oral dosage form, 750 mg of lithium carbonate would be given every 12 hours.

When lithium dosage alterations are needed, lithium serum concentrations should be measured within 1-2 weeks after the change. During lithium maintenance therapy, steady-state lithium serum concentrations should be repeated every 3-6 months. This time period should be altered to every 6-12 months for patients whose mood is stable or every 1-2 months for patients with frequent mood alterations.

7. *Answer to problem 7.*

Cooper Nomogram

1. *Administer 600 mg lithium carbonate test dose and measure 24 hour postdose lithium concentration. Use Cooper nomogram to recommend lithium carbonate maintenance dose.*

After the test dose was given, the 24-hour lithium concentration was 0.21 mmol/L. The recommended lithium carbonate maintenance dose is 300 mg three times daily. The doses would be given at 0900 H, 1500 H and 2100 H to allow a 12-hour window after the evening dose so that lithium serum concentration measurements can be made.

Upon initiation of therapy, serum concentrations can be measured every 2-3 days for safety reasons in patients that are predisposed to lithium toxicity even though steady-state has not yet been achieved. Once the desired steady-state lithium concentration has been achieved, lithium concentrations should be rechecked every 1-2 weeks for approximately 2 months or until concentrations have stabilized.

Bayesian Pharmacokinetic Computer Program

1. *Enter the patient's demographic, drug-dosing, and serum concentration/time data into the computer program.*

   Lithium doses must be entered into DrugCalc as mmoles of lithium ion; 600 mg of lithium carbonate provides 16.2 mmol of lithium ion: 600 mg (8.12 mmol Li^+/300 mg lithium carbonate) = 16.2 mmol Li^+.

2. *Compute pharmacokinetic parameters for the patient using Bayesian pharmacokinetic computer program.*

   The pharmacokinetic parameters computed by the program are a volume of distribution of 44 L, a half-life equal to 25 hours, and a clearance equal to 1.2 L/h.

3. *Compute dose required to achieve the desired lithium serum concentrations.*

   The one-compartment first-order absorption equations used by the program to compute doses indicates that a dose of 8 mmol Li^+ every 8 hours will produce a steady-state concentration of 0.8 mmol/L. This dose is equivalent to 296 mg of lithium carbonate [8 mmol (300 mg lithium carbonate/8.12 mmol Li^+) = 296 mg lithium carbonate]. Rounding this dose to an amount available as an oral dosage form, 300 mg of lithium carbonate would be given at 0900 H, 1500 H and 2100 H to allow a 12-hour window after the evening dose so that lithium serum concentration measurements can be made.

   Upon initiation of therapy, serum concentrations can be measured every 2-3 days for safety reasons in patients that are predisposed to lithium toxicity even though steady-state has not yet been achieved. Once the desired steady-state lithium concentration has been achieved, lithium concentrations should be rechecked every 1-2 weeks for approximately 2 months or until concentrations have stabilized.

8. *Answer to problem 8.*

Linear Pharmacokinetics Method

1. *Compute new dose to achieve the desired serum concentration.*

   Using linear pharmacokinetics, the new dose to attain the desired concentration should be proportional to the old dose (1800 mg/d) that produced the measured concentration:

   $$D_{new} = (C_{ss,new}/C_{ss,old})D_{old} = (1\ mmol/L\ /\ 1.5\ mmol/L)1800\ mg/d = 1200\ mg/d$$

   The patient would be administered 600 mg of lithium carbonate every 12 hours.

   When lithium dosage alterations are needed, lithium serum concentrations should be measured within 1-2 weeks after the change. During lithium maintenance therapy, steady-state lithium serum concentrations should be repeated every 3-6 months. This time period should be altered to every 6-12 months for patients whose mood is stable or every 1-2 months for patients with frequent mood alterations.

Bayesian Pharmacokinetic Computer Program

1. *Enter the patient's demographic, drug-dosing, and serum concentration/time data into the computer program.*

   Lithium doses must be entered into DrugCalc as mmoles of lithium ion; 600 mg of lithium carbonate provides 16.2 mmol of lithium ion: 600 mg (8.12 mmol Li^+/300 mg lithium carbonate) = 16.2 mmol Li^+. In this case, the concentration after the test dose (problem 7) as well as the concentration just before the 12th dose can be used in the program.

2. *Compute pharmacokinetic parameters for the patient using Bayesian pharmacokinetic computer program.*

   The pharmacokinetic parameters computed by the program are a volume of distribution of 44 L, a half-life equal to 25 hours, and a clearance equal to 1.2 L/h.

3. *Compute dose required to achieve the desired lithium serum concentrations.*

   The one-compartment first-order absorption equations used by the program to compute doses indicates that a dose of 16 mmol Li^+ every 12 hours will produce a steady-state concentration of 1 mmol/L. This dose is equivalent to 591 mg of lithium carbonate [16 mmol (300 mg lithium carbonate/8.12 mmol Li^+) = 591 mg lithium carbonate]. Rounding this dose to an amount available as an oral dosage form, 600 mg of lithium carbonate would be given every 12 hours.

   When lithium dosage alterations are needed, lithium serum concentrations should be measured within 1-2 weeks after the change. During lithium maintenance therapy, steady-state lithium serum concentrations should be repeated every 3-6 months. This time period should be altered to every 6-12 months for patients whose mood is stable or every 1-2 months for patients with frequent mood alterations.

9. *Answer to problem 9.*

Perry Method

1. *Administer lithium carbonate test dose and measure 12- and 36-hour postdose lithium concentrations. Compute the lithium elimination rate constant and accumulation ratio for the patient.*

   The lithium elimination rate constant is computed using the two serum concentrations: $k_e = (\ln C_{12h} - \ln C_{36h})/\Delta t = [\ln (0.42$ mmol/L$) - \ln (0.28$ mmol/L$)]/24$ h $= 0.0169$ h^{-1}. The lithium accumulation ratio is computed using the elimination rate constant and desired lithium dosage interval of 12 hours: $R = 1/(1 - e^{-k_e\tau}) = 1/(1 - e^{-(0.0169h^{-1})(12h)}) = 5.4$.

2. *Compute the estimated lithium concentration at steady state for the test dose that was given. Use this relationship to compute the dosage regimen for the patient.*

   Using the lithium concentration at 12 hours, the steady-state lithium concentration for 1200 mg every 12 hours can be computed: $C_{ss,t} = R \bullet C_{SD,t} = 5.4 \bullet 0.42$ mmol/L $= 2.3$ mmol/L. Linear pharmacokinetic principles can be used to compute the dose required to achieve the target lithium steady-state serum concentration: $D_{new} = (1$ mmol/L$/2.3$ mmol/L$)1200$ mg $= 522$ mg, rounded to 600 mg every 12 hours of lithium carbonate.

   Upon initiation of therapy, serum concentrations can be measured every 2-3 days for safety reasons in patients that are predisposed to lithium toxicity even though steady-state has not yet been achieved. Once the desired steady-state lithium concentration has been achieved, lithium concentrations should be rechecked every 1-2 weeks for approximately 2 months or until concentrations have stabilized. Because patients with acute mania can have increased lithium clearance, lithium concentrations should be remeasured in these patients once the manic episode is over and clearance returns to normal.

Bayesian Pharmacokinetic Computer Program

1. *Enter the patient's demographic, drug-dosing, and serum concentration/time data into the computer program.*

   Lithium doses must be entered into DrugCalc as mmoles of lithium ion; 1200 mg of lithium carbonate provides 32.5 mmol of lithium ion: 1200 mg (8.12 mmol Li^+/300 mg lithium carbonate) = 32.5 mmol Li^+.

2. *Compute pharmacokinetic parameters for the patient using Bayesian pharmacokinetic computer program.*

   The pharmacokinetic parameters computed by the program are a volume of distribution of 67 L, a half-life equal to 41 hours, and a clearance equal to 1.13 L/h.

3. *Compute dose required to achieve the desired lithium serum concentrations.*

   The one-compartment first-order absorption equations used by the program to compute doses indicates that a dose of 14 mmol Li^+ every 12 hours will produce a steady-state concentration of 1 mmol/L. This dose is equivalent to 517 mg of lithium carbonate [14 mmol (300 mg lithium carbonate/8.12 mmol Li^+) = 517 mg lithium carbonate]. Rounding this dose to an amount available as an oral dosage form, 600 mg of lithium carbonate would be given every 12 hours.

   Upon initiation of therapy, serum concentrations can be measured every 2-3 days for safety reasons in patients that are predisposed to lithium toxicity even though steady-state has not yet been achieved. Once the desired steady-state lithium concentration has been achieved, lithium concentrations should be rechecked every 1-2 weeks for approximately 2 months or until concentrations have stabilized.

10. *Answer to problem 10.*

Perry Method

1. *Administer lithium carbonate test dose and measure 12- and 36-hour postdose lithium concentrations. Compute the lithium elimination rate constant and accumulation ratio for the patient.*

   The lithium elimination rate constant is computed using the two serum concentrations: k_e = $(\ln C_{12h} - \ln C_{36h})/\Delta t$ = [ln (0.3 mmol/L) − ln (0.11 mmol/L)]/24 h = 0.0418 h^{-1}. The lithium accumulation ratio is computed using the elimination rate constant and the desired lithium dosage interval of 12 hours: $R = 1/(1 - e^{-k_e\tau}) = 1/(1 - e^{-(0.0418h^{-1})(12h)})$ = 2.5.

2. *Compute the estimated lithium concentration at steady-state for the test dose that was given. Use this relationship to compute the dosage regimen for the patient.*

   Using the lithium concentration at 12 hours, the steady-state lithium concentration for 900 mg every 12 hours can be computed: $C_{ss,t} = R \bullet C_{SD,t}$ = 2.5 • 0.3 mmol/L = 0.75 mmol/L. Linear pharmacokinetic principles can be used to compute the dose required to achieve the target lithium steady-state serum concentration: D_{new} = (1 mmol/L / 0.75 mmol/L)900 mg = 1200 mg every 12 hours of lithium carbonate.

   Upon initiation of therapy, serum concentrations can be measured every 2-3 days for safety reasons in patients that are predisposed to lithium toxicity even though steady-state has not yet been achieved. Once the desired steady-state lithium concentration has been achieved, lithium concentrations should be rechecked every 1-2 weeks for approximately 2 months or until concentrations have stabilized. Because patients with acute mania can have increased lithium clearance, lithium concentrations should be remeasured in these patients once the manic episode is over and clearance returns to normal.

Bayesian Pharmacokinetic Computer Program

1. *Enter the patient's demographic, drug dosing, and serum concentration/time data into the computer program.*

    Lithium doses must be entered into DrugCalc as mmoles of lithium ion; 900 mg of lithium carbonate provides 24.4 mmol of lithium ion: 900 mg (8.12 mmol Li^+/300 mg lithium carbonate) = 24.4 mmol Li^+.

2. *Compute pharmacokinetic parameters for the patient using Bayesian pharmacokinetic computer program.*

    The pharmacokinetic parameters computed by the program are a volume of distribution of 47 L, a half-life equal to 17 hours, and a clearance equal to 1.94 L/h.

3. *Compute dose required to achieve the desired lithium serum concentrations.*

    The one-compartment first-order absorption equations used by the program to compute doses indicates that a dose of 31 mmol Li^+ every 12 hours will produce a steady-state concentration of 1 mmol/L. This dose is equivalent to 1145 mg of lithium carbonate [31 mmol (300 mg lithium carbonate/8.12 mmol Li^+) = 1145 mg lithium carbonate]. Rounding this dose to an amount available as an oral dosage form, 1200 mg of lithium carbonate would be given every 12 hours.

    Upon initiation of therapy, serum concentrations can be measured every 2-3 days for safety reasons in patients that are predisposed to lithium toxicity even though steady-state has not yet been achieved. Once the desired steady-state lithium concentration has been achieved, lithium concentrations should be rechecked every 1-2 weeks for approximately 2 months or until concentrations have stabilized.

11. *Answer to problem 11.*

Ritschel Method

1. *Administer lithium carbonate test doses and measure lithium concentrations. Compute the lithium elimination rate constant and accumulation ratio for the patient.*

    The lithium elimination rate constant is computed using the two serum concentrations: $k_e = \{\ln [C_1/(C_2 - C_1)]\}/\tau, = \ln [(0.19 \text{ mmol/L})/(0.31 \text{ mmol/L} - 0.19 \text{ mmol/L})]/12 \text{ h} = 0.0383 \text{ h}^{-1}$. The lithium accumulation ratio is computed using the elimination rate constant and desired lithium dosage interval of 12 hours: $R = 1/(1 - e^{-k_e\tau}) = 1/(1 - e^{-(0.0383h^{-1})(12h)}) = 2.7$.

2. *Compute the estimated lithium concentration at steady-state for the test dose that was given. Use this relationship to compute the dosage regimen for the patient.*

    Using the lithium concentration at 12 hours, the steady-state lithium concentration for 900 mg every 12 hours can be computed: $C_{ss,t} = R \bullet C_{SD,t} = 2.7 \bullet 0.19$ mmol/L = 0.5 mmol/L. Linear pharmacokinetic principles can be used to compute the dose required to achieve the target lithium steady-state serum concentration: D_{new} = (1 mmol/L / 0.5 mmol/L)900 mg = 1800 mg every 12 hours of lithium carbonate. Because the dose exceeds 1200 mg per administration time, the total daily dose of 3600 mg/d would be split into three equal doses of 1200 mg and given at 0900 H, 1500 H, and 2100 H.

    Upon initiation of therapy, serum concentrations can be measured every 2-3 days for safety reasons in patients that are predisposed to lithium toxicity even though steady-state has not yet been achieved. Once the desired steady-state lithium concentration has been achieved, lithium concentrations should be rechecked every 1-2 weeks for approximately 2 months or until concentrations have stabilized. Because patients with acute mania can have increased lithium clearance, lithium concentrations should be remeasured in these patients once the manic episode is over and clearance returns to normal.

Bayesian Pharmacokinetic Computer Program

1. *Enter the patient's demographic, drug-dosing, and serum concentration/time data into the computer program.*

   Lithium doses must be entered into DrugCalc as mmoles of lithium ion; 900 mg of lithium carbonate provides 24.4 mmol of lithium ion: 900 mg (8.12 mmol Li^+/300 mg lithium carbonate) = 24.4 mmol Li^+.

2. *Compute pharmacokinetic parameters for the patient using Bayesian pharmacokinetic computer program.*

   The pharmacokinetic parameters computed by the program are a volume of distribution of 79 L, a half-life equal to 19 hours, and a clearance equal to 2.89 L/h.

3. *Compute dose required to achieve the desired lithium serum concentrations.*

   The one-compartment first-order absorption equations used by the program to compute doses indicates that a dose of 27 mmol Li^+ every 8 hours will produce a steady-state concentration of 1 mmol/L. This dose is equivalent to 998 mg of lithium carbonate [27 mmol (300 mg lithium carbonate/8.12 mmol Li^+) = 998 mg lithium carbonate]. Rounding this dose to an amount available as an oral dosage form, 900 mg of lithium carbonate would be given at 0900 H, 1500 H, and 2100 H.

   Upon initiation of therapy, serum concentrations can be measured every 2-3 days for safety reasons in patients that are predisposed to lithium toxicity even though steady-state has not yet been achieved. Once the desired steady-state lithium concentration has been achieved, lithium concentrations should be rechecked every 1-2 weeks for approximately 2 months or until concentrations have stabilized.

12. *Answer to problem 12.*

Ritschel Method

1. *Administer lithium carbonate test doses and measure lithium concentrations. Compute the lithium elimination rate constant and accumulation ratio for the patient.*

   The lithium elimination rate constant is computed using the two serum concentrations: k_e = $\{\ln [C_1/(C_2 - C_1)]\}/\tau$, = $\ln [(0.11 \text{ mmol/L})/(0.2 \text{ mmol/L} - 0.11 \text{ mmol/L})]/12 \text{ h} = 0.0167 \text{ h}^{-1}$. The lithium accumulation ratio is computed using the elimination rate constant and desired lithium dosage interval of 12 hours: $R = 1/(1 - e^{-k_e\tau}) = 1/(1 - e^{-(0.0167h^{-1})(12h)}) = 5.5$.

2. *Compute the estimated lithium concentration at steady-state for the test dose that was given. Use this relationship to compute the dosage regimen for the patient.*

   Using the lithium concentration at 12 hours, the steady-state lithium concentration for 300 mg every 12 hours can be computed: $C_{ss,t} = R \bullet C_{SD,t} = 5.5 \bullet 0.11 \text{ mmol/L} = 0.6 \text{ mmol/L}$. This is the desired steady-state concentration, so 300 mg every 12 hours of lithium carbonate would be prescribed.

   Upon initiation of therapy, serum concentrations can be measured every 2-3 days for safety reasons in patients that are predisposed to lithium toxicity even though steady-state has not yet been achieved. Once the desired steady-state lithium concentration has been achieved, lithium concentrations should be rechecked every 1-2 weeks for approximately 2 months or until concentrations have stabilized. Because patients with acute mania can have increased lithium clearance, lithium concentrations should be remeasured in these patients once the manic episode is over and clearance returns to normal.

Bayesian Pharmacokinetic Computer Program

1. *Enter the patient's demographic, drug-dosing, and serum concentration/time data into the computer program.*

Lithium doses must be entered into DrugCalc as mmoles of lithium ion; 300 mg of lithium carbonate provides 8.12 mmol of lithium ion: 300 mg (8.12 mmol Li$^+$/300 mg lithium carbonate) = 8.12 mmol Li$^+$.

2. *Compute pharmacokinetic parameters for the patient using Bayesian pharmacokinetic computer program.*

The pharmacokinetic parameters computed by the program are a volume of distribution of 61 L, a half-life equal to 65 hours, and a clearance equal to 0.65 L/h.

3. *Compute dose required to achieve the desired lithium serum concentrations.*

The one-compartment first-order absorption equations used by the program to compute doses indicates that a dose of 5 mmol Li$^+$ every 12 hours will produce a steady-state concentration of 0.6 mmol/L. This dose is equivalent to 185 mg of lithium carbonate [5 mmol (300 mg lithium carbonate/8.12 mmol Li$^+$) = 185 mg lithium carbonate]. Rounding this dose to an amount available as an oral dosage form, 150 mg of lithium carbonate would be given every 12 hours. Because of the long lithium half-life for this patient, a dose of 300 mg every day could also be prescribed.

Upon initiation of therapy, serum concentrations can be measured every 2-3 days for safety reasons in patients that are predisposed to lithium toxicity even though steady-state has not yet been achieved. Once the desired steady-state lithium concentration has been achieved, lithium concentrations should be rechecked every 1-2 weeks for approximately 2 months or until concentrations have stabilized.

REFERENCES

1. Meyer JM. Pharmacotherapy of psychosis and mania. In: Brunton L, Chabner B, Knollman B, eds. *The Pharmacological Basis of Therapeutics*. 12th ed. New York, NY: McGraw-Hill; 2011:417-452.
2. Drayton SJ. Bipolar disorder. In: DiPiro JT, Talbert RL, Yee GC, Matzke GR, Wells BG, Posey LM, eds. *Pharmacotherapy*. 12th ed. New York, NY: McGraw-Hill; 2011:1191-1208.
3. Weber SS, Saklad SR, Kastenholz KV. Bipolar affective disorders. In: Koda-Kimble MA, Young LY, Kradjan WA, Guglielmo BJ, eds. *Applied Therapeutics*. 5th ed. Vancouver, WA: Applied Therapeutics; 1992:51-58.
4. Perry PJ, Alexander B, Liskow BI, DeVane CL. *Psychotropic Drug Handbook*. 8th ed. Philadelphia, PA: Lippincott Williams & Wilkins; 2007.
5. Amdisen A. Serum level monitoring and clinical pharmacokinetics of lithium. *Clin Pharmacokinet.* 1977;2(2):73-92.
6. Thornhill DP, Field SP. Distribution of lithium elimination rates in a selected population of psychiatric patients. *Eur J Clin Pharmacol.* 1982;21(4):351-354.
7. Nielsen-Kudsk F, Amdisen A. Analysis of the pharmacokinetics of lithium in man. *Eur J Clin Pharmacol.* 1979;16:271-277.
8. Goodnick PJ, Meltzer HL, Fieve RR, Dunner DL. Differences in lithium kinetics between bipolar and unipolar patients. *J Clin Psychopharmacol.* 1982;2(1):48-50.
9. Mason RW, McQueen EG, Keary PJ, James NM. Pharmacokinetics of lithium: elimination half-time, renal clearance and apparent volume of distribution in schizophrenia. *Clin Pharmacokinet.* 1978;3(3):241-246.
10. Vertrees JE, Ereshefsky L. Lithium. In: Schumacher GE, ed. *Therapeutic Drug Monitoring*. Stamford, CT: Appleton & Lange; 1995:493-526.
11. Hardy BG, Shulman KI, Mackenzie SE, Kutcher SP, Silverberg JD. Pharmacokinetics of lithium in the elderly. *J Clin Psychopharmacol.* 1987;7(3):153-158.
12. Chapron DJ, Cameron IR, White LB, Merrall P. Observations on lithium disposition in the elderly. *J Am Geriatr Soc.* 1982;30(10):651-655.
13. Caldwell HC, Westlake WJ, Schriver RC, Bumbier EE. Steady-state lithium blood level fluctuations in man following administration of a lithium carbonate conventional and controlled-release dosage form. *J Clin Pharmacol.* 1981;21(2):106-109.
14. Meinhold JM, Spunt AL, Trirath C. Bioavailability of lithium carbonate: in vivo comparison of two products. *J Clin Pharmacol.* 1979;19(11-12):701-703.
15. Williams PJ, Browne JL, Patel RA. Bayesian forecasting of serum lithium concentrations. Comparison with traditional methods. *Clin Pharmacokinet.* 1989;17(1):45-52.

16. Vitiello B, Behar D, Malone R, Delaney MA, Ryan PJ, Simpson GM. Pharmacokinetics of lithium carbonate in children. *J Clin Psychopharmacol.* 1988;8(5):355-359.

17. Lauritsen BJ, Mellerup ET, Plenge P, Rasmussen S, Vestergaard P, Schou M. Serum lithium concentrations around the clock with different treatment regimens and the diurnal variation of the renal lithium clearance. *Acta Psychiatr Scand.* 1981;64(4):314-319.

18. Schou M. Lithium treatment during pregnancy, delivery, and lactation: an update. *J Clin Psychiatry.* 1990;51(10):410-413.

19. Pringuey D, Yzombard G, Charbit JJ, et al. Lithium kinetics during hemodialysis in a patient with lithium poisoning. *Am J Psychiatry.* 1981;138(2):249-251.

20. Zetin M, Plon L, Vaziri N, Cramer M, Greco D. Lithium carbonate dose and serum level relationships in chronic hemodialysis patients. *Am J Psychiatry.* 1981;138(10):1387-1388.

21. Golper TA, Marx MA. Drug dosing adjustments during continuous renal replacement therapies. *Kidney Int Suppl.* May 1998;66: 165S –168S.

22. Golper TA. Update on drug sieving coefficients and dosing adjustments during continuous renal replacement therapies. *Contrib Nephrol.* 2001;(132):349-353.

23. Hansten PD, Horn JR. *Drug Interactions Analysis and Management.* St. Louis, MO: Wolters Kluwer; 2014.

24. Bennett WM, Aronoff GR, Morrison G, et al. Drug prescribing in renal failure: dosing guidelines for adults. *Am J Kidney Dis.* 1983;3(3):155-193.

25. Swan SK, Bennett WM. Drug dosing guidelines in patients with renal failure. *West J Med.* 1992;156(6):633-638.

26. Bennett WM, Muther RS, Parker RA, et al. Drug therapy in renal failure: dosing guidelines for adults. Part II: sedatives, hypnotics, and tranquilizers; cardiovascular, antihypertensive, and diuretic agents; miscellaneous agents. *Ann Intern Med.* 1980;93(2):286-325.

27. Bennett WM, Muther RS, Parker RA, et al. Drug therapy in renal failure: dosing guidelines for adults. Part I: Antimicrobial agents, analgesics. *Ann Intern Med.* 1980;93(1):62-89.

28. Tschudy MM, Arcara KM. *The Harriet Lane Handbook: A Manual for Pediatric House Officers.* 19th ed. Philadelphia, PA: Mosby; 2012.

29. Zetin M, Garber D, Cramer M. A simple mathematical model for predicting lithium dose requirement. *J Clin Psychiatry.* 1983; 44(4):144-145.

30. Zetin M, Garber D, De Antonio M, et al. Prediction of lithium dose: a mathematical alternative to the test-dose method. *J Clin Psychiatry.* 1986;47(4):175-178.

31. Cooper TB, Bergner PE, Simpson GM. The 24-hour serum lithium level as a prognosticator of dosage requirements. *Am J Psychiatry.* 1973;130(5):601-603.

32. Cooper TB, Simpson GM. The 24-hour lithium level as a prognosticator of dosage requirements: a 2-year follow-up study. *Am J Psychiatry.* 1976;133(4):440-443.

33. Perry PJ, Prince RA, Alexander B, Dunner FJ. Prediction of lithium maintenance doses using a single point prediction protocol. *J Clin Psychopharmacol.* 1983;3(1):13-17.

34. Perry PJ, Alexander B, Prince RA, Dunner FJ. The utility of a single-point dosing protocol for predicting steady-state lithium levels. *Br J Psychiatry.* 1986;148:401-405.

35. Perry PJ, Alexander B, Dunner FJ, Schoenwald RD, Pfohl B, Miller D. Pharmacokinetic protocol for predicting serum lithium levels. *J Clin Psychopharmacol.* 1982;2(2):114-118.

36. Ritschel WA, Banarer M. Lithium dosage regimen design by the repeated one-point method. *Arzneimittelforschung.* 1982;32(2): 98-102.

37. Marr MA, Djuric PE, Ritschel WA, Garver DL. Prediction of lithium carbonate dosage in psychiatric inpatients using the repeated one-point method. *Clin Pharm.* 1983;2(3):243-248.

38. Wandell M, Mungall D. Computer assisted drug interpretation and drug regimen optimization. *Amer Assoc Clin Chem.* 1984;6:1-11.

22 Theophylline

INTRODUCTION

Theophylline is a methylxanthine compound that is used for the treatment of asthma, chronic obstructive pulmonary disease (COPD; chronic bronchitis and emphysema), and premature apnea. The bronchodilatory effects of theophylline are useful primarily for patients with asthma because bronchospasm is a key component of that disease state.[1] The use of theophylline in patients with chronic obstructive pulmonary disease is more controversial because these diseases have different pathophysiologic profiles, although some patients do exhibit a mixed disease profile with a limited reversible airway component. Even COPD patients without significant bronchospasm demonstrate clinical improvement when taking theophylline.[2-4] Theophylline is also a central nervous system stimulant which explains its usefulness in the treatment of premature apnea.

In the chronic management of asthma or chronic obstructive pulmonary disease patients, theophylline is now considered to be adjunctive therapy.[5-8] Asthma is now recognized as an inflammatory disease, and inhaled corticosteroids are considered the mainstay of therapy.[5,7] Inhaled selective β_2-agonists are used as bronchodilators in asthmatic patients. Other drugs that are useful in patients with asthma are cromolyn, nedocromil, oral corticosteroids, inhaled anticholinergics, leukotriene modifiers, and omalizumab.[5,7] Inhaled bronchodilators are the preferred treatment for COPD patients with selective β_2-agonists or anticholinergics considered first-line agents.[6,8] Theophylline is considered for use in asthmatic patients and chronic obstructive pulmonary disease patients after their respective therapies have commensed.[5-8] Theophylline is also useful in these patients when they are unable or unwilling to use multiple metered dose inhaler (MDI) devices or if an intravenous drug is needed. For the treatment of premature apnea, most clinicians prefer to use caffeine, a related methylxanthine agent, instead of theophylline because of smoother apnea control and reduced adverse effects.

The bronchodilatory response via smooth muscle relaxation in the lung to theophylline is postulated to occur due to several mechanisms.[9] Of these, the two predominate mechanisms of action are inhibition of cyclic nucleotide phosphodiesterases which increases intracellular cyclic AMP and cyclic GMP, and antagonism of adenosine receptors. In addition to bronchodilation, theophylline increases diaphragmatic contractility, increases mucociliary clearance, and exerts some anti-inflammatory effects. Theophylline is a general central nervous system stimulant and specifically stimulates the medullary respiratory center. These are the reasons why it is a useful agent in the treatment of premature apnea.

THERAPEUTIC AND TOXIC CONCENTRATIONS

The general accepted therapeutic ranges for theophylline are 10-20 µg/mL for the treatment of asthma or chronic obstructive pulmonary disease, or 6-13 µg/mL for the treatment of premature apnea. Clinical guidelines suggest that for initial treatment of pulmonary disease, clinical response to theophylline concentrations between 5 and 15 µg/mL should be assessed before higher concentrations are used.[7,8] Many patients requiring chronic theophylline therapy will derive sufficient bronchodilatory response with a low likelihood of adverse effects at concentrations of 8-12 μg/mL. However, theophylline therapy must be individualized for each patient in order to achieve optimal responses and minimal side effects.

In the upper end of the therapeutic range (>15 μg/mL) some patients will experience minor caffeine-like side effects due to theophylline treatment.[1] These adverse effects include nausea, vomiting, dyspepsia, insomnia, nervousness, and headache. Theophylline concentrations exceeding 20-30 μg/mL can cause various tachyarrhythmias including sinus tachycardia. At theophylline concentrations above 40 μg/mL, serious life-threatening adverse effects including ventricular arrhythmias (premature ventricular contractions, ventricular tachycardia, or fibrillation) or seizures can occur. Theophylline-induced seizures are an ominous sign as they respond poorly to antiepileptic therapy and can result in postseizure neurologic sequelae or death. Unfortunately, minor side effects do not always occur before severe, life-threatening adverse effects are manifested. Also, seizures due to theophylline therapy have been reported to occur in patients at theophylline concentrations as low as 25 μg/mL. Because of these reasons, serum concentration monitoring is mandatory for patients receiving theophylline. Clinicians should understand that all patients with "toxic" theophylline serum concentrations in the listed ranges will not exhibit signs or symptoms of theophylline toxicity. Rather, theophylline concentrations in the ranges given increase the likelihood that an adverse effect will occur.

CLINICAL MONITORING PARAMETERS

Measurement of pulmonary function tests are an important component of assessing response to bronchodilator therapy in patients with asthma or chronic obstructive pulmonary disease.[5,9] Forced expiratory volume over 1 second (FEV_1) should be measured on a regular basis for asthmatic patients, and peak-flow meter monitoring can be routinely performed by these individuals at home. Successful bronchodilator therapy will increase both of these values. In addition to the use of FEV_1 to monitor bronchodilator drug effect, other spirometric tests useful for patients with chronic obstructive pulmonary disease include vital capacity (VC), total lung capacity (TLC), forced vital capacity (FVC), and forced expiratory flow over the middle 50% of the expiratory curve ($FEF_{25\%-75\%}$ or $FEF_{50\%}$). Patients should also be monitored for clinical signs and symptoms of their disease states including frequency and severity of following events: dyspnea, coughing, wheezing, impairment of normal activity. During acute exacerbations or in severe cases of either pulmonary disease state, arterial blood gases may be determined and used as a monitoring parameter. When theophylline is used to treat premature infants with apnea, the frequency of apneic events are monitored as a measure of therapeutic effect.

Theophylline serum concentration monitoring is mandatory in patients receiving the drug. If a patient is experiencing clinical signs or symptoms that could be due to a theophylline adverse effect, a theophylline serum concentration should be obtained at that time to rule out drug-induced toxicity. For dose adjustment purposes, theophylline serum concentrations should be measured at steady-state after the patient has received a consistent dosage regimen for 3-5 drug half-lives. Theophylline half-life varies from 3-5 hours in children and tobacco-smoking individuals to 50 hours or more in patients with severe heart or liver failure. If the theophylline is given as a continuous intravenous infusion, it can take a considerable amount of time for some patients to achieve effective concentrations so an intravenous loading dose is commonly administered to patients (Figure 22-1). The ideal situation is to administer an intravenous loading dose that will achieve the desired concentration immediately, then start an intravenous continuous infusion that will maintain that concentration (see Figure 22-1). In order to derive this perfect situation, the theophylline volume of distribution (V in L) would have to be known to compute the loading dose (LD in mg): LD = Css • V, where Css is the desired theophylline concentration in mg/L. However, this pharmacokinetic parameter is rarely, if ever, known for a patient, so a loading dose based on a population average volume of distribution is used to calculate the amount of theophylline needed. Since the patient's own, unique volume of distribution will most

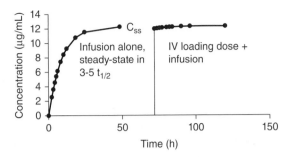

FIGURE 22-1   When intravenous theophylline or aminophylline is administered to a patient as a continuous infusion, it will take 3-5 half-lives for serum theophylline concentrations to reach steady-state levels. Because of this, maximal drug response will take time to achieve. To hasten onset of drug action, loading doses are given to attain effective theophylline concentrations immediately.

likely be greater (resulting in too low of a loading dose) or less (resulting in too large of a loading dose) than the population average volume of distribution used to compute the loading dose, the desired steady-state theophylline concentration will not be achieved. Because of this, it will still take 3-5 half-lives for the patient to reach steady-state conditions while receiving a constant intravenous infusion rate (Figure 22-2). Thus, theophylline intravenous loading doses do not usually achieve steady-state serum concentrations immediately, but, hopefully, they do result in therapeutic concentrations and response sooner than simply starting an intravenous infusion alone. If oral theophylline-containing products are used to treat a patient, steady-state predose, or "trough," concentrations should be used to monitor therapy after the patient has received a stable dosage regimen for 3-5 half-lives.

After an efficacious theophylline dosage regimen has been established for a patient, theophylline serum concentrations remain fairly stable in patients receiving long-term therapy. In these cases, theophylline dosage requirements and steady-state serum concentrations should be reassessed on a yearly basis. In patients with congestive heart failure or liver cirrhosis, theophylline dosage requirements can vary greatly according to the

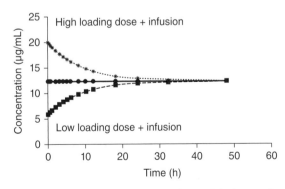

FIGURE 22-2   If the patient's own, unique theophylline volume of distribution (V) is known, the exact loading dose (LD) of intravenous theophylline or aminophylline to immediately achieve steady-state theophylline concentrations (Css) can be calculated (LD = Css • V). However, the volume of distribution for the patient is rarely known when loading doses need to be administered, and, for practical purposes, an average population volume of distribution for theophylline is used to estimate the parameter for the patient (V = 0.5 L/kg, use ideal body weight if >30% overweight). Because of this, the computed loading dose will almost always be too large or too small to reach the desired steady-state theophylline concentration, and it will still take 3-5 half-lives to attain steady-state conditions.

status of the patient. For example, if a patient with compensated heart failure is receiving a stable dose of theophylline, but experiences an exacerbation of their heart disease, it is very likely that they will need to have their theophylline dosage requirements reassessed to avoid theophylline toxicity. Also, acute viral diseases, especially in children, have been associated with theophylline adverse effects in patients previously stabilized on effective, nontoxic theophylline dosage regimens.[10,11] Methods to adjust theophylline doses using serum concentrations are discussed later in this chapter.

BASIC CLINICAL PHARMACOKINETIC PARAMETERS

Theophylline is primarily eliminated by hepatic metabolism (>90%). Hepatic metabolism is mainly via the CYP1A2 enzyme system with a smaller amount metabolized by CYP3A and CYP2E1. About 10% of a theophylline dose is recovered in the urine as unchanged drug.[12,13] Strictly speaking, theophylline follows nonlinear pharmacokinetics.[14-16] However, for the purposes of clinical drug dosing in patients, linear pharmacokinetic concepts and equations can be effectively used to compute doses and estimate serum concentrations. Occasionally, theophylline serum concentrations increase in a patient more than expected after a dosage increase for an unidentifiable reason, and nonlinear pharmacokinetics may explain the observation.[14-16]

Three different forms of theophylline are available. Aminophylline is the ethylenediamine salt of theophylline, and anhydrous aminophylline contains about 85% theophylline while aminophylline dihydrate contains about 80% theophylline. Oxtriphylline is the choline salt of theophylline and contains about 65% theophylline. Theophylline and aminophylline are available for intravenous injection and oral use. Oxtriphylline is available only for oral use. The oral bioavailability of all three theophylline-based drugs is very good and generally equals 100%. However, some older sustained-release oral dosage forms have been reported to exhibit incomplete bioavailability and loss of slow release characteristics under certain circumstances due to their tablet or capsule design. Theophylline plasma protein binding is only 40%.[17,18]

The recommended dose of theophylline or one of its salt forms is based on the concurrent disease states and conditions present in the patient that can influence theophylline pharmacokinetics. Theophylline pharmacokinetic parameters used to compute doses are given in the following section for specific patient profiles.

EFFECTS OF DISEASE STATES AND CONDITIONS ON THEOPHYLLINE PHARMACOKINETICS AND DOSING

Normal adults without the disease states and conditions given later in this section with normal liver function have an average theophylline half-life of 8 hours (range: 6-12 hours) and volume of distribution of 0.5 L/kg (range: 0.4-0.6 L/kg; Table 22-1).[19-21] Most disease states and conditions that change theophylline pharmacokinetics and dosage requirements alter clearance, but volume of distribution remains stable at ~0.5 L/kg in these situations. Tobacco and marijuana smoke causes induction of hepatic CYP1A2 which accelerates the clearance of theophylline.[19-24] In patients who smoke these substances, the average theophylline half-life is 5 hours. When patients stop smoking these compounds, theophylline clearance slowly approaches its baseline level for the patient over a 6- to 12-month period if the patient does not encounter "second-hand" smoke produced by other users.[25] If the patient inhales a sufficient amount of second-hand smoke, theophylline clearance for the exsmoker may remain in the fully induced state or at some intermediate induced state.[26]

Patients with liver cirrhosis or acute hepatitis have reduced theophylline clearance which results in a prolonged average theophylline half-life of 24 hours.[20,27-29] However, the effect that liver disease has on theophylline pharmacokinetics is highly variable and difficult to accurately predict. It is possible for a patient with liver disease to have relatively normal or grossly abnormal theophylline clearance and half-life.

TABLE 22-1   **Disease States and Conditions That Alter Theophylline Pharmacokinetics**

Disease State/Condition	Half-Life	Volume of Distribution	Comment
Adult, normal liver function	8 h (range: 6-12 h)	0.5 L/kg (range: 0.4-0.6 L/kg)	
Adult, tobacco or marijuana smoker	5 h	0.5 L/kg	Tobacco and marijuana smoke induces CYP1A2 enzyme system and accelerates theophylline clearance.
Adult, hepatic disease (liver cirrhosis or acute hepatitis)	24 h	0.5 L/kg	Theophylline is metabolized >90% by hepatic microsomal enzymes (primary: CYP1A2; secondary: CYP3A, CYP2E1), so loss of functional liver tissue decreases theophylline clearance. Pharmacokinetic parameters highly variable in liver disease patients.
Adult, mild heart failure (NYHA CHF classes I or II)	12 h	0.5 L/kg	Decreased liver blood flow secondary to reduced cardiac output due to heart failure reduces theophylline clearance.
Adult, moderate-severe heart failure (NYHA CHF classes III or IV) or cor pulmonale	24 h	0.5 L/kg	Moderate-severe heart failure reduces cardiac output even more than mild heart failure, resulting in large and variable reductions in theophylline clearance. Cardiac status must be monitored closely in heart failure patients receiving theophylline since theophylline clearance changes with acute changes in cardiac output.
Adult, obese (>30% over ideal body weight (IBW)	According to other disease states/ conditions that affect theophylline pharmacokinetics	0.5 L/kg IBW[a]	Theophylline doses should be based on ideal body weight for patients who weight more that 30% above their IBW.
Children, 1-9 years, normal cardiac and hepatic function	3.5 h	0.5 L/kg	Children have increased theophylline clearance. When puberty is reached, adult doses can be used taking into account disease states and conditions that alter theophylline pharmacokinetics.
Elderly, >65 years	12 h	0.5 L/kg	Elderly individuals with concurrent disease states/conditions known to alter theophylline clearance should be dosed using those specific recommendations.

[a]IBW; ideal body weight.

For example, a liver disease patient who also smokes cigarettes could have a theophylline half-life equal to 5 hours if some liver parenchyma is present and tobacco-induced enzyme induction occurred, or 50 hours if little or no liver tissue remains. An index of liver dysfunction can be gained by applying the Child-Pugh clinical classification system to the patient (Table 22-2). Child-Pugh scores are completely discussed in Chapter 3 (Drug Dosing in Special Populations: Renal and Hepatic Disease, Dialysis, Heart Failure, Obesity, and Drug Interactions), but will be briefly discussed here. The Child-Pugh score consists of five laboratory tests or clinical symptoms: serum albumin, total bilirubin, prothrombin time, ascites, and hepatic encephalopathy. Each of

TABLE 22-2   Child-Pugh Scores for Patients With Liver Disease[77]

Test/Symptom	Score 1 Point	Score 2 Points	Score 3 Points
Total bilirubin (mg/dL)	<2.0	2.0-3.0	>3.0
Serum albumin (g/dL)	>3.5	2.8-3.5	<2.8
Prothrombin time (seconds prolonged over control)	<4	4-6	>6
Ascites	Absent	Slight	Moderate
Hepatic encephalopathy	None	Moderate	Severe

Mild liver disease, 5-6 points; moderate liver disease, 7-9 points; severe liver disease: 10-15 points.

these areas is given a score of 1 (normal) to 3 (severely abnormal; see Table 22-2), and the scores for the five areas are summed. The Child-Pugh score for a patient with normal liver function is 5 while the score for a patient with grossly abnormal serum albumin, total bilirubin, and prothrombin time values in addition to severe ascites and hepatic encephalopathy is 15. A Child-Pugh score greater than 8 is grounds for a decrease in the initial daily drug dose for theophylline ($t_{1/2} = 24$ hours). As in any patient with or without liver dysfunction, initial doses are meant as starting points for dosage titration based on patient response and avoidance of adverse effects. Theophylline serum concentrations and the presence of adverse drug effects should be monitored frequently in patients with liver cirrhosis.

Heart failure causes reduced theophylline clearance because of decreased hepatic blood flow secondary to compromised cardiac output.[20,30-33] Venous stasis of blood within the liver may also contribute to the decrease in theophylline clearance found in heart failure patients. Patients with mild heart failure (New York Heart Association or NYHA Class I or II, Table 22-3) have an average theophylline half-life equal to 12 hours (range: 5-24 hours) while those with moderate to severe heart failure (NYHA Class III or IV) or cor pulmonale have an average theophylline half-life of 24 hours (5-50 hours). Obviously, the effect that heart failure has on theophylline pharmacokinetics is highly variable and difficult to accurately predict. It is possible for a patient with heart failure to have relatively normal or grossly abnormal theophylline clearance and half-life. For heart failure patients, initial doses are meant as starting points for dosage titration based on patient response and avoidance of adverse effects. Theophylline serum concentrations and the presence of adverse drug effects should be monitored frequently in patients with heart failure.

TABLE 22-3   New York Heart Association (NYHA) Functional Classification for Heart Failure[78]

NYHA Heart Failure Class	Description
I	Patients with cardiac disease but without limitations of physical activity. Ordinary physical activity does not cause undue fatigue, dyspnea, or palpitation.
II	Patients with cardiac disease that results in slight limitations of physical activity. Ordinary physical activity results in fatigue, palpitation, dyspnea, or angina.
III	Patients with cardiac disease that results in marked limitations of physical activity. Although patients are comfortable at rest, less than ordinary activity will lead to symptoms.
IV	Patients with cardiac disease that results in an inability to carry on physical activity without discomfort. Symptoms of congestive heart failure are present even at rest. With any physical activity, increased discomfort is experienced.

Obese patients (>30% above ideal body weight or IBW) should have volume of distribution estimates based on ideal body weight.[34-37] Theophylline half-life should be based on the concurrent disease states and conditions present in the patient. If weight-based dosage recommendations (mg/kg/d or mg/kg/h) are to be used, ideal body weight should be used to compute doses for obese individuals.

Patient age has an effect on theophylline clearance and half-life. Newborns have decreased theophylline clearance because hepatic drug–metabolizing enzymes are not yet fully developed at birth. Premature neonates have average theophylline half-lives equal to 30 hours 3-15 days after birth and 20 hours 25-57 days after birth.[38-40] Full-term infants have average theophylline half-lives of 25 hours 1-2 days after birth, and 11 hours 3-30 weeks after birth.[41-43] Children between the ages of 1 and 9 years have accelerated theophylline clearance rates resulting in an average half-life of 3.5 hours (range: 1.5-5 hours).[44-46] As children achieve puberty, their theophylline clearance and half-life approach the values of an adult. For elderly patients over the age of 65, some studies indicate that theophylline clearance and half-life are the same as in younger adults while other investigations have found that theophylline clearance is slower and half-life is longer (average half-life = 12 hours, range: 8-16 hours).[47-51] A confounding factor found in theophylline pharmacokinetic studies conducted in older adults is the possible accidental inclusion of subjects that have subclinical or mild cases of the disease states associated with reduced theophylline clearance (heart failure, liver disease, etc). Thus, the pharmacokinetics of theophylline in elderly individuals is somewhat controversial.

Febrile illnesses can temporarily decrease the clearance of theophylline and require an immediate dosage decrease to avoid toxicity.[10,11] The mechanism of this acute change in theophylline disposition is unclear, but probably involves decreased clearance due to the production of interleukins. Children seem to be at an especially high risk of theophylline adverse reactions since febrile illnesses are prevalent in this population and high theophylline doses (on a mg/kg/d basis) are prescribed.

Because only a small amount of theophylline is eliminated unchanged in the urine (<10% of a dose), dosage adjustments are not necessary in patients with renal impairment.[12,13] Theophylline is removed by hemodialysis, and, if possible, doses should be held until after the dialysis procedure is complete.[52-57] If a pulmonary exacerbation occurs due to decreased theophylline concentrations, individualized supplemental doses of theophylline may need to be given during or after the procedure is complete. The hemoperfusion sieving coefficient for theophylline is 0.80, which indicates significant removal by these techniques.[58,59] Theophylline is not appreciably removed by peritoneal dialysis.[55]

Hypothyroid patients have decreased basal metabolic rates, and require smaller theophylline doses until a euthyroid condition is established.[60] The breast milk to serum ratio for theophylline is 0.7.[61]

DRUG INTERACTIONS

Drug interactions with theophylline are common and occur with a variety of medications.[62] Serious inhibition drug interactions are those that decrease theophylline clearance more than 30%. Clinicians should consider an arbitrary decrease in theophylline dose of 30%-50% for patients receiving these agents until the actual degree of hepatic enzyme inhibition can be assessed using theophylline serum concentration monitoring. Patients should also be actively monitored for the signs and symptoms of theophylline toxicity. It should be emphasized that the magnitude of hepatic enzyme inhibition drug interactions is highly variable so some patients may require even larger theophylline dosage decreases while others will exhibit no drug interaction at all. Cimetidine given at higher doses (≥1000 mg/d) on a multiple daily dosage schedule decreases theophylline clearance by 30%-50%. Other cimetidine doses (≤800 mg/d) given once or twice daily decrease theophylline clearance by 20% or less.[63,64] Ciprofloxacin and enoxacin, both quinolone antibiotics, and troleandomycin, a macrolide antibiotic, also decrease theophylline clearance by 30%-50%. Estrogen and estrogen-containing oral contraceptives, propranolol, metoprolol, mexiletine, propafenone, pentoxifylline, ticlopidine, tacrine, thiabendazole, disulfiram, nefazodone, interferon, zileuton, and fluvoxamine can also decrease theophylline clearance by this extent.

Moderate-sized inhibition drug interactions are those that decrease theophylline clearance by 10%-30%. For this magnitude of drug interaction, many clinicians believe that a routine decrease in theophylline dose is unnecessary for patients with steady-state theophylline concentrations less than 15 µg/mL, but should be considered on a case-by-case basis for those with concentrations above this level. Should a decrease be warranted in a patient, theophylline doses can be cut by 20% to avoid adverse effects. Again, patients should be actively monitored for the signs and symptoms of theophylline toxicity. The calcium channel blockers, verapamil and diltiazem, have been reported to cause decreases in theophylline clearance of 15%-25%. Clarithromycin and erythromycin, both macrolide antibiotics, and norfloxacin, a quinolone antibiotic, can also decrease theophylline clearance by this magnitude. At doses of 600 mg/d or above, allopurinol has been reported to decrease theophylline clearance by 25%.

Theophylline elimination is also subject to induction of hepatic microsomal enzymes which increases theophylline clearance. Because hepatic microsomal enzyme induction is quite variable in patients, some individuals may require theophylline dosage increases while others will require no alteration in dosage requirements. Also, hepatic microsomal enzyme induction takes time to occur, and maximal effects may not be seen for 2-4 weeks of treatment with enzyme inducers. Patients treated with a drug that increases theophylline clearance need to be carefully monitored for the signs and symptoms of their respective disease state, and steady-state theophylline concentrations should be measured. Disease exacerbations may be due to decreased theophylline concentrations, and a dosage increase may be warranted in some patients. Phenytoin, carbamazepine, phenobarbital, rifampin, and moricizine all increase theophylline clearance.

INITIAL DOSAGE DETERMINATION METHODS

Several methods to initiate theophylline therapy are available. The *Pharmacokinetic Dosing method* is the most flexible of the techniques. It allows individualized target serum concentrations to be chosen for a patient, and each pharmacokinetic parameter can be customized to reflect specific disease states and conditions present in the patient. *Literature-based recommended dosing* is a very commonly used method to prescribe initial doses of theophylline. Doses are based on those that commonly produce steady-state concentrations in the lower end of the therapeutic range, although there is a wide variation in the actual concentrations for a specific patient.

Pharmacokinetic Dosing Method

The goal of initial dosing of theophylline is to compute the best dose possible for the patient given their set of disease states and conditions that influence theophylline pharmacokinetics and the pulmonary disorder being treated. In order to do this, pharmacokinetic parameters for the patient will be estimated using average parameters measured in other patients with similar disease state and condition profiles.

Half-Life and Elimination Rate Constant Estimate

Theophylline is predominately metabolized by liver. Unfortunately, there is no good way to estimate the elimination characteristics of liver-metabolized drugs using an endogenous marker of liver function in the same manner that serum creatinine and estimated creatinine clearance are used to estimate the elimination of agents that are renally eliminated. Because of this, a patient is categorized according to the disease states and conditions that are known to change theophylline half-life, and the half-life previously measured in these studies is used as an estimate of the current patient's half-life. For example, for a patient with COPD who currently smokes tobacco-containing cigarettes, theophylline half-life would be assumed to equal 5 hours. Alternatively, for a patient with moderate heart failure (NYHA CHF class III), theophylline half-life would be assumed to equal 24 hours, while a patient with severe liver disease (Child-Pugh score = 12) would be assigned an estimated half-life of 24 hours. To produce the most conservative theophylline doses in patients with multiple concurrent disease states or conditions that affect theophylline pharmacokinetics, the disease state or condition with the longest half-life should be used to compute doses. This approach will avoid accidental overdosage as much as currently possible. For instance, for a patient with asthma who currently smokes tobacco-containing cigarettes and has severe liver disease, an estimated theophylline half-life of 24 hours would be used to compute initial dosage requirements. Once the correct half-life is identified for the patient, it can be converted into the theophylline elimination rate constant (k) using the following equation: $k = 0.693/t_{1/2}$.

Volume of Distribution Estimate

Theophylline volume of distribution is relatively stable in patients regardless of the disease states and conditions that are present. Volume of distribution is assumed to equal 0.5 L/kg for nonobese patients. For obese patients (>30% above ideal body weight), ideal body weight is used to compute theophylline volume of distribution. Thus, for an 80-kg patient, the estimated theophylline volume of distribution would be 40 L: $V = 0.5$ L/kg • 80 kg = 40 L. For a 150-kg obese patient with an ideal body weight of 60 kg, the estimated theophylline volume of distribution is 30 L: $V = 0.5$ L/kg • 60 kg = 30 L.

Selection of Appropriate Pharmacokinetic Model and Equations

When given by continuous intravenous infusion or orally, theophylline follows a one-compartment pharmacokinetic model (Figures 22-1, 22-3, 22-4). When oral therapy is required, most clinicians utilize a sustained-release dosage form that has good bioavailability (F = 1), supplies a continuous release of theophylline into the gastrointestinal tract, and provides a smooth theophylline serum concentration-time curve that emulates an intravenous infusion after once or twice daily dosing. Because of this, a very simple pharmacokinetic equation that computes the average theophylline steady-state serum concentration (Css in µg/mL = mg/L) is widely used and allows maintenance dosage calculation: Css = [F • S (D/τ)]/Cl or D = (Css • Cl • τ)/(F • S), where F is the bioavailability fraction for the oral dosage form (F = 1 for most oral theophylline sustained-release products); S is the fraction of the theophylline salt form that is active theophylline (S = 1 for theophylline, S = 0.85 for anhydrous aminophylline, S = 0.80 for aminophylline dihydrate, S = 0.65 for oxtriphylline); D is the dose of theophylline salt in mg; and τ is the dosage interval in hours. Cl is theophylline clearance in L/h and is computed using estimates of theophylline elimination rate constant (k) and volume of distribution: Cl = kV. For example, for a patient with an estimated elimination rate constant equal to 0.139 h⁻¹ and an estimated volume of distribution equal to 35 L, the estimated clearance would equal 4.87 L/h: Cl = 0.139h⁻¹ • 35 L = 4.87 L/h.

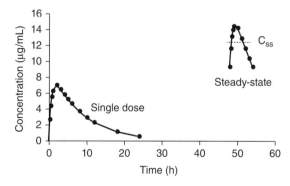

FIGURE 22-3   Serum concentration-time profile for rapid-release theophylline or aminophylline oral dosage forms after a single dose and at steady-state (given every 6 hours). The curves shown would be typical for an adult cigarette smoker receiving theophylline 300 mg. The steady-state serum concentration (Css) expected from an equivalent theophylline or aminophylline continuous infusion is shown by the dotted line in the steady-state concentrations.

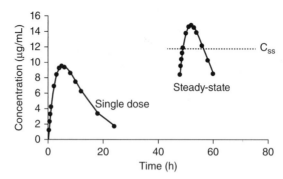

FIGURE 22-4   Serum concentration-time profile for sustained-release theophylline or aminophylline oral dosage forms after a single dose and at steady-state (given every 12 hours). The curves shown would be typical for an adult cigarette smoker receiving theophylline 600 mg. The steady-state serum concentration (Css) expected from an equivalent theophylline or aminophylline continuous infusion is shown by the dotted line in the steady-state concentrations.

When intravenous therapy is required, a similar pharmacokinetic equation that computes the theophylline steady-state serum concentration (Css in μg/mL = mg/L) is widely used and allows dosage calculation for a continuous infusion: Css = [S • k_0]/Cl or k_0 = (Css • Cl)/S, where S is the fraction of the theophylline salt form that is active theophylline (S = 1 for theophylline, S = 0.85 for anhydrous aminophylline, S = 0.80 for aminophylline dihydrate) and k_0 is the dose of theophylline salt in mg. Cl is theophylline clearance in L/h and is computed using estimates of theophylline elimination rate constant (k) and volume of distribution: Cl = kV.

The equation used to calculate an intravenous loading dose (LD in mg) is based on a simple, one-compartment model: LD = (Css • V)/S, where Css is the desired theophylline steady-state concentration in μg/mL which is equivalent to mg/L, V is the theophylline volume of distribution, and S is the fraction of the theophylline salt form that is active theophylline (S = 1 for theophylline, S = 0.85 for anhydrous aminophylline, S = 0.80 for aminophylline dihydrate). Intravenous theophylline loading doses should be infusions over at least 20-30 minutes.

Steady-State Concentration Selection

The generally accepted therapeutic ranges for theophylline are 10-20 μg/mL for the treatment of asthma or chronic obstructive pulmonary disease, or 6-13 μg/mL for the treatment of premature apnea. Recent guidelines suggest that for initial treatment of pulmonary disease, clinical response to theophylline concentrations between 5 and 15 μg/mL should be assessed before higher concentrations are used.[65] Many patients requiring chronic theophylline therapy will derive sufficient bronchodilatory response with a low likelihood of adverse effects at concentrations of 8-12 μg/mL. However, theophylline therapy much be individualized for each patient in order to achieve optimal responses and minimal side effects.

EXAMPLE 1 ▶▶▶

LK is a 50-year-old, 75-kg (height = 5 ft 10 in) male with chronic bronchitis who requires therapy with oral theophylline. He currently smokes two packs of cigarettes daily, and has normal liver and cardiac function. Suggest an initial theophylline dosage regimen designed to achieve a steady-state theophylline concentration equal to 8 μg/mL. (Note: μg/mL = mg/L and this concentration unit was substituted for Css in the calculations so that unnecessary unit conversion was not required.)

1. *Estimate half-life and elimination rate constant according to disease states and conditions present in the patient.*
    Cigarette smoke induces the enzyme systems responsible for theophylline metabolism, and the expected theophylline half-life ($t_{1/2}$) is 5 hours. The elimination rate constant is computed using the following formula: $k = 0.693/t_{1/2} = 0.693/5\ h = 0.139\ h^{-1}$.

2. *Estimate volume of distribution and clearance.*
    The patient is not obese, so the estimated theophylline volume of distribution will be based on actual body weight: $V = 0.5\ L/kg \bullet 75\ kg = 38\ L$. Estimated theophylline clearance is computed by taking the product of the volume of distribution and the elimination rate constant: $Cl = kV = 0.139\ h^{-1} \bullet 38\ L = 5.28\ L/h$.

3. *Compute dosage regimen.*
    Oral sustained-release theophylline tablets will be prescribed to this patient ($F = 1$, $S = 1$). Because the patient has a rapid theophylline clearance and short half-life, the initial dosage interval (τ) will be set to 8 hours. (Note: $\mu g/mL = mg/L$ and this concentration unit was substituted for Css in the calculations so that unnecessary unit conversion was not required.) The dosage equation for oral theophylline is: $D = (Css \bullet Cl \bullet \tau)/(F \bullet S) = (8\ mg/L \bullet 5.28\ L/h \bullet 8h)/(1 \bullet 1) = 338\ mg$, rounded to 300 mg every 8 hours.

    A steady-state trough theophylline serum concentration should be measured after steady-state is attained in 3-5 half-lives. Since the patient is expected to have a half-life equal to 5 hours, the theophylline steady-state concentration could be obtained any time after the first day of dosing (5 half-lives = $5 \bullet 5\ h = 25\ h$). Theophylline serum concentrations should also be measured if the patient experiences an exacerbation of their lung disease, or if the patient develops potential signs or symptoms of theophylline toxicity.

EXAMPLE 2 ▶▶▶

OI is a 60-year-old, 85-kg (height = 6 ft 1 in) male with emphysema who requires therapy with oral theophylline. He has liver cirrhosis (Child-Pugh score = 11) and normal cardiac function. Suggest an initial theophylline dosage regimen designed to achieve a steady-state theophylline concentration equal to 10 $\mu g/mL$.

1. *Estimate half-life and elimination rate constant according to disease states and conditions present in the patient.*
    Patients with severe liver disease have highly variable theophylline pharmacokinetics and dosage requirements. Hepatic disease destroys liver parenchyma where hepatic drug–metabolizing enzymes are contained, and the expected theophylline half-life ($t_{1/2}$) is 24 hours. The elimination rate constant is computed using the following formula: $k = 0.693/t_{1/2} = 0.693/24\ h = 0.029\ h^{-1}$.

2. *Estimate volume of distribution and clearance.*
    The patient is not obese, so the estimated theophylline volume of distribution will be based on actual body weight: $V = 0.5\ L/kg \bullet 85\ kg = 43\ L$. Estimated theophylline clearance is computed by taking the product of the volume of distribution and the elimination rate constant: $Cl = kV = 0.029\ h^{-1} \bullet 43\ L = 1.25\ L/h$.

3. *Compute dosage regimen.*
    Oral sustained-release theophylline tablets will be prescribed to this patient ($F = 1$, $S = 1$). The initial dosage interval (τ) will be set to 12 hours. (Note: $\mu g/mL = mg/L$ and this concentration unit was substituted for Css in the calculations so that unnecessary unit conversion was not required.) The dosage equation for oral theophylline is: $D = (Css \bullet Cl \bullet \tau)/(F \bullet S) = (10\ mg/L \bullet 1.25\ L/h \bullet 12\ h)/(1 \bullet 1) = 150\ mg$ every 12 hours.

    A steady-state trough theophylline serum concentration should be measured after steady-state is attained in 3-5 half-lives. Since the patient is expected to have a half-life equal to 24 hours, the theophylline steady-state concentration could be obtained any time after the fifth day of dosing (5 half-lives = $5 \bullet 24\ h = 120\ h$ or 5 days).

Theophylline serum concentrations should also be measured if the patient experiences an exacerbation of their lung disease, or if the patient develops potential signs or symptoms of theophylline toxicity.

To illustrate the differences and similarities between oral and intravenous theophylline dosage regimen design, the same cases will be used to compute intravenous theophylline loading doses and continuous infusions.

EXAMPLE 3 ▶▶▶

LK is a 50-year-old, 75-kg (height = 5 ft 10 in) male with chronic bronchitis who requires therapy with intravenous theophylline. He currently smokes two packs of cigarettes daily, and has normal liver and cardiac function. Suggest an initial intravenous aminophylline dosage regimen designed to achieve a steady-state theophylline concentration equal to 8 μg/mL.

1. *Estimate half-life and elimination rate constant according to disease states and conditions present in the patient.*
   Cigarette smoke induces the enzyme systems responsible for theophylline metabolism, and the expected theophylline half-life ($t_{1/2}$) is 5 hours. The elimination rate constant is computed using the following formula: $k = 0.693/t_{1/2} = 0.693/5\,h = 0.139\,h^{-1}$.

2. *Estimate volume of distribution and clearance.*
   The patient is not obese, so the estimated theophylline volume of distribution will be based on actual body weight: $V = 0.5\,L/kg \bullet 75\,kg = 38\,L$. Estimated theophylline clearance is computed by taking the product of the volume of distribution and the elimination rate constant: $Cl = kV = 0.139\,h^{-1} \bullet 38\,L = 5.28\,L/h$.

3. *Compute dosage regimen.*
   Theophylline will be administered as the aminophylline dihydrate salt form (S = 0.8). (Note: μg/mL = mg/L and this concentration unit was substituted for Css in the calculations so that unnecessary unit conversion was not required.) Therapy will be started by administering an intravenous loading dose of aminophylline to the patient: $LD = (Css \bullet V)/S = (10\,mg/L \bullet 38\,L)/0.8 = 475\,mg$, rounded to 500 mg intravenously over 20-30 minutes.

   An aminophylline continuous intravenous infusion will be started immediately after the loading dose has been administered. (Note: μg/mL = mg/L and this concentration unit was substituted for Css in the calculations so that unnecessary unit conversion was not required.) The dosage equation for intravenous aminophylline is: $k_0 = (Css \bullet Cl)/S = (10\,mg/L \bullet 5.28\,L/h)/0.8 = 66\,mg/h$, rounded to 65 mg/h.

   A steady-state theophylline serum concentration should be measured after steady-state is attained in 3-5 half-lives. Since the patient is expected to have a half-life equal to 5 hours, the theophylline steady-state concentration could be obtained any time after the first day of dosing (5 half-lives = $5 \bullet 5\,h = 25\,h$). Theophylline serum concentrations should also be measured if the patient experiences an exacerbation of their lung disease, or if the patient develops potential signs or symptoms of theophylline toxicity.

EXAMPLE 4 ▶▶▶

OI is a 60-year-old, 85-kg (height = 6 ft 1 in) male with emphysema who requires therapy with intravenous aminophylline. He has liver cirrhosis (Child-Pugh score = 11) and normal cardiac function. Suggest an initial intravenous aminophylline dosage regimen designed to achieve a steady-state theophylline concentration equal to 10 μg/mL.

1. *Estimate half-life and elimination rate constant according to disease states and conditions present in the patient.* Patients with severe liver disease have highly variable theophylline pharmacokinetics and dosage requirements. Hepatic disease destroys liver parenchyma where hepatic drug–metabolizing enzymes are contained, and the expected theophylline half-life ($t_{1/2}$) is 24 hours. The elimination rate constant is computed using the following formula: $k = 0.693/t_{1/2} = 0.693/24\ h = 0.029\ h^{-1}$.

2. *Estimate volume of distribution and clearance.* The patient is not obese, so the estimated theophylline volume of distribution will be based on actual body weight: $V = 0.5\ L/kg \bullet 85\ kg = 43\ L$. Estimated theophylline clearance is computed by taking the product of the volume of distribution and the elimination rate constant: $Cl = kV = 0.029\ h^{-1} \bullet 43\ L = 1.25\ L/h$.

3. *Compute dosage regimen.* Theophylline will be administered as the aminophylline dihydrate salt form (S = 0.8). (Note: µg/mL = mg/L and this concentration unit was substituted for Css in the calculations so that unnecessary unit conversion was not required.) Therapy will be started by administering an intravenous loading dose of aminophylline to the patient: $LD = (Css \bullet V)/S = (10\ mg/L \bullet 43\ L)/0.8 = 538\ mg$, rounded to 500 mg intravenously over 20-30 minutes.

   An aminophylline continuous intravenous infusion will be started immediately after the loading dose has been administered. (Note: µg/mL = mg/L and this concentration unit was substituted for Css in the calculations so that unnecessary unit conversion was not required.) The dosage equation for oral theophylline is: $k_0 = (Css \bullet Cl)/S = (10\ mg/L \bullet 1.25\ L/h)/0.8 = 16\ mg/h$, rounded to 15 mg/h.

   A steady-state theophylline serum concentration should be measured after steady-state is attained in 3-5 half-lives. Since the patient is expected to have a half-life equal to 24 hours, the theophylline steady-state concentration could be obtained any time after the fifth day of dosing (5 half-lives = 5 • 24 h = 120 h or 5 days). Theophylline serum concentrations should also be measured if the patient experiences an exacerbation of their lung disease, or if the patient develops potential signs or symptoms of theophylline toxicity.

Literature-Based Recommended Dosing

Because of the large amount of variability in theophylline pharmacokinetics, even when concurrent disease states and conditions are identified, many clinicians believe that the use of standard theophylline doses for various situations is warrented.[20,66,67] The original computation of these doses was based on the pharmacokinetic dosing method described in the previous section, and subsequently modified based on clinical experience. In general, the expected theophylline steady-state serum concentration used to compute these doses was 10 µg/mL. Suggested theophylline maintenance doses stratified by disease states and conditions known to alter theophylline pharmacokinetics are given in Table 22-4.[67] For obese individuals (>30% over

TABLE 22-4   Theophylline Dosage Rates for Patients With Various Disease States and Conditions[67]

Disease State/Condition	Mean Dose (mg/kg/h)
Children 1-9 y	0.8
Children 9-12 y or adult smokers	0.7
Adolescents 12-16 y	0.5
Adult nonsmokers	0.4
Elderly nonsmokers (>65 years)	0.3
Decompensated CHF, cor pulmonale, cirrhosis	0.2

ideal body weight), ideal body weight should be used to compute doses.[34-37] Because the doses are given in terms of theophylline, doses for other theophylline salt forms need to be adjusted accordingly (S = 1 for theophylline, S = 0.85 for anhydrous aminophylline, S = 0.8 for aminophylline dihydrate, S = 0.65 for oxtriphylline). If theophylline is to be given orally, the dose given in Table 22-4 (in mg/kg/h) must be multiplied by the appropriate dosage interval for the dosage form being used: D = (theophylline dose • Wt • τ)/S, where Wt is patient weight, τ is the dosage interval, and S is the appropriate salt form correction factor for aminophylline or oxtriphylline. If theophylline is to be given as a continuous intravenous infusion the following equation is used to compute the infusion rate: k_0 = (theophylline dose • Wt)/S, where Wt is patient weight and S is the appropriate salt form correction factor for aminophylline. When more than one disease state or condition is present in a patient, choosing the lowest dose suggested by Table 22-4 will result in the safest, most conservative dosage recommendation. If an intravenous loading dose is necessary, theophylline 5 mg/kg or aminophylline 6 mg/kg is used; ideal body weight is used to compute loading doses for obese patients (>30% over ideal body weight).

To illustrate the similarities and differences between this method of dosage calculation and the pharmacokinetic dosing method, the same examples used in the previous section will be used.

EXAMPLE 1 ▶▶▶

LK is a 50-year-old, 75-kg (height = 5 ft 10 in) male with chronic bronchitis who requires therapy with oral theophylline. He currently smokes two packs of cigarettes daily, and has normal liver and cardiac function. Suggest an initial theophylline dosage regimen for this patient.

1. *Choose theophylline dose based on disease states and conditions present in the patient.*
   A theophylline dose of 0.7 mg/kg/h is suggested by the table for an adult cigarette smoker.

2. *Compute dosage regimen.*
   Oral sustained-release theophylline tablets will be prescribed to this patient (F = 1, S = 1). Because the patient has a rapid theophylline clearance and half-life, the initial dosage interval (τ) will be set to 8 hours: D = (theophylline dose • Wt • τ)/S = (0.7 mg/kg/h • 75 kg • 8 h)/1 = 420 mg, rounded to 400 mg every 8 hours. This dose is similar to that suggested by the Pharmacokinetic Dosing method of 300 mg every 8 hours.

   A steady-state trough theophylline serum concentration should be measured after steady-state is attained in 3-5 half-lives. Since the patient is expected to have a half-life equal to 5 hours, the theophylline steady-state concentration could be obtained any time after the first day of dosing (5 half-lives = 5 • 5 h = 25 h). Theophylline serum concentrations should also be measured if the patient experiences an exacerbation of their lung disease, or if the patient develops potential signs or symptoms of theophylline toxicity.

EXAMPLE 2 ▶▶▶

OI is a 60-year-old, 85-kg (height = 6 ft 1 in) male with emphysema who requires therapy with oral theophylline. He has liver cirrhosis (Child-Pugh score = 11) and normal cardiac function. Suggest an initial theophylline dosage regimen for this patient.

1. *Choose theophylline dose based on disease states and conditions present in the patient.*
   A theophylline dose of 0.2 mg/kg/h is suggested by the table for an adult with cirrhosis.

2. *Compute dosage regimen.*
   Oral sustained-release theophylline tablets will be prescribed to this patient (F = 1, S = 1). The initial dosage interval (τ) will be set to 12 hours: D = (theophylline dose • Wt • τ)/S = (0.2 mg/kg/h • 85 kg • 12 h)/1 = 204 mg, rounded to 200 mg every 12 hours. This dose is similar to that suggested by the Pharmacokinetic Dosing method of 150 mg every 12 hours.

A steady-state trough theophylline serum concentration should be measured after steady-state is attained in 3-5 half-lives. Since the patient is expected to have a half-life equal to 24 hours, the theophylline steady-state concentration could be obtained any time after the fifth day of dosing (5 half-lives = 5 • 24 h = 120 h or 5 d). Theophylline serum concentrations should also be measured if the patient experiences an exacerbation of their lung disease, or if the patient develops potential signs or symptoms of theophylline toxicity.

To illustrate the differences and similarities between oral and intravenous theophylline dosage regimen design, the same cases will be used to compute intravenous theophylline loading doses and continuous infusions.

EXAMPLE 3 ▶▶▶

LK is a 50-year-old, 75-kg (height = 5 ft 10 in) male with chronic bronchitis who requires therapy with intravenous theophylline. He currently smokes two packs of cigarettes daily, and has normal liver and cardiac function. Suggest an initial theophylline dosage regimen for this patient.

1. *Choose theophylline dose based on disease states and conditions present in the patient.*
   A theophylline dose of 0.7 mg/kg/h is suggested by the table for an adult smoker.

2. *Compute dosage regimen.*
   Theophylline will be administered as the intravenous drug (S = 1): k_0 = (theophylline dose • Wt)/S = (0.7 mg/kg/h • 75 kg)/1 = 53 mg/h, rounded to 55 mg/h. A loading dose of theophylline 5 mg/kg will also be prescribed for the patient: LD = 5 mg/kg • 75 kg = 375 mg, rounded to 400 mg of theophylline infused over 20-30 minutes. These are similar to the doses that were suggested by the Pharmacokinetic Dosing method.

   A theophylline serum concentration should be measured after steady-state is attained in 3-5 half-lives. Since the patient is expected to have a half-life equal to 5 hours, the theophylline steady-state concentration could be obtained any time after the first day of dosing (5 half-lives = 5 • 5 h = 25 h). Theophylline serum concentrations should also be measured if the patient experiences an exacerbation of their lung disease, or if the patient develops potential signs or symptoms of theophylline toxicity.

EXAMPLE 4 ▶▶▶

OI is a 60-year-old, 85-kg (height = 6 ft 1 in) male with emphysema who requires therapy with intravenous theophylline. He has liver cirrhosis (Child-Pugh score = 11) and normal cardiac function. Suggest an initial intravenous aminophylline dosage regimen for this patient.

1. *Choose theophylline dose based on disease states and conditions present in the patient.*
   A theophylline dose of 0.2 mg/kg/h is suggested by the table for an adult with cirrhosis.

2. *Compute dosage regimen.*
   Theophylline will be administered as the aminophylline dihydrate salt form (S = 0.8): D = (theophylline dose • Wt)/S = (0.2 mg/kg/h • 85 kg)/0.8 = 21 mg/h, rounded to 20 mg/h. A loading dose of aminophylline 6 mg/kg will also be prescribed for the patient: LD = 6 mg/kg • 85 kg = 510 mg, rounded to 500 mg of aminophylline infused over 20-30 minutes. These doses are similar to that suggested by the Pharmacokinetic Dosing method of a 500-mg loading dose followed by a 15-mg/h continuous infusion.

A steady-state theophylline serum concentration should be measured after steady-state is attained in 3-5 half-lives. Since the patient is expected to have a half-life equal to 24 hours, the theophylline steady-state concentration could be obtained any time after the fifth day of dosing (5 half-lives = 5 • 24 h = 120 h or 5 days). Theophylline serum concentrations should also be measured if the patient experiences an exacerbation of their lung disease, or if the patient develops potential signs or symptoms of theophylline toxicity.

USE OF THEOPHYLLINE SERUM CONCENTRATIONS TO ALTER DOSES

Because of the large amount of pharmacokinetic variability among patients, it is likely that doses computed using patient population characteristics will not always produce theophylline serum concentrations that are expected or desirable. Because of pharmacokinetic variability, the narrow therapeutic index of theophylline, and the severity of theophylline adverse side effects, measurement of theophylline serum concentrations is mandatory for patients to ensure that therapeutic, nontoxic levels are present. In addition to theophylline serum concentrations, important patient parameters (pulmonary function tests, clinical signs and symptoms of the pulmonary disease state, potential theophylline side effects, etc) should be followed to confirm that the patient is responding to treatment and not developing adverse drug reactions.

When theophylline serum concentrations are measured in patients and a dosage change is necessary, clinicians should seek to use the simplest, most straightforward method available to determine a dose that will provide safe and effective treatment. In most cases, a simple dosage ratio can be used to change theophylline doses assuming the drug follows *linear pharmacokinetics*. Although it has been clearly demonstrated in research studies that theophylline follows nonlinear pharmacokinetics,[14-16] in the clinical setting most patients' steady-state serum concentrations change in proportion to theophylline dose below and within the therapeutic range, and assuming linear pharmacokinetics is adequate for dosage adjustments in most patients.

Sometimes, it is useful to compute theophylline pharmacokinetic constants for a patient and base dosage adjustments on these. In this case, it may be possible to calculate and use *pharmacokinetic parameters* to alter the theophylline dose. In some situations, it may be necessary to compute theophylline clearance for the patient during a continuous infusion before steady-state conditions occur using the *Chiou method* and utilize this pharmacokinetic parameter to calculate the best drug dose.

Finally, computerized methods that incorporate expected population pharmacokinetic characteristics (*Bayesian pharmacokinetic computer programs*) can be used in difficult cases where serum concentrations are obtained at suboptimal times or the patient was not at steady-state when serum concentrations were measured. An additional benefit of this method is that a complete pharmacokinetic workup (determination of clearance, volume of distribution, and half-life) can be done with one or more measured concentrations that do not have to be at steady-state.

Linear Pharmacokinetics Method

Because theophylline follows linear, dose-proportional pharmacokinetics in most patients with concentrations within and below the therapeutic range, steady-state serum concentrations change in proportion to dose according to the following equation: $D_{new}/C_{ss,new} = D_{old}/C_{ss,old}$ or $D_{new} = (C_{ss,new}/C_{ss,old})D_{old}$, where D is the dose, Css is the steady-state concentration, old indicates the dose that produced the steady-state concentration that the patient is currently receiving, and new denotes the dose necessary to produce the desired steady-state concentration. The advantages of this method are that it is quick and simple. The disadvantages are steady-state concentrations are required, and the assumption of linear pharmacokinetics may not be valid in all patients. When steady-state serum concentrations increase more than expected after a dosage increase or decrease less than expected after a dosage decrease, nonlinear theophylline pharmacokinetics is a possible explanation for the observation. Because of this, suggested dosage increases greater than 75% using this method should be scrutinized by the prescribing clinician, and the risk versus benefit for the patient assessed before initiating large dosage increases (>75% over current dose).

EXAMPLE 1 ▶▶▶

LK is a 50-year-old, 75-kg (height = 5 ft 10 in) male with chronic bronchitis who is receiving 300 mg every 8 hours of an oral theophylline sustained-release tablet. He currently smokes two packs of cigarettes daily, and has normal liver and cardiac function. The current steady-state theophylline concentration equals 8 μg/mL. Compute a theophylline dose that will provide a steady-state concentration of 12 μg/mL.

1. *Compute new dose to achieve the desired serum concentration.*

The patient smokes tobacco-containing cigarettes and would be expected to achieve steady-state conditions after the first day (5 $t_{1/2}$ = 5 • 5 h = 25 h) of therapy.

Using linear pharmacokinetics, the new dose to attain the desired concentration should be proportional to the old dose that produced the measured concentration (total daily dose = 300 mg/dose • 3 doses/d = 900 mg/d):

$$D_{new} = (C_{ss,new}/C_{ss,old})D_{old} = (12 \ \mu g/mL \ / \ 8 \ \mu g/mL) \ 900 \ mg/d = 1350 \ mg/d$$

The new suggested dose would be 1350 mg/d or 450 mg every 8 hours of theophylline sustained-release tablets to be started at the next scheduled dosing time.

A steady-state trough theophylline serum concentration should be measured after steady-state is attained in 3–5 half-lives. Since the patient is expected to have a half-life equal to 5 hours, the theophylline steady-state concentration could be obtained any time after the first day of dosing (5 half-lives = 5 • 5 h = 25 h). Theophylline serum concentrations should also be measured if the patient experiences an exacerbation of their lung disease, or if the patient develops potential signs or symptoms of theophylline toxicity.

EXAMPLE 2 ▶▶▶

OI is a 60-year-old, 85-kg (height = 6 ft 1 in) male with emphysema who is receiving 200 mg every 12 hours of an oral theophylline sustained-release tablet. He has liver cirrhosis (Child-Pugh score = 11) and normal cardiac function. The current steady-state theophylline concentration equals 15 μg/mL, and he is experiencing some minor caffeine-type adverse effects (insomnia, jitteriness, nausea). Compute a theophylline dose that will provide a steady-state concentration of 10 μg/mL.

1. *Compute new dose to achieve the desired serum concentration.*

The patient has severe liver disease and would be expected to achieve steady-state conditions after 5 days (5 $t_{1/2}$ = 5 • 24 h = 120 h or 5 d) of therapy.

Using linear pharmacokinetics, the new dose to attain the desired concentration should be proportional to the old dose that produced the measured concentration (total daily dose = 200 mg/dose • 2 doses/d = 400 mg/d):

$$D_{new} = (C_{ss,new}/C_{ss,old})D_{old} = (10 \ \mu g/mL \ / \ 15 \ \mu g/mL) \ 400 \ mg/d = 267 \ mg/d$$

The new suggested dose would be 267 mg/d or 134 mg every 12 hours, rounded to 150 every 12 hours of theophylline sustained-release tablets, to be started after holding one to two doses until adverse effects have subsided.

A steady-state trough theophylline serum concentration should be measured after steady-state is attained in 3-5 half-lives. Since the patient is expected to have a half-life equal to 24 hours, the theophylline steady-state concentration could be obtained any time after the fifth day of dosing (5 half-lives = 5 • 24 h = 120 h or 5 days). Theophylline serum concentrations should also be measured if the patient experiences an exacerbation of their lung disease, or if the patient develops potential signs or symptoms of theophylline toxicity.

To illustrate the differences and similarities between oral and intravenous theophylline dosage regimen design, the same cases will be used to compute altered intravenous theophylline continuous infusions using steady-state serum concentrations.

EXAMPLE 3 ▶▶▶

LK is a 50-year-old, 75-kg (height = 5 ft 10 in) male with chronic bronchitis who is receiving an aminophylline constant intravenous infusion at a rate of 50 mg/h. He currently smokes two packs of cigarettes daily, and has normal liver and cardiac function. The current steady-state theophylline concentration equals 8 μg/mL. Compute an aminophylline infusion rate that will provide a steady-state concentration of 12 μg/mL.

1. *Compute new dose to achieve the desired serum concentration.*

The patient smokes tobacco-containing cigarettes and would be expected to achieve steady-state conditions after the first day (5 $t_{1/2}$ = 5 • 5 h = 25 h) of therapy.

Using linear pharmacokinetics, the new infusion rate to attain the desired concentration should be proportional to the old infusion rate that produced the measured concentration:

$$D_{new} = (C_{ss,new}/C_{ss,old})D_{old} = (12 \ \mu g/mL / 8 \ \mu g/mL) \ 50 \ mg/h = 75 \ mg/h$$

The new suggested infusion rate would be 75 mg/h of aminophylline.

A steady-state theophylline serum concentration should be measured after steady-state is attained in 3-5 half-lives. Since the patient is expected to have a half-life equal to 5 hours, the theophylline steady-state concentration could be obtained any time after the first day of dosing (5 half-lives = 5 • 5 h = 25 h). Theophylline serum concentrations should also be measured if the patient experiences an exacerbation of their lung disease, or if the patient develops potential signs or symptoms of theophylline toxicity.

EXAMPLE 4 ▶▶▶

OI is a 60-year-old, 85-kg (height = 6 ft 1 in) male with emphysema who is receiving a 20-mg/h continuous infusion of theophylline. He has liver cirrhosis (Child-Pugh score = 11) and normal cardiac function. The current steady-state theophylline concentration equals 15 μg/mL, and he is experiencing some minor caffeine-type adverse effects (insomnia, jitteriness, nausea). Compute a theophylline dose that will provide a steady-state concentration of 10 μg/mL.

1. *Compute new dose to achieve the desired serum concentration.*

The patient has severe liver disease and would be expected to achieve steady-state conditions after 5 days (5 $t_{1/2}$ = 5 • 24 h = 120 h or 5 d) of therapy.

Using linear pharmacokinetics, the new infusion rate to attain the desired concentration should be proportional to the old infusion rate that produced the measured concentration:

$$D_{new} = (C_{ss,new}/C_{ss,old})D_{old} = (10\ \mu g/mL\ /\ 15\ \mu g/mL)\ 20\ mg/h = 13\ mg/h, \text{round to } 15\ mg/h$$

The new suggested dose would be 15 mg/h of theophylline as a continuous infusion. If necessary, the infusion could be temporarily stopped for 12-24 hours until theophylline adverse effects subsided.

A steady-state trough theophylline serum concentration should be measured after steady-state is attained in 3-5 half-lives. Since the patient is expected to have a half-life equal to 24 hours, the theophylline steady-state concentration could be obtained any time after the fifth day of dosing (5 half-lives = 5 • 24 h = 120 h or 5 days). Theophylline serum concentrations should also be measured if the patient experiences an exacerbation of their lung disease, or if the patient develops potential signs or symptoms of theophylline toxicity.

Pharmacokinetic Parameter Method

The Pharmacokinetic Parameter method of adjusting drug doses was among the first techniques available to change doses using serum concentrations. It allows the computation of an individual's own, unique pharmacokinetic constants and uses those to calculate a dose that achieves desired theophylline concentrations. The Pharmacokinetic Parameter method requires that steady-state has been achieved and uses only a steady-state theophylline concentration (Css). During a continuous intravenous infusion, the following equation is used to compute theophylline clearance (Cl): $Cl = [S • k_0]/Css$, where S is the fraction of the theophylline salt form that is active theophylline (S = 1 for theophylline, S = 0.85 for anhydrous aminophylline, S = 0.80 for aminophylline dihydrate) and k_0 is the dose of theophylline salt in mg/h. If the patient is receiving oral theophylline therapy, theophylline clearance (Cl) can be calculated using the following formula: $Cl = [F • S (D/\tau)]/Css$, where F is the bioavailability fraction for the oral dosage form (F = 1 for most oral theophylline sustained-release products), S is the fraction of the theophylline salt form that is active theophylline (S = 1 for theophylline, S = 0.85 for anhydrous aminophylline, S = 0.80 for aminophylline dihydrate, S = 0.65 for oxtriphylline), D is the dose of theophylline salt in mg, Css is the steady-state theophylline concentration, and τ is the dosage interval in hours.

Occasionally, theophylline serum concentrations are obtained before and after an intravenous loading dose. Assuming a one-compartment model, the volume of distribution (V) is calculated using the following equation: $V = (S • D)/(C_{postdose} - C_{predose})$ where S is the fraction of the theophylline salt form that is active theophylline (S = 1 for theophylline, S = 0.85 for anhydrous aminophylline, S = 0.80 for aminophylline dihydrate), D is the dose of theophylline salt in mg, $C_{postdose}$ is the post-loading dose concentration in mg/L, and $C_{predose}$ is the concentration before the loading dose was administered in mg/L (both concentrations should be obtained within 30-60 minutes of dosage administration). If the predose concentration was also a steady-state concentration, theophylline clearance can also be computed. If both clearance (Cl) and volume of distribution (V) have been measured using these techniques, the half-life $[t_{1/2} = (0.693 • V)/Cl]$ and elimination rate constant $(k = 0.693/t_{1/2} = Cl/V)$ can be computed. The clearance, volume of distribution, elimination rate constant, and half-life measured using these techniques are the patient's own, unique theophylline pharmacokinetic constants and can be used in one-compartment model equations to compute the required dose to achieve any desired serum concentration. Because this method also assumes linear pharmacokinetics, theophylline doses computed using the Pharmacokinetic Parameter method and the Linear Pharmacokinetic method should be identical.

EXAMPLE 1 ▶▶▶

LK is a 50-year-old, 75-kg (height = 5 ft 10 in) male with chronic bronchitis who is receiving 300 mg every 8 hours of an oral theophylline sustained-release tablet. He currently smokes two packs of cigarettes daily, and has normal liver and cardiac function. The current steady-state theophylline concentration equals 8 μg/mL. Compute a theophylline dose that will provide a steady-state concentration of 12 μg/mL.

1. *Compute pharmacokinetic parameters.*

   The patient smokes tobacco-containing cigarettes and would be expected to achieve steady-state conditions after the first day (5 $t_{1/2}$ = 5 • 5 h = 25 h) of therapy.

   Theophylline clearance can be computed using a steady-state theophylline concentration: Cl = [F • S (D/τ)]/Css = [1 • 1 (300 mg/8 h)]/ (8 mg/L) = 4.69 L/h. (Note: μg/mL = mg/L and this concentration unit was substituted for Css in the calculations so that unnecessary unit conversion was not required.)

2. *Compute theophylline dose.*

   Theophylline clearance is used to compute the new dose: D = (Css • Cl • τ)/(F • S) = (12 mg/L • 4.69 L/h • 8h)/ (1 • 1) = 450 mg every 8 hours.

   The new theophylline dosage regimen would be instituted at the next dosage time.

   A steady-state trough theophylline serum concentration should be measured after steady-state is attained in 3-5 half-lives. Since the patient is expected to have a half-life equal to 5 hours, the theophylline steady-state concentration could be obtained any time after the first day of dosing (5 half-lives = 5 • 5 h = 25 h). Theophylline serum concentrations should also be measured if the patient experiences an exacerbation of their lung disease, or if the patient develops potential signs or symptoms of theophylline toxicity.

EXAMPLE 2 ▶▶▶

OI is a 60-year-old, 85-kg (height = 6 ft 1 in) male with emphysema who is receiving 200 mg every 12 hours of an oral theophylline sustained-release tablet. He has liver cirrhosis (Child-Pugh score = 11) and normal cardiac function. The current steady-state theophylline concentration equals 15 μg/mL, and he is experiencing some minor caffeine-type adverse effects (insomnia, jitteriness, nausea). Compute a theophylline dose that will provide a steady-state concentration of 10 μg/mL.

1. *Compute pharmacokinetic parameters.*

   The patient has severe liver disease and would be expected to achieve steady-state conditions after 5 days (5 $t_{1/2}$ = 5 • 24 h = 120 h or 5 d) of therapy.

   Theophylline clearance can be computed using a steady-state theophylline concentration: Cl = [F • S (D/τ)]/ Css = [1 • 1 (200 mg/12 h)]/ (15 mg/L) = 1.11 L/h. (Note: μg/mL = mg/L and this concentration unit was substituted for Css in the calculations so that unnecessary unit conversion was not required.)

2. *Compute theophylline dose.*

   Theophylline clearance is used to compute the new dose: D = (Css • Cl • τ)/(F • S) = (10 mg/L • 1.11 L/h • 12 h)/ (1 • 1) = 133 mg, rounded to 150 mg every 12 hours.

   The new dose would be started after holding one to two doses until adverse effects have subsided.

   A steady-state trough theophylline serum concentration should be measured after steady-state is attained in 3-5 half-lives. Since the patient is expected to have a half-life equal to 24 hours, the theophylline steady-state concentration could be obtained any time after the fifth day of dosing (5 half-lives = 5 • 24 h = 120 h or 5 days). Theophylline serum concentrations should also be measured if the patient experiences an exacerbation of their lung disease, or if the patient develops potential signs or symptoms of theophylline toxicity.

To illustrate the differences and similarities between oral and intravenous theophylline dosage regimen design, the same cases will be used to compute altered intravenous theophylline continuous infusions using steady-state serum concentrations.

EXAMPLE 3 ▶▶▶

LK is a 50-year-old, 75-kg (height = 5 ft10 in) male with chronic bronchitis who is receiving an aminophylline constant intravenous infusion at a rate of 50 mg/h. He currently smokes two packs of cigarettes daily, and has normal liver and cardiac function. The current steady-state theophylline concentration equals 8 μg/mL. Compute an aminophylline infusion rate that will provide a steady-state concentration of 12 μg/mL.

1. *Compute pharmacokinetic parameters.*

The patient smokes tobacco-containing cigarettes and would be expected to achieve steady-state conditions after the first day (5 $t_{1/2}$ = 5 • 5 h = 25 h) of therapy.

Theophylline clearance can be computed using a steady-state theophylline concentration Cl = [S • k_0]/Css = (0.8 • 50 mg/h) / (8 mg/L) = 5 L/h. (Note: μg/mL = mg/L and this concentration unit was substituted for Css in the calculations so that unnecessary unit conversion was not required).

2. *Compute theophylline dose.*

Theophylline clearance is used to compute the new aminophylline infusion rate: k_0 = (Css • Cl)/S = (12 mg/L • 5 L/h)/(0.8) = 75 mg/h.

The new aminophylline infusion rate would be instituted immediately.

A steady-state theophylline serum concentration should be measured after steady-state is attained in 3-5 half-lives. Since the patient is expected to have a half-life equal to 5 hours, the theophylline steady-state concentration could be obtained any time after the first day of dosing (5 half-lives = 5 • 5 h = 25 h). Theophylline serum concentrations should also be measured if the patient experiences an exacerbation of their lung disease, or if the patient develops potential signs or symptoms of theophylline toxicity.

EXAMPLE 4 ▶▶▶

OI is a 60-year-old, 85-kg (height = 6 ft 1 in) male with emphysema who is receiving a 20-mg/h continuous infusion of theophylline. He has liver cirrhosis (Child-Pugh score = 11) and normal cardiac function. The current steady-state theophylline concentration equals 15 μg/mL, and he is experiencing some minor caffeine-type adverse effects (insomnia, jitteriness, nausea). Compute a theophylline dose that will provide a steady-state concentration of 10 μg/mL.

1. *Compute pharmacokinetic parameters.*

The patient has severe liver disease and would be expected to achieve steady-state conditions after 5 days (5 $t_{1/2}$ = 5 • 24 h = 120 h or 5 d) of therapy.

Theophylline clearance can be computed using a steady-state theophylline concentration Cl = [S • k_0]/Css = (1 • 20 mg/h) / (15 mg/L) = 1.33 L/h. (Note: μg/mL = mg/L and this concentration unit was substituted for Css in the calculations so that unnecessary unit conversion was not required.)

2. *Compute theophylline dose.*

Theophylline clearance is used to compute the new theophylline infusion rate: k_0 = (Css • Cl)/S = (10 mg/L • 1.33 L/h)/(1) = 13 mg/h, round to 15 mg/h.

The new suggested dose would be 15 mg/h of theophylline as a continuous infusion. If necessary, the infusion could be temporarily stopped for 12-24 hours until theophylline adverse effects subsided.

A steady-state theophylline serum concentration should be measured after steady-state is attained in 3-5 half-lives. Since the patient is expected to have a half-life equal to 24 hours, the theophylline steady-state concentration could be obtained any time after the fifth day of dosing (5 half-lives = $5 \cdot 24$ h = 120 h or 5 days). Theophylline serum concentrations should also be measured if the patient experiences an exacerbation of their lung disease, or if the patient develops potential signs or symptoms of theophylline toxicity.

EXAMPLE 5 ▶▶▶

PP is a 59-year-old, 65-kg (height = 5 ft 8 in) male with emphysema who is receiving an aminophylline constant intravenous infusion at a rate of 15 mg/h. He currently smokes two packs of cigarettes daily and has normal liver function. However, he also has heart failure (NYHA CHF Class IV). The current steady-state theophylline concentration equals 6 μg/mL. Compute an aminophylline infusion rate that will provide a steady-state concentration of 10 μg/mL. Additionally, in an attempt to boost theophylline concentrations as soon as possible, an aminophylline intravenous bolus of 300 mg over 30 minutes was given before the infusion rate was increased. The theophylline serum concentration after the additional bolus dose was 12 μg/mL.

1. *Compute pharmacokinetic parameters.*

   The patient has severe heart failure and would be expected to achieve steady-state conditions after 5 days ($5 \, t_{1/2} = 5 \cdot 24$ h = 120 h or 5 d) of therapy.

   Theophylline clearance can be computed using a steady-state theophylline concentration: $Cl = [S \cdot k_0]/Css = (0.8 \cdot 15 \text{ mg/h}) / (6 \text{ mg/L}) = 2$ L/h. (Note: μg/mL = mg/L and this concentration unit was substituted for Css in the calculations so that unnecessary unit conversion was not required.)

   Theophylline volume of distribution can be computed using the prebolus dose (Css = 6 μg/mL) and postbolus dose concentrations: $V = (S \cdot D)/(C_{postdose} - C_{predose}) = (0.8 \cdot 300 \text{ mg})/(12 \text{ mg/L} - 6 \text{ mg/L}) = 40$ L. (Note: μg/mL = mg/L and this concentration unit was substituted for Css in the calculations so that unnecessary unit conversion was not required.)

   Theophylline half-life ($t_{1/2}$) and elimination rate constant (k) can also be computed: $t_{1/2} = (0.693 \cdot V)/Cl = (0.693 \cdot 40 \text{ L})/(2 \text{ L/h}) = 14$ h; $k = Cl/V = (2 \text{ L/h})/(40 \text{ L}) = 0.05 \text{ h}^{-1}$.

2. *Compute theophylline dose.*

   Theophylline clearance is used to compute the new aminophylline infusion rate: $k_0 = (Css \cdot Cl)/S = (10 \text{ mg/L} \cdot 2 \text{ L/h})/(0.8) = 25$ mg/h.

   The new aminophylline infusion rate would be instituted immediately after the additional loading dose was given.

   A theophylline serum concentration should be measured after steady-state is attained in 3-5 half-lives. Since the patient has a half-life equal to 14 hours, the theophylline steady-state concentration could be obtained after 3 days of continuous dosing (5 half-lives = $5 \cdot 14$ h = 70 h). Theophylline serum concentrations should also be measured if the patient experiences an exacerbation of their lung disease, or if the patient develops potential signs or symptoms of theophylline toxicity.

CHIOU METHOD

For some patients, it is desirable to individualize theophylline infusion rates as rapidly as possible before steady-state is achieved. Examples of these cases include patients with heart failure or hepatic cirrhosis who have variable theophylline pharmacokinetic parameters and long theophylline half-lives. In this situation, two theophylline serum concentrations obtained at least 4-6 hours apart during a continuous infusion can be used to compute theophylline clearance and dosing rates.[68-70] In addition to this requirement, the only way theophylline can be entering the patient's body must be via intravenous infusion. Thus, the last dose of sustained-release theophylline must have been administered no less than 12-16 hours before this technique is used, or some residual oral theophylline will still be absorbed from the gastrointestinal tract and cause computation errors.

The following equation is used to compute theophylline clearance (Cl) using the theophylline concentrations:

$$Cl = \frac{2 \bullet S \bullet k_0}{C_1 + C_2} + \frac{2V(C_1 - C_2)}{(C_1 + C_2)(t_2 - t_1)}$$

where S is the fraction of the theophylline salt form that is active theophylline (S = 1 for theophylline, S = 0.85 for anhydrous aminophylline, S = 0.80 for aminophylline dihydrate), k_0 is the infusion rate of the theophylline salt, V is theophylline volume of distribution (assumed to equal 0.5 L/kg; use ideal body weight for obese patients >30% overweight), C_1 and C_2 are the first and second theophylline serum concentrations, and t_1 and t_2 are the times that C_1 and C_2 were obtained. Once theophylline clearance (Cl) is determined, it can be used to adjust the theophylline salt infusion rate (k_0) using the following relationship: k_0 = (Css • Cl)/S, where S is the fraction of the theophylline salt form that is active theophylline (S = 1 for theophylline, S = 0.85 for anhydrous aminophylline, S = 0.80 for aminophylline dihydrate).

EXAMPLE 1 ▶▶▶

JB is a 50-year-old, 60-kg (height = 5 ft 7 in) male with heart failure (NYHA CHF class III) started on a 50 mg/h aminophylline infusion after being administered an intravenous loading dose. The theophylline concentration was 15.6 µg/mL at 1000 H and 18.3 µg/mL at 1400 H. What aminophylline infusion rate is needed to achieve Css = 15 µg/mL?

1. *Compute theophylline clearance and dose.*

$$Cl = \frac{2 \bullet S \bullet k_0}{C_1 + C_2} + \frac{2V(C_1 - C_2)}{(C_1 + C_2)(t_2 - t_1)}$$

$$Cl = \frac{2[0.8(50\ mg/h)]}{15.6\ mg/L + 18.3\ mg/L} + \frac{2(0.5\ L/kg \bullet 60\ kg)(15.6\ mg/L - 18.3\ mg/L)}{(15.6\ mg/L + 18.3\ mg/L)\ 4\ h} = 1.17\ L/h$$

(Note: µg/mL = mg/L and this concentration unit was substituted for concentrations so that unnecessary unit conversion was not required. Additionally, the time difference between t_2 and t_1 was determined and placed directly in the calculation.)

k_0 = (Css • Cl)/S = (15 mg/L • 1.17 L/h)/0.8 = 22 mg/h, round to 20 mg/h of aminophylline

EXAMPLE 2 ▶▶▶

YU is a 64-year-old, 80-kg (height = 5 ft 9 in) male with COPD who smokes 1½ packs of cigarettes per day. He is started on a 40 mg/h theophylline infusion after being administered an intravenous loading dose at 0900 H. The theophylline concentration was 11.6 µg/mL at 1000 H and 8.1 µg/mL at 1600 H. What theophylline infusion rate is needed to achieve Css = 10 µg/mL?

1. *Compute theophylline clearance and dose.*

$$Cl = \frac{2 \cdot S \cdot k_0}{C_1 + C_2} + \frac{2V(C_1 - C_2)}{(C_1 + C_2)(t_2 - t_1)}$$

$$Cl = \frac{2[1(40 \text{ mg/h})]}{11.6 \text{ mg/L} + 8.1 \text{ mg/L}} + \frac{2(0.5 \text{ L/kg} \cdot 80 \text{ kg})(11.6 \text{ mg/L} - 8.1 \text{ mg/L})}{(11.6 \text{ mg/L} + 8.1 \text{ mg/L})6 \text{ h}} = 6.43 \text{ L/h}$$

(Note: μg/mL = mg/L and this concentration unit was substituted for concentrations so that unnecessary unit conversion was not required. Additionally, the time difference between t_2 and t_1 was determined and placed directly in the calculation.)

$$k_0 = (Css \cdot Cl)/S = (10 \text{ mg/L} \cdot 6.43 \text{ L/h})/1 = 64 \text{ mg/h, round to 65 mg/h of theophylline}$$

BAYESIAN PHARMACOKINETIC COMPUTER PROGRAMS

Computer programs are available that can assist in the computation of pharmacokinetic parameters for patients. The most reliable computer programs use a nonlinear regression algorithm that incorporates components of Bayes theorem. Nonlinear regression is a statistical technique that uses an iterative process to compute the best pharmacokinetic parameters for a concentration/time data set. Briefly, the patient's drug dosage schedule and serum concentrations are input into the computer. The computer program has a pharmacokinetic equation preprogrammed for the drug and administration method (oral, intravenous bolus, intravenous infusion, etc). Typically, a one-compartment model is used, although some programs allow the user to choose among several different equations. Using population estimates based on demographic information for the patient (age, weight, gender, liver function, cardiac status, etc) supplied by the user, the computer program then computes estimated serum concentrations at each time there are actual serum concentrations. Kinetic parameters are then changed by the computer program, and a new set of estimated serum concentrations are computed. The pharmacokinetic parameters that generated the estimated serum concentrations closest to the actual values are remembered by the computer program, and the process is repeated until the set of pharmacokinetic parameters that result in estimated serum concentrations that are statistically closest to the actual serum concentrations are generated. These pharmacokinetic parameters can then be used to compute improved dosing schedules for patients. Bayes theorem is used in the computer algorithm to balance the results of the computations between values based solely on the patient's serum drug concentrations and those based only on patient population parameters. Results from studies that compare various methods of dosage adjustment have consistently found that these types of computer dosing programs perform at least as well as experienced clinical pharmacokineticists and clinicians and better than inexperienced clinicians.

Some clinicians use Bayesian pharmacokinetic computer programs exclusively to alter drug doses based on serum concentrations. An advantage of this approach is that consistent dosage recommendations are made when several different practitioners are involved in therapeutic drug monitoring programs. However, since simpler dosing methods work just as well for patients with stable pharmacokinetic parameters and steady-state drug concentrations, many clinicians reserve the use of computer programs for more difficult situations. Those situations include serum concentrations that are not at steady-state, serum concentrations not obtained at the specific times needed to employ simpler methods, and unstable pharmacokinetic parameters. Many Bayesian pharmacokinetic computer programs are available to users, and most should provide answers similar to the one used in the following examples. The program used to solve problems in this book is DrugCalc written by Dr Dennis Mungall.[71]

EXAMPLE 1 ▶▶▶

LK is a 50-year-old, 75-kg (height = 5 ft 10 in) male with chronic bronchitis who is receiving 300 mg every 8 hours of an oral theophylline sustained-release tablet. He currently smokes two packs of cigarettes daily, and has normal liver (bilirubin = 0.7 mg/dL, albumin = 4.0 g/dL) and cardiac function. The current steady-state theophylline concentration equals 8 μg/mL. Compute a theophylline dose that will provide a steady-state concentration of 12 μg/mL.

1. *Enter the patient's demographic, drug-dosing, and serum concentration/time data into the computer program.*
2. *Compute pharmacokinetic parameters for the patient using Bayesian pharmacokinetic computer program.*
   The pharmacokinetic parameters computed by the program are a volume of distribution of 37 L, a half-life equal to 5.9 h, and a clearance equal to 4.33 L/h.
3. *Compute dose required to achieve the desired theophylline serum concentrations.*
   The one-compartment model first-order absorption equations used by the program to compute doses indicates that a dose of 450 mg every 8 hours will produce a steady-state theophylline concentration of 12 μg/mL. Using the Linear Pharmacokinetics and Pharmacokinetic Parameter methods previously described in the chapter produced the same answer for this patient.

EXAMPLE 2 ▶▶▶

HJ is a 62-year-old, 87 kg (height = 6 ft 1 in) male with emphysema who is given a new prescription of 300 mg every 12 hours of an oral theophylline sustained-release tablet. He has liver cirrhosis (Child-Pugh score = 12, bilirubin = 3.2 mg/dL, albumin = 2.5 g/dL) and normal cardiac function. The theophylline concentration after the sixth dose equals 15 μg/mL, and he is experiencing some minor caffeine-type adverse effects (insomnia, jitteriness, nausea). Compute a theophylline dose that will provide a steady-state concentration of 10 μg/mL.

1. *Enter the patient's demographic, drug-dosing, and serum concentration/time data into the computer program.*
   In this patient case, it is unlikely that the patient is at steady-state so the Linear Pharmacokinetics method cannot be used.
2. *Compute pharmacokinetic parameters for the patient using Bayesian pharmacokinetic computer program.*
   The pharmacokinetic parameters computed by the program are a volume of distribution of 38 L, a half-life equal to 19 h, and a clearance equal to 1.41 L/h.
3. *Compute dose required to achieve the desired theophylline serum concentrations.*
   The one-compartment first-order absorption equations used by the program to compute doses indicates that a dose of 200 mg every 12 hours will produce a steady-state concentration of 11 μg/mL.

EXAMPLE 3 ▶▶▶

JB is a 50-year-old, 60-kg (5 ft 7 in) male with heart failure (NYHA CHF class III) started on a 50-mg/h aminophylline infusion after being administered an intravenous loading dose of aminophylline 500 mg at 0800 H over 20 minutes. The theophylline concentration was 15.6 μg/mL at 1000 H and 18.3 μg/mL at 1400 H. What aminophylline infusion rate is needed to achieve Css = 15 μg/mL?

1. *Enter the patient's demographic, drug-dosing, and serum concentration/time data into the computer program.*
   In this patient case, it is unlikely that the patient is at steady-state so the Linear Pharmacokinetics method cannot be used. DrugCalc requires doses to be entered in terms of theophylline, so aminophylline doses must be converted to theophylline doses for entry into the program (LD = 500 mg aminophylline • 0.8 = 400 mg theophylline, k_0 = 50 mg/h aminophylline • 0.8 = 40 mg/h theophylline).

2. *Compute pharmacokinetic parameters for the patient using Bayesian pharmacokinetic computer program.*
   The pharmacokinetic parameters computed by the program are a volume of distribution of 29 L, a half-life equal to 21 h, and clearance equal to 0.98 L/h.
3. *Compute dose required to achieve the desired theophylline serum concentrations.*
   The one-compartment model intravenous infusion equations used by the program to compute doses indicates that a dose of aminophylline 20 mg/h will produce a steady-state concentration of 16 μg/mL. Using the Chiou method previously described in the chapter produced a comparable answer for this patient (20 mg/h to produce a steady-state concentration of 15 μg/mL).

DOSING STRATEGIES

Initial dose and dosage adjustment techniques using serum concentrations can be used in any combination as long as the limitations of each method are observed. Some dosing schemes link together logically when considered according to their basic approaches or philosophies. Dosage strategies that follow similar pathways are given in Table 22-5.

USE OF THEOPHYLLINE BOOSTER DOSES TO IMMEDIATELY INCREASE SERUM CONCENTRATIONS

If a patient has a subtherapeutic theophylline serum concentration in an acute situation, it may be desirable to increase the theophylline concentration as quickly as possible. In this setting, it would not be acceptable to simply increase the maintenance dose and wait 3-5 half-lives for therapeutic serum concentrations to be established in the patient. A rational way to increase the serum concentrations rapidly is to administer a booster dose of theophylline, a process also known as "reloading" the patient with theophylline, computed using pharmacokinetic techniques. A modified loading dose equation is used to accomplish computation of the booster dose (BD) which takes into account the current theophylline concentration present in the patient: $BD = [(C_{desired} - C_{actual})V]/S$, where $C_{desired}$ is the desired theophylline concentration, C_{actual} is the actual current theophylline concentration for the patient, S is the fraction of the theophylline salt form that is active theophylline (S = 1 for theophylline, S = 0.85 for anhydrous aminophylline, S = 0.80 for aminophylline dihydrate), and V is the volume of distribution for theophylline. If the volume of distribution for theophylline is known for the patient, it can be used in the calculation. However, this value is not usually known and is assumed to equal the population average of 0.5 L/kg (ideal body weight used for patients >30% overweight).

TABLE 22-5   Dosing Strategies

Dosing Approach/Philosophy	Initial Dosing	Use of Serum Concentrations to Alter Doses
Pharmacokinetic parameter/equations	Pharmacokinetic Dosing method	Pharmacokinetic Parameter method or Chiou method (IV infusion before steady-state)
Literature-based concept	Literature-based Recommended Dosing method	Linear Pharmacokinetics method
Computerized	Bayesian computer program	Bayesian computer program

Concurrent with the administration of the booster dose, the maintenance dose of theophylline is usually increased. Clinicians need to recognize that the administration of a booster dose does not alter the time required to achieve steady-state conditions when a new theophylline dosage rate is prescribed. It still requires 3-5 half-lives to attain steady-state when the dosage rate is changed. However, usually the difference between the post-booster dose theophylline concentration and the ultimate steady-state concentration has been reduced by giving the extra dose of drug.

EXAMPLE 1 ▶▶▶

BN is a 22-year-old, 50-kg (height = 5 ft 2 in) female with asthma who is receiving therapy with intravenous theophylline. She does not smoke cigarettes and has normal liver and cardiac function. After receiving an initial loading dose of aminophylline (300 mg) and a maintenance infusion of aminophylline equal to 20 mg/h for 16 hours, her theophylline concentration is measured at 5.6 μg/mL and her pulmonary function tests are worsening. Compute a booster dose of aminophylline to achieve a theophylline concentration equal to 10 μg/mL.

1. *Estimate volume of distribution according to disease states and conditions present in the patient.*
   In the case of theophylline, the population average volume of distribution equals 0.5 L/kg and this will be used to estimate the parameter for the patient. The patient is nonobese, so her actual body weight will be used in the computation: V = 0.5 L/kg • 50 kg = 25 L.

2. *Compute booster dose.*
   The booster dose is computed using the following equation: $BD = [(C_{desired} - C_{actual})V]/S = [(10 \text{ mg/L} - 5.6 \text{ mg/L})25 \text{ L}]/0.8 = 138$ mg, rounded to 150 mg of aminophylline infused over 20-30 minutes. (Note: μg/mL = mg/L and this concentration unit was substituted for Css in the calculations so that unnecessary unit conversion was not required.) If the maintenance dose was increased, it will take an additional 3-5 estimated half-lives for new steady-state conditions to be achieved. Theophylline serum concentrations should be measured at this time.

CONVERSION OF THEOPHYLLINE DOSES FROM INTRAVENOUS TO ORAL ROUTE OF ADMINISTRATION

Occasionally there is a need to convert a patient stabilized on theophylline therapy from the oral route of administration to an equivalent continuous infusion or vice versa.[72] In general, oral theophylline dosage forms, including most sustained-release tablets and capsules, have a bioavailability equal to one. Assuming that equal theophylline serum concentrations are desired, this makes conversion between the intravenous $[k_0 = (Css \bullet Cl)/S]$ and oral $[D = (Css \bullet Cl \bullet \tau)/(F \bullet S)]$ routes of administration simple since equivalent doses of drug (corrected for theophylline salt form) are prescribed: $k_0 = D_{po}/(24 \text{ h/d} \bullet S_{iv})$ or $D_{po} = S_{iv} \bullet k_0 \bullet 24 \text{ h/d}$, where k_0 is the equivalent intravenous infusion rate for the theophylline salt in mg/h, D_{po} is equivalent dose of oral theophylline in mg/d, and S_{iv} is the fraction of the intravenously administered theophylline salt form that is active theophylline.

EXAMPLE 1 ▶▶▶

JH is currently receiving oral sustained-release theophylline 600 mg every 12 hours. She is responding well to therapy, has no adverse drug effects, and has a steady-state theophylline concentration of 14.7 μg/mL. Suggest an equivalent dose of aminophylline given as an intravenous infusion for this patient.

1. *Calculate equivalent intravenous dose of aminophylline.*
   The patient is currently receiving 600 mg every 12 hours or 1200 mg/d (600 mg/dose • 2 doses/d = 1200 mg/d) of theophylline. The equivalent intravenous aminophylline dose would be: $k_0 = D_{po}/(24 \text{ h/d} • S_{iv}) = (1200 \text{ mg/d})/(24 \text{ h/d} • 0.8) = 62.5$ mg/h, rounded to 65 mg/h of aminophylline as a continuous intravenous infusion.

EXAMPLE 2 ▶▶▶

LK is currently receiving a continuous infusion of aminophylline at the rate of 40 mg/h. He is responding well to therapy, has no adverse drug effects, and has a steady-state theophylline concentration of 11.3 μg/mL. Suggest an equivalent dose of sustained-release oral theophylline for this patient.

1. *Calculate equivalent oral dose of theophylline.*
   The patient is currently receiving 40 mg/h of intravenous aminophylline as a constant infusion. The equivalent oral sustained-release theophylline dose would be: $D_{po} = S_{iv} • k_0 • 24 \text{ h/d} = 0.8 • 40 \text{ mg/h} • 24 \text{ h/d} = 768$ mg/d, rounded to 800 mg/d. The patient would be prescribed theophylline sustained-release tablets 400 mg orally every 12 hours.

REMOVAL OF THEOPHYLLINE BODY STORES IN MANAGEMENT OF THEOPHYLLINE OVERDOSE

In addition to supportive care, treatment of seizures with anticonvulsant agents, and treatment of cardiac arrhythmias with antiarrhythmic agents, removal of theophylline from the body should be considered in cases of acute and chronic overdoses.[66] Extracorporeal methods to remove theophylline in emergency situations include hemodialysis[52-57] and charcoal hemoperfusion.[73,74] Hemoperfusion is a technique similar to hemodialysis except the blood is passed through a column of activated charcoal instead of through an artificial kidney. Charcoal hemoperfusion is very effective in removing theophylline from the blood with an extraction ratio across the column in excess of 90%, but theophylline serum concentrations can rebound 5-10 μg/mL upon discontinuation of the procedure as theophylline in the tissues come into equilibrium with the blood.[73,74] Theophylline serum concentrations should be closely monitored when charcoal hemoperfusion is instituted. Other complications of charcoal hemoperfusion include hypotension, hypocalcemia, platelet consumption, and bleeding.

Theophylline can also be removed from the body using oral doses of activated charcoal.[75,76] This method to reduce theophylline body stores is about as effective as hemodialysis removal. Activated charcoal physically adsorbs theophylline, rendering it nonabsorbable from the gastrointestinal tract. If the patient is vomiting, appropriate antiemetic therapy must be instituted so that the charcoal is retained in the stomach. Phenothiazine antiemetics should be avoided as they may decrease the seizure threshold. In an acute theophylline overdose, oral activated charcoal (0.5 g/kg up to 20 g, repeated at least once in 1-2 hours) will bind theophylline that has not yet been absorbed and hold it in the gastrointestinal tract. Oral activated charcoal will also enhance the clearance of theophylline by binding theophylline secreted in gastrointestinal juices and eliminating the drug in the stool. When used in this fashion, oral activated charcoal (0.5 g/kg up to 20 g) is given every 2 hours. In both cases, a dose of oral sorbitol should be given to hasten the removal of charcoal-bound theophylline from the intestine.

After acute and chronic theophylline overdoses, a single dose of oral activated charcoal is recommended if the theophylline serum concentration is 20-30 μg/mL. For theophylline serum concentrations >30 μg/mL, multiple doses of oral activated charcoal should be used. Patients should be monitored for signs and symptoms of theophylline toxicity and treated appropriately. Theophylline serum concentrations should be measured every 2-4 hours in order to guide further therapy.

PROBLEMS

The following problems are intended to emphasize the computation of initial and individualized doses using clinical pharmacokinetic techniques. Clinicians should always consult the patient's chart to confirm that current pulmonary therapy, including inhaled bronchodilators and steroids, is appropriate. Additionally, all other medications that the patient is taking, including prescription and nonprescription drugs, should be noted and checked to ascertain if a potential drug interaction with theophylline exists.

1. NJ is a 67-year-old, 72-kg (height = 6 ft 1 in) male with chronic bronchitis who requires therapy with oral theophylline. He currently smokes three packs of cigarettes daily and has normal liver and cardiac function. Suggest an initial oral theophylline dosage regimen designed to achieve a steady-state theophylline concentration equal to 10 μg/mL.

2. Patient NJ (see problem 1) was prescribed theophylline sustained-release tablets 500 mg orally every 8 hours. The current steady-state theophylline concentration equals 18 μg/mL. Compute a new oral theophylline dose that will provide a steady-state concentration of 12 μg/mL.

3. GF is a 56-year-old, 81-kg (height = 5 ft 9 in) male with emphysema who requires therapy with oral theophylline. He has liver cirrhosis (Child-Pugh score = 12) and normal cardiac function. Suggest an initial theophylline dosage regimen designed to achieve a steady-state theophylline concentration equal to 8 μg/mL.

4. Patient GF (see problem 3) was prescribed theophylline sustained-release tablets 100 mg orally every 12 hours. The current steady-state theophylline concentration equals 8 μg/mL. Compute a new oral theophylline dose that will provide a steady-state concentration of 12 μg/mL.

5. YU is a 71-year-old, 60-kg (height = 5 ft 2 in) female with chronic obstructive pulmonary disease who requires therapy with oral theophylline. She has severe heart failure (NYHA CHF Class IV) and normal liver function. Suggest an initial theophylline dosage regimen designed to achieve a steady-state theophylline concentration equal to 8 μg/mL.

6. Patient YU (see problem 5) was prescribed theophylline sustained-release tablets 200 mg orally every 12 hours. A theophylline serum concentration was obtained just before the sixth dose of this regimen and equaled 19.5 μg/mL. Assuming the theophylline concentration was zero before the first dose, compute a new oral theophylline dose that will provide a steady-state concentration of 12 μg/mL.

7. WE is a 24-year-old, 55-kg (height = 5 ft 5 in) female with asthma who requires therapy with oral theophylline. She does not smoke cigarettes and has normal liver and cardiac function. Suggest an initial oral theophylline dosage regimen designed to achieve a steady-state theophylline concentration equal to 12 μg/mL.

8. Patient WE (see problem 7) was prescribed theophylline sustained-release tablets 400 mg orally every 12 hours. A theophylline serum concentration was obtained just before the third dose of this regimen and equaled 13.5 μg/mL. Assuming the theophylline concentration was zero before the first dose, compute a new oral theophylline dose that will provide a steady-state concentration of 10 μg/mL.

9. IO is a 62-year-old, 130-kg (height = 5 ft 11 in) male with chronic obstructive pulmonary disease who requires therapy with oral theophylline. He has mild heart failure (NYHA CHF Class I) and normal liver function. Suggest an initial theophylline dosage regimen designed to achieve a steady-state theophylline concentration equal to 8 μg/mL.

10. Patient IO (see problem 9) was prescribed theophylline sustained-release tablets 200 mg orally every 12 hours. A theophylline serum concentration was obtained just before the sixth dose of this regimen and equaled 6.2 μg/mL. Assuming the theophylline concentration was zero before the first dose, compute a new oral theophylline dose that will provide a steady-state concentration of 10 μg/mL.

11. LG is a 53-year-old, 69-kg (height = 5 ft 10 in) male with chronic bronchitis who requires therapy with intravenous theophylline. He currently smokes two packs of cigarettes daily, and has normal liver and cardiac function. Suggest an initial aminophylline dosage regimen designed to achieve a steady-state theophylline concentration equal to 8 μg/mL.

12. Patient LG (see problem 11) was prescribed intravenous aminophylline 50 mg/h. A theophylline serum concentration was obtained after 24 h of this regimen and equaled 7.4 μg/mL. Compute a new intravenous aminophylline infusion and an aminophylline booster dose that will provide a steady-state concentration of 11 μg/mL.

13. CV is a 69-year-old, 90-kg (height = 6 ft 1 in) male with emphysema who requires therapy with intravenous theophylline. He has liver cirrhosis (Child-Pugh score = 11) and normal cardiac function. Suggest an initial intravenous aminophylline dosage regimen designed to achieve a steady-state theophylline concentration equal to 10 μg/mL.

14. Patient CV (see problem 13) was prescribed intravenous aminophylline 25 mg/h and administered a loading dose of aminophylline 400 mg over 30 minutes before the continuous infusion began. A theophylline serum concentration was obtained after 72 h of the infusion and equaled 25.2 μg/mL. Compute a new intravenous aminophylline infusion that will provide a steady-state concentration of 15 μg/mL.

15. PE is a 61-year-old, 67-kg (height = 5 ft 6 in) female with chronic obstructive pulmonary disease who requires therapy with intravenous theophylline. She has severe heart failure (NYHA CHF Class IV) and normal liver function. Suggest an initial intravenous aminophylline dosage regimen designed to achieve a steady-state theophylline concentration equal to 8 μg/mL.

16. Patient PE (see problem 15) was prescribed intravenous aminophylline 20 mg/h and administered a loading dose of aminophylline 350 mg over 20 minutes before the continuous infusion began. Theophylline serum concentrations were obtained 12 h and 24 h after the infusion began and equaled 14.2 μg/mL and 18.6 μg/mL, respectively. Compute a new intravenous aminophylline infusion that will provide a steady-state concentration of 18 μg/mL.

17. ZQ is a 7-year-old, 20-kg (height = 4 ft 7 in) female with asthma who requires therapy with oral theophylline. She has normal liver and cardiac function. Suggest an initial oral theophylline dosage regimen designed to achieve a steady-state theophylline concentration equal to 6 μg/mL.

18. Patient ZQ (see problem 17) was prescribed theophylline sustained-release tablets 100 mg orally every 8 hours. A theophylline serum concentration was obtained after 3 days of this regimen and equaled 4 μg/mL just before the seventh dose was administered. Suggest a new oral theophylline dose that will provide a steady-state concentration of 6 μg/mL.

ANSWERS TO PROBLEMS

1. *Answer to problem 1.*

   The initial theophylline dose for patient NJ would be calculated as follows:

Pharmacokinetic Dosing Method

1. *Estimate the half-life and elimination rate constant according to disease states and conditions present in the patient.*

Cigarette smoke induces the enzyme systems responsible for theophylline metabolism, and the expected theophylline half-life ($t_{1/2}$) is 5 hours. The elimination rate constant is computed using the following formula: $k = 0.693/t_{1/2} = 0.693/5 \text{ h} = 0.139 \text{ h}^{-1}$.

2. *Estimate volume of distribution and clearance.*

The patient is not obese, so the estimated theophylline volume of distribution will be based on actual body weight: $V = 0.5 \text{ L/kg} \bullet 72 \text{ kg} = 36 \text{ L}$. Estimated theophylline clearance is computed by taking the product of the volume of distribution and the elimination rate constant: $Cl = kV = 0.139 \text{ h}^{-1} \bullet 36 \text{ L} = 5.0 \text{ L/h}$.

3. *Compute dosage regimen.*

Oral sustained-release theophylline tablets will be prescribed to this patient ($F = 1, S = 1$). Because the patient has a rapid theophylline clearance and half-life, the initial dosage interval (τ) will be set to 8 hours. (Note: µg/mL = mg/L and this concentration unit was substituted for Css in the calculations so that unnecessary unit conversion was not required.) The dosage equation for oral theophylline is: $D = (Css \bullet Cl \bullet \tau)/(F \bullet S) = (10 \text{ mg/L} \bullet 5.0 \text{ L/h} \bullet 8h)/(1 \bullet 1) = 400 \text{ mg}$ every 8 hours.

A steady-state trough theophylline serum concentration should be measured after steady-state is attained in 3-5 half-lives. Since the patient is expected to have a half-life equal to 5 hours, the theophylline steady-state concentration could be obtained any time after the first day of dosing (5 half-lives = $5 \bullet 5$ h = 25 h). Theophylline serum concentrations should also be measured if the patient experiences an exacerbation of their lung disease, or if the patient develops potential signs or symptoms of theophylline toxicity.

Literature-Based Recommended Dosing

1. *Choose theophylline dose based on disease states and conditions present in the patient.*

A theophylline dose of 0.7 mg/kg/h is suggested by the table for an adult smoker.

2. *Compute dosage regimen.*

Oral sustained-release theophylline tablets will be prescribed to this patient ($F = 1, S = 1$). Because the patient has a rapid theophylline clearance and half-life, the initial dosage interval (τ) will be set to 8 hours: $D = (\text{theophylline dose} \bullet Wt \bullet \tau)/S = (0.7 \text{ mg/kg/h} \bullet 72 \text{ kg} \bullet 8 \text{ h})/1 = 403 \text{ mg}$, rounded to 400 mg every 8 hours. This dose is identical to that suggested by the Pharmacokinetic Dosing method.

A steady-state trough theophylline serum concentration should be measured after steady-state is attained in 3-5 half-lives. Since the patient is expected to have a half-life equal to 5 hours, the theophylline steady-state concentration could be obtained any time after the first day of dosing (5 half-lives = $5 \bullet 5$ h = 25 h). Theophylline serum concentrations should also be measured if the patient experiences an exacerbation of their lung disease, or if the patient develops potential signs or symptoms of theophylline toxicity.

2. *Answer to problem 2.*

The revised theophylline dose for patient NJ would be calculated as follows:

Linear Pharmacokinetics Method

1. *Compute new dose to achieve the desired serum concentration.*

The patient smokes tobacco-containing cigarettes and would be expected to achieve steady-state conditions after the first day (5 $t_{1/2}$ = $5 \bullet 5$ h = 25 h) of therapy.

Using linear pharmacokinetics, the new dose to attain the desired concentration should be proportional to the old dose that produced the measured concentration (total daily dose = 500 mg/dose • 3 doses/d = 1500 mg/d):

$$D_{new} = (C_{ss,new}/C_{ss,old})D_{old} = (12 \text{ μg/mL} / 18 \text{ μg/mL}) \ 1500 \text{ mg/d} = 1000 \text{ mg/d}$$

The new suggested dose would be rounded to 900 mg/d or 300 mg every 8 hours of theophylline sustained-release tablets to be started at the next scheduled dosing time.

A steady-state trough theophylline serum concentration should be measured after steady-state is attained in 3-5 half-lives. Since the patient is expected to have a half-life equal to 5 hours, the theophylline steady-state concentration could be obtained any time after the first day of dosing (5 half-lives = 5 • 5 h = 25 h). Theophylline serum concentrations should also be measured if the patient experiences an exacerbation of their lung disease, or if the patient develops potential signs or symptoms of theophylline toxicity.

Pharmacokinetic Parameter Method

1. *Compute pharmacokinetic parameters.*

   The patient smokes tobacco-containing cigarettes and would be expected to achieve steady-state conditions after the first day (5 $t_{1/2}$ = 5 • 5 h = 25 h) of therapy.

   Theophylline clearance can be computed using a steady-state theophylline concentration: Cl = [F • S (D/τ)]/Css = [1 • 1 (500 mg/8 h)]/(18 mg/L) = 3.47 L/h. (Note: μg/mL = mg/L and this concentration unit was substituted for Css in the calculations so that unnecessary unit conversion was not required.)

2. *Compute theophylline dose.*

   Theophylline clearance is used to compute the new dose: D = (Css • Cl • τ)/(F • S) = (12 mg/L • 3.47 L/h • 8 h)/(1 • 1) = 333 mg, rounded to 300 mg every 8 hours.

   The new theophylline dosage regimen would be instituted at the next dosage time.

   A steady-state trough theophylline serum concentration should be measured after steady-state is attained in 3-5 half-lives. Since the patient is expected to have a half-life equal to 5 hours, the theophylline steady-state concentration could be obtained any time after the first day of dosing (5 half-lives = 5 • 5 h = 25 h). Theophylline serum concentrations should also be measured if the patient experiences an exacerbation of their lung disease, or if the patient develops potential signs or symptoms of theophylline toxicity.

3. *Answer to problem 3.*

   The initial theophylline dose for patient GF would be calculated as follows:

Pharmacokinetic Dosing Method

1. *Estimate half-life and elimination rate constant according to disease states and conditions present in the patient.*

   Patients with severe liver disease have highly variable theophylline pharmacokinetics and dosage requirements. Hepatic disease destroys liver parenchyma where hepatic drug–metabolizing enzymes are contained, and the expected theophylline half-life ($t_{1/2}$) is 24 hours. The elimination rate constant is computed using the following formula: k = 0.693/$t_{1/2}$ = 0.693/24 h = 0.029 h^{-1}.

2. *Estimate the volume of distribution and clearance.*

   The patient is not obese, so the estimated theophylline volume of distribution will be based on actual body weight: V = 0.5 L/kg • 81 kg = 41 L. Estimated theophylline clearance is computed by taking the product of the volume of distribution and the elimination rate constant: Cl = kV = 0.029 h^{-1} • 41 L = 1.19 L/h.

3. *Compute dosage regimen.*

Oral sustained-release theophylline tablets will be prescribed to this patient (F = 1, S = 1). The initial dosage interval (τ) will be set to 12 hours. (Note: μg/mL = mg/L and this concentration unit was substituted for Css in the calculations so that unnecessary unit conversion was not required.) The dosage equation for oral theophylline is: D = (Css • Cl • τ)/(F • S) = (8 mg/L • 1.19 L/h • 12 h)/(1 • 1) = 114 mg, rounded to 100 mg every 12 hours.

A steady-state trough theophylline serum concentration should be measured after steady-state is attained in 3-5 half-lives. Since the patient is expected to have a half-life equal to 24 hours, the theophylline steady-state concentration could be obtained any time after the fifth day of dosing (5 half-lives = 5 • 24 h = 120 h or 5 days). Theophylline serum concentrations should also be measured if the patient experiences an exacerbation of their lung disease, or if the patient develops potential signs or symptoms of theophylline toxicity.

Literature-Based Recommended Dosing

1. *Choose theophylline dose based on disease states and conditions present in the patient.*

A theophylline dose of 0.2 mg/kg/h is suggested by the table for an adult with cirrhosis.

2. *Compute dosage regimen.*

Oral sustained-release theophylline tablets will be prescribed to this patient (F = 1, S = 1). The initial dosage interval (τ) will be set to 12 hours: D = (theophylline dose • Wt • τ)/S = (0.2 mg/kg/h • 81 kg • 12 h)/1 = 194 mg, rounded to 200 mg every 12 hours. This dose is similar to that suggested by the Pharmacokinetic Dosing method of 100 mg every 12 hours.

A steady-state trough theophylline serum concentration should be measured after steady-state is attained in 3-5 half-lives. Since the patient is expected to have a half-life equal to 24 hours, the theophylline steady-state concentration could be obtained any time after the fifth day of dosing (5 half-lives = 5 • 24 h = 120 h or 5 days). Theophylline serum concentrations should also be measured if the patient experiences an exacerbation of their lung disease, or if the patient develops potential signs or symptoms of theophylline toxicity.

4. *Answer to problem 4.*

The revised theophylline dose for patient GF would be calculated as follows:

Linear Pharmacokinetics Method

1. *Compute new dose to achieve the desired serum concentration.*

The patient has liver disease and would be expected to achieve steady-state conditions after the fifth day (5 $t_{1/2}$ = 5 • 24 h = 120 h or 5 d) of therapy.

Using linear pharmacokinetics, the new dose to attain the desired concentration should be proportional to the old dose that produced the measured concentration (total daily dose = 100 mg/dose • 2 doses/d = 200 mg/d):

$$D_{new} = (C_{ss,new}/C_{ss,old})D_{old} = (12 \ \mu g/mL \ / \ 8 \ \mu g/mL) \ 200 \ mg/d = 300 \ mg/d$$

The new suggested dose would be 300 mg/d or 150 mg every 12 hours of theophylline sustained-release tablets to be started at the next scheduled dosing time.

A steady-state trough theophylline serum concentration should be measured after steady-state is attained in 3-5 half-lives. Since the patient is expected to have a half-life equal to 24 hours, the theophylline steady-state concentration could be obtained any time after the fifth day of dosing (5 half-lives = 5 • 24 h = 120 h or 5 d). Theophylline serum concentrations should also be measured if the patient experiences an exacerbation of their lung disease, or if the patient develops potential signs or symptoms of theophylline toxicity.

Pharmacokinetic Parameter Method

1. *Compute pharmacokinetic parameters.*

   The patient has liver disease and would be expected to achieve steady-state conditions after the fifth day (5 $t_{1/2}$ = 5 • 24 h = 120 h or 5 d) of therapy.

   Theophylline clearance can be computed using a steady-state theophylline concentration: Cl = [F • S (D/τ)]/Css = [1 • 1 (100 mg/12 h)]/ (8 mg/L) = 1.04 L/h. (Note: μg/mL = mg/L and this concentration unit was substituted for Css in the calculations so that unnecessary unit conversion was not required).

2. *Compute theophylline dose.*

   Theophylline clearance is used to compute the new dose: D = (Css • Cl • τ)/(F • S) = (12 mg/L • 1.04 L/h • 12 h)/(1 • 1) = 150 mg every 12 hours.

   The new theophylline dosage regimen would be instituted at the next dosage time.

   A steady-state trough theophylline serum concentration should be measured after steady-state is attained in 3-5 half-lives. Since the patient is expected to have a half-life equal to 24 hours, the theophylline steady-state concentration could be obtained any time after the fifth day of dosing (5 half-lives = 5 • 24 h = 120 h or 5 d). Theophylline serum concentrations should also be measured if the patient experiences an exacerbation of their lung disease, or if the patient develops potential signs or symptoms of theophylline toxicity.

5. *Answer to problem 5.*

   The initial theophylline dose for patient YU would be calculated as follows:

Pharmacokinetic Dosing Method

1. *Estimate half-life and elimination rate constant according to disease states and conditions present in the patient.*

   Patients with severe heart failure have highly variable theophylline pharmacokinetics and dosage requirements. Heart failure patients have decreased cardiac output which leads to decreased liver blood flow, and the expected theophylline half-life ($t_{1/2}$) is 24 hours. The elimination rate constant is computed using the following formula: k = $0.693/t_{1/2}$ = 0.693/24 h = 0.029 h^{-1}.

2. *Estimate volume of distribution and clearance.*

   The patient is not obese, so the estimated theophylline volume of distribution will be based on actual body weight: V = 0.5 L/kg • 60 kg = 30 L. Estimated theophylline clearance is computed by taking the product of the volume of distribution and the elimination rate constant: Cl = kV = 0.029 h^{-1} • 30 L = 0.87 L/h.

3. *Compute dosage regimen.*

   Oral sustained-release theophylline tablets will be prescribed to this patient (F = 1, S = 1). The initial dosage interval (τ) will be set to 12 hours. (Note: μg/mL = mg/L and this concentration unit was substituted for Css in the calculations so that unnecessary unit conversion was not required.) The dosage equation for oral theophylline is: D = (Css • Cl • τ)/(F • S) = (8 mg/L • 0.87 L/h • 12 h)/(1 • 1) = 84 mg, rounded to 100 mg every 12 hours.

   A steady-state trough theophylline serum concentration should be measured after steady-state is attained in 3-5 half-lives. Since the patient is expected to have a half-life equal to 24 hours, the theophylline steady-state concentration could be obtained any time after the fifth day of dosing (5 half-lives = 5 • 24 h = 120 h or 5 days). Theophylline serum concentrations should also be measured if the patient experiences an exacerbation of their lung disease, or if the patient develops potential signs or symptoms of theophylline toxicity. Theophylline pharmacokinetic parameters can change as the patient's cardiac status changes. If heart failure improves, cardiac output will increase resulting in increased liver blood flow and theophylline clearance.

Alternatively, if heart failure worsens, cardiac output will decrease further resulting in decreased liver blood flow and theophylline clearance. Thus, patients with heart failure receiving theophylline therapy must be monitored very carefully.

Literature-Based Recommended Dosing

1. *Choose theophylline dose based on disease states and conditions present in the patient.*

   A theophylline dose of 0.2 mg/kg/h is suggested by the table for an adult with severe heart failure.

2. *Compute dosage regimen.*

   Oral sustained-release theophylline tablets will be prescribed to this patient (F = 1, S = 1). The initial dosage interval (τ) will be set to 12 hours: D = (theophylline dose • Wt • τ)/S = (0.2 mg/kg/h • 60 kg • 12 h)/1 = 144 mg, rounded to 150 mg every 12 hours. This dose is similar to that suggested by the Pharmacokinetic Dosing method of 100 mg every 12 hours.

   A steady-state trough theophylline serum concentration should be measured after steady-state is attained in 3-5 half-lives. Since the patient is expected to have a half-life equal to 24 hours, the theophylline steady-state concentration could be obtained any time after the fifth day of dosing (5 half-lives = 5 • 24 h = 120 h or 5 days). Theophylline serum concentrations should also be measured if the patient experiences an exacerbation of their lung disease, or if the patient develops potential signs or symptoms of theophylline toxicity. Theophylline pharmacokinetic parameters can change as the patient's cardiac status changes. If heart failure improves, cardiac output will increase resulting in increased liver blood flow and theophylline clearance. Alternatively, if heart failure worsens, cardiac output will decrease further resulting in decreased liver blood flow and theophylline clearance. Thus, patients with heart failure receiving theophylline therapy must be monitored very carefully.

6. *Answer to problem 6.*

   The revised theophylline dose for patient YU would be calculated as follows:

   The patient has severe heart failure and would be expected to achieve steady-state conditions after the fifth day (5 $t_{1/2}$ = 5 • 24 h = 120 h or 5 d) of therapy. Because the serum theophylline serum concentration was obtained on the third day of therapy, it is unlikely that steady-state has been attained, so the Linear Pharmacokinetics or Pharmacokinetic Parameter methods cannot be used.

Bayesian Pharmacokinetic Computer Programs Method

1. *Enter the patient's demographic, drug-dosing, and serum concentration/time data into the computer program.*

2. *Compute pharmacokinetic parameters for the patient using Bayesian pharmacokinetic computer program.*

   The pharmacokinetic parameters computed by the program are a volume of distribution of 24.5 L, a half-life equal to 26.6 h, and a clearance equal to 0.64 L/h.

3. *Compute the dose required to achieve the desired theophylline serum concentrations.*

   The one-compartment model first-order absorption equations used by the program to compute doses indicates that a dose of 100 mg every 12 hours will produce a steady-state theophylline concentration of 12.4 µg/mL.

7. *Answer to problem 7.*

   The initial theophylline dose for patient WE would be calculated as follows:

Pharmacokinetic Dosing Method

1. *Estimate half-life and elimination rate constant according to disease states and conditions present in the patient.*

    The expected theophylline half-life ($t_{1/2}$) is 8 hours. The elimination rate constant is computed using the following formula: $k = 0.693/t_{1/2} = 0.693/8 \text{ h} = 0.087 \text{ h}^{-1}$.

2. *Estimate volume of distribution and clearance.*

    The patient is not obese, so the estimated theophylline volume of distribution will be based on actual body weight: $V = 0.5 \text{ L/kg} \bullet 55 \text{ kg} = 28 \text{ L}$. Estimated theophylline clearance is computed by taking the product of the volume of distribution and the elimination rate constant: $Cl = kV = 0.087 \text{ h}^{-1} \bullet 28 \text{ L} = 2.44 \text{ L/h}$.

3. *Compute dosage regimen.*

    Oral sustained-release theophylline tablets will be prescribed to this patient (F = 1, S = 1), and the initial dosage interval (τ) will be set to 12 hours. (Note: μg/mL = mg/L and this concentration unit was substituted for Css in the calculations so that unnecessary unit conversion was not required.) The dosage equation for oral theophylline is: $D = (Css \bullet Cl \bullet \tau)/(F \bullet S) = (12 \text{ mg/L} \bullet 2.44 \text{ L/h} \bullet 12 \text{ h})/(1 \bullet 1) = 351 \text{ mg}$, rounded to 300 every 12 hours. (Note: dose rounded down because of the narrow therapeutic index for theophylline.)

    A steady-state trough theophylline serum concentration should be measured after steady-state is attained in 3-5 half-lives. Since the patient is expected to have a half-life equal to 8 hours, the theophylline steady-state concentration could be obtained any time after the second day of dosing (5 half-lives = $5 \bullet 8 \text{ h} = 40 \text{ h}$). Theophylline serum concentrations should also be measured if the patient experiences an exacerbation of their lung disease, or if the patient develops potential signs or symptoms of theophylline toxicity.

Literature-Based Recommended Dosing

1. *Choose theophylline dose based on disease states and conditions present in the patient.*

    A theophylline dose of 0.4 mg/kg/h is suggested by the table for an adult without other disease states or conditions that alter theophylline dosing.

2. *Compute dosage regimen.*

    Oral sustained-release theophylline tablets will be prescribed to this patient (F = 1, S = 1), and the initial dosage interval (τ) will be set to 12 hours: $D = (\text{theophylline dose} \bullet Wt \bullet \tau)/S = (0.4 \text{ mg/kg/h} \bullet 55 \text{ kg} \bullet 12 \text{ h})/1 = 264 \text{ mg}$, rounded to 300 mg every 12 hours. This dose is identical to that suggested by the Pharmacokinetic Dosing method.

    A steady-state trough theophylline serum concentration should be measured after steady-state is attained in 3-5 half-lives. Since the patient is expected to have a half-life equal to 8 hours, the theophylline steady-state concentration could be obtained any time after the second day of dosing (5 half-lives = $5 \bullet 8 \text{ h} = 40 \text{ h}$). Theophylline serum concentrations should also be measured if the patient experiences an exacerbation of their lung disease, or if the patient develops potential signs or symptoms of theophylline toxicity.

8. *Answer to problem 8.*

    The revised theophylline dose for patient WE would be calculated as follows:

    The patient has normal cardiac and hepatic function and would be expected to achieve steady-state conditions after the second day (5 $t_{1/2}$ = $5 \bullet 8 \text{ h} = 40 \text{ h}$) of therapy. Because the serum theophylline serum concentration was obtained before the third dose, it is unlikely that the serum concentration was obtained at steady-state so the Linear Pharmacokinetics or Pharmacokinetic Parameter methods cannot be used.

Bayesian Pharmacokinetic Computer Programs Method

1. *Enter the patient's demographic, drug-dosing, and serum concentration/time data into the computer program.*

2. *Compute pharmacokinetic parameters for the patient using Bayesian pharmacokinetic computer program.*

    The pharmacokinetic parameters computed by the program are a volume of distribution of 24.6 L, a half-life equal to 15 h, and a clearance equal to 1.14 L/h.

3. *Compute the dose required to achieve the desired theophylline serum concentrations.*

    The one-compartment model first-order absorption equations used by the program to compute doses indicates that a dose of 150 mg every 12 hours will produce a steady-state theophylline concentration of 10 μg/mL.

9. *Answer to problem 9.*

    The initial theophylline dose for patient IO would be calculated as follows:

Pharmacokinetic Dosing Method

1. *Estimate half-life and elimination rate constant according to disease states and conditions present in the patient.*

    Patients with mild heart failure have highly variable theophylline pharmacokinetics and dosage requirements. Heart failure patients have decreased cardiac output which leads to decreased liver blood flow, and the expected theophylline half-life $(t_{1/2})$ is 12 hours. The elimination rate constant is computed using the following formula: $k = 0.693/t_{1/2} = 0.693/12 \text{ h} = 0.058 \text{ h}^{-1}$.

2. *Estimate volume of distribution and clearance.*

    The patient is obese [IBW_{male} (in kg) = 50 kg + 2.3(Ht − 60) = 50 kg + 2.3(71 in − 60) = 75 kg, patient >30% over ideal body weight], so the estimated theophylline volume of distribution will be based on ideal body weight: V = 0.5 L/kg • 75 kg = 38 L. Estimated theophylline clearance is computed by taking the product of the volume of distribution and the elimination rate constant: $Cl = kV = 0.058 \text{ h}^{-1} • 38 \text{ L} = 2.20 \text{ L/h}$.

3. *Compute dosage regimen.*

    Oral sustained-release theophylline tablets will be prescribed to this patient (F = 1, S = 1). The initial dosage interval (τ) will be set to 12 hours. (Note: μg/mL = mg/L and this concentration unit was substituted for Css in the calculations so that unnecessary unit conversion was not required.) The dosage equation for oral theophylline is: $D = (Css • Cl • \tau)/(F • S) = (8 \text{ mg/L} • 2.20 \text{ L/h} • 12 \text{ h})/(1 • 1) = 211$ mg, rounded to 200 mg every 12 hours.

    A steady-state trough theophylline serum concentration should be measured after steady-state is attained in 3-5 half-lives. Since the patient is expected to have a half-life equal to 12 hours, the theophylline steady-state concentration could be obtained any time after the third day of dosing (5 half-lives = 5 • 12 h = 60 h). Theophylline serum concentrations should also be measured if the patient experiences an exacerbation of their lung disease, or if the patient develops potential signs or symptoms of theophylline toxicity. Theophylline pharmacokinetic parameters can change as the patient's cardiac status changes. If heart failure improves, cardiac output will increase resulting in increased liver blood flow and theophylline clearance. Alternatively, if heart failure worsens, cardiac output will decrease further resulting in decreased liver blood flow and theophylline clearance. Thus, patients with heart failure receiving theophylline therapy must be monitored very carefully.

Literature-Based Recommended Dosing

1. *Choose theophylline dose based on disease states and conditions present in the patient.*

   A theophylline dose of 0.2 mg/kg/h is suggested by the table for an adult with heart failure. Because the patient is obese [IBW_{male} (in kg) = 50 kg + 2.3(Ht − 60) = 50 kg + 2.3(71 in − 60) = 75 kg, patient >30% over ideal body weight], ideal body weight will be used to compute doses.

2. *Compute dosage regimen.*

   Oral sustained-release theophylline tablets will be prescribed to this patient (F = 1, S = 1). The initial dosage interval (τ) will be set to 12 hours: D = (theophylline dose • Wt • τ)/S = (0.2 mg/kg/h • 75 kg • 12 h)/1 = 180 mg, rounded to 200 mg every 12 hours. This dose is the same as that suggested by the Pharmacokinetic Dosing method.

   A steady-state trough theophylline serum concentration should be measured after steady-state is attained in 3-5 half-lives. Since the patient is expected to have a half-life equal to 12 hours, the theophylline steady-state concentration could be obtained any time after the third day of dosing (5 half-lives = 5 • 12 h = 60 h). Theophylline serum concentrations should also be measured if the patient experiences an exacerbation of their lung disease, or if the patient develops potential signs or symptoms of theophylline toxicity. Theophylline pharmacokinetic parameters can change as the patient's cardiac status changes. If heart failure improves, cardiac output will increase resulting in increased liver blood flow and theophylline clearance. Alternatively, if heart failure worsens, cardiac output will decrease further resulting in decreased liver blood flow and theophylline clearance. Thus, patients with heart failure receiving theophylline therapy must be monitored very carefully.

10. *Answer to problem 10.*

    The revised theophylline dose for patient IO would be calculated as follows:

    The patient has mild heart failure and would be expected to achieve steady-state conditions after the third day (5 $t_{1/2}$ = 5 • 12 h = 60 h) of therapy. Since the serum theophylline serum concentration was obtained on the third day of therapy, it is possible that the serum concentration was obtained at steady-state, but half-life can vary widely in patients with heart failure. Because of this, the Linear Pharmacokinetics or Pharmacokinetic Parameter methods were not used for this patient.

Bayesian Pharmacokinetic Computer Programs Method

1. *Enter the patient's demographic, drug-dosing, and serum concentration/time data into the computer program.*

2. *Compute pharmacokinetic parameters for the patient using Bayesian pharmacokinetic computer program.*

   The pharmacokinetic parameters computed by the program are a volume of distribution of 39.4 L, a half-life equal to 12.4 h, and a clearance equal to 2.20 L/h.

3. *Compute the dose required to achieve the desired theophylline serum concentrations.*

   The one-compartment model first-order absorption equations used by the program to compute doses indicates that a dose of 300 mg every 12 hours will produce a steady-state theophylline concentration of 10.2 μg/mL.

   A steady-state trough theophylline serum concentration should be measured after steady-state is attained in 3-5 half-lives. Since the patient is expected to have a half-life equal to 12 hours, the theophylline steady-state concentration could be obtained any time after the third day of dosing (5 half-lives = 5 • 12 h = 60 h). Theophylline serum concentrations should also be measured if the patient experiences an exacerbation of their lung disease, or if the patient develops potential signs or symptoms of theophylline toxicity. Theophylline pharmacokinetic parameters can change as the patient's cardiac status changes. If heart failure improves, cardiac output will increase resulting in increased liver blood flow and theophylline clearance. Alternatively, if heart failure worsens, cardiac output will decrease further resulting in decreased liver blood flow and theophylline clearance. Thus, patients with heart failure receiving theophylline therapy must be monitored very carefully.

11. *Answer to problem 11.*
    The initial theophylline dose for patient LG would be calculated as follows:

Pharmacokinetic Dosing Method

1. *Estimate half-life and elimination rate constant according to disease states and conditions present in the patient.*

    Cigarette smoke induces the enzyme systems responsible for theophylline metabolism, and the expected theophylline half-life ($t_{1/2}$) is 5 hours. The elimination rate constant is computed using the following formula: $k = 0.693/t_{1/2} = 0.693/5 \text{ h} = 0.139 \text{ h}^{-1}$.

2. *Estimate volume of distribution and clearance.*

    The patient is not obese, so the estimated theophylline volume of distribution will be based on actual body weight: $V = 0.5 \text{ L/kg} \bullet 69 \text{ kg} = 35 \text{ L}$. Estimated theophylline clearance is computed by taking the product of the volume of distribution and the elimination rate constant: $Cl = kV = 0.139 \text{ h}^{-1} \bullet 35 \text{ L} = 4.87 \text{ L/h}$.

3. *Compute dosage regimen.*

    Theophylline will be administered as the aminophylline dihydrate salt form (S = 0.8). (Note: μg/mL = mg/L and this concentration unit was substituted for Css in the calculations so that unnecessary unit conversion was not required.) Therapy will be started by administering an intravenous loading dose of aminophylline to the patient: $LD = (Css \bullet V)/S = (8 \text{ mg/L} \bullet 35 \text{ L})/0.8 = 350 \text{ mg}$ intravenously over 20-30 minutes.

    An aminophylline continuous intravenous infusion will be started immediately after the loading dose has been administered. (Note: μg/mL = mg/L and this concentration unit was substituted for Css in the calculations so that unnecessary unit conversion was not required.) The dosage equation for intravenous aminophylline is: $k_0 = (Css \bullet Cl)/S = (8 \text{ mg/L} \bullet 4.87 \text{ L/h})/0.8 = 49 \text{ mg/h}$, rounded to 50 mg/h.

    A steady-state theophylline serum concentration should be measured after steady-state is attained in 3-5 half-lives. Since the patient is expected to have a half-life equal to 5 hours, the theophylline steady-state concentration could be obtained any time after the first day of dosing (5 half-lives = $5 \bullet 5 \text{ h} = 25 \text{ h}$). Theophylline serum concentrations should also be measured if the patient experiences an exacerbation of their lung disease, or if the patient develops potential signs or symptoms of theophylline toxicity.

Literature-Based Recommended Dosing

1. *Choose theophylline dose based on disease states and conditions present in the patient.*
    A theophylline dose of 0.7 mg/kg/h is suggested by the table for an adult cigarette smoker.

2. *Compute dosage regimen.*
    Theophylline will be administered as the aminophylline dihydrate salt form (S = 0.8): $k_0 = $ (theophylline dose $\bullet$ Wt)/S = (0.7 mg/kg/h $\bullet$ 69 kg)/0.8 = 60 mg/h. A loading dose of aminophylline 6 mg/kg will also be prescribed for the patient: $LD = 6 \text{ mg/kg} \bullet 69 \text{ kg} = 414 \text{ mg}$, rounded to 400 mg of aminophylline infused over 20-30 minutes. Similar doses were suggested by the Pharmacokinetic Dosing method.

A theophylline serum concentration should be measured after steady-state is attained in 3-5 half-lives. Since the patient is expected to have a half-life equal to 5 hours, the theophylline steady-state concentration could be obtained any time after the first day of dosing (5 half-lives = 5 • 5 h = 25 h). Theophylline serum concentrations should also be measured if the patient experiences an exacerbation of their lung disease, or if the patient develops potential signs or symptoms of theophylline toxicity.

12. *Answer to problem 12.*

The revised theophylline dose for patient LG would be calculated as follows:

Linear Pharmacokinetics Method

1. *Compute new dose to achieve the desired serum concentration.*

The patient smokes tobacco-containing cigarettes and would be expected to achieve steady-state conditions after the first day (5 $t_{1/2}$ = 5 • 5 h = 25 h) of therapy.

Using linear pharmacokinetics, the new infusion rate to attain the desired concentration should be proportional to the old infusion rate that produced the measured concentration:

$$D_{new} = (C_{ss,new}/C_{ss,old})D_{old} = (11 \text{ µg/mL} / 7.4 \text{ µg/mL}) 50 \text{ mg/h} = 74.3 \text{ mg/h},$$
rounded to 75 mg/h

The new suggested infusion rate would be 75 mg/h of aminophylline.

A booster dose of aminophylline would be computed using an estimated volume of distribution for the patient (0.5 L/kg • 69 kg = 35 L): BD = $[(C_{desired} - C_{actual})V]/S = [(11 \text{ mg/L} - 7.4 \text{ mg/L}) 35L]/0.8$ = 157 mg, rounded to 150 mg of aminophylline over 20-30 minutes. The booster dose would be given to the patient before the infusion rate was increased to the new value.

A steady-state trough theophylline serum concentration should be measured after steady-state is attained in 3-5 half-lives. Since the patient is expected to have a half-life equal to 5 hours, the theophylline steady-state concentration could be obtained any time after the first day of dosing (5 half-lives = 5 • 5 h = 25 h). Theophylline serum concentrations should also be measured if the patient experiences an exacerbation of their lung disease, or if the patient develops potential signs or symptoms of theophylline toxicity.

Pharmacokinetic Parameter Method

1. *Compute pharmacokinetic parameters.*

The patient smokes tobacco-containing cigarettes and would be expected to achieve steady-state conditions after the first day (5 $t_{1/2}$ = 5 • 5 h = 25 h) of therapy.

Theophylline clearance can be computed using a steady-state theophylline concentration Cl = $[S • k_0]/Css = [0.8 • 50 \text{ mg/h})]/(7.4 \text{ mg/L}) = 5.41 \text{ L/h}$. (Note: µg/mL = mg/L and this concentration unit was substituted for Css in the calculations so that unnecessary unit conversion was not required.)

2. *Compute theophylline dose.*

Theophylline clearance is used to compute the new aminophylline infusion rate: $k_0 = (Css • Cl)/S = (11 \text{ mg/L} • 5.41 \text{ L/h})/(0.8) = 74 \text{ mg/h}$, rounded to 75 mg/h.

A booster dose of aminophylline would be computed using an estimated volume of distribution for the patient (0.5 L/kg • 69 kg = 35 L): BD = $[(C_{desired} - C_{actual})V]/S = [(11 \text{ mg/L} - 7.4 \text{ mg/L}) 35L]/0.8$ = 157 mg, rounded to 150 mg of aminophylline over 20-30 minutes. The booster dose would be given to the patient before the infusion rate was increased to the new value.

A steady-state trough theophylline serum concentration should be measured after steady-state is attained in 3-5 half-lives. Since the patient is expected to have a half-life equal to 5 hours, the theophylline steady-state concentration could be obtained any time after the first day of dosing (5 half-lives = 5 • 5 h = 25 h). Theophylline serum concentrations should also be measured if the patient experiences an exacerbation of their lung disease, or if the patient develops potential signs or symptoms of theophylline toxicity.

13. *Answer to problem 13.*
    The initial theophylline dose for patient CV would be calculated as follows:

Pharmacokinetic Dosing Method

1. *Estimate half-life and elimination rate constant according to disease states and conditions present in the patient.*

   Patients with severe liver disease have highly variable theophylline pharmacokinetics and dosage requirements. Hepatic disease destroys liver parenchyma where hepatic drug–metabolizing enzymes are contained, and the expected theophylline half-life ($t_{1/2}$) is 24 hours. The elimination rate constant is computed using the following formula: $k = 0.693/t_{1/2} = 0.693/24\ h = 0.029\ h^{-1}$.

2. *Estimate the volume of distribution and clearance.*

   The patient is not obese, so the estimated theophylline volume of distribution will be based on actual body weight: V = 0.5 L/kg • 90 kg = 45 L. Estimated theophylline clearance is computed by taking the product of the volume of distribution and the elimination rate constant: $Cl = kV = 0.029\ h^{-1} \cdot 45\ L = 1.31\ L/h$.

3. *Compute dosage regimen.*

   Theophylline will be administered as the aminophylline dihydrate salt form (S = 0.8). (Note: μg/mL = mg/L and this concentration unit was substituted for Css in the calculations so that unnecessary unit conversion was not required.) Therapy will be started by administering an intravenous loading dose of aminophylline to the patient: LD = (Css • V)/S = (10 mg/L • 45 L)/0.8 = 562 mg, rounded to 550 mg intravenously over 20-30 minutes.

   An aminophylline continuous intravenous infusion will be started immediately after the loading dose has been administered. (Note: μg/mL = mg/L and this concentration unit was substituted for Css in the calculations so that unnecessary unit conversion was not required.) The dosage equation for oral theophylline is: k_0 = (Css • Cl)/S = (10 mg/L • 1.31 L/h)/0.8 = 16 mg/h, rounded to 15 mg/h.

   A steady-state theophylline serum concentration should be measured after steady-state is attained in 3-5 half-lives. Since the patient is expected to have a half-life equal to 24 hours, the theophylline steady-state concentration could be obtained any time after the fifth day of dosing (5 half-lives = 5 • 24 h = 120 h or 5 days). Theophylline serum concentrations should also be measured if the patient experiences an exacerbation of their lung disease, or if the patient develops potential signs or symptoms of theophylline toxicity.

Literature-Based Recommended Dosing

1. *Choose theophylline dose based on disease states and conditions present in the patient.*

   A theophylline dose of 0.2 mg/kg/h is suggested by the table for an adult with cirrhosis.

2. *Compute dosage regimen.*

   Theophylline will be administered as the aminophylline dihydrate salt form (S = 0.8):
   D = (theophylline dose • Wt)/S = (0.2 mg/kg/h • 90 kg)/0.8 = 23 mg/h, rounded to 20 mg/h.

A loading dose of aminophylline 6 mg/kg will also be prescribed for the patient: LD = 6 mg/kg • 90 kg = 540 mg, rounded to 550 mg of aminophylline infused over 20-30 minutes. These doses are similar to that suggested by the Pharmacokinetic Dosing method of a 550-mg loading dose followed by a 15 mg/h continuous infusion.

A steady-state trough theophylline serum concentration should be measured after steady-state is attained in 3-5 half-lives. Since the patient is expected to have a half-life equal to 24 hours, the theophylline steady-state concentration could be obtained any time after the fifth day of dosing (5 half-lives = 5 • 24 h = 120 h or 5 d). Theophylline serum concentrations should also be measured if the patient experiences an exacerbation of their lung disease, or if the patient develops potential signs or symptoms of theophylline toxicity.

14. *Answer to problem 14.*

The revised theophylline dose for patient CV would be calculated as follows:

The patient has liver cirrhosis and would be expected to achieve steady-state conditions after the fifth day (5 $t_{1/2}$ = 5 • 24 h = 120 h or 5 d) of therapy. Because the serum theophylline serum concentration was obtained after 72 h of therapy, it is unlikely that the serum concentration was obtained at steady-state even though a loading dose was given so the Linear Pharmacokinetics or Pharmacokinetic Parameter methods cannot be used.

Bayesian Pharmacokinetic Computer Programs Method

1. *Enter the patient's demographic, drug-dosing, and serum concentration/time data into the computer program.*

In this patient case, it is unlikely that the patient is at steady-state so the Linear Pharmacokinetics method cannot be used. DrugCalc requires doses to be entered in terms of theophylline, so aminophylline doses must be converted to theophylline doses for entry into the program (LD = 400 mg aminophylline • 0.8 = 320 mg theophylline, k_0 = 25 mg/h aminophylline • 0.8 = 20 mg/h theophylline).

2. *Compute the pharmacokinetic parameters for the patient using Bayesian pharmacokinetic computer program.*

The pharmacokinetic parameters computed by the program are a volume of distribution of 37 L, a half-life equal to 38 h, and a clearance equal to 0.67 L/h.

3. *Compute the dose required to achieve the desired theophylline serum concentrations.*

The one-compartment model infusion equations used by the program to compute doses indicates that an aminophylline infusion of 13 mg/h will produce a steady-state theophylline concentration of 15 μg/mL. This dose would be started after holding the infusion for 40 hours (~1 half-life) to allow theophylline serum concentrations to decrease by one-half.

15. *Answer to problem 15.*

The initial theophylline dose for patient PE would be calculated as follows:

Pharmacokinetic Dosing Method

1. *Estimate half-life and elimination rate constant according to disease states and conditions present in the patient.*

Patients with severe heart failure have highly variable theophylline pharmacokinetics and dosage requirements. Heart failure patients have decreased cardiac output which leads to decreased liver blood flow, and the expected theophylline half-life ($t_{1/2}$) is 24 hours. The elimination rate constant is computed using the following formula: $k = 0.693/t_{1/2} = 0.693/24\ h = 0.029\ h^{-1}$.

2. *Estimate the volume of distribution and clearance.*

The patient is not obese, so the estimated theophylline volume of distribution will be based on actual body weight: V = 0.5 L/kg • 67 kg = 34 L. Estimated theophylline clearance is computed by taking the product of the volume of distribution and the elimination rate constant: Cl = kV = 0.029 h^{-1} • 34 L = 0.99 L/h.

3. *Compute dosage regimen.*

Theophylline will be administered as the aminophylline dihydrate salt form (S = 0.8). (Note: μg/mL = mg/L and this concentration unit was substituted for Css in the calculations so that unnecessary unit conversion was not required.) Therapy will be started by administering an intravenous loading dose of aminophylline to the patient: LD = (Css • V)/S = (8 mg/L • 34 L)/0.8 = 340 mg, rounded to 350 mg intravenously over 20-30 minutes.

An aminophylline continuous intravenous infusion will be started immediately after the loading dose has been administered. (Note: μg/mL = mg/L and this concentration unit was substituted for Css in the calculations so that unnecessary unit conversion was not required.) The dosage equation for intravenous aminophylline is: k_0 = (Css • Cl)/S = (8 mg/L • 0.99 L/h)/0.8 = 9.9 mg/h, rounded to 10 mg/h.

A steady-state theophylline serum concentration should be measured after steady-state is attained in 3-5 half-lives. Since the patient is expected to have a half-life equal to 24 hours, the theophylline steady-state concentration could be obtained any time after the fifth day of dosing (5 half-lives = 5 • 24 h = 120 h or 5 days). Theophylline serum concentrations should also be measured if the patient experiences an exacerbation of their lung disease, or if the patient develops potential signs or symptoms of theophylline toxicity. Theophylline pharmacokinetic parameters can change as the patient's cardiac status changes. If heart failure improves, cardiac output will increase resulting in increased liver blood flow and theophylline clearance. Alternatively, if heart failure worsens, cardiac output will decrease further resulting in decreased liver blood flow and theophylline clearance. Thus, patients with heart failure that receive theophylline therapy must be monitored very carefully.

Literature-Based Recommended Dosing

1. *Choose theophylline dose based on disease states and conditions present in the patient.*

A theophylline dose of 0.2 mg/kg/h is suggested by the table for an adult with severe heart failure.

2. *Compute dosage regimen.*

Theophylline will be administered as the aminophylline dihydrate salt form (S = 0.8): D = (theophylline dose • Wt)/S = (0.2 mg/kg/h • 67 kg)/0.8 = 17 mg/h, rounded to 15 mg/h. A loading dose of aminophylline 6 mg/kg will also be prescribed for the patient: LD = 6 mg/kg • 67 kg = 402 mg, rounded to 400 mg of aminophylline infused over 20-30 minutes. These doses are similar to that suggested by the Pharmacokinetic Dosing method.

A steady-state trough theophylline serum concentration should be measured after steady-state is attained in 3-5 half-lives. Since the patient is expected to have a half-life equal to 24 hours, the theophylline steady-state concentration could be obtained any time after the fifth day of dosing (5 half-lives = 5 • 24 h = 120 h or 5 days). Theophylline serum concentrations should also be measured if the patient experiences an exacerbation of their lung disease, or if the patient develops potential signs or symptoms of theophylline toxicity. Theophylline pharmacokinetic parameters can change as the patient's cardiac status changes. If heart failure improves, cardiac output will increase resulting in increased liver blood flow and theophylline clearance. Alternatively, if heart failure worsens, cardiac output will decrease further resulting in decreased liver blood flow and theophylline clearance. Thus, patients with heart failure that receive theophylline therapy must be monitored very carefully.

16. *Answer to problem 16.*

   The revised theophylline dose for patient PE would be calculated as follows:

   The patient has severe heart failure and would be expected to achieve steady-state conditions after the fifth day (5 $t_{1/2}$ = 5 • 24 h = 120 h or 5 d) of therapy. Because the serum theophylline serum concentrations were obtained after 12 h and 24 h of therapy, it is unlikely that the serum concentrations were obtained at steady-state even though a loading dose was given so the Linear Pharmacokinetics or Pharmacokinetic Parameter methods cannot be used.

Chiou Method

1. *Compute theophylline clearance.*

$$Cl = \frac{2 \bullet S \bullet k_0}{C_1 + C_2} + \frac{2V(C_1 - C_2)}{(C_1 + C_2)(t_2 - t_1)}$$

$$Cl = \frac{2[0.8(20 \text{ mg/h})]}{14.2 \text{ mg/L} + 18.6 \text{ mg/L}} + \frac{2(0.5 \text{ L/kg} \bullet 67 \text{ kg})(14.2 \text{ mg/L} - 18.6 \text{ mg/L})}{(14.2 \text{ mg/L} + 18.6 \text{ mg/L}) \, 12 \text{ h}} = 0.23 \text{ L/h}$$

   (Note: μg/mL = mg/L and this concentration unit was substituted for concentrations so that unnecessary unit conversion was not required. Additionally, the time difference between t_2 and t_1 was determined and placed directly in the calculation.)

$$k_0 = (Css \bullet Cl)/S = (18 \text{ mg/L} \bullet 0.23 \text{ L/h})/0.8 = 5 \text{ mg/h of aminophylline}$$

Bayesian Pharmacokinetic Computer Programs Method

1. *Enter the patient's demographic, drug-dosing, and serum concentration/time data into the computer program.*

   In this case, the patient is not at steady-state so the Linear Pharmacokinetics method cannot be used. DrugCalc requires doses to be entered in terms of theophylline, so aminophylline doses must be converted to theophylline doses for entry into the program (LD = 350 mg aminophylline • 0.8 = 280 mg theophylline, k_0 = 20 mg/h aminophylline • 0.8 = 16 mg/h theophylline).

2. *Compute pharmacokinetic parameters for the patient using Bayesian pharmacokinetic computer program.*

   The pharmacokinetic parameters computed by the program are a volume of distribution of 26 L, a half-life equal to 31 h, and a clearance equal to 0.59 L/h.

3. *Compute the dose required to achieve the desired theophylline serum concentrations.*

   The one-compartment model infusion equations used by the program to compute doses indicates that an aminophylline infusion of 14 mg/h will produce a steady-state theophylline concentration of 18 μg/mL.

17. *Answer to problem 17.*

   The initial theophylline dose for patient ZQ would be calculated as follows:

Pharmacokinetic Dosing Method

1. *Estimate the half-life and elimination rate constant according to disease states and conditions present in the patient.*

   The expected theophylline half-life ($t_{1/2}$) is 3.5 hours. The elimination rate constant is computed using the following formula: k = 0.693/$t_{1/2}$ = 0.693/3.5 h = 0.198 h^{-1}.

2. *Estimate volume of distribution and clearance.*

The estimated theophylline volume of distribution is: V = 0.5 L/kg • 20 kg = 10 L. Estimated theophylline clearance is computed by taking the product of the volume of distribution and the elimination rate constant: Cl = kV = 0.198 h^{-1} • 10 L = 1.98 L/h.

3. *Compute dosage regimen.*

Oral sustained-release theophylline tablets will be prescribed to this patient (F = 1, S = 1), and the initial dosage interval (τ) will be set to 8 hours because children have rapid clearance rates. (Note: µg/mL = mg/L and this concentration unit was substituted for Css in the calculations so that unnecessary unit conversion was not required.) The dosage equation for oral theophylline is: D = (Css • Cl • τ)/(F • S) = (6 mg/L • 1.98 L/h • 8 h)/(1 • 1) = 95 mg, rounded to 100 every 8 hours.

A steady-state trough theophylline serum concentration should be measured after steady-state is attained in 3-5 half-lives. Since the patient is expected to have a half-life equal to 3.5 hours, the theophylline steady-state concentration could be obtained any time after the first day of dosing (5 half-lives = 5 • 3.5 h = 17.5 h). Theophylline serum concentrations should also be measured if the patient experiences an exacerbation of their lung disease, or if the patient develops potential signs or symptoms of theophylline toxicity.

Literature-Based Recommended Dosing

1. *Choose theophylline dose based on disease states and conditions present in the patient.*

A theophylline dose of 0.8 mg/kg/h is suggested by the table for a child of this age.

2. *Compute dosage regimen.*

Oral sustained-release theophylline tablets will be prescribed to this patient (F = 1, S = 1), and the initial dosage interval (τ) will be set to 8 hours because children have rapid clearance rates: D = (theophylline dose • Wt • τ)/S = (0.8 mg/kg/h • 20 kg • 8 h)/1 = 128 mg, rounded to 100 mg every 12 hours (note: dose rounded down to avoid potential theophylline side effects). This dose is identical to that suggested by the Pharmacokinetic Dosing method.

A steady-state trough theophylline serum concentration should be measured after steady-state is attained in 3-5 half-lives. Since the patient is expected to have a half-life equal to 3.5 hours, the theophylline steady-state concentration could be obtained any time after the first day of dosing (5 half-lives = 5 • 3.5 h = 17.5 h). Theophylline serum concentrations should also be measured if the patient experiences an exacerbation of their lung disease, or if the patient develops potential signs or symptoms of theophylline toxicity.

18. *Answer to problem 18.*

The revised theophylline dose for patient ZQ would be calculated as follows:

Linear Pharmacokinetics Method

1. *Compute new dose to achieve the desired serum concentration.*

The patient would be expected to achieve steady-state conditions after the first day (5 t$_{1/2}$ = 5 • 3.5 h = 17.5 h) of therapy.

Using linear pharmacokinetics, the new dose to attain the desired concentration should be proportional to the old dose that produced the measured concentration (total daily dose = 100 mg/dose • 3 doses/d = 300 mg/d):

$$D_{new} = (C_{ss,new}/C_{ss,old})D_{old} = (6 \ \mu g/mL \ / \ 4 \ \mu g/mL) \ 300 \ mg/d = 450 \ mg/d$$

The new suggested dose would be 450 mg/d or 150 mg every 8 hours of theophylline sustained-release tablets to be started at the next scheduled dosing time.

A steady-state trough theophylline serum concentration should be measured after steady-state is attained in 3-5 half-lives. Since the patient is expected to have a half-life equal to 3.5 hours, the theophylline steady-state concentration could be obtained any time after the first day of dosing (5 half-lives = 5 • 3.5 h = 17.5 h). Theophylline serum concentrations should also be measured if the patient experiences an exacerbation of their lung disease, or if the patient develops potential signs or symptoms of theophylline toxicity.

Pharmacokinetic Parameter Method

1. *Compute pharmacokinetic parameters.*

   The patient would be expected to achieve steady-state conditions after the first day (5 $t_{1/2}$ = 5 • 3.5 h = 17.5 h) of therapy.

   Theophylline clearance can be computed using a steady-state theophylline concentration: Cl = [F • S (D/τ)]/Css = [1 • 1 (100 mg/8 h)]/(4 mg/L) = 3.13 L/h. (Note: μg/mL = mg/L and this concentration unit was substituted for Css in the calculations so that unnecessary unit conversion was not required.)

2. *Compute theophylline dose.*

   Theophylline clearance is used to compute the new dose: D = (Css • Cl • τ)/(F • S) = (6 mg/L • 3.13 L/h • 8 h)/(1 • 1) = 150 mg every 8 hours.

   The new theophylline dosage regimen would be instituted at the next dosage time.

   A steady-state trough theophylline serum concentration should be measured after steady-state is attained in 3-5 half-lives. Since the patient is expected to have a half-life equal to 3.5 hours, the theophylline steady-state concentration could be obtained any time after the first day of dosing (5 $t_{1/2}$ = 5 • 3.5 h = 17.5 h). Theophylline serum concentrations should also be measured if the patient experiences an exacerbation of their lung disease, or if the patient develops potential signs or symptoms of theophylline toxicity.

Bayesian Pharmacokinetic Computer Programs Method

1. *Enter the patient's demographic, drug-dosing, and serum concentration/time data into the computer program.*

2. *Compute pharmacokinetic parameters for the patient using Bayesian pharmacokinetic computer program.*

   The pharmacokinetic parameters computed by the program are a volume of distribution of 9.9 L, a half-life equal to 2.8 h, and a clearance equal to 2.45 L/h.

3. *Compute the dose required to achieve the desired theophylline serum concentrations.*

   The one-compartment model, first-order absorption equations used by the program to compute doses indicates that a dose of 150 mg every 8 hours will produce a steady-state theophylline concentration of 6.1 μg/mL.

REFERENCES

1. Weinberger M, Hendeles L. Drug Therapy: Theophylline in asthma. *N Engl J Med.* 1996;334(21):1380-1388.
2. Anon. In chronic obstructive pulmonary disease, a combination of ipratropium and albuterol is more effective than either agent alone. An 85-day multicenter trial. COMBIVENT Inhalation Aerosol Study Group. *Chest.* 1994;105(5):1411-1419.

3. Vaz Fragoso CA, Miller MA. Review of the clinical efficacy of theophylline in the treatment of chronic obstructive pulmonary disease. *Am Rev Respir Dis.* 1993;147(6, pt 2):40S–47S.

4. Wesseling G, Mostert R, Wouters EF. A comparison of the effects of anticholinergic and beta 2-agonist and combination therapy on respiratory impedance in COPD. *Chest.* 1992;101(1):166-173.

5. Kelly HW, Sorkness CA. Asthma. In: DiPiro JT, Talbert RL, Yee GC, Matzke GR, Wells BG, Posey LM, eds. *Pharmacotherapy.* 12th ed. New York, NY: McGraw-Hill; 2011:439-469.

6. Williams DM, Bourdet SV. Chronic obstructive pulmonary disease. In: DiPiro JT, Talbert RL, Yee GC, Matzke GR, Wells BG, Posey LM, eds. *Pharmacotherapy.* 12th ed. New York, NY: McGraw-Hill; 2011:471-495.

7. Anon. Expert Panel Report 3: Guidelines for the Diagnosis and Management of Asthma. *National Heart, Lung, and Blood Institute and National Asthma Education and Prevention Program.* http://www.nhlbi.nih.gov/guidelines/asthma/asthgdln.pdf. Accessed May 15, 2014.

8. Anon. Global strategy for the diagnosis, management, and prevention of chronic obstructive pulmonary disease (updated 2013). *Global Initiative for Chronic Obstructive Lung Disease.* http://www.goldcopd.org/uploads/users/files/GOLD_Report_2013_Feb20.pdf. Accessed May 15, 2014.

9. Barnes PJ. Pulmonary pharmacology. In: Brunton L, Chabner B, Knollman B, eds. *The Pharmacological Basis of Therapeutics.* 12th ed. New York, NY: McGraw-Hill; 2011:1031-1066.

10. Chang KC, Bell TD, Lauer BA, Chai H. Altered theophylline pharmacokinetics during acute respiratory viral illness. *Lancet.* 1978;1(8074):1132-1133.

11. Koren G, Greenwald M. Decreased theophylline clearance causing toxicity in children during viral epidemics. *J Asthma.* 1985;22(2):75-79.

12. Levy G, Koysooko R. Renal clearance of theophylline in man. *J Clin Pharmacol.* 1976;16(7):329-332.

13. Bauer LA, Bauer SP, Blouin RA. The effect of acute and chronic renal failure on theophylline clearance. *J Clin Pharmacol.* 1982;22(1):65-68.

14. Sarrazin E, Hendeles L, Weinberger M, Muir K, Riegelman S. Dose-dependent kinetics for theophylline: observations among ambulatory asthmatic children. *J Pediatr.* 1980;97(5):825-828.

15. Weinberger M, Ginchansky E. Dose-dependent kinetics of theophylline disposition in asthmatic children. *J Pediatr.* 1977;91(5):820-824.

16. Tang-Liu DD, Williams RL, Riegelman S. Nonlinear theophylline elimination. *Clin Pharmacol Ther.* 1982;31(3):358-369.

17. Vallner JJ, Speir WA Jr, Kolbeck RC, Harrison GN, Bransome ED Jr. Effect of pH on the binding of theophylline to serum proteins. *Am Rev Respir Dis.* 1979;120(1):83-86.

18. Shaw LM, Fields L, Mayock R. Factors influencing theophylline serum protein binding. *Clin Pharmacol Ther.* 1982;32(4):490-496.

19. Hunt SN, Jusko WJ, Yurchak AM. Effect of smoking on theophylline disposition. *Clin Pharmacol Ther.* 1976;19(5, pt 1):546-551.

20. Jusko WJ, Gardner MJ, Mangione A, Schentag JJ, Koup JR, Vance JW. Factors affecting theophylline clearances: age, tobacco, marijuana, cirrhosis, congestive heart failure, obesity, oral contraceptives, benzodiazepines, barbiturates, and ethanol. *J Pharm Sci.* 1979;68(11):1358-1366.

21. Jusko WJ, Schentag JJ, Clark JH, Gardner M, Yurchak AM. Enhanced biotransformation of theophylline in marihuana and tobacco smokers. *Clin Pharmacol Ther.* 1978;24(4):405-410.

22. Jenne H, Nagasawa H, McHugh R, MacDonald F, Wyse E. Decreased theophylline half-life in cigarette smokers. *Life Sci.* 1975;17(2):195-198.

23. Grygiel JJ, Birkett DJ. Cigarette smoking and theophylline clearance and metabolism. *Clin Pharmacol Ther.* 1981;30(4):491-496.

24. Powell JR, Thiercelin JF, Vozeh S, Sansom L, Riegelman S. The influence of cigarette smoking and sex on theophylline disposition. *Am Rev Respir Dis.* 1977;116(1):17-23.

25. Lee BL, Benowitz NL, Jacob Pd. Cigarette abstinence, nicotine gum, and theophylline disposition. *Ann Intern Med.* 1987;106(4):553-555.

26. Matsunga SK, Plezia PM, Karol MD, Katz MD, Camilli AE, Benowitz NL. Effects of passive smoking on theophylline clearance. *Clin Pharmacol Ther.* 1989;46(4):399-407.

27. Mangione A, Imhoff TE, Lee RV, Shum LY, Jusko WJ. Pharmacokinetics of theophylline in hepatic disease. *Chest.* 1978;73(5):616-622.

28. Staib AH, Schuppan D, Lissner R, Zilly W, von Bomhard G, Richter E. Pharmacokinetics and metabolism of theophylline in patients with liver diseases. *Int J Clin Pharmacol Ther Toxicol.* 1980;18(11):500-502.

29. Piafsky KM, Sitar DS, Rangno RE, Ogilvie RI. Theophylline disposition in patients with hepatic cirrhosis. *N Engl J Med.* 1977;296(26):1495-1497.

30. Piafsky KM, Sitar DS, Rangno RE, Ogilvie RI. Theophylline kinetics in acute pulmonary edema. *Clin Pharmacol Ther.* 1977;21(3):310-316.

31. Vicuna N, McNay JL, Ludden TM, Schwertner H. Impaired theophylline clearance in patients with cor pulmonale. *Br J Clin Pharmacol.* 1979;7(1):33-37.

32. Jenne JW, Chick TW, Miller BA, Strickland RD. Apparent theophylline half-life fluctuations during treatment of acute left ventricular failure. *Am J Hosp Pharm.* 1977;34(4):408-409.

33. Powell JR, Vozeh S, Hopewell P, Costello J, Sheiner LB, Riegelman S. Theophylline disposition in acutely ill hospitalized patients. The effect of smoking, heart failure, severe airway obstruction, and pneumonia. *Am Rev Respir Dis.* 1978;118(2):229-238.

34. Gal P, Jusko WJ, Yurchak AM, Franklin BA. Theophylline disposition in obesity. *Clin Pharmacol Ther.* 1978;23(4):438-444.

35. Blouin RA, Elgert JF, Bauer LA. Theophylline clearance: effect of marked obesity. *Clin Pharmacol Ther.* 1980;28(5):619-623.

36. Slaughter RL, Lanc RA. Theophylline clearance in obese patients in relation to smoking and congestive heart failure. *Drug Intell Clin Pharm.* 1983;17(4):274-276.

37. Rohrbaugh TM, Danish M, Ragni MC, Yaffe SJ. The effect of obesity on apparent volume of distribution of theophylline. *Pediatr Pharmacol.* 1982;2(1):75-83.

38. Hilligoss DM, Jusko WJ, Koup JR, Giacoia G. Factors affecting theophylline pharmacokinetics in premature infants with apnea. *Dev Pharmacol Ther.* 1980;1(1):6-15.

39. Giacoia G, Jusko WJ, Menke J, Koup JR. Theophylline pharmacokinetics in premature infants with apnea. *J Pediatr.* 1976;89(5):829-832.

40. Aranda JV, Sitar DS, Parsons WD, Loughnan PM, Neims AH. Pharmacokinetic aspects of theophylline in premature newborns. *N Engl J Med.* 1976;295(8):413-416.

41. Rosen JP, Danish M, Ragni MC, Saccar CL, Yaffe SJ, Lecks HI. Theophylline pharmacokinetics in the young infant. *Pediatrics.* 1979;64(2):248-251.

42. Simons FE, Simons KJ. Pharmacokinetics of theophylline in infancy. *J Clin Pharmacol.* 1978;18(10):472-476.

43. Nassif EG, Weinberger MM, Shannon D, et al. Theophylline disposition in infancy. *J Pediatr.* 1981;98(1):158-161.

44. Zaske DE, Miller KW, Strem EL, Austrian S, Johnson PB. Oral aminophylline therapy. Increased dosage requirements in children. *JAMA.* 1977;237(14):1453-1455.

45. Loughnan PM, Sitar DS, Ogilvie RI, Eisen A, Fox Z, Neims AH. Pharmacokinetic analysis of the disposition of intravenous theophylline in young children. *J Pediatr.* 1976;88(5):874-879.

46. Ginchansky E, Weinberger M. Relationship of theophylline clearance to oral dosage in children with chronic asthma. *J Pediatr.* 1977;91(4):655-660.

47. Bauer LA, Blouin RA. Influence of age on theophylline clearance in patients with chronic obstructive pulmonary disease. *Clin Pharmacokinet.* 1981;6(6):469-474.

48. Antal EJ, Kramer PA, Mercik SA, Chapron DJ, Lawson IR. Theophylline pharmacokinetics in advanced age. *Br J Clin Pharmacol.* 1981;12(5):637-645.

49. Cusack B, Kelly JG, Lavan J, Noel J, O'Malley K. Theophylline kinetics in relation to age: the importance of smoking. *Br J Clin Pharmacol.* 1980;10(2):109-114.

50. Crowley JJ, Cusack BJ, Jue SG, Koup JR, Park BK, Vestal RE. Aging and drug interactions. II. Effect of phenytoin and smoking on the oxidation of theophylline and cortisol in healthy men. *J Pharmacol Exp Ther.* 1988;245(2):513-523.

51. Nielsen-Kudsk F, Magnussen I, Jakobsen P. Pharmacokinetics of theophylline in ten elderly patients. *Acta Pharmacol Toxicol (Copenh).* 1978;42(3):226-234.

52. Blouin RA, Bauer LA, Bustrack JA, Record KE, Bivins BA. Theophylline hemodialysis clearance. *Ther Drug Monit.* 1980;2(3):221-223.

53. Slaughter RL, Green L, Kohli R. Hemodialysis clearance of theophylline. *Ther Drug Monit.* 1982;4(2):191-193.

54. Levy G, Gibson TP, Whitman W, Procknal J. Hemodialysis clearance of theophylline. *JAMA.* 1977;237(14):1466-1467.

55. Lee CS, Peterson JC, Marbury TC. Comparative pharmacokinetics of theophylline in peritoneal dialysis and hemodialysis. *J Clin Pharmacol.* 1983;23(7):274-280.

56. Lee CS, Marbury TC, Perrin JH, Fuller TJ. Hemodialysis of theophylline in uremic patients. *J Clin Pharmacol.* 1979;19(4):219-226.

57. Kradjan WA, Martin TR, Delaney CJ, Blair AD, Cutler RE. Effect of hemodialysis on the pharmacokinetics of theophylline in chronic renal failure. *Nephron.* 1982;32(1):40-44.

58. Golper TA, Marx MA. Drug dosing adjustments during continuous renal replacement therapies. *Kidney Int Suppl.* May 1998;66:165S–168S.

59. Golper TA. Update on drug sieving coefficients and dosing adjustments during continuous renal replacement therapies. *Contrib Nephrol.* 2001;(132):349-353.

60. Pokrajac M, Simic D, Varagic VM. Pharmacokinetics of theophylline in hyperthyroid and hypothyroid patients with chronic obstructive pulmonary disease. *Eur J Clin Pharmacol.* 1987;33(5):483-486.

61. Yurchak AM, Jusko WJ. Theophylline secretion into breast milk. *Pediatrics.* Apr 1976;57(4):518-520.

62. Hansten PD, Horn JR. *Drug Interactions Analysis and Management.* St. Louis, MO: Wolters Kluwer; 2014.

63. Loi CM, Parker BM, Cusack BJ, Vestal RE. Aging and drug interactions. III. Individual and combined effects of cimetidine and cimetidine and ciprofloxacin on theophylline metabolism in healthy male and female nonsmokers. *J Pharmacol Exp Ther.* 1997;280(2):627-637.

64. Nix DE, Di Cicco RA, Miller AK, et al. The effect of low-dose cimetidine (200 mg twice daily) on the pharmacokinetics of theophylline. *J Clin Pharmacol.* 1999;39(8):855-865.

65. National Heart, Lung, and Blood Institute, National Asthma Education and Prevention Program. Expert Panel Report 2: *Guidelines for the Diagnosis and Management of Asthma (Publication # 97-4051).* 2nd ed. Bethesda, MD: US Department of Health and Human Services, National Institutes of Health. 1997.

66. Hendeles L, Jenkins J, Temple R. Revised FDA labeling guideline for theophylline oral dosage forms [see comments]. *Pharmacotherapy.* 1995;15(4):409-427.

67. Edwards DJ, Zarowitz BJ, Slaughter RL. Theophylline. In: Evans WE, Schentag JJ, Jusko WJ, Relling MV, eds. *Applied Pharmacokinetics.* 3rd ed. Vancouver, WA: Applied Therapeutics; 1992.

68. Anderson G, Koup J, Slaughter R, Edwards WD, Resman B, Hook E. Evaluation of two methods for estimating theophylline clearance prior to achieving steady state. *Ther Drug Monit.* 1981;3(4):325-332.

69. Chiou WL, Gadalla MA, Peng GW. Method for the rapid estimation of the total body drug clearance and adjustment of dosage regimens in patients during a constant-rate intravenous infusion. *J Pharmacokinet Biopharm.* 1978;6(2):135-151.

70. Pancorbo S, Davies S, Raymond JL. Use of a pharmacokinetic method for establishing doses of aminophylline to treat acute bronchospasm. *Am J Hosp Pharm.* 1981;38(6):851-856.

71. Wandell M, Mungall D. Computer assisted drug interpretation and drug regimen optimization. *Amer Assoc Clin Chem.* 1984;6:1-11.

72. Stein GE, Haughey DB, Ross RJ, Vakoutis J. Conversion from intravenous to oral dosing using sustained-release theophylline tablets. *Ann Pharmacother.* 1982;16:772-774.

73. Ehlers SM, Zaske DE, Sawchuk RJ. Massive theophylline overdose. Rapid elimination by charcoal hemoperfusion. *JAMA.* 1978; 240(5):474-475.

74. Russo ME. Management of theophylline intoxication with charcoal-column hemoperfusion. *N Engl J Med.* 1979;300(1):24-26.

75. Sintek C, Hendeles L, Weinberger M. Inhibition of theophylline absorption by activated charcoal. *J Pediatr.* 1979;94(2):314-316.

76. Davis R, Ellsworth A, Justus RE, Bauer LA. Reversal of theophylline toxicity using oral activated charcoal. *J Fam Pract.* 1985;20(1): 73-74.

77. Pugh RN, Murray-Lyon IM, Dawson JL, Pietroni MC, Williams R. Transection of the oesophagus for bleeding oesophageal varices. *Br J Surg.* 1973;60(8):646-649.

78. Parker RB, Cavallari LH. Systolic heart failure. In: J.T. D, Talbert RL, Yee GC, Matzke GR, Wells BG, Posey LM, eds. *Pharmacotherapy.* New York, NY: McGraw-Hill; 2011:137-172.

Index

Note: Page numbers followed by *f* or *t* indicate figures or tables, respectively.